QUICK Access

QUICK Access

Professional Guide to Conditions, Herbs & Supplements

INTEGRATIVMEDICINE

Integrative Medicine Communications
www.onemedicine.com

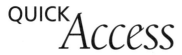

Professional Guide to Conditions, Herbs & Supplements

First edition 2000
Printed in the United States of America
ISBN 0-9670772-5-7
Library of Congress Catalog Card Number 99-096339

Integrative Medicine Communications
1029 Chestnut St., Newton, MA 02464
Phone: 617-641-2300
Fax: 617-641-2301
www.onemedicine.com

Disclaimer

No responsibility is assumed by the publisher for any injury and/or damage to any person or property as a matter of product liability, negligence, or otherwise, or from any use or operation of any methods, products, instructions, or ideas contained in any material herein. This publication contains information relating to general principles of medical care that should not in any event be construed as specific instructions for individual patients. The reader is advised to check product information (including package inserts) for changes and new information regarding dosage, precautions, and contraindications before administering any drug. No claim or endorsements are made for any drug or compound currently in investigative use.

ADVISORY BOARD

Robert A. Anderson, M.D.
Bastyr University
Bothell, Washington

Dennis Awang, Ph.D.
President, MediPlant Consulting
    Services
Ottawa, Ontario
Canada

Shiva Barton, N.D.
Naturopathy
Wellspace
Cambridge, Massachusetts

Stuart Bell, M.D.
Internal Medicine
Attending Physician, University of
    Maryland Hospital
Baltimore, Maryland

**Lawrence J. Cheskin, M.D.,
    F.A.C.P.**
Associate Professor of Medicine
Director, The Johns Hopkins Weight
    Management Center
Johns Hopkins School of Medicine
Director, Division of Gastroenterology
Johns Hopkins Bayview Medical
    Center
Baltimore, Maryland

Steven Dentali, Ph.D.
Senior Director, Botanical Sciences
Rexall Sundowne, Inc.
Boca Raton, Florida

Rainer Engle, M.D.
Associate Professor of Urology
Johns Hopkins Medical Institute
Maryland Urology Associates
Baltimore, Maryland

Constance Grauds, R.Ph.
Pharmacy
President, Association of Natural
    Medicine Pharmacists
San Rafael, California

**Gary M. Guebert, D.C.,
    D.A.C.B.R.**
Chiropractic
Login Chiropractic College
St. Louis, Missouri

Yan Qiu He, M.D., O.M.D, L.Ac.
Chinese Medicine and Acupuncture
American WholeHealth, Inc.
Chevy Chase, Maryland

Peter Hinderberger, M.D.
Internal Medicine/Homeopathy
Medical Director, Ruscombe
    Mansion Community Health
    Center
Baltimore, Maryland

Dahlia Hirsch, M.D.
Ophthalmology
Fellow, American College of
    Surgeons
Associate Professor, University of
    Maryland Medical Center
American Holistic Medical
    Association
Baltimore, Maryland

**William H.B. Howard, M.D.,
    F.A.C.S., F.A.C.P.E.**
Surgery/Sports Medicine
Attending Surgeon, Johns Hopkins
    Hospital
Baltimore, Maryland

Joel A. Kahn, M.D.
Chief Medical Officer, InteliHealth
Blue Bell, Pennsylvania

Joseph Lamb, M.D.
Senior Clinician
American WholeHealth, Inc.
Alexandria, Virginia

Lonnie Lee, M.D.
Internal Medicine
Silver Spring, Maryland

Richard A. Lippin, M.D.
Corporate Medical Director,
    Lyondell Chemical Company
Newtown Square, Pennsylvania

Bill Manahan, M.D.
Assistant Professor, Family
    Medicine
University of Minnesota
Mankato, Minnesota

Anne McClenon, N.D.
Naturopathy/Midwifery
Compass Family Health Center
Plymouth, Massachusetts

Marc S. Micozzi, M.D., Ph.D.
Adjunct Professor, Department of
    Medicine
University of Pennsylvania School of
    Medicine
Philadelphia, Pennsylvania

Sherif H. Osman, M.D.
President Elect, Medical Staff
Fallston General Hospital
Bel Air, Maryland

David Perlmutter, M.D.
Neurology
Director, Perlmutter Health Center,
    Inc.
Naples, Florida

Paul T. Rogers, M.D.
Facility Medical Director
Bright Oaks Pediatrics
Bel Air, Maryland

Eric Serejski, L.Ac., Dipl.Ac.
Acupuncture/Chinese Medicine
American WholeHealth, Inc.
Chevy Chase, Maryland

Scott Shannon, M.D.
Integrative Psychiatry
Lutheran Hospital System
Fort Collins, Colorado

R. Lynn Shumake, P.D.
Medicinal Herbs/Nutrition
American Herbalist Guild
Glenwood, Maryland

Pamela Stratton, M.D.
Associate Professor, Obstetrics and
    Gynecology
Uniformed Services University of the
    Health Sciences
Bethesda, Maryland

John B. Sullivan, Jr., M.D.
Associate Director, Arizona Poison
    Center
Associate Dean, University of
    Arizona Health Sciences Center
Tucson, Arizona

Eric Wellons, M.D.
House Officer
Union Memorial Hospital
Baltimore, Maryland

David Winston
Herbalist AHG
President, Herbalist and Alchemist
Washington, New Jersey

**Leonard A. Wisneski, M.D.,
    F.A.C.P.**
Clinical Professor of Medicine
George Washington University
    Medical Center
Chevy Chase, Maryland

Thomas Wolfe
Professional Member, American
    Herbalists Guild
Smile Herb Shop
College Park, Maryland

Elizabeth Wotton, N.D., L.M.
Naturopathy/Midwifery
Compass Family Health Center
Plymouth, Massachusetts

**Terry Yochum, D.C., D.A.C.B.R.,
    F.C.C.R.(C), F.I.C.C.**
Director, Rocky Mountain
    Chiropractic Radiological Center
Instructor, Department of Radiology
University of Colorado School of
    Medicine
Denver, Colorado

David Zeiger, D.O., A.B.F.P.
Adjunct Clinical Professor
Midwestern University
    Medical School
Chicago, IL

WELCOME TO QUICK ACCESS!

Let us tell you something about us, and this important product.

OUR COMPANY: This valuable information product has been developed by Integrative Medicine Communications (IMC), a company founded by people with a wealth of experience in professional and consumer publishing and information management, serving the continuing needs of modern health care providers. IMC strives to be the recognized source of high quality and scientifically sound information integrating conventional medicine with safe and efficacious complementary and alternative therapies.

OUR PRODUCT: In developing *Quick Access*, we undertook to build an information base that would allow health professionals from various educational and philosophical backgrounds access to a complete armamentarium of approaches used to maintain health, treat disease, or manage conditions. Building such a reference requires a respect for the evidence to support the use of "conventional" and "non-conventional" therapeutic modalities, and the ability to utilize the talents of advisors, researchers, writers, fact checkers, proofreaders, and project managers in synthesizing the information into a tightly formatted and well-balanced final work. We are quite proud of this work, and look forward to updating, adapting, and expanding it for the ongoing needs of those in the front lines of health care delivery.

OUR FOCUS: Our intention was to develop essential, accurate, practical, referenced, and formatted information—not to provide theory. Whether it be with conditions, herbs, or dietary supplements, health care providers can be assured that each monograph reflects a consistent organization and scope, aiding the initiated user who requires a quick review of the facts or the uninitiated user who seeks an overview of the subject matter. We sought to first achieve breadth of coverage, then depth of coverage as space allowed, as each monograph is designed to fill just a few printed pages. We believe we have created a quick review of therapeutic options, from various schools of healing and health promotion.

HOW TO USE Quick ACCESS: The work contains integrated monographs that allow quick answers to a wide range of questions. This monograph system is comprised of the following three broad categories.

1) Condition Monographs—allow the health professional to review a standard medical model of diagnosis and treatment protocols based on a known or suspected condition, with additional information on nutritional support and the use of alternative and complementary modalities. We include what the best evidence allows as safe and productive adjuncts to conventional medical care. As a result, herbs and dietary supplements receive a relatively larger share of coverage.

2) Herb Monographs—allow the health professional to consider the best evidence to support the use of herbs in maintaining health or in treating conditions. The user may be searching for a particular herb, and use this section first, or may be looking here for more substance, having seen reference to the herb's use in a condition monograph.

3) Supplement Monographs—provide substantive and well-referenced information on the use of dietary supplements in maintaining health or in support of condition management. Vitamins, minerals, trace elements, micro-nutrients, and food supplements are included.

A comprehensive CROSS-REFERENCE GUIDE allows for a quick search of category lists drawn from the ACCESS monographs. At a glance, you can review the herbs or supplements used in treating a particular condition, the contraindications of using a particular herb or supplement, and much more. Once you have found what you are looking for in the CROSS-REFERENCE GUIDE, refer to the appropriate monograph for detail. There are 13 separate lists that can be searched in this CROSS-REFERENCE GUIDE, allowing easy and targeted access to the information you are looking for:

- **CONDITIONS: By Medical Category**
- **CONDITIONS: By Signs and Symptoms**
- **CONDITIONS: By Herb or Supplement Treatment Options**
- **HERBS: By Uses/Indications**
- **HERBS: By Warnings, Precautions, Contraindications**
- **HERBS: By Side Effects**
- **HERBS: By Interactions With Other Drugs, Herbs, Supplements**

- **HERBS: By Taxonomic Cross Reference**
- **SUPPLEMENTS: By Uses/Indications**
- **SUPPLEMENTS: By Warnings, Precautions, Contraindications**
- **SUPPLEMENTS: By Side Effects**
- **SUPPLEMENTS: By Interactions With Other Drugs, Herbs, Supplements**
- **COMBINED HERB/SUPPLEMENT TREATMENTS BY CONDITION**

PRODUCT INTEGRITY: All of the information in *Quick Access* is well researched, succinctly presented, and consistently formatted. References are current and clinically significant, tracking the relevant and excluding the irrelevant. A panel of health professionals representing the intended audience of pharmacists, physicians, nurses and nurse practitioners, nutritionists, dietitians, chiropractors, herbalists, naturopathic physicians, and other health practitioners have, and will continue, to help us shape the product and review the information for appropriateness.

We have built this product for you, and pledge to be responsive to your existing and future information needs. We welcome your feedback. Good reading!

CONDITIONS

CONDITIONS CONTINUED

HERBS

SUPPLEMENTS CONTINUED

APPENDICES

QUICK Access

MEDICAL CONDITIONS

Allergic Rhinitis
Alopecia
Amenorrhea
Anemia
Angina
Anorexia Nervosa
Anxiety
Asthma
Atherosclerosis
Attention Deficit
Hyperactivity Disorder
Benign Prostatic Hyperplasia
Bronchitis
Burns
Bursitis
Candidiasis
Chronic Fatigue Syndrome
Chronic Obstructive Pulmonary
Disease
Cirrhosis Of The Liver
Common Cold
Congestive Heart Failure
Conjunctivitis
Constipation
Cough
Cutaneous Drug Reactions
Dementia
Depression
Dermatitis
Diabetes Mellitus
Diarrhea
Dysmenorrhea
Dysphagia
Eczema

Edema
Endocarditis
Endometriosis
Fever Of Unkown Orgin
Fibromyalgia
Food Allergy
Gallbladder Disease
Gastritis
Gastroesophageal Reflux Disease
Gout
Headache, Migraine
Headache, Sinus
Headache, Tension
Hemorrhoids
Hepatitis, Viral
Herpes Simplex Virus
Herpes Zoster (Varicella-Zoster) Virus
HIV and AIDS
Hypercholesterolemia
Hyperkalemia
Hypertension
Hyperthyroidism
Hypoglycemia
Hypothyroidism
Infantile Colic
Influenza
Insect Bites and Stings
Insomnia
Intestinal Parasites
Irritable Bowel Syndrome
Laryngitis
Low Back Pain
Menopause
Motion Sickness

Myocardial Infarction
Obesity
Osteoarthritis
Osteomyelitis
Osteoporosis
Otitis Media
Parkinson's Disease
Peptic Ulcer Disease
Pericarditis
Pertussis
Pharyngitis
Preeclampsia
Primary Pulmonary Hypertension
Prostatitis
Psoriasis
Pulmonary Edema
Raynaud's Phenomenon
Reiter's Syndrome
Rheumatoid Arthritis
Roseola
Seizure Disorders
Sexual Dysfunction
Sinusitis
Sleep Apnea
Sprains and Strains
Tendinitis
Thyroiditis
Ulcerative Colitis
Urethritis
Urinary Incontinence
Urinary Tract Infections In Women
Urolithiasis
Vaginitis
Warts

■ ALLERGIC RHINITIS
OVERVIEW
Definition
Allergic rhinitis (hay fever) is a reaction to airborne allergens. It affects between 1:6 and 1:10 Americans and is an IgE-mediated disorder of the immune system; 70% of cases occur before age 30. Symptoms resemble those of viral rhinitis but persist and show seasonal variation. This most common form of allergy involves the entire respiratory system—nasal cavity, mouth, throat, bronchi, lungs, and diaphragm. There is an inherited tendency, with a child having a 50% chance of developing such allergy if one parent is allergic and a 75% chance if both parents are allergic.

Etiology
The cause is an interaction of IgE on mast cells and basophils in the nasal mucosa with antigenic substances, especially pollens, grasses, or ragweed, which produce a seasonal variation; animal fur; dust, insect debris, household mites; inhaled irritants; changes in temperature or humidity.

Risk Factors
The following conditions can lead to allergic rhinitis.
- Tendency to produce large quantities of IgE
- Repeated exposure to allergen(s), which can be almost anything inhaled, eaten, touched, or injected into the body
- Sufficient potency and duration of exposure
- Other allergies
- Familial predisposition
- Smoking or prolonged exposure to second-hand smoke

Signs and Symptoms
- Nasal obstruction, increased secretions, sneezing
- Itching of mucous membranes of nose, eyes, posterior pharynx, conjunctivae
- Sinus symptoms: headache, pressure behind the eyes, pain in the frontal area, tenderness over cheekbones, aching teeth
- Ear infections
- Stomach cramps
- Skin rashes or hives
- Urinary frequency or diarrhea

DIFFERENTIAL DIAGNOSIS
- Viral, bacterial, or fungal infections
- Sinusitis
- Rhinitis medicamentosa
- Vasomotor rhinitis
- Obstruction of the septum
- Bronchitis
- Nasal polyps
- Swollen adenoids
- Systemic diseases—Wegener's granulomatosis, hypothyroidism (rare)
- Chronic rhinitis

DIAGNOSIS
Physical Examination
Turbinate mucosa is usually pale or blue and swollen, with nasal obstruction and copious secretions, sneezing, and itching of eyes, nose, and throat. Nasal polyps are uncommon, but serous otitis media occurs often, especially in young children. Cervical lymphadenopathy.

Laboratory Tests
- Microscopic examination of nasal smear shows high numbers of eosinophils.
- Increased IgE level

Pathological Findings
- Submucosal edema
- Congested mucous glands

Imaging
Sinus X rays for differential diagnosis

Other Diagnostic Procedures
On referral to an allergist, the following tests may be done.
- Skin testing—Diluted extracts of allergens are injected under the skin or applied to scratches on the back or upper arm. Positive results are indicated by raised welts surrounded by redness and high serum levels of IgE antibodies.
- Radioallergosorbent test (RAST)—Blood test to determine IgE levels
- ELISA allergy testing for IgE and IgG

TREATMENT OPTIONS
Treatment Strategy
Eliminate rhinitis by maintaining an allergen-free environment.
- Cover pillows and mattresses with plastic covers.
- Use synthetic materials (foam mattresses, acrylics) instead of animal products (wool, horsehair).
- Minimize dust-collecting household items (i.e., carpets, drapes)

Use of an air purifier/dust filter may help. When the allergen(s) is known, desensitization therapy can be done, which involves gradually increasing subdermal exposure to identified allergens; results vary.

Drug Therapies
- Oral decongestants—such as pseudoephedrine (Sudafed, 60 to 120 mg orally tid to qid); have systemic effects.
- Antihistamines—such as chlorpheniramine (Chlor-Trimeton; 4 mg orally every 6 to 8 hours, or 8 to 12 mg orally every 8 to 12 hours as sustained-release tablet), clemastine (Tavist; 1.34 to 2.67 mg orally bid; side effect of sedation often unacceptable).
- Nonsedating antihistamines (histamine-receptor antagonists)—such as astemizole (Hismanal; 10 mg orally daily), loratadine (Claritin; 10 mg orally daily), cetirizine (zyrtec; 10mg orally daily), fexofenadine (allegra; 60 mg orally bid), terfenadine (60 mg orally bid); although expensive and by prescription, are especially helpful in those patients who are intolerant of drowsiness; astemizole is associated with sudden death from presumed QT prolongation, especially in those receiving erythromycin or ketoconazole concomitantly; liver disease, hypokalemia are contraindications.
- Nasal corticosteroid sprays—such as beclomethasone (Beconase AQ, Vancenase AQ, 42 mcg/spray), fluticasone (Flonase, two sprays in each nostril once daily, decreasing to one spray each day, based on response), budesonide (Rhinocort, two sprays in each nostril bid or four sprays in each nostril every morning), and flunisolide (Nasalide, 25 mcg/spray); effective if used appropriately—two activations in each nostril bid for one month; improvement takes one to two weeks.
- Intranasal steroids—such as nasal cromolyn (Nasalcrom, one spray in each nostril tid to qid); used in seasonal allergies to shrink nasal polyps; must be started 24 to 36 hour before symptoms develop and must be used four to six times daily.
- Alpha-adrenergic agents—applied to nasal mucosa; come in short-term and long-acting forms; continued use for more than a few days

leads to rebound nasal congestion and rhinitis medicamentosa.
- Systemic steroids—in severe cases and for short duration only.

Complementary and Alternative Therapies

Allergic rhinitis may be successfully treated with alternative therapies. Begin with nutrition guidelines. Use the tincture and homeopathic remedies for acute exacerbations.

NUTRITION
- Eliminate all known food allergens.
- Minimize pro-inflammatory and highly allergenic foods such as saturated fats (meats and dairy products), refined foods, eggs, citrus, bananas, chocolate, peanuts, wheat, shellfish, food coloring, preservatives, caffeine, alcohol, tobacco, and sugar.
- Increase intake of whole foods including fresh fruits and vegetables, whole grains, nuts, seeds.
- Drink plenty of water and include fresh juices, especially carrot, celery, parsley, and pineapple.
- Vitamin A (10,000-15,000 IU/day), zinc (20-30 mg/day), vitamin B_6 (50-100 mg/day), and vitamin B_5 (50-75mg/day) for immune support
- Vitamin C (1,000 mg tid to qid) to reduce inflammation, stabilize mast cells to decrease histamine release
- Vitamin E (400 IU/day) for proper immune function
- N-acetylcysteine (200 mg tid) to reduce mucous formation

HERBS

Herbs are generally a safe way to strengthen and tone the body's systems. Ascertain a diagnosis before pursuing treatment. Herbs may be used as dried extracts (capsules, powders, teas), glycerites, or tinctures (alcohol extracts). Unless otherwise indicated, teas should be made with 1 tsp. herb per cup of hot water. Steep covered 10 to 20 minutes and drink 2 to 4 cups/day. Tinctures may be used singly or in combination as noted.

- Plants high in bioflavonoids (quercetin, curcuma, rose hips, bilberry) are especially useful as they reduce histamine release and stabilize connective tissue. Rose hips *(Rosa canina)* can be used as an infusion or solid extract. Nettles *(Urtica urens)* are traditionally used for hayfever and may be drunk as an infusion, two cups a day.
- Quercetin 250 mg bid to tid to reduce inflammation.
- A tincture of equal parts of coneflower *(Echinacea angustifolia)*, goldenseal *(Hydrastis canadensis)*, cleavers *(Gallium asparine)*, eyebright *(Euphrasia officinalis)*, ginger root *(Zingiber officinalis)*, and elderberry *(Sambucus nigra)* will support immune function and lymphatic drainage, as well as increase circulation and tonify the respiratory system. Take 30 drops bid to tid.

HOMEOPATHY

An experienced homeopath should assess individual constitutional types and severity of disease to select the correct remedy and potency. For acute prescribing use 3 to 5 pellets of a 12X to 30C remedy every one to four hours until acute symptoms resolve.

Allium cepa—for copious, acrid nasal discharge with bland eye lacrimation that is better outdoors.
Euphrasia—for bland nasal discharge with acrid lacrimation that is relieved by lying down at night.
Sabadilla—for sneezing with watery discharge from nose and eyes.
Wyethia—for marked itching of the nose, throat, and soft palate.
Several OTC combination homeopathics are available for hayfever.

PHYSICAL MEDICINE
- Contrast hydrotherapy. Alternating hot and cold applications brings nutrients to the site and diffuses metabolic waste from inflammation. The overall effect is decreased inflammation, pain relief, and enhanced healing. Alternate three minutes hot with one minute cold. Repeat three times. This is one set. Do two to three sets/day.
- Nasal lavage. Mix salt and water to taste like tears. Rinse nostrils by holding head over sink and letting water run from upper nostril to lower nostril. Keep nostrils lower than throat to prevent salt water draining into back of throat. Shrinks membranes and increases drainage.

ACUPUNCTURE

Treatment with acupuncture can help promote both immunity and lymphatic drainage while minimizing the effects of allergic rhinitis.

MASSAGE

Therapeutic massage is an excellent way to assist local lymphatic drainage.

Patient Monitoring

Tolerance to substances changes over the lifetime, and emotional stress, viral illness, fatigue, exposure to chemical irritants, overexertion, or severe weather conditions can increase reactivity. Eliminating these things can raise the threshold, as can age (the immune system is less efficient, so IgE antibodies are less involved with challenging allergens).

OTHER CONSIDERATIONS
Prevention
- If there is a family history of allergy, eliminate the usual allergens when possible before symptoms develop.
- Breastfed children have healthier immune systems and fewer allergies.

Complications/Sequelae
- Development of nonallergic rhinitis medicamentosa from use of nasal sprays more than twice daily for three consecutive days.
- With use of cortisone—cataracts, glaucoma, increased blood pressure, ulcers, diabetes, edema, loss of bone density, avascular necrosis of bone and suppression of adrenal gland function.
- Use of antihistamines or oral steroids may actually increase sensitivity.
- Secondary infections
- Compromised pulmonary function

Prognosis
Symptomatic relief is generally achieved.

Pregnancy
High levels of vitamins A and C are contraindicated in pregnancy.

REFERENCES
The Burton Goldberg Group. *Alternative Medicine: The Definitive Guide.* Tiburon, Calif: Future Medicine Publishing, Inc; 1997.

Ferri FF. *Ferri's Clinical Advisor: Instant Diagnosis and Treatment.* St Louis, Mo: Mosby-Year Book; 1999.

Fisher C. Nettles: an aid to the treatment of allergic rhinitus. *Eur J Herbal Med.* p. 34–35.

Morrison R. *Desktop Guide to Keynotes and Confirmatory Symptoms.* Albany, Calif: Hahnemann Clinic Publishing; 1993.

Noble J, ed. *Textbook of Primary Care Medicine.* 2nd ed. St Louis, Mo: Mosby-Year Book; 1996.

Tierney LM Jr, McPhee SJ, Papadakis MA, eds. *Current Medical Diagnosis and Treatment* 1994. Norwalk, Conn: Appleton & Lange; 1994.

■ ALOPECIA

OVERVIEW

Definition

Alopecia is the absence or thinning of hair in an area of the body where hair formerly grew. It may be caused by physical damage to the hair itself or to the hair follicles, but is most often the result of changes in the natural hair growth cycle.

The average scalp has about 100,000 hairs. Most of these hairs are in the anagen, or growing, phase, which may last as long as five years. In the catagen, or transitional, phase, the hair stops growing and the follicle begins to shrink. The hair then falls out and the follicle lies dormant in the telogen, or resting, phase until a new anagen phase begins. About 10% of the hair follicles on the normal scalp are in the transitional or resting phases, and about 100 hairs are lost every day. In some types of alopecia, the growth cycle is disrupted by some temporary situation such as a chemical imbalance or stress; often the problem may be resolved when the precipitating condition is alleviated. However, 95% of cases of hair loss in both men (male pattern baldness) and women (female diffuse baldness) are genetic in origin. This is called androgenetic alopecia.

Etiology

Androgenetic alopecia is caused by a genetic predisposition for certain hair follicles to produce the enzyme 5-alpha reductase, which combines with the testosterone in the follicle and transforms it into dihydrotestosterone (DHT). DHT accumulation eventually shuts down the follicle. In the interim, the hairs produced by the follicle gradually become shorter and finer. Female diffuse baldness progresses more slowly than male pattern baldness because of the small amount of testosterone in a woman's body. Androgenetic alopecia may be exacerbated by a hormone imbalance.

Many temporary forms of hair loss result from telogen effluvium, in which approximately 30% of the hair follicles go into the resting phase at once. Any shock to the body's systems, including starvation, systematic infection, childbirth, thyroid or immunologic disorders, drugs, or stress may precipitate such an episode. In anagen effluvium, the growth phase is suddenly halted and all or most of the hair falls out in clumps within a few weeks. The most common cause of this condition is chemotherapy for cancer.

In cicatricial, or scarring alopecia, hair follicles are destroyed by scarring from burns or other trauma, severe scalp infections, X-ray therapy, or skin disorders. Physical damage may also result from tight hairstyles maintained over a long period of time, called traction alopecia. Chemical treatments such as hair coloring or permanents can cause hair loss, as can trichotillomania, the habitual pulling out of the hair. Tinea capitis, or "ringworm of the scalp," a fungal condition, also results in hair loss. Except for scarring alopecia, these conditions are generally temporary.

The causes of alopecia areata, or patchy hair loss, are not well understood. There appears to be a genetic component, and it is sometimes associated with an autoimmune disorder. Onset tends to occur in times of stress. Since white hairs are less affected by alopecia areata than pigmented ones, a patient with this condition may report that areas of hair appear to have "turned gray overnight."

Risk Factors
- Male gender
- Advancing age
- Close family member with hair loss
- Hormone imbalance
- Stress
- Eczema, asthma or hay fever, thyroid disease, or vitiligo
- Autoimmune disorders such as lupus erythematosus
- Down's syndrome

Signs and Symptoms
- In male pattern baldness—thinning or absence of hair at the hairline and crown; normal hair growth remains in a "horseshoe" pattern around the sides and back of the scalp.
- In female diffuse baldness—a gradual thinning of hair, especially on the crown; hairline generally remains intact
- Broken hairs, or hairs easily removed
- One or more round or oval bald patches

DIFFERENTIAL DIAGNOSIS

Determine the type of alopecia and treat accordingly.

DIAGNOSIS

Physical Examination

Thin short hairs, tapering at their base ("exclamation point hairs"), easily pulled out, are seen in and near the bald patch or among hairs which have shed. Look for other patches of alopecia on eyebrows, eyelashes, beard or body hair. In alopecia areata, nails may be pitted or deformed.

Laboratory Tests

Thyroid function tests and complete blood count to rule out immunologic disorder

Pathological Findings

Biopsy will support diagnosis of several forms of alopecia.

TREATMENT OPTIONS

Treatment Strategy

Appropriate treatment options depend upon the type of alopecia. Aggressiveness of the treatment depends on the patient's attitude toward what is fundamentally a cosmetic problem and must be weighed against potential side effects. In many temporary forms of alopecia, the condition will begin to normalize without treatment upon removal of the cause. Surgery may be indicated for highly motivated patients with male pattern baldness for whom medical therapies are contraindicated or ineffective. Options include hair transplants, scalp reduction, and strip or flap grafts.

Drug Therapies
- Male pattern baldness—Topical minoxidil (Rogaine), 2% to 5% applied bid. Alternatively, finasteride (Propecia), 1 mg/day orally. Either drug must be used indefinitely to maintain regrown hair. Monitor for potential side effects.
- Female diffuse baldness—Topical minoxidil (Rogaine), 2% applied bid. Must be used indefinitely to maintain regrown hair. Monitor for potential side effects.
- Alopecia areata—Intralesional injections of aqueous corticosteroids, triamcinolone suspension 5 mg/ml, 0.05 to 0.1 ml at intervals of 1 to 2 cm. Injections should not be repeated at the same site for three months. Topical steroids (0.5% triamcinolone cream) may be used for children.
- Tinea capitis—Antifungal such as griseovulfin, orally for eight weeks, in combination with antifungal shampoo two to three times per week for eight weeks. Complete entire course of treatment to prevent relapse.

Complementary and Alternative Therapies

Alopecia is a multi-factorial condition. Correcting the underlying cause is the primary goal of treatment. Complementary therapies have limited success in treating male pattern baldness in men.

NUTRITION

- Optimizing diet by reducing intake of pro-inflammatory foods (saturated fats, dairy, and other animal products) and increasing fresh vegetables, whole grains, essential fatty acids, and, in particular, protein will help to provide essential nutrients for normal hair growth.
- Biotin (300 mcg/day) may be helpful in relieving alopecia. Trace minerals, such as those found in blue green algae (2 to 6 tablets/day), are also needed for hair growth.
- For androgenetic alopecia: Vitamin B_6 (50 to 100 mg/day), zinc (30 mg/day), and GLA (1,000 mg bid) helps to inhibit 5-alpha reductase. Hormone imbalance: Essential fatty acids (1,000 mg bid), B_6 (50 to 100 mg/day), vitamin E (400 IU/day) and magnesium (200 mg bid) enhance hormone production.

HERBS

Herbs are generally a safe way to strengthen and tone the body's systems. As with any therapy, it is important to ascertain a diagnosis before pursuing treatment. Herbs may be used as dried extracts (capsules, powders, teas), glycerites (glycerine extracts), or tinctures (alcohol extracts). Unless otherwise indicated, teas should be made with 1 tsp. herb per cup of hot water. Steep covered 5 to 10 minutes for leaf or flowers, and 10 to 20 minutes for roots. Drink 2 to 4 cups/day. Tinctures may be used singly or in combination as noted.

- Herbs that support circulation may aid in bringing nutrients to the scalp. Combine the following herbs in equal parts and use as tea (2 to 3 cups/day) or tincture (20 to 30 drops bid to tid). Ginkgo *(Ginkgo biloba)*, rosemary *(Rosemarinus officinalis)*, prickly ash bark *(Xanthoxylum clava-herculis)*, black cohosh *(Cimicifuga racemosa)*, yarrow *(Achillia millefolium)*, and horsetail *(Equisetum arvense)*. Ginkgo should be used with close supervision if pharmaceutical circulatory (anti-coagulation) agents are employed (e.g., coumadin or aspirin).
- Androgenetic alopecia: Green tea *(Camelia sinensis)*, 2 cups/day, and saw palmetto *(Serenoa repens)*, 100 mg bid, have anti-androgenic effects.
- Hormone imbalance: Chaste tree *(Vitex agnus-cactus)*, 200 to 300 mg/day, has a normalizing effect on the pituitary and may help correct hormonal imbalances.
- Viral or immune etiology: Herbs that support the immune function are helpful to treat the underlying cause of this type of alopecia. Echinacea *(Echinacea angustifolia)*, astagalus *(Astragalus membranaceus)*, and siberian ginseng *(Eluthrococcus senticosus)* may be helpful.

PHYSICAL MEDICINE

Effective stress reduction techniques are helpful to reduce stress, which will lead to increased blood flow to the scalp.

MASSAGE

Therapeutic massage increases circulation and reduces stress by enhancing overall sense of well-being.

Scalp massage using essential oils of rosemary, lavender, sage, thyme, and cedarwood may be helpful in increasing circulation. Add 3 to 6 drops of essential oil to 1 tbsp. of jojoba and/or grapeseed oils. Massage into scalp daily. Essential oils may also alleviate cases of tinnea capitis.

Patient Monitoring

Patients on minoxidil should be cautioned to use as directed, to prevent possible side effects from systemic absorption (uncommon). More likely side effects include irritation of the scalp. A small percentage of men using finasteride may experience decreased libido, difficulty in achieving an erection, or a decrease in ejaculate volume. Tinea capitis may be transmitted among family members. Support groups may help patients deal with the emotional effects of alopecia.

OTHER CONSIDERATIONS

Complications/Sequelae

Twenty four percent of adults and 54% of children diagnosed with alopecia areata progress to alopecia totalis, the loss of all scalp hair. Alopecia universalis, the loss of all body hair, is rare.

Prognosis

Minoxidil and finasteride result in reduced hair loss and/or new hair growth within a few months if they are going to be effective in the patient with androgenetic alopecia. In alopecia areata, the onset of the condition is generally sudden. The more extensive the hair loss, the less likely that recovery will be complete. However, in most cases, hair begins to regrow within a few months to a few years. With corticosteroid injections hair regrowth should occur in four to six weeks. New hair growth is fine and sometimes unpigmented, but normalizes over time.

Pregnancy

Treatment should be delayed until after pregnancy.

REFERENCES

Guendert DV. *Management of Alopecia.* February 1, 1995. Department of Otolaryngology, UTMB. Accessed at Neuropathy Research at the Medical College of Georgia, http://npntserver.mcg.edu/html/alopecia/documents/BALDNESS_95.html on January 13, 1999.

Hay IC, Jamieson M, Ormerod AD. Randomized trial of aromatherapy: successful treatment for alopecia areata. Arch Dermatol. 1998;134:1349–1352.

Lebwohl M. New treatments for alopecia areata. Lancet. 1997;349:222–223.

Whiting DA. The Diagnosis of Alopecia. Dallas, Tex: University of Texas. Baylor Hair Research and Treatment Center. Accessed at Neuropathy Research at the Medical College of Georgia, http://npntserver.mcg.edu/html/alopecia/documents/DiagnosisAA.html on January 13, 1999.

■ AMENORRHEA

OVERVIEW

Definition
Amenorrhea is the absence of menses. Primary amenorrhea is defined as the failure of menses to begin once a woman reaches 16 years of age, whether or not other pubertal changes such as breast development/pubic or axillary hair are present. Secondary amenorrhea is the absence of menses for the length of time equal to three consecutive normal menstrual cycles in a woman who has previously experienced cyclical menses. Interference with hypothalamic/pituitary functioning plays a major role in the disorder, and the resultant "hypoestrogenemic amenorrhea" may play a role in the development of cardiovascular disease, osteoporosis, and infertility. Amenorrhea may be present with other conditions or abnormalities, including hirsutism, obesity, and galactorrhea. Incidence of primary amenorrhea in U.S. is 2.5% of female population.

Etiology
Generally, the causes of amenorrhea include certain genetic defects, anatomic abnormalities, ovarian failure, or hypothalamic, pituitary, or other endocrine dysfunction.

- Pregnancy—high hCG: (Primary—even in denial of intercourse/Secondary)
- Hypothalamic/pituitary dysfunction—low-normal follicle-stimulating hormone (FSH): Interferes with GnRH production, therefore pituitary gonadotropin secretion (Primary/Secondary)
- Ovarian—high FSH: Dysfunction/dayysgenesis of ovaries (Primary); premature ovarian failure (before the age of 40) (Secondary)
- Hyperandrogenism—low-normal FSH: Secretion of excessive testosterone (Primary/Secondary)
- Pseudohermaphroditism—high luteinizing hormone (LH): Defective testosterone synthesis with excessive testosterone levels (Primary)
- Uterine—normal FSH: Absent or malformed uterus (Primary); intrauterine infection, endometritis (Secondary)
- Menopause—high FSH: Beginning as early as age 40 (Secondary)
- Normal delayed onset (Primary)

Related causes:
- Breast-feeding
- After stopping oral contraceptive use
- Diabetes mellitus
- Tuberculosis
- Stress
- Psychological disorders
- Brain disease
- Genetic defect
- Testicular Feminization Syndrome
- Malnutrition/extreme weight loss (anorexia)
- Strenuous exercise of long duration
- Extreme obesity
- Drug abuse
- Cyanotic congenital heart disease
- Drug therapies—steroids, danazol
- Turner's Syndrome

Risk Factors
- Genetic deficiencies
- Endocrine system disorders
- Extreme athletic training
- Psychological stresses

Signs and Symptoms
In addition to the obvious absence of menses, there may be other symptoms related to the particular cause of the amenorrhea. They include:

- Primary: Headaches, blood pressure/visual field abnormalities, acne, short stature (Turner's syndrome), tall stature (eunuchoidism/gigantism)
- Secondary: Nausea, breast enlargement, hot flushes, headaches, visual field abnormalities, thirst, polyuria, goiter, skin darkening, anorexia, alcoholism, Cushing's syndrome, cirrhosis, renal failure

DIFFERENTIAL DIAGNOSIS
- Primary and/or sexual infantilism: Differentiate between gonadal dysgenesis and hypopituitarism.
- Rule out pregnancy.
- Anatomical variants or tumor mass through examination

DIAGNOSIS

Physical Examination
- Breasts may or may not be developed; pubic and axillary hair may or may not be present; external genitalia/reproductive organs may be abnormal or absent.
- History and physical examination should determine the cause of amenorrhea.

Laboratory Tests
- Pregnancy test (serum or urine hCG)
- Cervical mucus/endometrium analysis
- Serum analysis: GnRH, LH, FSH, Thyroid-stimulating hormone (TSH), T_3, T_4, prolactin, estrogen, testosterone levels
- Renal/hepatic function
- Plasma potassium

Pathological Findings
- Dependent upon underlying disorder

Imaging
Frequently not necessary. Imaging studies could include:
- CT/MRI of head for brain/pituitary disease
- MRI of hypothalamus if high PRL levels
- Pelvic ultrasound

Other Diagnostic Procedures
- Detailed medical history, including prior menstrual cycles
- Physical examination to determine degree of breast development; presence of pubic and axillary hair in pubescent girls
- Examine external genitalia/reproductive organs: presence of uterus
- Chromosome analysis
- Trial period—usually 10 days—with progesterone and/or MPA or estrogen. If bleeding follows withdrawal, reproductive system is functional.

TREATMENT OPTIONS

Treatment Strategy
Treat according to underlying cause.
- Pituitary tumors: Bromocriptine to inhibit prolactin secretion; surgical removal; radiation therapy
- Developmental abnormalities: Hormone therapy; surgery; psychosocial counseling and support
- Oral contraceptives or hormones to artificially induce menses
- Estrogen replacement therapy for hypogonadism/hysterectomy/post menopause

Drug Therapies

- Estrogen replacement therapy: Greatly reduces risk of cardiovascular disease and inhibits osteoporosis. Conjugated estrogens 0.625 to 1.25 mg/day; or on days 1 to 25 of calendar month (0.3 mg/day prevents bone loss). Women with intact uterus should receive progestin to reduce risk of estrogen-induced endometrial carcinoma.
- Medroxyprogesterone acetate (MPA)—progestin of choice— is given at 5 to 10 mg/day on days 16 to 25 of calendar month
- Alternative estrogen replacement: Includes ethinyl estradiol (20 or 50 mcg); estradiol (0.5, 1, 2 mg); Selective Estrogen Receptor Modulators (SERMs) such as raloxifene and Evista for patients refusing estrogen but at-risk for osteoporosis
- Progesterone: For ovarian cysts or some intrauterine disorders (if no pregnancy desired)
- Pulsatile GnRH: To stimulate reproductive function
- Long-acting GnRH analogs: To suppress reproductive function
- Specific drugs to treat underlying disorders

Complementary and Alternative Therapies

Treating amenorrhea with alternative therapies may be effective in aiding the body to metabolize hormones efficiently while ensuring that the nutritional requirements for hormone production are met. Begin with nutritional support, vitamins and minerals, and essential fatty acids. Herbal treatment should begin with *Vitex* alone. Other herbs may be added according to underlying etiology. Minimum length of treatment is three months.

NUTRITION

Minimize refined foods, as they deplete the body of magnesium and other essential nutrients which are needed for normal hormone production. Limit animal products, as they are a source of saturated fats and exogenous estrogens. Limit the Brassica family of vegetables (cabbage, broccoli, brussel sprouts, cauliflower, kale) because they inhibit thyroid function. Eliminate methylxanthines (coffee, chocolate), as they place a burden on the liver and may compromise appropriate hormone ratios. Include whole grains, organic vegetables, and omega-3 fats (cold-water fish, nuts, and seeds).

- Calcium (1,000 mg/day), magnesium (600 mg/day), vitamin D (200 to 400 IU/day), vitamin K (1 mg/day), and Boron (1 to 3 mg/day) help to optimize bone density and are needed for hormone production.
- Iodine (up to 600 mcg/day), tyrosine (200 mg one to two times/day), zinc (30 mg/day), vitamin E (800 IU/day), vitamin A (10,000 to 15,000 IU/day), vitamin C (1,000mg tid), and selenium (200 mcg/day) are needed for thyroid health and hormone balance.
- B_6 (200 mg/day) is a specific therapy which may reduce high prolactin levels caused by pituitary tumors.
- Essential fatty acids: Flaxseed, evening primrose, or borage oil (1,000 to 1,500 mg one to two times/day) to enhance hormone production

HERBS

Herbs are generally a safe way to strengthen and tone the body's systems. As with any therapy, it is important to ascertain a diagnosis before pursuing treatment. Herbs may be used as dried extracts (capsules, powders, teas), glycerites (glycerine extracts), or tinctures (alcohol extracts). Unless otherwise indicated, teas should be made with 1 tsp. herb per cup of hot water. Steep covered 5 to 10 minutes for leaf or flowers, and 10 to 20 minutes for roots. Drink 2 to 4 cups/day. Tinctures may be used singly or in combination as noted.

Amenorrhea needs to be treated with a well-balanced formula that supports pituitary function and hormone activity, as well as addressing the underlying cause. Balancing hormones should be undertaken with the supervision of a qualified practitioner.

- Chaste tree *(Vitex agnus-cactus)* helps to normalize pituitary function but must be taken long term (12 to 18 months) for maximum effectiveness. To be used only under physician supervision with hormone therapy.
- Black cohosh *(Cimicifuga racemosa)*, licorice *(Glycyrrhiza glabra)*, and squaw vine *(Mitchella repens)* help to balance estrogen levels. Licorice is contraindicated in hypertension.
- Chaste tree, wild yam *(Dioscorea villosa)*, and lady's mantle *(Alchemilla vulgaris)* help to balance progesterone levels.
- Kelp *(Nereocystis luetkeana)*, bladderwrack *(Fucus vesiculosis)*, oatstraw *(Avena sativa)*, and horsetail *(Equisetum arvense)* are rich in minerals that support the thyroid.
- Milk thistle *(Silybum marianum)*, dandelion root *(Taraxecum officinalis)*, and vervain *(Verbena hastata)* support the liver and may help restore hormone ratios.
- Sage *(Salvia officinalis)* is a specific herb for reducing high prolactin levels due to pituitary tumors.

HOMEOPATHY

Constitutional homeopathic support can be very effective in addressing underlying causes of amenorrhea. This should be done by an experienced homeopathic practitioner.

PHYSICAL MEDICINE

The following methods help to increase circulation and relieve pelvic congestion.

- Castor oil pack. Used externally, castor oil is a powerful anti-inflammatory. Apply oil directly to skin, cover with a clean soft cloth (e.g., flannel) and plastic wrap. Place a heat source (hot water bottle or heating pad) over the pack and let sit for 30 to 60 minutes. For best results, use for three consecutive days.
- Contrast sitz baths. Use two basins that can be comfortably sat in. Fill one with hot water, one with cold water. Sit in hot water for three minutes, then in cold water for one minute. Repeat this three times to complete one set. Do one to two sets per day three to four days per week.

ACUPUNCTURE

Treatment of amenorrhea with acupuncture may be beneficial for normalizing hormone production and endocrine function. In some cases it may restore regular menstrual cycles.

MASSAGE

Therapeutic massage may be helpful in relieving the effects of stress and improving endocrine function.

Patient Monitoring

Track progress of therapy

OTHER CONSIDERATIONS

Although the mechanism is not known, the fat cell hormone, "leptin," is necessary for a healthy reproductive system

Prevention

- When cause is unknown, prevention is not possible
- Attention to nutrition/appropriate body weight/alcohol and drug abuse
- Stress-relieving techniques
- Avoid extreme exercise regimens

Complications/Sequelae

- Emotional and psychological distress, particularly in congenital defects and if pregnancy is desired and unattainable
- Hot flushes, mood changes, depression, and vaginal dryness in estrogen deficiency
- Long-term estrogen replacement increases risk of breast cancer, melanoma, seizures; 10-fold increased risk of endometrial carcinoma if unopposed with progestin. May cause weight gain, tender breasts, edema, and—rarely—venous thrombosis, and hypertriglyceridemia

Prognosis

- Not detrimental to overall health
- Prognosis is good where underlying disorders are correctly diagnosed and treated (normal delay of onset, weight issues, chronic illnesses, benign tumors, ovarian cysts, hormone imbalances, and similar causes; poor for congenital abnormalities, testicular feminization syndrome, true hermaphroditism, cystic fibrosis, Prader-Willi syndrome, and similar disorders

- After pregnancy and breast-feeding cease: Menses usually return spontaneously
- Discontinuation of oral contraceptives: Menses usually rectify spontaneously within 24 months
- Post-menopause/hysterectomy: Menses cease
- Irreversible amenorrhea: Where this causes emotional distress, induction of pseudo-menstruation may be possible through drug therapy if uterus is present

Pregnancy

- Impossible in certain congenital abnormalities
- Fertility may be affected
- Complications such as incomplete spontaneous abortion, ectopic pregnancy, trophoblastic disease

REFERENCES

Mowrey DB. *The Scientific Validation of Herbal Medicine.* New Canaan, Conn: Keats Publishing; 1988.

National Institutes of Health: Accessed at www.nih.gov on January 16, 1999.

Tierney LM, McPhee SJ, Papadakis MA, eds. *Current Medical Diagnosis & Treatment 1999.* 38th ed. Stamford, Conn: Appleton & Lange; 1999.

Tyler VE. *Herbs of Choice.* New York, NY: Pharmaceutical Products Press; 1994.

Ullman D. *Discovering Homeopathy.* Berkeley, Calif: North Atlantic Books; 1991.

■ ANEMIA

OVERVIEW

Definition

Anemia is characterized by a reduction in either the hematocrit (red blood cell [RBC] volume <42% in men and <36% in women) or the concentration of hemoglobin (<14.0 g/dL in men and <12 g/dL in women). The prevalence of anemia is highest among menstruating women (5.8%), infants (5.7%), and the elderly (12%). Anemias can be distinguished morphologically based on the size of the RBCs or the mean corpuscular volume.

- Microcytic anemias are characterized by small RBCs (mean corpuscular volume <80 fL) and include iron deficiency anemia, anemia of chronic disease, thalassemias, and sideroblastic anemias.
- Macrocytic anemias are characterized by large RBCs (mean corpuscular volume >98 fL) and include megaloblastic anemias (e.g., from vitamin B_{12} [pernicious anemia] and folic acid deficiencies), myelodysplastic anemias (e.g., from cancer chemotherapy), and liver disease (e.g., alcoholism).
- Normocytic anemias are characterized by RBCs within the normal size range (mean corpuscular volume, 80 to 98 fL) and include anemias of acute blood loss, acquired and inherited hemolytic anemias (e.g., sickle cell anemia), mixed micro-macrocytic anemias, and anemias related to renal failure and bone marrow disease.

Etiology

Anemia is caused by decreased production of RBCs resulting from deficiencies in the elemental ingredients necessary for RBC production, by increased destruction of RBCs (hemolysis) from defects in the RBC or environmental stressors, and from excessive bleeding.

Decreased production of RBC is caused by the following:

- Menstruation (monthly iron losses, 20 to 30 mg/month)
- Pregnancy (iron losses from increased needs and losses at the time of delivery) and lactation
- Iron, folic acid, vitamin B_{12}, or erythropoietin deficiencies
- Chronic disease states (e.g., rheumatoid arthritis, inflammatory bowel disease, renal failure)
- Inherited anomalies (e.g., thalassemias)
- Gastrointestinal blood loss (e.g., ulcers, cancer, parasites)
- Genitourinary blood loss (e.g., pregnancy, uterine bleeding, menstruation)
- Overt blood loss (e.g., after surgery, chronic ingestion of nonsteroidal anti-inflammatory drugs [NSAIDS], or regular blood donations)
- Malabsorption syndromes (e.g., celiac disease)
- Neoplasia
- Alcohol ingestion

Increased destruction of RBC is caused by the following:

- Inherited anomalies (e.g., membrane, enzyme, or hemoglobin anomalies)
- Environmental stresses (e.g., antibody deposition, parasitic infection)
- Oxidant drugs (e.g., antibiotics, antimalarials, analgesics)—specific to patients with glucose-6-phosphate dehydrogenase (G6PD) deficiency

Risk Factors

- Family history of anemia
- African American with G6PD deficiency
- Mediterranean ancestry (thalassemia)
- Women in the reproductive years
- Inflammatory disease or advanced malignancy
- Drugs that injure the gastric or intestinal mucosa
- Parasitic infestation (e.g., malaria and babesiosis)
- Malnutrition
- Alcoholism
- Low-income elderly with poor diets

Signs and Symptoms

There is tremendous variability among individuals in the clinical manifestations of anemia, which depend on the cause, severity, onset, and any underlying disease process. Generally symptoms occur when there is an acute drop in hemoglobin to 7 to 8 g/dL. However, if anemia develops slowly, patients, may be able to tolerate hemoglobin levels as low as 6 to 7 g/dL before becoming symptomatic.

- Fatigue
- Headache
- Dyspnea (shortness of breath)
- Lightheadedness
- Pain in the abdomen and back
- Palpitations and angina
- Episodic jaundice and dark urine (i.e., hemoglobinuria)—specific to sideroblastic anemia
- Pica (cravings for strange foods) and koilonychia (thin, concave nails)—specific to iron deficiency anemia
- Glossitis, jaundice, loss of vibratory and position sense, and neurologic symptoms, which may be permanent—specific to pernicious anemia (i.e., vitamin B_{12} deficiency)

DIFFERENTIAL DIAGNOSIS

Many disorders, including congestive heart failure and hypersplenism.

DIAGNOSIS

Physical Examination

Because anemia is often the result of an underlying disease process, the history and physical examination are extremely important. Anemic patients are often pale and may appear confused, frail, unsteady, and short of breath. The presenting symptom may be chest pain or syncope. Vital sign abnormalities include hypotension or tachycardia. Anemia is defined by the laboratory values and these values and the clinical picture are necessary for a definitive diagnosis.

Laboratory Tests

- Complete blood count (CBC)
- Peripheral blood smear
- Reticulocyte count
- Stool for occult blood
- Serum iron studies
- Platelet count
- Blood test for B_{12} and folic acid

Pathological Findings

- Low, normal, or high mean corpuscular volume defines microcytosis, normocytosis, or macrocytosis, respectively.
- Poilkilocytosis (abnormal variation in shape of RBCs) as described by the red cell distribution width
- Hypochromia (decreased hemoglobin content of RBCs)
- Reticulocytosis (increased number of reticulocytes [immature RBCs]) is an important distinguishing characteristic of hemolytic anemia.
- A decreased number of reticulocytes is an important distinguishing characteristic of hypoproliferative anemia.
- Iron accumulation is specific to sideroblastic anemia.
- Low serum iron is specific to iron deficiency anemia.
- Pancytopenia.
- Sickled RBCs are specific to sickle cell anemia.

- Elevated blood urea nitrogen and serum creatinine are specific to anemia of chronic renal failure.

Imaging
May need abdominal sonogram to check spleen size.

Other Diagnostic Procedures
- Coulter counter (for CBC)
- Radioimmunoassay (to measure vitamin B_{12} levels)
- Bone marrow examination
- Gene mapping for alpha and beta chains (for thalassemias) and for sickle cell disease
- Schilling test
- Coombs antiglobulin test
- Hemoglobin electrophoresis
- Erythrocyte sedimentation rate
- Creatinine levels
- Liver function tests
- Thyroid profile
- GI exam for source of bleeding

TREATMENT OPTIONS
Treatment Strategy
Therapy for anemia depends on the cause and the severity of the anemia. In some anemias, the therapy is well established; in others the therapy is largely expectant, depending on the successful treatment of the underlying disease (e.g., anemia of chronic disease). Avoid oxidant medications in patients with G6PD deficiency.
Other treatment options include the following.

- Supportive care (e.g., transfusions), folic acid, and fluids— for patients with sickle cell anemia
- Supportive care (e.g., transfusions), symptomatic therapy, bone marrow transplantation, and splenectomy—for the alpha and beta thalassemias
- Splenectomy—for hereditary spherocytosis

Drug Therapies
- Erythropoietin plus iron—for anemia of chronic renal failure
- Steroids (e.g.,prednisone), splenectomy, cytotoxic agents (e.g., azathioprine), or transfusions—for autoimmune hemolytic anemia
- Analgesics (for painful crises)—for sickle cell anemia
- Cessation of offending drugs—for acquired forms of sideroblastic anemia
- Iron replacement
- Transfusions
- Treatment of underlying disorders

Complementary and Alternative Therapies
Most cases of macrocytic and microcytic anemias may respond well to nutritional therapy. Patients need to be counseled that excess iron is toxic and should not be taken unless indicated by abnormal lab values. Herbal and dietary treatments may be helpful as adjunctive therapies.

NUTRITION
- Ferrous fumerate, glycerate or glycinate (100 mg/day for three to six months) are the most absorbable forms of iron. Ferrous sulfate (325 mg/day) is poorly absorbed and more frequently causes problems with GI upset and/or constipation. Dietary sources of iron include meat, beans, green leafy vegetables, beet greens, blackstrap molasses, almonds, and brewer's yeast.

- Vitamin C—for pernicious anemia, up to 1,000 mg tid will aid in absorption of iron.
- Vitamin B_{12}—cyanocobalamine, 1,000 IU intramuscular injection bid for one week, then weekly for one month, then every two to three months. (Note that dosing varies depending on individual case.) Dietary sources include organ meats, meats, eggs, fish and cheese.
- Folic acid (1 to 2 mg/day)—for folic acid deficiency and hereditary spherocytosis. Good food sources include green leafy vegetables and grains.
- Omega-3 and omega-6 essential fatty acids (1,000 to 1,500 IU) have been shown to decrease the frequency of sickle cell crisis. EFAs can increase clotting times so may need to be checked in people on anti-coagulants.

HERBS
Herbs are generally a safe way to strengthen and tone the body's systems. As with any therapy, it is important to ascertain a diagnosis before pursuing treatment. Herbs may be used as dried extracts (capsules, powders, teas), glycerites (glycerine extracts), or tinctures (alcohol extracts). Unless otherwise indicated, teas should be made with 1 tsp. herb per cup of hot water. Steep covered 5 to 10 minutes for leaf or flowers, and 10 to 20 minutes for roots. Drink 2 to 4 cups/day. Tinctures may be used singly or in combination as noted.

Patients may be treated for one to three months and then reassessed.
- Blackstrap molasses, also known as pregnancy tea (1 tbsp./day in a cup of hot water), is a good source of iron, B vitamins, minerals, and is also a very gentle laxative.
- Spirulina, or blue green algae has been used successfully to treat both microcytic and macrocytic anemias. Dose is 1 heaping tsp./day.
- Alfalfa (*Medicago sativa*), dandelion (*Taraxacum officinale*) root or leaf, burdock (*Arctium lappa*), and yellow dock (*Rumex crispus*) have long been used to fortify and cleanse the blood. For mild cases of anemia, they may help to bring lab values into normal range. Dosage is 1 tbsp./cup of water. Simmer roots for 20 minutes and leaves for five minutes. A single herb, or a combination of these four herbs, may be used.

HOMEOPATHY
An experienced homeopath should assess individual constitutional types and severity of disease to select the correct remedy and potency. Use *Ferrum phosphoricum* 12C once a day for iron deficiency anemia

Patient Monitoring
The frequency of checking the CBC for anemia depends on its cause and severity. Patients should be counseled to maintain a normal balanced diet containing all of the nutrients necessary for blood formation and on the potential adverse gastric effects of certain drugs. Vegetarians need to pay close attention to sources of vitamin B_{12} and iron, and may need to take supplements.

OTHER CONSIDERATIONS
Prevention
It can take three to five years to develop a vitamin B_{12} deficiency. Folic acid is more rapidly depleted, and deficiency can manifest within a few months. B_{12} requires sufficient hydrochloric acid for proper utilization. Macrocytic anemia treated with only folate may mask a B_{12} deficiency—leading to rare cases of permanent nerve damage. Therefore, B_{12} should be given with folate.

Complications/Sequelae

Complications for anemia can range from loss of productivity due to weakness and fatigue to myocardial infarction and death.

Prognosis

The expected course and prognosis is dependent on the type of anemia and the treatment.

Pregnancy

Pregnant women need three to four times as much iron as normal (10 mg/day); thus, the increased demands of pregnancy and blood loss at the time of delivery can lead to iron deficiency anemia, (iron, B_{12}, and/or folate). Iron-deficiencey anemia can result in premature labor, post-partum hemorrhage, low-birth-weight infants, perinatal mortality and can contribute to post-partum depression. A folic acid deficiency during pregnancy, but most importantly in the three months prior to conception, increases the risk of neural tube defects in the infant.

REFERENCES

Branch Jr WT. *Office Practice of Medicine.* Philadelphia, Pa: WB Saunders Company; 1994.

Fauci AS, Braunwald E, Isselbacher KJ et al, eds. *Harrison's Principles of Internal Medicine.* 14th ed. New York, NY: McGraw-Hill; 1998.

Kelley WN, ed. *Textbook of Internal Medicine.* 3rd ed. Philadelphia, Pa: Lippincott-Raven; 1997.

Varro TE. *The Honest Herbal: A Sensible Guide to the Use of Herbs and Related Remedies.* 3rd ed. New York, NY: Pharmaceutical Products Press; 1993.

■ ANGINA

OVERVIEW

Definition

Angina pectoris, or angina, is chest pain caused by underlying coronary heart disease resulting in myocardial ischemia. Different types include the following.

- Stable angina ("classic") occurs with exercise, emotional stress, or extreme temperatures. It seldom is associated with permanent damage to the heart muscle.
- Unstable angina occurs even at rest. Patients may present with symptoms resembling a myocardial infarction but with no evidence of heart muscle damage. Unstable angina may progress to acute myocardial infarction and should be treated as an emergency.
- Prinzmetal's or variant angina is a rare condition that occurs at rest and is caused by coronary artery spasm with electrocardiographic changes. This type of angina should be treated as a medical emergency, because it is often associated with acute myocardial infarction, ventricular tachycardia and fibrillation, and sudden cardiac death.
- Microvascular angina is chest pain in patients with no apparent coronary artery blockages and is caused by poor functioning of smaller blood vessels.

Etiology

Coronary atherosclerosis and/or coronary artery spasms are usually the root causes of angina. Episodes may be precipitated by exertion, emotional stress, smoking, extreme temperatures, overeating, alcohol, or a combination of these. Unstable angina is associated with inflammatory markers indicating possible immune system involvement.

Risk Factors

- Older age
- Male gender
- Postmenopausal women
- Family history of angina
- Diabetes
- Smoking
- Elevated blood cholesterol
- Hypertension
- Obesity
- Sedentary lifestyle
- Emotional stress

Signs and Symptoms

- Pressing or squeezing pain under the breastbone, or less often, in the shoulders, arms, neck, jaws, or back, generally brought on by exertion and relieved within a few minutes by rest and/or medication (e.g., nitroglycerin).
- Abnormal electrocardiogram (ECG) including transient abnormality during pain, QRS notching or slurring, ST-segment depression, and T-wave inversion

DIFFERENTIAL DIAGNOSIS

- Chest wall musculoskeletal conditions
- Aortic stenosis
- Hypertrophic obstructive cardiomyopathy
- Esophagitis
- Gastritis
- Pulmonary embolus
- Panic attack
- Hiatal hernia

DIAGNOSIS

Physical Examination

Blood pressure monitoring.

Laboratory Tests

Measure serum cholesterol, test for diabetes (blood glucose), test for underlying anemia (hemoglobin), measure thyroid function to detect underlying thyroid disease, CPK isoenzymes if myocardial infarction must be ruled out or in unstable angina.

Pathological Findings

- Atherosclerosis
- A recent study indicates elevated levels of basic fibroglast growth factor (BFGF) in urine are associated with exercise-induced ischemia.

Imaging

- Thallium stress test involves injecting radioactive thallium into a vein during a treadmill stress test. Radiation detectors are then used to evaluate the pattern of uptake into the heart muscle.
- Stress echocardiography involves imaging heart contractions during a stress test.
- Ultrafast CT scan can image calcium in atherosclerotic plaque.
- Coronary arteriography, to determine the need for angioplasty or coronary artery bypass, involves injecting liquid dye that is opaque to X rays into coronary arteries. X ray video is then used to detect blockages in the arteries.

Other Diagnostic Procedures

Resting 12-lead electrocardiography should be performed. Approximately 15% of patients with coronary artery disease have a normal ECG. Since stable angina manifests itself during exertion, a stress test (treadmill or bicycle) often is performed if a patient has a normal ECG.

TREATMENT OPTIONS

Treatment Strategy

The goals of managing angina are to relieve pain, increase exercise tolerance before the onset of pain, and treat any underlying coronary heart disease (and/or retard its development or progression). One or more of the following are recommended.

- Surgical treatment—Transcatheter revascularization, balloon angioplasty, stent, rotoblator
- Coronary artery bypass surgery—Surgery presents a larger initial risk but is more effective in relieving angina and preventing recurrence. Surgery improves survival in patients with coronary disease involving the left main coronary artery, multivessel disease involving the proximal left anterior descending artery, or three-vessel disease with impaired left ventricular systolic performance.

Drug Therapies

For chronic stable angina:

- Nitrates: Vasodilators. Glyceryl trinitrate in sublingual spray or tablets (10 mg), or buccal preparations, is used to treat pain or before performing activities that bring on pain. Also used as regular symptomatic treatment in the form of isosorbide mononitrate (40 to 180 mg/day). Transdermal glyceryl nitrate (10 to 20 mg patch) is effective if used intermittently; tolerance effects are likely with continuous use.
- Beta-blockers, used for regular symptomatic treatment of angina, inhibit the action of adrenaline, and thereby reduce blood pressure, heart rate, and pumping force. If beta-blockers are stopped suddenly, coronary events have been shown to increase fourfold over the subse-

quent month. Thus, patients using beta-blockers must be warned not to run out. If the drugs must be stopped, a gradual reduction over a period of two to four weeks should be done. Common beta-blockers are metoprolol (100 to 200 mg/day), atenolol (50 to 100 mg/day) and carvedilol (50 mg/day).

- Calcium-channel blockers, used for regular symptomatic treatment of angina, reduce blood pressure and heart pumping force; some also reduce heart rate. Common calcium-channel blockers include nicardipine (90 mg/day), nifedipine (30 to 120 mg/day), isradipine (5 to 10 mg/day), amlodipine (2.5 to 10 mg/day), and diltiazem (60 to 480 mg/day).

For patients taking beta-blockers, calcium-channel blockers or nitrates may be added as second-line agents for increased effectiveness. Aspirin (75 to 300 mg/day) is generally used for its antiplatelet properties as a secondary prophylaxis. Other antiplatelet drugs such as heparin or eptifibatide may be given during an episode of unstable angina to reduce the risk of myocardial infarction or sudden death. Cholesterol-lowering medications are often prescribed to retard the process of atherosclerosis.

Complementary and Alternative Therapies

Specific herbs and nutrients can be helpful in strengthening the contractility of the heart and increasing oxygenation of tissues. Meditation, yoga, and relaxation techniques may be helpful in reducing stress, increasing circulation, and reducing frequency and severity of angina episodes.

NUTRITION

- Minimize intake of saturated animal fats (meat and dairy products), refined foods, caffeine, and alcohol.
- Increase fresh vegetables, whole grains, and essential fatty acids (cold-water fish, nuts, and seeds).
- Coenzyme Q10 (50 to 100 mg one to two times/day) helps to oxygenate tissues and strengthen cardiac muscle.
- L-Carnitine (330 mg bid to tid) enhances the contractility of cardiac muscle.
- Vitamin E (400 to 800 IU/day) inhibits platelet aggregation.
- Essential fatty acids (1,000 to 1,500 mg one to two times/day) to reduce inflammation and lower cholesterol.
- L-Taurine (100 mg bid) and magnesium (200 mg bid to tid) help to normalize cardiac muscle contractility.
- Vitamin C (1,000 mg bid to tid) helps to support connective tissue and is an antioxidant.
- Bromelain (400 to 1,000 mg/day) reduces platelet aggregation and relieves symptoms.

HERBS

Herbs are generally a safe way to strengthen and tone the body's systems. As with any therapy, it is important to ascertain a diagnosis before pursuing treatment. Herbs may be used as dried extracts (capsules, powders, teas), glycerites (glycerine extracts), or tinctures (alcohol extracts). Unless otherwise indicated, teas should be made with 1 tsp. herb per cup of hot water. Steep covered 5 to 10 minutes for leaf or flowers, and 10 to 20 minutes for roots. Drink 2 to 4 cups/day. Tinctures may be used singly or in combination as noted.

Hawthorn (Crataegus oxyacantha), linden flowers (Tilia cordata), and motherwort (Leonorus cardiaca) may be used as teas long-term with a high degree of safety. The rest of the herbs listed in this section should be used only with the supervision of a qualified practitioner as their use may produce toxic side effects.

A cardiac tonic that contains herbs to stimulate circulation and strengthen the cardiovascular system includes hawthorn, ginkgo (Ginkgo biloba), linden flowers, mistletoe (Viscum album), Indian tobacco (Lobelia inflata), and motherwort. A tincture made from equal parts of these herbs should be taken 20 drops tid.

For acute relief of symptoms use a tincture made from equal parts of the following herbs: yellow jasmine (Gelsemium sempervirens), Indian tobacco (Lobelia inflata), monkshood (Aconite napellus), night-blooming cereus (Cactus grandiflorus), and ginger (Zingiber officinalis). Take 10 to 20 drops every 15 minutes when necessary, up to eight consecutive doses.

HOMEOPATHY

An experienced homeopath should assess individual constitutional types and severity of disease to select the correct remedy and potency. For acute prescribing use 3 to 5 pellets of a 12X to 30C remedy every one to four hours until acute symptoms resolve.

- *Aconite* for panic and fear of death with tachycardia
- *Cactus* for constriction in chest and pains that shoot down the left arm
- *Glonoine* for rapid pulse, violent palpitations, cardiac pains that radiate to arms, and waves of pounding headache

ACUPUNCTURE

Helpful for some patients with angina. Acupuncture may be useful for both symptomatic relief and addressing underlying or concurrent pathologies.

MASSAGE

Therapeutic massage has been shown to be effective in reducing stress and improving general well-being. Massage also helps to improve circulation and nourishment to peripheral tissues.

Patient Monitoring

Patients and their providers should monitor the pattern of angina for changes in symptoms, frequency, length, and response to medication, which may indicate imminent myocardial infarction. Patients who have undergone coronary-artery bypass surgery must be monitored for the redevelopment of atherosclerosis in the graft; likewise, after transmyocardial revascularization, irritation may result in restenosis.

OTHER CONSIDERATIONS

Prevention

Lifestyle changes (such as quitting smoking, reducing stress, and eating a low-fat diet) should be recommended as necessary to slow the progression of the underlying disease. Studies have shown that eating an extremely low-fat diet coupled with exercise and meditation (the Ornish program) reduces cardiac events and coronary artery stenosis as compared to the normally recommended diet. Hormone replacement therapy for post-menopausal women seems to mitigate their increased risk of atherosclerosis.

Complications/Sequelae

Coronary heart disease may progress to arrhythmias and acute myocardial infarction, with resultant damage to the heart muscle and the risk of sudden death.

Prognosis

A patient with angina is at greater than average risk for myocardial infarction and other coronary events. The most reliable predictors of mortality are the number of diseased coronary arteries and the left ventricular contraction pattern. In the stress test, ST-segment depression greater than 1 mm, decreased ejection fraction, or angina pain during exercise, and exercise tolerance less than 120 watts are indicative of a higher risk. Annual mortality is 3% to 4% overall.

Pregnancy

Hawthorn, linden, and motherwort are safe in pregnancy. Stronger herbs should not be used without physician supervision.

REFERENCES

Ballegard S, et al. Acupuncture in angina pectoris: does acupuncture have a specific effect? *J Intern Med.* 1991; 229:357–362.

Caligiuri G, et al. Immune system activation follows inflammation in unstable angina: pathogenetic implications. *J Am Coll Cardiol.* 1998;32:1295–1304.

Cohen M, et al. A comparison of low-molecular weight heparin with unfractionated heparin for unstable coronary artery disease. *N Engl J Med.* 1997;337:447–452.

Kruzel T. *The Homeopathic Emergency Guide.* Berkeley, Calif: North Atlantic Books; 1992:58–60.

Werbach M. *Nutritional Influences on Illness.* New Canaan, Conn: Keats Publishing; 1988:40–77.

Zhou XP, Liu JX. Metrological analysis for efficacy of acupuncture on angina pectoris [in Chinese]. *Chung-Kuo Chung His I Chieh Ho Tsa Chih.* 1993;13:212–214.

■ ANOREXIA NERVOSA
OVERVIEW
Definition
An emotional disorder characterized by severe and potentially life-threatening weight loss through self-induced reduction in total food intake. More than 90% of reported cases occur in women in industrialized countries where thin bodies are considered attractive, though anorexia now occurs in a growing number of men. Although seldom appearing prior to puberty, associated mental disturbances are usually more severe when it does. Mean onset is 17 years; it rarely begins after age 40; onset is often associated with a stressful event; prevalence is 0.5% to 1.0% when full diagnostic criteria is met—higher for subthreshold diagnosis (Eating Disorders Not Otherwise Specified). Death may result—usually caused by starvation, suicide, heart failure, or electrolyte imbalance.

Two subtypes:
- Restricting Type: Dieting, fasting, or excessive exercise
- Binge-Eating/Purging Type: Regular binge-eating, and/or purging by self-induced vomiting and/or misuse of laxatives, enemas, and/or diuretics. Binge-eating may not occur; purging is common even after small amounts of food have been eaten.

Full diagnostic criteria:
- Refusal to maintain minimum body weight for age and height
- Unrealistic fear of weight gain
- Distorted perception of personal body shape and/or size; denial of seriousness of low body weight
- Amenorrhea

Etiology
- Psychopathological fear of biological and psychological maturity
- Severe trauma during puberty or pre-puberty (death of a loved one; sexual abuse)
- Abnormalities with neurotransmitters (dopamine, serotonin, norepinephrine, and endogenous opioids)

Risk Factors
- Heredity in 20% of cases compared to 6% in other psychiatric illnesses. Incidence higher among first-degree relatives (2% to 10% among mothers and sisters of anorectic women); and monozygotic twins (9 of 16) as opposed to dizygotic twins (1 of 14)
- Co-morbid depression in most patients
- Obsessive-compulsive and/or sensitive-avoidant personalities more vulnerable
- Significant increase in risk among normal dieters
- Societal attitudes place some individuals at higher risk:
  - Dancers
  - Runners
  - Models
  - Jockeys
  - Wrestlers
  - Actresses/actors

Signs and Symptoms
- Significant weight loss, or emaciation
- Depressive symptoms (depression, social withdrawal, irritability, insomnia, diminished sex drive)
- Obsessive-compulsive behavior related to eating or other activities
- Denial
- Distorted perception of physical self
- Preoccupation with body size, image, weight control
- Preoccupation with food (collecting recipes; hoarding food)
- Reluctance to eat in public
- Feelings of ineffectiveness
- Excessive need to control personal environment
- Rigid thinking
- Limited social spontaneity
- Excessively restrained initiative and emotional expression

DIFFERENTIAL DIAGNOSIS
- Physical disorders
- Tumors
- Bulimia
- Superior Mesenteric Artery Syndrome
- Major Depressive Disorder
- Schizophrenia
- Social Phobia
- Obsessive-Compulsive Disorder
- Body Dysmorphic Disorder

DIAGNOSIS
Physical Examination
- Substantial weight loss unexplainable medically
- Emaciation
- Hypothermia
- Hypotension
- Hypocaratenemia
- Constipation
- Abdominal pain
- Cold intolerance
- Lethargy
- Excess energy
- Lanugo on trunk
- Brachycardia
- Eroded tooth enamel (from vomiting)
- Scars/calluses on dorsum of hand (from teeth during induction of vomiting)
- Dry skin, thinning hair

Laboratory Tests
Abnormal findings are primarily due to starvation:
- Hematology: leukopenia, mild anemia and—rarely—thrombocytopenia
- Chemistry: dehydration, hypercholesterolemia, elevated liver function tests, metabolic alkalosis, hypochloremia, hypokalemia, metabolic acidosis, low levels of serum thyroxine and triiodothyronine, hyperadrenocorticism, and low serum estrogen/testosterone
- Electrocardiography: sinus bradycardia and arrhythmias
- Electroencephalography: abnormalities caused by fluid and electrolyte disturbances
- Resting energy expenditure: may be significantly reduced

Pathological Findings
- Hypotension and bradycardia
- Peripheral edema

Other Diagnostic Procedures
Evaluation of signs and symptoms after eliminating depressive disorders and/or medical conditions as primary

TREATMENT OPTIONS
Treatment Strategy
Treatment is lengthy and challenging; relapse is common and preoccupa-

tion with dieting and weight usually continues. The greater the time between symptom onset and treatment commencement, and/or presence of personality disorders, the less likelihood of success. Controlling the fear of abnormal body weight and relieving feeding anxiety must be central and awareness of potential medical risks is important. Treatment must be tailored to the individual an integrated treatment is most beneficial. Patients are at greater risk of osteoporosis and lifelong problems with depression/anxiety. Many patients with anorexia may be quite accomplished at carrying extra weight on their bodies when being weighed and are addicted to the heightened sensations of starvation. Support groups may actually be damaging if the patient is competitive and attends groups to get ideas on deceiving care givers. Other general treatment strategies may include the following.

- Cognitive-behavioral/educational approaches—psychoeducational principles focusing on personal, inter-relational, and social conflicts; fears/misconceptions about eating; supervised exercise programs; body image therapy
- Psychodynamic, feminist, and family approaches—self-psychological methods; consultation and therapeutic engagement; family therapy
- Special issues—managing medical/comorbid medical consequences and/or substance abuse/dependence; traumas and/or sexual abuse; refusal of treatment; group psychotherapy; self-help
- Inpatient and/or partial hospitalization in severe cases

Drug Therapies
- Antidepressants appear to be helpful only after intensive psychotherapy, attainment of normal weight, and development of good eating patterns

Complementary and Alternative Therapies
Alternative therapies may be especially helpful in patients who have fixated on avoiding anything "artificial". Treatment is long with frequent setbacks. Herbs can be effective in both calming anxiety and stimulating digestion. "Systematic desensitization" through muscle relaxation with visual imagery can be helpful.

NUTRITION
- Zinc (15 mg/day increased to 50 mg bid)—may improve mood and appetite, may be most useful at increasing the accuracy of body image
- Protein supplements (1 to 3 servings a day)—will help insure sufficient amino acids and prevent wasting. Some protein supplements are low in calories, which may make the patient more willing to consider this therapy.
- Multi-vitamin—A well-rounded multi-vitamin will help to compensate for dietary deficiencies. Due to ease of assimilation, a vitamin made from whole food concentrates is more effective in eating disorders.

HERBS
Herbs are generally a safe way to strengthen and tone the body's systems. As with any therapy, it is important to ascertain a diagnosis before pursuing treatment. Herbs may be used as dried extracts (capsules, powders, teas), glycerites (glycerine extracts), or tinctures (alcohol extracts). Unless otherwise indicated, teas should be made with 1 tsp. herb per cup of hot water. Steep covered 5 to 10 minutes for leaf or flowers, and 10 to 20 minutes for roots. Drink 2 to 4 cups/day. Tinctures may be used singly or in combination as noted.

- Goldenseal (*Hydrastis canadensis*): a strong digestive stimulant, and tonic to the digestive tract, is a specific to anorexia nervosa
- Condurango (*Marsdenia condurango*): alterative and digestive stimulant, where there is diminished appetite or dietary abuse is a specific to anorexia nervosa

- Licorice (*Glycyrrhiza glabra*): antidepressant effects, heals mucous membranes of the digestive tract, regulates cortisol release, modulates estrogen effects; Contra-indicated in hypertension, may cause peripheral edema (pseudoaldosteronism), which resolves when licorice is discontinued
- Wild yam (*Dioscorea villosa*): hormone balancing, antidepressant, supports adrenals, antispasmodic
- Valerian (*Valeriana officinalis*): sedative, digestive bitter and appetite stimulant
- Lemon balm (*Melissa officinalis*): mild sedative, spasmolytic, may gently help regulate TSH and thyroid function
- Oatstraw (*Avena sativa*): nerve tonic, anti-depressant, demulcent, historically used for general debility with nervous exhaustion; this herb is slow to start acting but long lasting.
- St. John's Wort (*Hypericum perforatum*): restorative nervous system tonic specific in use in depression or anxiety states that have led to fatigue and adrenal exhaustion
- Fenugreek (*Trigonella foenum-graecum*): nutritive and digestive tonic used where there is digestive debility and poor nutrition; traditionally used in muscle wasting states or where there is great weight loss; saw palmetto can be used as an alternative to fenugreek.
- Saw Palmetto (*Serenoa repens, S. serrulatta, S. serrullatum*): digestive tonic and connective tissue rebuilder; traditionally used to prevent muscle wasting and general debility
- Siberian ginseng (*Eleutherococcus senticosis*): a supportive adaptogen used to improve vitality and stamina

HOMEOPATHY
Acute homeopathics may be helpful during acute illness. For appropriate constitutional prescribing, which can be helpful, consult a homeopath.

ACUPUNCTURE
May be helpful in restoring energy and reducing stress.

MASSAGE
May be helpful if patient is willing to be touched. Essential oils (lavender, rosemary, verbena) can be added to the massage to increase its effect.

Patient Monitoring
- Long-term monitoring and support is necessary, particularly in severe cases. Prognosis deteriorates significantly without long-term follow-up care.
- Follow daily activity patterns, rituals

OTHER CONSIDERATIONS
- Intravenous nutritional supplements, multivitamins, and potassium may be necessary in severe cases.
- Because the disorder is primary psychological and not simply appetite loss, psychotherapy is usually necessary to establish normal eating patterns.
- Seek professional care from specialists in eating disorders

Prevention
- Education about serious related medical problems
- Intervention programs
- Developing skills to cope with social fixation on thinness and dieting
- Sufficient zinc intake/absorption

Complications/Sequelae
- See Laboratory subhead
- Starved patients have greater sensitivity to medications in general

- Cardiac arrhythmia and arrest
- Necrotizing colitis
- Hypokalemia

Prognosis

- Prognosis is variable
- Long-term (4 to 30 years) mortality rate is more than 10%
- Manifestation in early adolescence usually indicates a more optimistic prognosis.
- Long-term studies show 50% to 70% of patients are no longer clinically anorectic but many (presumably those doing the poorest) drop out; 25% show poor outcomes and chronic illness; and, in a given 10-year period, 5% die—usually from complications, suicide, or cardiac arrest.

Pregnancy

Possible problems include:

- Difficulty conceiving/carrying to term
- Miscarriage
- Parental malnourishment as fetus grows, particularly calcium
- Exacerbation of medical complications
- Retarded, slow, weaker, and smaller offspring at risk of inheriting the disorder
- Stress of pregnancy and/or parenthood may trigger a relapse

REFERENCES

Balch JF, Balch PA. *Prescription for Nutritional Healing*. 2nd ed. Garden City Park, NY: Avery Publishing Group; 1997.

Diagnostic and Statistical Manual of Mental Disorders. 4th ed. Washington, DC: American Psychiatric Association; 1994.

Garner DM, Garfinkel PE, eds. *Handbook of Treatment for Eating Disorders*. 2nd ed. New York, NY: The Guilford Press; 1997.

The Harvard Mental Health Letter. October & November, 1997.

Kalasky KL, ed. *The Alternative Health & Medicine Encyclopedia*. 2nd ed. Detroit, MI: Gale Research; 1998.

Kaplan AS, Garfinkel PE, eds. *Medical Issues and the Eating Disorders—The Interface*. New York, NY: Brunner/Mazel Publishers; 1993.

Shils ME, Olson JA, Shike M, ed. *Modern Nutrition in Health and Disease*. 8th ed. Philadelphia, Pa: Lea & Febiger; 1994:2.

Werbach MR. *Nutritional Influences on Illness*. New Canaan, Conn: Keats Publishing Inc; 1987.

■ ANXIETY
OVERVIEW
Definition
Generalized anxiety disorder recognized by DSM-IV, a chronic psychiatric condition of excessive worry or fear, is distinct from anxiety related to depression, medications, or other causes. Symptoms typically begin in the teens or twenties and, while persisting, tend to fluctuate considerably over time. The condition occurs in up to 5% to 15% of general medical outpatients, more commonly in women. Significant adjustments can be noted in motor tension, autonomic hyperactivity, and hypervigilance.

Etiology
Anxiety may result from medications or drugs, medical conditions, or specific life situations. Generalized anxiety not associated with any specific physiological cause is poorly understood. Genetic or neurochemical factors may play a role, possibly along with behavioral and developmental factors.

Risk Factors
- Traumatic early life experiences
- Anxious mother
- Stress, depression, other psychiatric conditions
- Life situations (social or financial problems)

Signs and Symptoms
- Muscle tension
- Tachycardia
- Hypervigilance
- Dyspnea
- Dizziness/Near-syncope
- Palpitations
- Trembling
- Sweating
- Feelings of unreality
- Fatigue
- Impaired concentration
- Irritability
- Excessive worry/sense of impending doom
- Sighing respiration
- Sleep disturbances

DIFFERENTIAL DIAGNOSIS
- Situation-related anxiety
- Adjustment disorder with anxiety
- Phobic anxiety
- Panic disorder
- Depression with anxiety
- Post-traumatic stress disorder
- Medical conditions that may cause or contribute to anxiety, including angina pectoris, cardiac arrhythmias, asthma, congestive heart failure, limbic lobe epilepsy, hyperthyroidism, hypoglycemia, valvular heart disease, nutritional deficiencies
- Anxiety caused by medications, including psychostimulants, sympathomimetic agents, theophylline, and indomethacin
- Caffeine, alcohol, or cocaine

DIAGNOSIS
Physical Examination
The patient may appear nervous, irritable, or tense. With generalized anxiety disorder, there will be no specific findings on physical exam.

Laboratory Tests
To rule out other conditions, test thyroid function and calcium levels. Use a general laboratory screen if the patient has physical symptoms. Laboratory findings are negative in cases of generalized anxiety disorder.

Other Diagnostic Procedures
Conduct a detailed medical history, focusing on substance use, and life stresses. The DSMIV states six diagnostic criteria, which are listed below.
- Excessive anxiety and worry occurring more often than not for months
- Patient cannot control the worry.
- Anxiety is associated with at least three of the following six symptoms for 6 months: restlessness; fatigue; difficulty concentrating; irritability; muscle tension; and sleep disturbance.
- The focus of the anxiety is not confined to features of other Axis I disorders (panic disorder, social phobia, separation anxiety disorder, anorexia nervosa, etc.).
- The anxiety or symptoms cause significant distress or impairment in social, occupational, or other functioning.
- The anxiety is not due to direct effects of a substance or a medical condition and does not occur exclusively with a mood disorder, psychotic disorder, or pervasive developmental disorder.

Having the patient hyperventilate may reproduce the symptoms and differentiate the disorder from cardiac and neurologic conditions.
- Special tests: EEG for patients over 40 to rule out other conditions; EEG for patients with prominent episodic neurological symptoms

TREATMENT OPTIONS
Treatment Strategy
If no specific known etiology, treatment focuses on eliminating or reducing the symptoms. Except in severe cases, counseling and relaxation therapies may be tried first, with pharmacologic therapy used as needed.
- Short-term counseling can assist the patient in restoring self-esteem, problem solving, and coping with life stresses.
- Patients can be instructed in self-treating techniques to control anxiety; many patients require no pharmacological treatment and succeed with self-regulation techniques, including deep breathing.
- If symptoms of hypervigilance, autonomic hyperactivity, and muscle tension persist, a short course of therapeutics may be helpful—even necessary—while the patient undergoes counseling and learns self-control techniques.

Drug Therapies
Benzodiazepines depress subcortical levels of the CNS; side effects include dizziness or drowsiness, constipation or nausea and vomiting, EEG changes, and orthostatic hypotension; contraindicated with narrow-angle glaucoma, psychosis, or pregnancy. Some benzodiazepines, which should be used for one to two months as needed, are listed below.
- Alprazolam (Xanax), 0.25 to 1 mg
- Chlordiazepoxide (Librium), 5 to 25 mg
- Clonazepam (Klonopin), 3.75 to 22.5 mg
- Clorazepate dipotassium (Tranxene), 3.75 to 22.5 mg
- Diazepam (Valium), 2 to 15 mg
- Halazepam (Paxipam), 20 to 40 mg
- Lorazepam (Ativan), 0.5 to 2 mg
- Oxazepam (Serax), 10 to 30 mg
- Prazepam (Centrax), 5 to 10 mg
- Hydroxyzine (Vistaril, Atarax), 10 to 25 mg as needed, may be used for a patient at risk of abusing a benzodiazepine; side effects include dizziness or drowsiness, dry mouth; contraindicated in pregnancy.

- A tricyclic antidepressant may be used for a patient with persistent cognitive symptoms of apprehension. It inhibits the action of serotonin. Side effects include dizziness, headache, stimulation, insomnia, nervousness, numbness, incoordination, tremors, nausea, diarrhea, constipation, tachycardia, palpitations, sore throat, tinnitus, blurred vision, and muscle pain or weakness. Some tricyclic antidepressants are listed below.
- Buspirone (Buspar), 5 to 10 mg
- Imipramine, 10 mg
- Nortriptyline, 10 mg

Complementary and Alternative Therapies

Supporting the nervous system with mind-body techniques, nutrition, and herbs may be an effective way to minimize and resolve anxiety. Progressive muscle relaxation, diaphragmatic breathing, biofeedback, meditation, and self-hypnosis can help induce the relaxation response and alleviate anxiety.

NUTRITION

Avoid caffeine, alcohol, sugar, refined foods, and all known food allergens. Fresh vegetables, whole grains, and protein nourish the nervous system. Calcium (1,000 mg/day), magnesium (400 to 600 mg/day), and B-complex (50 to 100 mg/day) help support the nervous system and minimize the effects of stress.

HERBS

Herbs are generally a safe way to strengthen and tone the body's systems. As with any therapy, it is important to ascertain a diagnosis before pursuing treatment. Herbs may be used as dried extracts (capsules, powders, teas), glycerites (glycerine extracts), or tinctures (alcohol extracts). Unless otherwise indicated, teas should be made with 1 tsp. herb per cup of hot water. Steep covered 5 to 10 minutes for leaf or flowers, and 10 to 20 minutes for roots. Drink 2 to 4 cups/day. Tinctures may be used singly or in combination as noted.

- A tea (3 to 4 cups/day) or tincture (10 to 20 drops four to six times/day) from the following herbs will help to reduce anxiety and strengthen the nervous system.
- Kava kava *(Piper methysticum)* for mild to moderate anxiety.
- St. John's wort *(Hypericum perforatum)* for anxiety associated with depression.
- Passionflower *(Passiflora incarnata)* for anxiety with insomnia.
- Oatstraw *(Avena sativa)* nourishes the nervous system.
- Lemon balm *(Melissa officinalis)* for anxiety with depression and heart palpitations.
- Lavender *(Lavendula officinalis)* for nervous exhaustion and restoring the nervous system.
- Skullcap *(Scutellaria laterifolia)* relaxes and revitalizes the nervous system.
- Kava kava (100 to 200 mg bid to qid) and St. John's wort (300 mg bid to tid) may be taken as dried extracts to maximize effectiveness in moderate anxiety.

Essential oils of lemon balm, bergamot, and jasmine are calming and may be used as aromatherapy. Place several drops in a warm bath, atomizer, or cotton ball.

HOMEOPATHY

An experienced homeopath should assess individual constitutional types and severity of disease to select the correct remedy and potency. For acute prescribing use 3 to 5 pellets of a 12X to 30C remedy every one to four hours until acute symptoms resolve.

- *Aconite* for anxiety with palpitations, shortness of breath, and fear

of death.
- *Arsenicum album* for anxiety with restlessness, especially after midnight.
- *Phosphorus* for anxiety when alone and fear that something bad will happen.

ACUPUNCTURE

Acupuncture can be very effective in reducing anxiety.

MASSAGE

Therapeutic massage can be very effective in reducing anxiety and alleviating stress.

Patient Monitoring

Patients learning self-regulatory techniques generally require multiple training sessions and periodic follow-up to ensure the technique is successful. Patients using benzodiazepines are not likely to experience tolerance, but physical and psychological dependence may occur with higher doses used frequently. Monitor the patient for signs of dependence or abuse; discontinuation requires tapering to prevent withdrawal symptoms.

OTHER CONSIDERATIONS

Hormonal balancing for cyclic anxiety

Prevention

- Caffeine can produce or aggravate symptoms
- Avoid stimulants
- Avoid refined sugar-containing foods
- Daily exercise helps prevent or reduce anxiety symptoms

Complications/Sequelae

The condition of the patient with anxiety is often complicated with other psychiatric or behavioral problems. The treatment of underlying or associated conditions is necessary along with symptomatic relief of anxiety. Anxiety in many patients may be complicated by substance abuse or dependence.

Prognosis

Variable prognosis: milder disorders may resolve with self-regulation treatment; more severe conditions may continue and become chronic or become a relapsing-remitting pattern. Psychotherapy may be necessary if other techniques fail or as an adjunct to other therapies for symptom relief. For patients on drug therapy, attempt gradual withdrawal every three to six months; in some cases a chronic maintenance dose may be required.

Pregnancy

Care should be taken in prescribing certain drugs, listed below, for the pregnant patient.

- Benzodiazepines contraindicated (U.S. FDA safety category D)
- Hydroxyzine contraindicated (U.S. FDA safety category C)
- Buspirone with precaution (U.S. FDA safety category B)
- Imipramine and nortriptyline with precaution (U.S. FDA safety category C)

While the herbal tea earlier described is safe in pregnancy, the dried extracts of kava kava and St. John's wort should be avoided.

REFERENCES
American Council on Collaborative Medicine. *Dr. Victor Bagnall's Nutritional Therapy.* Accessed at: http://www.nutrimed.com/anxiety.htm on December 2, 1998.

American Psychiatric Association. *Diagnostic and Statistical Manual of Mental Disorders*. 4th ed. Washington, DC: American Psychiatric Association; 1994.

Andreoli TE, Bennett JC, Carpenter CCJ. *Cecil Essentials of Medicine*. 3rd ed. Philadelphia, Pa: WB Saunders; 1993.

Barker LR, Burton JR, Zieve PD, eds. *Principles of Ambulatory Medicine*. 4th ed. Baltimore, Md: Williams & Wilkins; 1995:139–154.

Blumenthal M, ed. *The Complete German Commission E Monographs*. Boston, Mass: Integrative Medicine Communications; 1998:422, 463–464.

Dr. Bower's Complementary and Alternative Medicine Home Page. Available at: http://avery.med.virginia.edu/~pjb3s.

Goldberg RJ. Anxiety reduction by self-regulation: theory, practice, and evaluation. *Ann Intern Med*. 1982;96:483.

Health and Healing News. Accessed at: http://hhnews.com/kava_update.htm on December 2, 1998.

Herbal Alternatives. Accessed at: http://herbalalternatives.com/kava.htm on December 2, 1998.

Jussofie A, Schmiz A, Hiernke C. Kavapyrone enriched extract from *Piper methysticum* as modulator of the GABA binding site in different regions of the rat brain. *Psychopharmacology*. 1994;116:469–474.

Kinzler E, Kromer J, Lehmann E. Effect of a special kava extract in patients with anxiety-, tension-, and excitation states of non-psychotic genesis. Double blind study with placebos over four weeks [in German]. *Arzneimforsch*. 1991;41:584–588.

Lehmann E, et al. Efficacy of special kava extract *(Piper methysticum)* in patients with states of anxiety, tension and excitedness of non-mental origin-A double blind placebo controlled study of four weeks treatment. *Phytomedicine*. 1996;3:113–119.

Lindenberg Von D, Pitule-Schodel H. D, L-Kavain in comparison with oxazepam in anxiety states. Double-blind clinical trial. *Forschr Med*. 1990;108:50–54.

Morrison R. *Desktop Guide to Keynotes and Confirmatory Symptoms*. Albany, Calif: Hahnemann Clinic Publishing; 1993:4, 40, 293.

Stein JH, ed. *Internal Medicine*. 4th ed. St. Louis, Mo: Mosby-Year Book; 1994.

Volz HP, Kieser M. Kava kava extract WS 1490 versus placebo in anxiety disorders-a randomized placebo controlled 25 week outpatient trial. *Pharmacopsychiatry*. 1997;30:1–5.

■ ASTHMA
OVERVIEW
Definition
Asthma is chronic inflammation of the airways associated with excess swelling and mucus, resulting in obstructed airflow. The airways may be further blocked when an irritant, or trigger, causes bronchial spasms to occur. Asthma symptoms are characteristically worse during sleep and may be intensified by emotion.

Etiology
- Hypersensitivity to aeroallergens (including dust mites; cockroaches; dog, cat, or other animal proteins; fungal spores; pollens; dusts; and fumes)
- Respiratory infections
- Gastroesophageal reflux
- Air pollutants, such as tobacco, aerosols, perfumes, fresh newsprint, diesel particles, sulfur dioxide, elevated ozone levels, and fumes from chemical-cleaning agents and gas stoves
- Meteorological changes in temperature and humidity
- Exercise
- Emotional behaviors that alter breathing such as laughing, shouting, or crying

Risk Factors
- Family history of allergies or asthma
- Genetic predisposition to immunoglobulin E (IgE) and genes located on chromosomes 5, 6, and 11 to 14
- Exposure to aeroallergens and pollutants
- Viral respiratory illness
- Exposure to tobacco smoke
- Exposure to irritants
- Low socioeconomic status
- African- and Hispanic-American race, for both prevalence and severity
- Age and sex—older women and children

Signs and Symptoms
- Shortness of breath or dyspnea
- Wheezing
- Chest tightness or constriction
- Cough (can be the only symptom)
- Cyanosis
- Flattened diaphragm and hyperinflated chest

DIFFERENTIAL DIAGNOSIS
- Mechanical obstruction of air passages
- Functional disorders of the extrathoracic airway, especially of the larynx
- Chronic obstructive pulmonary diseases (COPD), such as chronic bronchitis or emphysema
- Cardiac asthma as a result of myxoma and left ventricle or mitral valve disease
- Pulmonary embolism, although few have bronchoconstriction and wheezing
- Eosinophilic lung diseases
- Carcinoid tumors, especially with wheezing accompanied by flushing, facial rash, or diarrhea
- Congestive heart failure
- Tuberculosis
- Hyperventilation

DIAGNOSIS
Physical Examination
Physical signs of asthma may include tachypnea, tachycardia, exaggerated normal inspiratory fall of systolic blood pressure, hyperinflation of chest, diaphoresis, prolonged expiration, musical-sonorous rhonchi, and wheezing during auscultation.

Laboratory Tests
- CBC normal
- Blood test to determine eosinophil levels for diagnosis
- Blood leukocyte and red blood cell count, (limited usefulness in diagnosis)
- To distinguish from chronic bronchitis, a sputum or "wet prep" test to reveal bronchial epithelium, eosinophils, Charcot-Leyden crystals, and Curschmann's spirals

Pathological Findings
- Serum test that indicates elevated IgE antibody levels
- Increased eosinophil level
- Mucous plugs
- Mucosal edema

Imaging
- Chest radiographs and computerized tomographs to rule out abnormalities or other disease
- Sinus X rays for differential diagnosis

Other Diagnostic Procedures
- The diagnosis of asthma is best confirmed by spirometric measurement of lung volume and flow rate improvement after use of a bronchodilator. Decrease in forced expiratory volume in one second (FEV_1) by 20% occurs after inhalation of methacholine (25 mg/ml) in 95% of asthmatics.
- Bronchoprovocation tests for patients in remission and to determine the extent of aeroallergens and occupational exposure can be helpful but risky.
- Sophisticated tests of lung mechanics are occasionally used.
- For severe asthma, measurements of arterial blood tensions of oxygen and carbon dioxide as well as pH are indicated.
- PPD yearly
- Exercise tolerance tests
- Electrocardiograms: may show sinus tachycardia as well as right axis shift and P pulmonale, which is indicative of negative tidal pleural pressure and increased right side heart transmural pressure

TREATMENT OPTIONS
Treatment Strategy
- Controlling environmental stimuli or triggers
- Anti-inflammatory drugs to promote relaxation of the bronchial smooth muscle
- Bronchodilator drugs to stimulate the beta 2-adrenergic agonist receptors during an attack
- Antibiotics, when precipitated by bacterial infection
- Combination of these treatments for severe attacks, in addition to oxygen and injected epinephrine in emergencies

Drug Therapies
- Nonsteroidal anti-inflammatory inhalers, such as cromolyn sodium (Intal); prevents mediator release from airway mast cells; dose dependent on severity; may cause coughing

- Corticosteroids, such as methylprednisolone (60 to 80 mg intravenous push each six to eight hours for 36 to 48 hours), for severe attacks; prevents migration and activation of inflammatory cells
- Corticosteroid inhalers, such as beclomethasone dipropionate (Beclovent, Vanceril, or Asthmacort), 1 to 5 puffs two to four times a day; side effects: include cough, hoarseness, oral candidiasis (thrush); chronic adverse side effects rare

Bronchodilators:

- Beta 2-adrenergic agonists, such as albuterol (more than 8 puffs three to four times a week warrants reassessment), administer by metered dose inhalers (MDI) or by nebulizer in the hospital (every one to two hours); stimulate adrenaline or epinephrine receptors; side effects include: rapid or irregular heartbeat, insomnia, shakiness, nervousness.
- Anticholinergic agents, such as ipratropium bromide (Atrovent), inhibit the parasympathetic nervous system; by inhaler (dose varies); side effects include: dry mouth, cough, headaches, urinary retention, worsening of glaucoma.
- Methylxanthines, such as aminophylline and theophylline, are now used only intravenously for severe attacks and for nighttime asthma because of side effects, which include: nausea, vomiting, headaches, insomnia, tremor, seizures, abnormal heart rhythms, death.

Complementary and Alternative Therapies

Discerning and eliminating triggers are key in treating asthma. Suspect food allergy if asthma develops in childhood, if there is a positive family history, if atopic dermatitis is present, or with poorly controlled asthma with elevated total serum IgE levels. Following nutritional guidelines and using herbal support as needed may be effective in reducing inflammation and hypersensitivity reactions.

Hypersensitivity reactions may be associated with stress and anxiety. Mind-body techniques such as diaphragmatic breathing, meditation, tai chi, yoga, and stress management may help reduce frequency, duration, and severity of symptoms.

NUTRITION

Note: Lower doses are for children.

- Eliminate all food allergens from the diet. The most common allergenic foods are dairy, soy, citrus, peanuts, wheat, fish, eggs, corn, food colorings, and additives. An elimination/challenge trial may be helpful in uncovering sensitivities, or an IgG Elisa food allergy test may be used. Remove suspected allergens from the diet for at least two weeks. Re-introduce foods at the rate of one food every three days. Watch for reactions which may include gastrointestinal upset, mood changes, headaches, and exacerbation of asthma. Warning:
  Do not challenge peanuts, or any other food, if there is history of anaphylaxis.
- Reduce pro-inflammatory foods in the diet including saturated fats (meats, especially poultry, and dairy), refined foods, and sugar. Patients sensitive to antibiotics should eat only organic meats to avoid antibiotic residues.
- Increase intake of fresh vegetables, whole grains, legumes, onions, and garlic if not sensitive to those foods.
- Vitamin C (250 to 1,000 mg bid to qid) inhibits histamine release and increases prostacyclin production which promotes vasodilation. Vitamin C from rose hips or palmitate is citrus-free and hypoallergenic. Vitamin C taken one hour before exposure to allergen may reduce reactions. This also applies to exercise-induced asthma.
- B_6 (50 to 200 mg/day) may improve symptoms, particularly in children with a defect in tryptophan metabolism. Use caution with high dose (usually above 500 mg per day in adults). If neuropathy develops, discontinue immediately. Pyridoxal-5-phosphate (P5P) is an activated form of B_6 that may be more readily bio-utilized.
- Magnesium (200 mg bid to tid) relaxes bronchioles. Magnesium may cause loose stools in sensitive patients.
- Consider hydrochloric acid supplementation as deficiency is believed to increase the number and severity of food sensitivities and impair micronutrient absorption.
- B_{12} is linked to hypochlorhydria and a deficiency may increase reactivity to sulfites. Dr. Jonathan Wright's protocol for childhood asthma: Hydroxycobalamin 1cc (1,000 mcg) IM every day for 30 days, then three times weekly for two weeks, two times weekly for two weeks, then once weekly (according to response). Oral B_{12}, 1 mg per day, has also been shown to be helpful.
- N-acetyl cysteine (50 to 200mg tid) and selenium (50 to 200 mcg/day) increase glutathione peroxidase activity and protect lung tissue from oxidative damage.

HERBS

Herbs are generally a safe way to strengthen and tone the body's systems. As with any therapy, it is important to ascertain a diagnosis before pursuing treatment. Herbs may be used as dried extracts (capsules, powders, teas), glycerites (glycerine extracts), or tinctures (alcohol extracts). Unless otherwise indicated, teas should be made with 1 tsp. herb per cup of hot water. Steep covered 5 to 10 minutes for leaf or flowers, and 10 to 20 minutes for roots. Drink 2 to 4 cups/day. Tinctures may be used singly or in combination as noted.

Green tea (Camellia sinensis) is a powerful antioxidant and contains theophylline. Drink 1 to 2 cups/day.

For long-term lung support, combine equal parts of the following herbs in a tea and drink 3 to 4 cups/day. Licorice root (Glycyrrhiza glabra), coltsfoot (Tussilago farfara), wild cherry bark (Prunus serotina), elecampane (Inula helenium), plantain (Plantago major), and skullcap (Scutellaria laterifolia). Licorice root is contraindicated in hypertension. If given, blood pressure should be checked every six weeks. Coltsfoot contains pyrrolizidine alkaloids that can be hepatotoxic with prolonged use. Pyrrolizidine alkaloid-free coltsfoot products still have the desired therapeutic effect. The rest of the herbs in this section should be used only under the supervision of a physician.

For a stronger formula to be used during periods of exacerbation, combine the following herbs in a tincture, 20 to 60 drops tid to qid. Ginkgo (Ginkgo biloba), thyme leaf (Thymus vulgarus), skunk cabbage (Symphlocarpus factida), khella (Ammi visnaga), grindelia (Grindelia robusta), and valerian (Valeriana officinalis). Caution should be used when combining ginkgo with anti-coagulant therapies. Ginkgo may reduce platelet aggregation.

For acute antispasmodic action combine the following herbs in a tincture, 5 to 10 drops every 15 minutes up to eight doses. Indian tobacco (Lobelia inflata) two parts, thyme leaf (Thymus vulgaris) one part, ginger root (Zingiber officinalis) one part, gelsemium (Gelsemium sempiverens) one part, ma huang (Ephedra sinica) $1/2$ part, and belladonna (Atropa belladonna) $1/2$ part. These herbs may produce toxic side effects and should be used under physician supervision and with caution.

Essential oils that may be helpful are elecampane, frankincense, lavender, mint, and sage. Add 4 to 6 drops in a bath, atomizer, or humidifier.

HOMEOPATHY

An experienced homeopath should assess individual constitutional types and severity of disease to select the correct remedy and potency. For acute prescribing use 3 to 5 pellets of a 12X to 30C remedy every one to four hours until acute symptoms resolve.

- *Arsenicum album* for asthma with restlessness, anxiety, and fear of death
- *Ipecac* for constant constriction in chest with incessant cough that may lead to vomiting
- *Pulsatilla* for asthma with pressure in chest and air hunger. Patient may be thirstless and weepy
- *Sambucus* for asthma that wakes patient at midnight with sensation of suffocation

PHYSICAL MEDICINE

Cold applications to the chest during acute attack may lessen severity.

Contrast hydrotherapy may be tonifying to the lungs. Alternating hot and cold applications brings nutrients to the site and diffuses metabolic waste from inflammation. The overall effect is decreased inflammation, pain relief, and enhanced healing. If possible, immerse the part being treated (as with an extremity). Alternate three minutes hot with one minute cold. Repeat three times. This is one set. Do two to three sets/day.

Castor oil pack. Used externally, castor oil is a powerful anti-inflammatory. Apply oil directly to skin, cover with a clean soft cloth (e.g., flannel) and plastic wrap. Place a heat source (hot water bottle or heating pad) over the pack and let sit for 30 to 60 minutes. For best results, use for three consecutive days.

ACUPUNCTURE

Acupuncture may be helpful for reducing frequency and intensity of asthma attacks.

MASSAGE

Therapeutic massage may help reduce stress which exacerbates hypersensitivity reactions.

Patient Monitoring

Patient education and compliance with inhaler and drug administration are designed to prevent asthma attacks. A peak-flow meter should be used at home; instruct patient to notify provider if it drops below 70% of baseline.

OTHER CONSIDERATIONS

Prevention

Conservative introduction of solid foods as child is weaning may help prevent hypersensitivity conditions. If there is a strong family history of allergies or atopic conditions and/or if the child's immunity has been compromised in infancy, delay the introduction of highly allergenic foods, such as grains and dairy, until one year or older.

Prognosis

Good with attention to health and proper use of medications

Pregnancy

There are perinatal complications such as preeclampsia, perinatal mortality, preterm births, and low-birth-weight infants, especially in mothers with severe or uncontrolled asthma who are steroid-dependent or who have not received close monitoring. Upper respiratory infections are the most common precipitant. High doses of vitamins are contraindicated in pregnancy. Small amounts of vitamin C (500 to 1,000 mg bid to tid) may alleviate symptoms. Magnesium may also be used during pregnancy. Follow nutritional guidelines. Herbal support should be undertaken only with physician supervision.

REFERENCES

Bartram T. *Encyclopedia of Herbal Medicine.* Dorset, England: Grace Publishers; 1995:40–41.

Hope BE, Massey DB, Fournier-Massey G. Hawaiian materia medica for asthma. *Hawaii Med J.* 1993;52:160–166.

Kruzel T. *The Homeopathic Emergency Guide.* Berkeley, Calif: North Atlantic Books; 1992:21–27.

Middleton E, ed. *Allergy: Principles and Practice.* 5th ed. St. Louis, Mo: Mosby-Year Book, Inc; 1998.

Monteleone CA, Sherman AR. Nutrition and asthma. *Arch Intern Med.* 1997;157:23–24.

Murray MT, Pizzorno JE. *Encyclopedia of Natural Medicine.* Rocklin, Calif: Prima Publishing; 1998:150–155.

Rakel RE, ed. *Conn's Current Therapy.* 50th ed. Philadelphia, Pa: WB Saunders; 1998.

■ ATHEROSCLEROSIS

OVERVIEW

Definition

Atherosclerosis (hardening of the arteries) is the most common form of arteriosclerosis, a class of diseases in which the walls of a person's artery become thicker and less elastic. In atherosclerosis, fatty material (atheromas) accumulates under the inner lining of arterial walls. It can affect medium and large arteries in the brain, heart, kidneys, other vital organs, and arms and legs. When it develops in the carotid arteries, atherosclerosis can lead to stroke. In the coronary arteries, it can result in heart attack.

The disease develops slowly. It shows few symptoms until the arteries have narrowed severely or have actually become obstructed. Nevertheless, atherosclerosis is the leading cause of illness and death in the United States and most other Western countries. It causes about one million deaths per year in the United States alone, double the number of deaths from cancer.

Treatment should start before symptoms appear, with preventive measures. Recommended measures include lowering cholesterol and blood pressure, ceasing cigarette smoking, losing excess weight, and starting physical activity. When symptoms emerge, treatment focuses on the complications of atherosclerosis, such as angina pectoris, heart failure, kidney failure, stroke, and peripheral arterial occlusion.

Etiology

Some degree of the condition is normal with aging. Researchers have advanced two main theories. The lipid hypothesis is that low-density lipoprotein (LDL) leaks into the arterial walls when its plasma level increases. As a result, LDL accumulates in smooth muscle cells and foam cells, and is oxidized in such a way that it becomes more reactive. This causes the appearance of streaks of fat-containing cells that, as they grow, invade the deeper levels of the arterial walls. These large accumulations, or plaques, cause the artery to narrow and harden.

The chronic endothelial injury hypothesis suggests that injury to the endothelium, the innermost layer of the arterial wall, starts the process. As the injury heals, the endothelium takes up more LDL, which builds up into plaque. Some researchers believe that both processes occur simultaneously. However the atherosclerotic plaque arises, it grows slowly over the years, gradually narrowing the artery, and making the patient vulnerable to thrombosis.

Risk Factors

- Male gender
- Menopause in women
- Hypertension
- Elevated levels of low-density lipoprotein (LDL)
- Decreased levels of high-density lipoprotein (HDL)
- Cigarette smoking
- Diabetes
- Obesity
- Familial atherosclerosis
- Sedentary lifestyle
- Increasing age
- High sucrose intake
- Hyperhomocysteinemia
- Elevated fibrinogen levels
- Deficiency of Coenzyme Q10, L-carnitine
- Air pollution
- Stress
- Sleep deficiency
- Social isolation
- High degrees of negative attitudes (such as hostility and cynical distrust)
- Excessive experience of negative emotions (such as depression, anger, and anxiety)
- High ration of free radical markers to antioxidants

Signs and Symptoms

- Pain and cramps at the site of the narrowed artery, such as chest pain or leg cramps when walking
- Gradual or sudden increase in the extent of the above
- Hardened feel, like small, hard pipes, of arteries in forearms or carotid arteries in the neck
- Clinical signs and symptoms include aneurysm, thrombosis, embolus, and stenosis
- Lowered or absent pulses
- Circulation of a bruit over a narrowed vessel
- In more severe cases muscle atrophy, ulcer, or gangrene

DIFFERENTIAL DIAGNOSIS

- Hypothyroidism
- Poorly controlled diabetes
- Kidney failure
- Malnutrition

DIAGNOSIS

Physical Examination

Listen for a bruit during your stethoscope examination of the patient's neck, abdomen, or groin area. The sound may indicate turbulence in the blood flow caused by a narrowing of the arteries. Check blood pressure. Estimate blood flow by feeling for pulsations in the wrists, legs, and feet; a decrease in pulsations may indicate partly obstructed blood flow. The ankle-arm index (systolic blood pressure at the ankle divided by the brachial systolic blood pressure in the arm) of less that .9 is a highly accurate quantitative indicator of significant arteriosclerosis.

Laboratory Tests

Check blood sugar level for diabetes. Take blood for fasting serum cholesterol, LDL, HDL, and triglycerides.

Pathological Findings

- Streaks of lipid in arteries
- Plaque with associated fibrosis and calcification
- Neovascularization
- Arterial obstruction

Imaging

Conventional X-rays of the chest and blood vessels provide limited diagnostic information. Ultrasound or computed tomography can help to locate the presence and measure the extent of decreased blood flow. Arteriography of the appropriate organ or limb can locate the site of damage more precisely.

Other Diagnostic Procedures

- Family and personal history
- Blood pulsations check
- A stress test will indicate the state of the patient's heart, which may be affected by atherosclerosis.

TREATMENT OPTIONS

Treatment Strategy

Persuade patients that prevention is the best form of treatment. Eliminate controllable risk factors: high blood cholesterol, high blood pressure, obesity, lack of exercise, cigarette smoking.

Drug Therapies

Several prescription medications can reduce blood cholesterol and other fats.

- Cholestyramine and colestipol (12 to 32 g in two to four divided doses) bind bile acids in the intestinal tract, thereby causing the liver to increase its manufacture of bile acids and reduce production of cholesterol. May cause constipation and bloating.
- Nicotinic acid (2 to 6 g daily in divided doses), taken in large quantities, reduces triglycerides and LDL cholesterol, while increasing HDL cholesterol. Side effects may include flushing and changes in liver function.
- Gemfibrozil (600 mg bid) has effects similar to nicotinic acid and is more convenient to take. It may have adverse intestinal effects.
- Probucol (500 mg bid) lowers total cholesterol, but also reduces HDL.
- Statins, such as lovastatin (20 to 80 mg daily), pravastatin, simvastatin, and fluvastatin, interfere directly with the manufacture of cholesterol and may promote the resorption of cholesterol deposits.
- Aspirin lessens the likelihood that blood clots will form. Recommend 325 mg per day unless contraindicated for patients at risk of stroke or heart attack.
- Anticoagulants in crescendo and unstable angina are thought to forestall thrombotic events resulting from rupture of atherosclerotic plaques.

Surgical Procedures

Endarterectomy removes the plaque from inside of the arteries. It is used particularly for the carotid artery, at the point where it divides into internal and external branches; plaque at that junction commonly causes transient ischemic attacks or ischemic stroke. After removing the plaque, the surgeon closes the junction, a procedure that may require a patch of synthetic material. Surgeons must restore blood flow carefully to prevent clots. Reblockage is uncommon. In fact, the surgery has a high success rate, although it carries some risks.

Complementary and Alternative Therapies

Lifestyle changes, diet, and exercise should be an integral part of any treatment plan. Nutritional supplements can be very effective. Hawthorn has an important role in both treating and preventing atherosclerosis. Mind/body techniques, such as yoga, meditation, relaxation, and biofeedback show promise in increasing cardiovascular health. Counseling strategies and behavioral techniques help patients to manage stress, move toward more positive attitudes, and establish broader, supportive social relationships. There is increasing evidence that elevated levels of homocystiene may be important in the genesis of atherosclerosis and cardio-vascular disease, and that nutrition can be helpful at modifying those levels.

NUTRITION

- Vegetarian diet promotes stabilization or possible reversal of the atherogenic process.
- Antioxidants: vitamin C (1,000 mg tid), vitamin E (400 IU/day), coenzyme Q10 (30 to 50 mg tid), selenium (200 mcg/day), lipoic acid (recycles vitamins E and C when they've been used, 50 mg bid)
- Essential fatty acids high in omega-3 fatty acids (1,500 mg bid): While there has been much emphasis on low fat diets, there are some intriguing studies that show that a low fat diet may actually increase LDLs and that it may be more important to alter the fats in the diet, decreasing saturated fats and trans fatty acids, and replacing them with poly- and mono-unsaturated fats. Hydrogenated oils are at least, if not more, as atherogenic as saturated fats.
- Diet: Garlic, ginger and onions all have a beneficial effect on platelet aggregation. Increase fiber (especially water-soluble), fruits, vegetables, and vegetarian sources of protein.
- Homocystiene metabolism: Folic acid (800 mcg/day), B$_6$ (50 mg/day), B$_{12}$ (400 mg/day), betaine (200 to 1,000 mg/day)
- Chromium (200 mcg/day): deficient in AS, supplementation may result in plaque regression
- Magnesium (500 mg): decreases arrhythmias, angina, and death rates following infarction, especially when given with potassium
- Bromelian (150 to 250 mg qid away from meals): inhibits platelet aggregation and breaks down plaque
- Carnitine (750 to 1,500 mg bid): important in fatty acid metabolism, depleted in cardiac muscle during acute infarctions

HERBS

Herbs are generally a safe way to strengthen and tone the body's systems. As with any therapy, it is important to ascertain a diagnosis before pursuing treatment. Herbs may be used as dried extracts (capsules, powders, teas), glycerites (glycerine extracts), or tinctures (alcohol extracts). Unless otherwise indicated, teas should be made with 1 tsp. herb per cup of hot water. Steep covered 5 to 10 minutes for leaf or flowers, and 10 to 20 minutes for roots. Drink 2 to 4 cups/day. Tinctures may be used singly or in combination as noted.

- Hawthorn (Crataegus oxycantha): Proanthocyanadins stabilize collagen to prevent cholesterol deposits on arterial walls, prevents free radical damage, reduces peripheral vascular resistance, angina, cholesterol, and increases coronary and myocardial perfusion; historic use in congestive heart failure; dose is 3 to 5 g as either dried herb, solid extract, or liquid extract.
- Ginkgo (Ginkgo biloba): peripheral arterial occlusion, intermittent claudication, platelet aggregation, watch with thrombolytic therapy (250 mg tid)
- Mistletoe (Viscum album): atherosclerosis, possible anti-hypertensive, historically for exhaustion and nervousness, yet a strong potential for toxicity
- Linden (Tilia cordata): atherosclerosis, historic use as a hypotensive, especially with digestive problems and nervousness
- Rosemary (Rosemariana officinalis): increases coronary artery blood flow, historically used to stimulate digestion and relieve nervous tension
- Gentian (Gentiana lutea): bitter, digestive tonic, historic use to aid in smoking cessation, avoid with ulcers

Hawthorn and/or ginkgo are recommended. Concentrated extracts may be required to achieve the recommended doses. In addition, a tincture (30 to 60 drops tid) or tea (1 cup tid) of one to four of the above herbs, taken before meals, may be helpful.

HOMEOPATHY

Constitutional treatment may be helpful in stimulating overall vitality and should be prescribed by an experienced practitioner.

ACUPUNCTURE

May be helpful in decreasing tension, stimulating proper digestion and elimination, and increasing a sense of well-being.

MASSAGE
May be helpful at relieving tension and increasing overall sense of well-being.

Patient Monitoring
Emphasize preventive measures.

OTHER CONSIDERATIONS
Prevention
Careful lifestyle choices represent the first line of attack on incipient atherosclerosis.

Approaches include:

- Achieving and maintaining normal weight
- Controlling high blood pressure, diabetes, and other disorders that may contribute to the buildup of plaque in arteries
- Eating a diet low in saturated and hydrogenated fats and cholesterol, and high in starches, fiber, fruits, and vegetables
- Exercising for 15 minutes or more three to four times per week
- Avoiding cigarette smoking and second-hand smoke

Complications/Sequelae
- Coronary artery disease
- Congestive heart failure
- Cardiac arrythmias
- Stroke
- Myocardial infarction
- Ischemia and pre-gangrene of the lower limgs
- Premature renal failure

Prognosis
Focus on prevention—it is the best treatment with the best results. Treat complications if they emerge.

REFERENCES
Bartram T. *Encyclopedia of Herbal Medicine.* Dorset, England: Grace Publishers; 1995:41–42, 198–199, 215, 270.

Berkow R, ed. *Merck Manual of Diagnosis and Therapy.* 16th ed. Rahway, NJ: The Merck Publishing Group; 1992.

Berkow R, Beers MH, Fletcher AJ, eds. *Merck Manual, Home Edition.* Rahway, NJ: Merck & Co; 1997.

Blumenthal M, ed. *The Complete German Commission E Monographs.* Boston, Mass: Integrative Medicine Communications; 1998:71–72, 135–138, 142–143, 197.

Fauci AS, Braunwald E, Isselbacher KJ et al, eds. *Harrison's Principles of Internal Medicine.* 14th ed. New York, NY: McGraw-Hill; 1998.

Gruenwald J, Brendler T, Jaenicke C et al, eds. *PDR for Herbal Medicines.* Montvale, NJ: Medical Economics Company; 1998:871–873,1219–1222.

Larson DE, ed. *Mayo Clinic Family Health Book.* 2nd ed. New York, NY: William Morrow and Company; 1996.

Miller Alan. Cardiovascular Disease: Toward a unified approach. *Alternative Medicine Review.* September 1996;1:132–147.

Murray MT. *The Healing Power of Herbs: The Enlightened Person's Guide to the Wonders of Medicinal Plants.* Rocklin, Calif: Prima Publishing; 1998:107–113, 118–131.

Murray MT, Pizzorno JE. *Encyclopedia of Natural Medicine.* Rocklin, Calif: Prima Publishing; 1998:156–170.

Raloff J. Why cutting fats may harm the heart. *Science News.* March 20, 1999;155:181.

Ravitsky M. Herbs: Atherosclerosis. *Newlife Magazine.* Jan/Feb 1997:19.

Werbach M. *Nutritional Influences on Illness.* New Canaan, Conn: Keats Publishing; 1988:40–78.

■ ATTENTION-DEFICIT/ HYPERACTIVITY DISORDER

OVERVIEW

Attention-deficit hyperactivity disorder (ADHD) is a complex, controversial, neurobehavioral disorder. Characterized by excessive, long-term, and pervasive behavior appearing before the age of 7 years, the disorder presents as distractibility, impulsivity, and hyperactivity. The condition may present without the hyperactivity component. Often misdiagnosed because symptoms overlap with other physical or psychological illnesses, it is the most prevalent behavioral disorder in the juvenile population, affecting 3% to 5% of children—90% of whom are boys. Fully 60% experience significant symptoms throughout their lifetime, causing extreme difficulties across educational, vocational, home, and social settings. Accurate diagnosis is essential and challenging; early intervention is key.

Definition

Diagnostic criteria is fully defined in the Diagnostic and Statistical Manual of Mental Disorders, Fourth Edition (DSM-IV), although many primary health providers do not rely on rigid diagnostic criteria.
Either (1) or (2):
1. Six (or more) symptoms of inattention (see Signs and Symptoms) persistent for at least six months to a maladaptive degree inconsistent with developmental level
2. Six (or more) symptoms of hyperactivity-impulsivity (see Signs and Symptoms) persistent for at least six months to a maladaptive degree inconsistent with developmental level
   - Some symptoms of 1 or 2 present before the age of 7 years
   - Some impairment from symptoms present in two or more settings (e.g., school/work, and home)
   - Clear evidence of clinically significant impairment in functioning
   - Symptoms not exclusively present during other mental disorders
Specific types are:
- Combined: if both A1 and A2 are met
- Predominantly inattentive: if A1 is met but A2 is not
- Predominantly hyperactive-impulsive: if A2 is met but A1 is not

Etiology

There are several factors known or suspected to have a role in the development of ADHD.
- Biological influences on neurotransmitter activity
- Environmental factors (associative), poor prenatal health, low birth weight, hypoxia at birth, in vivo exposure to toxins, including lead, mercury, alcohol, cocaine, nicotine
- Genetic predisposition (possibly as high as 80%); one-third of fathers with childhood ADHD may bear ADHD children; concordance rate in monozygotic twins vs. dizygotic twins up to 60%
- Nutritional (controversial): allergies to food/food coloring/additives, heavy metal intoxification, nutrient deficiencies

Risk Factors

- Presence in a family member
- Maternal drug, cigarette, and alcohol use
- Poor prenatal nutrition
- Communication/learning disabilities
- Conduct disorder/oppositional defiant disorder (present in 40% of ADHD children)
- Tourette's syndrome (half of Tourette's patients have ADHD)

Signs and Symptoms

Criteria A(1)—Inattention:
- Fails to give close attention to details or makes careless mistakes
- Difficulty sustaining attention in tasks or play activities
- Does not seem to listen when spoken to directly
- Does not follow through on instructions and fails to finish schoolwork, chores, or duties in the workplace
- Difficulty organizing tasks and activities
- Avoids, dislikes, or is reluctant to engage in tasks that require sustained mental effort
- Loses things necessary for tasks or activities
- Easily distracted by extraneous stimuli
- Forgetful in daily activities
Criteria A(2)—Hyperactivity-Impulsivity:
- Fidgets with hands or feet or squirms in seat
- Leaves seat in situations where remaining seated is expected
- Runs or climbs excessively in appropriate situations (in adolescents or adults, may be limited to subjective feelings of restlessness)
- Difficulty playing or engaging in leisure activities quietly
- Acts as if "driven by a motor"
- Talks excessively
Impulsivity:
- Blurts out answers before questions are completed
- Difficulty awaiting turn
- Interrupts or intrudes on others

DIFFERENTIAL DIAGNOSIS

- Age-appropriate behavior in active children
- Mental retardation/learning, hearing, vision disorder
- Pervasive developmental disorder
- Psychotic disorder
- Understimulating environments
- Oppositional behavior
- Lead poisoning/mercury toxicity
- Substance-related disorder not otherwise specified
- Dysfunctional family

DIAGNOSIS

Physical Examination

- Restlessness: difficulty paying attention, easily distracted
- Motor tics in some cases
- Assessment for ADHD criteria
- Nutritional history—caffeine stimulants, sugar, preservatives

Laboratory Tests

- Hair analysis to eliminate heavy metal toxicity
- Five-hour fasting glucose tolerance tests—abnormal curves in 74% of people with ADHD indicates connection to poor carbohydrate metabolism
- Thyroid function studies to rule out hyperthyroidism
- Test for food allergies, wheat gluten sensitivity, lactose intolerance, red dye sensitivity

Pathological Findings

- Low levels of dopamine
- Low levels of MHPG (breaks down norepinephrine)
- Differences in brain structure

Imaging

Not required for diagnosis.
- PET scans to determine brain metabolism/activity
- MRI to view brain structure

Other Diagnostic Procedures

- Extensive, detailed history from parent, teachers, baby-sitters, grandparents; synthesize information
- Observe behavior in environment comfortable to the child, e.g., in playroom
- Review report cards for comments pertaining to inattention, hyperactivity, disruptive behavior

In adults:
- Wechsler Intelligence Test to measure IQ
- Conners' Continuous Performance Test and Rey-Osterrieth Complex Figure Test to measure neuropsychological functioning

In children:
- Conners' Parent and Teacher Rating Scales
- McLean Test to measure both attention and body movement

TREATMENT OPTIONS

Treatment Strategy

Multimodal treatment most effective with some allowance and adaptability to the special needs of the patient required. Treatments include:

- Pharmacological, to reduce inattention, hyperactivity, impulsivity
- Behavioral modification/cognitive/psychodynamic therapies, to aid social/vocational skills; for example:
- Positive stimuli to change undesirable behavior
- Specific, positive incentives/rewards (eliminate negative/physical punishment)
- Exercises and activities to improve cognitive deficits
- Parent/teacher cooperation to design individualized education program
- Esteem-raising activities such as sports or other special interests
- Elimination/challenge diet, or food allergy testing, to detect possible allergic underpinnings
- Regimented work and play schedules

Drug Therapies

- Methylphenidate (Ritalin): 70% to 80% positive impact on hyperactivity, 0.3 to 0.7 mg/kg/day up to 60 mg/day; sustained release form available
- Pemoline (Cylert), 18.75 to 112.5 mg/day
- Dextroamphetamine (Dexedrine) 0.1 to 0.5 mg/kg/day

In more severe cases:
- Beta-blockers (propranolol/nadolol) to reduce jitters
- Antidepressants (imipramine/bupropion) when severe symptoms coupled with low self-esteem

Complementary and Alternative Therapies

Many parents seek alternative treatment for ADHD, because of concerns with side effects from pharmacotherapy, and initiating chronic drug therapy in young children. Some, but not all, children respond dramatically to dietary manipulation. Herbal treatment can be very effective, as can homeopathic treatment. Behavioral optometry has been found to be quite helpful in certain cases. The doses listed are for children. For adults, increase the dose by 1 1/2 to 2 times.

NUTRITION

- Essential fatty acids help regulate inflammation and nervous irritability. Dietary manipulation includes reducing animal fats and increasing fish and vegetable oil intake, especially olive and grapeseed oils. A mix of omega-6 (evening primrose) and omega-3 (flaxseed) may be most optimum (2 tbsp. oil/day or 1,000 to 1,500 mg bid). For pre-pubescent children under 10, cod liver oil may be the most effective (1 tsp./day).

- Diet: Some children respond dramatically to food additives, artificial colorings, and flavorings. Avoid processed foods. Decrease soda and red meat intake. Foods containing salicylates (almonds, apples, berries, tomatoes, oranges) may be another dietary factor. A possible mechanism is related to prostaglandin metabolism. The most common food sensitivities are dairy, corn, wheat, soy and eggs. An elimination/challenge diet will help identify offending foods.
- Vitamins: C (1,000 mg bid), E (400 IU/day), B-complex (50 to 100 mg/day)
- Minerals: Calcium/magnesium (250/500 mg/day) especially before bed

HERBS

Herbs are generally a safe way to strengthen and tone the body's systems. As with any therapy, it is important to ascertain a diagnosis before pursuing treatment. Herbs may be used as dried extracts (capsules, powders, teas), glycerites (glycerine extracts), or tinctures (alcohol extracts). Unless otherwise indicated, teas should be made with 1 tsp. herb per cup of hot water. Steep covered 5 to 10 minutes for leaf or flowers, and 10 to 20 minutes for roots. Drink 2 to 4 cups/day. Tinctures may be used singly or in combination as noted. The focus for herbal treatment is calming the nervous and digestive systems.

- Lemon balm *(Melissa officinalis):* mild sedative, carminative, spasmolytic, especially with insomnia
- Lavender *(Lavendula angustifolia):* mild sedative, cholagogue, especially with restlessness
- Chamomile *(Matricaria recutita):* anti-inflammatory, antispasmodic
- Passionflower *(Passiflora incarnata):* nervous gastrointestinal complaints
- Linden *(Tilia cordata):* mild sedative, antispasmodic
- Catnip *(Nepeta cataria):* sedative, spasmolytic
- Kava Kava *(Piper methysticum):* anti-anxiety

A combination of four to six of the above herbs (1 cup tea bid to tid, or 30 to 60 drops tincture) can be helpful. A cup of tea before homework or bed often provides a nice structure.

HOMEOPATHY

Homeopathic remedies may be very helpful for ADHD. An experienced homeopath should assess individual constitutional types and severity of disease to select the correct remedy and potency. For acute prescribing use 3 to 5 pellets of a 12X to 30C remedy every one to four hours until acute symptoms resolve.

- *Chamomilla* for irritability with great sensitivity to any stimuli, especially if one cheek is red and the other is pale
- *Arsenicum album* for anxiety, especially with stomach pains and insomnia or restless sleep
- *Argentum nitricum* for anxious children that may be very cheerful, but do not control their impulses

ACUPUNCTURE

Adults, and some children, respond well to acupuncture.

MASSAGE

May be quite helpful. Parents can be taught massage techniques to use on their children.

Patient Monitoring

- Ensure stimulants are effective; if not, diagnosis may be inaccurate.
- Monitor cardiovascular side effects; increased blood pressure; tachycardia.

- Monitor for headache, abdominal pain, insomnia, poor eating habits, and poor growth.
- Behavior/cognitive therapies are usually only effective while ongoing.

OTHER CONSIDERATIONS

Complications/Sequelae
Antisocial behavior, poor self-esteem, and poor school/work performance if left untreated.

Prognosis
- Long-term condition that may become more manageable with increasing age.
- May be effectively controlled.
- Adolescents and adults may develop adaptive measures to aid daily functioning.

Pregnancy
Good prenatal care and avoidance of toxins may have a positive impact. Avoid sugar excesses, particularly to avoid fluctuating blood sugar levels related to glucose intolerance.

REFERENCES

Balch JF, Balch PA. *Prescription for Nutritional Healing.* Garden City Park, NY: Avery Publishing Group; 1997.

Bartram T. *Encyclopedia of Herbal Medicine.* Dorset, England: Grace Publishers; 1995:270, 238.

Blumenthal M, ed. *The Complete German Commission E Monographs.* Boston, Mass: Integrative Medicine Communications; 1998:160, 107.

Gruenwald J, Brendler T et al, eds. *PDR for Herbal Medicines.* Montvale, NJ: Medical Economics Company; 1998:929, 961–963, 967–968, 991–992, 1015–1016.

Morrison R. *Desktop Guide to Keynotes and Confirmatory Symptoms.* Albany, Calif: Hahnemann Clinic Publishing; 1993:33–36, 39–44, 115–117.

Murray MT, Pizzorno JE. *Encyclopedia of Natural Medicine.* Rocklin, Calif: Prima Publishing; 1998:372–377.

Werbach M. *Nutritional Influences on Illness.* New Canaan, Conn: Keats Publishing; 1988:221–226.

■ BENIGN PROSTATIC HYPERPLASIA

OVERVIEW

Definition

Benign prostatic hyperplasia (BPH) is noncancerous growth of the prostate gland that gradually narrows the urethra. The clamping effect eventually obstructs the flow of urine. As a result, the bladder fails to empty completely. Urine remaining in the bladder stagnates, leaving the patient vulnerable to infections, formation of bladder stones, and kidney damage. The condition usually presents itself gradually, via increased difficulty in urinating. Not infrequently, however, a patient suddenly suffers acute urinary retention, finding himself completely unable to urinate. BPH rarely causes symptoms in men under age 40, but affects many males over age 50. Four out of every five men who reach age 80 develop some symptoms of BPH. Some studies, so far unconfirmed, suggest that BPH occurs more frequently in married men than single men, and more often in the United States than in Europe.

Etiology

So far the causes are unknown. Three major theories involve different facets of the aging process in men. As men age, the amount of active testosterone in the blood decreases, resulting in a higher proportion of estrogen in the blood. Animal studies suggest that this excess estrogen increases the activity of promoters of cell growth in the prostate. Another theory targets dihydrotestosterone, a derivative of testosterone that may accumulate in the prostate and encourage the growth of cells there. The third theory suggests that cells in parts of the prostate "reawaken" in later life and direct other cells to grow or to become more sensitive to hormonal growth promoters.

Risk Factors

- Age over 50
- Partial urethral obstruction which can escalate to acute urinary retention as a result of sympathomimetic drugs or alcohol, exposure to cold temperatures, or a long period of immobility

Signs and Symptoms

- Need to urinate frequently
- Inability to sleep through the night without getting up to urinate
- Difficulty starting urine stream
- Decreased strength and force of the stream
- Dribbling after urination
- Blood in the urine, caused by bursting of small veins in the urethra and bladder
- Burning sensation during urination, sometimes the result of bladder infections caused by urine backup
- Not infrequently, complete inability to urinate, sometimes after taking sympathomimetic remedies, leading to a feeling of fullness in the bladder, followed by severe pain in the lower abdomen.

DIFFERENTIAL DIAGNOSIS

- Acute prostatitis
- Prostate cancer
- Urethral blockage/stricture
- Neurogenic bladder

DIAGNOSIS

Physical Examination

Rectal examination indicates whether or not the prostate is enlarged. Nodules detected in the examination may indicate cancer. Tenderness suggests infection.

Laboratory Tests

- Urine and blood tests serve to differentiate between BPH, infections such as acute prostatitis, and prostate cancer.
- Analysis of urine sample identifies bacteria, if any, responsible for infection.
- Blood tests for kidney function eliminate the kidney as a source of the problems.
- Elevated level of prostate-specific antigen (PSA) in the blood indicates further evaluation of the patient for prostate cancer.

Imaging

- Transrectal ultrasound measures the size of the prostate and indicates whether any abnormalities represent malignancies.
- An intravenous pyelogram reveals any obstruction or blockage in the urinary tract.
- A cystoscope inserted through the urethra images the prostate and checks for blockages of urine flow not caused by the prostate.

Other Diagnostic Procedures

- Ask the patient to complete a prostate symptoms score questionnaire.
- Post-void catheterization to determine amount of residual urine.

TREATMENT OPTIONS

Treatment Strategy

The choice among a variety of treatments depends on the age and overall health of the patient, the extent of prostate enlargement, and its effect on urination. Several recent studies suggest watchful waiting, rather than any specific treatment, for patients with mildly enlarged prostates. Regular checkups monitor the condition's progress and point the way to targeted treatment when symptoms worsen. Treatment should start once problems become truly bothersome or present a health risk. The choice among medical therapy, nonsurgical intervention, or surgery will depend on the extent of the discomfort and the risk.

Drug Therapies

- Antibiotics of choice clear up infections prior to BPH treatment.
- Alpha-adrenergic drugs such as terazosin (Hytrin) and doxazosin (Cardura) can relieve symptoms by relaxing tissues in the area of the prostate.
- Finasteride (Proscar) inhibits production of the male hormone involved in prostate enlargement. It can shrink the prostate in some patients. However, it can take up to three months to relieve symptoms.

Surgical Procedures

- Balloon urethroplasty, carried out as an outpatient procedure, widens the urethra, thus easing the flow of urine. Its long-term effectiveness remains unclear.
- Transurethral microwave therapy, performed on an outpatient basis without anesthesia, uses microwaves to destroy excess prostate tissue.
- Transurethral hyperthermia, under investigation by researchers, uses a series of heat treatments to shrink enlarged tissue. The procedure can cause such side effects as irritation and bleeding of the urethra.
- Prostatic stents, under study in Europe, widen the urethra from the inside by pushing back prostatic tissue. Used only if other measures can not be utilized or are not effective.
- Transurethral resection of the prostate (TURP) is the operation performed in 90% BPH surgeries. About 5% of patients retain some urinary incontinence after surgery.
- Transurethral incision of the prostate, a less invasive form of TURP, widens the urethra by making small cuts in the bladder neck and

the prostate. Its advantages and long-term side effects remain to be established.

- Open prostatectomy, approached through an external incision instead of the urethra, offers an alternative for a greatly enlarged prostate or in cases of bladder damage.
- Laser surgery vaporizes obstructing prostate tissue, without causing as much nerve damage as TURP. Today used infrequently.

Complementary and Alternative Therapies

May be very helpful to add to watchful waiting management of BPH. Saw palmetto is widely used in Europe. Saw palmetto in conjunction with nutrition may be very effective.

NUTRITION

- Zinc (60 mg/day)—has been shown to reduce the size of the prostate.
- Selenium (200 mcg/day)—anti-oxidant concentrated in the prostate
- Essential fatty acids (1,000 to 1,500 IU one to two times/day)— anti-inflammatory, for optimum prostaglandin concentrations
- B_6 (100 to 250 mg/day)—reduces the elevated levels of prolactin found in BPH
- Amino acids glycine, glutamic acid, and alanine (200 mg/day of each)—provide symptomatic relief
- Avoid alcohol, especially beer, and saturated fats.
- Pumpkin seeds have been used historically to help maintain a healthy prostate.

HERBS

Herbs are generally a safe way to strengthen and tone the body's systems. As with any therapy, it is important to ascertain a diagnosis before pursuing treatment. Herbs may be used as dried extracts (capsules, powders, teas), glycerites (glycerine extracts), or tinctures (alcohol extracts). Unless otherwise indicated, teas should be made with one teaspoon herb per cup of hot water. Steep covered 5 to 10 minutes for leaf or flowers, and 10 to 20 minutes for roots. Drink 2 to 4 cups/day. Tinctures may be used singly or in combination as noted.

- Saw palmetto (Serenoa ripens)—studies suggest this can be as effective as Proscar. Dose of 160 mg bid is difficult to achieve in tea or tincture; extract standardized for 85% to 95% of fatty acids and sterols is recommended.
- Stinging nettle root (Urticae radix)—for BPH stages 1 and 2. Increases urinary flow and volume. Daily dose of 4 to 6 g of drug or equivalent preparation.

HOMEOPATHY

An experienced homeopath should assess individual constitutional types and severity of disease to select the correct remedy and potency. For acute prescribing use three to five pellets of a 12X to 30C remedy every one to four hours until acute symptoms resolve.

- *Chimaphila umbellata* is specific for retention of urine with an enlarged prostate

- *Conium* for BPH with a feeling of heaviness in the perineum, especially with premature ejaculation
- *Pareira* for urinary retention with BPH, especially with painful urging or pain in the bladder
- *Selenium* for BPH with dribbling, impotence and constipation
- *Thuja occidentalis* for BPH, specifically if there is a forked stream of urine and/or genital condyloma

PHYSICAL MEDICINE

- Kegel exercises increase pelvic circulation and improve muscle tone.
- Contrast sitz baths. Fill one basin with hot water, one with cold water. Sit in hot water for three minutes, then in cold water for one minute. Repeat three times to complete one set. One to two sets per day, three to four days per week. Increases pelvic circulation and relieves congestion.

Patient Monitoring

Rectal examination of patients at least annually following prostate surgery. Encourage postsurgical patients to drink plenty of water to flush the bladder, eat a balanced diet to prevent constipation, avoid caffeine, heavy lifting, and straining during bowel movements.

OTHER CONSIDERATIONS

Complications/Sequelae

- Patients may also experience bladder stones or prostatitis.
- Occasionally, scar tissue around the bladder opening or in the urethra, resulting from surgery, requires treatment within a year of surgery.

Prognosis

Ineffectiveness of medical treatments may indicate the need for surgery, which usually offers about 15 years of relief from BPH. Ten percent of men who undergo surgery eventually need a second operation for enlargement; most of these patients had their first surgery at an early age. Less than 33% of men with BPH have occult prostate cancer.

REFERENCES

Berkow R, Beers MH et al, eds. *Merck Manual of Medical Information: Home Edition.* Whitehorse Station, NJ: The Merck Publishing Group; 1997.

Blumenthal M, ed. *The Complete German Commission E Monographs.* Boston, Mass: Integrative Medicine Communications; 1998:201.

Morrison R. *Desktop Guide to Keynotes and Confirmatory Symptoms.* Albany, Calif: Hahnemann Clinic Publishing; 1993:119, 141, 286, 341, 388–389.

Murray MT, Pizzorno JE. *Encyclopedia of Natural Medicine.* Rocklin, Calif: Prima Publishing; 1998:480–486.

Prostate Enlargement: Benign Prostatic Hyperplasia. The National Kidney and Urologic Diseases Information Clearinghouse. NIH publication no. 91:3012.

Werbach, M. *Nutritional Influences on Illness.* New Canaan, Conn: Keats Publishing; 1988:82–84.

■ BRONCHITIS

OVERVIEW

Definition

Bronchitis is a respiratory tract infection (viral or bacterial) that causes inflammation of the mucous lining of the bronchial tubes. It can be acute or chronic. Acute bronchitis generally is reversible. Chronic bronchitis, referred to as smoker's cough, is one of several destructive pulmonary diseases and is not usually reversible.

Etiology

Acute bronchitis is usually viral but can be bacterial and is generally community-acquired. The main causes of chronic bronchitis are cigarette smoking and prolonged exposure to air pollution or other bronchial irritants such as dust, grain, and mined products.

Risk Factors

- Winter
- Cigarette smoking
- Air pollutants and irritants
- Male gender and over 50
- Severe pneumonia early in life

Signs and Symptoms

Acute bronchitis:
- Cough that produces mucus
- Burning sensation in the chest
- Sore throat and fever
- Fatigue/weight gain
- Cyanosis
- Wheezing

Chronic bronchitis:
- Chronic cough that produces excessive amounts of mucus or pus
- Wheezing, shortness of breath
- Present for at least three months a year, two years in a row

DIFFERENTRIAL DIAGNOSIS

- Pneumonia
- Emphysema, tuberculosis, cystic fibrosis, asthma, Legionnaires' disease, pertussis
- Lung tumor
- Congestive heart failure
- Pulmonary embolus
- Sleep apnea

DIAGNOSIS

Bronchitis must be considered a diagnosis of exclusion because of serious, life-threatening lower respiratory diseases also associated with cough.

Physical Examination

Auscultation may reveal wheezing and rhonchi.

Laboratory Tests

Acute bronchitis (distinguish between viral and bacterial causes):
- Sputum culture, which is diagnostic for pneumonia and tuberculosis
- White blood cell count
- Increase in serum antibody titers
- Gamma M immunoglobulin-specific conjugate, which detects current infection
- Moderate to severe hypoxia

Chronic bronchitis (in addition to above):
- Spirometry for large airway obstruction and closing volume; maximal midexpiratory flow rate determinations for small airway obstruction

Imaging

- Chest X ray to rule out pneumonia, heart failure, or pneumothorax complications
- Chest X ray for bronchovascular markings with chronic bronchitis
- Bronchoscopy or computed tomography for exclusion of endo-bronchial lesion or localized bronchiectasis

Other Diagnostic Procedures

Bronchitis is diagnosed by the exclusion of other disease(s).
- Pulmonary function test
- ABGs
- Chest exam
- Electrocardiogram for differential diagnosis of chest pain
- Pulmonary function tests

TREATMENT OPTIONS

Treatment Strategy

Eliminating risk factors, preventing or treating infection, controlling bronchospasm, mobilizing secretions, and preventing chronic hypoxemia.

Drug Therapies

- Beta-sympathomimetic and anticholinergic bronchodilators for bronchospasm (e.g., from 2 to 4 to 6 to 12 puffs a day of albuterol)
- Corticosteroids (e.g., 20 to 40 mg/day of prednisone or 100 to 200 mcg, 2 to 4 puffs/day of inhaled beclomethasone) to reduce mucus and inflammation
- Symptomatic treatment: humidifier to loosen secretions; cough uppressants (only with dry cough or to allow sleep; not with bacterial infections); hydration
- Expectorant medication (e.g., 10 to 12 drops tid of potassium iodide) or tracheal suction
- Antibiotics with bacterial infection (e.g., 250 to 500 mg of penicillin or tetracycline every six hours for 10 days), sometimes given pro-phylactically
- Oxygen for hypoxia: more than 12 hours/day required to be effective

Complementary and Alternative Therapies

While acute bronchitis due to severe underlying pathology requires pharmacologic treatment, alternative therapies can be useful in treating bronchitis secondary to viral agents, allergens, and environmental irritants.

NUTRITION

- Eliminate known allergenic foods, food coloring, preservatives, and additives. Reduce intake of mucus-producing foods such as dairy, citrus, wheat, and bananas. Increase fresh vegetables, fruits, and whole grains. Onions and garlic should be eaten liberally to thin mucus.
- Vitamin C (1,000 mg tid to qid), zinc (30 mg/day), and beta-carotene (50,000 to 100,000 IU/day) support the immune system and help to restore the integrity of the respiratory tract. Some studies have suggested that beta-carotene is contraindicated in smokers. N-acetyl cysteine (200 mg bid between meals) protects lung tissue from oxidative damage and is a mucolytic agent.

HERBS

Herbs are generally a safe way to strengthen and tone the body's systems. As with any therapy, it is important to ascertain a diagnosis before pursuing treatment. Herbs may be used as dried extracts (capsules, powders, teas), glycerites (glycerine extracts), or tinctures (alcohol extracts). Infusions are made with 1 heaping tsp. herb per cup of hot water, steeped covered for 10 minutes, and drunk 3 to 4 cups/day. Tinctures may be used singly or in combination, 30 drops tid to qid.

A well-balanced formula contains herbs to increase the effectiveness of the cough (by stimulating expectoration or calming an irritable cough reflex), soothe irritated tissues, and support immune function. Licorice root should be avoided in hypertension; substitute grindelia (*Grindelia robusta*).

- Acute Bronchitis: Thyme leaf (*Thymus vulgaris*), licorice root (*Glycyrrhiza glabra*), coneflower (*Echinacea purpura*), ginger (*Zingiber officinalis*), and linden flowers (*Tilia cordata*). Smokers should substitute Indian tobacco (*Lobelia inflata*) for the linden flowers. White horehound (*Marrabium vulgare*) is a gentle stimulating expectorant and circulatory tonic that relaxes spasms of the bronchi. Sundew (*Drosera rotundifolia*) is a relaxing expectorant and antispasmodic with antimicrobial and mucolytic qualities.
- Chronic Bronchitis: Pleurisy root (*Asclepias tuberosa*), Indian tobacco, elecampane (*Inula helenium*), licorice root, lungwort (*Sticta pulmonaria*), and lomatium (*Lomatium dissectum*). Boneset (*Eupatorium perfoliatum*), a diaphoretic and antispasmodic herb, has traditionally been used for chronic bronchitis. Pill Bearing Spurge (*Euphorbia hirta*), an antispasmodic and mucolytic herb, is a specific for bronchial conditions.
- Garlic (*Allium sativum*)/ginger tea can be used long-term to relieve bronchitis and support immune function. Use 2 cloves of garlic and 2 to 3 slices of ginger root. Simmer in 1 cup of water for 10 to 15 minutes. Drink 3 to 4 cups/day. May add honey or lemon to flavor.

HOMEOPATHY

An experienced homeopath should assess individual constitutional types and severity of disease to select the correct remedy and potency. For acute prescribing use 3 to 5 pellets of a 12X to 30C remedy every one to four hours until acute symptoms resolve. It is imperative that the underlying condition be addressed; however, homeopathic remedies can be helpful in acute coughs or chronic coughs that fail to resolve.

- Antimonium tart for rattling cough with dizziness
- Hepar sulphuricum for later stages of bronchitis with wheezing, scant expectoration, and coughing that comes on when any part of the body gets cold.
- Ipecacuanha for first stages of bronchitis with deep, wet cough and gagging from the cough.
- Phosphorus for painful cough in patients who are thirsty and chilly.

PHYSICAL MEDICINE

- Castor oil pack. Used externally, castor oil is a powerful anti-inflammatory. Apply oil directly to skin, cover with a clean soft cloth (e.g., flannel) and plastic wrap. Place a heat source (hot water bottle or heating pad) over the pack and let sit for 30 to 60 minutes. For best results, use for three consecutive days.
- Chest rubs with 3 to 6 drops of essential oil in 1 tbsp. of food grade oil (olive, flax, sesame, almond, etc.). Thyme, eucalyptus, and pine oils can be applied to ease bronchial spasm and help thin mucus. May combine this treatment with the castor oil pack.
- Running a humidifier with essential oils such as eucalyptus, tea tree, or marjoram at night may help thin mucus and ease cough.
- Postural drainage can be of great help in relieving congestion and removing mucus from the chest.

ACUPUNCTURE

Acupuncture can bring relief to bronchial spasm and enhance immune function. Smoking cessation through acupuncture can be very successful.

MASSAGE

Therapeutic massage can increase circulation. Tapotement (striking with the side of the hand), can be helpful in loosening mucus and aiding expectoration.

Patient Monitoring

For acute presentation, closely follow temperature, respiratory rate, and white blood cell count. Altered mental status, infection, serious shortness of breath, and electrolyte abnormality warrant hospitalization.

OTHER CONSIDERATIONS

Prevention

Avoiding causative environmental pollutants. Smoking cessation, annual influenza vaccinations, and a polyvalent pneumococcal vaccination (once in a lifetime or every five years if spleen has been removed) prevent complications and, possibly, irreversible progression.

Complications/Sequelae

- Lowered resistance to bronchopulmonary infection
- Pulmonary hypertension
- Pneumonia
- Inappropriate antibiotic use may cause resistance

Prognosis

Acute bronchitis: This condition takes one to eight weeks to resolve (with no complications).

Chronic bronchitis: Progressive airway damage, worsening exercise tolerance, acute respiratory failure, resting tachycardia, cor pulmonale, and comorbidity are indicators of poor prognosis

Pregnancy

Avoiding fetal hypoxia is essential in treating respiratory disorders during pregnancy. Ventilator support is sometimes required. Medications used for bronchodilation or for infection need to be carefully selected, as many have deleterious effects (e.g., use of albuterol has not been associated with congenital abnormalities, but tachyphylaxis can occur with prolonged use in late pregnancy). High doses of vitamins and herbal support should not be undertaken without physician supervision.

REFERENCES

Allan H, Goroll MD, et al, eds. *Primary Care Medicine.* 3rd ed. Philadelphia, Pa: Lippincott-Raven Publishers; 1995:252–260, 285–294.
Bartram T. *Encyclopedia of Herbal Medicine.* Dorset, England: Grace Publishers; 1995:72–73.
Bone RC, ed. *Pulmonary and Critical Care Medicine.* St. Louis, Mo: Mosby-Year Book, Inc; 1998:G3 1–6.
Cecil RL, Plum F, Bennett JC, eds. *Cecil Textbook of Medicine.* 20th ed. Philadelphia, Pa: WB Saunders Company; 1996:382–389.
Kruzel T. *The Homeopathic Emergency Guide.* Berkeley, Calif: North Atlantic Books; 1992:40–43.
Rakel RE, ed. *Conn's Current Therapy.* 50th ed. Philadelphia, Pa: WB Saunders Company; 1998:211–212.

■ BURNS

OVERVIEW

Definition

About 80% of thermal injuries (burns) occur in the home, and 5% (one million per year) require hospitalization. Included among thermal injuries are sunburns (most common), direct heat, scalding (a moist burn), electrical burns, and chemical burns. The severity of the burn, based on depth, duration of exposure, and extent, determines appropriate management.

Etiology

Fires, hot water or steam, sun overexposure, electricity, and certain chemicals produce burns.

Risk Factors

- Hot water heater set above 120° F
- Careless smoking
- Unsafe storage of flammable or caustic materials
- Microwaved foods/containers
- Wood stoves or exposed heating sources or electrical cords
- Sun overexposure, especially for older and fair-skinned people

Signs and Symptoms

- Superficial partial-thickness burns (first degree)—epidermis only; red, painful but intact; no blisters
- Deep partial-thickness burns (second degree)—epidermis only; red, painful, blisters, oozing
- Full-thickness burns (third degree)—all layers of dermis and epidermis plus deeper layers; skin charred, pale, or brownish yellow and leathery, often without pain or blisters; also injuries that involve the face, neck, shoulders, elbows, hands, perineum, popliteal fossa, ankles, or feet (where skin is thin). Requires specialist in burn care.

DIFFERENTIAL DIAGNOSIS

Infections or drug reactions causing toxic epidermal necrolysis (scalded skin syndrome)

DIAGNOSIS

Physical Examination

Evaluate depth and extent of injury using the rule of nines (Lund-Browder chart): surface area estimated as each arm 9%, each leg 18%, front of torso 18%, back of trunk 18%, head 9%, and groin 1%. For infants and small children, as above but head is 18% and legs 13.5%. Determine the cause to see if smoke inhalation is a possibility. Check for localized edema impeding circulation.

TREATMENT OPTIONS

Treatment Strategy

For thermal injuries:

- Cool the area with cold water.
- Gently debride and cleanse the wound.
- Give oral analgesics for pain; IV medications for major burns.
- Open blisters and excise dead skin.
- Cover with bacteriostatic cream and apply soft bulky dressing, which should be changed and medication reapplied twice a day.
- Review status of tetanus prophylaxis and update.
- Do not give systemic antibiotics.
- Fluid resuscitation.

For chemical burns:

- Remove patient's clothing.
- Irrigate area copiously with water, especially if the eyes are involved.

For electrical burns:

- Damage depends on resistance, type of current, amperage, voltage, duration of exposure, and pathway. Areas most affected are neurovascular bundles and muscles.
- Because cardiorespiratory arrest is common, patient may require CPR and advanced cardiac life support.
- Characteristic lesions are most intense at port of entry and exit.
- Evaluate for other injuries.
- May need early decompressive fasciotomies and debridement to assess the extent of damage; the incidence of major amputation with electrical burns is 33%.
- Transfer to a specialized center after patient's condition is stabilized.
- ECG monitoring for 24 hours.

Hospitalization required for: second-degree burns over 10% of body; third-degree burns; burns on hands, feet, face, or genitals; electrical/chemical burns; smoke inhalation.

Burn center required for: second- or third-degree burns over 10% of body in patients under 10 years or over 50 years; second- or third-degree burns over 20% of body.

Drug Therapies

- Silver sulfadiazine (Silvadene). Topical antibiotic applied to burned area, effective against most *Pseudomonas,* fairly good eschar penetration. Some microorganisms are resistant. Side effects are leukopenia or fever and delay in epithelialization.
- Mafenide. Penetrates eschar better than silver sulfadiazine, more effective against *Pseudomonas;* recommended for burns over cartilage and deep burns. Side effects are (in 10% solution) carbonic anhydrase inhibition, causing metabolic acidosis, delay in epithelialization, pain; can be lessened in 5% solution. Limit use to no more than 10% of total body surface.
- Povidone-iodine (Betadine). Especially useful against *Candida* and gram-positive and gram-negative microorganisms, but poor eschar penetration. Side effects are desiccation of wound surface, pain, high blood iodine levels.

Complementary and Alternative Therapies

Herbal support, both internally and externally, can facilitate wound healing, reduce the risk for infection by stimulating the immune system, and may help prevent scarring. Homeopathic remedies can provide excellent pain relief and reduction of symptoms.

NUTRITION

- Hydration is of primary importance in managing moderate to severe burns. Fresh vegetable and fruit juices, water, and electrolyte replacement drinks should be used liberally.
- Vitamin C (1,000 to 1,500 mg tid), zinc (30 to 50 mg/day), and beta-carotene (100,000 IU/day) supports immune function and enhances dermal healing.
- Vitamin E (1,200 IU d-alpha tocopherols tid) is a strong anti-oxidant and reduces scarring.
- Bromelain (250 to 500 mg qid between meals) is a proteolytic enzyme that decreases inflammation. Use with turmeric (*Curcuma longa,* 500 mg qid) to potentiate effects.
- L-glutamine (3 to 10 g tid) provides amino acids to the gut that may be necessary to prevent damage secondary to severe burns.

HERBS

Herbs are generally a safe way to strengthen and tone the body's systems. As with any therapy, it is important to ascertain a diagnosis before pursuing treatment. Herbs may be used as dried extracts (capsules, powders, teas), glycerites (glycerine extracts), or tinctures (alcohol extracts). Unless otherwise indicated, teas should be made with 1 tsp. herb per cup of hot water. Steep covered 5 to 10 minutes for leaf or flowers, and 10 to 20 minutes for roots. Drink 2 to 4 cups/day. Tinctures may be used singly or in combination as noted.

- To mobilize the immune system and minimize risk of infection during the acute phase, combine equal parts of tinctures of coneflower (*Echinacea purpura*) and goldenseal (*Hydrastis canadensis*). Take 30 to 60 drops every three to four hours.
- Gotu kola (*Centella asiatica*) has been used in patients with second- to third-degree burns with great success. Daily topical application prevented or limited shrinking and swelling of the skin, inhibited scar formation, increased healing, and decreased fibrosis.
- Herbs that enhance circulation to the skin can facilitate the delivery of nutrients and elimination of metabolic waste. Combine equal parts of the following in a tea (1 cup four to six times/day) or tincture (30 to 60 drops tid to qid). Yarrow (*Achillea millefolium*), cleavers (*Gallium aparine*), prickly ash bark (*Xanthoxyllum clava-herculis*), marigold (*Calendula officinalis*), plantain (*Plantago major*), and ginger root (*Zingiber officinalis*).
- For acute pain relief combine equal parts of tincture of Jamaican dogwood (*Piscidia erythrina*), valerian (*Valeriana officinalis*), St. John's wort (*Hypericum perforatum*), and California poppy (*Escholzia californica*) with one-half part of gelsemium (*Gelsemium sempivirens*). Take 10 to 15 drops every 15 minutes up to eight doses, acutely. For general pain relief, take 30 drops tid to qid.
- Aloe vera: Cut a fresh leaf and apply the gel to skin, or peel leaf, blend pulp, then apply to skin.
- Comfrey leaf (*Symphytum officinalis*): Make a strong tea with 1 heaping tsp. herb/cup. Use as a wash. Do not use internally for prolonged periods due to potential for liver damage.
- Combine powders of slippery elm (*Ulmus rubra*), marshmallow root (*Althea officinalis*), goldenseal, and comfrey root. Apply to burns to speed healing and reduce risk for infection.

HOMEOPATHY

An experienced homeopath should assess individual constitutional types and severity of disease to select the correct remedy and potency. For acute prescribing, use 3 to 5 pellets of a 12X to 30C remedy every one to four hours until acute symptoms resolve.

- *Cantharis* for burns and scalds with cutting, burning, or smarting pains that are relieved with cold applications. Specifically for extensive burns causing renal involvement.
- *Carbolic acid* for rapid prostration following a burn, with coldness of the skin and rapidly progressing to shock and collapse.
- *Carbo vegetabilis* for burns with great prostration and sluggishness of circulation. Patient has air hunger and wishes to be fanned even though they are chilly.

Topical homeopathic preparations for burns may provide acute pain relief. Do not apply over broken skin.

Patient Monitoring

Patient should return 72 hours after injury, then every five to seven days until the wound is healed.

- If excessive swelling: Assess circulation and instruct patient to keep injured area elevated to avoid developing a compartment syndrome, wherein the injury progresses to full-thickness burn.
- If superficial infection: Do wound culture and sensitivity.
- If systemic signs of sepsis (fever, leukocytosis, extensive erythema): Manage aggressively with systemic antibiotics.
- If moderate swelling and erythema: Use elevation and warm moist dressings.
- For itching: Use moisturizing cream.
- To prevent functional disability, refer to physical therapist or reconstructive surgeon.

OTHER CONSIDERATIONS

Prevention

- Safety inspection of home by fire department.
- Plan fire/emergency escape route.
- Keep hot water heater set at maximum of 120° F.

Complications/Sequelae

- Local edema: maintain adequate circulation
- Functional or cosmetic defects (risk greater with partial-thickness burns)
- Burn sepsis
- Carcinoma developing in burn site

Prognosis

Partial-thickness burns generally heal in three to five weeks. Third-degree burns require skin graft.

Pregnancy

Topical applications and homeopathic remedies may provide excellent support in pregnancy.

REFERENCES

Bartram T. *Encyclopedia of Herbal Medicine*. Dorset, England: Grace Publishers; 1995:77.

Blumenthal M, ed. *The Complete German Commission E Monographs*. Boston, Mass: Integrative Medicine Communications; 1998:423.

Castro M. *The Complete Homeopathy Handbook*. New York, NY: St. Martin's Press; 1991.

Foley D, Nechas E, Perry S, Salmon DK. *The Doctor's Book of Home Remedies for Children*. Emmaus, Pa: Rodale Press; 1994.

Forgey WW, ed. *Wilderness Medical Society Practice Guidelines for Wilderness Emergency Care*. Merrillville, Ind: ICS Books, Inc; 1995.

Kruzel T. *The Homeopathic Emergency Guide*. Berkeley, Calif: North Atlantic Books; 1992:48–50.

Lynn SG, Weintraub P. *Medical Emergency! The St. Luke's-Roosevelt Hospital Center Book of Emergency Medicine*. New York, NY: Hearst Books; 1996.

Noble J, ed. *Textbook Of Primary Care Medicine*. St. Louis, Mo: Mosby-Year Book; 1996.

Tierney Jr LM, McPhee SJ, Papadakis MA, eds. *Current Medical Diagnosis and Treatment*. Norwalk, Conn: Appleton & Lange; 1994.

Tyler VE. *Herbs of Choice: The Therapeutic Use of Phytomedicinals*. New York, NY. Pharmaceutical Products Press; 1994.

■ BURSITIS
OVERVIEW
Definition
Bursitis is the inflammation of a bursa, a sac lined by a synovial membrane, filled with fluid, and located between bones and tendons or muscles. Commonly affected bursae are the subdeltoid, olecranon, prepatellar, trochanteric, iliopsoas, ischial, anserine, Achilles, calcaneal, and radio-humeral. Bursae exist where joint friction occurs, helping lubricate and cushion the joint. Bursitis seldom occurs in patients before adulthood and is more common in middle and old age. Bursitis can be acute or chronic. Septic bursitis is an infection of the bursa.

Etiology
- Chronic overuse or repetitive use
- Traumatic injury
- Bacterial infection
- Gout, pseudogout
- Rheumatoid arthritis

Risk Factors
Repetitive activities putting strain on the joint (e.g., athletic, occupational).

Signs and Symptoms
- Localized pain aggravated by movement
- Abrupt onset of pain in acute bursitis
- Localized swelling
- Localized tenderness
- Erythema
- Fever, swelling, and increased temperature of the overlying skin (septic bursitis)

DIFFERENTIAL DIAGNOSIS
- Arthritis
- Gout or pseudogout
- Tendinitis
- Sprain or strain

For shoulder pain:
- Referred cardiac pain
- Referred cervical nerve root compression
- Referred gallbladder pain
- Injury to the rotator cuff

DIAGNOSIS
Physical Examination
Physical signs of bursitis are pain or tenderness and swelling that can be localized to the bursa rather than the entire joint, except in cases of deep bursae.

Laboratory Tests
For infection:
- White blood count
- Gram stain and culture of bursal fluid

To rule out gout:
- Analysis of bursal fluid for crystals

To rule out rheumatic and connective tissue disease:
- CBC
- ESR
- Serum protein electrophoresis
- Rheumatoid factor
- Serum uric acid
- Calcium
- Phosphorus
- Alkaline phosphatase
- VDRL

Pathological Findings
- Distended bursa filled with serous fluid
- In chronic cases, thickened bursal wall
- Very high white blood counts in septic bursitis

Imaging
X-ray to rule out arthritic conditions.

Other Diagnostic Procedures
Bursitis can often be diagnosed by the history and physical assessment. The absence of pain on passive motion may help differentiate bursitis from arthritis. A swollen, inflamed bursa should be aspirated to rule out infection; crystals in the fluid usually indicate gout. EKG if necessary to rule out referred cardiac pain.

TREATMENT OPTIONS
Treatment Strategy
In most cases of nonseptic bursitis, conservative treatment with rest is sufficient to allow the inflammation to resolve. Rarely, in severe chronic cases is surgical excision of the bursa necessary.

Acute bursitis:
- Rest the joint, and elevate if possible
- Ice application
- Immobilization and or compression of the joint
- Ultrasound therapy helpful in some cases
- NSAIDs for pain
- In more severe cases, local anesthetic and corticosteroid injected into the bursa
- Oral corticosteroids
- Rarely, aspiration is indicated

Septic bursitis:
- Drain bursal fluid
- Antibiotics

Chronic bursitis:
- Repeated corticosteroid injections with physical therapy to restore joint function

Drug Therapies
- Nonsteroidal anti-inflammatory drugs for pain; continue four to five days to prevent recurrence; side effects include gastrointestinal bleeding, abdominal pain, nausea, vomiting, possible renal damage with chronic use.
- Corticosteroids and local anesthetic, such as a combination of 2 to 3 ml of 1% to 2% lidocaine with 20 to 40 mg of a depoglucocorticoid (Celestone, Aristocort, Kenalog), by injection of 1 to 3 ml using a 22-gauge needle for more severe acute and chronic inflammation; wait two weeks before repeat injection to rule out iatrogenic sepsis; side effects of corticosteroids include blurred vision, frequent urination, increased thirst.
- Antibiotics for septic bursitis; the drug of choice depends on the results of the Gram stain and culturing; most cases caused by *Staphylococcus aureus.*

Complementary and Alternative Therapies
Alternative therapies may be useful in reducing the pain and inflammation of bursitis while supporting healthy connective tissue.

NUTRITION

Minimize pro-inflammatory foods, especially arachidonic acid from saturated fats (dairy and animal products). Include anti-inflammatory oils such as found in cold-water fish, nuts, and seeds.

- Glucosamine sulfate (500 mg bid to tid), for connective tissue support
- Omega-3 oils (1,000 mg bid to tid), such as flaxseed oil, for anti-inflammatory support
- Vitamin C with bioflavanoids (1,000 mg tid), for connective tissue repair
- Proteolytic enzymes such as bromelain (250 mg bid), to reduce inflammation

HERBS

Herbs are generally a safe way to strengthen and tone the body's systems. As with any therapy, it is important to ascertain a diagnosis before pursuing treatment. Herbs may be used as dried extracts (capsules, powders, teas), glycerites, or tinctures (alcohol extracts). Unless otherwise indicated, teas should be made with 1 tsp. herb per cup of hot water. Steep covered 10 to 20 minutes and drink 2 to 4 cups/day. Tinctures may be used singly or in combination as noted.

- Anti-inflammatory herbs include meadowsweet *(Filipendula ulmaria)*, white willow *(Salix alba)*, Jamaican dogwood *(Piscidia erythrina)*, and turmeric *(Curcuma longa)*. A tincture of one, or a combination of these, may be taken at 15 drops every 15 minutes up to four doses for acute pain relief, or 30 drops qid. Turmeric helps potentiate the effects of bromelain.
- For concurrent muscle spasm, add valerian *(Valeriana officinalis)*.
- For chronic bursitis, add hawthorn *(Crataegus oxyanthoides)* to help restore the integrity of the connective tissue.

HOMEOPATHY

An experienced homeopath should assess individual constitutional types and severity of disease to select the correct remedy and potency. For acute prescribing use 3 to 5 pellets of a 12X to 30C remedy every one to four hours until acute symptoms resolve.

- *Arnica* gel applied topically (as directed) gives excellent short-term pain relief.

Acute remedies to be considered include the following.

- *Arnica* for post-trauma bursitis
- *Ruta graveolons* for rheumatic pains in the joint
- *Bellis perennis* for injury with much bruising
- *Rhus toxicodendron* for pain that is relieved with movement
- "Traumeel" injections as an alternative to corticosteroids

ACUPUNCTURE

Can be helpful in resolving swelling and inflammation, especially for pain relief.

MASSAGE

Contraindicated in septic bursitis. Otherwise, massage (especially myofascial release therapy) can be used for general relaxation and to reduce discomfort from holding patterns secondary to pain and compensating for an injured part.

Patient Monitoring

Monitor the patient for rare allergic reaction to corticosteroids. Educate the patient to discontinue use of NSAIDs as soon as possible to reduce the risk of side effects. If the pain does not resolve within two weeks, have the patient return for reexamination and, if necessary, a second corticosteroid injection.

OTHER CONSIDERATIONS

Prevention

Most acute and chronic bursitis can be prevented by avoiding overuse of the joint, by resting between periods of activity, and by adequately warming up and stretching before strenuous activity.

Complications/Sequelae

Infection or inflammation at the injection site; instruct patient to report redness or swelling that occurs at this site. Atrophy may occur if the injection enters the skin. Possible motion or activity restrictions in chronic cases.

Prognosis

Bursitis usually resolves within a one to two weeks but may recur with repeated overuse of joint. Recurring acute bursitis can progress to chronic bursitis.

Pregnancy

Use glucocorticoids with caution in pregnancy (U.S. FDA pregnancy safety category C).

REFERENCES

Andreoli TE, Bennett JC, Carpenter CCJ. *Cecil Essentials of Medicine.* 3rd ed. Philadelphia, Pa: W.B. Saunders; 1993.

Barker LR, Burton JR, Zieve PD, eds. *Principles of Ambulatory Medicine.* 4th ed. Baltimore, Md: Williams & Wilkins; 1995:885–894.

Dambro MR, ed. *Griffith's 5 Minute Clinical Consult 1999.* Baltimore, Md: Lippincott Williams & Wilkins; 1999.

Murray MT. *The Healing Power of Herbs: The Enlightened Person's Guide to the Wonders of Medicinal Plants.* Rocklin, Calif: Prima Publishing; 1998.

Stein JH, ed. *Internal Medicine.* 4th ed. St. Louis, Mo: Mosby-Year Book; 1994:2400–2404.

■ CANDIDIASIS

OVERVIEW

Definition

Candidiasis is a yeast, or fungal, infection caused by several species of candida, the most predominant being *Candida albicans*. Although approximately 80% of healthy individuals will have normal colonization in the mouth, gastrointestinal tract, vagina, and rectum, most produce bacterial flora to protect against infections. Clinical manifestations vary according to subtype and range from superficial to severe infections. Candidiasis is the fourth leading cause of nosocomial infectious disease. Approximately 75% of women will contract candidiasis of the vagina during their lifetime, and 90% of people diagnosed with HIV/AIDS will develop a Candida infection. The primary subtypes are:

- Oral candidiasis (thrush)
- Perlèche (candidal angular chelitis)
- Cutaneous disease
- Vulvovaginitis
- Disseminated candidiasis (can affect lungs, liver, spleen, kidneys, heart, brain, and eyes)
- Gastrointestinal candidiasis
- Urinary tract candidiasis
- Candidal endocarditis (often due to damaged or prosthetic cardiac valves or long-term intravenous catheter use)
- Central nervous system candidiasis (extremely rare)
- Chronic candidiasis (occurs predominantly in immunosuppressed patients)

Etiology

Biological factors (e.g., immunologic defects); physical influences (e.g., excessive moisture in groin and inframammary folds); pharmaceutical therapies (e.g., broad-spectrum antibacterials); and genetic predisposition (e.g., chronic mucocutaneous candidiasis) are factors in the etiology of candidiasis.

Risk Factors

- Dermatitis (e.g., contact or primary irritant, seborrheic, atopic)
- Prolonged neutropenia
- Psoriasis
- Bacterial infection
- Cushing's disease
- Obesity
- Histiocytosis
- Pregnancy
- Diabetes
- HIV infection
- Intravenous drug abuse
- Surgery
- Intravascular catheter
- Long-term antibiotic use

Signs and Symptoms

- Fever, malaise
- Hypotension
- Creamy white patches overlying erythematous buccal mucosa (thrush)
- Painful, macerated fissures at the corners of the mouth (perlèche)
- Erythematous skin lesion found most commonly in the groin, between fingers and toes, under the female breast, and in the axilla (cutaneous disease)
- Vulvar erythema, edema, and pruritus; usually includes a curdlike discharge (vulvovaginitis)

- Large abscesses and diffuse microabscesses (disseminated candidiasis)
- Erosive lesions of the distal esophagus and stomach (gastrointestinal candidiasis)
- Urinary tract infection (urinary tract candidiasis)

DIFFERENTIAL DIAGNOSIS

- Herpes simplex virus
- Acquired immunodeficiency syndrome (AIDS)
- Contact or primary irritant (e.g., diaper rash), seborrheic, or atopic dermatitis
- Psoriasis
- Bacterial infection
- Acrodermatitis enteropathica
- Histiocytosis

DIAGNOSIS

Physical Examination

The physical presentations of candidiasis vary according to subtype. They may include white patches in the mouth or throat; peeling skin on hands; swollen nail folds; itchy, shiny rash that is pink with scaly or blistered edges; vaginal redness and swelling of the vulva accompanied by thick white discharge; and red patches and blisters on penis.

Laboratory Tests

Because candida is commonly found in healthy individuals, caution is recommended in diagnosis based on laboratory findings alone. Laboratory tests include culture analysis for yeast and pseudohyphae, antibiotic susceptibility testing, blood culture, candida antibody and candida antigen tests, and analysis of the cerebrospinal fluid.

Pathological Findings

Histologic response is often purulent and may resemble infectious bacterial lesions; abscesses or microabscesses may be present; occasional response is granulomatous; budding yeast, pseudohyphae, and true hyphae may be found in tissue.

Imaging

CT scans of the abdomen may show hepatosplenomegaly with low-density liver defects in disseminated disease; esophagoscopy may be used in candidiasis patients with swallowing difficulties and the absence of thrush or who do not respond to antifungal therapy.

Other Diagnostic Procedures

- Physical examination—assess appearance and clinical symptoms; tissue biopsy or evidence of retinal disease required for diagnosis of invasive systemic disease
- Clinician interview—evaluate for intravenous drug use, recent surgery or hospitalization, and chronic antibiotic use
- Lysis/centrifuge of blood cultures to isolate causative organism

TREATMENT OPTIONS

Treatment Strategy

A number of topical and systemic antifungal agents are available for treating the subtypes of candidiasis.

Topical agents include oral rinses, oral tablets (troches), vaginal tablets or suppositories, and creams. Fluid and electrolyte therapy may be required for more serious cases.

Drug Therapies

- Imidazole antibiotics, such as fluconazole (Difulcan), ketoconazole (Nizoral—topical), and itraconazol (Sporanox), are effective in treating several subtypes of candidiasis; dosages vary depending on subtype; some isolates of candida species are developing resistance to imidazoles; recommended dosages include the following examples:

- fluconazole or itraconazol (100 mg/day) for oral candidiasis
- fluconazole (150 mg once) for vulvovaginal candidiasis
- flucytosine (150 mg/kg/day) or fluconazole (200 to 400 mg/day intravenously) for disseminated candidiasis
- Other antifungals, such as amphotericin B (topical, infusion, or liquid form), are also available to treat more severe or recalcitrant cases or where esophagitis is present; side effects include irreversible kidney damage, allergic reaction (preventable with steroids), and lowering of blood potassium and magnesium levels; may be contraindicated if patient is taking other medications such as antineoplastics, interferon, or AZT.
- Topical azole preparations, such as vaginal tablet clotrimazole (100 mg once a day for seven days) and the vaginal suppository miconazole (200 mg once a day for three days); creams are sometimes combined with low-strength corticosteroid for anti-inflammatory and antipruritic action.

Complementary and Alternative Therapies

Many patients may present with a self-diagnosis of intestinal candida. Stool culture or candida antigen (serum) may be the preferred methods for testing in this population. However, neither test is perfect. Many people without symptoms will test positive. The "candida diet" allows no alcohol, no simple sugars, and very limited refined foods. Many people may feel better due to the diet alone. The thrust of alternative therapies for candida is to "starve" the yeast present and use natural anti-fungals.

NUTRITION

- Vitamin C (500 to 1,000 mg/day), vitamin E (200 to 400 IU/day), and selenium (200 mcg/day) anti-inflammatory
- Essential fatty acids: anti-inflammatory, a mix of omega-6 (evening primrose) and omega-3 (flaxseed) may be most optimum (2 tbsp. oil/day or 1,000 to 1,500 mg bid). Dietary manipulation includes reducing animal fats and increasing fish and nuts.
- Biotin: (300 mcg) inhibits the pseudo-hyphae form of candida, which is the most irritating to membranes.
- B-complex: B_1 (50 to 100 mg), B_2 (50 mg), B_3 (25 mg); B_5 (100 mg); B_6 (50 to 100 mg), B_{12} (100 to 1,000 mcg), folate (400 mcg/day) should be yeast free
- Calcium (1,000 to, 1,500 mg/day) to correct deficiency often found in yeast infections and magnesium (750 to 1,000 mg/day) to balance calcium intake.
- Lactobacillus acidophilus (2 to 5 million organisms tid) to help restore normal balance of bowel and mucous membranes. Many European physicians routinely prescribe acidophilus when they prescribe antibiotics. Studies showed saccromyces boulardii effectively treats antibiotic-induced diarrhea.
- Caprylic acid: (1 g with meals) anti-fungal fatty acid
- Avoid simple carbohydrates including fruit juice, yeast and fermented foods, limit fruit to 1 serving/day, increase garlic (fungicidal), nuts (essential fatty acids), whole grains (B vitamins), oregano, cinnamon, sage, and cloves (anti-fungal spices)

HERBS

Herbs are generally a safe way to strengthen and tone the body's systems. As with any therapy, it is important to ascertain a diagnosis before pursuing treatment. Herbs may be used as dried extracts (capsules, powders, teas), glycerites (glycerine extracts), or tinctures (alcohol extracts). Unless otherwise indicated, teas should be made with 1 tsp. herb per cup of hot water. Steep covered 5 to 10 minutes for leaf or flowers, and 10 to 20 minutes for roots. Drink 2 to 4 cups/day. Tinctures may be used singly or in combination as noted.

- Pau d'arco bark (lapacho or taheebo): anti-fungal, best used as a tea (2 tbsp. boiled in 1 quart of water; 3 to 6 cups/day), or use the cooled tea as a vaginal douche
- Goldenseal (Hydrastis canadensis), Oegon grape root (Mahonia Nervosa), and barberry (Berberis vulgaris) are bitter, digestive, and immune stimulants. Chamomile (Matricaria recicuta) and licorice (Glycyrrhiza glabra) are anti-inflammatory and soothing to mucous membranes. Use a tea or tincture of the four herbs listed above (1 cup tea tid or 30 to 60 drops tincture tid) for six weeks.
- Topical treatments include tea tree oil (Melaleuca alternifolia) or lavender essential oil (Lavendula species) bid to tid; apply full strength to skin infections, discontinue if skin irritation develops; marigold (Calendula officinalis) apply three to five times/day in a salve for rashes, soothing to skin and mucous membranes
- Fireweed (Epilobium parviflorum): quite effective as a tea for oral, vaginal, and intestinal candidias.

HOMEOPATHY

An experienced homeopath should assess individual constitutional types and severity of disease to select the correct remedy and potency. For acute prescribing use 3 to 5 pellets of a 12X to 30C remedy every one to four hours until acute symptoms resolve.

- Borax for bleeding oral mucosa, especially with diarrhea
- Belladonna for bright red, inflamed skin that is not raw or oozing, but is painful, especially with irritability
- Chamomilla for "diaper" rash that is bright red, especially with irritability
- Arsenicum album for burning, itching rashes, especially with anxiety
- Graphites for thick, cracked skin (corners of mouth or heels) that oozes
- Kreosotum for leukorrhea that causes itching, swelling, and extreme excoriation

ACUPUNCTURE

May be helpful to stimulate immune system, digestion, and relieve stress.

Patient Monitoring

Almost all AIDS patients will have some form of mucosal candidiasis; underlying predisposing factor(s) should be addressed in all forms of invasive disease. Monitor closely patients who are on daily amphotericin B therapy. Repeat blood cultures until negative.

OTHER CONSIDERATIONS

Prevention

When taking anti-biotics, supplement with lactobacillus acidophilus; avoid broad-spectrum antibiotics unless necessary; practice good hygiene, including oral hygiene and thorough cleansing of genital areas; maintain appropriate weight; wear cotton or silk underwear; women should avoid douches (unless medically indicated), vaginal deodorants and bubble baths; limit sweets and alcohol intake; diabetics should adhere to treatments; wear rubber gloves if occupation requires keeping hands in water; keep skin dry.

Complications/Sequelae

- Secondary bacterial infections (e.g., in the vagina); drug side effects and interactions may range from severe irreversible kidney damage (amphotericin) and liver toxicity (fluconazole) to milder bouts of nausea, vomiting, headache, abdominal pain, and diarrhea.

- Endocarditis, myocarditis, pericarditis
- CNS infection

Prognosis

Most cases of candidiasis are curable, often responding to treatment within days; people with immune deficiencies or taking immunosuppressants require long-term monitoring. Overall mortality associated with hematogenously disseminated candidiasis is significant.

Pregnancy

Animal studies have shown that ketoconazole can cause birth defects, although this side effect has not been studied in pregnant women.

REFERENCES

Bartram T. *Encyclopedia of Herbal Medicine*. Dorset, England: Grace Publishers; 1995:263, 417.

Berkow R, Fletcher AJ, eds. *The Merck Manual of Diagnosis and Therapy*. Rahway, NJ: Merck & Company Inc; 1992.

Blumenthal M, ed. *The Complete German Commission E Monographs*. Boston, Mass: Integrative Medicine Communications; 1998:463.

Coeugniet E, Kühnast R. Recurrent candidiasis: Adjutant immunotherapy with different formulations of Echinacin®. *Therapiewoche*. 1986;36:3352–3358.

Conn RB, Borer WZ, Snyder JW, eds. *Current Diagnosis 9*. Philadelphia, Pa: WB Saunders; 1996.

Gruenwald J, Brendler T, Jaenicke C et al, eds. *PDR for Herbal Medicines*. Montvale, NJ: Medical Economics Company; 1998:728.

Henry JR. *Clinical Diagnosis and Management by Laboratory Methods*. Philadelphia, Pa: WB Saunders Company; 1996.

Morrison R. *Desktop Guide to Keynotes and Confirmatory Symptoms*. Albany, Calif: Hahnemann Clinic Publishing; 1993:68, 115–117, 171–172, 210.

Thierney Jr LM, McPhee SJ, Papadakis MA, eds. *Current Medical Diagnosis and Treatment 1999*. 38th ed. Stamford, Conn: Appleton & Lange; 1999.

■ CHRONIC FATIGUE SYNDROME
OVERVIEW
Definition
Chronic fatigue syndrome (CFS) involves fatigue that is sufficiently intense and persistent to reduce normal daily activities by at least 50% for a minimum of six months. Women account for 70% of cases of CFS, with the typical patient being a Caucasian woman in her mid-20s to late 40s. The prevalence is 4 to 10 formally diagnosed cases per 100,000 U.S. adults (18 years or older). Women are affected almost twice as often as men.

Etiology
Although not conclusive, CFS may be precipitated by infectious agents (for example, *Borrelia burgdorferi*), herpesviruses, *Candida albicans*, and parasitic agents. This may very well be a multifactorial pathologic entity with lifestyle and constitutional/psychological makeup a factor.

Risk Factors
- Stressed immune system caused by recent acute illness, chronic health problems, emotional factors (anxiety, depression), or poor nutrition
- Possibly environmental pollutants and contaminants

Signs and Symptoms
- Sudden onset of severe fatigue, developing over a few hours to a few days and often after an acute viral illness
- Low-grade fever (less than 100.4°F) and chills
- Sore throat
- Lymphadenopathy
- Myalgias and arthralgias
- Headaches
- Sleep disturbances
- Decreased ability to concentrate or remember
- Allergies
- General muscle weakness

DIFFERENTIAL DIAGNOSIS
Rule out conditions producing fatigue.
- Fibromyalgia
- Psychiatric: extreme anxiety, depression
- Endocrine or metabolic: hypothyroidism, diabetes, pituitary insufficiency, hypoparathyroidism, hypercalcemia, Addison's disease, chronic renal failure
- Pharmacologic: use of sleeping pills, antihypertensives, or tranquilizers
- Infectious: subacute bacterial endocarditis, hepatitis, AIDS, syphilis, Lyme disease, intestinal parasites, tuberculosis, cytomegalovirus, toxoplasmosis, fungal disease
- Musculoskeletal disorders, neoplastic or hematologic conditions.
- Cardiopulmonary: chronic congestive heart failure, chronic obstructive pulmonary disease
- Immunologic: systemic lupus erythematosus, hypogammaglobulinemia
- Toxic disorders: lead or mercury poisoning
- Inadequate sleep or sleep apnea

DIAGNOSIS
Physical Examination
The patient may appear exhausted and obviously ill, eyes with dark circles, ecchymosis in the throat, swollen tonsils, and enlarged lymph nodes in the neck. However, physical appearance may be normal.

Laboratory Tests
No tests are specifically diagnostic for CFS. The minimal battery of tests should include all of the following (with further tests indicated on an individual basis).
- complete blood count with leukocyte differential
- erythrocyte sedimentation rate
- serum alanine aminotransferase, total protein, albumin, globulin, calcium, alkaline phosphastase, phosphorus, glucose, blood urea nitrogen, electrolytes, and creatinine
- glucose tolerance test
- thyroid-stimulating hormone assay
- urinalysis
- lyme disease titer and c-reactive protein

Other Diagnostic Procedures
- Clinical interview should note any recent history of mononucleosis, hepatitis, or long-lasting influenza and family history of infectious diseases, allergies, anergy, asthma, and cancer.
- Review of lifestyle issues/medical history (include diet, drug use—alcohol, tobacco, and recreational drugs plus current medications such as antibiotics, steroids, birth control pills, and chemotherapy).
- Review of symptoms should note the occurrence of frequent sore throats and swollen glands, colds, or other infections; hormonal imbalances; menstrual irregularities; hypoglycemia; energy level; functional abnormalities of the digestive system (indigestion, gas, abdominal pain), the respiratory system (shortness of breath), and cardiovascular system (palpitations); and the mental and emotional state (foggy, confused, emotionally unstable).
- It may be helpful to test for viral infections such as Lyme disease, and for rheumatoid factor, allergies, hepatitis A and B antibodies, and HIV.

TREATMENT OPTIONS
Treatment Strategy
Patients require both symptomatic and emotional support.

Drug Therapies
Antidepressant and other psychoactive drugs appear to be most successful.
- The tricyclic antidepressants doxepin (Sinequan) and amitriptyline (Elavil) relieve depression, insomnia, muscle tension and pain, general fatigue, nasal congestion, gastritis, and neurologic symptoms. Side effects include dry mouth, drowsiness, constipation, tachycardia (elevated heart rate), and weight gain. Start at one-tenth to one-fourth the usual clinical dose.
- Fluoxetine (Prozac) is another antidepressant that increases brain serotonin levels, may improve energy level, and relieves fatigue but not sleep disorders. Its side effects include increased insomnia and anxiety, rashes, digestive upsets, and impaired sexual functioning.
- Benzodiazepines, such as alprazolam (Xanax), clonazepam (Klonopin), or lorazepam (Ativan), are used to treat anxiety. Their side effects are sedation, amnesia, and withdrawal symptoms (insomnia, abdominal and muscle cramps, vomiting, sweating, tremors, and convulsions).
- Aspirin, nonsteroidal anti-inflammatory drugs, or acetaminophen relieve muscle and joint pains, headache, and fever. Side effects include possible renal damage, gastrointestinal bleeding, abdominal pain, nausea, and vomiting.
- Nonsedating antihistamines relieve allergy symptoms. These include astemizole (Hismanal) and loratadine (Claritin). Side effects are drowsiness, fatigue, and headache.
- Histamine blockers, such as cimetidine (Tagamet) and ranitidine (Zantac), block production of stomach acid, stimulate T-cell function, and improve energy.

- For antihypotensive therapy, fludrocortisone (Florinef) is currently being tested in clinical trials; side effects are elevated blood pressure, and fluid retention.
- Gammaglobulin therapy is given intramuscularly two to three times per month for passive immunity. It is expensive (as much as $1,000 per treatment), with no clear evidence of efficacy. Side effects are nausea, dizziness, transient flu-like symptoms, headache, and low blood pressure.
- Transfer factor triggers an active immune response.
- Alpha-interferon enhances immune function.
- Ampligen is a synthetic nucleic acid product that stimulates interferon production. It is experimental.

Complementary and Alternative Therapies

Following nutritional guidelines and using herbs and homeopathic remedies as needed, may be effective in alleviating the debilitating symptoms of chronic fatigue and strengthening overall vitality. Counseling, support groups, meditation, yoga, and progressive muscle relaxation are stress management techniques that may be helpful for people with CFS.

NUTRITION

- Avoid refined foods, sugar, caffeine, alcohol, saturated fats, dairy products, and gluten-containing grains.
- Increase fresh vegetables, legumes, whole grains (non-gluten), protein, and essential fatty acids (nuts, seeds, and cold-water fish).
- Beta carotene (50,000 IU/day) to strengthen immune function.
- Vitamin C (1,000 mg three to six times/day) to increase endurance.
- B complex (50 to 100 mg/day or 2 ml IM one to two times/week) with additional B_6 (100 mg/day) and B_5 (100 to 250 mg/day) to reduce the effects of stress.
- Pantothenic acid (4 to 7 mg/day)
- Magnesium aspartate (400 to 1,000 mg/day) to support energy production.
- L-Carnitine (330 mg one to three times/day) supports energy production in the cells.

HERBS

Herbs are generally a safe way to strengthen and tone the body's systems. As with any therapy, it is important to ascertain a diagnosis before pursuing treatment. Herbs may be used as dried extracts (capsules, powders, teas), glycerites (glycerine extracts), or tinctures (alcohol extracts). Unless otherwise indicated, teas should be made with 1 tsp. herb per cup of hot water. Steep covered 5 to 10 minutes for leaf or flowers, and 10 to 20 minutes for roots. Drink 2 to 4 cups/day. Tinctures may be used singly or in combination as noted.

A tincture of adaptogenic herbs may help increase resistance to stress and strengthen the immune system. These herbs include Siberian ginseng *(Eleuthrococcus senticosus)*, schizandra berry *(Schizandra chinensis)*, ashwaganda root *(Withania somnifera)*, gotu kola *(Centella asiatica)*, and astragalus root *(Astragalus membranaceus)*. Take 20 to 30 drops bid to tid. Adaptogens are generally safe to take long-term and may need to be taken for four to six months for maximum benefit. Some may require several days respite from Ginseng after several weeks of use.

Herbs that support overall vitality and relieve the effects of exhaustion include the following: Licorice root *(Glycyrrhiza glabra)*, lomatium root *(Lomatium dissectum)*, skullcap *(Scutellaria laterifolia)*, passionflower *(Passiflora incarnata)*, lavender *(Lavendula officinalis)*, and rosemary leaf *(Rosemariana officinalis)*. Take 20 to 30 drops bid to tid. Licorice root is contraindicated in hypertension.

Essential oils of jasmine, peppermint, and rosemary are calming and restorative and may be used in aromatherapy. Place several drops in a warm bath, an atomizer, or cotton ball.

HOMEOPATHY

An experienced homeopath should assess individual constitutional types and severity of disease to select the correct remedy and potency.

ACUPUNCTURE

Chronic fatigue syndrome is related to deficiencies in multiple organ systems which can be addressed with acupuncture treatment. It could be used with custom formulations of Chinese herbs.

MASSAGE

Therapeutic massage is helpful in reducing stress-related symptoms, improving circulation and increasing the overall sense of well-being.

Patient Monitoring

Schedule follow-up visits every three to six months or whenever there is an exacerbation of the condition or new symptoms. Patients taking psychoactive drugs or speculative therapies should be monitored closely.

OTHER CONSIDERATIONS

Complications/Sequelae

- Depression
- Continuing morbidity

Prognosis

One-third of patient presentations recover quickly (within months), one-third recover within two years, and one-third suffer at least some degree of long-term disability.

Pregnancy

The effects of herbs in pregnancy have not been fully investigated and treatment should be undertaken only with physician supervision. High doses of vitamin C should be avoided.

REFERENCES

Castro M. *The Complete Homeopathy Handbook*. New York, NY: St. Martin's Press; 1990.

Fukuda K, et al. The chronic fatigue syndrome: a comprehensive approach to its definition and study. *Ann Intern Med*. 1994;121:953–959.

Management of CFS: Pharmacologic therapy and nonpharmacologic therapy. Centers for Disease Control and Prevention. Accessed at www.cdc.gov/ncidod/diseases/cfs/mgmt1.htm on January 4, 1999.

Noble J, ed. *Textbook of Primary Care Medicine*. 2nd ed. St Louis, Mo: Mosby-Year Book, Inc; 1996:918–922.

Scalzo R. *Naturopathic Handbook of Herbal Formulas*. Durango, Colo: 2nd ed. Kivaki Press; 1994:S/A18–S/A19.

Werbach M. *Nutritional Influences on Illness*. New Canaan, Conn: Keats Publishing; 1988:418–421.

■ CHRONIC OBSTRUCTIVE PULMONARY DISEASE
OVERVIEW
Definition
Chronic obstructive pulmonary disease (COPD) refers to a clinical syndrome of chronic dyspnea as a result of expiratory airflow obstruction due to chronic bronchitis or emphysema (often both). Chronic bronchitis is defined clinically and is associated with chronic cough, resulting from excessive tracheobronchial mucus production and impaired mucus elimination, lasting for at least three months of the year for more than two consecutive years. Emphysema is defined anatomically and is characterized by enlarged air spaces distal to the terminal bronchioles with destruction of the alveolar walls; there is also a loss of elastic recoil in the lung. In the United States, COPD affects an estimated 15 million people and is the fifth leading cause of death.

Etiology
- Smoking is the number one cause of COPD. Obstruction of airflow in the small airways has been shown to be the earliest detrimental effect of smoking.
- Exposure to environmental air pollutants
- Alpha$_1$-antitrypsin deficiency, the only known inherited form of the disease

Risk Factors
- History of smoking or passive smoke exposure
- History of working with high levels of airborne particulates (e.g., dusts), gases, and fumes (such as coal and gold miners; farmers; and cement, cadmium, and cotton workers)
- Low socioeconomic status
- Male gender
- Allergy and airway hyper-responsiveness (e.g., asthma)
- Women in undeveloped countries exposed to open fires for cooking and heating
- Living in heavily industrialized urban areas
- Recurrent respiratory illnesses
- Family history of chronic bronchitis and emphysema (e.g., alpha$_1$-antitrypsin deficiency)
- Emotional stress and repressed emotions have also been shown to contribute

Signs and Symptoms
Patients with emphysema present with a long history of dyspnea on exertion. Patients with chronic bronchitis present with chronic cough productive of sputum.
- Cough
- Cyanosis
- Weight gain
- Dyspnea on exertion (and eventually at rest)
- Excessive sputum production
- Wheezing
- Recurrent bronchial infections
- Weight loss in late stages
- Peripheral edema secondary to cor pulmonale

DIFFERENTIAL DIAGNOSIS
- Asthma
- Bronchiolitis obliterans
- Pneumonia
- Lung cancer
- Cystic fibrosis
- Congestive heart failure
- Interstitial lung disease
- Primary pulmonary hypertension
- Acute viral infection

DIAGNOSIS
Physical Examination
There is considerable variability in the clinical presentation of COPD, which can range from simple chronic bronchitis (cough without airway obstruction) to severe respiratory disability and fatal respiratory failure. The classic patient with emphysema is often very thin and barrel chested and shows obvious difficulty breathing, manifesting tachypnea (rapid respirations) with prolonged expiration through pursed lips. Patients often assume a "tripod" position, leaning forward while sitting, bracing with the arms. Cyanosis is not present so the patient is considered a "pink puffer." The classic patient with bronchitis is often overweight, even obese, and appears cyanotic. The respiratory rate is normal, and there is no obvious distress. These patients are called "blue bloaters." In reality most patients with COPD have a combination of chronic bronchitis and emphysema.

Laboratory Tests
Shown moderate to severe hypoxia

Pathological Findings
In bronchitis:
- Hyperplastic and hypertrophied mucous glands in the submucosa of large bronchi
- Increased Reid index (ratio of bronchial gland thickness to bronchial wall thickness)
- Small airways: mucus plugging, goblet-cell metaplasia, airway thickening, peribronchial fibrosis, mucosal and submucosal inflammatory changes, increased smooth muscle, and accumulation of macrophages and neutrophils in respiratory bronchioles
- Large airways: mucous gland enlargement, goblet cell hyperplasia, and squamous metaplasia

In emphysema:
- Enlargement of air spaces distal to the nonrespiratory bronchioles
- Destruction of the alveolar walls

Imaging
- Chest X ray may show hyperinflation (flattened diaphragm, increased retrosternal air space, outwardly bowed lower ribs), bulbous or cystic change, especially in upper lung, and wide pulmonary diameter (due to pulmonary hypertension).
- High-resolution CT can show areas of anatomic emphysema, bronchiectasis, and allow measurement of pulmonary artery diameter.
- Echocardiography (two-dimensional, M-mode, or transesophageal) may show characteristic changes of cor pulmonale, right atrial and ventricular hypertrophy, and tricuspid regurgitation. It may allow estimation of the severity of pulmonary hypertension.

Other Diagnostic Procedures
- Pulmonary function tests define the physiologic abnormalities of COPD. Spirometry before and after bronchodilator administration confirms airflow obstruction and helps in assessing the severity and reversibility of lung damage. Lung volume measurements (e.g., plethysmography) show characteristic overinflation. Diffusion capacity is impaired in COPD.
- Arterial blood gases may show hypoxemia, hypercapnea, or both.
- Exercise testing (i.e., on a treadmill or stationary bicycle, 6- or 12-minute tests) will show reduced exercise tolerance and exercise-induced hypoxemia.

TREATMENT OPTIONS

Treatment Strategy

Smoking cessation is the key to preventing exacerbations and progression. Management is dependent on the degree of obstruction, the severity of disability, and reversibility of the illness. Respiratory infections must be treated aggressively.

Drug Therapies

- Alpha$_1$-antitrypsin replacement therapy
- Supplemental oxygen (1 to 3 L/min)—dosage should be appropriate to relieve hypoxemia (i.e., to maintain a PaO$_2$ of 55 to 60 mm Hg)
- Bronchodilators—to increase airflow and reduce dyspnea
- Anticholinergic agents (e.g., ipratropium, 0.18 mg, 2 puffs qid)
- Beta2-adrenergic agonists (e.g., metaproterenol, terbultaline, or albuterol, 2 to 6 puffs every three to six hours)
- Theophylline (200 to 400 mg bid)—requires frequent blood monitoring for toxicity
- Corticosteroids (e.g., prednisone, 40 mg/day for two weeks then reduce to 0 to 10 mg every day or on alternate days)
- Broad-spectrum antibiotics (e.g., ampicillin or amoxicillin, 2 g/day; erythromycin, 2 g/day; or trimethoprim-sulfamethoxazole, 1 double-strength capsule/day)—for treatment of exacerbations
- Acetylcysteine—for mucolytic therapy; however, it may cause bronchospasm
- Magnesium can also be markedly helpful as an IV infusion of 5 to 10 grams of elemental magnesium over 6 to 10 hours.

Complementary and Alternative Therapies

May be very helpful at decreasing the symptoms and preventing infections. Since smoking cessation is very important, the alternative treatments for this will be listed. Psychotherapy and support groups can be very helpful in learning to cope with chronic disease.

NUTRITION

- Dairy products and bananas increase mucous buildup and should be avoided. Garlic, onions, and horseradish may actually decrease mucous production. IgG Elisa food allergy testing can determine other foods that can cause inflammation in the lungs.
- Some essential fatty acids are anti-inflammatory, dose is 1,000 to 2,000 IU, mixed omega-3 and omega-6 oils (flax, fish, borage, and/or evening primrose oil; avoid vegetable oils and saturated fats)
- Coenzyme Q$_{10}$ prevents fatty acid oxidation and increases exercise tolerance as a cardio-protective antioxidant. Dose is 10 to 50 mg tid.
- Other important antioxidants: selenium (200 micrograms/day), vitamin E (400 IU/day), vitamin C (1,000 mg tid), L-carnitine (750 mg bid). Note that beta-carotene increases the risk of lung cancer in smokers.
- Bromelain is a mucolytic, 250 to 500 mg tid away from meals. People with pineapple allergy may be sensitive to this product. Bromelain may also aggravate gastritis.
- N-acetyl cysteine is a mucolytic, 400 mg tid.
- Magnesium promotes muscle relaxation in bronchial smooth muscle and blood vessels (100 to 500 mg bid). Magnesium may cause diarrhea in some sensitive individuals.

HERBS

Herbs are generally a safe way to strengthen and tone the body's systems. As with any therapy, it is important to ascertain a diagnosis before pursuing treatment. Herbs may be used as dried extracts (capsules, powders, teas), glycerites (glycerine extracts), or tinctures (alcohol extracts). Unless otherwise indicated, teas should be made with 1 tsp. herb per cup of hot water. Steep covered 5 to 10 minutes for leaf or flowers, and 10 to 20 minutes for roots. Drink 2 to 4 cups/day. Tinctures may be used singly or in combination as noted.

- Mullein *(Verbascum thaspis):* expectorant, soothes irritation
- Ginger *(Zingiber officinalis):* dissolves secretions, relieves bronchial spasms
- Fennel *(Foeniculum fructus):* dissolves secretions, mild antispasmodic, calming digestive stimulant
- Colts foot *(Tussilago farfara):* anticatarrh, demulcent. Prolonged use may cause liver damage due to pyrrolizidine alkaloids.
- Licorice *(Glycyrrhiza glabra):* antiviral, antidepressant, soothing, anticatarrh, contraindicated in hypertension
- Hawthorne *(Cretaegus oxycanthus):* protective of blood vessels, increases cardiac output without increasing cardiac load
- Mix equal parts of herb, or tincture of four to six of the above herbs. Dose is 1 cup tea tid, or 30 to 60 drops tincture tid.
- Essential oils: eucalyptus, thyme, rosemary, and/or lavender: place 3 to 5 drops in 2 cups of water in a humidifier to prevent infection.

HOMEOPATHY

Constitutional treatment by a homeopathic prescriber may help with symptoms and address underlying emotional issues that will aid patients in smoking cessation.

PHYSICAL MEDICINE

- Castor oil pack: Used externally, castor oil is a powerful anti-inflammatory. Apply oil directly to skin, cover with a clean soft cloth (e.g., flannel) and plastic wrap. Place a heat source (hot water bottle or heating pad) over the pack and let sit for 30 to 60 minutes. For best results use three consecutive days in one week. When placed over the lungs, castor oil packs decrease inflammation and stimulate drainage.
- Postural drainage, yogic breathing, and pulmonary rehabilitation programs may all be helpful.

ACUPUNCTURE

Has been shown to have great benefit in smoking cessation.

Patient Monitoring

Serial monitoring of pulmonary function is performed annually or as symptoms dictate. If patient is unstable or if home oxygen is required, more frequent visits are needed.

OTHER CONSIDERATIONS

Prevention

Cessation of smoking is the single best way to prevent disease progression. Respirators of the appropriate type can reduce the risk to workers exposed to dusts, fumes, and gases.

Negative air ion generators are frequently helpful. Electronic air cleaners and HEPA filters are helpful in highly polluted environments and for persons who have a marked allergic basis for their chronic bronchitis contribution to COPD.

Complications/Sequelae

The most common complication of COPD is pulmonary infection. Prophylactic influenza vaccination (annually) and pneumococcal vaccination (every six to eight years) can be effective. Patients on steroid therapy are at risk for steroid-related complications—adrenal suppression, capillary fragility, easy bruisability, glucose intolerance, weight gain in the face, and muscle wasting.

Prognosis

By the time dyspnea develops with simple daily activity, patients may have lost two-thirds of their pulmonary function. The diagnosis is often made very late in the course of the disease. Thus, the mortality rate after diagnosis is high (>50% after 10 years).

Pregnancy

With the exception of patients with alpha$_1$-antitrypsin deficiency, women are usually diagnosed with COPD well beyond the reproductive years.

REFERENCES

Blumenthal M, ed. *The Complete German Commission E Monographs.* Boston, Mass: Integrative Medicine Communications; 1998:423, 468.

Bordow RA, Moser KM. *Manual of Clinical Problems in Pulmonary Medicine.* 4th ed. Boston, Mass:Little, Brown; 1996:212–215.

Celli BR. Pulmonary rehabilitation in patients with COPD. *Am J Respir Crit Care Med.* 1995;152:861–864.

Duke JA. *The Green Pharmacy.* Emmaus, Pa: Rodale Press; 1997:93–95, 179–183.

Fauci AS, Braunwald E, Isselbacher KJ et al, eds. *Harrison's Principles of Internal Medicine.* 14th ed. New York, NY: McGraw-Hill; 1998:1451–1457.

Ferguson GT, Cherniack RM. Management of chronic obstructive pulmonary disease. *N Engl J Med.* 1993;328:1017–1022.

Snider GL. *Standards for the Diagnosis and Care of Patients with Chronic Obstructive Pulmonary Disease.* Washington Crossing, Pa: Scientific Frontiers; l996:1–12.

Woodley M, Whelan A. *Manual of Medical Therapeutics.* 27th ed. Boston, Mass: Little, Brown; 1992:200–202.

■ CIRRHOSIS OF THE LIVER

OVERVIEW

Definition

Cirrhosis is characterized by irreversible chronic injury of the liver manifested by hepatic fibrosis and small regenerative nodules; it is often a subclinical condition diagnosed on the basis of the history, physical examination, and biochemical and serologic tests. Approximately 10% of cases have no known etiology (cryptogenic cirrhosis). Between 5% to 10% of people in the U .S. are alcoholics; of these, 10% to 15% will develop liver disease.

Etiology

- Average daily consumption of alcohol (32 to 48 oz. of beer, 4 to 8 oz. of liquor, 16 to 32 oz. of wine) for 10 years or more is associated with an increased incidence of alcoholic cirrhosis. The amount and duration of alcohol ingestion are more important than the type of alcoholic beverage ingested.
- Drugs and toxins (e.g., alcohol, methotrexate, isoniazid, methyldopa)
- Infectious diseases (e.g., hepatitis B and C, brucellosis, echinococcus, schistosomiasis, toxoplasmosis)
- Inherited and metabolic disorders (e.g., Wilson's disease, hemochromatosis, protoporphyria, galactosemia, glycogen storage disease, alpha1-antitrypsin deficiency, tyrosinosis, hereditary fructose intolerance)
- Biliary obstruction (e.g., carcinoma, chronic pancreatitis, sclerosing cholangitis)
- Cardiovascular diseases (e.g., chronic right heart failure, Budd-Chiari syndrome, veno-occlusive disease)
- Miscellaneous causes (e.g., sarcoidosis, jejunoileal bypass)

Risk Factors

Excessive ingestion of alcohol, exposure to toxins and infectious agents.

Signs and Symptoms

The clinical manifestations of cirrhosis can range from an absence of symptoms (10% to 20% of patients) to hepatic failure.

- Hepatomegaly and splenomegaly
- Jaundice
- Peripheral edema
- Weakness, malaise
- Anorexia and weight loss
- Abdominal pain or gastrointestinal complaints
- Gastroesophageal varices and bleeding
- Hepatic encephalopathy
- Ascites with portal hypertension
- Spider angiomas and palmar erythema
- Testicular atrophy and gynecomastia (in men)
- Menstrual irregularities (in women)
- Parotid enlargement

DIFFERENTIAL DIAGNOSIS

- Nodular regenerative hyperplasia
- Congenital hepatic fibrosis
- Acute or chronic viral hepatitis
- Diabetes mellitus
- Biliary obstruction, lymphatic obstruction
- Drug toxicity
- Bacterial infections
- Primary biliary or cardiac cirrhosis
- Wilson's disease

- Hemochromatosis
- Hepatic Schistosomiasin

DIAGNOSIS

Physical Examination

The three most common hepatic findings in alcoholics are fatty liver, alcoholic hepatitis, and cirrhosis. Patients with fatty liver may have abdominal pain, mild icterus, or gastrointestinal symptoms but they may also present asymptomatically. Patients with alcoholic hepatitis may present with anorexia, nausea, vomiting, weight loss, abdominal pain, hepatomegaly, splenomegaly, ascites, and jaundice. Patients with alcoholic cirrhosis may present asymptomatically (10% to 20%) or with signs of chronic liver disease such as ascites, gastrointestinal bleeding, encephalopathy, spider angiomas, palmar erythema, parotid enlargement, testicular atrophy, gynecomastia, menstrual disorders, and muscle wasting.

Laboratory Tests

A patient with significant liver injury may have normal results.

- Elevated serum aspartate aminotransferase
- Hyperbilirubinemia, hypoalbuminemia, and hyperglobulinemia
- Elevated alkaline phosphatase
- Prolonged prothrombin time
- Hypomagnesemia, hypophosphatemia, and hypokalemia
- Respiratory alkalosis
- Anemia (from folic acid and vitamin B_{12} deficiency), gastrointestinal blood loss, or toxic effects of alcohol on bone marrow

Pathological Findings

- Fibrosis and regenerative nodules
- With fatty liver—large droplets of fat in the hepatocyte
- With alcoholic hepatitis—hepatocellular necrosis, alcoholic hyalin (Mallory bodies), increased intralobular connective tissue in the space of Disse, central vein sclerosis, infiltration by polymorphonuclear leukocytes
- With alcoholic cirrhosis—portal and central areas are linked by dense bands of connective tissue, severe scarring in the central areas, hypersplenism or bone marrow suppression, leading to thrombocytopenia, leukopenia, and anemia

Imaging

- Ultrasonography—to exclude biliary obstruction, confirm hepatosplenomegaly, and detect textural abnormalities
- Endoscopic retrograde cholangiopancreatography (ERCP)—to rule out biliary tract disease by determining patency of the biliary tree
- Computed tomography—to determine severity of hepatic encephalopathy, liver size, and density in hemochromatosis

Other Diagnostic Procedures

- Percutaneous needle biopsy—to distinguish the severity of the liver damage and to evaluate patients who do not drink but present with clinical manifestations of liver disease
- Paracentesis—to diagnose cirrhotic ascites, ruling out other disorders
- Cholangiography for duct obstruction
- Laparoscopic liver biopsy

TREATMENT OPTIONS

Treatment Strategy

Remove/reduce the effects of the cause, prevent further damage if possible, and prevent/manage complications. Surgery is limited to procedures for portal hypertension and complete liver transplantation.

- Well-balanced diet (2,000 to 3,000 kcal/day)—for malnutrition
- Protein restriction—to reduce ammonia production in colon in patients with hepatic encephalopathy, yet ensure adequate protein
- Salt and water restriction—to help manage ascites (no more than 1.2 g of sodium and 1 liter of water per day)

Drug Therapies

- Colchicine (0.6 mg bid)—to slow progression of disease
- Diuretics—for ascites (e.g., spironolactone (Aldactone) 100 to 400 mg/day; furosemide, 40 to 120 mg/day). Caution must be used with diuretics so as not to cause electrolyte abnormalities, hypovolemia, and death.
- Neomycin (1 g every six hours)—to reduce ammonia production in intestine that causes encephalopathy
- Lactulose (65 g/dL every two hours)—to reduce serum ammonia levels and improve hepatic encephalopathy
- Other specific drugs based on complications and etiology

Complementary and Alternative Therapies

Effective either alone or as adjunctive therapy.

NUTRITION

- B-complex: B_1 (50 to 100 mg), B_2 (50 mg), B_3 (25 mg); B_5 (100 mg); B_6 (50 to 100 mg), B_{12} (100 to 1,000 mcg), folate (400 mcg/day) to prevent deficiencies common in liver disease
- Anti-oxidants: vitamin C (1,000 to 3,000 mg/day), vitamin E (400 to 800 IU/day), and selenium (200 mcg/day) reduce toxic effects of alcohol/drugs and prevent fatty acid oxidation.
- Essential fatty acids are anti-inflammatory; dietary manipulation includes reducing animal fats and increasing fish and nuts. A mix of omega-6 (evening primrose) and omega-3 (flax seed) may be best (one tbsp. oil/day or 1,000 to 1,500 mg/day). Watch clotting times.
- Choline, lecithin, methionine (1 g each/day) for fat absorption
- Carnitine (300 mg/day) prevents fatty liver.
- Glutathione (500 mg bid) helps remove ammonia from the brain, a complication of cirrhosis.
- Vitamin K is necessary for blood clotting; often depleted in cirrhosis
- Desiccated liver (500 mg tid) helps to provide nutrition to promote liver repair.
- Protein restriction to 45 g/day without development of negative nitrogen balance as long as a minimum of 400 g of carbohydrates is ingested daily.
- A change from animal to vegetable protein may be helpful.

HERBS

Ascertain a diagnosis before pursuing treatment. Herbs may be used as dried extracts (capsules, powders, teas), glycerites (glycerine extracts), or tinctures (alcohol extracts). Unless otherwise indicated, teas should be made with 1 tsp. herb per cup of hot water. Steep covered 5 to 10 minutes for leaf or flowers, and 10 to 20 minutes for roots. Drink 2 to 4 cups/day. Tinctures may be used singly or in combination as noted.

Due to the high doses required and the need to avoid alcohol, the preferred form of these herbs is powdered.

- Milk thistle (*Silybum marianum*): 100 mg tid prevents free radical damage in the liver, stimulates regeneration of hepatocytes, aids in digestion of fats, effective in treating cirrhosis
- Barberry (*Berberis vulgaris*): 250 to 500 mg/day corrects metabolic abnormalities in liver cirrhosis
- Catechin (*Uncaria gambir*): 400 mg tid, is antioxidant, antiviral, and helps to regenerate liver tissue

HOMEOPATHY

May offer relief of symptoms, but needs to be prescribed by an experienced practitioner.

PHYSICAL MEDICINE

Castor oil pack. Used externally, castor oil is a powerful anti-inflammatory. Apply oil directly to skin, cover with a clean soft cloth (e.g., flannel) and plastic wrap. Place a heat source (hot water bottle or heating pad) over the pack and let sit for 30 to 60 minutes. For best results, use for three consecutive days. Apply pack over liver. Preliminary study shows immune enhancement in healthy patients, historic use to stimulate hepatic function.

ACUPUNCTURE

May be helpful to alleviate symptoms and increase physiological functioning.

MASSAGE

May help alleviate stress and lymph congestion.

Patient Monitoring

Patients need long-term management because of the serious/life-threatening complications associated with cirrhosis. Repeated liver tests are necessary, with frequency based on the relative stability of the patient.

OTHER CONSIDERATIONS

Prevention

The incidence of alcoholic cirrhosis is directly related to the ingestion of alcohol. Approximately 10% to 20% of alcoholics develop cirrhosis. To prevent some other forms of cirrhosis, patients must practice safe sex and avoid IV drug use.

Complications/Sequelae

- Portal hypertension and its subsequent complications due to collateral flow from the portal venous system
- Bleeding esophageal varices
- Hypersplenism
- Ascites
- Hepatorenal syndrome
- Hepatic encephalopathy
- Liver failure
- Hepatocellular carcinoma
- Bacterial peritonitis
- Other infections

Prognosis

Dependent on etiology, extent of damage, and success of intervention

Pregnancy

Cirrhosis can jeopardize the chances for a healthy infant.

REFERENCES

Bartram T. *Encyclopedia of Herbal Medicine.* Dorset, England: Grace Publishers; 1995:295.

Bone K. *Clinical Applications of Ayurvedic and Chinese Herbs.* Queensland, Australia: Phytotherapy Press; 1996:69.

Branch WT. *Office Practice of Medicine.* 3rd ed. Philadelphia, Pa: WB Saunders; 1994:326–338.

Fauci AS, Braunwald E, Isselbacher KJ et al, eds. *Harrison's Principles of Internal Medicine.* 14th ed. New York, NY: McGraw-Hill; 1998:1704–1710.

Ferenci P, Dragosics B, Dittrich H, et al. Randomized controlled trial of silymarin treatment in patients with cirrhosis of the liver. *J Hepatol.* 1989;9:105–113.

Gruenwald J, Brendler T et al, eds. *PDR for Herbal Medicines.* Montvale, NJ: Medical Economics Company; 1998:1138–1139.

Marshall AW, Graul RS, Morgan MY, Sherlock S. Treatment of alcohol-related liver disease with thioctic acid: a six month radomized double-blind trial. *Gut.*1982;23:1088–1093.

Mowrey DB. *The Scientific Validation of Herbal Medicine.* New Canaan, Conn: Keats Publishing; 1986:179.

Murray MT, Pizzorno *JE. Encyclopedia of Natural Medicine.* 2nd ed. Rocklin, Calif:

Prima Publishing; 1998:211–220.

Walker LP, Brown EH. *The Alternative Pharmacy.* Paramus, NJ: Prentice Hall; 1998:394.

Wyngaarden JB, Smith Jr LH, Bennett JC, eds. *Cecil Textbook of Medicine.* 19th ed. Philadelphia, Pa: WB Saunders; 1992:786–795.

■ COMMON COLD
OVERVIEW
Definition
The common cold is a viral upper respiratory infection. It accounts for at least one-half of all human illnesses. In the United States, adults average between 3 and 5.6 colds a year, while children have as many as 8.3.

Etiology
More than 200 possible serologically different viruses cause colds. They are transmitted by respiratory droplets, hand-to-hand, or by object contact. Exposure to cold and fatigue do not increase susceptibility, although psychological stress may.

Risk Factors
- Day care centers and office buildings
- Large family size
- Poor hygiene
- Psychological stress—can increase rate and severity

Signs and Symptoms
- Rhinorrhea, sneezing, nasal congestion
- Sore throat, cough, or hoarseness
- Fever (uncommon in adults, usually indicates flu or bacterial infection)
- In children, sudden onset of fever (lasting two to three days), irritability, restlessness, and sneezing
- Headache

DIFFERENTIAL DIAGNOSIS
- Asthma
- Sinusitis
- Pneumonia
- Bronchitis, bronchiolitis
- Flu
- Allergic rhinitis
- Children—initial symptoms of measles or pertussis; intranasal foreign body
- Infants—choanal atresia or congenital syphilis

DIAGNOSIS
Physical Examination
The patient may be sneezing, have a runny nose, look fatigued, and complain of sore throat, rarely of diarrhea or vomiting.

Laboratory Tests
Cultures are rarely done for diagnostic purposes but are performed for research.

Pathological Findings
- Cultures determine the type of infection:
- Rhinoviruses—15% to 40% of colds; grows at 33 to 34°C (temperature of the nasal passages); one subtype, 100 serotypes
- Coronaviruses—10% to 20% of colds; three subgroups
- Adenoviruses—3% to5% of children's colds, less than 2% of adults, six subgenera (A to F) and 47 serotypes
- Respiratory syncytial virus and parainfluenza viruses—can cause colds but more likely to cause lower respiratory tract infections, especially in children
- Edematous and hyperemic mucosa; hyperactive mucus glands
- Inflammatory cells include neutrophils, lymphocytes, plasma cells, and eosinophils.

Imaging
Computed tomography scans may show bilateral abnormalities in the ethmoid and maxillary sinuses, with residual density possible in the maxillary sinus two weeks after resolution.

Other Diagnostic Procedures
- Self-diagnosis is generally accurate.
- Diagnosis can be made only by isolation of the virus (e.g., by nasal wash), which is done almost exclusively for research purposes (e.g., rhinoviruses—grown in human embryonic lung fibroblasts).
- Antibodies for rhinovirus receptors are currently being researched.
- Experimental serotype vaccines are available but of little use given the large number of possible serotypes.

TREATMENT OPTIONS
Treatment Strategy
There is no known antiviral treatment for the common cold, which is generally benign and self-limited. Live vaccines exist for adenovirus types 4 and 7, primarily for use in the military. Antibiotics should not be given unless there are bacterial complications. Antihistamines are inappropriate and may increase and/or prolong congestion. Treatment is primarily to relieve symptoms.

Drug Therapies
- Nasal decongestants: may aid in preventing sinus and eustachian tube obstruction (e.g., pseudoephrine 60 mg tid); general vasoconstriction may cause high blood pressure
- Nasal sprays: localized decongestant; rebound effect after three to five days
- Analgesics: can be used for malaise; may delay immune response or increase nasal symptoms; aspirin can cause Reye's syndrome in children
- Adequate hydration: loosens secretions
- Warm fluids and steam inhalation: provide symptom relief by increasing the rate of mucous flow
- Reduced activity: helps avoid complications

Complementary and Alternative Therapies
Alternative therapies offer effective symptom relief. General measures for treating infection are to get plenty of fluids and rest.

NUTRITION
- Vitamin C (1,000 mg three to six times/day) enhances immune function (may affect interferon and interleukin), some studies show that it shortens the duration and ameliorates the symptoms of the common cold.
- Zinc (23 mg lozenges taken every two hours) may shorten the duration of a cold, and may also protect against the development of symptoms. This high a dose is for short-term use only.
- Vitamin A (25,000 IU/day) maintains integrity of mucous membranes and stimulates antibody response. Use high a dose short-term only.
- Beta-carotene (200,000 IU/day) stimulates the immune system and is an anti-oxidant; safe in women of childbearing years
- Avoid dairy and bananas, foods that increase mucous production.
- Garlic and onions are antivirals that can be included in the diet.

HERBS
Herbs are generally a safe way to strengthen and tone the body's systems. As with any therapy, it is important to ascertain a diagnosis before pursuing treatment. Herbs may be used as dried extracts (capsules, powders, teas), glycerites (glycerine extracts), or tinctures (alcohol extracts). Unless oth-

erwise indicated, teas should be made with 1 tsp. herb per
cup of hot water. Steep covered 5 to 10 minutes for leaf or flowers,
and 10 to 20 minutes for roots. Drink 2 to 4 cups/day. Tinctures may
be used singly or in combination as noted.

- Coneflower *(Echinacea angustifolia):* immunomodulating, increases
  phagocytosis; controversy exists whether to use for longer than two
  to six weeks at a time and whether to use in autoimmune conditions
  or AIDS.
- Goldenseal *(Hydrastis canadensis):* antiviral, antibacterial
- Astragulus *(Astragulus membraneceus):* increases interferon
  to shorten duration of colds
- Licorice *(Glycyrrhiza glabra):* antiviral, soothing to mucous
  membranes
- Elderberry *(Sambuccus canadensis):* antiviral, increases bronchial
  secretions

A mix of the above every two to four hours (1 cup tea or 30 to 60 drops
tincture)

HOMEOPATHY

An experienced homeopath should assess individual constitutional types
and severity of disease to select the correct remedy and potency. For acute
prescribing use 3 to 5 pellets of a 12X to 30C remedy every one to four
hours until acute symptoms resolve.

- *Allium cepa* for colds with profuse watery discharge that burns
  and/or irritates the nostrils
- *Euphrasia* for colds with profuse watery discharge that is irritating
  to the eyes
- *Aconite* for colds that come on suddenly, with fever and anxiety
- *Mercurius* for profuse discharge that is irritating everywhere;
  patient feels weak

ACUPUNCTURE

Acupuncture for increased circulation, particularly helpful with Chinese
herbal formulas.

Patient Monitoring

Patients must learn that antibiotics cannot cure colds. High fever, sinus tenderness, purulent sputum, dyspnea, and chest pain are indications
they should seek medical attention.

OTHER CONSIDERATIONS

Children get colds more often than adults do. Day care centers and schools
increase exposure to and frequency of illness.

Prevention

Colds are transmitted by small aerosol particles, airborne droplets, or
secretions transferred by hand with subsequent self-inoculation. Careful
hand washing and avoiding contact with the eyes and nose is the best
prevention for nonaerosol types of infection. Interferon intranasal sprays
are moderately prophylactic (especially for rhinovirus) but may cause
localized nasal irritation or damage (e.g., oxymetazoline 0.05%, two sprays
to each nostril bid for five days). High doses of vitamin C and
zinc lozenges may be no more effective in preventing a cold than
placebo, depending on the study.

Complications/Sequelae

Secondary bacterial infections can cause complication in viral colds.

- Otitis media: in 5% of preschoolers
- Asthma and chronic pulmonary disease
- Sinusitis: in 0.5% of colds; suspect when cold persists 7 to 10 days
  past onset
- Bronchitis: more likely with coronavirus
- Pneumonia, bronchiolitis, diarrhea, and keratoconjunctivitis: more
  common with adenovirus

Prognosis

Colds usually last five to seven days in adults and 10 to 14 days in children.
Without complications, they are benign and self-limiting.

Pregnancy

Goldenseal is contraindicated in pregnancy because of its ability to
stimulate oxytocin and uterine contractions. Alpha-adrenergic compounds
and epinephrine (except in cases of anaphalaxis) should be avoided.
Dextromethorphan should not be prescribed for cough. The most
conservative treatment for colds in pregnancy is rest and fluids.

REFERENCES

Behrman RE, ed. *Nelson Textbook of Pediatrics.* 15th ed. Philadelphia, Pa: WB
   Saunders; 1996.

Cummings S, Ullman D. *Homeopathic Medicines.* Los Angeles, Calif: Jeremy P. Tarcher,
   Inc; 1984.

Dorn M, Knick E, Lewith G. Placebo-controlled, double-blind study of *Echinacea
   pallidae radix* in upper respiratory tract infections. *Complementary Therapies in
   Medicine.* 1997;5:40–42.

Eby GA. Zinc ion availability—the determinant of efficacy in zinc lozenge treatment of
   common colds. *J Antimicrob Chemother.* 1997;40:483–493.

Fauci AS, Braunwald E, Isselbacher KJ et al, eds. *Harrison's Principles of Internal
   Medicine.* 14th ed. New York, NY: McGraw-Hill; 1998.

Garland ML, Hagmeyer KO. The role of zinc lozenges in treatment of the common cold.
   Ann Pharmacother. 1998;32:63–69.

Gruenwald J, Brendler T, Jaenicke C et al, eds. *PDR for Herbal Medicines.* Montvale, NJ:
   Medical Economics Company; 1998:817.

Hoheisel O, Sandberg M, Bertram S, Bulitta M, Schäfer M. Echinagard treatment shortens
   the course of the common cold: a double-blind, placebo-controlled clinical trial. *Eur J
   Clin Res.* 1997;9:261–269.

Melchart D, Walther E, Linde K, Brandmeier R, Lersch, C. Echinacea root extracts for the
   prevention of upper respiratory tract infections. *Archives of Family Medicine.*
   1998;7:541–545.

Morrison R. *Desktop Guide to Keynotes and Confirmatory Symptoms.* Albany, Calif:
   Hahnemann Clinic Publishing; 1993:3–6, 13–14, 158, 244–246.

Sazawal S, Black RE, Jalla S, et al. Zinc supplementation reduces the incidence of acute
   lower respiratory infections in infants and preschool children: a double-blind, controlled trial. *Pediatrics.* 1998;102(part 1):1–5.

Scaglione, et al. Efficacy and safety of the standardized ginseng extract G115 for potentiating vaccination against common cold and/or influenza syndrome. *Drugs Exp Clin Res.*
   1996;22:65–72.

Schöneberger D. The influence of immune-stimulating effects of pressed juice from
   Echinacea purpurea on the course and severity of colds. *Forum Immunol.*
   1992;8:2–12.

CONGESTIVE HEART FAILURE

OVERVIEW

Definition

Congestive heart failure (CHF) occurs when the heart cannot pump out an adequate supply of blood to meet the metabolic needs of the body. This condition results in ventricular dysfunction that correlates with reduced exercise capacity. Any form of heart disease may lead to CHF. End-stage CHF is characterized by a large dilated heart, elevated left ventricular (LV) filling pressure, reduced cardiac output, and peripheral and pulmonary edema. It is the most common cause of death for people over 65 years, affecting 10% of the geriatric U.S. population.

Etiology

- Hypertension
- Coronary artery disease
- Systolic dysfunction, diastolic dysfunction, or both
- Congenital heart disease
- Pericardial disease
- Tricuspid stenosis
- Pulmonary embolism
- Valvular function defects
- Myocardial infarction
- Myocarditis
- Arrhythmias
- Cardiomyopathy
- Anemia
- Thyrotoxicosis

Risk Factors

- Smoking
- High fat diet, excess body weight
- Alcohol abuse
- High sodium intake
- Influenza, pneumonia
- Noncompliance with prescribed medications or diet

Signs and Symptoms

- Dyspnea
- Fatigue, exercise intolerance
- Pulmonary edema—audible rales
- Hemoptysis—rust-colored sputum
- Distended neck veins
- Orthopneic cough
- Nocturia
- Proteinuria
- Insomnia
- Nausea, vomiting
- Anorexia
- Anxiety
- Peripheral edema

DIFFERENTIAL DIAGNOSIS

- Cirrhosis
- Nephrotic syndrome
- Venous occlusive disease

DIAGNOSIS

Physical Examination

No physical finding can confirm a diagnosis of CHF. Patients typically appear pale and present with fatigue and dyspnea. Echocardiography is therefore essential for early diagnosis.

Laboratory Tests

- Blood tests may indicate elevated serum creatinine, blood urea nitrogen (BUN), erythrocyte sedimentation rate, enzymes
- Serial blood gas measurements may indicate carbon dioxide retention with pulmonary edema

Pathological Findings

- Hypoperfusion
- Sodium and nitrogen retention from diminished renal perfusion
- Inadequate tissue oxygen delivery
- Endothelial dysfunction
- Orthopenea from elevated jugular venous pressure
- Pulmonary edema—excessive elevation of filling pressures results in aveolar flooding and gas exchange disturbance

Resulting adaptive mechanisms include:

- Renin–angiotensin and adrenergic systems activate causing arterial and venous vasoconstriction; arterial vasoconstriction increases the afterload, venous vasoconstriction increases preload
- Increased LV mass (hypertrophy) and volume (dilation)—contribute to dyspnea
- Increased sympathetic nervous system activity, resulting in systemic vascular resistance increase

Imaging

- X rays—show increased heart size and blood flow; indicates pulmonary, vascular, interstitial, and alveolar edema
- Radionuclide ventriculography—assesses ventricular function

Other Diagnostic Procedures

Diagnoses focus on identifying etiology and precipitating factors. Procedures include blood tests and ECG.

- Electrocardiogram (ECG)—measures heart's electrical activity; may be normal, or suggest ventricular dysrhythmias, left ventricular hypertrophy/damage, and inadequate blood flow
- Echocardiogram—assesses ventricular function; wall and valvular abnormalities; LV hypertrophy and abnormal filling pressures suggest diastolic dysfunction, pericardial disease, and valvular disease.
- Cardiac catherization—definitive diagnoses of extent of damage
- Angiography—diagnoses coronary occlusion and wall abnormalities
- Exercise stress test—assess blood pressure, heart rate and rhythm, and oxygen consumption while exercising

TREATMENT OPTIONS

Treatment Strategy

Immediate relief of the precipitating event. Typically, combined drug therapy (e.g., vasodilator, diuretic, digitalis glycoside) is prescribed for CHF. Mechanical or surgical therapies are added with severe CHF. Heart valve surgery, revascularization, or cardiac transplantation as required and as available. Bed rest and reduced activity are recommended until condition is stabilized. Oxygen relieves dyspnea and pulmonary vasoconstriction.

Drug Therapies

- Vasodilators—reduce arterial and venous vasoconstriction (afterload/preload); shifts blood volume from the arterial to the venous side of circulation; cornerstone of treatment; gradually titrate

Oral vasodilators:

- Angiotensin-converting enzyme (ACE) inhibitors (e.g., enalapril, 2.5 to 5.0 mg bid to qid); side effects—acute renal failure (avoid potassium-sparing diuretics), cough, angioedema, hypotension
- Angiotensin II receptor antagonists (e.g., Losartan, 12.5 mg qid titrated to 50 mg qid); monitor blood pressure

- Nitrates may relieve venous and pulmonary congestion
- Calcium channel blockers and alpha- and beta-adrenergic receptor antagonists—variable effects and potential serious adverse effects
- Parenteral vasodilators:
- Nitroglycerin—10 to 100 mg/min; tolerance problems with long-term use
- Sodium nitroprusside—5 to 150 mg/min per kg; thiocyanate and cyanide toxicity
- For fluid control and sodium retention
- Restriction of dietary fluid and sodium (< 2 g/day) reduces need for diuretics.
- Maximum daily net fluid loss—0.5 to 1.0 liter/day to avoid serious complications (e.g., oliguria, impaired renal function)
- Thiazide diuretics (e.g., chlorothiazide 500 to 100 mg/day); loop diuretics (e.g., furosemide 20 to 600 mg/day); potassium-sparing diuretics (e.g., spironolactone 25 to 200 mg/day)
- Mechanical removal of fluid—phlebotomy, thoracentesis, dialysis, paracentesis
- Digitalis glycosides—increase myocardial contractile function; prevent rhythm disturbances by increasing cardiac output and lowering filling pressures; digoxin—monitor closely for toxicity (5% to 15% of patients) and drug interactions; 0.25 to 0.5 mg/day then 0.25 mg every six hours to 1.0 to 1.5 mg
- Inotropic agents—for CHF unresponsive to other therapies; poor long-term benefit (e.g., dopamine 1 to 3 mg/kg/min; milrinone 50 mg/kg/min then 0.375 to 0.750 mg/kg/min); closely monitor for tachycardia and arrhythmia

Complementary and Alternative Therapies

The true goal is to prevent the pathologies leading to congestive heart failure. Nutrition and herbal medicine can play an important role in increasing the strength of the heart without also increasing the workload. In addition, treating the lungs with herbs and physical medicine may increase the comfort of the patient and decrease pulmonary pathology. Mind/body techniques, such as yoga, meditation, relaxation, and biofeedback show promise in increasing cardiovascular health and increasing a sense of well-being.

NUTRITION

- Antioxidants: vitamin C (1,000 mg tid), vitamin E (400 IU/day), selenium (200 mcg/day)
- Coenzyme Q10: (30 to 50 mg tid) antioxidant, increases oxygenation of tissue, including heart muscle
- Essential fatty acids: (1,500 mg bid) antiinflammatory
- Garlic, ginger and onions all have a beneficial effect on platelet aggregation. Increase fiber (especially water-soluble), fruits, vegetables, and vegetarian sources of protein. Increase potassium and decrease sodium in the diet.
- Homocystiene metabolism: Folic acid (800 mcg/day), B$_6$ (50 mg/day), B$_{12}$ (400 mg/day), betaine (200 to 1,000 mg/day)
- Magnesium: (500 mg) mild vasodilation, decreases vascular resistance
- Taurine: (500 mg bid) enhances cardiac efficiency, mild diuretic
- Carnitine: (750 to 1,500 mg bid) important in fatty acid metabolism, increases efficiency of cardiac function

HERBS

Herbs are generally a safe way to strengthen and tone the body's systems. As with any therapy, it is important to ascertain a diagnosis before pursuing treatment. Herbs may be used as dried extracts (capsules, powders, teas),

glycerites (glycerine extracts), or tinctures (alcohol extracts). Unless otherwise indicated, teas should be made with 1 tsp. of herb per cup of hot water. Steep covered 5 to 10 minutes for leaf or flowers, and 10 to 20 minutes for roots. Drink 2 to 4 cups/day. Tinctures may be used singly or in combination as noted.

- Hawthorn (*Crataegus oxyacantha*): stabilizes collagen and increases blood vessel integrity, prevents free radical damage, reduces peripheral vascular resistance, and increases coronary and myocardial perfusion without increasing cardiac load; historic use in CHF; dose is 3 to 5 g. This dose is difficult to achieve in tea or tincture. Supplements or solid extract are used.
- Mistletoe (*Viscum album*): mild antihypertensive, antiatherosclerotic, historically for exhaustion and nervousness
- Linden (*Tilia cordata*): historic use as a hypotensive, especially with digestive problems and nervousness
- Rosemary (*Rosemariana officinalis*): increases coronary artery blood flow, historically used to stimulate digestion and relieve nervous tension
- Mother wort (*Leonorus cardiaca*): chronotropic, arrythmias, especially with nervousness
- Dandelion (*Taraxacum officinalis*): potassium-sparing diuretic, can be used as a coffee substitute
- Indian tobacco (*Lobelia inflata*): anti-spasmodic, stimulates respiratory function, used in smoking cessation. May be toxic if used above recommended doses.
- Lily of the valley (*Convallaria majalis*): specific for cardiac insufficiency; exceeding recommended doses may lead to nausea, vomiting, headache, stupor. Use no more than 30 drops/day.
- Horsetail herb (*Equisetum arvense*): diuretic

Hawthorn should be included in any treatment. In addition, use a combination of four to six of the above herbs at 1 cup tea tid or 30 to 60 drops tincture tid.

HOMEOPATHY

Constitutional homeopathy may be helpful for stimulating overall vitality and should be prescribed by an experienced homeopath.

PHYSICAL MEDICINE

Castor oil pack. Used externally, castor oil is a powerful anti-inflammatory. Apply oil directly to chest, cover with a clean soft cloth (e.g., flannel) and plastic wrap. Place a heat source (hot water bottle or heating pad) over the pack and let sit for 30 to 60 minutes. For best results use three consecutive days. Applied over the lungs, this will increase pulmonary function stimulating drainage.

Contrast hydrotherapy. Alternating hot and cold applications to the chest brings nutrients to the lungs and diffuses metabolic waste from inflammation. The overall effect is decreased inflammation, pain relief, and enhanced healing. Alternate three minutes hot with one minute cold and repeat three times. This is one set. Do two to three sets/day. For debilitated patients, use cool and warm applications to decrease the contrast.

ACUPUNCTURE

May be helpful for increasing circulation, diuresis, and cardiac strength.

MASSAGE

May be helpful to increase lymphatic drainage and reduce edema.

Patient Monitoring

Close and frequent monitoring (X rays, blood levels) may reduce the need for hospitalization.

OTHER CONSIDERATIONS

Prevention

Every effort must be made to prevent progression of disease. Avoiding risks (see above) and isometric exercise may help prevent CHF.

Complications/Sequelae

- Pulmonary edema—medical emergency
- Electrolyte disturbances
- Arrhythmias

Prognosis

- 50% of patients die in four to five years
- 50% of those with advanced CHF live < 1 year
- Diastolic dysfunction has better prognosis than systolic
- Independent predictors include:
- Elevated ventricular filling
- Extent of ventricular function impairment
- Reduced cardiac index
- Exercise capacity

Pregnancy

Diuretics and sodium restriction are indicated. Anemia, infection, and preeclampsia increase cardiac workload and must be treated vigorously. The first two weeks postpartum is particularly dangerous for CHF.

REFERENCES

Bartram T. *Encyclopedia of Herbal Medicine.* Dorset, England: Grace Publishers; 1995:218–219.

Blumenthal M, ed. *The Complete German Commission E Monographs.* Boston, Mass: Integrative Medicine Communications; 1998:120,142–144,162–163,171–172,197.

Brady JA, Rock CL, Horneffer MR. Thiamin status, diuretic medications, and the management of congestive heart failure. *J Am Diet Assoc.* 1995;95:541–544.

Cecil RL, Plum F, Bennett JC, eds. *Cecil Textbook of Medicine.* 20th ed. Philadelphia, Pa: WB Saunders; 1996.

Gruenwald J, Brendler T, Jaenicke C et al, eds. *PDR for Herbal Medicines.* Montvale, NJ: Medical Economics Company; 1998:779–781,932–923,1101–1103,1175–1176,1185–1187,1219–1221.

Murray MT. *Encyclopedia of Nutritional Supplements.* Rocklin, Calif: Prima Publishing; 1996:378–379.

Schmidt U, Kuhn U, Ploch M, Hubner WD. Efficacy of the hawthorn (Crataegus) preparation LI 132 in 78 patients with chronic congestive heart failure defined as NYHA functional class II. *Phytomedicine.* 1994;1:17-24.

Washington University School of Medicine, Department of Medicine. *Washington Manual of Medical Therapeautics.* 29th ed. Philadelphia, Pa: Lippincott-Raven Publishers; 1998.

Werbach MR. *Nutritional Influences on Illness.* New Canaan, Conn: Keats Publishing, Inc; 1987:40–78,136–139,227–240.

■ CONJUNCTIVITIS
OVERVIEW
Definition
Conjunctivitis is inflammation of the palpebral and/or bulbar conjunctiva, the mucous membrane covering the inside of the eyelids and the outer part of the eye. There are several types of conjunctivitis.

- Viral conjunctivitis
- Bacterial conjunctivitis
- Allergic conjunctivitis
- Contact conjunctivitis
- Giant papillary conjunctivitis
- Traumatic conjunctivitis

Etiology
- Viral infection: Most common. Generally rhinovirus or adenovirus, often as a result of a respiratory infection spread to the eye via contaminated fingers, towels, or handkerchiefs. May start in one eye and spread to the other.
- Bacterial infection: Generally *Staphylococcus aureus, Staphylococcus pneumoniae,* or *Haemophilus influenzae;* occasionally *Pseudomonas, Neisseria,* or *Chlamydia.* Neonatal conjunctivitis may be caused by gonorrhea or chlamydia transmitted from the mother.
- Exposure to chemical irritants such as cigarette smoke, chlorine from swimming pools, and cosmetics.
- Giant papillary conjunctivitis is caused by long-term contact lens use. There is some controversy over the specific etiology. The condition may result from hypersensitivity to protein buildup on the lens, or from cumulative physical irration/trauma to the eye.

Risk Factors
- Recent upper-respiratory infection
- Allergies
- Group day-care situations
- Contact lens use, or other foreign body contact
- Exposure to severe wind, heat, or cold

Signs and Symptoms
Conjunctivitis produces the following in one or both eyes.
- Redness
- Itching, tearing, burning
- Discharge (watery or purulent)
- Overnight crusting
- Sensitivity to light
- Gritty sensation

DIFFERENTIAL DIAGNOSIS
- Foreign body
- Blepharitis
- Scleritis and episcleritis
- UV keratitis
- Herpes simplex keratitis
- Subconjunctival hemorrhage
- Iritis or iridocyclitis
- Acute angle closure glaucoma

DIAGNOSIS
Physical Examination
Examine conjunctiva while having patient look up, down, right, and left. Evert eyelids. The redness of conjunctivitis is non-specific, as opposed to the localized appearance of a subconjunctival hemorrhage. Palpable preau-

ricular lymph nodes and a clear discharge are indicative of viral conjunctivitis. Bilateral presentation, itching, and a clear or absent discharge without lymph node enlargement is generally indicative of allergic conjunctivitis. A thick purulent discharge is seen in bacterial conjunctivitis. In giant papillary conjunctivitis, enlarged papillae (0.3 mm in diameter or greater) will have formed on the superior palpebral conjunctiva due to the eruption of subepithelial collagen. Check for corneal abrasions or other defects using a slit lamp and fluorescein staining.

Laboratory Tests
Cultures may be done to determine infectious organism if necessary. The appearance of cells stained with gram stain or giamsa may indicate the presence of eosinophils, supporting the diagnosis of allergic conjunctivitis.

Other Diagnostic Procedures
Visual acuity may be tested with Snellen chart if necessary for diagnosis. Reduced visual acuity is not common with conjunctivitis and may be a sign of iritis or iridocyclitis, acute angle closure glaucoma, or herpes simplex keratitis. Intraocular pressure significantly elevated from the normal 10 to 20 mm mercury would not result from conjunctivitis and may be a sign of glaucoma. Culture and immunofluorescence for herpes simplex.

TREATMENT OPTIONS
Treatment Strategy
Viral conjunctivitis does not respond to antibiotics and is generally self-limiting. Treatment such as vasoconstrictive drops and/or cool compresses ease symptoms. For bacterial conjunctivitis, local antibiotics are indicated.

Drug Therapies
- Viral conjunctivitis: Cool compresses tid for one to three weeks; may also use antihistamines to relieve inflammation. Trifluridine 1% drops, every two hours. Acyclovir oral and topical as indicated.
- Allergic conjunctivitis: Attempt to eliminate contact with allergen. Treat with cool compresses, OTC or topical antihistamines, mast cell stabilizers such as cromolyn sodium, NSAIDs (particularly ketorolac). Vasoconstrictor/antihistamine combination of naphazoline 0.05%/antazoline 0.5%. Possibly mild corticosteroids.
- Bacterial conjunctivitis: Polytrim drops (trimethoprim sulfate, polymixin B sulfate, Allergan), 1 drop tid for one week, or polymixin B-bacitracin ointment (Polysporin). Fluoroquinolones as second-line therapy. 0.3% tobramycin or gentamicin as drops, or 10% sodium sulfacetamide as drops, every four hours.
- Giant papillary conjunctivitis: Avoid use of lenses until condition clears up and then consider prescribing a different material or design. The NSAID suprofen has been shown to be helpful in treatment, as are antihistamines. A short course of low-dosage topical corticosteroids may be necessary initially to reduce inflammation.

Complementary and Alternative Therapies
Mild to moderate cases of conjunctivitis may respond well to alternative treatment. Antibiotics may be needed for bacterial infections. For mild cases, begin with compresses. For moderate infection, use an eyewash as well. In the case of chronic or recurrent infection, nutritional support is suggested. Homeopathic remedies may be used for symptomatic relief.

NUTRITION
Doses listed are for adults. Decrease by one-half to two-thirds for children. Vitamin A (10,000 IU/day), vitamin C (1,000 mg tid to qid), and zinc (30 to 50 mg/day) enhance the immune response and promote healing.

HERBS

Herbs are generally a safe way to strengthen and tone the body's systems. As with any therapy, it is important to ascertain a diagnosis before pursuing treatment. Herbs may be used as dried extracts (capsules, powders, teas), glycerites (glycerine extracts), or tinctures (alcohol extracts). Unless otherwise indicated, teas should be made with 1 tsp. herb per cup of hot water. Steep covered 5 to 10 minutes for leaf or flowers, and 10 to 20 minutes for roots. Drink 2 to 4 cups/day. Tinctures may be used singly or in combination as noted.

Compresses and eye washes are external treatments. A compress is made with a clean cloth, gauze pads, or cotton balls soaked in a solution then applied over eyes. Washes may be used with an eye cup, or sterile dropper.

Compress:
Use 5 drops of tincture in 1/4 cup water or steep 1 tsp. herb in 1 cup hot water for 5 to 10 minutes and strain. Soak compress in solution and apply for 10 minutes, tid to qid.
- Eyebright *(Euphrasia officinalis):* antimicrobial, astringent, specific for eyes
- Chamomile *(Matricaria recutita):* antimicrobial, astringent, vulnerary, calming
- Fennel seed *(Foeniculum vulgare):* antimicrobial, astringent, vulnerary, soothing
- Marigold *(Calendula officinalis):* soothing vulnerary
- Plantain *(Plantago lanceolata, P. Major):* antimicrobial, astringent, and demulcent. Plantago lanceolata is specific to inflammation in the eye. The fresh leaves are superior in action.
- Flax *(Linum usitatissimum)* as a soothing poultice made with 1 oz of bruised flax seed steeped for 15 minutes in 4 oz of water, wrapped in cheesecloth then applied directly to the affected eye. Reheated poultice can be applied many times.
- Grated fresh potato has astringent properties. Wrap in cheesecloth and apply.

Eyewash: Use above herbs singly or in combination: Mix equal parts together then steep 1 tsp. herb in 1 cup of hot water to make a tea.

Goldenseal *(Hydrastis canadensis)* and boric acid: 10 drops of goldenseal tincture with 1 tsp. of boric acid mixed in 1 cup of water.

HOMEOPATHY

An experienced homeopath should assess individual constitutional types and severity of disease to select the correct remedy and potency. For acute prescribing use 3 to 5 pellets of a 12X to 30C remedy every one to four hours until acute symptoms resolve.
- *Aconite* for after exposure to wind or cold; thin discharge
- *Apis mellifica* for red, burning and swollen eyelids that feel better with cold applications
- Combination remedies containing *Apis, Euphrasia,* and *Sabadilla* may be effective for allergic conjunctivitis.
- *Allium cepa* for red, burning, tearing eyes that are sensitive to light.

ACUPUNCTURE

Treatment may be administered for pain relief and resolving congestion.

Patient Monitoring

Viral and bacterial conjunctivitis are both very contagious. Patients should be advised to take appropriate steps such as frequent handwashing and using separate towels, and family members should be monitored for signs of infection. Children are generally excluded from school and daycare situations while infection is active. In giant papillary conjunctivitis, monitoring is especially important once contact lens use has been resumed, in order to avoid recurrence. Any patient on corticosteroids must be carefully monitored for increase in intraocular pressure, infections, and incipient cataracts.

OTHER CONSIDERATIONS

Prevention

General hygiene is important in the prevention and treatment of conjunctivitis, especially in the use of contact lenses. Contact lens patients who have had giant papillary conjunctivitis should avoid heat disinfection and thimerosal in their cleaning regimen.

To prevent neonatal gonococcal conjunctivitis, silver nitrate is administered to the eyes of infants shortly after birth.

Complications/Sequelae

Allergic conjunctivitis is uncomplicated in most cases. However, some patients who are hypersensitive to allergens and develop atopic disorders such as asthma, hay fever, urticaria, or eczema may present with a severe form, called atopic keratoconjunctivitis, generally bilateral. Chronic marginal blepharitis and corneal ulcers or perforations are possible with bacterial conjunctivitis. Corneal scars are possible with viral conjunctivitis.

Prognosis

Patients with infectious conjunctivitis should assume they will be contagious for approximately seven days. Bacterial conjunctivitis will resolve in one to two weeks without treatment, two to five days with treatments. Some minor effects, such as dryness, irritation and discomfort with contact lenses, may linger for a few weeks. If symptoms have not improved or get worse, contact an opthamologist.

Pregnancy

High doses of vitamin A and vitamin C are contraindicated in pregnancy.

REFERENCES

Abelson MB, Casey R. How to manage atopic keratoconjunctivitis. *Rev Ophthalmol.* May 1996.

Abelson MB, McGarr, P. How to diagnose and treat inclusion conjunctivitis. *Rev Ophthalmol.* March 1997.

Abelson MB, Richard KP. What we know and don't know about GPC. *Rev Ophthalmol.* August 1994.

Abelson MB, Welch D. How to treat bacterial conjunctivitis. *Rev Ophthalmol.* December 1994.

Acute conjunctivitis. Acupuncture.com. Accessed at www.acupuncture.com/Clinical/Conjunct.htm on January 29, 1999.

Clinical imperatives of ocular infection. *Primary Care Optometry News.* Roundtable. March 1996. Available at www.slackinc.com/eye/pcon/199603/impera.htm.

Friedlaender MH. Update on allergic conjunctivitis. *Rev Ophthalmol.* March 1997.

Homeopathic drops for allergy: ready or not? *Primary Care Optometry News.* May 1996.

Infectious Diseases and Immunization Committee. Canadian Pediatric Society. Recommendations for the prevention of neonatal ophthalmia. *Can Med Assoc J.* 1983; 129:554–555.

Morrison R. *Desktop Guide to Keynotes and Confirmatory Symptoms.* Albany, Calif: Hahnemann Clinic Publishing; 1993:5, 28.

Pascucci S, Shovlin J. How to beat giant papillary conjunctivitis. *Rev Ophthalmol.* June 1994.

Rapoza PA, Francesconi CM. How to diagnose chronic red eye. *Rev Ophthalmol.* October 1997.

■ CONSTIPATION
OVERVIEW
Definition
Constipation, a condition in which a person has difficult or infrequent passage of feces, can be a symptom of an underlying pathology or an acute or chronic condition in itself, lasting days, months, or years. Normal bowel movements occur from two or three times a week to two or three a day. Constipation usually results from a delay in transit within the colon from a wide variety of causes. Constipation can occur at any age, and most people have constipation sometime in life, but it is more frequent in infancy and old age.

Etiology
Most cases of constipation result from changes in diet or physical activity, including inadequate fluid intake. Psychological factors, particularly depression, may cause acute or chronic constipation. Chronic abuse of laxatives or cathartics can also lead to chronic constipation. Psychogenic constipation may be the patient's misunderstanding of what constitutes abnormal bowel movements and an overreaction to less frequent bowel movements or changes in feces. The following may cause constipation.
Drugs:
- Aluminum and calcium antacids
- Anticholinergics
- Antidepressants
- Calcium supplements
- Calcium channel blockers
- Cholestyramine
- Narcotics
- Sympathomimetics, including pseudoephedrine
- Tranquilizers and sedatives

Structural abnormalities:
- Anorectal fissures or thrombosed hemorrhoids
- Strictures
- Tumors

Endocrine or metabolic disorders or changes:
- Hypothyroidism
- Hypercalcemia
- Hypokalemia
- Pregnancy

Neurological disorders:
- Parkinson's disease
- Cerebrovascular events
- Spinal cord tumors
- Trauma

Smooth muscle or connective tissue disorders:
- Amyloidosis
- Scleroderma

Congenital impairments:
- Aganglionic megacolon (Hirschsprung's disease)
- Neuromuscular bowel impairment
- Irritable bowel syndrome

Risk Factors
- Decrease in exercise or activity, often occurring with illness and travel
- Dietary changes
- Use of many medications
- Low fiber diet
- Caffeine use
- Diuretic use

Signs and Symptoms
- Infrequent, difficult passage of stools (< three times a week)
- Sudden and significant decrease in frequency of bowel movements
- Stools harder than normal, possibly impacted
- Sensation of incomplete bowel emptying
- Bloated sensation

DIFFERENTIAL DIAGNOSIS
Before the constipation is treated as a primary condition, underlying medical or psychogenic causes should be ruled out.

DIAGNOSIS
The history of bowel-elimination frequency and consistency is important, along with any changes in activity or diet. The medical history may reveal a patient with a misconception about normal elimination habits or neurotically preoccupied with bowel movements. Most systemic diseases that produce constipation as a symptom also result in other signs and symptoms. Intestinal problems such as strictures or tumors often present with other gastrointestinal symptoms, such as abdominal pain or bleeding. Idiopathic diet-induced or drug-induced constipation is not usually associated with such other signs and symptoms.

Physical Examination
Inspect and palpate for abdominal masses. Inspect the anorectal area for fissures, hemorrhoids, and stenosis or stricture secondary to surgery or inflammation. Rectal exam for possible masses or impacted stool.

Laboratory Tests
Lab tests are generally necessary only if a medical disorder is suspected or if patient is over 50 years of age:
- Test stool for occult blood
- CBC for anemia if colorectal neoplasm suspected
- Thyroid function tests
- Electrolytes and calcium levels
- Blood sugar

Pathological Findings
Constipation not related to a medical condition produces no pathological findings.
On physical examination:
- Gaping or asymmetrical anal opening may indicate a neurologic disorder.
- Masses may be found in abdomen or rectum, indicating further studies.
- Laboratory testing may detect occult blood in stool. If positive, follow with colonoscopy to rule out malignancy.

On endoscopy:
- Carcinoma or polyp
- Inflamed hemorrhoids or fissures, resulting from or promoting constipation
- Melanosis coli (brown pigmentation of the mucosa), indicating chronic laxative abuse

On rectal biopsy:
- Amyloidosis
- Ulcerative colitis
- Crohn's disease
- Hirschsprung's disease (The barium enema may reveal an obstructing tumor, stricture, or narrowed rectal segment characteristic of Hirschsprung's disease.)

Imaging

Barium enema may be performed if an obstructing lesion is
suspected.

Other Diagnostic Procedures

- Anoscopy and proctosigmoidoscopy or colonoscopy are performed
  in acute cases with unknown cause.
- Rectal biopsy may be performed if indicated for a suspected lesion.
- Colonic motility tests or transit studies are reserved for more severe
  cases in which conventional treatments fail.

TREATMENT OPTIONS

Treatment Strategy

Treatment focuses on the underlying disease or removing factors causing
the constipation. Chronic constipation can usually be prevented with a
combination of diet, fluid intake, exercise, and, when necessary, short-
term use of a laxative. Educate the patient about normal variations in
bowel movements and bowel retraining (consistent, unhurried elimination
practices). Discourage chronic use of laxatives.

In the absence of underlying pathology:

- Eliminate medications that may be causing the constipation.
- Increase fluid intake.
- Encourage a diet rich in fiber (whole-grain bread or cereal, bran,
  green vegetables, fruits).
- Check for food allergies.

Bowel retraining should emphasize a regular daily routine with sufficient
time for a bowel movement shortly after mealtime. Lukewarm tap water
enemas or bisocodyl suppositories (Dulcolax) may assist in starting the
retraining program.

Drug Therapies

Laxatives: Few comparative data are available for the different classes
of laxatives, and with more than 700 commercial products available, the
choice is often individual preference. Laxatives are contraindicated with any
bowel obstruction, acute intra-abdominal inflammation, or renal or heart
failure.

Bulk-forming agents are generally effective and work by stimulating
contractions of the large intestine, with low risk of adverse effects:

- Psyllium (Konsyl, Metamucil, Perdiem)
- Bran
- Calcium polycarbophil
- Methylcellulose (Citrucel)

Stool softeners increase the amount of water in the stool, increasing bulk
and stimulating natural contractions of the large intestine:

- Dioctyl sodium sulfosuccinate (Colace)

Saline laxatives, or osmotic laxatives, stimulate the release of cholecystokinin, which stimulates colonic motility; may result in hypermagnesemia
in cases of renal failure or hypocalcemia; magnesium compounds prevent
absorption of tetracyclines and reduce the effectiveness of digitalis and
phenothiazines.

- Milk of magnesia
- Magnesium citrate
- Sodium phosphate
- Lactulose (Chronulac)
- Sorbitol
- Alumina-magnesia (Maalox, Mylanta)

Stimulant laxatives, or irritant laxatives, alter electrolyte transport by
intestinal mucosa and increase intestinal activity; adverse effects include
impaired bowel motility or dependence with chronic use, hypokalemia,
protein-losing enteropathy, and salt overload:

- Anthraquinone derivatives (senna, aloe, cascara)
- Diphenylmethane compounds (phenolphthalein, bisacodyl)

Castor oil increases intraluminal fluid levels and thereby increases motility;
not recommended because of fluid and electrolyte alterations.

Complementary and Alternative Therapies

Lifestyle and dietary changes along with nutritional support can contribute
to the long-term resolution of constipation. Herbs can be used to help tonify and strengthen bowel function. Laxative herbs should be used with caution, as they may become less effective with habitual use. Mind-body techniques, such as meditation and yoga, may help reduce nervous tension that
may contribute to constipation.

NUTRITION

- Take time to eat in a relaxed atmosphere, breathing slowly and
  chewing food thoroughly.
- Eat smaller, more frequent meals and avoid overeating at one sitting.
- Eliminate refined foods, sugars, caffeine, alcohol, and dairy products.
- Decrease saturated fats (animal products) and increase essential fatty
  acids (cold-water fish, nuts, and seeds).
- Increase intake of fresh vegetables, whole grains, and water.
- Stewed or soaked prunes, 1 to 3 a day, have a slightly laxative effect.
- Flax meal, 1 heaping tsp. in 8 oz. of apple juice, provides fiber and
  essential fatty acids to help relieve constipation and promote normal
  motility within the digestive tract. Follow with an additional 8 oz. of
  water.
- Warm lemon water taken before meals stimulates digestion.
- Consider digestive enzymes for chronic constipation.
- Vitamin C 1,000 mg bid to tid.
- Magnesium 250 mg bid to tid.

HERBS

Herbs are generally a safe way to strengthen and tone the body's systems.
As with any therapy, it is important to ascertain a diagnosis before pursuing
treatment. Herbs may be used as dried extracts (capsules, powders, teas),
glycerites (glycerine extracts), or tinctures (alcohol extracts). Unless otherwise indicated, teas should be made with 1 tsp. herb per cup of hot
water. Steep covered 5 to 10 minutes for leaf or flowers, or 10 to
20 minutes for roots. Drink 2 to 4 cups/day. Tinctures may be used singly
or in combination as noted.

A combination of herbs to tonify digestion and relieve constipation includes
the following in equal parts as a tea or tincture: licorice root (*Glycyrrhiza
glabra*), cascara sagrada (*Rhamnus purshiana*), dandelion root
(*Taraxacum officinalis*), yellow dock (*Rumex crispus*), fennel seed
(*Foeniculum vulgare*), and ginger (*Zingiber officinalis*). A tea should be
steeped for 20 minutes. Drink 1 cup tid before meals. A tincture may be
taken tid, 15 to 20 drops before meals. For long-term use (more than two
weeks), eliminate cascara and substitute burdock (*Arctium lappa*).
Licorice root is contraindicated in hypertension.

HOMEOPATHY

An experienced homeopath should assess individual constitutional types
and severity of disease to select the correct remedy and potency. For acute
prescribing, use 3 to 5 pellets of a 12X to 30C remedy every one to four
hours until acute symptoms resolve.

- *Calcarea carbonica* for constipation without urge for stool
- *Nux vomica* for constipation with constant, ineffectual urging for stool
- *Silica* for constipation with the sensation that stool remains in the rectum after bowel movements

PHYSICAL MEDICINE

Castor oil packs to the abdomen may be useful in resolving constipation. Used externally, castor oil is a powerful anti-inflammatory. Apply oil directly to skin, and cover with a clean, soft cloth (e.g., flannel) and plastic wrap. Place a heat source (hot water bottle or heating pad) over the pack and let sit for 30 to 60 minutes. For best results, use three consecutive days in one week.

Contrast hydrotherapy may help to tonify and strengthen bowel function. Alternating hot and cold applications brings nutrients to the site and diffuses metabolic waste from inflammation. The overall effect may be decreased inflammation, pain relief, and enhanced function. Apply hot and cold towels to the abdomen. Alternate 3 minutes hot with 1 minute cold and repeat three times. This is one set. Do two to three sets/day.

ACUPUNCTURE

Constipation may be effectively treated with acupuncture, which can stimulate and tonify digestive function.

MASSAGE

Therapeutic massage can induce stress release and relieve constipation that is due to spasm and nervous tension. Massage of abdomen can also stimulate some increase in peristalsis.

Patient Monitoring

If constipation persists despite changes in diet, activity, and fluid intake, investigate further for underlying cause.

OTHER CONSIDERATIONS

Prevention

For patients with chronic tendencies toward constipation, emphasize the importance of including fiber in the daily diet, adequate fluid intake, exercise, and bowel retraining.

Complications/Sequelae

Megacolon may be acquired in severe cases that have either persisted a long time or have subsequently perforated. Chronic laxative abuse may lead to cathartic colon and fluid and electrolyte abnormalities. Frequent fecal impaction can lead to rectal ulceration. Fluid and electrolyte depletion may result.

Prognosis

In the absence of an underlying condition, constipation should resolve soon with medications if needed and not recur frequently with adequate diet, fluids, and exercise. Occasional constipation is generally harmless.

Pregnancy

Constipation is a common ailment in pregnancy and is usually relieved with dietary changes and increased water intake. Digestive enzymes may be safely taken to support digestion. Herbs that are stimulating to the digestive tract may have a reflexive reaction in uterine muscle and induce contractions. Laxative herbs should not be used in pregnancy without the supervision of a physician.

REFERENCES

Andreoli TE, Bennett JC, Carpenter CCJ. *Cecil Essentials of Medicine.* 3rd ed. Philadelphia, Pa: WB Saunders; 1993.

Ashraf W, Park F, Lof J, Quigley EM. Effects of psyllium therapy on stool characteristics, colon transit and anorectal function in chronic idiopathic constipation. *Aliment Pharmacol Ther.* 1995;9:639–647.

Barker LR, Burton JR, Zieve PD, eds. *Principles of Ambulatory Medicine.* 4th ed. Baltimore, Md: Williams & Wilkins; 1995:476–491.

Dambro MR. *Griffith's 5 Minute Clinical Consult 1999.* Baltimore, Md: Lippincott Williams & Wilkins; 1999.

Hobbs C. *Foundations of Health: The Liver and Digestive Herbal.* Capitola, Calif: Botanica Press; 1992:129–135.

McRorie JW, Daggy BP, Morel JG, Diersing PS, Miner PB, Robinson M. Psyllium is superior to docusate sodium for treatment of chronic constipation. *Aliment Pharmacol Ther.* 1998;12:491–497.

Morrison R. *Desktop Guide to Keynotes and Confirmatory Symptoms.* Albany, Calif: Hahnemann Clinic Publishing; 1993:85, 274, 281, 350.

Stein JH, ed. *Internal Medicine.* 4th ed. St. Louis, Mo: Mosby-Year Book; 1994.

■ COUGH

OVERVIEW

Definition

Cough is defined as explosive expiration providing a protective mechanism for clearing the tracheobronchial tree of secretions and foreign material and is necessary to aid normal oxygenation. Interruption of the cough reflex—as in certain neuromuscular disorders or excessive coughing, which can cause cerebral ischemia and thus interfere with respiration, can impair this process.

The cough is one of the most common reasons people seek medical attention. It can indicate a minor airway irritation or a serious underlying disorder. Coughs are generally diagnosed into one of two categories:

- Acute cough (less than three weeks duration)—usually from viral/bacterial upper respiratory tract infections (URIs)
- Chronic cough (more than three weeks duration)—attributable to underlying factors. One-fourth of patients have multiple contributing disorders, making systematic evaluation essential.

Etiology

- Viral or bacterial URI
- Inhaled irritants, such as cigarette smoke, airborne pollutants, or noxious fumes
- Gastroesophageal reflux disease (GERD)
- Asthma
- Bronchitis
- Upper-airway secretions
- Angiotensin-converting enzyme (ACE) inhibitors and beta-blockers
- Aspiration (bulimia, alcoholism, stroke)
- Congestive heart failure
- Stimulation of neural receptors in the pleura, pericardium, or ears (severe wax impaction) may cause chronic coughs.

Risk Factors

- Chronic cough—appears in 14% to 23% of adult nonsmokers and in 25% to 50% of adult smokers, increasing proportionately with the number of cigarettes smoked per day
- Occupational exposure to airborne environmental pollutants
- Immunosuppressive diseases
- IV drug user

Signs and Symptoms

A cough can be accompanied by the following symptoms/conditions:

- URI
- Postnasal drip
- Wheezing (cough variant asthma)
- Heartburn (GERD)
- Regurgitation (bulimia)
- Fever/chills/night sweats (pulmonary tuberculosis)
- Edema (congestive heart failure)
- Weight loss (cancer)

DIFFERENTIAL DIAGNOSIS

- Chronic bronchitis
- Pertussis (whooping cough)
- Asthma
- Granulomas
- GERD
- Bronchogenic carcinoma/carcinoid tumor
- Irritation of cough receptors in the ear
- Cystic fibrosis
- Congestive heart failure
- Parenchymal lung diseases (pneumonia, lung abscess)
- Compressed airways due to external masses

DIAGNOSIS

Physical Examination

Acute or persistent cough causing the patient concern or anxiety

Laboratory Tests

- Sputum analysis (for chronic bronchitis, pneumonia, lung abscess, endobronchial tumor)
- Esophageal pH monitoring (for GERD)
- Tuberculosis skin test (for those at high risk, including IV drug users, immunosuppressed individuals, homeless persons, prisoners, immigrants)

Pathological Findings

Dependent upon underlying disorder or cause

Imaging

- Chest/sinus radiography
- High resolution computed tomography (HRCT)

Other Diagnostic Procedures

Step-by-step evaluation, from most common cause to least common cause:

- Elicit careful and detailed history.
- Examine cough reflex receptor sites (nose, nasopharynx, lungs).
- Eliminate cigarette smoke and occupational or household exposure to airway irritants.
- Discontinue ACEs and beta-blockers; substitute alternative class of drug.
- Identify chronic bronchitis.
- Treat empirically according to etiologies to help avoid invasive and expensive diagnostic methods.
- Perform radiography, CT scans, bronchoscopy, or laboratory analyses to identify lung carcinoma, chronic lung infections, interstitial lung disease, or aneurysm if patient nonresponsive to treatments.
- Fiberoptic bronchoscopy
- Special tests include sweat chloride tests for cystic fibrosis in children who experience recurrent pneumonia and fail to thrive; barium swallow; and pulmonary function tests.

TREATMENT OPTIONS

Treatment Strategy

Treating the cough without treating the cause may be detrimental, as the cough reflex is necessary to keep airways clear. Symptomatic therapy becomes necessary when etiology is unknown, specific treatment is not possible, or the cough performs no useful purpose. Treatment, determined by underlying pathology, may include the following:

- Elimination therapy (of airway irritants or medications that trigger cough reflex)
- Pharmacotherapy
- Surgery
- Immunotherapy (allergy shots)
- Air humidification

Drug Therapies

- Antitussives—suppress cough reflex at the medullary cough center in the brain or the site of irritation. Oral (codeine [15 mg qid] or dextromethorphan [15 mg qid]), inhaled anticholinergic agent (ipratropium bromide [2 to 4 puffs qid]), inhaled glucocorticoids (beclomethasone or triamcinolone [8 to 16 puffs/day]), and Benzonanate peripherally acting anesthetic antitussive.

- Expectorants/bronchodilators—reduce viscosity of mucus, facilitating its movement from the tracheobronchial tree with antitussive effect (inhaled ipratropium [Atrovent])
- Antibiotics/antihistamines/decongestants—for URIs
- Antihistamines/decongestants: for postnasal drip; intranasal steroids if no improvement
- Antibiotics—for chronic sinusitis (amoxicillin-clavulanate potassium [Augmentin], trimethoprim-sulfamethoxazole [Bactrim, Septra], oral cephalosporin)
- Bronchodilators, beta-agonists, or corticosteroids—for asthma
- Intranasal steroids—for allergic rhinitis
- Antibiotics (often prolonged)—for *Haemophilus influenzae*
- High doses of proton-pump inhibitors (omeprazole) and H_2-blockers for complete suppression

Surgical Procedures
May be necessary to remove masses, carcinomas, aneurysms

Complementary and Alternative Therapies
While coughs due to severe underlying pathology require pharmacologic treatment, alternative therapies can be useful in treating coughs secondary to viral URI, allergens, irritants, and asthma. Alternative therapies can also be used concurrently with pharmacologic treatment to optimize recovery.

NUTRITION
- Eliminate known allergenic foods. IgG Elisa food allergy testing can help to determine food allergies.
- Reduce intake of mucus-producing foods, (i.e. dairy, citrus, wheat, and bananas). Increase fresh vegetables, fruits, and whole grains.
- Vitamin C (1,000 mg tid to qid), zinc (30 mg/day), and beta-carotene (100,000 IU/day) support the immune system.

HERBS
Herbs are generally a safe way to strengthen and tone the body's systems. As with any therapy, it is important to ascertain a diagnosis before pursuing treatment. Herbs may be used as dried extracts (capsules, powders, teas), glycerites (glycerine extracts), or tinctures (alcohol extracts). Unless otherwise indicated, teas should be made with 1 tsp. herb per cup of hot water. Steep covered 5 to 10 minutes for leaf or flowers, and 10 to 20 minutes for roots. Drink 2 to 4 cups/day. Tinctures may be used singly or in combination as noted.

Herbs can be used in combination for symptomatic relief and cough resolution while addressing the underlying etiology. A well-balanced formula contains herbs from several categories to increase the effectiveness of the cough (by stimulating expectoration or calming an irritable cough reflex), soothe irritated tissues, and support immune function. Tincture combinations should be taken at 30 drops tid to qid. Infusions are made with 1 heaping tsp. of herbal combination, steeped covered for 10 minutes, and drunk 3 to 4 cups/day. Licorice root should be avoided in hypertension.

- Strong expectorants: Horehound (*Marrubium vulgare*), thyme (*Thymus vulgaris*), and mullein (*Verbascum densiflorum*).
- Gentle expectorants: Fennel (*Foeniculum vulgare*), sweet violet (*Viola odorata*), ginger (*Zingiber officianalis*), and balm of Gilead (*Populus candicans*)
- Anti-tussives: Wild cherry bark (*Prunus serotina*), coltsfoot (*Tussilago farfara*), and linden flowers (*Tilia cordata*)

- Immune support: Purple coneflower (*Echinacea purpura*), licorice root, (*Glycyrrhiza glabra*), garlic (*Allium sativum*), and onion (*Allium cepa*)
- Tonification: Indian tobacco (*Lobelia inflata*) is especially useful for smokers; elderberry (*Sambucus nigra*), elecampane (*Inula helenium*), plantain (*Plantago lancelota*), and gumweed (*Grindelia camporum*).

Essential oils:
- Thyme, eucalyptus, and pine oils can be applied to ease bronchial spasm and help thin mucus.
- Chest rubs with 2 to 4 drops of essential oil in 1 tbsp. of food grade oil (e.g., olive, flax, sesame, almond oils)
- Castor oil pack with 4 to 6 drops of essential oil
- Chest poultice—flaxseed oil with baume de Canada, frankincense, mustard, oregano, or thyme oils

Note: Exposure to essential oils may antidote homeopathic remedies and their actions.

HOMEOPATHY
An experienced homeopath should assess individual constitutional types and severity of disease to select the correct remedy and potency. For acute prescribing use 3 to 5 pellets of a 12X to 30C remedy every one to four hours until acute symptoms resolve.

It is imperative that the underlying condition is addressed; however, homeopathic remedies can be helpful in acute coughs or chronic coughs that fail to resolve.
- *Aconite* for sudden onset of cough or croup
- *Spongia tosta* for harsh, barking cough
- *Drosera* for dry, spasmodic cough
- *Rumex crispus* for dry, shallow, ticklish cough
- *Ipecac* for deep, wet cough with gagging from the cough
- *Phosphorous* for tight chest with cough
- *Causticum* for cough with raw painful feeling in chest
- *Antimonium tart* for rattling cough with dizziness

ACUPUNCTURE
Acupuncture can be very helpful for acute and chronic coughs.

Patient Monitoring
Systematic evaluation and treatment applied in progressive steps is effective in managing patients with persistent, chronic cough.

OTHER CONSIDERATIONS
- Consider psychogenic cough if no pathology (nervous tic or attention-seeking device).
- Rib fractures may indicate presence of osteoporosis.

Prevention
- Elimination of airway irritants
- Exercise, ample rest, nutritious diet, vitamins, minerals, herbs, and other supplements (particularly C, A, zinc, echinacea, garlic) to boost immune system and decrease risk of viral/bacterial infections
- Immunization with pneumococcal vaccine; annual influenza vaccination

Complications/Sequelae
Sleep disruption, rib fractures, cerebral ischemia, bronchospasms, urinary incontinence

Prognosis

- Dependent upon etiology/underlying cause
- Acute cough usually dissipates upon recovery from infection but may persist for several weeks.

Pregnancy

Check for medication contraindications.

REFERENCES

American Academy of Family Physicians. Available at: http://www.aafp.org/.

Duke JA. *The Green Pharmacy.* Emmaus, Pa: Rodale Press; 1997.

Fauci AS, Braunwald E, Isselbacher KJ et al, eds. *Harrison's Principles of Internal Medicine.* 14th ed. New York, NY: McGraw-Hill; 1998.

Kruzel T. The Homeopathic Emergency Guide. Berkeley, Calif: North Atlantic Books; 1992.

Newall A, Anderson LA, Phillipson JD. *Herbal Medicines.* London, England: The Pharmaceutical Press; 1996.

Schulz V, Hänsel R, Tyler VE. *Rational Phytotherapy.* 3rd ed. Berlin, Germany: Springer-Verlag, 1998

Tierney Jr. LM, McPhee SJ, Papadakis MA, eds. *Current Medical Diagnosis & Treatment, 1999.* Stamford, Conn: Appleton & Lange; 1999.

Tyler VE. *Herbs of Choice.* Binghamton, NY: Pharmaceutical Products Press; 1994.

■ CUTANEOUS DRUG REACTIONS

OVERVIEW

Definition

Adverse drug reactions affect up to 30% of hospitalized patients. Cutaneous drug reactions are estimated at 2.2 per 100 inpatients and 3 per 1,000 drug courses. Penicillins, sulfonamides, and blood products account for two-thirds of these. Prevalence in outpatient settings is unknown. Reactions may be immunologic or nonimmunologic, the latter being more prevalent. Although most reactions are obvious with a week of drug-therapy initiation, some may take up to four weeks to manifest. Clinical effects range from acneiforms and phototoxicity to exfoliative dermatitis and toxic epidermal necrolysis (TEN). Most common reactions are exanthems and urticarial eruptions; however, multiple morphologic types may occur. Inpatient treatment should be considered for anaphylatic reactions, Stevens-Johnson syndrome, TEN, and widespread bullous reactions as they may be life-threatening. Risk of these reactions is 1 to 10 per 1,000,000. Causative drugs include sulfonamide antibiotics, aminopenicillins, phenytoin (and structurally related anticonvulsants), allopurinol, and oxicam nonsteroidal anti-inflammatories. Because many skin disorders mimic drug reactions and certain reactions are specific to drug type, accurate assessment is critical. Reactions specifically induced by drugs include fixed drug eruptions, argyria, and arsenical keratosis.

Etiology

Adverse reaction is either immunologic or nonimmunologic.

- Immunologic responses—defined as drug allergies—stem from activation of the host immunologic pathways, inducing the release of histamines.
- Nonimmunologic reactions—the more common type—can be attributed to several factors, including overdose, interaction between drugs, metabolic alterations, inherited protein or enzyme deficiencies, and cumulative toxicity.

Major causative drugs include:

- Allopurinol
- Androgens
- Aspirin
- Barbiturates
- Chemotherapeutic agents
- Corticosteroids
- Diuretics
- Heavy metals (gold, copper)
- Hydralazine
- NSAIDs
- Penicillins
- Phenothiazines
- Procainamide
- Sulfonamides
- Sulfonylureas
- Tetracyclines
- Certain hypertensive agents

Risk Factors

- 3 per 1,000 drug courses/2.2 per 100 patients
- Elderly more susceptible, otherwise unrelated to age
- Prevalence greater among women
- Previous drug reactions
- Drug interactions
- Genetic predisposition
- Drug therapy

Signs and Symptoms

- Acneiforms
- Lupus erythematosus with malar erythema
- Photosensitivity
- Urticaria
- Maculopapular eruptions
- Eczematous reaction
- Erythema multiforme/nodosum
- Fixed eruptions
- Lichenoid
- Vasculitis
- Dermal tissue necrosis

DIFFERENTIAL DIAGNOSIS

- Viral exanthem—fever and other systemic symptoms to rule out more common maculopapular eruptions
- Primary dermatosis—drug eruptions manifest as many types of dermatosis

DIAGNOSIS

Physical Examination

May include:

- Urticaria
- Erythema
- Facial edema
- Skin pain
- Epidermal detachment
- Dermal necrosis
- Blisters
- Swollen tongue
- Fever
- Enlarged lymph nodes
- Wheezing/hypotension

Laboratory Tests

Laboratory tests are generally nonspecific. These tests may be helpful.

- Eosinophilia (>1,000/mm3), indicates possible allergic reaction
- Lymphocytosis with atypical lymphocytes
- Abnormal liver function test
- Drug levels/possible overdose; nonallergic reaction
- Enzymes/metabolites
- Skin culture/biopsy
- CBC/differential

Pathological Findings

Although certain drugs will cause specific reactions, some general pathologies include:

- Urticaria: pruritic, red wheals ranging from small spots to large area; swelling of deep dermal/subcutaneous tissue indicates angioedema, which may involve mucous membranes
- Photosensitivity eruptions:

Phototoxic—resemble sunburn, are dose-related, may occur with first exposure to drug and exposure to light

Photoallergic—require drug immune response and light, often delayed reaction; eruptions range from lichenoid papules to eczematous changes.

- Pigmentation (type of change determined by type of drug): oral contraceptives—increase melanocytic activity; heavy metals (like inorganic arsenic, silver, gold)—drug deposition; zidovudine (AZT)—pigmentation in nails; nicotinic acid—brown pigmentation
- Cutaneous necrotizing vasculitis: palpable purpuric lesions, ulcers, hemorrhagic blisters (may involve organs)

- Phenytoin hypersensitivity reaction (from inherited deficiency of expoxide hydrolase): becomes purpuric—with fever, edema, tender lymphadenopathy, leukocytosis, hepatitis
- Warfarin skin necrosis: rare, usually in women; sharply demarcated erythematous; indurated, purpuric lesions (associated with protein C/vitamin K deficiency)

Other Diagnostic Procedures

Assessment of possible reaction includes:

- History of drug use—including OTCs, prescriptions, illegal drugs, herbs, vitamins—in prior four weeks
- Drug level/evidence of overdose
- Previous history (personal and populational) with the suspected causative agent
- Similar etiology to existing/new disease unrelated to drug (drug may, however, modify these reaction rates)
- Timing of reaction in relation to drug administration
- Discontinuation of medication or—if multiple medications in use—withdrawal of suspected agent based on its likelihood to cause the current reaction
- Response of symptoms to drug withdrawal
- Recurrence of symptoms with drug rechallenge
- Special tests: skin test for IgE-mediated reaction; IgG/IgM for drug-specific antibodies; prick/scratch/patch tests for allergic reaction

TREATMENT OPTIONS

Treatment Strategy

Choice of treatment will depend on:

- Type, severity, and natural history of eruption—urticaria, angioedema, and bullous lesions can be more serious and should be aggressively managed. Consider inpatient management for anaphylactic reactions and toxic epidermal necrolysis, and Stevens-Johnson syndrome extensive bullous reactions.
- Importance of drug in disease/disorder control
- Availability of pharmacologically similar yet chemically unrelated drugs
- Risk/benefit ratio of drug reaction compared to disease
- Consideration of overall patient management

Common therapies include the following.

- Cessation of suspect or proven offending drugs
- Alteration of dosage/administration route
- Pharmacotherapy
- Inpatient treatment for serious reactions
- Surgery (when necessary)

Drug Therapies

- Corticosteroids (systemic/IV): for anaphylaxis, severe urticaria, angioedema—prednisone 40 to 60 mg/day, 5 to 10 days
- Corticosteroids (topical): for limited eczematous or lichenoid eruptions (Group I to III)
- Antihistamines: for pruritic—diphenhydramine (Benadryl) 25 to 50 mg every six hours; hydroxyzine (Atarax) 10 to 25 mg every six to eight hours; for anaphylaxis/widespread urticaria—epinephrine (1;1,000, 0.01 ml/kg to 0.3 ml max. sq)
- Epinephrine: for severe respiratory/cardiovascular implications
- Topical antipruritics/lubricants/emollients: for eczematous reactions
- Baths (with or without additives)
- Special treatments: for severe reactions (depending upon severity)
- H_1 Blockers (i.e., tagamet): in severe cases

Surgical Procedures

Debridement of necrotic tissue in severe reactions

Complementary and Alternative Therapies

Severe cutaneous drug reactions require immediate medical attention. Mild to moderate reactions may be safely and effectively treated with alternative therapies. Begin with vitamin C, bioflavanoids, and anti-inflammatory herbs. Add other nutritional supplements and herbs as needed for pain relief and immune support.

NUTRITION

- Vitamin C (1,000 mg tid to qid) stabilizes mast cells and prevents the secretion and breakdown of histamines.
- B-complex with extra B_{12} (1,000 mcg) aids in overall dermal health, can ease nerve pain, and promotes normal skin growth.
- Vitamin E (400 to 800 IU/day) improves dermal circulation.
- Zinc (30 to 50 mg/day) supports the immune system and promotes healing.
- Bromelain (125 to 250 mg bid to tid) is a proteolytic enzyme that reduces inflammation.
- Magnesium (400 to 800 mg) may help prevent spasms in the bronchial passages.

HERBS

Herbs are generally a safe way to strengthen and tone the body's systems. As with any therapy, it is important to ascertain a diagnosis before pursuing treatment. Herbs may be used as dried extracts (capsules, powders, teas), glycerites, or tinctures (alcohol extracts). Unless otherwise indicated, teas should be made with 1 tsp. herb per cup of hot water. Steep covered 10 to 20 minutes and drink 2 to 4 cups/day. Tinctures may be used singly or in combination as noted.

Anti-inflammatory herbs help to stabilize mast cells and reduce inflammation. Those herbs include the following.

- Turmeric (*Curcuma longa*), 100 mg bid to tid potentiates bromelain when taken together.
- Quercetin (may be given up to 1,000 mg tid)
- Hesperidin (200 mg tid to qid)

An infusion of equal parts of coneflower (*Echinacea angustifolia*), yarrow (*Achillea millefolium*), chamomile (*Matricaria recutita*), peppermint (*Mentha piperata*), and red clover (*Trifolium pratense*) will give immune support, reduce inflammation, and aid in lymph drainage.

For urticaria:

- Skin wash—To provide symptomatic relief of itching use one or more of the following herbs brewed as a tea 1 tsp/cup, cooled, and applied as needed. Peppermint, chickweed (Stellaria media), and chamomile. To aid healing, add one or more of the following: marigold (*Calendula officinalis*), comfrey (*Symphytum officinale*), or coneflower (*Echinacea angustifolia*).
- Skin poultice—For open sores use powdered slippery elm (*Ulmus fulva*), goldenseal (*Hydrastis canadensis*), and marshmallow root (*Althea officinalis*). Add enough skin wash to make a paste. Apply as needed.
- Aloe vera gel applied topically can soothe burning inflammations.
- Oatmeal baths—Add powdered oatmeal (or 1 cup of oatmeal in a sock) to tepid bath.
- Skin balm—Flaxseed oil (2 tbsp.) plain or with 5 drops of oil of chamomile or marigold. Specifically for eczema-type reactions.

HOMEOPATHY

An experienced homeopath should assess individual constitutional types and severity of disease to select the correct remedy and potency. For acute prescribing use 3 to 5 pellets of a 12X to 30C remedy every one to four hours until acute symptoms resolve.

Cutaneous drug reactions may be life-threatening, and need immediate medical attention. Homeopathic remedies can be used successfully for symptomatic relief of itching, burning, and swelling.
- *Apis mellifica* for acute swelling with burning pains that are relieved by cold applications
- *Graphites* for eczema or urticaria with tremendous itching
- *Ledum palustre* for cellulitis or eczema with severe inflammation
- *Rhus toxicodendron* for burning and itching that are relieved by hot applications
- *Urtica urens* for burning and itching

Patient Monitoring
- Close physical follow-up/monitoring to ensure no progression of reaction
- Telephone contact until eruption completely cleared
- Inpatient observation in severe reactions
- Clearly indicate on patient records suspected causative agent/specific reaction

OTHER CONSIDERATIONS
Prevention
To minimize morbidity and mortality from drug reactions:
- Patient education: drugs to avoid, drugs to use; familial implication
- Medical alert jewelry identifying causative drugs

Complications/Sequelae
- Anaphylaxis, laryngeal edema, bone marrow suppression, future cross-reaction to chemically similar compounds

Prognosis
- Remission of symptoms within days of drug withdrawal
- Bullae, urticaria, angioedema potentially life-threatening

Pregnancy
- Drugs of any kind should be avoided unless absolutely necessary and safety to fetus is proven.

REFERENCES
American Academy of Dermatology. Guidelines of care for cutaneous adverse drug reactions. *J Am Acad Dermatol.* 1996;35:458-461. Available at www.aad.org/guide-linecutaneousdrug.html.

Balch JF, Balch PA. *Prescription for Nutritional Healing.* 2nd ed. Garden City Park, NY: Avery Publishing Group; 1997.

Dambro MR, ed. *Griffith's 5 Minute Clinical Consult.* Baltimore, Md: Lippincott, Williams & Wilkins; 1998.

Fauci AS, Braunwald E, Isselbacher KJ et al, eds. *Harrison's Principles of Internal Medicine.* 14th ed. New York, NY: McGraw-Hill; 1998.

Morrison R. *Desktop Guide to Keynotes and Confirmatory Symptoms.* Albany, Calif: Hahnemann Clinic Publishing; 1993.

Murray MT, Pizzorno JE. *Encyclopedia of Natural Medicines.* 2nd ed. Rocklin, Calif: Prima Publishing; 1998.

■ DEMENTIA
OVERVIEW
Definition
According to DSM-IV, dementia is characterized by multiple cognitive deficits that are severe enough to cause significant impairment in social or occupational functioning. These deficits must show evidence of decline from previous levels of functioning, include memory impairment, and at least one other cognitive disturbance (aphasia, apraxia, agnosia, or a disturbance in executive functioning). The rate of occurrence is higher in later life; the highest prevalence is above age 85. Dementia is classified as being progressive, static, or remitting. The subtypes of dementia are listed below.

- Dementia of the Alzheimer's type (DAT)—deterioration of higher cortical function (this is the most common form)
- Vascular dementia—one form is multi-infarct dementia (MID), which is secondary to atherosclerosis
- Dementia due to other general medical conditions, including infection with the human immunodeficiency virus (HIV), traumatic brain injury, Parkinson's disease, Huntington's disease, Pick's disease, Creutzfeldt-Jakob disease, normal-pressure hydrocephalus, hypothyroidism, brain tumor, and vitamin B deficiencies
- Substance-induced persisting dementia due to drug or alcohol abuse, medication, or toxin exposure

Etiology
Alzheimer's disease is the most common cause of dementia. Other causes include biologic factors (e.g., neurofibrillary tangles); nutritional deficiencies (e.g., the B vitamins); physiological effects of general medical conditions (e.g., Creutzfeld-Jakob disease); persisting effects of a substance (e.g., alcohol or medications); and multiple etiologies (e.g., the combination of Alzheimer's disease and cerebrovascular disease).

Risk Factors
- Family history of Alzheimer's disease and other dementias
- Down's syndrome
- Head trauma (especially with loss of consciousness)
- Other factors sometimes associated with dementia include age (onset at age 65 and above); late maternal age; history of depression; strokes, especially with a history of hypertension; alcohol or drug abuse; and history of CNS infection.

Signs and Symptoms
- Memory impairment
- Language deterioration (aphasia)
- Motor activities impairment (apraxia)
- Impaired ability to recognize objects (agnosia)
- Inability to think abstractly, i.e., to plan, initiate, sequence, monitor, and stop complex behavior (disturbances in executive functioning)
- Spatial disorientation
- Suicidal behavior
- Motor disturbances
- Disinhibited behavior
- Anxiety, mood, and sleep disturbances
- Hallucinations
- Increased susceptibility to physical stressors such as illness or bereavement that worsen intellectual deficits and other problems
- Incontinence
- Tremor
- Seizures

DIFFERENTIAL DIAGNOSIS
- Mental retardation
- Other cognitive disorders (delirium, amnestic disorder)
- Substance abuse
- Psychiatric disorders (e.g., schizophrenia)
- Major depressive disorder
- Malingering and factitious disorder
- Aging (e.g., age-related cognitive decline)

DIAGNOSIS
Laboratory Tests
There is no accepted diagnostic test for Alzheimer's disease available in blood, cerebrospinal fluid, or other tissue. Underlying medical conditions (e.g., cerebellar atrophy focal or focal brain lesions) may be determined via neurological imaging. The "gold standard" for diagnosing dementia is neuropathological findings made at autopsy. However, there are potential biomarkers for Alzheimer's disease, including characteristics of the beta-amyloid protein found in senile plaques.

Routine laboratory evaluations should include CBC count, sedimentation rate, stool for occult blood, thyroid functions, electrolytes, BUN, calcium, phosphorus, urinalysis and culture, B_{12} liver function, blood sugar, syphilis serology, chest radiograph, and electrocardiogram.

Pathological Findings
Several microscopic changes in brain tissue have been identified in Alzheimer's disease, principally the formation of senile or neuritic plaques and neurofibrillary tangles.

Imaging
Neuroimaging, including CT, MRI, PET, or SPECT scans, may aid in the differential diagnosis of dementia.

Other Diagnostic Procedures
There are no objective tests, but the Dementia Questionnaire is often applied.

- Clinician interview—assessment of symptoms and degree of severity of dementia; includes (1) focused history emphasizing mode of onset (abrupt versus gradual); (2) progression (stepwise versus continuous decline; worsening versus fluctuating versus improving), duration of symptoms; (3) medical history; (4) family history; (5) social and cultural history; (6) medication history; and (7) informant reports
- Neurological assessment—CT scan; EEG for suspected seizure disorder or Creutzfeldt-Jakob disease; MRI scan for suspected Huntington's disease; Genetic Testing—Recent studies show that genetic testing may be useful, especially for the ApoE-E4 allele and mutations in the presenilin 1 gene in Alzheimer's disease.
- Use of standardized instruments such as the Dementia Mood Assessment Scale developed for Alzheimer's patients

TREATMENT OPTIONS
Treatment Strategy
Treatments are aimed at the arrest and reversal of the disease or the reduction of symptoms, including those listed below.

- Pharmacotherapy
- Psychotherapy, including psychosocial, interpersonal, environmental, and psychoeducational interventions
- Environmental interventions (e.g., fostering a secure and predictable environment with a minimum of sensory stimulation)
- Medication management

Drug Therapies

- Acetycholinesterase inhibitors (antidementia treatment), such as tacrine (Cognex, 10 to 40 mg qid) and donepezil (Aricept, 5 to 10 mg/day) increase precursor substances and acetylcholine in synapses; slow degradation of acetylcholine, direct activation of the postsynaptic receptor, and deactivation of inhibiting impulses on cholinergic systems; side effects include elevated serum alanine aminotrasterase levels; contraindicated for patients who currently have or have a history of liver disease
- Neuroleptics (behavior problems), such as haloperidol (Haldol, 0.5 to 5 mg/day) and trifluoperazine (Stelazine, 1 to 20 mg/day); side effects, even at low doses, include extrapyramidal signs (e.g., parkinsonism and akathisia)
- Benzodiazepines (agitation), such as lorazepam (Ativan, 0.5 to 2 mg, one to three/day) and clonazepam (Klonopin, 0.5 to 1 mg bid); side effects include sedation and falls.
- Selective serotonin reuptake inhibitors (SSRIs) (depressive symptoms), such as paroxetine (Paxil, 10 to 40 mg/day) and sertraline (Zoloft, 25 to 200 mg/day) block serotonin reuptake. Anticholinergic side effects include dry mouth, constipation, urinary retention, atrioventricular conduction delay, and orthostatic hypotension.
- Estrogen therapy may help to maintain connections between neurons and reduce development of Alzheimer's disease in postmenopausal women.

Complementary and Alternative Therapies

Alternative therapies may offer great promise in treating dementia without the side effects of the commonly prescribed pharmaceuticals. Treatment with nutrition can provide rapid results in those with deficiencies. Herbal treatment is widely used in Europe with promising results.

NUTRITION

- Anti-oxidants are a key component, with emphasis on both water and fat soluble antioxidants—vitamin E (400 to 800 IU/day), vitamin C (1,000 mg tid), and coenzyme Q10 (10 to 50 mg tid)
- Vitamins: Biotin (300 mcg); B vitamins are often depleted in dementia; B_1 (50 to 100 mg), B_2 (50 mg), B_6 (50 to 100 mg), B_{12} (100 to 1,000 mcg). B_{12} may need to be administered IM for optimum results.
- Minerals: calcium/magnesium (1,000/500 mg/day), zinc (30 to 50 mg/day); excess of manganese and copper can increase the risk for dementia
- IV chelating agents such as ethylenediaminetetraacetic acid (EDTA) may help to restore normal circulation in the brain, remove calcium plaques and heavy metals from brain arteria.
- Essential fatty acids regulate platelet aggregation, stabilize arterial walls and are anti-inflammatory. Dietary manipulation includes reducing animal fats and increasing fish.

HERBS

Herbs are generally a safe way to strengthen and tone the body's systems. As with any therapy, it is important to ascertain a diagnosis before pursuing treatment. Herbs may be used as dried extracts (capsules, powders, teas), glycerites (glycerine extracts), or tinctures (alcohol extracts). Unless otherwise indicated, teas should be made with 1 tsp. herb per cup of hot water. Steep covered 5 to 10 minutes for leaf or flowers, and 10 to 20 minutes for roots. Drink 2 to 4 cups/day. Tinctures may be used singly or in combination as noted.

Choose four to six herbs from the most appropriate category and use 1 cup or 30 to 60 drops tid.

- Ginkgo (*Ginkgo biloba*) is specific for preventing and treating Alzheimer's and senile dementia from cerebral vascular insufficiency; regulates platelets, may exacerbate peripheral edema, clotting times may need to be checked. May be taken as a single herb in a standardized extract of 40 to 50 mg tid. Monitor carefully with concurrent use of anti-coagulants.
- Hawthorn (*Crataegus oxyacantha*)—circulatory stimulant, cardiac tonic
- Rosemary (*Rosemariana officinalis*)—circulatory stimulant, digestive bitter, anti-depressant
- Siberian ginseng (*Eleuthrococcus senticosus*)—increases endurance, increases cerebral circulation, may be contra-indicated in hypertension.
- Lemon balm (*Melissa officinalis*)—carminative, spasmolytic; anti-anxiety, insomnia
- Ginger (*Zingiber officinale*)—carminative, vasodilator; general weakness
- St. John's wort (*Hypericum perforatum*)—depression, anxiety

HOMEOPATHY

An experienced homeopath should assess individual constitutional types and severity of disease to select the correct remedy and potency. For acute prescribing use 3 to 5 pellets of a 12X to 30C remedy every one to four hours until acute symptoms resolve.

- *Alumina* for dullness of mind, vagueness, slow answers to questions, especially with constipation
- *Argentum nitricum* for dementia with irritability, especially when lack pf control over impulses
- *Cicuta* for dementia after head injuries, especially with convulsions
- *Helleborus* for stupefaction, person answers questions slowly and stares vacantly
- *Silica* for mental deterioration with anxiety over small details

Patient Monitoring

Patients should be monitored closely due to the combination of age and presence of neurologic disorder, which drastically increases sensitivity to the side effects of pharmacologic agents. Smaller initial doses, longer titration intervals, and lower final doses are recommended.

OTHER CONSIDERATIONS

Prevention

Preventive measures for specific dementias are effective (e.g., abstinence for alcoholic dementia; safety measures for postconcussive dementia; lowering blood pressure, treating cardiac disease, and preventing atherosclerosis or embolization for multi-infarct dementia). Caregiver and patient education focusing on knowledge of the disease, health, and the patient's well-being result in better patient care. Exercise, both physical and mental, may prevent or slow dementia.

Complications/Sequelae

- Drug interactions or drug overdose can be severe.
- Malnutrition
- General hygiene problems

Prognosis

Dementia may be progressive, static, or remitting. The underlying pathology and application of effective treatment in a timely manner plays a large role in its reversibility and manageability.

REFERENCES

American Psychiatric Association. *Diagnostic and Statistical Manual of Mental Disorders*. 4th ed. Washington, DC: American Psychiatric Association; 1994.

Bartram T. *Encyclopedia of Herbal Medicine*. Dorset, England: Grace Publishers; 1995:214, 376.

Blumenthal M, ed. *The Complete German Commission E Monographs*. Boston, Mass: Integrative Medicine Communications; 1998:136, 138, 197.

Gruenwald J, Brendler T, Jaenicke C et al, eds. *PDR for Herbal Medicines*. Montvale, NJ: Medical Economics Company; 1998:967–968, 1101–1102, 1219–1220, 1229–1230.

Hofferberth B. The efficacy of EGb 761 in patients with senile dementia of the Alzheimer type; A double-blind, placebo-controlled study on different levels of investigation. *Hum Psychopharmacol*. 1994;9:215–222.

Kanowski S, Hermann WM, Stephan K, Wierich W, Horr R. Proof of efficacy of the Ginkgo biloba special extract EGb 761 in outpatients suffering from mild to moderate dementia of the Alzheimer's type or multi-infarct dementia. *Pharmacopsychiatry*. 1996;29:47–56.

Le Bars, et al. A placebo-controlled, double-blind, randomized trial of an extract of Gingko biloba for dementia. *JAMA*. 1997;278:1327–1332.

Maurer K. et al. Clinical efficacy of Gingko biloba special extract EGb 761 in dementia of the Alzheimer type. *J Psychiatr Res*. 1997;31:645–655.

Morrison R. *Desktop Guide to Keynotes and Confirmatory Symptoms*. Albany, Calif: Hahnemann Clinic Publishing; 1993:17–17, 32–33, 124–125, 176–177, 248–249.

Morris JC, ed. *Handbook of Dementing Illnesses*. New York, NY: Marcel Dekker Inc; 1994.

National Institutes of Health. Available at http://text.nlm.nih.gov/.

Perry EK, Pickering AT, Wang WW, Houghton P, Perry NS. Medicinal plants and Alzheimer's disease: Integrating ethnobotanical and contemporary scientific evidence. *J Altern Complement Med*. 1998;4:419–428.

Rai GS, Shovlin C, Wesnes KA. A double-blind, placebo controlled study of Ginkgo biloba extract in elderly patients with mild to moderate memory impairment. *Curr Med Res Opin*. 1991;12:350–355.

Rakel RE. *Conn's Current Therapy 1997: Latest Approved Methods of Treatment for the Practicing Physician*. Philadelphia, Pa: WB Saunders; 1997.

Werbach, M. *Nutritional Influences on Illness*. New Canaan, Conn: Keats Publishing; 1988:149–154.

■ DEPRESSION

OVERVIEW

Definition

Unipolar depressive disorder is a mood disorder state where life experiences of loss, anger, upset, and frustration outweigh a person's ability to effectively cope with daily experiences. It is characterized by one or more major depressions (requiring at least four or more additional symptoms) without mania and lasting at least two weeks (but typically longer). It involves emotional, cognitive, behavioral, and somatic disturbances. Depression is rated in terms of severity (mild, moderate, severe) and is classified by frequency (single episode, recurrent, or chronic [i.e., lasting more than two years]). There are three subtypes.

- Major depressive disorder—one or more major depressions with or without interepisodic recovery
- Dysthymic disorder—chronic (at least two years), low-grade depression without a major depressive episode
- Depression not otherwise specified—PMS; depressions with psychotic, melancholic, catatonic, or atypical features; and depressions that briefly recur or with postpartum or seasonal patterns

Etiology

Psychodynamic influences (e.g., chronic stress, especially early childhood loss or deprivation), biologic factors (e.g., alteration of neurotransmitters), and genetic predisposition are factors in the etiology of depression.

Risk Factors

- Prior episodes of depression
- Family history of depression
- Prior suicide attempt(s)
- Female gender (lifetime risk, 20% to 25% for women and 7% to 12% for men)
- Age (rate of occurrence is highest from age 25 to 44)
- Postpartum period
- Medical comorbidity
- Stressful life events, especially loss
- Lack of social support system
- Current or past alcohol or drug abuse

Signs and Symptoms

Significantly depressed mood, diminished interest or pleasure in activities (including reduced sexual functioning), and at least four of the following.

- Feelings of worthlessness, self-reproach, inappropriate guilt
- significant weight loss or weight gain
- insomnia or hypersomnia (especially early morning awakening)
- hyperactivity or inactivity
- fatigue/loss of energy
- poor concentration, restlessness, irritability, withdrawal
- recurrent thoughts of death or suicide

DIFFERENTIAL DIAGNOSIS

- Bipolar I and II mood disorders (manic or hypomanic)
- Schizoaffective disorder
- Substance abuse or withdrawal (e.g., cocaine, amphetamines, caffeine)
- Medical illness (e.g., endocrine dysfunctions such as hypothyroidism, pancreatic cancer, other malignant neoplasms, central nervous system lesions, diabetes mellitus, vitamin deficiency)
- Normal life stress (e.g., bereavement)
- Delusional, adjustment, or anxiety disorder
- Dementia or malnutrition in the elderly

DIAGNOSIS

Physical Examination

The facial expression and demeanor may appear withdrawn, sad, exhausted, or agitated. The physical appearance may include weight loss or gain.

Laboratory Tests

A variety of laboratory tests can be abnormal with depression.

- Determine underlying medical conditions.
- Screen for biologic abnormalities (e.g., the dexamethasone suppression test to differentiate psychotic depression from schizophrenia; sleep EEG to differentiate sleep apnea from depression).
- Blood tests (e.g., measure neurotransmitter levels; screen for amino acid or folate deficiency).

Other Diagnostic Procedures

The Hamilton Rating Scale for Depression (HAM-D) or Beck's Depression Inventory (BDI) are used to assess symptoms and severity of depression.

- Assess symptoms/degree of severity. This may include a clinician-completed rating scale, such as the HAM-D; a psychological test, such as the Minnesota Multiphasic Personality Inventory (MMPI); or a mental status examination, such as the Global Assessment Functioning Scale.
- Evaluate for concurrent substance abuse, medical conditions, or nonmood psychiatric conditions.
- Self-reported questionnaire, e.g., Beck Depression Inventory (BDI).

TREATMENT OPTIONS

Treatment Strategy

Depending on the type, number, severity, and duration of episodes one or more of the following are recommended.

- Pharmacotherapy
- Psychotherapy, including interpersonal and cognitive–behavioral psychotherapies
- Bright light treatment, for seasonal depression
- Nutritional support
- Yoga, exercise, meditation, massage and Tai chi may be helpful
- Hospitalization if suicide is possible

Drug Therapies

- Selective serotonin reuptake inhibitors (SSRIs) such as fluoxetine (Prozac; 10 to 80 mg once a day) or sertraline (Zoloft; 50 to 200 mg once a day) block serotonin reuptake. Side effects are generally fewer than for MAOIs and tricyclic antidepressants but can include gastrointestinal upset, sedation, sexual dysfunction, and headache with a three day to two-week onset. SSRIs can be combined with tricyclics.
- Monoamine oxidase inhibitors (MAOIs) such as phenelzine (Nardil; 15 to 90 mg once a day) increase intrasynaptic norepinephrine levels. Severe side effects (e.g., hypertension) require a tyramine-free diet. Use of other antidepressants is contraindicated.
- Tricyclic antidepressants such as amitriptyline (Elavil; 50 to 300 mg once a day) increase the activity of norepinephrine. Side effects include xerostomia, constipation, and orthostatic hypotension with a two-week onset.
- Atypical antidepressants include drugs such as bupropion (Wellbutrin; 200 to 450 mg bid), a dopamine reuptake blocker; heterocyclics; and newer medications, such as venlafaxine (Effexor; 75 to 375 mg bid or tid), or mirtazapine (Remeron; 15 to 45 mg once a day).

Complementary and Alternative Therapies

Usually a combination of relaxation techniques, nutrition, and herbs provide the greatest relief.

NUTRITION

- B$_{12}$ and folate: Even with normal serum values, some patients respond well to supplementation. Particularly the elderly are at risk for deficiency, since proper digestion is required for good utilization. Dose is 800 mcg/day for folate and 100 to 500 mcg/day for B$_{12}$.
- Other vitamins shown to be low in depression are vitamin C (1,000 mg tid), biotin (300 mcg), B$_1$ (50 to 100 mg), B$_2$ (50 mg), B$_6$ (50 to 100 mg). Minerals shown to be deficient are calcium (800 to 1,200 mg), iron (15 to 30 mg), magnesium (400 to 800 mg). A good multi-vitamin can efficiently address these deficiencies. In addition, chromium (200 to 500 mcg) helps to stabilize mood changes associated with hypoglycemia.
- Essential fatty acids: depleted in depression (1,000 to 1,500 IU/day)
- Vanadium: Excess vanadium is associated with depression.

HERBS

Herbs are generally a safe way to strengthen and tone the body's systems. As with any therapy, it is important to ascertain a diagnosis before pursuing treatment. Herbs may be used as dried extracts (capsules, powders, teas), glycerites (glycerine extracts), or tinctures (alcohol extracts). Unless otherwise indicated, teas should be made with 1 tsp. herb per cup of hot water. Steep covered 5 to 10 minutes for leaf or flowers, and 10 to 20 minutes for roots. Drink 2 to 4 cups/day. Tinctures may be used singly or in combination as noted.

- St. John's wort *(Hypericum perforatum):* Numerous studies support its use in mild to moderate depression; side effects may include photosensitization, gastric upset, headaches, and rash. Dose is 1 to 4 ml tincture/day, or 250 mg tid when taken as the only herb. It may take four to six weeks to become effective. Do not use concomitantly with an antidepressant agent.
- Valerian *(Valeriana officinalis):* sedative, with digestive problems
- Black Cohosh *(Cimicifuga racemosa):* chronic depression, especially with a hormonal component
- Ginkgo *(Ginkgo biloba):* circulatory stimulant, especially with decreased circulation and/or memory loss
- Oat straw *(Avena sativa):* nerve tonic, gentle, slow acting
- Siberian ginseng *(Eleuthrococcus senticosus):* improves ability to withstand stress
- Licorice *(Glycyrrhiza glabra):* antidepressant, especially for long-term stress with a digestive and/or hormonal component. (Contraindicated in hypertension.)
- Passionflower *(Passiflora incarnata):* especially for emotional upheaval with nervousness and insomnia
- Lemon balm *(Melissa officinalis):* mild sedative and spasmolytic, especially with a "nervous stomach"

A combination of equal parts of four to six herbs (1 cup tea tid, or 30 to 60 drops tincture) listed above can be very helpful.

HOMEOPATHY

Although homeopathics can be very helpful, an experienced homeopath should be consulted for appropriate treatment based on constitutional type.

ACUPUNCTURE

Recent studies show that acupuncture can be effective at relieving symptoms, at times statistically comparable to antidepressants or psychotherapy.

MASSAGE

Therapeutic massage has been shown to be effective in increasing circulation and promoting general well-being.

Patient Monitoring

Patients should be closely monitored for compliance, comorbidity, and side effects. Concurrent psychotherapy should be encouraged.

OTHER CONSIDERATIONS

Prevention

Education that compliance with regimen decreases the chance of relapse. Cognitive or psychotherapy directed at coping skills may help prevent relapses. Sleep, exercise, and good diet are important self-care steps that should be encouraged. Biofeedback, meditation, visualization techniques, and Tai chi are effective ways to prevent or reduce the symptoms associated with depression.

Complications/Sequelae

- Drug interactions (e.g., combining of MAOIs and SSRIs) or drug overdose (e.g., tricyclics) can be severe or fatal.
- 20% to 25% rate of associated medical problems with depression.
- 15% of patients with major depressive disorder die from suicide.

Prognosis

The course of recurrence is variable. Fifty percent of patients who have suffered an initial episode suffer a second major depressive disorder, 70% of those suffer a third, and 90% of those suffer a fourth episode. Twenty-five percent of patients with depression develop a bipolar disorder. Untreated episodes of depression last 6 to 24 months. The need for pharmacologic and psychologic treatment is greater with subsequent episodes.

Pregnancy

Preschool children whose mothers took tricyclic antidepressant drugs or fluoxetine during pregnancy showed no significant difference in global IQ or language and behavioral development.

REFERENCES

Blumenthal M, ed. *The Complete German Commission E Monographs.* Boston, Mass: Integrative Medicine Communications; 1998:422, 425.

Diagnostic and Statistical Manual of Mental Disorders. 4th ed. Washington, DC: American Psychiatric Association; 1994.

Gruenwald J, Brendler T et al, eds. *PDR for Herbal Medicines.* Montvale, NJ: Medical Economics Company; 1998:967–968, 1015.

Hippius H. St John's wort *(Hypericum perforatum)*—a herbal antidepressant. *Curr Med Res Opin.* 1998;14:171–184. In process.

Kaplan HW, ed. *Comprehensive Textbook of Psychiatry.* 6th ed. Baltimore, Md: Williams & Wilkins; 1995.

Linde K, Ramirez G, Mulrow CD, et al. St. John's wort for depression—an overview and meta-analysis of randomized clinical trials. *Br Med J.* 1996;313:253–258.

Rakel RE, ed. *Conn's Current Therapy.* 50th ed. Philadelphia, Pa: WB Saunders Company; 1998.

Reuter HD. St. John's wort as a herbal antidepressant. *Eur J Herbal Med.* Part 1. 1995;1(3):19–24. Part 2. 1995;1(4):15–21.

■ DERMATITIS

OVERVIEW

Definition

Dermatitis, sometimes referred to as eczema, is an inflammation of the skin that occurs in acute, subacute, and chronic stages. The cardinal feature is itching. There are numerous types of dermatitis, ranging from mild to chronic and affecting approximately 10% of children and from 7% to 24% of adults.

Etiology

Dermatitis is caused by allergic contact (e.g., poison ivy), irritant contact (e.g., factors promoting water loss such as low humidity, organic solvents, or alkaline soaps), chemicals (e.g., nickel, cobalt, or detergent), or allergies (especially those associated with dairy products). Acute dermatitis may progress to subacute dermatitis, and chronic dermatitis either results from subacute dermatitis or appears as lichen simplex chronicus. Atopic dermatitis and dermatitis herpetiformis do not have clear etiology, but both have genetic links. Atopic dermatitis is associated with asthma and allergic rhinitis.

Risk Factors

- Genetic risk factors (for atopic dermatitis and dermatitis herpetiformis)
- Occupation (e.g., cleaners, hair dressers, jobs requiring repeated hand-wetting)
- Allergic or irritant contact
- Gender (female, for contact dermatitis)
- Skin infections

Signs and Symptoms

- Mild to intense pruritus, pain, stinging, or burning
- Vesicles, blisters, scales, fissuring, thickened and lichenified skin, excoriations
- Mildly to intensely red skin

DIFFERENTIAL DIAGNOSIS

- Psoriasis
- Fungal infection
- Skin eruption from reaction to drugs, including botanicals
- Scabies
- Human immunodeficiency virus–associated dermatitis
- Cutaneous T-cell lymphoma
- Mycosis fungoides
- Exfoliative erythroderma
- Photosensitivity

DIAGNOSIS

Physical Examination

The skin appears red and inflamed with serum-filled vesicles, lesions, or blisters. Excoriation causes accumulation of serum, crust, and/or purulent material. There is thickened and lichenified skin with chronic dermatitis.

Laboratory Tests

- Patch testing can determine the type of allergic dermatitis, especially for environmental allergens.
- Biopsy can rule out spongiosis and lymphoma.
- Cultures reveal bacterial infections (e.g., *Staphylococcus aureus*).
- Blood testing may reveal elevated serum immunoglobulin E levels, which are seen in about 80% of cases of atopic dermatitis, especially those involving food allergens.

Pathological Findings

When the protective properties of the stratum corneum epidermidis are diminished, the skin decompensates and becomes eczematous. Epidermis becomes thickened.

Other Diagnostic Procedures

- Rash is recognized as eczematous and not psoriasiform or lichenoid.
- Determine allergic, irritant, or endogenous source.
- The diagnosis for atopic dermatitis, in addition to itchy skin, includes flexural dermatitis, history of hay fever or asthma, and rash before the age of 2.

TREATMENT OPTIONS

Treatment Strategy

In addition to avoiding the triggering agent (if applicable), treatment may include one or more of the following.

- control of symptoms
- control of external stresses that may exacerbate the condition
- drugs (corticosteroids, nonsteroidal immunomodulators, antihistamines, and antibiotics)
- ultraviolet light, including photochemotherapy that combines psoralen and UVA light (PUVA)

Compresses are a good choice for controlling symptoms. Cool wet compresses cause vasoconstriction and decrease serum production, reducing inflammation and itching. The patient should replace the soaked cloth after 30 minutes. Burrow's solution (Domeboro) added to the compress reduces bacterial growth. Doak Tar and Complex 15 lotions or colloidal oatmeal (Aveeno) baths help to decrease itching.

Drug Therapies

Corticosteroids: Systemic corticosteroids reduce inflammation (e.g., prednisone 20 to 30 mg bid for 7 to 30 days, tapered gradually, depending on severity), side effects, and rebound effects. Topical corticosteroids cannot penetrate vesicles but decrease pruritus, preventing further complications (e.g., 1% to 2.5% hydrocortisone, twice daily on affected areas, decreasing the strength as the conditions improves). Side effects with more potent brands include atrophy, telangiectasia, striae, and adrenal axis suppression.

Nonsteroidal immunomodulators (e.g., tacrolimus [FK-506], phosphodiesterase inhibitors) are newer topical ointments.

Antihistamines: Antihistamines relieve itching but do not change the course of the disease (e.g., diphenhydramine [Benadryl], every 4 hours, as needed; hydroxyzine [Atarax], every four hours, as needed or 10 to 100 mg three hours before sleep for soporific effect). Newer, less sedating antihistamines include cetirizine (Zyrtec) and loratadine (Claritin).

Antibiotics: Systemic antibiotics (e.g., erythromycin, 250 mg qid for 7 to 10 days), treat secondary infections, which usually involve staphylococcus (in 90% of patients). Infections of the hand frequently occur with atopic dermatitis. Topical antibiotics are less effective than systemic antibiotics.

Complementary and Alternative Therapies

Discerning and eliminating exposure to the causative factor is of primary importance in treating dermatitis. Following nutritional guidelines and using herbal support as needed may be effective in reducing inflammation, hypersensitivity reactions, and relieving dermatitis.

Hypersensitivity reactions may be associated with stress and anxiety. Mind-body techniques such as meditation, tai chi, yoga, and stress management may help reduce reactivity.

NUTRITION
Note: Lower doses are for children.
- Eliminate or reduce exposure to all known environmental or food allergens. The most common allergenic foods are dairy, soy, citrus, peanuts, wheat (may be intolerant to all gluten-containing grains), fish, eggs, corn, and tomatoes.
- Reduce pro-inflammatory foods in the diet including saturated fats (meats, especially poultry, and dairy), refined foods, and sugar.
- Increase intake of fresh vegetables, whole grains, and essential fatty acids (cold-water fish, nuts, and seeds).
- Flax seed, borage, or evening Primrose oil (1,000 to 1,500 mg one to two times/day) are anti-inflammatory. Children should be supplemented with cod liver oil (1 tsp./day). Excessive omega-6 oils may increase inflammation. In this case, omega-3 (fish oils) are more effective.
- Beta-carotene (25,000 to 100,000 IU/day), zinc (10 to 30 mg/day), and vitamin E (200 to 800 IU/day) support immune function and dermal healing.
- Vitamin C (1,000 mg bid to qid) inhibits histamine release. Vitamin C from rose hips or palmitate are citrus-free and hypoallergenic.
- Selenium (100 to 200 mcg/day) helps to regulate fatty acid metabolism and is a co-factor in liver detoxification.
- Bromelain (100 to 250 mg bid to qid) is a proteolytic enzyme that reduces inflammation.

HERBS
Herbs are generally a safe way to strengthen and tone the body's systems. As with any therapy, it is important to ascertain a diagnosis before pursuing treatment. Herbs may be used as dried extracts (capsules, powders, teas), glycerites (glycerine extracts), or tinctures (alcohol extracts). Unless otherwise indicated, teas should be made with 1 tsp. herb per cup of hot water. Steep covered 5 to 10 minutes for leaf or flowers, and 10 to 20 minutes for roots. Drink 2 to 4 cups/day. Tinctures may be used singly or in combination as noted.

Flavanoids, a constituent found in dark berries and some plants, have anti-inflammatory properties, strengthen connective tissue, and help reduce hypersensitivity reactions. The following are bioflavanoids that may be taken in dried extract form as noted.
- Catechin (25 to 150 mg bid to tid), quercetin (50 to 250 mg bid to tid), hesperidin (50 to 250 mg bid to tid), and rutin (50 to 250 mg bid to tid).
- Rose hips (Rosa canina) are also high in bioflavanoids and may be used as a tea. Drink 3 to 4 cups/day.

Herbs that support dermal healing and lymphatic drainage are useful for relieving dermatitis. Use the following herbs in combination as a tincture (15 to 30 drops tid) or tea (2 to 4 cups/day). Peppermint (Mentha piperita), red clover (Trifolium pratense), cleavers (Gallium aparine), yarrow (Achillea millefolium), and prickly ash bark (Xanthoxylum clava-herculis).

Sarsaparilla (Smilax species) helps heal hot, red, inflamed skin, and gotu kola (Centella asiatica) is good for dry, scaly, crusty skin. Use 3 ml sarsaparilla and 2 ml gotu kola tincture daily, or 3 cups tea per day.

Oregon grape (Mahonia aquafolium) or red alder bark (Alnus rubra) can be taken as tincture (20 to 30 drops tid) to help liver eliminate waste.

Topical applications of creams and salves containing one or more of the following herbs may help relieve itching, burning, and promote healing. Chickweed (Stellaria media), marigold (Calendula officinalis), comfrey (Symphytum officinale), and chamomile (Matricaria recutita).

A tea made from peppermint leaf (Mentha piperita) may be cooled and applied via spray bottle to relieve itching and burning. An external ointment containing menthol can also be applied.

HOMEOPATHY
An experienced homeopath should assess individual constitutional types and severity of disease to select the correct remedy and potency. For acute prescribing use 3 to 5 pellets of a 12X to 30C remedy every one to four hours until acute symptoms resolve.
- *Apis mellifica* for hot, swollen vesicles that are relieved with cold applications.
- *Rhus toxicodendron* for intense itching and burning relieved with hot applications.
- *Urtica urens* for burning, stinging pains.

ACUPUNCTURE
Acupuncture may help restore normal immune function and reduce the hypersensitivity response.

MASSAGE
Therapeutic massage may help reduce stress which exacerbates dermatitis.

Patient Monitoring
Dermatitis worsens with pruritus and excoriation. Monitoring control of symptoms aids resolution.

OTHER CONSIDERATIONS
Prevention
Avoiding the irritating agent can prevent recurrence. Controlling symptoms can prevent scratching, thus avoiding further complications.

Complications/Sequelae
Uncontrolled pruritus and excoriations cause infection and scarring. Psychological problems (e.g., anxiety, anger, self-esteem) may occur. Ocular complications that may occur with atopic dermatitis include keratoconjunctivitis.

Prognosis
With causes of irritation removed, excoriation controlled, and no secondary infection, inflammation can be resolved without scarring. The disease can progress to being self-perpetuating and chronic. Atopic dermatitis cannot be cured, but symptoms and appearance can be controlled. Compliance with treatment ensures a more successful prognosis.

Pregnancy
Types of pregnancy-induced dermatitis include pemphigoid gestationis, polymorphic eruption of pregnancy, prurigo of pregnancy, and pruritic folliculitis of pregnancy. Symptoms usually clear postpartum. Pemphigoidal gestation is associated with a risk of premature births and low birth weight; however, there is no correlation to spontaneous abortion or fetal mortality.

High-risk drugs during pregnancy and lactation include isotretinoin, antineoplastic agents (e.g., methotrexate), antipruritic medications (e.g., doxepin), antibiotics (e.g., tetracycline, ciprofloxacin), and nonsteroidal antiinflammatory drugs. Analgesics and topical corticosteroids (except povidone-iodine and podophyllin) are lower risk drugs during pregnancy, and penicillins are comparatively safe antibiotics. Maternal antigen avoidance diets do not reduce the risk of giving birth to an infant with atopic dermatitis and may adversely affect fetal birth weight.

High doses of vitamin A are contraindicated during pregnancy. Nutritional support, rose hips tea, and topical herbal applications are safe supportive treatment of dermatitis in pregnancy.

REFERENCES

Bartram T. *Encyclopedia of Herbal Medicine.* Dorset, England: Grace Publishers; 1995:144.

Habif TP. *Clinical Dermatology.* 3rd ed. St. Louis, Mo: Mosby-Year Book; 1996.

Middleton E, ed. *Allergy: Principles and Practice.* 5th ed. St. Louis, Mo: Mosby-Year Book; 1998.

Morrison R. *Desktop Guide to Keynotes and Confirmatory Symptoms.* Albany, Calif: Hahnemann Clinic Publishing; 1993:29, 326, 394.

Rakel RE, ed. *Conn's Current Therapy.* 50th ed. Philadelphia, Pa: WB Saunders; 1998.

Scalzo R. *Naturopathic Handbook of Herbal Formulas.* Durango, Colo: 2nd ed. Kivaki Press; 1994:36.

Schulpis KH, Nyalala JO, Papakonstantinou ED, et al. Biotin recycling impairment in phenylketonuric children with seborrheic dermatitis. *Int J Dermatol.* 1998;37:918-921.

Stewart JCM, et al. Treatment of severe and moderately severe atopic dermatitis with evening primrose oil (Epogam): a multi-center study. *J Nut Med.* 1991;2:9-16.

■ DIABETES MELLITUS

OVERVIEW

Definition

Diabetes mellitus results from the body's failure to regulate blood glucose levels adequately. It is a common endocrine disease, with more than 600,000 new cases diagnosed in the United States each year. It affects men and women of all ages, races, and income levels. Among those over 40, it affects 1:15 Caucasians and 1:10 to 1:8 African-Americans and Hispanics. Among those over 65, 1 of every 5 persons has diabetes and up to 50% of patients are undiagnosed. There is a strong familial susceptibility to the condition. Two major forms are seen:

- Type I (insulin-dependent diabetes mellitus [IDDM]): usually occurs before age 30, most likely between ages 11 and 13; accounts for about 10% of cases.
- Type II (non-insulin-dependent diabetes mellitus [NIDDM]): usually occurs in those over age 40; accounts for about 90% of cases; 30% to 40% need insulin.

Gestational diabetes (GDM) can occur in pregnant women. Diabetes can be secondary to pancreatic disease, the use of chemicals or drugs, various genetic syndromes (Turner's syndrome, myotonic dystrophy, or Prader-Willi syndrome), rare abnormalities in the cellular receptor for insulin, or an autosomal dominant inherited disorder.

Etiology

Unknown, but most likely a combination of genetic predisposition, viral infection, lifestyle, nutrition and diet, obesity, autoimmune disorders, and exposure to toxic agents. Type I probably results when pancreatic beta cells are attacked and destroyed by an autoimmune process triggered by a viral infection in a genetically susceptible individual. Type II develops in older, overweight individuals whose insulin production is insufficient to meet body needs or whose response to insulin is diminished by a loss of insulin receptors on the surface membranes of target cells.

Risk Factors

Type I:
- Family history of diabetes, thyroid disease, or other endocrinopathies
- Family history of autoimmune diseases such as Hashimoto's thyroiditis, Graves' disease, myasthenia gravis, or pernicious anemia
- Cow's milk consumption in infancy

Type II:
- Obesity and age over 40 years
- Family history of diabetes, thyroid disease, or other endocrinopathies
- Sedentary lifestyle with diet high in fats and calories
- African-American, Hispanic, American Indian, or Asian or Pacific Island-American

Signs and Symptoms

- Polyuria, polydipsia, rapid weight loss, and hyperglycemia
- Glycosuria
- Increased susceptibility to infection
- Dehydration
- Polyphagia
- Fatigue or weakness
- Blurred vision
- Stiffness in the shoulder and upper back
- Pruritus, numbness, and tingling in the hands and feet
- Leg cramps
- Hyperlipidemia
- Ketoacidosis

DIFFERENTIAL DIAGNOSIS

- Polydipsia-medication side effect, psychogenic factors, diabetes insipidus
- Polyuria-hypercalcemia, medication side effect, renal wasting, urologic or prostate conditions
- Blurred vision-myopia, presbyopia
- Fatigue or weakness-thyroid disorder, anemia, adrenal insufficiency, depression
- Pruritus-allergy, renal failure
- Cushing's disease
- Corticosteroid use

DIAGNOSIS

Physical Examination

Patient may present with fatigue, lethargy, poor concentration, and atypical thirst for liquids.

Laboratory Tests

- Two or more fasting plasma glucose levels over 140 mg/dL or one level over 200 mg/dL plus other signs and symptoms.
- Oral glucose tolerance test values 120 to 140 mg/dL
- Glycosylated hemoglobin test showing consistently elevated values.
- Glycosylated hemoglobin is used to track treatment efficacy, not to diagnose DM.

Pathological Findings

Elevated blood sugar levels with weight loss, decreased blood pressure, nonhealing wounds (especially on the extremities), recurrent cutaneous infections, decreased extremity sensation, retinal abnormalities or cataract formation, carotid bruits, abdominal tenderness, dry skin, and hair loss over lower leg and foot.

Other Diagnostic Procedures

Blood glucose testing.

TREATMENT OPTIONS

Treatment Strategy

- Control blood sugar levels; helps reduce complications.
- Requires patients to be self-disciplined, able to concentrate, able to maintain a positive attitude, and honest with self and physician.
- Components are diet, exercise, blood glucose self-monitoring, oral hypoglycemic agents (Type II), and insulin (Type I).
- Because diabetes affects so many body systems, treatment planning must include a whole-body approach.

Treatment specific to Type I:
- Diet—consistent timing/content (same gram amount of carbohydrates, protein, and fat at each meal); consult dietitian for meal planning.
- Exercise—daily; wear proper shoes and protective equipment; avoid extreme heat or cold; check feet daily and after exercise; suspend exercise when blood glucose control is poor.
- Self-monitoring—teach the patient to use a home glucose meter and make needed adjustments in diet, exercise, and/or insulin.86

Treatment specific to Type II:
- Diet—use moderation; lose weight by decreasing calories while increasing activity; base choices on USDA Food Pyramid.
- Exercise—as for Type I; do moderate aerobic exercise (50% to 70% of VO$_2$ max) for 20 to 45 minutes at least three days a week; include low-intensity warm-up and cool-down exercises.
- Self-monitoring—as for Type I, with adjustments in diet, exercise, and/or oral hypoglycemic agent as needed.

Drug Therapies

Insulin (used for Type I and occasionally Type II [30% to 40%]). Taken subcutaneously, with dose and type individualized to the patient's condition. Possible treatment regimens:

- Three-injections/day, doses adjusted to variations in control
- Long-acting and short-acting preparations taken at meals for stable background levels
- External insulin pump for tight control
- Single injection/day for those with some pancreatic function

Sulfonylureas (Type II only). Oral hypoglycemic agents used when diet and exercise are ineffective or in conjunction with diet and exercise. Doses individualized to the patient's condition. Side effects include hypoglycemia, nausea, heartburn, stomach fullness; intolerance and allergy (<2% of patients). Use with caution in persons with liver or kidney impairment and those with sulfa allergy. Approved agents:

- Acetohexamide (Dymelor)—250 to 1,500 mg; slight diuretic effect
- Chlorpropamide (Diabinese, Glucamide)—100 to 750 mg; very long duration of action, antidiuretic effect
- Tolazamide (Tolinase)—100 to 1,000 mg; slight diuretic effect
- Tolbutamide (Orinase)—500 to 3,000 mg; usually taken in two to three doses/day
- Glipizide (Glucotrol)—5 to 40 mg; take on empty stomach
- Glipizide-extended release (Glucotrol XL)—20 mg; do not break tablet, take once/day
- Glyburide (Diabeta, Micronase)—1.25 to 30 mg
- Glyburide-micronized (Glynase)—12 mg/day; not equivalent in action to glyburide
- Glimepiride (Amaryl)—8 mg/day
- Metformin (Glucophage)—Used as a supplement to or substitute for sulfonylureas. Side effects include weight loss, nausea, abdominal discomfort, and diarrhea. Use with caution in persons with conditions leading to lactic acid buildup (congestive heart failure, severe vascular disease, kidney or liver disease). Discontinue 24 to 48 hours before surgery or radiographic dye study. Dose: 1 to 2.5 g/day in two to three doses; available in 500 and 850 mg tablets; take before meals
- Acarbose (Precose)—Slows absorption of carbohydrate into blood, acts locally in the intestine. Take at the beginning of a meal for immediate action. Major side effect is increased gas production (up to 75% of users). Dose: 50 to 100 mg depending on results and side effects
- Troglitazone (Rezulin)—In trials for use with insulin; liver damage reported
- Repaglinide (Prandin)—Meglitinide class; use in Type II disease

Complementary and Alternative Therapies

Treatments stabilize blood sugars. Also, alternative therapies have an important role in preventing vascular damage and some of the serious complications that may be involved with DM. A combination of herbs and nutrition, along with lifestyle changes, can be quite helpful. Regular exercise is extrememly important. Ten minutes/day of exercise has been shown to have an effect on glucose tolerance, although a minimum of 30 minutes three times/week is required to see significant changes. Extended exercise is desired. Short bursts of activity may actually increase glucose levels.

NUTRITION

- Diet: the classic diet for DM is high in complex carbohydrates and fiber. Some people, however, achieve better glucose control with a high-protein diet with very few carbohydrates. If the classic diet does not stabilize blood sugar, a trial of high-protein diet may be indicated.
- Essential fatty acids: anti-inflammatory, decrease insulin resistance, and prevent cardiovascular and neurological complications of DM. Evening primrose oil (2,000 mg bid) or fish oil (1,200 mg bid) rather than flax or borage may be required, since a greater percentage of diabetics are lacking enzymes required for utilization of flax and/or borage oil.
- OPCs (Oligomericprocyanidins) such as pycnogenol or grape seed extracts help to support vascular health and prevent oxidation side effects associated with diabetes
- B-complex: biotin (300 mcg), B_1 (50 to 100 mg), B_2 (50 mg), B_3 (100 mg), B_6 (50 to 100 mg), B_{12} (100 to 1,000 mcg), folate (400 mcg/day) help prevent neuropathy, control glucose levels, and prevent nephropathy
- Vitamin C (2 to 3 g/day) may prevent microangiopathy and hypertriglyceridemia
- Vitamin E (400 IU/day) may reduce insulin requirements so should start at 100 IU and gradually increase the dose; enhances healing of ulcers, and is a cardio-protective antioxidant
- Brewer's yeast: contains chromium, which may improve glucose tolerance, and glutathione, an antioxidant (9 g or 3 tbsp. brewer's yeast/day and/or 200 mcg chromium)
- Magnesium: (400 mg/day) low in diabetics, may help prevent the calcium deposition in arterial walls
- Manganese: (500 to 1,000 mcg) low in diabetics, may help stabilize glucose levels
- Zinc: (30 mg/day) may decrease fasting glucose levels and help prevent fatty acid oxidation
- Coenzyme Q10: (50 to 100 mg bid) depleted by oral hypoglycemic agents, prevents fatty acid oxidation
- Vanadium: (5 to 10 mg/day) to normalize serum cholesterol and triglycerides
- Some feel that chromium picolinate (200 mcg) helps normalize sugar metabolism.

HERBS

Herbs are generally a safe way to strengthen and tone the body's systems. Ascertain a diagnosis before pursuing treatment. Herbs may be used as dried extracts (capsules, powders, teas), glycerites (glycerine extracts), or tinctures (alcohol extracts). Unless otherwise indicated, teas should be made with 1 tsp. herb per cup of hot water. Steep covered 5 to 10 minutes for leaf or flowers, and 10 to 20 minutes for roots. Drink 2 to 4 cups/day. Tinctures may be used singly or in combination as noted.

- Garlic *(Allium sativum)* increases fibrolysis, inhibits platelet aggregation, lowers lipids
- Onion *(Allium cepa)* lowers lipids and blood pressure, inhibits thrombocyte aggregation
- Bilberry *(Vaccinium myrtillus)* is a bioflavonoid, historic use in DM, especially to prevent diabetic retinopathy
- Fenugreek *(Trigonella foenum-graecum)* historically used to stabilize blood sugar
- Garlic and onions should be consumed liberally in the diet; bilberry and fenugreek, equal parts, can be used as 1 cup tea tid or 30 to 60 drops tincture tid
- Cayenne *(Capsicum annum):* 0.075% capsaicin cream topically, decreases pain in peripheral neuropathy after two to four weeks of use

HOMEOPATHY

An experienced homeopath should assess individual constitutional types and severity of disease to select the correct remedy and potency. Constitutional homeopathy may be helpful.

ACUPUNCTURE

May be helpful in both symptomatic relief and increasing overall vitality.

MASSAGE

May be helpful in relieving stress, which decreases cortisol and stabilizes blood sugar, and for maintaining healthy circulation in the extremities.

Patient Monitoring

- Patients taking insulin-daily fingerstick to measure blood sugar levels, weight, and skin evaluation (redness indicating allergy to insulin, edema, or cellulitis)
- Electrocardiogram at initial visit
- Thyroid-stimulating hormone and thyroid antibody screening for high-risk patients at initial visit and then as indicated by antibody tests and physical examination
- Lipid profile four to six weeks after beginning therapy and three months later
- Every three months: glycosylated hemoglobin or hemoglobin A, urine dipstick, LFT
- Yearly: 24-hour urine collection to measure microalbumin, protein, creatinine clearance rate; electrolytes, BUN, dilated funduscopic examination
- Yearly: opthalmology exam, foot exam

OTHER CONSIDERATIONS

Prevention

Avoid weight gain and obesity. Maintain regular physical activity.

Complications/Sequelae

- Diabetic ketoacidosis
- Hyperosmolar coma
- Arteriosclerosis—cardiac, peripheral vascular, or cerebrovascular disease
- Diabetic eye disease—glaucoma, cataracts, blindness
- Diabetic kidney disease—nephropathy, failure
- Diabetic neuropathy—peripheral symmetrical polyneuropathy, autonomic neuropathies, mononeuropathies
- Foot ulcers/infections
- Skin changes—bruising, hypertrophy, or lipoatrophy at injection site, dryness, fungal infections, vitiligo, necrobiosis lipoidica diabeticorum, pruritus, alopecia, scleroderma adultorum, xanthomas, xanthelasma, acanthosis nigricans, gangrene, skin ulcers
- Musculoskeletal problems—stiff joints, tendon contractures of the hands, bursitis

Prognosis

Prevent and/or slow development of complications by maintaining blood glucose averages around 155 mg/dL. Complications usually begin 10 to 20 years after onset of disease.

Pregnancy

Women of child-bearing age with diabetes should consult an endocrinologist about the benefits of tight glucose control before attempting conception. Target blood glucose concentrations are:

- Fasting: 60 to 90 mg/dL (3.3 to 5 mmol/L)
- Preprandial: 60 to 105 mg/dL (3.3 to 5.8 mmol/L)
- Two hours postprandial: 90 to 120 mg/dL (5 to 6.7 mmol/L)

Women with gestational diabetes should be treated to normalize glucose levels and reduce the risk of complications (developmental malformations, perinatal morbidity/mortality). Modify diet to improve glucose values. If this fails, use insulin therapy; oral hypoglycemic agents are contraindicated during pregnancy. Subsequent pregnancies can be affected, and risk of developing type II diabetes is increased. If maternal glucose levels uncontrolled, infant can suffer CNS defects, macrosomia, organomegaly, cardiac or renal anomalies, situs inversus, stillbirth, asphyxia, respiratory distress, increased blood volume, hyperviscosity, congestive heart failure, hypocalcemia, hypomagnesemia, hypoglycemia, or hyperbilirubinemia.

REFERENCES

Anderson RA, Cheng N, Bryden NA, et al. Elevated intakes of supplemental chromium improve glucose and insulin variables in individuals with type 2 diabetes. *Diabetes.* 1997;46:1786–1791.

Blumenthal M, ed. *The Complete German Commission E Monographs.* Boston, Mass: Integrative Medicine Communications; 1998:134, 176.

Boden G, Chen X, Igbal N. Acute lowering of plasma fatty acids lowers basal insulin secretion in diabetic and nondiabetic subjects. *Diabetes.* 1998;47:1609–1612.

Cohen N, Halberstam M, Shlimovich P, Chang CJ, Shamoon H, Rossetti L. Oral vanadyl sulfate improves hepatic and peripheral insulin sensitivity in patients with with non-insulin-dependent diabetes mellitus. *J Clin Invest.* 1995;95:2501–2509.

Gruenwald J, Brendler T, Jaenicke C, et al, eds. *PDR for Herbal Medicines.* Montvale, NJ: Medical Economics Company; 1998:1201.

Hirsch IB, Atchley DH, Tsai E, et al. Ascorbic acid clearance in diabetic nephropathy. *J Diabet Complications.* 1998;12:259–263.

Koutsikos D, Agroyannis B, Tzanatos-Exarchou H. Biotin for diabetic peripheral neuropathy. *Biomed Pharmacother.* 1990;44:511–514.

Noble J. *Textbook of Primary Care Medicine.* 2nd ed. St Louis, Mo: Mosby-Year Book; 1996.

Perossini M, et al. Diabetic and hypertensive retinopathy therapy with Vaccinum myrtillus anthocyanosides (Tegens): double blind placebo controlled clinical trial. *Annali di Ottalmaologia e Clinica Ocaulistica.* 1987;CXII.

Poucheret P, Verma S, Grynpas MD, McNeill JH. Vanadium and diabetes. *Mol Cell Biochem.* 1998;188:73–80.

Tandan R, et al. Topical capsaicin in painful diabetic neuropathy. Controlled study with long-term follow-up. *Diabetes Care.* 1992;15:8–14.

Thibodeau GA, Patton KT. *Anatomy and Physiology.* 4th ed. St Louis, Mo: Mosby-Year Book; 1999.

Tierney Jr LM, McPhee SJ, Papadakis MA, eds. *Current Medical Diagnosis and Treatment.* 33rd ed. Norwalk, Conn: Appleton & Lange; 1994.

Ziegler D, Hanefeld M, Ruhnau KJ, et al. Treatment of symptomatic diabetic peripheral neuropathy with the anti-oxidant slpha-lipoic acid. A 3-week randomized controlled trial. *Diabetologia.* 1995;38:1425–1433.

Ziegler D, Schatz H, Conrad F, Gries FA, Ulrich H, Reichel G. Effects of treatment with the antioxidant alpha-lipoic acid on cardiac autonomic neuropathy in NIDDM patients. A 4-month randomized controlled multicenter trial. *Diabetes Care.* 1997;20:369–373.

■ DIARRHEA

OVERVIEW

Definition

Diarrhea is characterized by unformed, watery stools (>200 to 250 g/day) and increased bowel movement frequency, often accompanied by fever, chills, malaise. The symptom of an underlying condition or conditions, diarrhea is considered to be acute at onset, and chronic after two to three weeks. Although diarrhea is a common condition and usually self-limiting (two to three days), complications can be serious, even fatal, in infants and elderly patients, consequently it is important to attempt to determine the cause(s).

Diarrhea has four primary classifications.
- Osmotic: reduced solute absorption
- Secretory: increased electrolyte and water secretion
- Exudative: loss of fluid and protein from intestinal mucosa
- Motility disorder: intestinal transit alterations

Etiology

Common causes include viral, bacterial, and parasitic infection (often spread person-to-person), inflammation, drugs, and psychogenic causes. In particular:

Acute:
- Infection (primary)
- Inflammatory bowel disease (primary)
- Iatrogenic causes
- Poisoning

Chronic:
- Malabsorption (notably lactose intolerance)
- Inflammatory bowel disease
- Colitis
- Irritable bowel syndrome
- Food allergies
- *Giardia*
- Chronic constipation
- AIDS and other immune disorders

Chronic subdivisions (multiple types of diarrhea may be present):

Osmotic diarrhea:
- Malabsorption
- Low sugar absorption (lactose intolerance)
- Antacids

Secretory diarrhea:
- Bacterial infections (e.g., cholera)
- Collagenous colitis
- Crohn's disease
- Celiac sprue
- Laxative abuse (common with chronic diarrhea)
- Tumors
- Hyperthyroidism

Exudative diarrhea:
- Bacterial infections (e.g., *Shigella, Salmonella*)
- Ulcerative colitis
- Inflammatory bowel disease

Motility disorder diarrhea:
- Irritable bowel syndrome
- Scleroderma
- Diabetes
- Surgical procedures
- Laxatives
- Hyperthyroidism

Risk Factors
- Dairy products, some fruits and legumes
- Sugar substitutes (hexitols, sorbitol, mannitol)
- Hospitalization/surgery (iatrogenic)
- Foreign travel
- Hiking, camping, fishing trips
- Exposure to infected persons
- Medications (e.g., antibiotics, antacids, diuretics, antihypertensives, anti-inflammatories, and cardiovascular medications)
- Stress
- Recent antibiotic therapy

Signs and Symptoms
- Loose stools, with or without blood and mucus
- Frequent need to defecate
- Abdominal pain, cramping
- Fever, chills, malaise
- Weight loss

DIFFERENTIAL DIAGNOSIS
- Crohn's disease
- Colitis, ulcerative colitis
- Whipple's disease
- Inflammatory bowel disease
- Irritable bowel syndrome
- Reiter's syndrome
- Zollinger-Ellison syndrome
- Over-the-counter medications
- Various rare intestinal tumors (ganglioneuroblastoma, mucinous cystadenoma, and intestinal lipoblastoma)
- Congenital microvillous atrophy
- Congenital chloride diarrhea
- Magnesium or Vitamin C supplementation

DIAGNOSIS

Physical Examination

For most patients, diarrhea is relatively benign and self-limiting. A few patients, however, have an underlying illness that should be diagnosed and treated—in particular, patients with diarrhea that has persisted for longer than three days or with blood in the feces (suggesting exudative diarrhea). Determining the mechanism (osmotic, secretory, exudative, or motility) helps direct treatment.

Because patients will not be capable of reporting stool weight/day, patient history plays a major role in diagnosing diarrhea.
- Confirm that the condition is diarrhea, not fecal incontinence.
- Determine the volume type of diarrhea.
- Determine if diarrhea is acute (generally related to infection) or chronic.
- Note signs and symptoms.
- Ask patient about risk factors, lactose intolerance, antibiotics use, sexual orientation, and surgery.
- Explore the effect of diet. (Osmotic diarrhea generally ends when fasting. Secretory diarrhea generally does not end when fasting. Lactase deficiency generally is an accurate diagnosis if symptoms improve with the elimination of milk and dairy products).

Assess:
- Hydration
- Abdominal tenderness
- Bowel sounds
- Rectum (carcinoma, fecal impactions)

Laboratory Tests
- Stool sample
- CBC
- Serum electrolytes
- BUN
- d-xylose
- Pancreatic function
- Urinalysis

Pathological Findings
Blood:
- Leukocytosis
- Pathogens
- Anemia
- Biochemical deficiencies

Endoscopy:
- Mucosal abnormalities
- Bleeding
- Ulcers

Stool:
- Blood (generally exudative diarrhea)
- Weight/volume
- Fecal fat
- Electrolytes
- Osmolality
- Parasites

Imaging
- Small-bowel radiography
- Barium enema

Other Diagnostic Procedures
In addition to patient history and physical assessment, endoscopy, laboratory tests (including stool analysis), and rectal biopsy (occasionally) can help determine the cause—and thus the treatment—of diarrhea.

TREATMENT OPTIONS
Treatment Strategy
Because diarrhea is a symptom, treatment should be dictated by the cause (or causes). For acute, uncomplicated diarrhea, it may be sufficient to reassure patients that the diarrhea is benign and will resolve in a couple of days and simply treat the symptoms.

For some chronic diarrhea, dietary change can be sufficient without additional evaluation.

Serious acute bloody diarrhea and chronic diarrhea will require evaluation and treatment of underlying cause(s). Hospitalization should be considered with dehydration; in any case, replacement of fluids (clear fluids without caffeine and rehydration fluids) and electrolytes—particularly with very young and very old patients—is critical.

Drug Therapies
Because some medications prescribed for diarrhea can delay resolution of certain infectious diarrhea conditions (as well as other contraindications), diarrhea should be diagnosed before drug therapy is undertaken. Common drug therapies (many OTC) include the following.
- Opioid derivatives: diphenoxylate-atropine (Lomotil) and loperamide (Imodium). May have CNS effect.
- Adsorbents: bismuth salts (Pepto-Bismol), kolin, and pectin

(Kaopectate), aluminum hydroxide (Amphojel), cholestyramine (Questran)
- Bulk-forming medications: psyllium (Metamucil, Konsyl)

Specific guidelines include:
- Bismuth salts for traveler's diarrhea
- Cholestyramine for bile-acid-induced diarrhea

Complementary and Alternative Therapies
Severe diarrhea can be life-threatening, and it is imperative that the underlying etiology be assessed before initiating any treatment other than fluid replacement. Nutrition suggestions should be followed for all types of diarrhea.

NUTRITION
- Avoid coffee, chocolate, dairy products, strong spices, and solid foods. Introduce clear soup, crackers and white bread, rice, potatoes, apple-sauce, and bananas as diarrhea begins to resolve. Sips of black tea may help settle the stomach when nausea is present.
- To restore and maintain fluid and electrolyte balance, consider rice and/or barley water, fresh vegetable juices (especially carrot and celery), miso broth, or other clear broths. Rice and barley water are made using 1 cup of grain to 1 quart of boiling water. Let steep for 20 minutes. Strain and drink throughout the day.
- Lactobacillus species taken as powder or in capsules helps to normalize bowel flora and may help resolve diarrhea. Take as directed, or one dose with each meal. Sacromyces bolardii and brewer's yeast are specific for treating antibiotic-induced diarrhea that has caused c. difficile overgrowth.
- Vitamin C (1,000 mg tid to qid) and vitamin A (10,000 to 20,000 IU/day) support immune function. High doses of vitamin C may cause diarrhea. High doses of vitamin A should not be taken long-term without physician supervision.
- Glutamine (3,000 mg tid) is helpful to treat diarrhea that is caused by mucosal irritation rather than infection, such as chemotherapy-induced diarrhea.

HERBS
Herbs are generally a safe way to strengthen and tone the body's systems. As with any therapy, it is important to ascertain a diagnosis before pursuing treatment. Herbs may be used as dried extracts (capsules, powders, teas), glycerites (glycerine extracts), or tinctures (alcohol extracts). Unless otherwise indicated, teas should be made with 1 tsp. herb per cup of hot water. Steep covered 5 to 10 minutes for leaf or flowers, and 10 to 20 minutes for roots. Drink 2 to 4 cups/day. Tinctures may be used singly or in combination as noted.

Do not initiate anti-diarrheal therapy if the diarrhea is secondary to an infectious agent. Herbs can be used as anti-inflammatories, antimicrobials, or antidiarrheals. Choose one or two from each category as needed. They are best used as teas unless otherwise noted.

Anti-inflammatory herbs:
- Quercetin (250 to 500 mg bid to qid)
- Chamomile *(Matricaria recutita)* is a soothing anti-spasmodic.
- Marshmallow root *(Althea officinalis)* is best prepared as cold-water tea. Soak 2 tbsp. root in one quart of water overnight. Strain and drink throughout the day.

Antimicrobial herbs:
- Barberry *(Berberis vulgaris),* 250 to 500 mg tid
- Goldenseal *(Hydrastis canadensis),* 250 to 500 mg tid
- Licorice root *(Glycyrrhiza glabra)* (contraindicated in hypertension)

Antidiarrheal herbs:
- Blackberry leaf *(Rubus fruticosus)* or raspberry leaf *(Rubus idaeus)*—use 1 heaping tsp./cup. Drink 1/2 cup per hour.
- Carob powder—use 4 tsp. per 4 oz. of water or mix in applesauce. Take 1/2 to 1 tsp. every 30 to 60 minutes.
- Slippery elm powder *(Ulmus rubra)* or marshmallow root powder— use 1 oz. powder to 1 quart of water. Make a paste with the powder and a small amount of water. Gradually add in the rest of the water and then simmer down to one pint. Take 1 tsp. every 30 to 60 minutes.

HOMEOPATHY

An experienced homeopath should assess individual constitutional types and severity of disease to select the correct remedy and potency. For acute prescribing use 3 to 5 pellets of a 12X to 30C remedy every one to four hours until acute symptoms resolve.
- *Arsenicum album* when patient is weak, chilly, anxious, and restless with diarrhea.
- *Podophyllum* for yellow, explosive, gushing, gurgling, painless diarrhea
- *Chamomilla* for greenish, frothy stool with severe colicky pains; stool smells like rotten eggs.
- *Mercurius vivus* for strong urging with offensive, bloody diarrhea.
- *Aloe* for colicky, cramping pains before and during stool. Weak and sweaty after diarrhea.
- *Veratrum album* for diarrhea and vomiting, collapsed states.

Patient Monitoring

Dehydrated patients and infant and elderly patients with serious signs and symptoms should be monitored carefully. Patients with acute diarrhea should report conditions that do not resolve in three to five days. Follow up with chronic patients as required.

OTHER CONSIDERATIONS

Prevention
Avoid risk factors as possible.

Complications/Sequelae
- Dehydration
- Syncope, arrhythmias (from loss of electrolytes)
- Anemia

Prognosis
- Acute: generally resolves in two to three days
- Chronic, idiopathic diarrhea: generally self-limiting, although it may continue indefinitely

Pregnancy

Dehydration can cause preterm labor. Gastrointestinal spasm may have reflexive action on uterine muscle and induce contractions. Goldenseal *(Hydrastic canadensis)* and barberry *(Berberis vulgaris)* should be avoided in pregnancy as they may stimulate contractions. High doses of vitamin A may be teratogenic and should be avoided.

REFERENCES

Andreoli TE, Bennett JC, Carpenter CCJ. *Cecil Essentials of Medicine.* 3rd ed. Philadelphia, Pa: WB Saunders; 1993:271–277.

Barker LR, Burton JR, Zieve PD, eds. *Principles of Ambulatory Medicine.* 4th ed. Baltimore, Md: Williams & Wilkins; 1995:481–491.

Bartram T. *Encyclopedia of Herbal Medicine.* Dorset, England: Grace Publishers; 1995:147.

Bensky D, Gamble A. *Chinese Herbal Medicine.* Seattle, Wash: Eastland Press; 1986:47–49.

Blumenthal M, ed. *The Complete German Commission E Monographs.* Boston, Mass: Integrative Medicine Communications; 1998:425, 464.

Berkow R. *The Merck Manual of Medical Information.* Whitehouse Station, NJ: Merck Research Laboratories; 1997:523–525.

Morrison R. *Desktop Guide to Keynotes and Confirmatory Symptoms.* Albany, Calif: Hahnemann Clinic Publishing; 1993:15, 42, 116, 246, 305.

Murray MT. *Encyclopedia of Nutritional Supplements.* Rocklin, Calif: Prima Publishing; 1996:431–439.

Dambro MR. *Griffith's 5-Minute Clinical Consult–1999.* Baltimore, Md: Lippincott Williams & Wilkins; 1999: 316–319.

Gruenwald J, Brendler T, Jaenicke C et al, eds. *PDR for Herbal Medicines.* Montvale, NJ: Medical Economics Company; 1998:617–618, 621–622, 763–766, 1047–1050, 1061–1063, 1078–1079, 1103–1104, 1201–1202, 1226–1227.

Stein JK, ed. *Internal Medicine.* 4th ed. St. Louis, Mo: Mosby-Year Book; 1994:436–440.

Stoller JK, Ahmad M, Longworth DL, eds. *The Cleveland Clinic Intensive Review of Internal Medicine.* Baltimore, Md: Williams & Wilkins; 1998:638–643.

Tyler VE. *Herbs of Choice.* Binghamton, NY: Haworth Press; 1994:51–54.

Walker LP, Brown EH. *The Alternative Pharmacy.* Paramus, NJ: Prentice Hall Press; 1998:147–150.

■ DYSMENORRHEA
OVERVIEW
Definition
Dysmenorrhea, pain associated with menses, is either Primary (Functional) or Secondary (Acquired). It is most common during adolescence and tends to decrease over time and after pregnancy. Pain results from myometrial uterine contractions stimulated by increased prostaglandin production in secretory endometrium. Treatment involves suppressing prostaglandin secretion and/or ovulation and addressing underlying disorders.

Primary dysmenorrhea is cyclical pain associated with menses during ovulatory cycles without demonstrable lesions affecting the reproductive structures. Secondary dysmenorrhea is pain with menses that is caused by demonstrable pathology. Dysmenorrhea causes more absenteeism from school and work than any other single factor. Up to 40% of female adults have some degree of menstrual pain.

Etiology
Primary:
- Contractions due to increased prostaglandin secretion
- Uterine ischemia
- Anxiety and stress
- Narrow cervical os
- Tissue expulsion through narrow cervix
- Displaced uterus

Secondary:
- Endometriosis
- Adenomyosis
- Narrow cervical os, cervical stemosis, other anatomic abnormalities
- Tissue expulsion through narrow cervix
- Extrauterine pregnancy
- Congenital abnormalities
- Endometrial polyp/submucosal fibroid expulsion
- Fibroids
- Uterine infections
- Chronic/acute PID
- Intrauterine device (IUD)

Risk Factors
- Ovulatory cycles
- IUD
- Stressful events
- Pelvic infection
- Abdominal surgery/ectopic pregnancy
- Sexually transmitted diseases

Signs and Symptoms
Symptoms and degree of pain vary from person to person.
Primary:
- Low abdominal cramping/dull ache
- Ache radiating to lower back, groin, legs
- Pain may begin before or at start of menses, usually peaks after 24 hours, and decreases after 48 hours
- Heavy menstrual flow
- Headache
- Nausea
- Constipation or diarrhea
- Frequent urination
- Vomiting (infrequently)
- Premenstrual syndrome

Secondary:
- Often vague, often continuous low abdominal pain/cramping
- Increased pain with menses
- Associated gastrointestinal upset, thigh pain

DIFFERENTIAL DIAGNOSIS
- PMS
- Gastrointestinal disorders
- Irritable bowel syndrome
- Sexually transmitted disease
- Chronic tubal inflammation
- Adhesions from previous abdominal surgery/ectopic pregnancy
- Enlarged uterus
- Urinary tract infection
- Endometriosis

DIAGNOSIS
Physical Examination
- Abdominal exam: Rule out any palpable mass; check for abnormal bowel sounds and tender or distended bladder.
- Pelvic exam: Uterine or ovarian pressure may result in extreme tenderness—suggestive of pelvic inflammatory disease.

Laboratory Tests
To exclude infection:
- White blood cell count/differential
- Elevated erythrocyte sedimentation rate (ESR)
- Urinalysis
- Cervical/vaginal cultures to rule out localized infection

Pathological Findings
- Enlarged uterus
- Adhesions
- Fibrous/ovarian tumors
- Abdominal surgery/ectopic pregnancy adhesions
- Uterine displacement/ prolapse

Imaging
- Pelvic ultrasound; pelvic CT may be necessary

Other Diagnostic Procedures
- Pain occurrence in relation to menstrual cycle (pain two to three days prior to and/or lasting two to three days following commencement of blood flow may indicate pathology, or relationship to bowel movements or urination)
- Presence and/or condition of intrauterine devices
- Psychological assessment (major life events, level of physical/emotional functioning, history of physical abuse)
- Laproscopy, cervical mucous/endometrium analysis

TREATMENT OPTIONS
Treatment Strategy
Prior to invasive diagnosis, trial therapeutic medical management is recommended. Exercise/relaxation can also be done. Studies indicate relief in 25% to 85% of patients without pathological disorders.

Drug Therapies
- Antiprostaglandins, anti-inflammatory (ibuprophen 800 mg to start; 400 to 600 mg every six hours) for primary disorder without pathological complications
- Gonadotropin-releasing hormone (GnRH) analogs/oral contraceptives

to suppress ovarian function (consider age/risk factors)
- Antibiotics for PID
- Estrogen/oral progestins for endometriosis (e.g., norethindrone for 12 months. Prognosis: 80% relief, 50% return of fertility.
- Diuretics, if edema present

Complementary and Alternative Therapies

Dysmenorrhea may be effectively treated with alternative therapies and mind-body techniques such as meditation, yoga, tai chi, and gentle exercise. Begin with nutritional support, magnesium, B₆, vitamin E, and red raspberry. A minimum of three months may be required to accurately assess the effects of treatment.

NUTRITION

Increase intake of essential fatty acids. These are anti-inflammatory and needed for hormone synthesis. Essential fatty acids are found in cold-water fish, nuts, and seeds. Reduce intake of saturated fats (meat products and dairy products) which are pro-inflammatory. Eliminate refined foods, sugar, dairy products, and methylxanthines (coffee and chocolate) which are pro-inflammatory and deplete the body of essential nutrients. Increase fresh fruits and vegetables, proteins, and whole grains.

- Magnesium (400 mg/day) with B₆ (100 mg/day) throughout cycle to promote hormone production and induce relaxation. Can be used at higher doses during menses (magnesium up to 600 mg/day, and B₆ up to 300 mg/day) for acute relief.
- Vitamin E (400 to 800 IU/day) to improve blood supply to muscles and promote oxygen utilization
- B-complex (50 to 100 mg/day) for reducing the effects of stress
- Flaxseed, evening primrose, or borage oil (1,000 to 1,500 mg one to two times/day), to reduce inflammation and support hormone production
- Niacinamide (50 mg bid) to reduce pain and inflammation. Begin seven days before menses and continue until the end of flow. Adding rutin (60 mg/day) and vitamin C (300 mg/day) will potentiate effects.

HERBS

Herbs are generally a safe way to strengthen and tone the body's systems. As with any therapy, it is important to ascertain a diagnosis before pursuing treatment. Herbs may be used as dried extracts (capsules, powders, teas), glycerites (glycerine extracts), or tinctures (alcohol extracts). Unless otherwise indicated, teas should be made with 1 tsp. herb per cup of hot water. Steep covered 5 to 10 minutes for leaf or flowers, and 10 to 20 minutes for roots. Drink 2 to 4 cups/day. Tinctures may be used singly or in combination as noted.

- Chaste tree *(Vitex agnus-cactus)* and black cohosh *(Cimicifuga racemosa)*, 30 drops each, bid, influence the pituitary to balance the estrogen:progesterone ratio and reduce dysmenorrhea.
- Red raspberry *(Rubus idaeus)* tea has tonifying properties and strengthens uterine tissue.
- Tea of chamomile *(Matricaria recutita)* and ginger root *(Zingiber officinalis)* can help reduce ovarian cyst pain.
- Tinctures of cramp bark *(Viburnum opulus)*, black cohosh, Jamaican dogwood *(Piscidia erythrina)*, and wild yam *(Dioscorea villosa)* can be used together in equal parts to relieve pain and cramping. Use 20 drops every half hour for four doses, then as needed up to eight doses/day for seven days.

HOMEOPATHY

An experienced homeopath should assess individual constitutional types and severity of disease to select the correct remedy and potency.

PHYSICAL MEDICINE

The following methods help to increase circulation and relieve pelvic congestion. Do one or both for maximum therapeutic effects.

- Castor oil pack: Used externally, castor oil is a powerful anti-inflammatory. Apply oil directly to skin, cover with a clean soft cloth (e.g., flannel) and plastic wrap. Place a heat source (hot water bottle or heating pad) over the pack and let sit for 30 to 60 minutes. For best results use three consecutive days in one week.
- Contrast sitz baths: Use two basins that can be comfortably sat in. Fill one with hot water, and one with cold water. Sit in hot water for three minutes, then in cold for one minute. Repeat this three times to complete one set. Do one to two sets per day three to four days per week.

ACUPUNCTURE

Dysmenorrhea may respond to acupuncture treatment, for pain relief and resolving deficiencies/excesses that may contribute to symptoms.

MASSAGE

Therapeutic massage is helpful in reducing the effects of the stress which may exacerbate dysmenorrhea.

Patient Monitoring

- Regular evaluation to determine effectiveness of treatments
- Patient to report additional symptoms/complaints or if treatment offers no relief

OTHER CONSIDERATIONS

- Patient's desire for pregnancy when determining treatment
- Allergies/adverse interactions to traditional/nontraditional medications

Prevention

- Avoid stress; caffeine, alcohol, and sugar prior to onset of menses.
- Regular exercise increases blood circulation.
- Relaxation reduces stress.
- Reduce risk of acquiring sexually transmitted diseases.

Complications/Sequelae

Infection from underlying pathology

Prognosis

- Most women experience dysmenorrhea at some time in their lives.
- Pregnancy often relieves primary dysmenorrhea.
- Prognosis is good when underlying causes accurately diagnosed and treated.

Pregnancy

- Certain drugs/underlying pathologies may interfere with pregnancy.

REFERENCES

Batchelder HJ, Scalzo R. Allopathic specific condition review: dysmenorrhea. *The Protocol Journal of Botanical Medicine.* 1995;1(1).

Berkow R, ed. *The Merck Manual of Diagnosis and Therapy.* 16th ed. Rahway, NJ: Merck Research Laboratories; 1992.

Branch WT, Jr. *Office Practice of Medicine.* 3rd ed. Philadelphia, Pa: WB Saunders Company; 1994.

Penland JG, Johnson PE. Dietary calcium and manganese effects on menstrual cycle symptoms. *Am J Obstet Gynecol.* 1993;168:1417–1423.

Werbach MR. *Nutritional Influences on Illness.* New Canaan, Conn: Keats Publishing Inc; 1987.

■ DYSPHAGIA
OVERVIEW
Definition
Generally defined as difficulty in swallowing (or the sensation of difficulty in swallowing), dysphagia reflects an esophageal or pharyngeal transport disorder, either from anatomical malformations or from a disruption of the physiological events in swallowing. Dysphagia can be subdivided into the following two distinct types, which can occur independently.

- Oropharyngeal dysphagia: Difficulty initiating the act of swallowing, of moving food from the mouth to the upper esophagus (generally from abnormalities of the pharynx and upper esophageal sphincter)
- Esophageal dysphagia: Difficulty moving food through the esophagus

The lifetime incidence of dysphagia is less than 10%. Although all ages are affected, the prevalence increases with age. No sex differentiation.

Etiology
The causes of oropharyngeal dysphagia (dysphagia for solids or liquids) include the following.

- CNS: cerebrovascular accident (CVA), Parkinson's disease, brainstem tumors
- Muscle: myasthenia, polymyositis, thyroid disease, systemic lupus erythematosus
- Structural: web, Zenker's diverticulum, extrinsic compression

The causes of esophageal dysphagia include the following.

- Dysphagia for solids only, intermittent: webs, rings, diverticulum, esophagitis
- Solids only, continuous/progressive: carcinoma (particularly under age 40), stricture
- Solids and liquids: motility disorder such as diffuse esophageal spasm, tumor, stricture, esophagitis

Dysphagia in children usually indicates the following.

- Congenital malformations: esophageal atresia, choanal atresia
- Acquired malformations: corrosive or herpetic esophagitis
- Neuromuscular/neurologic conditions: cerebral palsy, muscular dystrophy
- GERD

Dysphagia in adults usually indicates the following.

- Structural: tumors (benign and malignant), strictures, rings and webs, extrinsic compression
- Neuromuscular: achalasia, diffuse esophageal spasm, scleroderma, myasthenia gravis
- GERD

Risk Factors
- Smoking
- Recurrent or chronic GERD
- Medications (such as quinine, potassium chloride, vitamin C, tetracycline, NSAIDs)
- Poor dentition
- Ill-functioning dentures
- Excessive alcohol consumption
- Achalasia
- Esophageal cancer
- Plummer-Vinson syndrome
- Barrett's mucosa
- Hereditary or congenital malformations

Signs and Symptoms
Oropharyngeal dysphagia is characterized by the following.

- Difficulty initiating swallowing
- Inability to move food into the esophagus
- Choking or aspiration while swallowing
- Coughing while swallowing
- Regurgitation of liquid through the nose
- Aspiration with swallowing
- Weak voice
- Weight loss

Esophageal dysphagia is characterized by the following.

- Pressure sensation in mid-chest
- Sensation of food stuck in the esophagus
- Retrosternal fullness after swallowing
- Weight loss
- Chest pain and other Gastroesophageal reflux disorder (GERD) symptoms
- Extended period of time required for eating

DIFFERENTIAL DIAGNOSIS
- Cardiac-associated chest pain
- Globus hystericus
- Scleroderma

DIAGNOSIS
Because dysphagia is symptomatic of a structural or functional abnormality, determining the etiology is essential for effective treatment. Avoid dismissing the symptom as psychosomatic or "globus hystericus." Consult-ation with a gastroenterologist is advised.

Physical Examination
Determine precisely where the patient's symptoms are felt; whether symptoms appear with solids, liquids, or both; if the symptoms are intermittent or progressive. Also, question patients about length of time spent eating (i.e., unconsciously chewing food thoroughly). For infants/children, observe sucking and eating practices.

During evaluation, consider the following.

- Esophageal patency, inflammation
- Airway function
- Pulmonary function
- Cardiac disease
- Nutritional status
- Evidence of aspiration pneumonia
- Symptoms of heartburn

Pathological Findings
- Mass lesion, including squamous cell carcinoma and Adenocarcinoma
- Barrett's metaplasia
- Fibrous tissue from a ring, web, or stricture
- Heterotopic gastric mucosa
- Acute or chronic inflammatory change
- Deformities or scars

Imaging
For infants and children:

- X ray of neck, chest
- Contrast X ray

For adults:

- X ray of neck, chest, abdomen
- Barium swallow (cine/video esophagogram)
- Contrast X ray: esophogram, cine-esophogram, modified cine-esophogram
- CT scan

Other Diagnostic Procedures

In addition to physical assessment and history, these special tests may be done:

- Esophagoscopy: particularly relevant for patients with persistent difficulty swallowing solid food. Disruption of webs and rings during endoscopy can be therapeutic.
- Esophageal manometry: preferred procedure for esophageal motor function evaluation (affected by anticholinergics, calcium channel blockers, nitrates, prokinetics, sedatives)
- Endoscopic ultrasonography: to diagnose and stage benign and malignant esophageal neoplasms
- Infants and children: nasogastric tube assessment of esophagus patency

TREATMENT OPTIONS

Treatment Strategy

Outpatient care is appropriate for patients capable of maintaining nutrition and with low risk of complications. Hospitalization may be necessary for infants and children, and for adults with total or near-total obstruction of the esophageal lumen.

Treatment can include drug therapies, esophageal dilatation, and surgery.

Drug Therapies

Check manufacturers' profiles for possible drug interactions. Liquid forms of medications may be necessary.

For spasms:

- Nitrates: nitroglycerin, isosorbide (contraindications: early myocardial infarction, severe anemia, increased intracranial pressure)
- Anticholinergics: dicyclomine (Bentyl) or hyoscyamine sulfate (Lepsin) (contraindications: obstructive uropathy, glaucoma, myasthenia gravis, achalasia)
- Calcium channel blockers: nifedipine (Procardia), diltiazem (Cardizem)
- Sedatives/antidepressants: diazepam (Valium), trazodone (Desyrel), doxepin (Sinequan)
- Smooth-muscle relaxants: hydralazine

For esophagitis:

- H_2-blockers: cimetidine (Tagamet), ranitidine (Zantac), nizatidine (Axid), famotidine (Pepcid)
- Proton pump inhibitors (for failure of H_2-blockers or as initial therapy): omeprazole (Prilosec), lansoprazole (Prevacid)
- Prokinetic agents: metoclopramide (Reglan), cisapride (Propulsid); adjunct to acid-suppressive therapy

Complementary and Alternative Therapies

Herbs can be very effective at decreasing spasms and healing esophagitis. Homeopathics could be used concurrently for symptomatic relief.

HERBS

Herbs are generally a safe way to strengthen and tone the body's systems. As with any therapy, it is important to ascertain a diagnosis before pursuing treatment. Herbs may be used as dried extracts (capsules, powders, teas), glycerites (glycerine extracts), or tinctures (alcohol extracts). Unless otherwise indicated, teas should be made with 1 tsp. herb per cup of hot water. Steep covered 5 to 10 minutes for leaf or flowers, and 10 to 20 minutes for roots. Drink 2 to 4 cups/day. Tinctures may be used singly or in combination as noted.

- Licorice *(Glycyrrhiza glabra):* an anti-inflammatory, anti-spasmodic, and analgesic specific for the gastrointestinal tract. Glycyrrhetinic acid

has been shown in studies to aid healing of gastric, peptic, and mouth ulcers. In patients with hypertension, use deglycerinated licorice to prevent aggravating hypertension. Prolonged use may lead to pseudoaldosteronism, which resolves with discontinuation of the herb. The dose is 380 to 1,140 mg/day. Chewable lozenges may be the best form of licorice for treating GERD.

- Slippery elm *(Ulmus fulva):* demulcent (protects irritated tissues and promotes their healing); dose is 60 to 320 mg/day. One tsp. powder may be mixed with water tid to qid.

In addition, a combination of four of the following herbs may be used as either a tea or tincture. Use equal parts of the herbs, either 1 tsp. of each per cup of water and steep 10 minutes tid, or equal parts of tincture 30 to 60 drops tid.

- Valerian *(Valeriana officinalis):* bitter, sedative, especially where there is anxiety and/or depression and poor digestion
- Wild yam *(Dioscorea villosa):* anti-spasmodic, anti-inflammatory, especially where there is fatigue from long term stress or maldigestion
- St. John's wort *(Hypericum perforatum):* analgesic, anti-depressant, historically used to treat adhesions, especially where there is anxiety and/or pain
- Skullcap *(Scutellaria lateriflora):* anti-spasmodic, sedative, nervine, especially with disturbed sleep
- Linden flowers *(Tilea europea):* anti-spasmodic, mild diuretic, gentle bitter, especially with dyspepsia

HOMEOPATHY

An experienced homeopath should assess individual constitutional types and severity of disease to select the correct remedy and potency. For acute prescribing use 3 to 5 pellets of a 12X to 30C remedy every one to four hours until acute symptoms resolve.

- *Baptesia* for patients who can only swallow liquids and gag on the smallest amount of solids; especially with a red inflamed throat that is relatively pain free.
- *Baryta carbonica* for huge tonsils that make it difficult to swallow even liquids; especially with shyness
- *Carbo vegatabilis* for bloating and indigestion that is worse from lying down; especially with flatulence and fatigue
- *Ignatia imara* for "lump in the throat," back spasms, spasmodic cough; especially when symptoms appear after grieving
- *Lachesis* for difficulty swallowing, intolerance to touch around the throat, and tight clothes

Patient Monitoring

Discuss etiology and prognosis with patients, including possible need for repeat dilatations. Dysphagia should not require limits on patients' activities. Depending on the degree of obstruction, diet may have to be restricted.

OTHER CONSIDERATIONS

Prevention

Counsel patients (and/or caregivers) to do the following:

- Avoid exacerbating drugs
- Chew thoroughly
- Avoid extremely hot or cold foods
- Do not drink alcohol in excess
- Correct poorly fitting dentures
- Observe infants/children carefully when eating

Complications/Sequelae

- Aspiration
- Esophageal "asthma"

- Pneumonia
- Barrett's syndrome; esophageal cancer

Prognosis

Prognosis varies from good for relatively uncomplicated dysphagia (e.g., peptic strictures) to poor for dysphagia with cancer etiologies. Speech therapy may be appropriate for patients who need to learn swallowing techniques.

REFERENCES

Andreoli TE, Bennett JC, Carpenter CCJ. *Cecil Essentials of Medicine.* 3rd ed. Philadelphia, Pa: WB Saunders; 1993:284–285.

Barker LR, Burton JR, Zieve PD, eds. *Principles of Ambulatory Medicine.* 4th ed. Baltimore, Md: Williams & Wilkins; 1995:435–447.

Bartram T. *Encyclopedia of Herbal Medicine.* Dorset, England: Grace Publishers; 1995.

Dambro MR, ed. Griffith's 5-Minute Clinical Consult–1999. Baltimore, Md: Lippincott Williams & Wilkins; 1999:346–347.

Morrison R. *Desktop Guide to Keynotes and Confirmatory Symptoms.* Albany, Calif: Hahnemann Clinic Publishing; 1993.

Reynolds JEF. *Martindale: the Extra Pharmacopoeia.* 31st ed. London, England: Royal Pharmaceutical Society of Great Britain; 1996:1192.

Snow JA. *Glycyrrhiza glabra L.* (Leguminaceae). *The Protocol Journal of Botanical Medicine.* 1996;1:9.

Stein JK, ed. *Internal Medicine.* 4th ed. St. Louis, Mo: Mosby–Year Book; 1994:361–362.

Stoller JK, Ahmad M, Longworth DL eds. *The Cleveland Clinic Intensive Review of Internal Medicine.* Baltimore, Md: Williams & Wilkins; 1998:592–601.

■ ECZEMA
OVERVIEW
Definition
Eczema (or dermatitis) refers to a group of chronic skin disorders that primarily involve the epidermis and include atopic, contact, stasis, seborrheic, nummular, dyshidrotic, generalized, or localized scratch dermatitis. Type depends on cause and location on body, but treatment is generally the same. Family history of allergic rhinitis, asthma, or atopic dermatitis often exists. Neurodermatitis is used to describe eczematoid rashes that seem to have a major stress-related component.

Etiology
Eczema can be caused by allergies, allergies secondary to digestive disorders (hydrochloric acid deficiency, for example), drugs, environmental exposures, or be secondary to immune diseases, genetic metabolic disorders, or nutritional deficiencies.

Risk Factors
Inflammation exacerbated by:
- Stress or anxiety
- Allergies to ingestants (foods), inhalants, and contactants
- Lack of sleep
- Heredity
- Excessive consumption of fruit, especially citrus and sour types
- Underlying emotional problems, especially compulsive behaviors

Signs and Symptoms
- Itching
- Erythema
- Lesions usually appear on face, neck, trunk, and genital areas. May be characterized as: Papules, oozing and crusting vesicles (infants); Induration, scaling (adults, children)

DIFFERENTIAL DIAGNOSIS
Various types of eczema (dermatitis):
- Contact eczema: localized rash where offending agent touched skin; caused by irritants, allergens, light, chemicals, perfumes, metals
- Atopic eczema: patient often has a history of vitamin B_{12} problems, asthma, allergic respiratory problems (hay fever), allergies
- Seborrheic eczema: on face, chest, scalp
- Nummular eczema: chronic round red spots that crust and scale; accompanies dry skin in winter; often associated with emotional stress; usually found in people over the age of 35
- Stasis eczema: over lower legs; associated with poor venous return; skin turns brown
- Dyshidrotic eczema (pompholyx, vesicular dermatitis): 1 to 2 mm "tapioca"-like vesicles found on soles, palms, and sides of fingers that may merge to form multiloculated blisters; scaling and fissuring after blisters dry; itching, usually occurs after age 30 and will recur
- Localized scratch eczema: patches with whitish areas surrounded by increased pigmentation; more frequent in women age 20 to 50; allergic components, exacerbated by scratching.

Other noneczematous disorders:
- Inflammatory tinea pedis
- Vesicular tinea
- Herpes simplex virus infection
- Dermatophytosis
- Psoriasis

DIAGNOSIS
Physical Examination
Skin inflammation with blisters that itch, ooze, and crust over. Patient may have a family history of asthma or food or environmental allergies.

Laboratory Tests
If HSV infection suspected, a Tzanck smear is done.

Other Diagnostic Procedures
Obvious physical appearance is generally basis for diagnosis. Food allergy tests may be necessary if food allergy is suspected cause.

TREATMENT OPTIONS
Treatment Strategy
Lubricate skin with oil, moisturizers

Drug Therapies
- Topical and systemic corticosteroids—apply according to package directions for skin lesions; high-potency topical steroid applied early may stop the itching and the attack. One percent topical hydrocortisone for children; may use higher concentration in adults
- Disulfiram—recommended for nickel allergy or dyshidrotic eczema
- Oral cromolyn sodium—recommended for nickel allergy or dyshidrotic eczema
- Zinc oxide—apply locally for severe itching
- Topical psoralen with special UVA light sources—to treat hands and feet; response slow

Complementary and Alternative Therapies
Eliminating allergenic foods is key in treating eczema. Following nutritional guidelines and using herbal support as needed may be effective in reducing inflammation, and hypersensitivity reactions`.

Hypersensitivity reactions may be associated with stress and anxiety. Mind-body techniques such as meditation, Tai chi, yoga, and stress management may help reduce reactivity.

NUTRITION
Note: Lower doses are for children.
- Eliminate all food allergens from the diet. The most common allergenic foods are dairy, soy, citrus, peanuts, wheat, fish, eggs, corn, and tomatoes. An elimination/challenge trial may be helpful in uncovering sensitivities. Remove suspected allergens from the diet for two weeks. Reintroduce foods at the rate of one food every three days. Watch for reactions that may include gastrointestinal upset, mood changes, flushing, and exacerbation of eczema.
- A rotation diet, in which the same food is not eaten more than once every four days, may be helpful in chronic eczema.
- Reduce inflammatory foods in the diet including saturated fats (meats, especially poultry, and dairy), refined foods, and sugar. Patients with antibiotic sensitivity should eat only organic meats to avoid antibiotic residues. Avoid caffeine and alcohol.
- Increase intake of fresh vegetables, whole grains, and essential fatty acids (cold-water fish, nuts, and seeds).
- Flaxseed (3,000 mg bid), borage (1,500 mg bid), or evening primrose oil (1,500 mg bid) are anti-inflammatory. Children should be supplemented with 500 mg doses of these oils bid, or with cod liver oil ($^{1}/_{2}$ to 1 tsp. daily).
- Beta-carotene (25,000 to 100,000 IU/day), zinc (10 to 30 mg/day), and vitamin E (100 to 400 IU/day) support immune function and dermal healing.

- Zinc Spray can heal the tissue in a subset of patients.
- Vitamin C (250 to 1,000 mg bid to qid) inhibits histamine release. Vitamin C from rose hips is citrus-free and hypoallergenic.
- Selenium (50 to 200 mcg/day) helps to regulate fatty acid metabolism and is a co-factor in liver detoxification.
- Bromelain (250 mg bid to qid taken between meals) is a proteolytic enzyme that reduces inflammation.
- For eczema that is resistant to treatment consider oral supplementation with hydrochloric acid.
- If after six weeks there is no improvement, switch oils to omega-6/vegetable oils one to two times/day.

Bioflavanoids, a constituent found in dark berries and some plants, have anti-inflammatory properties, strengthen connective tissue, and help reduce hypersensitivity reactions. The following are bioflavanoids that may be taken in dried extract form as noted.

- Catechin (25 to 150 mg bid to tid), quercetin (100 to 250 mg bid to tid), hesperidin (100 to 250 mg bid to tid), and rutin (100 to 250 mg bid to tid).
- Rose hips (Rosa canina) are also high in bioflavonoids and may be used as a tea. Drink 3 to 4 cups/day.

HERBS

Herbs are generally a safe way to strengthen and tone the body's systems. As with any therapy, it is important to ascertain a diagnosis before pursuing treatment. Herbs may be used as dried extracts (capsules, powders, teas), glycerites (glycerine extracts), or tinctures (alcohol extracts). Unless otherwise indicated, teas should be made with 1 tsp. of herb per cup of hot water. Steep covered 5 to 10 minutes for leaf or flowers, and 10 to 20 minutes for roots. Drink 2 to 4 cups/day. Tinctures may be used singly or in combination as noted.

Herbs that support dermal healing and lymphatic drainage are useful for relieving eczema. Use the following herbs in combination as a tincture (15 to 30 drops tid) or tea (2 to 4 cups/day). Burdock root (Arctium lappa), yellow dock (Rumex crispus), red clover (Trifolium pratense), cleavers (Gallium aparine), yarrow (Achillea millefolium), peppermint (Mentha piperita), and nettles (Urtica dioica). To prepare a tea, steep the root elements for 10 minutes, then add the rest of the herbs and steep an additional 5 to 10 minutes.

Topical applications of creams and salves containing one or more of the following herbs may help relieve itching, burning, and promote healing. Chickweed (Stellaria media), marigold (Calendula officinalis), comfrey (Symphytum officinalis), and chamomile (Matricaria recutita).

Marshmallow root tea (Althea officinalis) may soothe and promote healing of gastrointestinal inflammation that is often found with this condition. Soak 1 heaping tbsp. of marshmallow root in 1 quart of cold water overnight. Strain and drink throughout the day.

HOMEOPATHY

An experienced homeopath should assess individual constitutional types and severity of disease to select the correct remedy and potency. The use of acute remedies may exacerbate eczema.

PHYSICAL MEDICINE

Starch, oatmeal, and other baths may temporarily relieve the symptoms.

ACUPUNCTURE

Acupuncture may help restore normal immune function and reduce the hypersensitivity response.

Patient Monitoring

- This chronic, recurring disorder can flare up with stress or exposure to offending agents. Lesions of the hands and feet can become severe and need prompt attention.
- With underlying psychopathologies, short- or long-term psychotherapy, hypnosis, behavioral therapy, or biofeedback techniques may help.

OTHER CONSIDERATIONS

Prevention

Conservative introduction of solid foods as child is weaning may help prevent hypersensitivity conditions. If there is a strong family history of allergies or atopic conditions and/or if the child's immunity has been compromised in infancy, delay the introduction of highly allergenic foods (especially dairy and grains) until 1 year or older.

Infants exclusively breast fed, have a lower risk of atopic eczema development, and develop symptoms at a later age. This may reflect later contact with cow's milk, a common sensitizer.

Complications/Sequelae

Continuing recurrences may accompany stress and increase levels of anxiety or depression. Overuse of topical cortiosteroids may atrophy skin.

Prognosis

Even moderate to severe cases of eczema are usually just an annoyance. Meticulous care will control most flare-ups. Eczema is a chronic disease that tends to lessen in severity or resolve with advancing age. Most children see resolution by puberty.

Pregnancy

Nutritional support and topical applications may safely relieve symptoms during pregnancy.

REFERENCES

The Burton Goldberg Group. *Alternative Medicine: The Definitive Guide.* Tiburon, Calif: Future Medicine Publishing Inc; 1997.

Morse PF, et al. Meta-analysis of placebo-controlled studies of the efficacy of Epogam in the treatment of atopic eczema: Relationship between plasma essential fatty acid changes and clinical response. *Br J Dermatol.* 1989;121:75–90.

Murray MT, Pizzorno JE. *Encyclopedia of Natural Medicine.* Rocklin, Calif: Prima Publishing; 1998:296–300.

Noble J, ed. *Textbook of Primary Care Medicine.* 2nd ed. St Louis, Mo: Mosby-Year Book; 1996:345–365, 368–375, 1064–1084.

Tierney LM Jr, McPhee SJ, Papadakis MA, eds. *Current Medical Diagnosis and Treatment.* Norwalk, Conn: Appleton & Lange; 1994.

Werbach, M. *Nutritional Influences on Illness.* New Canaan, Conn: Keats Publishing; 1988:186–188.

■ EDEMA
OVERVIEW
Definition
Edema (also known as dropsy or fluid retention) is the accumulation of excessive amounts of fluid in the interstitial space due to imbalance between hydrostatic and oncotic pressure. It is a symptom caused by an underlying disease or disorder. Edema may either be localized due to venous/lymphatic obstruction or increased vascular permeability, or systemic due to organ failure. It may be mild and cyclical, as in fluid retention associated with menses, or severe and life-threatening, as in angioneurotic or cerebral edema. Types of edema include the following.

- Angioneurotic edema (angioedema/Quincke's disease): recurrent swelling of skin, mucous membranes, viscera, or brain with sudden onset lasting from hours to days
- Blue edema: cyanosis of swollen extremity
- Brown edema: associated with chronic, passive congestion of the lungs
- Cardiac edema: associated with congestive heart failure
- Cerebral edema: affecting the neuropile and white matter—often associated with diabetic ketoacidosis (DKA)
- Corneal edema: swelling of the cornea
- Cystoid macular: swelling in posterior pole of the eye
- High Altitude Pulmonary Edema (HAPE): potentially life-threatening non-cardiogenic altitude illness
- Idiopathic leg edema: swollen legs with no apparent cause
- Lipedema edema: fat/fluid accumulation in legs
- Lymphedema: abnormal accumulation of lymph fluid
- Malignant edema: anthrax
- Menstrual edema: associated with hormonal cycle
- Nutritional edema: from excess fluid and salt intake and insufficient protein intake
- Pulmonary edema: affecting the lungs and most commonly due to cardiac disorders

Etiology
Vary according to age, gender, underlying disorders.

Cyclical/generally non-life-threatening disorders, often evident in lower extremities only, include the following causes.

- Sitting or standing for extended periods: reduces blood flow so blood "pools" in veins, inhibiting oncotic movement
- Heat: expands blood vessels, allowing greater hydrostatic effusion
- Medications (steroids, NSAIDs antidepressants, HRT): increased hydrostatic movement
- Menstruation/pregnancy: hormonal changes affect hydrostatic/oncotic pressure gradients
- Damage to lymphatic system
- Infection/injury: vein damage impairs fluid movement
- Obesity
- High salt intake
- Allergies (food, insect bites)
- Hypoalbuminemia
- Proteinuria

Chronic and/or potentially life-threatening underlying disorders, include the following causes.

- Renal, cardiac, hepatic, thyroid diseases
- Hypothyroidism
- High/low blood pressure
- Pregnancy
- Vascular and arterial diseases
- Thrombosis

- Weakened venous system/varicose veins
- Infection/inflammation
- Tumors
- Short-term exposure to altitude combined with heavy physical exertion
- DKA, head trauma, anoxia, exposure to toxic substances

Risk Factors
The underlying cause of life-threatening conditions must be identified. At higher risk are those with the following.

- Radiation to surgical sites following lymphadenectomy increases lymphedema risk
- Genetic lymphatic abnormalities
- Obesity
- High salt intake

Signs and Symptoms
Will vary according to disorder.

- Swollen extremities (possibly accompanied by pain, redness, heat, and open sores)
- Facial puffiness
- Abdominal bloating
- Shortness of breath, extreme difficulty breathing, coughing up blood (pulmonary/HAPE)
- Sudden change in mental status/abnormal neurological signs, respiratory arrest (cerebral edema associated with DKA)
- Muscular pain due to bloating and swelling

DIFFERENTIAL DIAGNOSIS
- Inflammatory diseases (gout, rheumatoid arthritis)
- Preeclampsia (toxemia)

DIAGNOSIS
Physical Examination
Varies according to underlying disorder; may include the following.
- Swelling in face, limbs, extremities, and/or trunk; weight gain
- Dermatological lesions may be present
- Pulmonary edema: fluid accumulation in pleural cavity
- Cerebral edema: intracellular (cytotoxic)—cellular swelling in grey matter; extracellular (vasogenic)—white matter moist and swollen; microscopically—micro-vacuolization/halos surrounding nuclei

Laboratory Tests
Reduced serum albumin; increased fecal loss of antiprotease

Pathological Findings
Excess fluid in intercellular tissue spaces due to the following.
- Increased hydrostatic pressure gradient, or elevated extracellular fluid volume
- Decrease in overall osmotic pressure gradient, or increase in capillary permeability to plasma protein

Imaging
- CT, MRI, X ray as appropriate to aid in diagnosis

Other Diagnostic Procedures
Because certain forms of edema are life-threatening, treating immediate symptoms may be necessary before diagnosis of underlying disorder is established.
Medical history/interview to determine:
- Time frame/longevity of symptoms
- Whether continuous, intermittent, or cyclical (e.g., with menses)

- Diet
- History of cardiac/renal/hepatic/thyroid disease
- Exposure to toxic fumes
- Allergic reactions

Physical examination:
- Location
- Degree of pitting (indentation remaining following application of pressure with finger)
- Cutaneous wounds/sores
- Varicose veins
- Blood clots
- Shortness of breath
- Determine underlying cause (e.g., pregnancy; cardiac, renal, hepatic, thyroid disease)

Special tests:
- Serum electrolyte/albumin tests
- Urinalysis
- ECG
- Echocardiography
- Liver Function Test

TREATMENT OPTIONS

Treatment Strategy
Treatment will depend upon underlying disorder. In pulmonary edema or HAPE, immediate hospitalization and/or treatment with oxygen, diuretics and/or medications are necessary.

To reduce swelling:
- Salt reduction diet
- Daily exercise
- Periodic elevation of legs above heart level
- Diuretics
- Support hose
- Massage
- Complete Decongestive Therapy (CDT): compression physical therapy (including sleeves, pumps) to move fluid through alternate lymph channels for reabsorption by the body, compression bandaging, skin care/manipulation.

Drug Therapies
Diuretics effectively reduce fluid levels; however, they also deplete potassium, magnesium, B vitamins, and calcium, which results in loss of bone mass.
- Loop/thiazide diuretics (heart failure, cirrhosis, nephrosis, renal failure, hypertension)
- Potassium-sparing diuretics (hypokalemia caused by other diuretics, hypertension)
- Carbonic anhydrase inhibitors (glaucoma, HAPE, heart failure)
- Osmotic diuretic (Mannitol—1/gm/kg at onset of neurologic symptoms in DKA-related edema)
- Morphine (in pulmonary disease reduces congestion/anxiety)
- Corticosteroid/immunosuppressives
- Medications appropriate for underlying disorder

Surgical Procedures
- Surgical removal of fat and fluid deposits in lipedema
- Attempt to reestablish lymph/blood flow

Complementary and Alternative Therapies
While following nutritional and herbal support guidelines may help alleviate edema, it is essential that the underlying cause be addressed. Edema is multi-factorial. Choose the appropriate guidelines according to the underlying cause.

NUTRITION
- Eliminating food allergens from the diet decreases inflammation edema secondary to inflammatory processes.
- A low-salt, high-protein diet may help resolve edema. High protein is contraindicated in renal involvement. Dietary intake of sugar and refined carbohydrates should also be reduced.
- Increase dietary potassium with diuretic use (e.g., bananas, apricots, and green leafy vegetables).
- Some foods are natural diuretics: asparagus, parsley, beets, grapes, green beans, leafy greens, pineapple, pumpkin, onion, leeks, and garlic. These foods also support kidney and liver function.
- Vitamin B_6 (50 to 100 mg/day) induces diuresis. Thiamine may be depleted with Lasix and should be supplemented (200 mg/day).
- Vitamins C (1,000 to 1,500 mg tid), E (400-800 IU/day), and coenzyme Q10 (50 to 100 mg bid) protect and strengthen blood vessels.
- Potassium aspartate (20 mg/day) may need to be supplemented if using diuretics.
- Magnesium (200 mg bid to tid) and calcium (1,000 mg/day) influence intra- and inter-cellular fluid exchange and may be depleted with diuretic use.

HERBS
Herbs are generally a safe way to strengthen and tone the body's systems. As with any therapy, it is important to ascertain a diagnosis before pursuing treatment. Herbs may be used as dried extracts (capsules, powders, teas), glycerites (glycerine extracts), or tinctures (alcohol extracts). Unless otherwise indicated, teas should be made with 1 tsp. herb per cup of hot water. Steep covered 5 to 10 minutes for leaf or flowers, and 10 to 20 minutes for roots. Drink 2 to 4 cups/day. Tinctures may be used singly or in combination as noted.

A general diuretic should contain herbs that support circulation and lymphatic drainage. They are best administered in a cooled tea (four to six cups/day), although a tincture may also be used (30-60 drops qid). Drinking the tea cool will support circulation and lymphatic drainage without increasing vasodilation. Combine three of these herbs with equal parts of two to three additional herbs from the following categories, as indicated: cleavers (*Gallium aparine*), yarrow (*Achillea millefolium*), oatstraw (*Avena sativa*), elder (*Sambucus canadensis*), red clover (*Trifolium pratense*), and red root (*Ceonothus americanus*).

Cyclic edema and idiopathic orthostatic edema:
- Ginkgo (*Ginkgo biloba*) strengthens the integrity of the vasculature and its use has improved cyclical edema associated with hormonal changes.
- Bilberry (*Vaccinium myrtillus*) is a gentle diuretic as well as a tonic for the vasculature.
- Topical applications of creams containing one or more of the following may be helpful in increasing vascular integrity in orthostatic edema: horse chestnut (*Aesculus hippocastanum*), butcher's broom (*Ruscus asuleatus*), sweet clover (*Melilotus officinalis*), and rue (*Ruta graveolens*).

Renal insufficiency:
Use caution in administering diuretics with renal failure. Herbal options include parsley (*Petrosilinum crispum*), dandelion leaves (*Taraxacum officinalis*), buchu (*Barosma betulina*), couchgrass (*Agropyron repens*), horsetail (*Euquisetum arvense*), and goldenrod (*Solidago virgaurea*)

Cardiac and/or pulmonary involvement:
- Hawthorn *(Crataegus oxyacantha)*, motherwort *(Leonorus cardiaca)*, rosemary *(Rosemariana officinalis)*, and linden *(Tilia cordata)*
- Lily of the valley *(Convalleria majalus)*, night blooming cereus *(Cactus grandiflorus)*, and broom *(Sarothamnus scoparius)* have toxic side effects but may be added to the cardiopulmonary formula under physician supervision

Hepatic involvement (may be used in conjunction with treatment for cyclic edema) may respond to milk thistle *(Silybum marianum)*, dandelion root *(Taraxacum officinalis)*, turmeric *(Curcuma longa)*, and artichoke leaves *(Cynara scolymus)*

HOMEOPATHY

Because of the many presentations of edema, remedies are best chosen by an experienced homeopath.

PHYSICAL MEDICINE

- Dry skin brushing. Before bathing, briskly brush the entire skin surface with a rough washcloth, loofa, or soft brush. Begin at the feet and work up. Always stroke in the direction of the heart. This helps facilitate lymphatic circulation. There is no need to press deeply as the lymph are superficial vessels.
- Cold compresses to the face or backs of the legs with yarrow tea may give temporary relief of edema.
- Contrast hydrotherapy involves alternating hot and cold application to bring nutrients to the site and to diffuse metabolic waste from inflammation. The overall effect is decreased inflammation, pain relief, and enhanced healing. Using this technique with hand and/or foot baths may help to improve circulation and lymphatic drainage. Alternate three minutes hot with one minute cold and repeat three times. This is one set. Do two to three sets/day. Use caution in areas of decreased sensation by ensuring that the hot application does not burn.

ACUPUNCTURE

Acupuncture may improve fluid balance and provide support in the treatment of underlying cause and improve circulation.

MASSAGE

Therapeutic massage can assist with lymph drainage and improve circulation.

Patient Monitoring

Monitor for:
- Fluid input/outflow.
- Potassium levels, electrolyte balance, blood pressure, allergic reactions, GI bleeding, CNS effects, muscle cramps, and other side effects of diuretic use.

OTHER CONSIDERATIONS

Daily exercise is highly beneficial in general, unless contraindicated by underlying condition.

Prevention

- Pulmonary edema: reduce risk by treating cardiac disorder
- Lymphedema: keep skin clean/supple, protect surgical site from injury; drainage-promoting exercises, elevation of affected limb
- Idiopathic disease: reduce salt intake; avoid constrictive clothing around legs and wrists

Complications/Sequelae

- Hypertensive disease
- Pulmonary edema/HAPE/cerebral edema are life-threatening
- Infection/ulceration of cutaneous lesions

Prognosis

- Life-threatening edema treatable and often curable with prompt attention combined with treatment for underlying disorder
- Effective reduction of swelling attainable with diuretics and compression therapies

Pregnancy

Orthostatic edema is common in pregnancy and can be safely addressed with leg elevation, hawthorn tea, and topical applications. Edema may also be a sign of preeclampsia and should be monitored closely.

REFERENCES

Balch JF, Balch PA. *Prescription for Nutritional Healing.* Garden City Park, NY: Avery Publishing Group; 1997.

Bartram T. *Encyclopedia of Herbal Medicine.* Dorset, England: Grace Publishers; 1995:73, 155, 156, 188.

Blumenthal M, ed. *The Complete German Commission E Monographs.* Boston, Mass: Integrative Medicine Communications; 1998:424, 425, 429.

Mayo Foundation for Medical Education and Research. Available at www.healthanswers.com

MDX Health Digest. Available at www.thriveonline.com

Mindell E, Hopkins V. *Prescription Alternatives.* New Canaan, Conn: Keats Publishing Inc; 1998.

Vanderbilt University Medical Center. Available at www.mc.vanderbilt.edu

Weiss RF. *Herbal Medicines.* Beaconsfield, England: Beaconsfield Publishers, Ltd; 1988:188–191, 241.

■ ENDOCARDITIS
OVERVIEW
Definition
Endocarditis, an infection and inflammation of the endocardium, usually affects the external lining of heart valves (valvular endocarditis), although it also can impact the lining of heart chambers (mural endocarditis). A complex condition with a variety of causes, often a potentially serious complication of prosthetic cardiac valve or tissue graft valve replacement. While endocarditis does have non-bacterial etiologies, the condition generally is related to bacterial infection and thus frequently is referred to as infective endocarditis, infectious endocarditis, or bacterial endocarditis.

For purposes of diagnosis:
- Acute endocarditis (acute bacterial endocarditis, acute infective endocarditis): begins abruptly, progresses aggressively, and is quite life-threatening. Usually caused by virulent organisms.
- Subacute endocarditis (subacute bacterial endocarditis, subacute infective endocarditis): often in patients with underlying cardiac condition (e.g., valves damaged by rheumatic fever); progresses slowly.
- Intravenous (IV) drug user endocarditis: common in IV drug users, usually with tricuspid valve involvement.
- Prosthetic valve endocarditis
  - Early: <60 days after implantation
  - Late: >60 days after implantation
- Culture-negative endocarditis: affects a small percentage of patients.

Etiology
Acute endocarditis:
- *Staphylococcus aureus*
- *Streptococcus* groups A, B, C, and G
- *Haemophilus influenzae* and *H. parainfluenzae*
- *Streptococcus pneumoniae*
- *Staphylococcus lugdunensis*
- *Enterococcus*
- *Neisseria gonorrhoeae*

Subacute endocarditis:
- Alpha-hemolytic streptococci (viridans streptococci)
- *Streptococcus bovis*
- *Enterococcus*
- *Haemophilus aphrophilus* and *H. paraphrophilus*
- *Actinobacillus actinomycetemcomitans*
- *Cardiobacterium hominis*
- *Eikenella corrodens*
- *Kingella kingae*
- *Staphylococcus aureus*

IV drug user endocarditis:
- *Staphylococcus aureus*
- *Pseudomonas aeruginosa*
- *Burkholderia cepacia*
- *Enterococcus*
- Candida

Prosthetic valve endocarditis:
Early (<60 days after implantation):
- *Staphylococcus aureus* and *S. epidermidis*
- Gram-negative bacilli
- Candida
- *Aspergillus*

Late (>60 days after implantation):
- Alpha-hemolytic streptococci (viridans streptococci)
- *Enterococcus*
- *Staphylococcus epidermidis*

- Candida
- *Aspergillus*

Culture-negative endocarditis:
- Antibiotics (side effects)
- *Bartonella quintana* and *B. henselae*
- *Brucella*
- Fungi
- *Coxiella burnetii* (Q fever)
- *Chlamydia trachomatis* and *C. psittaci*
- Libman-Sachs associated with systemic Lupus Erythematosus

Risk Factors
Risk factors include patient's susceptibility and medical procedures:
Predisposing conditions:
- Prosthetic cardiac valves
- Previous endocarditis
- Congenital cardiac malformations
- Degenerative heart disease
- Hypertrophic cardiomyopathy
- Mitral valve prolapse
- Dental and surgical procedures resulting in transient bacteremia
- Intravenous drug use

Signs and Symptoms
Remittent fever (high or low) is the most common symptom of endocarditis; often the only symptom in prosthetic valve endocarditis.

Other possible signs and symptoms include the following.
- Skin lesions (Janeway lesions)
- Chills, night sweats
- Malaise, fatigue
- Muscle, joint, and back pain; stiff neck
- Headache, delirium, seizures
- Myocardial infarction
- Aphasia
- Paralysis, hemiparesis, numbness, muscle weakness
- Cold, painful extremity
- Bloody urine or sputum
- Painful finger or toe tip (Osler node)
- Pulmonary infarction
- Shortness of breath
- Cough
- Pallor

DIFFERENTIAL DIAGNOSIS
- Cerebral embolus or hemorrhage
- Connective tissue disease
- Fever of unknown origin
- Glomerulonephritis
- Intra-abdominal infections
- Meningitis
- Myocardial infarction
- Osteomyelitis
- Pericarditis
- Salmonellosis
- Septic pulmonary infarcts
- Tuberculosis

DIAGNOSIS
Physical Examination
Common signs of endocarditis include cardiac murmur (generally new, possibly absent), an old valvular heart lesion, and embolisms.
Other physical signs include:
- Weight loss
- Neck vein distension
- Gallops
- Arrhythmia

- Pericardial rub
- Osler's nodes
- Rales
- Pleural friction rub
- Hemorrhagic or necrotic pustule
- Conjunctival hemorrhage
- Roth's spots
- Splenomegaly
- Splinter hemorrhages

Laboratory Tests
Hematologic, serologic, urine, and/or bacteremia tests may be required.

Pathological Findings
Repeated positive blood cultures are the primary indicator of endocarditis. (Antibiotics can make cultures falsely negative.)
- Elevated erythrocyte sedimentation rate
- Hematuria (gross or microscopic)
- Blood in sputum (from septic pulmonary emboli)
- Positive echocardiography for vegetations, abscess, valve dehiscence
- Emboli and/or infarction in body organs
- Abscesses and microabscesses in body organs
- Embolic and/or immune-complex glomerulonephritis in kidneys
- Valvular endocardium destruction
- Valve leaflet perforation
- Chordae tendineae rupture
- Myocardium abscesses
- Sinus of Valsalva rupture
- Pericarditis

Acute endocarditis:
- Leukocytosis

Subacute endocarditis:
- Anemia
- Leukopenia
- Decreased C3, C4, CH50
- Rheumatoid factor

Culture-negative endocarditis:
- *Chlamydia*, Q fever *(Coxiella)*, and *Bartonella*

Imaging
- Echocardiography (transesophageal/transthoracic)
- Pulmonary ventilation perfusion scan
- Cinefluoroscopy
- CAT scan
- Endoscopy

Other Diagnostic Procedures
- Cardiac catheterization
- Aortic root injection

TREATMENT OPTIONS
Treatment Strategy
Historically, endocarditis patients have been hospitalized for IV therapy (intensive care if critical and oxygen treatment, treatment for congestive heart failure, and hemodialysis is required). Oral and outpatient therapy for stable and reliable patients are being considered more frequently.

Drug Therapies
Drug treatment is generally two to six weeks of IV antibiotics. The drug of choice depends on the type of endocarditis (antibodies tested against the causal bacteria), the patient's medical conditions, and drug allergies.

Endocarditis caused by streptococci and *Streptococcus bovis* that responds to penicillin:
- Uncomplicated patients: Penicillin G plus gentamicin
- Patients older than 65 or with impairment of the eighth nerve, impairment of renal function, heart failure, or CNS complications: Penicillin G only
- Patients nutritionally deficient, in relapse, or with complications (e.g., shock, extracardiac focus): Penicillin G plus gentamicin
- Patients with penicillin allergy: Vancomycin or cefazolin

Endocarditis caused by strains of streptococci and *Streptococcus bovis* resistant to penicillin:
- Patients with prosthetic valve infection: Penicillin G plus gentamicin
- Patients with penicillin allergy who should avoid gentamicin: Vancomycin or cefazolin

Endocarditis caused by *Enterococci:*
- Uncomplicated patients: Penicillin G plus gentamicin
- Patients with penicillin allergy: Vancomycin and gentamicin

Endocarditis caused by *Staphylococcus aureus*
- Patients with methicillin-susceptible strain: Nafcillin and gentamicin
- Patients with methicillin-susceptible strain but significant renal impairment: Nafcillin
- Patients with methicillin-resistant strain or penicillin allergy: Vancomycin
- Patients with penicillin allergy: Cefazolin or oxacillin
- Patients with prosthetic valve infected with methicillin-susceptible strain: oxacillin or nafcillin and rifampin and gentamicin
- Patients with prosthetic valve infected with methicillin-resistant strain: vancomyein and rifampin and gentamicin

Endocarditis caused by coagulase-negative staphylococci or prosthetic valve infection:
- Patients with methicillin-susceptible strain: Nafcillin and rifampin and gentamicin
- Patients with methicillin-resistant strain: Vancomycin and rifampin and gentamicin
- Patients with methicillin-resistant strain and penicillin allergy: Vancomycin and rifampin and gentamicin

Endocarditis caused by HACEK organisms:
- Uncomplicated patients: Ampicillin and gentamicin
- Patients with penicillin allergy: Ceftriaxone

Complementary and Alternative Therapies
Endocarditis has serious ramifications and requires aggressive medical treatment. Alternative therapies may be used concurrently to help support immune function, reduce severity, duration, and progression of disease, as well as improve overall cardiac health.

NUTRITION
- Avoid foods that may compromise optimal health such as refined foods, sugar, and saturated fats (meat and dairy products).
- To support immune function, include vitamins C (1,000 mg up to tid), E (400 to 800 IU/day), A (10,000 IU/day) or beta carotene (100,000 IU/day), selenium (200 mcg/day), and zinc (30 mg/day).
- Coenzyme Q10 (100mg bid) is a powerful antioxidant and has cardio-protective properties.
- Magnesium (200 to 500 mg bid to tid) is essential for normal cardiac function. Magnesium is contraindicated if the patient has kidney damage.
- Bromelain (250 to 500 mg tid between meals) is a proteolytic enzyme which may increase the effectiveness of antibiotic therapy.

HERBS

Herbs are generally a safe way to strengthen and tone the body's systems. As with any therapy, it is important to ascertain a diagnosis before pursuing treatment. Herbs may be used as dried extracts (capsules, powders, teas), glycerites (glycerine extracts), or tinctures (alcohol extracts). Unless otherwise indicated, teas should be made with 1 tsp. of herb per cup of hot water. Steep covered 5 to 10 minutes for leaf or flowers, and 10 to 20 minutes for roots. Drink 2 to 4 cups/day. Tinctures may be used singly or in combination as noted. The goals of herbal therapies are to fight infection, enhance immune function, reduce cardiac damage, and restore the integrity of cardiac tissue.

- For long-term cardiac support combine the following herbs in a tea (3 cups/day) or tincture (30 to 60 drops tid): 2 parts of hawthorn (*Crataegus oxyacantha*) with 1 part each of motherwort (*Leonorus cardiaca*) and linden flowers (*Tilia cordata*). Use additional herbs from the following categories as needed.
- Cardiac arrhythmias: Add 1 part each of lily of the valley (*Convalleria majus*) and night-blooming cereus (*Cactus grandiflorus*) to the cardiac formula above. These herbs must be used with caution and under a health care provider's supervision. Side effects may include nausea, vomiting, headache, and cardiac arrhythmias.
- Hawthorne berry (*Crataegus laevigata*) can be helpful in promoting cardiac output and decreasing arrhythmias. Use $^1/_2$ tsp. of the solid extract, or 1,000 mg tid.
- Infection: Combine equal parts of four to six of the following herbs: coneflower (*Echinacea purpura*), goldenseal root (*Hydrastis canadensis*), wild indigo (*Baptisia tinctoria*), myrrh (*Commiphora molmol*), garlic (*Allium sativum*), rosemary (*Rosemariana officinalis*). For acute infection take 60 drops of tincture every 2 hours. For chronic infections or for prophylaxis, take 30 to 60 drops tid.
- Renal involvement: Combine equal parts of bearberry (*Arctostaphylos uva ursi*), cleavers (*Galium aparine*), dandelion leaf (*Taraxecum officinalis*), black cohosh (*Cimicifuga racemosa*), yarrow (*Achillea millefolium*), and corn silk (*Zea mays*). Drink as a tea 3 cups/day. Flax oil or fish oil (3 to 5 g bid) is also helpful to decrease inflammation in the kidney.

HOMEOPATHY

An experienced homeopath should assess individual constitutional types and severity of disease to select the correct remedy and potency. For acute prescribing use 3 to 5 pellets of a 12X to 30C remedy every one to four hours until acute symptoms resolve.

- *Aconite* if patient fears death, has tachycardia with full, hard bounding pulse of sudden onset.
- *Cactus grandiflorus* for endocarditis with mitral insufficiency. Patient has feeble, irregular pulse and feels a constriction as if an iron band is around the chest.
- *Digitalis* if patient has irregular pulse with a sensation as if the heart would stop if they moved. Pulse is quickened by the least movement and patient feels compelled to walk.
- *Spongia* if patient has a sensation of the heart swelling as if it would explode; especially for hypertrophy of the heart and valvular insufficiency.

ACUPUNCTURE

May improve immunity and strengthen cardiac function.

PATIENT MONITORING

Bedrest initially, ambulation after clinical improvement. Patient follow up is critical to assess for relapse, determine if another course of antibiotics (or surgery) is required, and avoid complications.

Blood levels should be performed if gentamicin is used for more than five days or with renal dysfunction, and BUN and serum creatine should be performed twice a week while the drug is being administered. For patients receiving vancomycin, blood levels should be performed with renal dysfunction. Audiometry baseline and periodic testing is advisable with long-term aminoglycoside therapy.

OTHER CONSIDERATIONS

Prevention
Prophylaxis antibiotics for medical procedures that could cause transient bacteremia (see "Risk Factors") may be advantageous, although the effectiveness of this practice is unproven. Also, discuss the importance of dental hygiene with endocarditis patients and avoid having dental caries treated during endocarditis treatment.

Complications/Sequelae
- Cardiologic: congestive heart failure, sinus of Valsalva aneurysm, aortic root abscesses, myocardial abscesses, myocardial infarction, pericarditis, cardiac arrhythmia, arterial emboli
- Neurologic: stroke, hemorrhage, brain abscesses, meningitis, cerebral emboli
- Other: septic pulmonary infarcts, splenic infarcts, glomerulonephritis, acute renal failure, mesenteric infarct

Prognosis
The prognosis of endocarditis depends on its complications. For streptococcal endocarditis, patients usually exhibit a negative blood culture quickly, with a clinical response within two days; for staphylococcal endocarditis, fever and positive blood culture may continue for up to 10 days after treatment begins. Endocarditis mortality is about 20%.

Pregnancy
Gentamicin should be avoided or used with caution during pregnancy. Herbs containing berberine (e.g., goldenseal) are not recommended during pregnancy.

REFERENCES

Barker LR, Burton JR, Zieve PD, eds. *Principles of Ambulatory Medicine.* 4th ed. Baltimore, Md: Williams & Wilkins; 1995:379–381.

Bartram T. *Encyclopedia of Herbal Medicine.* Dorset, England: Grace Publishers; 1995:99,167–168,220.

Dambro MR. *Griffith's 5-Minute Clinical Consult–1999.* Baltimore, Md: Lippincott Williams & Wilkins; 1999:358–361.

Endocarditis: a rare but serious disease. *Drug Ther Perspect.* 1998;12(4):6–9.

Gruenwald J, Brendler T, Jaenicke C et al, eds. *PDR for Herbal Medicines.* Montvale, NJ: Medical Economics Company; 1998:772–773, 1130–1131.

Kruzel T. *The Homeopathic Emergency Guide.* Berkeley, Calif: North Atlantic Books; 1992:58–61.

Murray MT. *Encyclopedia of Nutritional Supplements.* Rocklin, Calif: Prima Publishing; 1996:401,404, 463–464.

Snow JM. Hydrastis canadensis L. (Ranunculaceae). *The Protocol Journal of Botanical Medicine.* 1997;2:25–28.

Stein JK, ed. *Internal Medicine.* 4th ed. St. Louis, Mo: Mosby-Year Book; 1994:189–201.

Stoller JK, Ahmad M, Longworth DL, eds. *The Cleveland Clinic Intensive Review of Internal Medicine.* Baltimore, Md: Williams & Wilkins; 1998:137–141,299.

Walker LP, Brown EH. *The Alternative Pharmacy.* Paramus, NJ: Prentice Hall Press; 1998:239–240.

Werbach MR. *Nutritional Influences on Illness.* New Canaan, Conn: Keats Publishing, Inc; 1987:252–262.

■ ENDOMETRIOSIS

OVERVIEW

Definition

Endometriosis, in which functioning ectopic endometrial glands and stroma are present outside the uterine cavity, affects 5% of American women of childbearing age. Extrapelvic manifestations develop primarily in the 35-to-40 age group. Usually accompanied by chronic or acute pelvic pain which may radiate to the buttocks and perianal region, endometriosis develops gradually. The condition is underdiagnosed (often mistaken for dysmenorrhea) and is present in 30% of infertile women.

While etiology remains uncertain, retrograde menstruation, genetic predisposition, and immune system involvement are widely accepted theories. Because ectopic endometrial implants respond to exogenous and endogenous hormones, medical treatment aims at suppressing estrogen production to bring about amenorrhea, which halts retrograde menstruation and promotes decidualization and atrophy of implants.

Endometriosis is "staged" as either:
- Mild—small, localized implants
- Moderate—larger, more extensive implants; scar tissue may be present
- Severe—large, widespread implants; extensive scar tissue

Etiology

Etiology uncertain; three major theories are widely accepted:
- Immunoincompetence: increased macrophage, prostaglandin, and lymphokine action; decreased T- and NK-cell responsiveness. (Studies indicate that TCDD [dioxin], an environmental toxicant, alters the action of estrogen in reproductive organs and increases incidence of endometriosis.)
- Retrograde (or reflux) menstruation: transtubal dissemination of endometrial cells into pelvic cavity; lymphatic and/or vascular transportation to remote areas.
- Genetic predisposition/congenital defect: Cells intended to be part of the female reproductive system fail to migrate to the appropriate locations and become embedded in inappropriate locations. Under estrogen stimulation, they differentiate into functioning endometrial glands and stroma.

Risk Factors

- Genetic predisposition (daughters of mothers having the disorder)
- Reproductive age

Signs and Symptoms

Endometriosis is asymptomatic in one-third of cases. Symptoms typically begin several years after onset of menses, progress as ectopic endometrial deposits increase, and subside after menopause. Most common symptoms include:
- Pelvic pain cycling with menses (not always related to severity of disorder)
- Dysmenorrhea
- Dyspareunia
- Infertility
- Pain with bladder/bowel function
- Intestinal pain
- Tenderness when affected areas are palpated

DIFFERENTIAL DIAGNOSIS

- Abortion (including complete, incomplete, threatened, septic)
- Crohn's disease
- Irritable bowel
- Appendicitis
- Bowel obstruction, irritable bowel syndrome
- Dysmenorrhea
- Ectopic pregnancy
- Gastric/peptic ulcers
- Ovarian cysts/torsion
- Pelvic inflammatory disease (PID)
- Urinary obstruction, urinary tract infection (UTI)

DIAGNOSIS

Physical Examination

- Nonspecific pelvic/adnexal ovarian tenderness
- Nodular masses along uterosacral ligaments, posterior uterus
- Obliteration of cul-de-sac with fixed uterine retroversion (extensive disease)
- Ruptured ovarian endometriomas (acute abdomen)
- Adhesions/obstruction of rectum/GI tract

Laboratory Tests

For differential diagnosis:
- CBC/differentials: PID
- Urinalysis: UTI
- Cervical gram stain/culture: PID
- Beta HCG: ectopic pregnancy

Pathological Findings

Cyclic bleeding of ectopic endometrial tissue produces lesions/implants which have been found in every extrapelvic organ system except the spleen, including lungs, CNS, kidneys, GI tract. Also found in rectum, bladder, vagina, cervix, vulva, thigh, and arm. Most frequently involved sites are:
- Ovaries
- Fallopian tubes
- Broad and uterosacral ligaments
- Bladder
- Area between the vagina and rectum
- External surface of the uterus
- Cul-de-sac

Imaging

Ultrasound/MRI to detect pelvic masses (low sensitivity to detection of ectopic endometrial deposits, however).

Other Diagnostic Procedures

- Medical history
- Physical examination (exclude life-threatening etiology of abdominal pain)
- Laparoscopy (essential for confirmation)
- CA 125 (ineffective for screening, however).

TREATMENT OPTIONS

Treatment Strategy

Appropriate and early diagnosis and aggressive treatment prevent significant complications and sequelae.

Drug Therapies

Drug therapy is intended for pain relief and hormone suppression.
- NSAIDs/narcotics
- Combined oral contraceptives
- Estrogen/progestin androgens—suppress (FSH) and (LH) and endogenous estrogen production
- Progestational agents—acetate, norethynodrel, megestrol acetate,

dydrogesterone, norethisterone, lynestrenol (may cause irregular vaginal bleeding, bloating, or depression)

- Danazol (synthetic 3-isoxazole derivative of 17 ethinyl-testosterone)—most frequent choice for hormone suppression; reduces size/extent of lesions with 80% to 90% symptom relief and 20% to 35% recurrence rate after treatment cessation (unsafe for developing fetus; common side effects synonymous with menopause)
- Gonadotropin-releasing hormone agonist (GnRHa)—induces amenorrhea (loss of bone mineral precludes long-term therapy). Nafarelin (Synarel), Leuprolide (Lupron), Goserelin acetate implant.

Surgical Procedures

- Laparoscopic laser/electrocoagulating techniques—for destruction of implants, excision of ovarian endometriomas, and lysis of adhesions (10% to 50% recurrence rate within 12 months)
- Total hysterectomy/bilateral salphingo-oophorectomy—90% effective for pain relief (recommended only when essential and when child-bearing is no longer desired)

Complementary and Alternative Therapies

Providing liver support is the backbone of alternative treatment of endometriosis. Enhancing the liver's ability to metabolize hormones may help restore normal hormone ratios. Endometriosis is best treated early and alternative therapies alone may not be sufficient to eradicate this condition.

NUTRITION

- Eliminate all known food allergens. The most common allergens are dairy, wheat, citrus, corn, soy, and fish.
- Eliminate alcohol, caffeine, chocolate, refined foods, food additives, sugar, and saturated fats (meats and dairy products).
- Avoid exogenous estrogens found in estrogen-fed poultry and pesticide-sprayed fruits and vegetables. Eat only organic poultry and produce.
- Increase intake of whole grains, fresh vegetables, essential fatty acids (cold-water fish, nuts, and seeds), and vegetable proteins (legumes such as soy). Include liberal amounts of liver-supporting foods such as beets, carrots, onions, garlic, dark leafy greens, artichokes, apples, and lemons.
- Vitamin C (1,000 mg tid) decreases inflammation and supports immune function.
- Zinc (30 to 50 mg/day) and Beta carotene (50,000 to 100,000 IU/day) support immune function and enhance healing.
- Vitamin E (400 IU/day) is necessary for hormone production and is an antioxidant.
- Selenium (200 mcg/day) is needed for fatty acid metabolism.
- Iron supplementation may be necessary if bleeding is severe. Elemental iron (30 mg bid). Glycinate form is least constipating and 30% better absorbed than ferrous sulphate.
- Calcium (1,000 to 1,500 mg/day) and magnesium (200 mg bid to tid) are needed for hormone metabolism and to modulate inflammation.
- Essential fatty acids (1,000 to 1,500 mg bid) to support hormone production and decrease inflammation.

HERBS

Herbs are generally a safe way to strengthen and tone the body's systems. As with any therapy, it is important to ascertain a diagnosis before pursuing treatment. Herbs may be used as dried extracts (capsules, powders, teas), glycerites (glycerine extracts), or tinctures (alcohol extracts). Unless otherwise indicated, teas should be made with 1 tsp. herb per cup of hot water. Steep covered 5 to 10 minutes for leaf or flowers, and 10 to 20 min-

utes for roots. Drink 2 to 4 cups/day. Tinctures may be used singly or in combination as noted.

Chaste tree *(Vitex agnus-cactus)* helps to normalize pituitary function and balance estrogen/progesterone ratios. This herb may need to be taken long term (12 to 18 months) for maximum effectiveness. Combine 2 parts of chaste tree with 1 part of two herbs from each category. Herbs are listed in order of preference. Drink 3 cups of tea/day or take 30 to 60 drops of tincture/day.

For liver support (include milk thistle with one other herb from this section): Milk thistle *(Silybum marianum),* dandelion root *(Taraxacum officinalis),* vervain *(Verbena hastata),* and/or blue flag *(Iris versicolor)* support the liver and may help restore hormone ratios. Use vervain with nervousness and anxiety; blue flag, for poor fat digestion and liver congestion; dandelion, for fluid retention.

For reducing pelvic congestion: Squaw vine *(Mitchella repens),* motherwort *(Leonorus cardiaca),* red root (Ceonothus americanus), red raspberry *(Rubus idaeus).* Red raspberry may be used alone and drunk as a tea (2 to 3 cups/day) throughout treatment.

Herbal therapy may also be used to treat acute pain during menstruation. Combine equal parts of the following herbs in a tea ($^1/_2$ cup every three to four hours) or tincture (15 drops every 15 minutes for up to eight doses acutely or 30 to 60 drops tid to qid): black cohosh *(Cimicifuga racemosa),* wild yam *(Dioscorea villosa),* Jamaican dogwood *(Piscidia erythrina),* ginger root *(Zingiber officinalis),* cramp bark *(Viburnum opulus),* and valerian *(Valeriana officinalis).* In cases of excessive menstrual flow, substitute yarrow *(Achillea millefolium)* for ginger root.

For management of severe pain and extensive endometriosis, Turska's formula is the preferred combination and should only be used under physician supervision. The formula contains two parts of poke root *(Phytolacca americana),* and one part each of monkshood *(Aconitum nappelus),* gelsemium *(Gelsemium sempeverins),* and white bryony *(Bryonia alba).* These herbs have anodyne properties and may help shrink endometrial tissue. They have toxic side effects and are used at very low doses (10 to 15 drops bid).

HOMEOPATHY

An experienced homeopath should assess individual constitutional types and severity of disease to select the correct remedy and potency. For acute prescribing use 3 to 5 pellets of a 12X to 30C remedy every one to four hours until acute symptoms resolve.

- *Belladonna* for menstruation with sensation of heaviness and heat in abdomen. Patient may be restless, thirstless, and sensitive to drafts.
- *Calcarea phosphoricum* for excessive and too frequent menses with violent backache.
- *Chamomilla* for heavy menses with dark clotted blood and labor-like pains. Patient may be irritable, thirsty, and oversensitive to pains that radiate to the thighs.
- *Cimicifuga racemosa* for profuse, dark, coagulated menstrual blood with unbearable pain radiating from hip to hip.

PHYSICAL MEDICINE

Do not perform these therapies during menstrual flow.

- Contrast sitz baths may relieve symptoms and promote circulation, reducing pelvic congestion. You will need two basins that can be comfortably sat in. Fill one basin with hot water, one with cold water. Sit in hot water for three minutes, then in cold water for one minute. Repeat this three times to complete one set. Do one to two sets per day, three to four days per week.

- Castor oil pack. Used externally, castor oil is a powerful anti-inflammatory. Apply oil directly to abdomen, cover with a clean soft cloth (e.g., flannel) and plastic wrap. Place a heat source (hot water bottle or heating pad) over the pack and let sit for 30 to 60 minutes. For best results use three consecutive days. Adding a few drops of St. John's wort oil (*Hypericum perforatum,* four to six drops) may potentiate the pain-relieving effects. One or more essential oils (four to six drops) can be added to increase circulation and enhance relaxation. Essential oils to consider include clary sage, rose maroc, geranium, or nutmeg.
- Kegel excercises should be performed frequently, up to 100 times/day to improve pelvic tone.

ACUPUNCTURE

Chinese herbal formulas may have profound effects on liver function and hormone balance. Acupuncture may resolve excesses and deficiencies associated with endometriosis.

MASSAGE

Therapeutic massage not only increases the overall sense of well-being but it may help resolve pelvic congestion. To enhance the benefit of massage, add three to four drops of essential oils (see castor oil pack) to one tbsp. massage oil. Particular attention should be paid to the sacral area.

Patient Monitoring
- Monitoring for side effects/effectiveness of treatment
- Track bone density during hormone treatment

OTHER CONSIDERATIONS

Exercise, swimming, relaxation/meditation/visualization, yoga, polarity therapy, magnet therapy, reflexology, Schuessler tissue salts, and Kegel exercises may relieve symptoms of endometriosis.

Complications/Sequelae
- Infertility
- Chronic pelvic pain
- Infection from ruptured ovarian lesions
- Adhesions/obstructions
- Progression into infection/abscesses
- Drug therapy reactions

Prognosis
- Progressive after onset of menses
- Complete regression may be seen during pregnancy and following menopause

Pregnancy
- Pregnancy is postponed during hormonal therapy.
- Danazol unsafe for developing fetus
- Although no definite cause-effect relationship, other disease is present in 30% of infertile women.
- Endometriosis often resolves during pregnancy because of sustained, increased progesterone and decreased estrogen levels. Treatment should be delayed until after breastfeeding has been discontinued.

REFERENCES

Facts About Endometriosis. U.S. Department of Health and Human Services. National Institutes of Child Health and Human Development. NIH Publication no. 91-2413.

Kruzel T. *The Homeopathic Emergency Guide.* Berkeley, Calif: North Atlantic Books; 1992:112–114.

Medicines from the Earth. Harvard, Mass: Gaia Herbal Research Institute; 1997:182–183.

Protocol Journal of Botanical Medicine. 1996;1:30–46.

Tureck RW. Endometriosis: diagnosis and initial treatment. *Hospital Physician Obstetrics and Gynecology Board Review Manual.* April 1997;3:1–8.

■ FEVER OF UNKNOWN ORIGIN
OVERVIEW
Definition
By at least one definition, when a fever of more than 101°F (38.3°C) occurs on several occasions over three weeks without identification of its cause despite extensive investigation for at least a week, it becomes a fever of unknown origin (FUO). There are other definitions specific to institutional protocols, which include (a) 2 weeks of fever with either 3 days of inpatient assessment or 3 outpatient visits, and (b) fever on at least 4 occasions over a 2 week period and 2 weeks of illness. Difficult-to-diagnose fevers have several potential underlying causes, including infections, autoimmune diseases, and undiscovered cancers. Between 5% and 15% of FUOs remain undiagnosed.

To determine the underlying cause of a FUO, take careful note of the patient's history and symptoms. Recent travel to regions endemic for specific infections provides clues, as does a history of drinking contaminated water. The diagnostic path should include repeated physical examinations, laboratory evaluations, noninvasive methods such as sonography, and invasive diagnostic techniques such as biopsy.

The inability to diagnose FUO creates a dilemma regarding treatment. Experimental evidence suggests that elevated temperatures benefit patients by enhancing the body's defense mechanisms. However, clinical studies have not conclusively supported that position.

Treat fevers in children susceptible to febrile seizures. Also provide therapy to adults with cardiac or pulmonary conditions, as increases in body temperature reduce oxygen consumption.

Etiology
Unknown by definition, but most probably due to infection, neoplasm, vascular disease, or other endocrine, occupational, or environmental causes. Provider must rely on patient's present and previous symptoms and diseases, current medications, exposure to infections, recent travel, and other diagnostic clues. Efforts to identify the cause of any fever start with the patient's medical history and move on through physical examination, blood tests, noninvasive diagnostic techniques, and invasive methods.

Risk Factors
- Recent travel, especially overseas
- Exposure to malaria, which can cause fever every second or third day
- Exposure to certain fungi, such as coccidioidomycosis in the southwestern United States and histoplasmosis in the Ohio River and Mississippi River valleys
- Drinking contaminated water or consuming ice made from such water, which may indicate typhoid fever
- Working in a meat-packing plant, which can harbor brucellosis
- Use of medications that cause feverish adverse reactions
- Drug use or abuse
- AIDS

Signs and Symptoms
- Fever of more than 101°F (38.3°C), either continuous or intermittent, for at least two weeks
- Fever above 101°F whose identity remains unknown even after extensive diagnostic testing
- Accompanying headache, myalgia, and general malaise

DIFFERENTIAL DIAGNOSIS
There is a long list of potential causes, including the many forms of infection, neoplasms, vascular disease, endocrine disorders, and environmental or occupational insults.

DIAGNOSIS
Physical Examination
Concentrate on the skin, eyes, nail beds, lymph nodes, heart, and abdomen to obtain the best clues to the fever's origin. Repeat the examinations frequently as the fever progresses undiagnosed. Take a thorough history. Inquire about exposure to malaria. Determine whether the patient's workplace might harbor infective agents. Check whether the patient has drunk contaminated water. Consider the possibility that a medication has caused the fever.

Laboratory Tests
CBC for anemia, leukopenia, lymphocytosis, thrombocytosis. Liver function tests for obstructive diseases and inflammation. Blood cultures for aerobic or anaerobic pathogens. Other body fluids and tissue for bacteria, mycobacteria, and fungi. Urine analysis for infection or malignancy in urinary tract. Serology for CMV, infectious mononucleosis, HIV, toxoplasmosis, and chlamydia.

Pathological Findings
Dependent on etiology

Imaging
Ultrasound can reveal the presence of cardiac vegetations, as well as abnormalities in the pancreas, liver, and gallbladder. Computed tomography and magnetic resonance imaging can help detect intra-abdominal abscesses, abnormalities in the lymph nodes, and pathology of the spleen, liver, kidneys, adrenals, pancreas, heart, mediastinum, or pelvis. Scanning with radionuclide tracers (especially gallium) may identify localized areas of infection or inflammation.

Other Diagnostic Procedures
- Skin tests and sputum/urine cultures
- HIV antibody, thyroid, and rheumatoid factor tests
- Biopsy liver, bone marrow, or other suspected sites if other tests have failed to produce a definitive diagnosis.

TREATMENT OPTIONS
Treatment Strategy
Debate surrounds the issue of whether or not to treat fever, particularly when its source remains unknown. Advise rest, avoidance of rapid changes in ambient temperature, and drinking large amounts of fluids. Prescribe antipyretics for children who have suffered febrile seizures and adults with heart or lung insufficiencies, who can be endangered by the excess demand for oxygen brought on by the fever. Expect increased caloric and fluid demands. Also, treat patients with organic brain syndrome; fever can cause changes in their mental status. Wise treatment requires all possible efforts to identify the fever's origin.

Drug Therapies
Use appropriate antipyretics where necessary to control the fever:
- Acetaminophen
- Aspirin and other nonsteroidal anti-inflammatory drugs. Avoid prescribing aspirin for children and teenagers, because it increases the risk of Reye's syndrome.

If examination indicates the presence of infection, prescribe appropriate agents based on patient history. A wide variety of anti-infective drugs exists, tailored to specific types of infection. These include antibiotics, and antimicrobial, antifungal, and antiviral agents. Note that the drugs have less effect in patients with severely impaired immune systems. A steroid trial may be considered, although consider detrimental effects with certain undiagnosed conditions.

Complementary and Alternative Therapies

General immune support with nutrition and herbs may alleviate fevers of unknown origin. Homeopathic remedies may provide relief.

NUTRITION

- Eliminate alcohol, caffeine, refined foods, and sugar which have an immunosuppressive effect.
- Water and/or electrolyte replacement drinks should be increased to prevent dehydration.
- Vitamin C (250 to 1,000 mg bid to tid), beta-carotene (15,000 to 50,000 IU/day), and zinc (10 to 30 mg/day) enhance immunity and reduce inflammation.

HERBS

Herbs are generally a safe way to strengthen and tone the body's systems. As with any therapy, it is important to ascertain a diagnosis before pursuing treatment. Herbs may be used as dried extracts (capsules, powders, teas), glycerites (glycerine extracts), or tinctures (alcohol extracts). Unless otherwise indicated, teas should be made with one teaspoon herb per cup of hot water. Steep covered 5 to 10 minutes for leaf or flowers, and 10 to 20 minutes for roots. Drink 2 to 4 cups/day. Tinctures may be used singly or in combination as noted.

The following anti-pyretic herbs and immune supportive herbs may be helpful in reducing fever and improving immunity: Coneflower *(Echinacea purpura)*, yarrow *(Achillea millefolium)*, white willow bark *(Salix alba)*, lemon balm *(Melissa officinalis)*, spearmint *(Mentha spicata)*, catnip *(Nepeta cateria)*, and elder *(Sambucus canadensis)*. Combine one part of coneflower and one part white willow bark with equal parts of two or more herbs. Drink three to four cups/day, two to four ounces tid to qid for children.

HOMEOPATHY

An experienced homeopath should assess individual constitutional types and severity of disease to select the correct remedy and potency. For acute prescribing use three to five pellets of a 12X to 30C remedy every one to four hours until acute symptoms resolve.

- *Aconite* when fever comes on suddenly and alternates with chills, heat, and flushing of the face. There is thirst for cold drinks, with anxiety.
- *Apis mellifica* for fever with alternating sweats and dry heat.
- *Belladonna* for sudden onset of high fever with hot, red face, glassy eyes, thirstlessness, and hot body with cold hands.
- *Bryonia* for fever with marked aggravation from the slightest movement.

ACUPUNCTURE

Acupuncture may be helpful in supporting immune function.

Patient Monitoring

Continue to examine patient and take blood for culturing until the cause of the fever becomes evident. A thoughtful, individualized approach to the patient eventually identifies the cause in most cases.

OTHER CONSIDERATIONS

Prevention

Caution with international travel and exposure to obvious contaminants will reduce likelihood of acquiring certain causative pathogens.

Complications/Sequelae

Dependent on etiology. Before any surgeries, patient should inform staff of history of fever of unknown origin.

Prognosis

Dependent on etiology, patient age, and other compromise

Pregnancy

Left untreated, fever can be dangerous to the fetus. Nutritional, herbal, and homeopathic support for fevers are generally safe in pregnancy, yet use with caution.

REFERENCES

Bartram T. *Encyclopedia of Herbal Medicine.* Dorset, England: Grace Publishers; 1995:182.

Berkow R. *Merck Manual, Home Edition.* Rahway, NJ: The Merck Publishing Group; 1997.

Berkow R, Beers MH. *The Merck Manual of Diagnosis and Therapy.* Rahway, NJ: The Merck Publishing Group; 1992.

Blumenthal M, ed. *The Complete German Commission E Monographs.* Boston, Mass: Integrative Medicine Communications; 1998:427.

Duke JA. *The Green Pharmacy.* Emmaus, Pa: Rodale Press, 1997.

Morrison R. *Desktop Guide to Keynotes and Confirmatory Symptoms.* Albany, Calif: Hahnemann Clinic Publishing; 1993:6, 58, 62.

Walker LP, Hodgson Brown E. *The Alternative Pharmacy.* Paramus, NJ: Prentice Hall Press; 1996.

■ FIBROMYALGIA

OVERVIEW

Definition

Fibromyalgia syndrome (FMS) is characterized by three cardinal symptoms: widespread musculoskeletal pain that persists for at least three months with no evidence of inflammation or muscle abnormalities; disordered sleep patterns, especially stage 4 non-rapid eye movement (NREM) sleep; and multiple tender points (11 of 18 tender points of the American College of Rheumatology Criteria for Fibromyalgia). However, FMS is not simply a muscle pain syndrome as most patients present with an array of other symptoms. Long thought to be a psychosomatic condition, FMS is now regarded as a distinct clinical disorder. Patients should know that their disease is not deforming, degenerative, life-threatening, or imaginary, and that there will be flare-ups; however, treatment is available.

Etiology

Patients with FMS often attribute a precipitating event to the initial onset of symptoms. These events include: flu-like illness, human immunodeficiency virus, Lyme disease, parvovirus B19, persistent stress, chronic sleep disturbance, and physical trauma. Studies have proposed the causative mechanisms listed below.

- Disruption of stage 4 NREM sleep by alpha-wave intrusions, which results in impaired short-term memory (and perhaps low growth hormone levels)
- Low levels of somatomedin C (mediator of growth hormone function), which alters muscle homeostasis, predisposing the patient to muscle trauma and impaired healing
- A deficiency of serotonin, a neurotransmitter that regulates pain and NREM sleep
- Increased levels of substance P, a neurotransmitter, as a result of disordered capillary blood flow, which sensitizes peripheral nociceptors to previously harmless stimuli

Risk Factors

FMS is not unique to any country, ethnic group, or climate, although the tendency to develop it may be inherited. FMS is more common in women (2% to 5% of women) and is rare in men (0.5% of men); however, some researchers think that FMS may simply be underreported in men. The prevalence of FMS increases progressively from age 18 to 80; approximately 26% of patients with FMS are over 60 years of age. Many patients with FMS report a history of psychiatric problems, most often depression, anxiety, somatization, and hypochondriasis.

Signs and Symptoms

While chronic, widespread musculoskeletal pain that waxes and wanes is the primary symptom of FMS. Features commonly associated with FMS include those listed below.

- Fatigue
- Paresthesia
- Psychological disturbances
- Postexertional pain
- Allodynia
- Restless leg syndrome
- Irritable bowel syndrome
- Joint pain without erythema and swelling
- Morning stiffness
- Raynaud's phenomenon
- Memory lapses
- Headaches
- Sleep disorders
- Dizziness

DIFFERENTIAL DIAGNOSIS

- Chronic fatigue syndrome
- Polymyalgia rheumatica
- Myofascial pain syndrome
- Multiple chemical sensitivity syndrome
- Systemic lupus erythematosus
- Rheumatoid arthritis
- Malingering
- Hypothyroidism

DIAGNOSIS

Physical Examination

The careful patient history should be taken that focuses on the timing and the conditions surrounding the presentation of symptoms, and a physical examination should be performed to exclude other disorders.

Laboratory Tests

Laboratory tests are useful only to exclude some of the disorders listed above.

Other Diagnostic Procedures

Radiographs, blood tests, and a physical examination of the joints should be performed to show that there are no abnormalities. Because FMS does not have a recognizable patho-physiolgic basis, a patient is classified as having FMS if there is a history of the symptoms listed below.

- Widespread pain for at least three months
- Pain reproduced by digital palpation of tender points
- Persistent fatigue
- Generalized morning stiffness
- Nonrestorative sleep disturbance (patients often complain of being tired on awakening)

TREATMENT OPTIONS

Treatment Strategy

There is no single treatment protocol because of the variable patient presentations. The goal of treatment is simply to maximize functional status. The nonsteroidal anti-inflammatory drugs and salicylates do not provide complete or long-lasting pain relief, though they may transiently reduce pain in some patients during flare-ups. Because FMS is not an inflammatory condition, glucocorticoids are ineffective. Narcotics may work initially but should only be used for intense flare-ups and for short periods.

Drug Therapies

- Sleep disturbances are often treated successfully with low dosages of tricyclic antidepressants (e.g., amitriptyline, 10 to 35 mg; doxepin, 10 to 25 mg; cyclobenzaprine, 2.5 to 10 mg). Often many different tricyclics must be tried because of variable response and tolerance of side effects. Benzodiazapines (e.g., alprazolam) are used if tricyclics do not work but may result in drug dependence.
- Psychological disturbances can be treated with tricyclic antidepressants (e.g., fluoxetine, 20 mg) and sedative-hypnotics (e.g., alprazolam, 0.5 to 1 mg).
- Musculoskeletal pain may be treated palliatively by lidocaine (1%) or procaine injections into trigger points. Tramadol (Ultram, 50 to 400 mg) is a relatively new drug marketed as having a low addiction potential that inhibits pain neurons; however, as an opiate its use should be limited to flare-ups only. Capsaicin is a topical agent that can be applied to areas of localized pain. Ibuprofen (400 to 800 mg bid) along with amtriptyline or cyclobenzaprine are used to alleviate pain, depression, and insomnia.

Complementary and Alternative Therapies

Nutritional support, herbs, and mind-body techniques may be particularly helpful in reducing symptoms of fibromyalgia and minimizing exacerbations.

Cognitive-behavioral therapy, support groups, meditation, visualizations, progressive muscle relaxation, tai chi, yoga, and gentle exercise may alleviate concurrent depression and/or anxiety, as well as improve coping skills, sleep, and sense of well-being.

NUTRITION

Eliminate all food allergens from the diet. The most common allergenic foods are dairy, soy, citrus, peanuts, wheat, fish, eggs, corn, and tomatoes. An elimination/challenge trial may be useful in uncovering sensitivities. Remove suspected allergens from the diet for two weeks. Reintroduce foods at the rate of one food every three days. Watch for reactions that may include gastrointestinal upset, mood changes, flushing, fatigue, and exacerbation of symptoms.

A rotation diet, in which the same food is not eaten more than once every four days, may be helpful in reducing sensitivities.

Decrease overall intake of carbohydrates. Eat protein as part of each meal and include moderate amounts of fat. The ideal ratio is approximately 30/30/40 (protein/fat/carbohydrate). Eating this way will help improve insulin sensitivity and normalize metabolism. Eliminate inflammatory foods such as refined foods, sugar, saturated fats (meat and dairy products), alcohol, and caffeine. Eat whole foods such as vegetables, whole grains, fruits, protein, and essential fatty acids (cold-water fish, nuts, and seeds).

- Vitamin C (1,000 mg tid to qid) reduces inflammation and supports immune function.
- Coenzyme Q10 (50 to 100 mg one to two times/day) improves oxygenation of tissues and has anti-oxidant activity.
- Chromium picolinate (200 mcg with meals) may reduce reactive hypoglycemia which may exacerbate symptoms.
- Magnesium (200 mg bid to tid) with malic acid (1,200 mg one to two times/day) helps to relieve pain, tenderness, and fatigue.
- 5-Hydroxytryptophan (100 mg tid) is a precursor to L-tryptophan and may help alleviate concurrent depression and insomnia. May take up to one week to be effective.
- B vitamins help reduce the effects of stress: B-complex (50 to 100 mg/day), niacinamide (100 mg/day), and B6 (100 mg/day).
- Melatonin (0.5 to 3 mg one time before bed) is a neurotransmitter secreted by the pineal gland. It is a precursor to serotonin and is needed for sound sleep.
- Zinc (30 mg/day) essential for immune function.
- Phosphatidyl choline and phosphatidyl serine (300 mg/day) may counteract the stress-induced activation of the hypothalamic-pituitary-adrenal axis and improve depression and memory.

HERBS

Herbs are generally a safe way to strengthen and tone the body's systems. As with any therapy, it is important to ascertain a diagnosis before pursuing treatment. Herbs may be used as dried extracts (capsules, powders, teas), glycerites (glycerine extracts), or tinctures (alcohol extracts). Unless otherwise indicated, teas should be made with one teaspoon herb per cup of hot water. Steep covered 5 to 10 minutes for leaf or flowers, and 10 to 20 minutes for roots. Drink 2 to 4 cups/day. Tinctures may be used singly or in combination as noted.

Note: Herbs containing salicylates may exacerbate symptoms of fibromyalgia.

Some herbs, known as adaptogens, may help increase resistance to stress and strengthen the immune system. These herbs include Siberian ginseng (*Eleuthrococcus senticosus*), schizandra berry (*Schizandra chinensis*), ashwaganda root (*Withania somnifera*), gotu kola (*Centella asiatica*), and astragalus root (*Astragalus membranaceus*). Use ginseng alone or with equal parts of 2 to 3 herbs. Take 20 to 30 drops bid to tid.

Herbs that alleviate pain and nervous tension include the following: black cohosh (*Cimicifuga racemosa*), kava kava (*Piper methysticum*), skullcap (*Scutellaria laterifolia*), passionflower (*Passiflora incarnata*), lavender (*Lavendula officinalis*), and valerian (*Valeriana officinalis*). Combine equal parts and take as a tincture 20 to 30 drops bid to tid.

Essential oils of jasmine, lemon balm, rosemary, and clary sage relieve nervous exhaustion and may be used in aromatherapy. Place several drops in a warm bath, an atomizer, or cotton ball.

HOMEOPATHY

An experienced homeopath should assess individual constitutional types and severity of disease to select the correct remedy and potency.

PHYSICAL MEDICINE

Epsom salt baths: Adding two to four cups of Epsom salts to a warm bath can soothe aching muscles.

ACUPUNCTURE

Fibromyalgia may be related to deficiencies in multiple organ systems which can be addressed with acupuncture treatment that stimulates circulation and promotes a sense of well-being.

MASSAGE

Therapeutic massage is helpful in reducing stress-related symptoms, improving circulation, and increasing the overall sense of well-being.

Patient Monitoring

A multidisciplinary team approach is essential because management of patients with FMS is extremely demanding. The importance of self-help to maximize the benefit of any treatment should be emphasized. Support groups can help patients to take control of their lives and their condition.

OTHER CONSIDERATIONS

Prevention

Symptoms are worsened by emotional stress, anxiety, medical illness, trauma, cold damp weather, overexertion, and surgery.

Complications/Sequelae

Chronic FMS may predispose the patient to greater psychological disturbances, particularly depression, anxiety, panic attacks, and poor coping mechanisms.

Prognosis

The prognosis for a full recovery for most patients with FMS is generally poor, with the severity of the disease waxing and waning over time, and only rarely remitting completely. In some cases, simple treatment of poor sleep hygiene may bring positive results.

Pregnancy

Fibromyalgia may be exacerbated in pregnancy. Dietary changes may be safely followed in pregnancy, however, nutritional supplements and herbs should be used only with caution.

REFERENCES

Abraham GE, Flechas JG. Management of fibromyalgia: rationale for the use of magnesium and malic acid. *J Nutr Med.* 1992;3:49–59.

Caruso I, Sarzi Puttini P, Cazzola M, et al. Double-blind study of 5-hydroxytryptophan versus placebo in the treatment of primary fibromyalgia syndrome. *J Int Med Res.* 1990;18:201–209.

Chaitow L. *Fibromyalgia: the muscle pain epidemic.* Part I. Available at: www.healty.net/library/articles/chaitow/fibromy/fibro1.htm.

Fauci AS, Braunwald E, Isselbacher KJ et al, eds. *Harrison's Principles of Internal Medicine.* 14th ed. New York, NY: McGraw-Hill; 1998:1955–1957.

Holland NW, Gonzalez EB. Soft tissue problems in older adults. *Clin Geriatr Med.* 1998;14:601–603.

Kelley WN, ed. *Textbook of Rheumatology.* 5th ed. Philadelphia, Pa: WB Saunders; 1997:511–518.

Koopman WJ. *Arthritis and Allied Conditions: A Textbook of Rheumatology.* 13th ed. Baltimore, Md: Williams & Wilkins; 1993:1619–1635.

Nicolodi M, Sicuteri F. Fibromyalgia and migraine, two faces of the same mechanism. Serotonin as the common clue for pathogenesis and therapy. *Adv Exp Med Biol.* 1996;398:373–379.

Romano TJ, Stiller JW. Magnesium deficiency in fibromyalgia syndrome. *J Nutri Med.* 1994;4:165–167.

Russell IJ. Fibromyalgia syndrome: formulating a strategy for relief. *J Musculoskel Med.* 1998;November:4–21.

Starlanyl D, Copeland M. *Fibromyalgia and Chronic Myofascial Pain Syndrome: A Survival Manual.* Oakland, Calif: New Harbinger Publications Inc; 1996:215–224, 227–235.

Tyler VE. *Herbs of Choice: The Therapeutic Use of Phytomedicinals.* New York, NY: Haworth Press; 1994.

Wolfe F, Smyth HA, Yunus MB, et al. American College of Rheumatology 1990 Criteria for the Classification of Fibromyalgia: report of the Multicenter Criteria Committee. *Arthritis Rheum.* 1990;33:160–172.

■ FOOD ALLERGY
OVERVIEW
Definition
A food allergy occurs when the body's immune system responds to otherwise benign proteins (allergens) as though they threatened the health and integrity of the system. In a classic reaction, the immune system attempts to counter the food allergens by stimulating IgE antibodies. When these antibodies react with the allergen, histamine and other chemicals (mediators) are released. This process then gives rise to such allergic symptoms as itching, swelling, hives, and breathing difficulties. While most food allergies are mild, in some cases, they can cause anaphylactic shock. Because this type of reaction can be life threatening, food allergies must be taken seriously.

Approximately 5% of children younger than age 3 have food allergies. As many as two out of five Americans believe that they have allergies to certain foods. According to the National Institute of Allergy and Infectious diseases, fewer than 2%—about 4 million Americans—have true food allergies.

The majority of adverse reactions to food are caused by nonimmulogic mediated mechanisms. Also called food intolerance or food hypersensitivity, adverse food reactions can occur because a person lacks the enzymes needed for proper digestion, such as for the lactose in milk, or has a sensitivity to such common preservatives and additives as monosodium glutamate (MSG), sulfites, and gluten. Some adverse reactions are caused by food-borne microbial pathogens and toxins.

Etiology
Foods that most commonly cause allergic reactions include peanuts, tree nuts, milk, eggs, soy, fish, shellfish, wheat, some fruits, seeds, and chocolate. Food allergies arise when a genetic sensitivity is coupled with environmental exposure.

Risk Factors
- Family history of allergies, asthma, or atopic dermatitis
- Personal history of asthma, atopic dermatitis, or other allergies

Signs and Symptoms
- Patches of swelling (urticaria, angioedema), atopic dermatitis, hives
- Swelling or itching lips, tongue, and mouth
- Itching or tightness in the throat
- Runny and itchy nose
- Headache
- Nausea, cramping, vomiting, flatulence, diarrhea
- Respiratory distress

The following symptoms should be treated as a medical emergency.
- Immediate and extreme facial swelling and itching
- Breathing difficulties
- Rapid increase in heart rate
- Rapid drop in blood pressure
- Tightening of the throat
- Sudden hoarseness

DIFFERENTIAL DIAGNOSIS
- Food intolerance or food poisoning
- Seasonal or environmental allergies or asthma
- Mononucleosis
- Viral hepatitis
- Parasitic infection
- Urticarial vasculitis
- Skin malignancy
- Connective tissue disease

DIAGNOSIS
Physical Examination
Physical assessment includes noting characteristic symptoms, signs, and pattern of reaction, as well as a history of past exposures and reactions to related foods.

Laboratory Tests
The blood tests radioallergosorbent (RAST) and enzyme-linked immunosorbent assay (ELISA) are generally more useful in ruling out a food allergy than diagnosing one.

Pathological Findings
- Blood tests reveal elevated levels of IgE antibodies or the presence of eosinophilia.

Imaging
In rare cases of gastric inflammation, an upper GI series may be needed.

Other Diagnostic Procedures
Assess the likelihood of a more serious reaction through the examination, patient's history, and description of reaction pattern to certain foods. Further tests may be needed to assess patient's overall susceptibility to food and other allergies. Suggest that patient keep a food diary that tracks eating habits, medications, and adverse reactions.
- Elimination trial, supervised by health care provider. See "Nutrition" section.
- Skin tests that measure a person's reactions to superficial contact with suspected allergens can determine or rule out a food allergy.
- Challenge or provocative testing involves placing food extracts under the tongue or injecting them under the skin. However, this test tends to be expensive and unreliable. Provoking symptoms is not advised for patients who have experienced anaphylactic reactions to foods, insect stings, or medications.

TREATMENT OPTIONS
Treatment Strategy
There is no cure for food allergies. Managing them usually means avoiding offending foods and treating symptoms when they occur. If the problem involves food intolerance, a registered dietitian may be helpful in guiding the patient so that reactions are minimized, thus avoiding unnecessary food restrictions.

Usually, once the food is eliminated from the diet, symptoms will abate. However, avoidance may not always be possible. For example, the substance may be present as an unspecified additive within another food or "hidden" in another form. Other factors such as the amount of the food, which parts of the food are used, or the way in which it is prepared can influence the systemic response. Therefore, treatment may be necessary to address occasional allergic symptoms.

Drug Therapies
- Antihistamines—for mild itching, swelling, rash, runny nose, or headache; available both by prescription and over the counter in many cold, sinus, and allergy remedies. These include diphenhydramine (Benadryl), clemastine (Tavist), chlorpheniramine (Chlor-Trimeton), loratadine (Claritin), and astemizole (Hismanal). Possible side effects include drowsiness, irritability, dry mouth, and heart palpitations. Hismanal when used with erythromycin, clarithromycin, and antifungal medications such as Nizoral and Sporanox can cause irregular heartbeat, fainting, dizziness, and, rarely, cardiac arrest and death.

- Antispasmodics—such as hyoscyamine (Levsin, Anaspaz) for diarrhea, nausea, abdominal bloating, and cramping.
- Adrenaline (epinephrine injection)—for anaphylactic shock.

Complementary and Alternative Therapies

The key to treatment of food allergy is complete avoidance of allergens for four to six months. Reducing inflammation, minimizing hypersensitivity reactions, and restoring the integrity of the digestive tract are ways in which alternative therapies may help resolve food allergies.

Hypersensitivity reactions may be associated with stress and anxiety. Mind-body techniques such as meditation, tai chi, yoga, and stress management may help normalize immune function.

NUTRITION

Note: Lower doses are for children.

- Eliminate all food allergens from the diet. The most common allergenic foods are dairy, soy, citrus, peanuts, wheat, fish, eggs, corn, chocolate, and tomatoes.
- An elimination/challenge trial may be helpful in uncovering sensitivities. Remove suspected allergens from the diet for two weeks. Re-introduce foods at the rate of one food every three days. Watch for reactions which may include gastrointestinal upset, mood changes, headaches, and exacerbation of symptoms. Do not perform a challenge with peanuts if there is history of anaphylaxis.
- A rotation diet, in which the same food is not eaten more than once every four days, may be helpful in minimizing food allergies.
- Reduce pro-inflammatory foods in the diet including saturated fats (meats, especially poultry, and dairy), refined foods, and sugar. For those with sensitivities to antibiotics it is essential to eat only organic meats to avoid antibiotic residues.
- Increase intake of fresh vegetables, whole grains, and essential fatty acids (cold-water fish, nuts, and seeds).
- Flaxseed, borage, or evening primrose oil (1,000 to 1,500 mg one to two times/day) are anti-inflammatory. Children should be supplemented with cod liver oil ($^1/_2$ to 1 tsp./day).
- Zinc (10 to 30 mg/day) and beta-carotene (25,000 to 50,000 IU/day) support immune function and encourage healing of mucosal tissues.
- Vitamin C (250 to 1,000 mg bid to qid) inhibits histamine release. Vitamin C from rose hips or palmitate is citrus-free and hypoallergenic.
- B-complex vitamins (25 to 100 mg/day) help to reduce the effects of stress and normalize immune function.
- Selenium (50 to 200 mcg/day) helps to regulate fatty acid metabolism and is a co-factor in liver detoxification.
- Bromelain (100 to 250 mg between meals) is a proteolytic enzyme that decreases inflammation.
- Pancreatin (8X USP) one to two tablets with meals to enhance digestion.
- Pro-flora supplements (one to three capsules/day) can help to normalize bowel flora.

HERBS

Herbs are generally a safe way to strengthen and tone the body's systems. As with any therapy, it is important to ascertain a diagnosis before pursuing treatment. Herbs may be used as dried extracts (capsules, powders, teas), glycerites (glycerine extracts), or tinctures (alcohol extracts). Unless otherwise indicated, teas should be made with 1 tsp. herb per cup of hot water. Steep covered 5 to 10 minutes for leaf or flowers, and 10 to 20 minutes for roots. Drink 2 to 4 cups/day. Tinctures may be used singly or in combination as noted.

- Quercetin (100 to 250 mg tid before meals) minimizes reactions to food.
- Rose hips (*Rosa canina*) tea is anti-inflammatory, high in hypoallergenic vitamin C, and healing to the digestive tract. Drink three to four cups/day, four ounces tid to qid for children. This is particularly effective for children.
- Marshmallow root tea (*Althea officinalis*) may soothe and promote healing of gastrointestinal inflammation. Soak one heaping tbsp. of marshmallow root in one quart of cold water overnight. Strain and drink throughout the day.
- Dandelion (*Taraxacum officinale*), milk thistle (*Silybum marianum*), celandine (*Chelidonium majus*), and chicory (*Cichorium intybus*) stimulate liver function.
- Soothing carminative herbs will enhance digestion and reduce spasm. Choose three or more of the following to make a tea to sip before meals. Chamomile (*Matricaria recutita*), peppermint (*Mentha piperita*), passionflower (*Passiflora incarnata*), meadowsweet (*Filependula ulmaria*), fennel (*Foeniculum vulgare*), and catnip (*Nepeta cataria*).

HOMEOPATHY

An experienced homeopath should assess individual constitutional types and severity of disease to select the correct remedy and potency.

ACUPUNCTURE

Acupuncture may help restore normal immune function and reduce the hypersensitivity response.

MASSAGE

Therapeutic massage may help reduce the effects of stress.

Patient Monitoring

A diet based on vegetables, fruits, and high-fiber foods and one that is also low in fat and refined sugar is considered best when addressing any type of allergy. Because there seems to be a connection between the inflammatory process and animal fat, it may help to reduce consumption of animal products.

OTHER CONSIDERATIONS

Prevention

Conservative introduction of solid foods as child is weaning may help prevent hypersensitivity conditions. If there is a strong family history of allergies or atopic conditions and/or if the child's immunity has been compromised in infancy, delay the introduction of highly allergenic foods until one year or older.

Complications/Sequelae

Some research suggests a link between food allergies and celiac disease, arthritis, chronic infection, depression, anxiety, and chronic fatigue.

Prognosis

Most infants outgrow their sensitivity to food by 2 to 4 years. Adults with food allergies tend to retain them for years. While there is no cure for food allergies, prognosis for remaining symptom-free is excellent as long as offending foods are identified and avoided.

Pregnancy

Nutritional support may safely relieve symptoms during pregnancy.

REFERENCES

American College of Allergy, Asthma and Immunology. Accessed at www.allergy.mcg.edu on January 1, 1999.

Carey CF, Lee HH, Woeltje KF, eds. *The Washington Manual of Medical Therapeutics.* 29th ed. New York, NY: Lippincott-Raven; 1998:216–271, 223–225.

Dambro MD. *Griffith's 5 Minute Clinical Consult.* Philadelphia, Pa: Williams & Wilkins; 1998:400–401.

Fauci AS, Braunwald E, Isselbacher KJ et al, eds. *Harrison's Principles of Internal Medicine.* 14th ed. St. Louis, Mo: McGraw-Hill; 1997.

he Food Allergy Network. Accessed at www.foodallergy.org/ on January 1, 1999.

Klag MJ, ed. *Johns Hopkins Family Health Book.* Harper Resource; 1998.

Murray MT. *Encyclopedia of Nutritional Supplements.* Rocklin, Calif: Prima Health;1996:448–449.

Murray MT, Pizzorno JE. *Encyclopedia of Natural Medicine.* Rocklin, Calif: Prima Publishing; 1998:321.

TMurray MT, Pizzorno JE. *Encyclopedia of Natural Medicine.* 2nd ed. Rocklin, Calif: Prima Publishing; 1998:464–475.

National Institute of Allergy and Infectious Diseases. National Institute of Health. Accessed at www.niaid.nih.gov/ on January 1, 1999.

Sampson HA. Food allergy. *JAMA.* 1997; 278:1888–1894.

Werbach M. *Nutritional Influences on Illness.* New Canaan, Conn: Keats Publishing Inc; 1987:23–28.

■ GALLBLADDER DISEASE
OVERVIEW
Definition
Cholecystitis (gallbladder inflammation) or symptomatic gallbladder disease is associated with cholelithiasis (formation of gallstones) in 98% of cases. It affects about 20 million people or about 10% of the U.S. population. Most people with gallstones never develop symptoms. Types of gallstones include pigmented (20% to 30% prevalence, composed of calcium bilirubinate), cholesterol (70% to 80% prevalence, at least 70% cholesterol by weight), and rarely, calcium carbonate stone (chalky, white paste).

Etiology
Development of gallstones is a complicated process, and is not completely understood.
- Imbalance in the relative amounts of cholesterol, phospholipids, and bile salts
- Increased biliary secretion of cholesterol (e.g., from obesity, estrogen therapy, age)
- Decreased hepatic secretion of bile salts and phospholipids (e.g., from resection, ileal disease, long-term total parenteral nutrition)
- Nucleation of cholesterol monohydrate initiates the process of stone formation
- Stone formation requires cholesterol saturation, biliary stasis within the gallbladder, and a nucleating agent (either pronucleating or antinucleating), such as bacteria, calcium salts, proteins, pigments, or other substances
- First liquid then solid crystals form, then stones
- Biliary sludge
- Precursor to gallbladder disease
- Thick mucous material composed of bile containing cholesterol crystals, calcium bilirubinate, and mucoproteins forms in the gallbladder
- Gallbladder motor functioning impairment—delayed stasis and emptying
- Pigmented stones—excess of unconjugated bilirubin
- Black stones—associated with hemolysis and cirrhosis
- Brown stones—associated with biliary tract infection, bacteria (especially *E. coli*), or parasites

Risk Factors
- Demographic features, may relate largely to diet
- Obesity and extremely low-calorie diets
- Complications and incidence increase with age
- Female (2:1)
- Estrogen therapy
- Diabetes
- Crohn's disease
- Cystic fibrosis
- Ileal disease or resection
- Biliary parasites
- Cirrhosis
- Total parenteral nutrition
- Hemolytic disorders

Signs and Symptoms
Symptoms usually occur following cystic duct obstruction by a stone.
- Upper right quadrant epigastric pain radiating around mid-torso to infrascapular region
- Biliary colic
- Fluctuating intensity
- Pain following meals, intolerance of fatty foods
- Nausea, vomiting, anorexia

DIFFERENTIAL DIAGNOSIS
- Peptic ulcer
- Appendicitis
- Pneumonia
- Myocardial infarction
- Hepatitis
- Pancreatitis
- Gallbladder cancer

DIAGNOSIS
Physical Examination
Physical findings are present during an acute attack and include upper right quadrant epigastric tenderness and guarding (indicates peritoneal involvement) to palpation. Murphy's sign may be evident. There may be fever, tachycardia, and tachypnea from inflammation. Jaundice occurs with concurrent bile duct obstruction in 10% to 30% of cases.

Laboratory Tests
- Leukocytosis is usually present.

Pathological Findings
- Acute cholecystitis
- Gallbladder wall edema
- Mucosal necrosis
- Subserosal hemorrhaging
- Week 1—granuloma formation
- Week 2—collagen formation, fibroblast proliferation
- Chronic cholecystitis
- Gallbladder—distended
- Gallbladder walls are edematous, ischemic, and inflamed
- Deconjugated bile salts produce mucosal damage
- Leukocytic infiltration

Imaging
- Ultrasound—98% sensitivity and specificity for diagnosis
- Oral cholecystography—iopanoic acid (Telepaque) is administered before X ray; less accurate than ultrasound; used to confirm a negative ultrasound
- Computed tomography scan—results similar to ultrasound
- Hepatobiliary isotopic scan—better sensitivity for acute cystic duct obstruction
- Cholescintigraphy with technetium 99m-iminodiacetic acid (99mTc IDA)

Other Diagnostic Procedures
- Cholecystokinin is administered; samples of gallbladder bile examined for crystal; diagnostic for cholecystitis

TREATMENT OPTIONS
Treatment Strategy
Only patients with symptomatic stones are treated.

Drug Therapies
- Parenteral narcotic administration—relieves pain, relaxes gallbladder
- Nasogastric aspiration
- Intravenous fluid replacement
- Antibiotics
- Oral bile acids are used primarily for cholesterol stones; stone must be radiolucent, float on oral cholecystogram, and be <15 mm in diameter; 40% effective in 2 years; used when laparoscopic surgery is not an option.

- Chenodeoxycholic acid—250 mg bid for two weeks, then increase dose by 250 mg/day until 13 to 16 mg/kg/day is reached; side effects include diarrhea and possible liver damage.
- Ursodeoxycholic acid—8 to 10 mg/kg/day/bid to tid; few side effects
- Methyl tert-butyl ether—strong lipid solvent; 95% of mass is dissolved in 12.5 hours

Surgical Procedures

The following surgical methods are performed when the patient's condition deteriorates or there is a perforated gallbladder or serious complication.

- Laparoscopic cholecystectomy
- Comparable mortality (0% to 0.3%) and morbidity (1.3% to 11.2%) rates, less pain, and shorter hospital stays than open cholecystectomy
- Rate of common bile duct injury is slightly greater (0.4% to 0.5% compared to 0.1% to 0.2%) than open cholecystectomy
- Open cholecystectomy
- About 5% of cases convert to open technique—unclear anatomy, bleeding, bile leakage
- Asymptomatic cholecystectomy—can be preventive; controversial
- Cholecystostomy—planned alternative when biliary anatomy is obscured by inflammation; done under local anesthesia
- Lithotripsy shock wave procedure—not approved by the Food and Drug Administration; not effective for large or multiple stones

Complementary and Alternative Therapies

Imaging is imperative before beginning any alternative treatment. Herbs that are stimulating to the gallbladder may induce contraction triggering acute choleycystitis with a stone too large to pass. Follow dietary guidelines and consider herbs if indicated.

NUTRITION

- Decrease total fat intake, especially saturated fats (meat and dairy products).
- Eliminate food allergens. Eggs, in particular, may be irritating to the gallbladder and exacerbate spasm.
- Increase dietary fiber in order to promote secretion of bile acids and reduce bile saturation.
- Consider fiber supplements such as flax meal (1 tsp., one to three times a day). Combine 1 heaping tsp. of flax meal in 8 oz. of apple juice for a drink high in fiber and pectin.
- Lecithin (1,000 to 5,000 mg/day) emulsifies cholesterol and facilitates its excretion.
- Lipotropic agents such as choline (1,000 mg/day) and lipase (10,000 NF units with meals) stimulate gallbladder function.
- Vitamin E (400 to 800 IU/day) and vitamin C (1,000 mg bid to tid) promote bile production.

HERBS

Herbs are generally a safe way to strengthen and tone the body's systems. As with any therapy, it is important to ascertain a diagnosis before pursuing treatment. Herbs may be used as dried extracts (capsules, powders, teas), glycerites (glycerine extracts), or tinctures (alcohol extracts). Unless otherwise indicated, teas should be made with 1 tsp. herb per cup of hot water. Steep covered 5 to 10 minutes for leaf or flowers, and 10 to 20 minutes for roots. Drink 2 to 4 cups/day. Tinctures may be used singly or in combination as noted.

Choleretic herbs stimulate bile production and increase bile solubility. Especially useful are milk thistle (*Silybum marianum*), dandelion root (*Taraxecum officinalis*), greater celandine (*Chelidonium majus*), globe

artichoke (*Cynara scolymus*), and turmeric (*Curcuma longa*). Use these herbs singly or in combination as a tea or tincture (15 to 20 drops), bid to tid before meals.

Enteric-coated peppermint oil (*Mentha piperita*) may help to dissolve stones (0.2 to 0.4 ml tid between meals).

HOMEOPATHY

An experienced homeopath should assess individual constitutional types and severity of disease to select the correct remedy and potency. For acute prescribing use 3 to 5 pellets of a 12X to 30C remedy every 1 to 4 hours until acute symptoms resolve.

- *Colocynthis* for colicky abdominal pains that are ameliorated by pressure or bending double.
- *Chelidonium* for abdominal pain that radiates to right scapular region.
- *Lycopodium* for abdominal pain that is worse with deep inhalation.

PHYSICAL MEDICINE

Castor oil pack. Used externally, castor oil is a powerful anti-inflammatory. Apply oil directly to skin, cover with a clean soft cloth (e.g., flannel) and plastic wrap. Place a heat source (hot water bottle or heating pad) over the pack and let sit for 30 to 60 minutes. For best results, use for three consecutive days.

Apply to abdomen, especially the gallbladder area to help reduce inflammation.

ACUPUNCTURE

Acupuncture may prove especially beneficial in pain relief, reducing spasm, and facilitating bile flow and proper liver and gallbladder function.

Patient Monitoring

- Patients on oral therapy need to have liver enzymes monitored.
- Complications generally indicate need for immediate treatment.

OTHER CONSIDERATIONS

Prevention

- A vegetarian low-fat, high-fiber diet reduces absorption of deoxycholic acid and aids prevention.
- Patients should drink 6 to 8 glasses of water a day.
- Chenodeoxycholic acid naturally occurs in cereal fiber.
- Patients should avoid refined sugars, simple carbohydrates, fried foods, animal proteins, coffee, food that causes allergic symptoms, and high calorie intake.

Complications/Sequelae

- With previous biliary colic, complications after cholecystectomy increase .
- Cholangitis or common bile duct stone obstruction (with jaundice)
- Pneumocholecystitis (*Emphysematous cholecystitis*)—secondary infection by gas-forming organisms
- Gallbladder cancer—90% of patients who have gallbladder cancer have gallstones
- Diabetes—20% of patients with diabetes have perforation or gangrene of the gallbladder; elective cholecystectomy is highly recommended.
- Gallstone ileus—gallbladder forms a fistulous connection with adjacent bowel (usually duodenum), and a large gallstone passes into the small intestine, creating an acute obstruction in the terminal small bowel.

Prognosis

- Patients with asymptomatic stones may remain symptom-free by controlling their risks.
- Can take two years for stone to dissolve.
- Early cholecystectomy usually ends symptoms and recurrence; however, stones may recur in the bile duct.
- Mortality (0% to 0.3%) and morbidity (1.3% to 11.2%) rates are lower for elective surgery than for emergency surgery.

Pregnancy

- It is difficult to diagnose any intra-abdominal disease during pregnancy.
- Ultrasound is a safe diagnostic tool.
- Surgery is indicated if more conservative treatments fail.
- Choleretic herbs must be used with caution in pregnancy. Milk thistle and dandelion root are generally safe in pregnancy.

REFERENCES

Blumenthal M, ed. *The Complete German Commission E Monographs.* Boston, Mass: Integrative Medicine Communications; 1998:422, 427, 465

Fauci AS, Braunwald E, Isselbacher KJ et al, eds. *Harrison's Principles of Internal Medicine.* 14th ed. New York, NY: McGraw-Hill; 1998.

Morrison R. *Desktop Guide to Keynotes and Confirmatory Symptoms.* Albany, Calif: Hahnemann Clinic Publishing; 1993:118, 139, 230.

Murray MT, Pizzorno JE. *Encyclopedia of Natural Medicine.* 2nd ed. Rocklin, Calif: Prima Publishing, 1998.

Sabiston DC, Lyerly HK. *Textbook of Surgery.* 15th ed. Philadelphia, Pa: WB Saunders, 1998

Weiss RF; Meuss AR, trans. *Herbal Medicine.* Medicina Biologica; 82–89, 94–97.

■ GASTRITIS

OVERVIEW

Definition

Gastritis is inflammation of the gastric mucosa. It is a group of disorders, not a single disease entity. These disorders are distinguished by clinical features, histologic findings, anatomic distribution, and etiology.

- Erosive and hemorrhagic gastritis is generally associated with alcoholism, nonsteroidal anti-inflammatory drug (NSAID) injury, stress lesions in critically ill patients (e.g., intensive care unit [ICU] disease), trauma (e.g., nasogastric tube suction, retching, radiation, chemotherapy), and surgery (e.g., postgastrectomy).
- Nonerosive, nonspecific gastritis is generally associated with infectious etiologies (e.g., *Helicobactor pylori)*, aging, gastric or duodenal ulcers, autoimmune diseases (e.g., pernicious anemia, lymphocytic gastritis), and reactive gastropathies (e.g., postgastrectomy).
- Distinctive gastritis is generally associated with bacterial (e.g., syphilis, tuberculosis), viral (e.g., cytomegalovirus), fungal (e.g., *Candida),* and parasitic (e.g., cryptosporidiosis) infections; with chronic systemic inflammatory diseases (e.g., Crohn's disease, sarcoidosis), as well as with unknown localized disease of unknown causes (e.g., Menetrier's disease).

Etiology

- NSAID use
- Alcohol and tobacco
- Reflux injury (e.g., bile)
- Trauma (e.g., surgery, radiation, vomiting, foreign body)
- Bacterial infections (e.g., *H. pylori,* Treponema pallidum, Mycobacterium tuberculosis)
- Autoimmune etiologies
  (e.g., pernicious anemia)
- Viral, fungal, and parasitic infections
- Systemic disease (e.g.,
  Crohn's disease, sarcoidosis, graft-versus-host disease)
- Unknown causes (e.g., Menetrier's disease or other hypertrophic gastropathies)
- Stress lesions

Risk Factors

For erosive and hemorrhagic gastritis:

- Exposure to ulcerogenic drugs
- Alcoholism
- Severe illness or trauma

For nonerosive gastritis:

- Colonization with *H. pylori*
  in early childhood
- Familial contact infected
  with *H. pylori*
- Latino or African American ancestry
- Institutionalized individuals
- Low socioeconomic status
- Gastroenterologists (person-to-person transmission, especially from endoscopy)
- Age over 60 years
- History of pernicious anema
  or gastric lymphoma

Signs and Symptoms

Most patients are asymptomatic; even gastric erosions and hemorrhages are not usually associated with abdominal pain. Symptomatic patients often have other gastrointestinal conditions, and gastritis is diagnosed as an inci-

dental histologic finding. Presenting complaints may include the following.

- Dyspepsia
- Anorexia
- Abdominal pain often
  aggravated by eating
- Nausea with/without vomiting
- Gastrointestinal bleeding
  (e.g., hematemesis, melena)

DIFFERENTIAL DIAGNOSIS

- Nonulcerative dyspepsia
- Peptic ulcer disease
- Gastroesophageal reflux
- Gastric cancer
- Gastroenteritis
- Celiac disease
- Functional gastrointestinal
  disorder
- Pancreatic disease

DIAGNOSIS

Physical Examination

Unremarkable physical presentation unless the patient presents with abdominal pain, bleeding, vomiting, and anorexia, where the patient looks ill, pale, and in severe cases, cachectic (malnourished) or dehydrated.

Laboratory Tests

Usually unremarkable unless the patient presents with pernicious anemia. Blood or breath tests, as well as tissue examination, can detect *H. pylori* (the major cause of nonerosive gastritis).

- Histologic studies using the following stains: hematoxylin and eosin, modified Giemsa, Warthin-Starry, Gram
- Serologic studies using enzyme-linked immunosorbent assay (ELISA)
- Histologic studies using the rapid urease test *(H. pylori* produces increased quantities of urease)
- Urea carbon breath test using 13C- and 14C-labeled urea, given orally; it is hydrolyzed by the urease produced by *H. pylori,* creating ammonia and CO_2; CO_2 in patient's breath then measured
- Serologic studies using polymerase chain reaction (PCR)

Pathological Findings

For erosive and hemorrhagic gastritis:

- Erosions (breaks in the mucosa that do not extend beyond the muscularis mucosae) that appear as multiple lesions surrounded by erythema
- Hemorrhagic lesions that appear as bright red streaks or petechiae
- Epithelial abnormalities and hyperplasia
- Minimal inflammation

For nonerosive gastritis:

- Clumps of monuclear cells and neutophils
- Foveolar hypoplasia (abnormal pit epithelium)
- Intestinal metaplasia (epithelial cells resemble intestinal epithelium)
- Mucus gland metaplasia (fundic replaced by mucus glands)
- Endocrine cell hyperplasia
- *H. pylori* organisms

Imaging

Imaging studies such as an upper GI series are used to rule out conditions that mimic gastritis such as gastroesophageal reflux or gastric malignancy.

Other Diagnostic Procedures

Endoscopy with biopsy is the gold standard for diagnosing gastritis (several suspected areas must be biopsied because of patchy and irregular distribution). A complete blood count will detect anemia, and a guaiac test of stool or vomitus will detect gastrointestinal bleeding.

TREATMENT OPTIONS
Treatment Strategy
No specific treatment is required for gastritis even with atrophic changes in asymptomatic individuals; however, treat associated conditions in symptomatic patients.

Drug Therapies
To treat *H. pylori* infection: triple-drug therapy (for two weeks) to prevent antibiotic resistance, Pepto-Bismol, 2 tablets every six hours; metronidazole, 250 mg every eight hours; and tetracycline, 500 mg every eight hours; use amoxicillin (500 mg every eight hours) if tetracycline is not tolerated. Treatment of asymptomatic *H. pylori* infections is controversial; at present *H. pylori* is only treated if associated with duodenal and gastric ulcers and MALT lymphoma.

To treat peptic ulcer disease: triple-drug therapy (for one week) to reduce acid production—omeprazole, 20 mg bid; clarithromycin, 250 mg bid; and metronidazole, 500 mg bid.

Complementary and Alternative Therapies
Nutritional and herbal support help to heal gastric mucosa, fight infection, and reduce recurrence. In addition, mind-body techniques such as meditation, progressive muscle relaxation, tai chi, yoga, and stress management may reduce the frequency and severity of symptoms and enhance healing.

NUTRITION
- Avoid dairy, caffeine, alcohol, and sugar. Coffee, even decaffeinated, should be eliminated because of irritating oils.
- Eliminate any known food allergens.
- Include sulphur-containing foods such as garlic, onions, broccoli, cabbage, brussel sprouts, and cauliflower in the diet. Sulphur is a precursor to glutathione which provides antioxidant protection to the gastric mucosa. N-acetyl cysteine (200 mg bid between meals) is also a precursor to glutathione.
- Vitamin C (1,000 mg tid) decreases nitrosamines which are linked to stomach cancer.
- Zinc (30 to 50 mg/day) enhances healing.
- To treat pernicious anemia: lifelong regular parenteral vitamin B_{12}

HERBS
Herbs are generally a safe way to strengthen and tone the body's systems. As with any therapy, it is important to ascertain a diagnosis before pursuing treatment. Herbs may be used as dried extracts (capsules, powders, teas), glycerites (glycerine extracts), or tinctures (alcohol extracts). Unless otherwise indicated, teas should be made with 1 tsp. herb per cup of hot water. Steep covered 5 to 10 minutes for leaf or flowers, and 10 to 20 minutes for roots. Drink 2 to 4 cups/day. Tinctures may be used singly or in combination as noted.
- DGL (deglycyrrhizinated licorice), 250 mg qid 15 to 20 minutes before meals and one to two hours after last meal, increases circulation and healing to gastric mucosa. This preparation has the hypertensive factor in licorice root removed making it safe to take long-term and in cases of hypertension.
- Powders of slippery elm *(Ulmus fulva)* and marshmallow root *(Althea officinalis)* may be taken singly or together, 1 tsp. bid to tid, to decrease inflammation and encourage healing.
- Ginger root tea *(Zingiber officinalis)* is a warming carminative that increases circulation and enhances digestion. Drink 2 to 3 cups/day with meals.
- For *H. pylori,* bismuth subcitrate (120 mg qid for eight weeks) may be helpful in eradicating *H. pylori* and reducing recurrence. It is poorly absorbed which decreases the likelihood of side effects; however, it is associated with neurotoxicity if used long-term. Patient may still need antibiotics if *H. pylori* has not resolved after eight weeks.

HOMEOPATHY
An experienced homeopath should assess individual constitutional types and severity of disease to select correct remedy and potency. Consider three remedies, *Nux vomica, Arsenicum album,* and *Lycopodium.*

ACUPUNCTURE
Acupuncture may help in reducing stress and improving digestive function.

MASSAGE
Therapeutic massage can alleviate stress and increase sense of well-being.

Patient Monitoring
Symptomatic individuals must be treated and followed with repeat endoscopy or gastroscopy if symptoms persist.

OTHER CONSIDERATIONS
Prevention
Patients must be advised of the risks of continued alcohol, tobacco, and NSAID use. A high-fiber diet is recommended to decrease the incidence of digestive problems. *H. pylori* should be eradicated in symptomatic individuals.

Complications/Sequelae
- Epidemiolgic studies have linked the presence of *H. pylori* with the development of gastric cancer (a three- to six-fold increased risk).
- Chronic gastritis may lead to atrophic gastritis, gastric atrophy, and gastric metaplasia, which may result in gastric cancer.
- Acid-suppressive therapy alone may indirectly increase the risk of gastric cancer by increasing the development of gastric atrophy
- GI bleeding may result from advanced mucosal erosion/ulceration.

Prognosis
If the etiology of the gastritis is properly identified, most cases are successfully treated. Gastritis resulting from *H. pylori* infection may clear initially but require repeated treatment.

Pregnancy
Do not use bismuth subcitrate in pregnancy.

REFERENCES
Blumenthal M, ed. *The Complete German Commission E Monographs.* Boston, Mass: Integrative Medicine Communications; 1998:427.

Fauci AS, Braunwald E, Isselbacher KJ et al, eds. *Harrison's Principles of Internal Medicine.* 14th ed. New York, NY: McGraw-Hill; 1998: 941–943,1610–1614.

Murray MT, Pizzorno JE. *Encyclopedia of Natural Medicine.* Rocklin, Calif: Prima Publishing; 1998:522–523.

Sklar M, ed. Gastoenterologic problems. *Clinics in Geriatric Medicine.* 1991;7:235–238.

Sleisenger MH, Fordtran JS, Scharschmidt BF, et al. *Gastrointestinal Disease.* 5th ed. Philadelphia, Pa: WB Saunders; 1993:545–564.

■ GASTROESOPHAGEAL REFLUX DISEASE

OVERVIEW

Definition

Gastroesophageal reflux disease (GERD), a disorder associated with a range of clinical manifestations, results from the reflux of gastroduodenal contents into the esophagus. A common and often chronic condition, GERD affects a large percentage of healthy individuals, both male and female, many of whom have experienced symptoms for more than a decade. Heartburn, the primary symptom, is often exacerbated by lying down after eating. Complications are more common with older patients. Although nearly 20% of adults use indigestion aids at least weekly, only about one-quarter of those who experience true GERD seek medical attention.

GERD is generally not considered to be a disease unless the symptoms are severe and occur frequently or the esophageal mucosa is damaged. It is important to note that individual symptoms do not always reflect the severity of esophageal mucosal damage.

Etiology

- Lower esophageal sphincter (LES) dysfunction
- Peptic stricture
- Esophageal inflammation
- Peristaltic dysfunction
- Esophageal cancer
- Abnormal saliva
- Excessive acid production
- Delayed gastric emptying
- Reflux of bile salts
- Reflux of pancreatic enzymes
- Scleroderma
- Decreased LES pressure resulting from progestational hormones during pregnancy
- Chalasia in infants
- Heller's myotomy for achalasia

Risk Factors

- Esophageal clearance dysfunction (possibly hiatal hernia)
- Taking medications that lower LES pressure
- Eating foods that lower LES pressure
- Exposure to substances that irritate esophageal mucosa
- Smoking
- Alcohol or coffee consumption
- Chest trauma
- Indwelling nasogastric tube
- Elimination of *H. pylori* infection (controversial)
- Children: cerebral palsy, Down syndrome, mental retardation

Signs and Symptoms

- Heartburn
- Regurgitation
- Dysphagia
- Odynophagia
- Water brash
- Belching
- Retrosternal burning sensation
- Chest pain (similar to angina)
- Bronchospasm (asthma)
- Laryngitis
- Chronic cough
- Recurrent aspiration
- Pulmonary fibrosis
- Wheezing
- Hoarseness
- Sore throat
- Globus sensation in the neck
- Infants: apnea syndrome, failure to thrive, recurrent emesis

DIFFERENTIAL DIAGNOSIS

- Esophagitis
- Angina
- Respiratory ailments
- Ear, nose, and throat ailments
- Radiation exposure
- Crohn's disease
- Esophageal carcinoma
- Achalasia
- Ulcer disease

DIAGNOSIS

Physical Examination

Usually normal

Pathological Findings

- Abnormal peristalsis
- Poor LES tone
- Actual mucosal damage (including from cell damage), ranging from shallow, linear erosions to denudation
- Hyperplasia
- Barrett's epithelium changes
- Acute esophageal inflammation, including erosions, ulceration, and strictures

Imaging

- Barium swallow: reveals reflux, esophageal damage (not effective for mild esophagitis), and hiatal hernia; simple and inexpensive
- Radionuclide scintigraphy: reveals reflux

Other Diagnostic Procedures

Can be used to confirm GERD, determine if GERD resulted from acid reflux, determine if mucosal inflammation or other damage has resulted, and ascertain the severity of the condition.

- Esophageal manometry: indicates abnormal peristalsis and poor LES tone; does not show reflux
- Prolonged esophageal pH monitoring: enables comparison of symptoms to actual acid levels
- Acid perfusion (Bernstein) test: indicated for patients with atypical symptoms or treatment complications
- Endoscopy with biopsy: most effective assessment of reflux-induced mucosal damage; recommended with complications (e.g., stricture or Barrett's epithelium)
- Gastric analysis

TREATMENT OPTIONS

Treatment Strategy

The goal of GERD treatment depends on the severity of the condition:

- Patients without esophagitis: relieve symptoms
- Patients with esophagitis: relieve symptoms, treat damage, and prevent complications

GERD treatment is generally based on three levels of severity:

- Patients with mild symptoms but without esophagitis: modify lifestyle, prescribe PRN medications (H_2 antagonists, antacids, alginic acid, prokinetics), maintain with PRN medications

- Patients with moderate to severe symptoms but without significant esophagitis: modify lifestyle, prescribe daily medications (H_2 antagonists and prokinetics), maintain with same medications
- Patients with intractable symptoms and severe esophagitis and patients who have not responded to other drug therapy: modify lifestyle, prescribe daily medication (proton-pump inhibitor), maintain with proton-pump inhibitor, consider antireflux surgery

Drug Therapies

- Antacids and alginic acid—appropriate for mild and infrequent symptoms; ineffective for esophagitis. Gaviscon, 10 ml qid (30 minutes after meals and at bedtime).
- Prokinetics—effectively relieve heartburn; debatable effectiveness for esophagitis. Bethanechol, 10 to 15 mg qid or Metoclopramide (both 30 minutes before meals and at bedtime); frequent side effects in young and older patients. Cisapride, 10 mg qid (30 minutes before meals and at bedtime); increases LES pressure; minimal side effects; useful for maintenance therapy for symptoms and mild esophagitis; should be used cautiously with antifungal imidazole agents.
- H_2 antagonists—effectively relieve symptoms and generally heal mild-to-moderate esophagitis; can prevent relapse with mild GERD. Cimetidine or famotidine or nizatidine or ranitidine, once or twice/day; some interactions.
- Proton-pump inhibitors (PPIs)—potent, long-acting acid secretion inhibitors; relieve severe symptoms and heal esophagitis; provide effective maintenance therapy; minimal short-term side effects, long-term side effects unknown. Omeprazole or lansoprazole.

Complementary and Alternative Therapies

Dietary changes can be very important in decreasing the irritation of GERD. Herbs may be very effective at healing esophagitis. The correct homeopathic treatment may also be quite helpful.

NUTRITION

- Digestive enzymes may assist in decreasing the occurrence of heartburn.
- Avoid any known allergens. May be helpful to test for food allergies.
- Avoid sweets, oils, fats, and caffeine.

HERBS

Herbs are generally a safe way to strengthen and tone the body's systems. As with any therapy, it is important to ascertain a diagnosis before pursuing treatment. Herbs may be used as dried extracts (capsules, powders, teas), glycerites (glycerine extracts), or tinctures (alcohol extracts). Unless otherwise indicated, teas should be made with 1 tsp. herb per cup of hot water. Steep covered 5 to 10 minutes for leaf or flowers, and 10 to 20 minutes for roots. Drink 2 to 4 cups/day. Tinctures may be used singly or in combination as noted.

Herbs used as carminatives often contain volatile oils that may actually worsen relaxation of LES. Instead, digestive bitters are often astringent and tonifying to mucous membranes.

- Licorice (*Glycyrrhiza glabra*)—anti-inflammatory antispasmodic and analgesic specific for the gastrointestinal tract. Glycyrrhetinic acid has been shown in studies to aid healing of gastric, peptic, and mouth ulcers. In patients with hypertension, use deglycerinated licorice to prevent aggravating hypertension. Prolonged use may lead to pseudoaldosteronism, which resolves with discontinuation of the herb.

Chewable lozenges may be the best form for treating GERD, 380 to 1,140 mg/day.

- Slippery elm (*Ulmus fulva*)—demulcent (protects irritated tissues and promotes their healing), 60 to 320 mg/day; 1 tsp. powder may be mixed with water tid to qid.

In addition, a combination of four of the following herbs may be used as either a tea (1 cup tid) or tincture (30 to 60 drops tid):

- Valerian (*Valeriana officinalis*)—bitter, sedative, especially for anxiety or depression and poor digestion
- Wild yam (*Dioscorea villosa*)—antispasmodic, anti-inflammatory, especially for fatigue from long-term stress or maldigestion
- St. John's wort (*Hypericum perforatum*)—analgesic, antidepressant, historically used to treat adhesions and strictures, especially for anxiety or pain
- Skullcap (*Scutellaria laterifolia*)—antispasmodic, sedative, nervine, especially for disturbed sleep
- Linden flowers (*Tilia cordata*)—antispasmodic, mild diuretic, gentle bitter, especially for dyspepsia

HOMEOPATHY

An experienced homeopath should assess individual constitutional types and severity of disease to select the correct remedy and potency. For acute prescribing use 3 to 5 pellets of a 12X-to-30C remedy every one to four hours until acute symptoms resolve.

- *Arsenicum album* for burning pain that feels better with warmth, especially with anxiety
- *Carbo vegatabilis* for bloating and indigestion that is worse from lying down, especially with flatulence and fatigue
- *Lycopodium* for heartburn that feels worse with eating, and bloating that is relieved by eructation
- *Nux vomica* for heartburn with cramping and constipation, especially with irritability

ACUPUNCTURE

May be helpful to normalize digestion and alleviate stress

Patient Monitoring

Repeat endoscopy 6 to 12 weeks if symptoms not relieved. Annual endoscopy/biopsy for Barrett's esophagus. Attentive management when complications are present.

OTHER CONSIDERATIONS

Prevention

- Reduce LES pressure: avoid fats, chocolate, coffee, and carminatives. Avoid medications that lower LES pressure (e.g., calcium antidepressants, channel blockers, nitrates, progesterone, and theophylline).
- Avoid esophageal irritants: avoid spicy foods, tomato-based foods, and citrus. Avoid medications associated with drug-induced esophagitis.
- Improve acid clearance: change sleeping angle by elevating head of bed or upper body. Do not lie down after meals. Avoid voluntary eructation.
- Reduce gastric distension: avoid excessive eating. Avoid food and liquid two to three hours before bedtime or lying down. Lose weight. Avoid tight-fitting garments. Avoid bending and stooping.
- Maintenance drug therapy, if needed.
- Possible periodic dilation of peptic stricture.
- Surgery (primarily laparoscopic) as alternative to long-term drug therapy.

Complications/Sequelae

- Esophageal (peptic) stricture
- Esophageal ulcer
- Adenocarcinoma
- Pulmonary aspiration
- Upper GI hemorrhage
- Esophageal mucosa damage, possibly severe
- Ear, nose, and throat complications
- Loss of dental enamel
- Vocal cord granuloma
- Halitosis
- Pneumonia

Prognosis

A chronic condition, GERD lapses and relapses (generally when treatment concludes), producing symptoms with varying intensity over time.

Pregnancy

GERD is common in pregnancy, especially in the third trimester. Chewable papaya tablets may provide relief and are safe for pregnant women.

REFERENCES

Andreoli TE, Bennett JC, Carpenter CCJ. *Cecil Essentials of Medicine.* 3rd ed. Philadelphia, Pa: WB Saunders; 1993:285–287.

Barker LR, Burton JR, Zieve PD, eds. *Principles of Ambulatory Medicine.* 4th ed. Baltimore, Md: Williams & Wilkins; 1995:443–446.

Bartram T. *Encyclopedia of Herbal Medicine.* Dorset, England: Grace Publishers; 1995:217.

Dambro MR. *Griffith's 5 Minute Clinical Consult–1999.* Baltimore, Md: Lippincott Williams & Wilkins; 1999:422–423.

Kelley WN, ed. *Essentials of Internal Medicine.* Philadelphia, Pa: J.B. Lippincott Company; 1994:104–106.

Morrison R. *Desktop Guide to Keynotes and Confirmatory Symptoms.* Albany, Calif: Hahnemann Clinic Publishing; 1993:39–43, 102–103, 229–231, 272–275.

Stoller JK, Ahmad M, Longworth DL, eds. *The Cleveland Clinic Intensive Review of Internal Medicine.* Baltimore, Md: Williams & Wilkins; 1998:595–599.

Werbach MR. *Nutritional Influences on Illness.* New Canaan, Conn: Keats Publishing Inc; 1987:210.

■ GOUT

OVERVIEW

Definition

In gout, monosodium urate crystals are deposited in tissue, causing inflammation and sudden severe pain, usually in a single joint. It occurs in three or four out of 1,000 persons, and 90% to 95% of patients are men over age 30. One in four have a family history of gout. Once called a rich man's disease because of its association with overindulgence in food and alcohol, this metabolic disorder can be exacerbated by poor diet. Primary gout is the result of overproduction or underexcretion of uric acid. Secondary gout is the result of myeloproliferative diseases, lead poisoning, enzyme deficiencies, or renal failure. Left untreated, gout may lead to a chronic arthritis.

Etiology

Its reputation associates gout with overeating (especially meats), overindulgence in alcohol, and being overweight, but it can strike at any time and for no apparent reason. The mechanism is excessive uric acid production, decreased uric acid excretion, or both. Primary disease is an inborn error of metabolism attributed to several biochemical defects. Secondary disease is a complication of acquired disorders such as leukemia or the use of certain drugs.

Risk Factors

- Family history of gout
- Obesity
- Hypertension
- Stress resulting from a fracture or surgical procedure
- Thiazide diuretics
- Drinking alcohol
- Polynesian heritage
- Diabetes
- Renal failure

Signs and Symptoms

- Pain in a single joint, often at the base of the great toe, but can be in other joints of the feet, fingers, wrists, elbows, knees, and ankles
- "Exquisite" pain and tenderness
- Swelling, heat, and stiffness of joint
- Shiny red or purple coloration of joint
- Fever up to 39°C (102.2°F) with or without chills
- Begins in hours and may subside over a few days or up to three weeks
- In later attacks, may see tophi (accumulations of urate just beneath the skin) in hands, feet, olecranon, prepatellar bursa, and in external parts of ears
- Untreated, attacks will be more frequent and more severe

DIFFERENTIAL DIAGNOSIS

- Pseudogout
- Rheumatoid arthritis
- Osteoarthritis
- Cellulitis
- Infectious (acute pyogenic) arthritis
- Sarcoidosis
- Multiple myeloma
- Hyperparathyroidism
- Hand–Schüller–Christian disease
- Chronic lead intoxication
- Lead toxicity

DIAGNOSIS

Physical Examination

Metatarsophalangeal joint is most commonly affected and appears red, swollen, hot, and exquisitely painful to touch. History may reveal recent food and alcohol excess, surgery, infection, physical or emotional stress, use of diuretics, certain chemicals, or uricosuric drugs. Fever is common, along with tachycardia, local desquamation, and sometimes pruritus. Tophi may be found in later attacks, as can progressive functional loss and disability and possibly gross deformities. Hyperuricemia with typical history of monarticular acute arthritis is usually sufficient for diagnosis.

Laboratory Tests

- Serum uric acid level—Hyperuricemia greater than 7.5 mg/dL (unless uricosuric drugs are being taken) may be present but is not in itself diagnostic.
- Erythrocyte sedimentation rate (ESR) is elevated during attack.
- White blood cell count (WBC) is mildly elevated during attack.

Pathological Findings

- Urate crystals in synovial membrane
- Tophi present in some patients

Imaging

Plain radiograph to rule out other disorders; no typical findings in early disease, but late disease may show punched-out lesions (tophi) and joint destruction.

Other Diagnostic Procedures

Synovial aspirate is cloudy and markedly inflammatory, with urate crystals (needle-shaped and birefringent under polarized light).

Microscopic gout crystals seen in synovial fluid.

TREATMENT OPTIONS

Treatment Strategy

Gout is often completely controlled by proper treatment.

- Nonsteroidal anti-inflammatory drugs (NSAIDs) for pain and inflammation
- Abstinence from alcohol
- Dietary restrictions (avoid fat, alcohol, sardines, anchovies, scallops, organ meats, sweetbreads, cocoa, spinach, asparagus, eggs, oatmeal, and mushrooms)
- Medication to reduce the amount of uric acid produced or to promote its excretion

Drug Therapies

- NSAIDs—such as ibuprofen and indomethacin; I/M 50 mg every 8 hours until symptoms resolve (5 to 10 days); avoid if allergic or have active peptic ulcer disease or impaired renal function.
- Colchicine—0.5 to 0.6 mg orally every hour until pain is relieved or nausea or diarrhea appears, then stop drug; usual total dose, 4 to 8 mg; generally only effective for 24 to 48 hours; many side effects, but GI symptoms relieved by IV administration of initial dose of 1 to 2 mg in 10 to 20 ml saline solution; severe toxicity limits usefulness of IV colchicine. Can also be used to prevent future attacks.
- Corticosteroids—dramatic symptom relief in acute attack; best for clients who cannot take NSAIDs. For monarticular disease, give intra-articularly (e.g., triamcinolone 10 to 40 mg depending on size of joint). For polyarticular disease, give IV (e.g., methylprednisolone, 40 mg daily tapered over seven days) or orally (e.g., prednisone 40 to 60 mg daily tapered over seven days). Do joint aspiration and

Gram stain of synovial fluid before giving steroids.

- Analgesics—such as codeine or meperidine for severe pain. Avoid aspirin as salicylates may exacerbate the condition.
- Uricosuric agents—to reduce serum uric acid levels; probenecid (250 mg bid for one week, increased to 500 mg bid) or sulfinpyrazone (100 mg daily initially, gradually increased to 200 to 400 mg daily). Hypersensitivity is indicated by fever and rash (5% of cases) or GI complaints (10%). Maintain daily urine output of at least 2,000 ml and urine pH of at least 6.0; salicylates must be avoided.
- Allopurinol—to reduce serum uric acid levels; 100 mg daily for one week, increased as needed; normal levels often obtained with 200 to 300 mg daily. Use cautiously in renal insufficiency; do not use in asymptomatic hyperuricemia (may precipitate attack). May develop signs ranging from pruritic rash to toxic epidermal necrolysis (rare, yet potentially fatal).

Complementary and Alternative Therapies

A combination of therapies can be very effective at decreasing both the length and frequency of attacks. Alternative therapies are often most useful in decreasing the frequency and severity of attacks, but may not necessarily offer the best pain relief. Alternative therapies avoid the sometimes toxic effects of some pharmaceutical agents used for gout. Some nutrients may actually exacerbate the condition.

NUTRITION

- Avoid obesity. However, it is important to avoid crash dieting and rapid weight loss.
- Avoid alcohol, especially beer, which has a higher purine content than wine or spirits.
- Hydration—drink plenty of water, dehydration may exacerbate gout
- Restrict purines in diet—Purines increase lactate production which competes with uric acid for excretion. Foods with a high purine content are beef, goose, organ meats, sweetbreads, mussels, anchovies, herring, mackerel and yeast. Foods with a moderate amount of purines include meats, poultry, fish and shellfish not listed above. Spinach, asparagus, beans, lentils, mushrooms, and dried peas also contain moderate amounts of purines.
- Cherries—One half pound of cherries/day (fresh or frozen) for two weeks lowers uric acid and prevents attacks. Cherries and other dark red berries (hawthorn berries and blueberries) contain anthocyanadins that increase collagen integrity and decrease inflammation. 8 to 16 oz. of unadulterated cherry juice per day is also helpful. A lower maintenance dose can be continued for prevention.
- Vitamin C—8 g/day can lead to decreased serum uric acid levels. Note that there is a small subset of patients with gout who will actually get worse with this level of vitamin C.
- Folic acid—10 to 75 mg/day inhibits xanthine oxidase which is required for uric acid production. B_{12} levels need to be monitored to avoid masking a B_{12} deficiency.
- EPA (eicospentaenoic acid) inhibits pro-inflammatory leukotrienes. Dose is 1,500 mg/day.
- Niacin—Avoid niacin in doses greater than 50 mg/day. Nicotinic acid may precipitate an attack of gout by competing with uric acid for excretion.
- Vitamin A—There is some concern that elevated retinol levels may play a role in some attacks of gouty arthritis.

HERBS

Herbs are generally a safe way to strengthen and tone the body's systems. As with any therapy, it is important to ascertain a diagnosis before pursuing treatment. Herbs may be used as dried extracts (capsules, powders, teas), glycerites (glycerine extracts), or tinctures (alcohol extracts). Unless otherwise indicated, teas should be made with 1 tsp. herb per cup of hot water. Steep covered 5 to 10 minutes for leaf or flowers, and 10 to 20 minutes for roots. Drink 2 to 4 cups/day. Tinctures may be used singly or in combination as noted.

- Devil's claw (*Harpagophytum procumbens*)—analgesic and anti-inflammatory. Dose is 1 to 2 g tid of dried powdered root, 4 to 5 ml tid of tincture, or 400 mg tid of dry solid extract during acute attacks.
- Bromelain (*Ananas comosus*)—proteolytic enzyme (anti-inflammatory) when taken apart from food. Dose is 125 to 250 mg tid during acute attacks.

HOMEOPATHY

An experienced homeopath should assess individual constitutional types and severity of disease to select the correct remedy and potency. For acute prescribing use 3 to 5 pellets of a 12X to 30C remedy every one to four hours until acute symptoms resolve.

- *Aconite* for sudden onset of burning pain, anxiety, restlessness, and attacks that come after a shock or injury
- *Belladonna* for intense pain that may be throbbing; pain is made worse by any motion and better by pressure; joint is very hot.
- *Bryonia* for pain made much worse by any kind of motion; pain is better with pressure and with heat.
- *Colchicum* for pains made worse by motion and changes of weather, especially if there is any nausea associated with the attacks
- *Ledum* when joints become mottled, purple and swollen; pain is much better with cold applications and is worse from getting overheated.

PHYSICAL MEDICINE

- Hot and cold compresses—three minutes hot alternated with 30 seconds of cold compresses provide pain relief and increase circulation to the affected joint.
- Bed rest for 24 hours after acute attack. However, prolonged bed rest may exacerbate the condition.

Patient Monitoring

If joint destruction is present, refer patient for orthopedic consultation. Surgical intervention is occasionally needed. There is increased incidence of urolithiasis, with 80% of calculi being uric acid stones, and of hypertension, renal disease, diabetes mellitus, hypertriglyceridemia, and atherosclerosis.

OTHER CONSIDERATIONS

Prevention

Dietary measures and nutritional supplementation may help prevent attacks and decrease their frequency, thereby decreasing the risk for joint destruction.

Complications/Sequelae

- Renal disease or kidney stones are most common, but these develop slowly with no effect on life expectancy.
- Chronic tophaceous arthritis may occur after repeated attacks of acute gout, but only with inadequate treatment.
- Possible nerve or spinal cord impairment

Prognosis

Asymptomatic periods grow shorter as the disease progresses. Marked deformities are possible, but few patients become bedridden. The younger the client at onset, the greater the chance of progressive disease. Destructive arthropathy is rare in those whose first attack is after age 50. Appropriate treatment will suppress attacks and keep uric acid to normal levels.

Pregnancy
Because the disease affects mainly men and postmenopausal women, pregnancy is not usually impacted.

REFERENCES

The Burton Goldberg Group, compilers. *Alternative Medicine: The Definitive Guide.* Tiburon, Calif: Future Medicine Publishing; 1997.

Ferri FF. *Ferri's Clinical Advisor: Instant Diagnosis and Treatment.* St Louis, Mo: Mosby-Year Book; 1999.

Larson DE, ed. *Mayo Clinic Family Health Book.* 2nd ed. New York, NY: William Morrow and Company; 1996.

Murray MT, Pizzorno JE. *Encyclopedia of Natural Medicine.* 2nd ed. Rocklin, Calif: Prima Publishing; 1997.

Rose B. *The Family Health Guide To Homeopathy.* Berkeley, Calif: Celestial Arts Publishing; 1992.

Theodosakis J, Adderly B, Fox B. *The Arthritis Cure.* New York, NY: St Martin's Press; 1997.

Tierney LM Jr, McPhee SJ, Papadakis MA, eds. *Current Medical Diagnosis and Treatment 1994.* Norwalk, Conn: Appleton & Lange; 1994.

Werbach MR. *Nutritional Influences on Illness.* New Canaan, Conn: Keats Publishing Inc; 1987.

■ HEADACHE, MIGRAINE

OVERVIEW

Definition

A throbbing, recurring headache, typically affecting only one side of the head. Onset is sudden, and pain is usually severe. Visual, auditory, neurological, or gastrointestinal symptoms may appear 10 to 30 minutes before head pain or may accompany the headache. Duration may be from a few hours to several days. True migraine headaches affect approximately 11% of the population and are more common in females than males. True migraine is consistently present with aura, which provides warning of the upcoming attack. Migraines may begin at any age; they are most common between age 10 and 30 and may vanish after age 50 or, in women, after menopause.

Etiology

Blood vessels to the brain and scalp constrict and then dilate, irritating surrounding nerves and resulting in pulsating or pounding pain with blood flow. The underlying etiology is not known. Possible causes include the following.

- Abnormal blood levels of serotonin, a neurotransmitter that may precipitate vasoconstriction
- Vasoactive medications such as drugs to treat hypertension, angina, and arthritis
- Hypersensitivity to certain foods or odors, missed meals, excessive sun exposure, altered sleep patterns, alcohol consumption
- Menstruation, hormonal changes
- Stress
- Malformed cranial blood vessel (rare)

Risk Factors

- Female gender
- Family history of migraine
- History of motion sickness, recurrent vomiting spells
- Patients who chronically suffer from migraine headaches have levels of blood magnesium well below normal levels
- Smoking

Signs and Symptoms

The following symptoms may vary between patients but usually remain consistent in individuals.

- Aura preceding headache, irritability, restlessness, hearing or vision disturbances, numbness, weakness, or tingling sensations may precede head pain by 10 to 30 minutes or may be present with headache
- Severe, throbbing, usually unilateral headache
- Headache accompanied by increased sensitivity to light and noise
- Headache persists for hours and if untreated may last days
- Pounding pain worsens with movement or bending
- Nausea, vomiting
- Near-syncope, vertigo
- Feet and hands may be cold and cyanosed
- Scalp arteries may be prominent

DIFFERENTIAL DIAGNOSIS

- Brain tumor or brain abscess
- Systemic disease
- Meningitis or meningeal irritation
- Seizure disorder
- Encephalitis
- Subarachnoid hemorrhage
- Subdural hematoma
- Hypertension

DIAGNOSIS

Physical Examination

Patient describes migraine symptoms, without intracranial pathologic changes.

Laboratory Tests

No laboratory tests are available to diagnose migraine. Lumbar puncture to rule out meningitis/encephalitis. Assessment of thyroid function is essential. Headaches, menstrual cramps, constipation, and depression are some of the hidden symptoms of functional hypothyroid, even in the presence of normal thyroid function tests.

Pathological Findings

Intracranial blood flow changes.

Imaging

Usually not appropriate. Some migraines can mimic strokes, and cause one-sided numbness or paralysis. The first episode of these types of migraines should be evaluated with an MRI.

Other Diagnostic Procedures

- Careful patient history should note characteristics of headache, timing, frequency, duration, and possible triggers.
- Positive response to a migraine drug will confirm diagnosis of migraine.

TREATMENT OPTIONS

Treatment Strategies

Treatment varies according to the severity of the migraine attack. Proper use of analgesics should be explained to patients to help prevent rebound headaches from overuse. Cold compresses to forehead and eyes, complete immobility, and minimalization of light, noise, and odor are management approaches.

Drug Therapies

There is no simple drug of choice.

For mild migraines: Aspirin (600 to 1,000 mg every four hours), ibuprofen (800 mg followed by 400 mg every 4 hours), naproxen (500 mg), and codeine may be sufficient if taken early in attack.

For moderate migraines: NSAIDS, ergotamines (dihydroergotamine—DHE, particularly ergotamine combined with anti-emetic), ergotamoine suppositories (1/2 up to 2 suppositories per attack)

For severe migraines:

- First treatment: DHE by subcutaneous, intramuscular or intravenous injection, or sumatriptan (orally or subcutaneous injection); if an IV line is used, 10 mg IV metoclopramide is recommended. If ineffective after 20 minutes, 0.5 to 1.0 mg of DHE may be added intravenously up to a maximum dose of 2 mg over three hours.
- Other options include: chlorpromazine (0.1 mg/kg intravenously) may be given over 20 minutes and may be repeated after 15 minutes, to a maximum dose of 37.5 mg; saline (5 mL per kg of body weight or 50 mg intramuscularly) should be given to prevent hypotension; prochlorperazine may be given rectally (25 mg), intravenously or intramuscularly (5 to 10 mg); ketorolac (39 to 60 mg intramuscularly) or dexamethasone (12 to 20 mg intravenously) may be given in resistant cases.

Other treatment options include intranasal lidocaine.

Complementary and Alternative Therapies

These therapies may be quite useful in decreasing the frequency of migraines. Some homeopathics may be helpful in the acute stage, but most acute migraines require greater pain relief than alternative therapies have to offer. It is often helpful to differentiate migraines in treating them with complementary therapies. Diet and allergy elimination have offered great relief to some. Hormone balancing can be quite helpful for cyclic migraines. Just as the specific symptoms of a migraine are often unique to the individual, the specific treatments that are most effective may be a unique combination for each patient. A combination approach of drugs for pain relief and complementary therapies to reduce recurrence can offer effective management of migraines. Some patients receive significant relief with chiropractic treatment.

Biofeedback: to control vascular contraction and dilation and improve stress management; may influence both the frequency and the intensity of attacks.

NUTRITION

- Allergy identification and elimination: Elimination/challenge diets have been shown to effect a 30% to 93% decrease in migraines. Patient eliminates suspected food allergens for two weeks and then reintroduces the foods and/or additives, noting the response. Once the offending agents are identified, they generally need to be eliminated for six months, and then they may be reintroduced. While effective, elimination/challenge diets are more challenging in hormonally influenced migraines. Some common allergens are alcohol (especially red wine), cheese, chocolate, citrus, cow's milk, wheat, eggs, coffee, tea, beef, pork, corn, tomato, rye, yeast, and shellfish. Food additives (preservatives and coloring) and nitrates are also common irritants.
- Caffeine should be avoided due to its vasoactive effects.
- Essential fatty acids (1,500 and 3,000 mg/day) regulate platelet aggregation and arachadonic acid metabolites, and may be very helpful for all migraines. Dietary manipulation includes reducing animal fats and increasing fish. Supplementing with fish or flax oil (1 to 3 mg bid) may also be helpful.
- Magnesium (500 mg/day) minimizes nerve excitability and increases muscle relaxation. Since magnesium-deficient people are more subject to vascular headache, adequate intake from food or supplements is essential. Excess magnesium may cause diarrhea in sensitive individuals. The diarrhea resolves with cessation of magnesium. Patients with a heart block without a pacemaker should refrain from high doses of magnesium.
- Intravenous injection of one gram of magnesium by your physician can terminate an acute migraine headache within minutes (in up to nearly 100 percent of subjects in some reviews).
- IV injection of folic acid (15 mg) in one study achieved total subsidence of acute headache within one hour in 60 percent, with great improvement in another 30 percent. These two agents are strikingly successful.
- Omega-3 oils (EPA and DHA, average dose 14 grams daily) greatly reduce intensity and frequency of migraines.
- Vitamin B_2 (riboflavin) (400 mg/day for three months) has been shown to reduce migraine frequency by two-thirds.
- Vitamin C (2,000 mg/day), vitamin E (400 to 600 IU/day), vitamin B_6 (100 mg/day), choline (100 to 300 mg/day) and mixed bioflavonoids (1,000 mg/day) all inhibit the tendency to high platelet adhesion rates in migraine.
- 5-hydroxytryptophan (300 mg bid) works as well as methysergide for prevention of migraine, enhanced by taking with 25 mg of vitamin B_6.

HERBS

Herbs are generally a safe way to strengthen and tone the body's systems. As with any therapy, it is important to ascertain a diagnosis before pursuing treatment. Herbs may be used as dried extracts (capsules, powders, teas), glycerites (glycerine extracts), or tinctures (alcohol extracts). Unless otherwise indicated, teas should be made with 1 teaspoon herb per cup of hot water. Steep covered 5 to 10 minutes for leaf or flowers, and 10 to 20 minutes for roots. Drink 2 to 4 cups/day. Tinctures may be used singly or in combination as noted.

- Feverfew *(Tanacetum parthenium):* Studies show that feverfew cuts the frequency of migraines (25% to 70% in some studies); this may possibly be by suppressing the release of inflammatory prostaglandins and histamines. Feverfew also inhibits platelet aggregation. Feverfew helps with both frequency and intensity of migraines. Dose is two fresh leaves daily, dried herb capsules (250 to 300 mg bid), or 30 drops of tincture tid. It may take 2 months to show an effect. Feverfew may be taken in larger quantities to help reduce pain during a headache.
- Jamaican dogwood *(Piscidia erythrina):* anodyne, antispasmodic, anxiolytic, historic use is specifically for migraines
- Skullcap *(Scutellaria laterifolia):* sedative, antispasmodic, bitter digestive aid
- Gingko *(Gingko biloba):* inhibits lipid peroxidation, especially in the brain, prevents cerebral ischemia, stabilizes smooth muscle of blood vessels, affects platelet activating factor (watch with thrombolytics)
- Ginger *(Zingiber officinalis):* anti-inflammatory, anti-emetic, choleretic
- Meadowsweet *(Filipendula ulmaria):* anti-inflammatory, contains salicylic acid, anti-emetic, astringent
- Total herbal treatment could include feverfew by itself. In addition, a combination of the above herbs may be useful. Dose is equal parts dried herb as a tea—1 cup bid to qid, or a tincture of equal parts 60 drops bid to qid.

HOMEOPATHY

An experienced homeopath should assess individual constitutional types and severity of disease to select the correct remedy and potency. For acute prescribing use three to five pellets of a 12X to 30C remedy every one to four hours until symptoms resolve.

- *Iris versicolor* for periodic migraines that begin with blurred vision, especially after eating sweets or after relaxing from a mental strain
- *Lac defloratum* for frontal migraine preceded by an aura of dim vision, marked nausea, vomiting and chills, that may be brought on by milk
- *Natrum muriaticum* for migraines "like hammers beating the head," that are much better lying down alone in the quiet dark, especially if the migraines are associated with menstruation
- *Sanguinaria* for right sided migraines that begin in the neck and move up, migraines with vomiting, especially if the vomiting provides some relief

PHYSICAL MEDICINE

Appropriate regular aerobic exercise—brisk walking, gardening, low impact aerobics, and water aerobics—are among the options that reduce the frequency and intensity of migraine episodes. Chiropractic adjustments and/or cranio-sacral therapy may be helpful.

ACUPUNCTURE

May be very helpful, especially in migraines that are hormonally influenced. Acupuncture is one of the most effective treatments for migraines.

MASSAGE

Stretching, yoga, massage and other stress management techniques can be quite helpful. Massage may help release chronic neck and shoulder tension that may exacerbate migraines.

Patient Monitoring

Patient should seek medical assistance if headache begins after exercise, straining, coughing, or sexual activity, or is accompanied by changes in mental state or memory, confusion, or sleepiness. A sudden, severe headache may be caused by brain hemorrhage, or if accompanied by stiff neck and fever, meningitis or encephalitis.

OTHER CONSIDERATIONS

Prevention

- Patient should keep a headache diary to record migraine triggers. Identified triggers should be avoided.
- Antihypertensive drugs including beta blockers and calcium channel blockers help prevent attacks in some patients. Begin with low doses and increase if needed. Prophylactic antihypertensives are contraindicated with certain illnesses including asthma, chronic obstructive pulmonary disease, insulin-dependent diabetes mellitus, peripheral vascular disease, heart block or heart failure, hypotension, congestive heart failure, arrhythmias, and current or previous depressive illness. (propranolol hydrochloride 40 to 80 mg bid, increasing to 320 mg/day, with a maximum of 640 mg/day; atenolol 50 to 100 mg/day; metroprolol tartrate 100 mg/day, increasing to 400 mg/day; amitriptyline 75 mg/day, increasing to 150 mg/day.)

Complications/Sequelae

Severe migraine may be so incapacitating it requires emergency treatment.

Prognosis

Migraines start suddenly, sometimes waking patient from sleep, and then usually last several hours but can persist for days. Headaches may occur repeatedly over several weeks or months, then may disappear for weeks or months. Frequency and severity may decrease with age.

Pregnancy

Avoid prophylactic antihypertensive drugs and other medications or alternative remedies that are contraindicated during pregnancy.

REFERENCES

Berkow R. *The Merck Manual.* 15th ed. Rahway, NJ: Merck Sharp & Dohme Research Laboratories; 1987.

De Weerdt CJ, Bootsma HPR, Hendricks H. Herbal medicines in migraine prevention. Randomized double-blind placebo controlled crossover trial of a feverfew preparation. *Phytomedicine.* 1996;3:225–230.

Gruenwald J, Brendler T, Jaenicke C et al, eds. *PDR for Herbal Medicines.* Montvale, NJ: Medical Economics Company; 1998.

Minirth F. *The Headache Book: Prevention and Treatment for All Types of Headaches.* Nashville, Tenn: Thomas Nelson; 1994.

Morrison R. *Desktop Guide to Keynotes and Confirmatory Symptoms.* Albany, Calif: Hahnemann Clinic Publishing; 1993.

Murphy JJ, Heptinsall S, Mitchell JRA. Randomised double-blind placebo-controlled trial of feverfew in migraine prevention. *Lancet.* 1988;2:189–192.

Murray MT. *Encyclopedia of Nutritional Supplements.* Rocklin, Calif: Prima Publishing; 1996.

Palevitch D, Earon G, Carasso R. Feverfew (Tanacetum parthenium) as a prophylactic treatment for migraine: a double-blind controlled study. *Phytotherapy Res.* 1997;11:508–511.

Pryse-Phillips W. Guideline for the diagnosis and management of migraine in clinical practice. *Can Med Assoc J.* 1997;156:1273–1287.

Walker L, Brown E. *The Alternative Pharmacy: Break The Drug Cycle With Safe Natural Treatment For 200 Everyday Ailments.* Paramus, NJ: Prentice Hall; 1998.

■ HEADACHE, SINUS

OVERVIEW

Definition
An acute or subacute headache caused by sinus congestion and/or infection results in dull, deep, or severe pain in the front of the head, localized over the affected sinus. Found in patients with a previous history of upper respiratory infection with residual nasal congestion and discharge. Allergies that interfere with the body's protective mechanisms may precede the viral infection. Symptoms worsen in cold, damp conditions. Pain is greater in the morning and decreased by afternoon. Bending or leaning over worsens headache. Sinus headache may be a symptom of sinusitis, a bacterial infection. Some believe that true sinus headaches affect only 2 % of the population; the rest who believe they are experiencing sinus headache may instead have vascular headaches (migraine, cluster).

Etiology
After an acute viral respiratory tract infection, the patient develops a bacterial infection. Gram-negative rod or anaerobic microorganisms may worsen infection.
- Streptococci
- Pneumococci
- *Hemophilus influenzae*
- Staphylococci

Risk Factors
- Viral respiratory tract infections
- Sinusitis

Signs and Symptoms
- Dull or severe frontal headache
- Previous upper respiratory infection
- Purulent nasal discharge; yellow or green rhinorrhea
- Fever
- Red, turgescent nasal passages
- Pain may be worse in mornings, better in afternoons
- Bending or leaning over increases pain
- Pain is worse in cold and damp weather
- Pain may be localized to one part of the face

DIFFERENTIAL DIAGNOSIS
- Migraine, tension, or cluster headache
- Brain tumor or brain abscess
- Systemic disease or condition such as hypertension, allergy, anemia
- Meningitis or meningeal irritation
- Sensitivity to vasoactive substances, nitrites, carbon monoxide
- Seizure disorder
- Encephalitis
- Subdural hematoma
- Allergies

DIAGNOSIS

Physical Examination
Patient has history of upper respiratory infection and current swollen mucous membranes, tenderness on compression over affected sinus, and evidence of nasal obstruction. Eliminate vascular headaches masquerading as sinus headache: Patient complains of general malaise and presents with mild to moderate fever and apparent nasal congestion or discharge.

Laboratory Tests
- CBC
- Nasapharyngeal cultures

Imaging
- CT scan if headache is recent and cause is not immediately clear, especially if abnormal neurological signs are present
- Xray of sinuses, transillumination

Other Diagnostic Procedures
Patient history and examination, with emphasis on upper respiratory symptoms and previous infection. Patient history should note characteristics of headache, timing, frequency, duration and possible triggers.
- Try a migraine drug to see if it stops the headache.

TREATMENT OPTIONS

Treatment Strategy
Treatment should be directed at improving sinus drainage and eliminating infection. Patients will appreciate pain relief. Inhaling steam or using a vaporizer helps shrink mucous membrane blood vessels and improves drainage.

Drug Therapies
- Nasal vasoconstrictor spray medications such as phenylephrine 0.25% spray once every three hours are effective but must not be used longer than seven days.
- Systemic vasoconstrictors such as pseudoephedrine 30 mg orally (adult) every four to six hours may be helpful but are less reliable.
- Antibiotics for a minimum of 10 to 12 days. Ampicillin (2 g/day) or amoxicillin (1.5 g/day), active against s. pneumoniae and H. influenzae. Augmentin when beta-lactanase strains of influenzae. For patients allergic to penicillin, trimethoprimsuffamethoxazole and cefaclor. Nasal decongestants as supportive therapy.

Complementary and Alternative Therapies
Can be very helpful at minimizing the discomfort, treating the infection, stimulating the immune system, clearing the congestion, and decreasing the frequency of headaches/infections. A combination of physical medicine and herbal or homeopathic treatment is often very effective.

NUTRITION
- Use the same nutritional regimens as used in other treatments of acute infection—vitamin C (1,000 mg tid), zinc (30 to 60 mg/day for acute phase only), beta-carotene (15,000 IU/day).
- Use bromelain (1,200 to 1,800 mcu, 250 to 500 mg) between meals.

HERBS
Herbs are generally a safe way to strengthen and tone the body's systems. As with any therapy, it is important to ascertain a diagnosis before pursuing treatment. Herbs may be used as dried extracts (capsules, powders, teas), glycerites (glycerine extracts), or tinctures (alcohol extracts). Unless otherwise indicated, teas should be made with 1 tsp. herb per cup of hot water. Steep covered 5 to 10 minutes for leaf or flowers, and 10 to 20 minutes for roots. Drink 2 to 4 cups/day. Tinctures may be used singly or in combination as noted.
- Wild indigo (*Baptisia tinctoria*)—specific for upper respiratory and sinus infections
- Eyebright (*Euphrasia officinalis*)—stimulates drainage, warming and soothing
- Licorice (*Glycyrrhiza glabra*)—anti-viral, soothing, especially with exhaustion and/or heartburn, avoid with hypertension
- Coneflower (*Echinacea*)—stimulates the immune system, anti-viral
- Goldenseal (*Hydrastis canadensis*)—anti-viral, anti-bacterial, digestive tonic
- A combination of all of the above herbs, equal parts, may be very effec-

tive. Using dried herb—one tbsp./cup water, four to six cups/day. Using tincture—equal parts of tincture, 60 drops every two to four hours.

- Jamaican dogwood *(Piscidea piscipula)* or St. John's wort *(Hypericum perforatum),* in equal parts—may be added for pain relief
- Garlic *(Allium sativum)* and ginger *(Zingiber officinalis),* as a tea—Use 2 to 3 cloves of garlic and 2 to 3 slices of fresh ginger, steep 5 to 15 minutes and drink, breathing in the steam. Stimulates immune system and drainage, prevents sinus problems from extending into lungs.
- Essential oils may be used as a bath or as a steam. For a steam, place 2 to 5 drops in a pot, bring to a simmer and hold head over pot. For a bath, add 5 to 10 drops of oil to the bath. Eucalyptus, lavender and thyme are specific for upper respiratory infections. Lavender and rosemary are also very calming. All of these essential oils have antiseptic properties.

HOMEOPATHY

An experienced homeopath should assess individual constitutional types and severity of disease to select the correct remedy and potency. For acute prescribing use 3 to 5 pellets of a 12X to 30C remedy every one to four hours until acute symptoms resolve.

The goal of homeopathic remedies for sinus problems is to encourage drainage; patient should be advised that the resulting runny nose is helping to clear out bacteria. Peptostrep, a German homeopathic remedy, works well to clear sinuses and may be taken in 200X to 5X strength over the period of a month.

- *Arsenicum album* for sinusitis with thin, watery, excoriating discharge, especially with sneezing without any relief from the nasal stuffiness and restlessness and/or anxiety.
- *Kali bichromium* for sinusitis with post-nasal drip, especially with ulcerations of the septum and weakness.
- *Mercurius* for raw, ulcerated nostrils with swelling, may have bloody discharge and exhaustion.
- *Pulsatilla* for sinusitis with thick, bland discharges, especially with weepiness, a lack of thirst, and wanting to be constantly comforted/held

PHYSICAL MEDICINE

- Alternating hot and cold compresses. Three minutes hot compress/cloth across the sinus, alternating with 30 second cold compress. Repeat this cycle three times for a single treatment. Treatment may be repeated from two to six times/day. The hot compress brings blood, white blood cells, and therapeutic agents (herbs or antibiotics), into the area. Heat is also analgesic. The cold flushes the sinuses and relieves congestion, thereby relieving pain.
- Nasal lavage. Mix salt water to taste like tears. Rinse each nostril by holding head over sink and letting water run from upper nostril to the lower nostril. Keep nostrils lower than throat to prevent salt water draining into back of throat. This shrinks membranes and increases drainage.
- Cranio-sacral therapy can be very effective at decreasing the frequency of infections and headaches.

ACUPUNCTURE

May be useful to stimulate immune system and increase drainage.

Patient Monitoring

Use of nasal vasoconstriction sprays must be limited. Patients should be instructed on proper use of this medicine and the importance of limiting the time it is used.

Patient should return for treatment if a headache begins after exercise, straining, coughing, sexual activity, or is accompanied by changes in mental state or memory, confusion, or sleepiness. A sudden, severe headache may be caused by hemorrhage or bleeding in the brain; or if accompanied by stiff neck and fever, meningitis or meningoencephalitis.

OTHER CONSIDERATIONS
Prevention

- At higher risk for sinusitis are smokers and people who are repeatedly exposed to bacteria, such as school and health care workers, and those who have allergies or deformities of the nose such as a deviated septum.
- Avoid respiratory illnesses and infections.
- Treat respiratory illnesses promptly to prevent developing bacterial infection.
- Patients should be advised not to use over-the-counter decongestant nose drops or sprays that contain phenylephrine longer than three days because they can lead to addiction.

Complications/Sequelae

- If decongestant and antibiotic therapies are not effective, patient may need surgery to remove infected material from sinus.
- Poorly controlled diabetic or immunocompromised patients are at risk of developing potentially serious fungal infections.

Prognosis

Depending on severity of sinus infection, condition may take weeks to months to resolve. When sinus infection is eliminated, sinus headaches are eliminated also.

Pregnancy

Avoid medications or alternative remedies that are contraindicated during pregnancy.

REFERENCES

Berkow R. *The Merck Manual.* 15th ed. Rahway, NJ: Merck Sharp & Dohme Research Laboratories; 1987.

Gobel H, Schmidt G, Soyka D. Effect of Peppermint and Eucalyptus oil preparations on neurophysiological and experimental algesimetric headache parameters. *Cephalalgia.* 1994;14:228–234.

National Headache Foundation. Headache Topics: Sinus Headache. Accessed at www.headaches.org/sheets/sinus.html on January 30, 1999.

Pryse-Phillips W: Guideline for the diagnosis and management of migraine in clinical practice, *Canadian Medical Association Journal (CMAJ)* 1997, 156:1273-87

University of Michigan Health System. Health Topics A to Z: Sinus Headaches. Accessed at www.med.umich.edu/1libr/topics/hdache08.htm on January 30, 1999.

Walker L, Brown E. *The Alternative Pharmacy: Break the Drug Cycle With Safe Natural Treatment for 200 Everyday Ailments.* Paramus, NJ: Prentice Hall; 1998.

■ HEADACHE, TENSION
OVERVIEW

Definition
Tension headaches are frequent, intermittent, moderate headache pain originating occipitally or bifrontally. Tension headaches may be episodic or chronic, characterized by a dull, persistent sensation of tightness, pressure, or stiffness that may spread to both temples and the entire head. With chronic tension headache, muscles in the neck, shoulders, and jaw may be tight and sore. Duration ranges from 30 minutes to several days, or longer. Tension (also called muscle contraction) headaches account for the majority of all headaches. Most resolve spontaneously. Surveys indicate higher incidence in women, which might be explained by women's greater likelihood of seeking medical assistance.

Etiology
Prolonged contraction of shoulder, neck, face, and scalp muscles constricts blood vessels, which irritates surrounding nerves and triggers pain. Restricted circulation also causes oxygen deficiency in muscles, resulting in excessive accumulation and impaired circulatory removal of pain-producing toxins.

- Referred pain from forehead, scalp, mouth, throat, eyes, sinuses, and meninges serviced by the trigeminal nerve
- Prolonged sitting, sitting in an uncomfortable position, or immobility
- Anxiety or stress
- PMS, hypoglycemia, dehydration, food allergy, insomnia
- Depression

Risk Factors
- Family history of tension headache; although tension headaches are probably not inherited, family members may share personality traits, behavior patterns, and poor stress management skills
- Chronic stress or anxiety
- Depression
- Poor posture
- Irritability
- Excessive caffeine intake (including caffeine withdrawal)
- Fatigue, lack of sleep and overwork syndrome
- Deficient exercise pattern
- Eyestrain
- Temporomandibular joint dysfunction
- Cervical spine mechanical problems
- Hypothyroidism and low adrenal function
- Carbon monoxide exposures
- Artificial sweeteners (up to 14% incidence in aspartame [Nutrasweet] users)
- Trichloroethylene (industrial chemical) contamination of the water supply

Signs and Symptoms
- Originates bifrontally or occipitally, then spreads to entire head
- Often described as feeling as though one's head were being squeezed in a vise or constricted by a tight hatband
- Chronic or continuous headache lasting 30 minutes to days, or longer
- Morning or early afternoon onset with pain continuing through the day; headache may be present on waking but does not disrupt sleep
- Grinding teeth
- Insomnia
- Tight, sore muscles in neck, and shoulders
- Pain is not aggravated by routine physical activity
- Headache is often associated with emotional stress or depression, or may occur premenstrually in women

DIFFERENTIAL DIAGNOSIS
- Acute headache
- Brain tumor or brain abscess
- Eye lesions, eyestrain, iritis, glaucoma
- Toxic states, including infections, alcoholism, uremia, lead, arsenic, morphine, CO poisoning, encephalatides
- Overuse of caffeine
- Premenstrual syndrome
- Migraine or sinus headache

DIAGNOSIS
Rule out organic disease and cranial trauma.

Physical Examination
Patients are generally in good health. Patient may present with tight muscles in face, scalp, and neck.

Laboratory Tests
Diagnostic tests for tension headache are not available. Laboratory tests may be used to rule out other causes of headache symptoms.

TREATMENT OPTIONS
Treatment Strategy
Educate patient in stress avoidance and stress management to prevent recurrence of tension headaches. Physical fitness should be encouraged. Biofeedback, yoga, and relaxation techniques can be quite effective for both acute relief and decreasing headache frequency.

Drug Therapies
- Nonprescription analgesics are usually effective temporary remedies; to prevent rebound headaches, educate patient about proper use of analgesics. Caffeine enhances effect of analgesics for some people; excessive caffeine or caffeine withdrawal may itself cause headaches. Prescription analgesics containing codeine or oxycodone relieve severe headache.
- For acute attack, NSAIDS: naproxen (500 mg bid), ibuprofen (400 mg tid)
- As prophylaxis for chronic headache, antidepressants: amitriptyrine (50 to 100 mg/day), imipramine (50 to 100 mg/day).
- Beta-blockers as a prophylaxis: propanolol (80 mg/day), atenolol (50 to 100 mg/day)

Complementary and Alternative Therapies
The main emphasis of therapies is stress managment and muscle relaxation.

NUTRITION
- Micronutrients: Because tension headache is so often related to increased stress, replacement of micronutrients which are depleted in times of stress is essential; the most critical are vitamins C, E, beta-carotene, B-complex and minerals magnesium, potassium, calcium, zinc, manganese, and selenium. Magnesium (aspartate or glycinate, up to 750 mg/day) is especially critical because of its antispasmodic action.
- Avoid caffeine: Increased caffeine intake is correlated with increased incidence of headaches. Cessation of caffeine may lead to withdrawal

headaches that should resolve in two to four days.

- Essential fatty acids: regulate platelet aggregation and arachadonic acid metabolites. Dietary manipulation includes reducing animal fats and increasing fish. A mix of omega-6 (evening primrose) and omega-3 (flax seed) may be most optimum (2 tbsp. oil/day or 1,000 to 1,500 IU bid).
- Vitamin E: 400 to 800 IU/day may decrease muscle cramping.
- Elimination/challenge diet: The most common allergic foods are wheat, dairy, corn, soy, and chocolate. Avoid foods completely for two weeks, then reintroduce the foods one at a time, every three days, and note symptoms. Citrus, alcohol, red meat, flour products, spices, and carbonated drinks may also aggravate headaches.
- Calcium/magnesium: 1,000/500 mg/day may help to regulate muscle contraction and relaxation.

HERBS

Herbs are generally a safe way to strengthen and tone the body's systems. As with any therapy, it is important to ascertain a diagnosis before pursuing treatment. Herbs may be used as dried extracts (capsules, powders, teas), glycerites (glycerine extracts), or tinctures (alcohol extracts). Unless otherwise indicated, teas should be made with 1 tsp. herb per cup of hot water. Steep covered 5 to 10 minutes for leaf or flowers, and 10 to 20 minutes for roots. Drink 2 to 4 cups/day. Tinctures may be used singly or in combination as noted.

- Peppermint oil—a natural antispasmodic and diuretic, was shown in German studies to be as effective against tension as Extra-strength Tylenol. Add two drops of peppermint or lavender essential oil to one cup of water. Soak a cloth in the solution and apply as a compress.
- White willow bark *(Salix alba)*—contains salicin, the pain reliever in aspirin.
- Meadowsweet *(Filipendula ulmaria)*—contains salicylic acid. Relieves pain, reduces nausea and heartburn; particularly effective for tension with digestive effects
- Valerian *(Valeriana officinalis)*—sedative and anti-spasmodic, digestive bitter, particularly for tension with anxiety and/or digestive effects
- Jamaican dogwood *(Piscidia piscipula)*—sedative, pain reliever, anti-spasmodic
- Ginkgo *(Ginkgo biloba)*—increases circulation to the brain, regulates platelet aggregation, particularly for tension with difficulty concentrating or circulatory problems
- Combine white willow, meadowsweet and two of the above herbs. Use equal parts of either herb or tincture. Herbs: 1 tbsp. in 1 cup water tid. Tincture: 60 drops tid.
- Kava Kava *(Piper methysticum)*—45 to 60 mg of kavalactone content tid, has a calming effect if anxiety is prominent.

HOMEOPATHY

An experienced homeopath should assess individual constitutional types and severity of disease to select the correct remedy and potency. For acute prescribing use 3 to 5 pellets of a 12X to 30C remedy every one to four hours until acute symptoms resolve.

- *Aconite* for sudden onset tension headaches with anxiety that follow shock or are accompanied by a fever

- *Bryonia* for congestive headaches that feel worse with movement and better with pressure and/or eyes closed; headaches may start on the left and spread to the whole head
- *Gelsemium* for heavy feeling headaches and confusion, especially with blurry vision or vertigo
- *Belladonna* for throbbing headaches of sudden onset, that feel worse with motion, but the pain keeps the patient from being able to be still

PHYSICAL MEDICINE

During any of these therapies, patient should be instructed to practice deep breathing, visualization or relaxation techniques.

- Biofeedback helps patients learn to control muscle tension and to relax problem areas.
- Neck stretches can relieve pain. Gently stretch by moving the head to one side, then the other, resting it against the palm of the hand. Shoulder rolls will also help to relax the upper torso.
- Press an ice pack to the forehead to constrict swollen blood vessels and relieve pain.
- Acupressure points at the web between thumb and first finger. Press in small circular motions at the tender points.
- Regular exercise, with an emphasis on both upper and lower back and abdominal areas increases muscle tone, i.e. better contraction but also better relaxation.

ACUPUNCTURE

May be helpful for pain relief and decreasing frequency of headaches

MASSAGE

Gentle massage of shoulders and neck to loosen tight muscles and relieve tension can be very helpful.

Patient Monitoring

A sudden change in symptoms may indicate possible serious illness.

OTHER CONSIDERATIONS

Prevention

- Patient should learn to avoid stressors that trigger headaches.
- Psychological counseling may benefit patients whose headaches stem from suppressed emotions, depression, or anxiety.

Prognosis

Most tension headaches are self-limiting or rapidly remedied with patient education and analgesics. Underlying factors should be addressed to decrease frequency of occurrences.

Pregnancy

Care should be taken when using analgesics or alternative remedies during pregnancy. Some headaches resolve during pregnancy.

REFERENCES

Berkow R. *The Merck Manual.* 15th ed. Rahway, NJ: Merck Sharp & Dohme Research Laboratories; 1987.
Scalzo R. *Naturopathic Handbook of Herbal Formulas.* Durango, Colo: 2nd ed. Kivaki Press; 1994.
Walker L, Brown E. *The Alternative Pharmacy: Break the Drug Cycle With Safe Natural Treatment for 200 Everyday Ailments.* Paramus, NJ: Prentice Hall; 1998.

■ HEMORRHOIDS
OVERVIEW
Definition
Hemorrhoids are a varicosity of the rectal venous plexus, classified as either internal or external to the anal verge.
- External skin tags at the anal verge
- External hemorrhoids, possibly thrombosed
- Internal hemorrhoids: (first degree—bulging into anal canal and causing bleeding; second degree—prolapsing during defecation and reducing spontaneously; third degree—prolapsing and requiring manual reduction; thrombosed—prolapsing and may be strangulated)

Hemorrhoids are uncommon before age 25 (except in women who have been pregnant) and thereafter increase in prevalence by age. After age 50, about 50% of the population have asymptomatic hemorrhoids and 5% have symptomatic hemorrhoids.

Etiology
Hemorrhoids are caused by dilation of veins within the rectal venous plexus. Prolapse in internal hemorrhoids may be caused by shearing forces from passage of large, firm stool or urgent defecation; the prolapse may become entrapped by the internal anal sphincter.

Risk Factors
In most cases, there is no obvious predisposing factor. The following factors increase a patient's risk.
- Family history
- Age
- Irritable bowel syndrome
- Portal hypertension
- Pregnancy
- Constipation
- Obesity
- Regular prolonged sitting
- Congestive heart failure
- Pelvic inflammatory disease or neoplasms
- Carcinoma of the rectum

Signs and Symptoms
- Constipation
- Straining while defecating
- Anal fissures
- Stool mucus

External hemorrhoids:
- Discomfort, pain
- Tender perianal lump
- Possible bleeding
- Pruritus

Internal hemorrhoids:
- Intermittent or sustained bleeding
- Pain (if thrombosed or strangulated)
- Sensation of fullness (if prolapsed)

DIFFERENTIAL DIAGNOSIS
- Hypertrophied anal papillae from anal fissure, Crohn's disease, or other cause
- Anal skin tags from previous hemorrhoids or Crohn's disease
- Prolapsed rectal mucosa
- Rectal or anal tumors, polyps
- Endometriosis
- Condyloma

DIAGNOSIS
Physical Examination
External hemorrhoids appear as a mass outside the anal verge, which may be soft and painless or, if thrombosed, firm and tender with blue col-

oration. Internal hemorrhoids may be visualized with buttocks retracted and the patient straining. Sigmoidoscopy or colonoscopy may be performed when there is bleeding or if carcinoma is suspected as a cause of the hemorrhoids.

Imaging
In cases of significant or repeated bleeding, barium enema may be performed.

Other Diagnostic Procedures
Since hemorrhoids usually do not produce significant bleeding, question the patient carefully about any bleeding as well as about any constipation experienced. Assess the level of pain, as severe pain may indicate strangulation and the need for immediate surgical referral. Rectal examination. Sigmoidoscopy.

TREATMENT OPTIONS
Treatment Strategy
The goal is to alleviate symptoms and promote healing. Surgery may be needed in severe cases, but most cases respond well to other measures.
- Treating any underlying condition
- Preventing direct pressure (positional changes, sitting on an inflatable ring)
- Avoiding straining on defecation
- Limiting the amount of time sitting on the toilet
- Sitz baths with soapy water or Epsom salts 2 to 3 times daily for 15 to 20 minutes
- Stool softeners and high-fiber foods reduce straining and prolapse
- Topical preparations for pain or pruritus
- Analgesics (rectal or systemic) for pain

Drug Therapies
- Stool softeners, such as docusate (Docusate Calcium, 240 mg p.r.n.), help reduce straining and prevent hard stools; side effects include nausea, cramps, diarrhea; contraindicated in obstruction and fecal impaction.
- Bulk laxatives, such as psyllium (Effer-Syllium, Metamucil, 1 to 2 tsps. in water bid to tid, or premeasured packets), help prevent hard stools; side effects include nausea, vomiting, diarrhea; contraindicated in obstruction, abdominal pain, and fecal impaction.
- Rectal preparations, such as hydrocortisone (Anusol-HC cream, ProctoFoam-HC aerosol, or Wyanoids-HC ointment), relieve itching and discomfort; side effects include local irritation, burning, blistering.
- Topical anesthetics, such as dibucaine hydrochloride (Nupercainal, applied topically qid as needed) or lidocaine 2.5% (Xylocaine, applied topically tid to qid), relieve rectal discomfort; side effects include contact allergy symptoms.
- Systemic analgesics, such as oxycodone (Tylox, 5 to 10 mg every 6 hours), for severe pain of thrombosed hemorrhoids; side effects include drowsiness, dizziness, sedation, nausea, vomiting, constipation; contraindicated in addictive personality.

Surgical Procedures
Surgery is indicated if conservative measures fail or for persistent bleeding, severe pain with thrombosis, prolapse, strangulation, ulceration, or perianal infection. Surgical methods include the following.
- Excision hemorrhoidectomy
- Rubber band ligation
- Cryosurgery
- Injection of sclerosing agents
- Laser therapy
- Infrared photocoagulation

Complementary and Alternative Therapies

Nutritional support, topical preparations, and sitz baths may be effective in restoring the integrity of the vasculature, reducing hemorrhoids, and minimizing recurrence.

NUTRITION

- Take time to eat in a relaxed atmosphere, breathing and chewing food thoroughly.
- Eat smaller, more frequent meals and avoid over-eating at one sitting.
- Decrease low-fiber foods and foods and drinks that cause excess urination (refined foods, sugars, caffeine, alcohol, meat, and dairy products), which leads to harder stools. Increase foods that are high in fiber (fresh fruits and vegetables, whole grains) to soften stools. Increase water intake.
- Decrease saturated fats (animal products) and increase polyunsaturated fats (cold-water fish, nuts, and seeds).
- Stewed or soaked prunes, one to three/day have a slightly laxative effect and may help soften stools.
- Flax meal, 1 heaping tsp. in 8 oz. of apple juice, provides fiber and essential fatty acids to help relieve constipation and soothe the digestive tract. Follow with an additional 8 oz. of water. Flax meal can be made by grinding flax seeds in a blender.
- Vitamin C (1,000 mg bid to tid) supports the integrity of connective tissue.
- Vitamin E (400 to 800 IU/day) promotes normal clotting and healing.

HERBS

Herbs are generally a safe way to strengthen and tone the body's systems. As with any therapy, it is important to ascertain a diagnosis before pursuing treatment. Herbs may be used as dried extracts (capsules, powders, teas), glycerites (glycerine extracts), or tinctures (alcohol extracts). Unless otherwise indicated, teas should be made with 1 tsp. herb per cup of hot water. Steep covered 5 to 10 minutes for leaf or flowers, and 10 to 20 minutes for roots. Drink 2 to 4 cups/day. Tinctures may be used singly or in combination as noted.

Bioflavanoids, a constituent found in dark berries and some plants, help restore the integrity of the vasculature. The following are bioflavanoids that may be taken in dried extract form as noted.

- Catechin (150 mg bid to tid), quercetin (250 mg tid to qid), hesperidin (250 mg tid to qid), and rutin (250 mg tid to qid).
- Rose hips (*Rosa canina*) and green tea (*Camelia sinensis*) are also high in bioflavanoids and either one may be used as a tea. Drink 3 to 4 cups/day.
- Stone root (*Collinsonia canadensis*) and horse chestnut (*Aesculus hippocastanum*) can be used to strengthen blood vessel walls (60 drops tincture bid).

Topical applications may relieve itching and burning, as well as promote healing. Apply one of the following bid to qid.

- Witch hazel (*Hamamelis virginiana*) is an astringent that may reduce swelling (commercially available as Tuck's pads).
- A salve containing comfrey (*Symphytum officinalis*) and/or marigold (*Calendula officinalis*) soothes and promotes healing.
- A poultice made from grated potato is astringent and soothing.

HOMEOPATHY

An experienced homeopath should assess individual constitutional types and severity of disease to select the correct remedy and potency. For acute prescribing use 3 to 5 pellets of a 12X to 30C remedy every one to four hours until acute symptoms resolve.

- *Aesculus* for burning hemorrhoids with a sensation of a lump in anus and aggravations from walking
- *Aloe* for a sensation of pulsation in the rectum with large, external hemorrhoids
- *Collinsonia* for chronic, itchy hemorrhoids with obstinate constipation
- *Hamamelis* for large bleeding hemorrhoids with raw feeling in the anus

PHYSICAL MEDICINE

Contrast hydrotherapy: Contrast sitz baths may relieve symptoms and promote circulation, relieving pelvic vascular congestion. You will need two basins that can be comfortably sat in. Fill one basin with hot water, one with cold water. Sit in hot water for three minutes, then in cold water for one minute. Repeat this three times to complete one set. Do one to two sets per day three to four days per week.

ACUPUNCTURE

Acupuncture may be effective in resolving stagnant, congestive conditions.

Patient Monitoring

If the hemorrhoids do not resolve in one to two weeks, reevaluate the patient's condition and consider additional therapy.

OTHER CONSIDERATIONS

Patients with severe congestive heart failure, portal hypertension, or debilitating disease should consider options outside of surgery and be treated with general measures.

Prevention

A high-fiber diet and avoiding prolonged sitting may help prevent hemorrhoids in susceptible individuals.

Complications/Sequelae

- Secondary infection
- Ulceration
- Thrombosis

Prognosis

Untreated, the symptoms of hemorrhoids often resolve within days to weeks, though likely to recur. If a thrombosed hemorrhoid strangulates, however, it may ulcerate and cause infection.

Pregnancy

Nutritional support, topical herbal applications, and homeopathic remedies are safe in pregnancy. Hemorrhoids often resolve after childbirth.

REFERENCES

Balch JF. *Prescription for Nutritional Healing.* 2nd ed. Garden City Park, NY: Avery Publishing, 1997.

Barker LR, Burton JR, Zieve PD, eds. *Principles of Ambulatory Medicine.* 4th ed. Baltimore, Md: Williams & Wilkins; 1995:1,347–1,361.

Duke JA. *The Green Pharmacy.* Emmaus, Pa: Rodale Press; 1997.

Gruenwald J, Brendler T, Jaenicke C et al, eds. *PDR for Herbal Medicines.* Montvale, NJ: Medical Economics Company; 1998.

Kruzel T. *The Homeopathic Emergency Guide.* Berkeley, Calif: North Atlantic Books; 1992:181–183.

Murray MT, Pizzorno JE. *Encyclopedia of Natural Medicine.* Rocklin, Calif: Prima Publishing; 1998.

Olshevsky M, Noy S, Zwang M. *Manual of Natural Therapy: A Succinct Catalog of Complementary Treatments.* New York, NY: Facts on File; 1989.

Stein JH, ed. *Internal Medicine.* 4th ed. St. Louis, Mo: Mosby-Year Book; 1994:486–492.

United States Pharmacopeial Convention, Inc. *Advice for the Patient.* 15th ed. USPDI; 1995:2.

■ HEPATITIS, VIRAL

OVERVIEW

Definition

Hepatitis—inflammation of the liver—refers to a broad range of conditions with viral, toxic (including alcohol), pharmacologic, and immune-mediated etiologies. A systemic infection, hepatitis can be localized in the liver or be part of a generalized process. Viral hepatitis, the most common, can be subdivided into a number of types.

- Type A (HAV) or epidemic, infectious, MS-1, or short-incubation hepatitis
- Type B (HBV) or serum, long-incubation, or transfusion hepatitis
- Type C (HCV)
- Type D (HDV) or delta hepatitis
- Type E (HEV)
- Non-A, non-B hepatitis (NANB hepatitis)
- Non-A, non-B, non-C hepatitis (NANBNC hepatitis)

Hepatitis also is categorized by duration.

- Acute hepatitis: Less than six months
- Chronic hepatitis: Longer than six months - chronic persistent hepatitis, the most common, - chronic active hepatitis, the most serious

HAV, HBV, and HCV, the most prevalent, affect a half million Americans annually and millions worldwide.

- HAV, the most common, occurs both infrequently and in epidemics (autumn and winter), often affecting school children. Incubation is 15 to 50 days (infectivity two to three weeks near end of incubation). Not chronic.
- HBV, the most quickly growing hepatitis, affects all ages. Six-month incubation (infectivity during HBsAg positivity). Possibly chronic.
- HCV, the primary cause of NANB hepatitis, affects all ages, often as community-acquired hepatitis. Incubation is 30 to 90 days (infectivity during anti-HCV positivity). Possibly chronic.

Etiology

- HAV: 27-nm RNA virus transmitted via fecal-oral and ingestion of contaminated food and water
- HBV: 42-nm DNA virus transmitted via injection of contaminated blood/derivatives, IV drug use, and parenteral exchange of bodily fluids
- HCV: Flavivirus-like RNA agent transmitted via blood transfusion, IV drug use, and possibly sexual intercourse

Viral hepatitis also results from herpes, yellow fever, rubella, coxsackie, and adenovirus.

Risk Factors

HAV:

- Poor hygiene, unsanitary conditions
- Contaminated food and water
- Raw shellfish

HBV and HCV:

- Transfusions
- Employment as health care worker, medical laboratory technician, dialysis technician (needlestick)
- IV drug use
- Unprotected sex
- Infected parent (infant)
- Impaired immunity (leukemia, Down syndrome, dialysis patients)
- Tattoos
- Organ transplants

Signs and Symptoms

Symptoms range from mild to severe. Although HAV, HBV, and HCV symptoms are similar, HBV and HCV symptoms usually will be more severe. Importantly, patients with chronic active hepatitis may be asymptomatic. (Increased transaminase level may be the first sign.)

Symptoms include:

- Jaundice (most are anicteric)
- Malaise, fatigue, anorexia
- Nausea, vomiting, abdominal discomfort
- Dark urine, colorless stool
- Aversion to cigarettes
- Myalgia, arthralgia
- Headache, fever, flu

DIFFERENTIAL DIAGNOSIS

- Cytomegalic inclusion infection
- Mononucleosis
- Hepatic malignancy
- Ischemic hepatitis
- Leptospirosis
- Drug-induced hepatitis
- Alcoholic hepatitis
- Extrahepatic biliary obstruction
- Autoimmune hepatitis
- Wilson's disease

DIAGNOSIS

Physical Examination

Physical signs include:

- Enlarged and tender liver
- Posterior cervical lymphadenopathy
- Enlarged spleen

Laboratory Tests

- Serodiagnosis
- Urinalysis

Pathological Findings

Serodiagnosis reveals the presence of components of HBV and HCV viruses and of antibodies to HAV (IgM antibodies), HBV (HbsAG antigen and IgM antibodies), and HCV (not for a number of weeks), markers that help determine the type, severity, and status of the condition. Urinalysis reveals bilirubin and an increase in serum aminotransferases.

Other findings include:

- Hepatocellular damage (elevated transaminase levels)
- Elevated serum alkaline phosphatase
- Increase in serum aminotransferases
- Depressed white cell count
- Signs of cirrhosis (fibrous scarring and hepatic lobular architecture damage)
- Necrosis of periportal liver cells
- Lymphocytic and plasma cell infiltration
- Mild transient anemia, mild hemolytic anemia
- Granulocytopenia
- Lymphocytosis
- Increase in reticulocyte count

Imaging
Ultrasound can indicate ascites and obstruction.

Other Diagnostic Procedures
Diagnosis involves both physical assessment and laboratory work and may require biopsy. A detailed history can reveal risk factors as well as previous incidences of hepatitis. Liver biopsy may be needed to confirm chronic hepatitis (active or persistent) and to assess disease progression.

TREATMENT OPTIONS
Treatment Strategy
Treatment is usually outpatient, but hospitalization may be necessary for severe cases. Treatment regiment depends on condition severity and prognosis.

- Acute viral hepatitis: Treat with rest, aggressive hydration, and balanced nutrition. Base patient activity on fatigue limits. Mandate that patients avoid alcohol at least until liver enzymes are normal, perhaps longer. Use drug therapy to alleviate symptoms.
- Chronic active hepatitis: Generally treat with corticosteroids or immunomodulators, but only after liver biopsy.

Drug Therapies
Nausea:
- Oral benadryl (25 mg tid)
- Metoclopramide
- Compazine (10 mg bid to qid)
- Hydroxyzine

Abdominal discomfort: acetaminophen 500 mg qid

To treat chronic active hepatitis:
- Corticosteroids (generally not HBV, some controversy remains over corticosteroid use): prednisone or prednisolone 40 to 60 mg/day initially, tapered to 15 to 20 mg/day over one to three months, and 10 mg/day over six months.
- Azathioprine (possibly in combination with prednisone) 50 mg/day
- Interferon alpha-2b

Sedatives can precipitate hepatic encephalopathy and should be avoided. Transplantation may be necessary with fulminant active hepatitis and end-stage liver disease.

Complementary and Alternative Therapies
Fulminant active hepatitis and end-stage liver disease require immediate medical attention. Alternative therapies may be hepatoprotective, support liver function, minimize severity of the disease, and enhance healing.

NUTRITION
- Reduce or eliminate alcohol, caffeine, refined foods, sugar, food additives, and saturated fats (meat and dairy products).
- Small, frequent meals are suggested to optimize digestion and absorption, as well as to stabilize blood sugar. Hypo- and hyperglycemic conditions place undue strain on the liver.
- Increase intake of whole grains, fresh vegetables, fruits, vegetable proteins (legumes such as soy), and essential fatty acids (cold-water fish, nuts, and seeds). Include foods that are supportive to liver function, such as beets, artichokes, yams, onions, garlic, green leafy vegetables, apples, and lemons.
- Green tea is a powerful antioxidant and contains bioflavonoids that decrease inflammation. Drink 2 to 3 cups/day. Use decaffeinated, or caution with caffeinated.

- Acidophilus supplements (one capsule with meals) normalizes bowel flora, especially after antibiotic use. Vitamin K is synthesized by these beneficial bacteria and is essential for normal clotting activities of the liver. Vitamin K levels are often low in hepatitis and may be supplemented, 100 to 500 mg/day. Dark leafy green vegetables are high in vitamin K.
- Vitamin C (1,000 to 1,500 mg/day), beta-carotene (100,000 IU/day), vitamin E (400 to 800 IU/day), and zinc (30 to 50 mg/day) enhance immunity. B-complex (50 to 100 mg/day), especially folic acid (800 to 1,000 mcg/day) and B_{12} (1,000 mcg/day) are needed for optimum liver function and are hepatoprotective.
- Selenium (200 mcg/day) is needed for liver detoxification and fatty acid metabolism.
- Dessicated liver and thymus extracts may be considered to improve liver regeneration and immune function.
- Glutathione (500 mg bid) or N-acetyl cysteine (200 mg bid to tid, a precursor to glutathione) provide detoxification and antioxidant support.
- Consider lecithin, choline, and methionine to support fat metabolism.

HERBS
Herbs are generally a safe way to strengthen and tone the body's systems. As with any therapy, it is important to ascertain a diagnosis before pursuing treatment. Herbs may be used as dried extracts (capsules, powders, teas), glycerites (glycerine extracts), or tinctures (alcohol extracts). Unless otherwise indicated, teas should be made with 1 teaspoon herb per cup of hot water. Steep covered 5 to 10 minutes for leaf or flowers, and 10 to 20 minutes for roots. Drink 2 to 4 cups/day. Tinctures may be used singly or in combination as noted.

Many herbs have powerful liver-protective properties, aiding in detoxification and promoting bile production and flow, as well as nourishing and repairing liver tissue. For best results, three to four liver-supportive herbs should be combined with two to three anti-viral and immune-stimulating herbs. The herbal treatment of hepatitis can be complicated and should be administered under physician supervision. Choice of herbs is dependent on disease state and presentation of pathology. The high doses of single herbs suggested may be best administered via dried extracts (encapsulated) although tinctures (60 drops qid) and teas (4 to 6 cups/day) may also be used.

Herbs for liver support:
- Milk thistle (*Silybum marianum*, 200 to 250 mg tid) protects the liver parenchyma and may prevent necrotic changes. May also be used as phosphatidylcholine-bound silymarin (100 to 150 mg tid), which is more specific for hepatitis infections.
- Chinese thoroughwax (*Bupleurum falcatum*) contains steroid-like molecules that are potent anti-inflammatories. May induce nausea in sensitive individuals; decrease dose to ameliorate side effect.
- Globe artichoke (*Cynara scolymus*) promotes liver regeneration.
- Schizandra berry (*Schizandra chinensis*) is hepatoprotective and promotes liver regeneration and detoxification.
- Eclipta alba inhibits hepatitis B replication and is usually used with phyllanthus.
- *Phyllanthus amarus* (200 mg tid) is an ayurvedic herb shown to inhibit hepatitis B replication. Long-term use of a year or more may be necessary for optimum effectiveness.
- Turmeric (*Curcuma longa*, 250 to 500 mg tid) is a potent anti-inflammatory herb that is also hepatoprotective. Combine with bromelain (250 to 500 mg tid between meals), a proteolytic enzyme, to potentiate effects.

Immune support and anti-virals:

- Licorice root (*Glycyrrhiza glabra,* 250 to 500 mg tid), particularly its extract, glycyrrhizin, is hepatoprotective. Concurrent administration of glycine and cysteine appear to modulate glycyrrhizin's actions and prevent its aldosterone-like action.
- Astragalus root *(Astragalus membrinaceus)* augments NK cell activity and interferon response as well as promoting liver detoxification.
- Coneflower *(Echinacea purpurea)* is an anti-viral and immune-stimulating herb best used during acute infection.
- Goldenseal *(Hydrastis canadensis)* has antimicrobial and immune-stimulating properties, and also enhances liver function.

HOMEOPATHY

An experienced homeopath should assess individual constitutional types and severity of disease to select the correct remedy and potency.

PHYSICAL MEDICINE

Castor oil pack. Used externally, castor oil is a powerful anti-inflammatory. Apply oil directly to right upper abdomen over the liver, cover with a clean soft cloth (e.g. flannel) and plastic wrap. Place a heat source (hot water bottle or heating pad) over the pack and let sit for 30 to 60 minutes. For best results, use for three consecutive days. The addition of four to six drops of essential oil may enhance the beneficial effects. Consider essential oils of chamomile, cinnamon, eucalyptus, thyme, or patchouli.

ACUPUNCTURE

May be beneficial in modulating immune function and supporting liver function.

MASSAGE

Therapeutic massage may be helpful in reducing the effects of stress, which inhibits immune function.

Patient Monitoring

- Although patient isolation usually is not required during treatment, strict attention to hygiene is. Segregate food handlers with HAV and health care workers with HBV and HCV.
- Monitor patients at one- to three-week intervals; normal activities can resume when symptoms disappear and laboratory tests are normal. HBV patients with detectable surface antigen at six months should be managed with a heptologist.
- Patients with chronic persistent hepatitis may require a follow-up liver biopsy after two to three years to confirm the diagnosis.

OTHER CONSIDERATIONS

Prevention

- HAV: Attention to hygiene and immune serum globulin
- HBV: Attention to hygiene, blood-product screening, proper needle use/disposal, safe-sex practices, hepatitis B immune globulin, vaccine
- HCV: Attention to hygiene, blood-product screening, proper needle use/disposal, safe-sex practices, and possibly immune serum globulin

Complications/Sequelae

- Posthepatitis syndrome
- Cholestatic hepatitis
- Fulminant hepatitis (necrosis)
- Chronic hepatitis
- Cirrhosis
- Hepatocellular carcinoma

Prognosis

Acute:

- Self-limiting, generally resolves in one to three months
- Suspect chronic active liver disease after 10 weeks
- In rare cases, progresses to necrosis and possibly death in less than six months

Chronic:

- Persists for longer than six months
- Chronic persistent hepatitis is benign, generally asymptomatic, seldom results in cirrhosis, and generally resolves without progressing.
- Chronic active hepatitis can result in cirrhosis and liver failure.

Jaundice, if present, usually disappears in two to eight weeks. Fulminant hepatitis (more common in HBV) is the primary cause of death.

Morbidity and mortality are higher with HBV and HCV:

- HAV: Seldom fatal, but requires up to 30 days bed rest. Could recur after 90 days.
- HBV: Patients sometimes become asymptomatic carriers. Frequently slow to resolve, thus a common cause of chronic liver disease and cirrhosis.
- HCV: Virus remains in the blood for many years, thus a common cause of liver failure, liver cancer, and cirrhosis.

Pregnancy

Active viral hepatitis can be a serious complication in pregnancy. The safety of herbs in pregnancy has not been adequately investigated. Milk thistle (1 cup of tea tid) is safe to use as maintenance. Other herbs and high doses of vitamins should be used only under the supervision of a qualified practitioner.

REFERENCES

Andreoli TE, Bennett JC, Carpenter CCJ. *Cecil Essentials of Medicine.* 3rd ed. Philadelphia, Pa: WB Saunders; 1993:327–334.

Batchelder HJ. The Protocol Journal of Botanical Medicine. Ayer, MA: *Herbal Research Publications, Inc.;* 1995: Vol 1, No 2, 133–137.

Batchelder HJ, Hudson, T." *The Protocol Journal of Botanical Medicine.* 1995;1:138–140.

Barker LR, Burton JR, Zieve PD, eds. *Principles of Ambulatory Medicine.* 4th ed. Baltimore: Williams & Wilkins; 1995:507–515.

Dambro MR. *Griffith's 5-Minute Clinical Consult–1999.* Baltimore, Md: Lippincott Williams & Wilkins; 1999:408-409.

Dharmananda S. *The Protocol Journal of Botanical Medicine.* 1995: Vol 1, No 2: 151-158.

Ergil K. *The Protocol Journal of Botanical Medicine.* 1995:Vol 1, No 2:145–150.

Kiesewetter E, et al. Results of two double-blind studies on the effect of silymarin in chronic hepatitis. *Leber Magen Darm.* 1977;7:318–323.

Stein JK, ed. *Internal Medicine.* 4th ed. St. Louis: Mosby-Year Book; 1994:586–601.

Stoller JK, Ahmad M, Longworth DL, eds. *The Cleveland Clinic Intensive Review of Internal Medicine.* Baltimore, Md: Williams & Wilkins; 1998:573-756.

Scalzo R. *Therapeutic Botanical Protocol for Viral Hepatitis.* The Protocol Journal of Botanical Medicine. 1995:Vol 1, No 2, 159-160.

Sodhi V. *The Protocol Journal of Botanical Medicine.* 1995:Vol 1, No 2, 141-144.

Stedman's Medical Dictionary. 26th edition. Baltimore, Md: Williams & Wilkins; 1995:784-786.

Thyagarajan SP. Effect of Phyllanthus amarus on chronic carriers of hepatitis B virus. *Lancet.* October 1, 1988:764–766.

■ HERPES SIMPLEX VIRUS
OVERVIEW
Definition

Herpes simplex virus (HSV-1, HSV-2) infections are ubiquitous worldwide and have been described clinically since the 1700s. They usually present as painful vesicles on the skin and mucous membranes but may present as a disseminated infection. It has been reported that over 90% of adults have antibodies to HSV-1 and over 25% have antibodies to HSV-2. Transmission of the virus is through infected secretions: HSV-1, through contact with oral secretions (oral-facial herpes) and HSV-2, through contact with genital secretions (genital herpes); however, both HSV-1 and HSV-2 can cause genital and oral-facial infections. The virus can be transmitted from active lesions or shed from asymptomatic individuals. Recurrent infections usually indicate a reactivation of the initial virus, but reinfection is possible. Reactivation appears to be triggered by ultraviolet light, fever, menstruation, emotional stress, immunosuppression, infections by other organisms, and trauma to the skin or ganglia. Disseminated herpes infections in neonates and the immunocompromised, as well as ophthalmic herpes, are emergencies requiring aggressive treatment.

Etiology

HSV is caused by exposure to a symptomatic or asymptomatic individual infected with HSV-1 or HSV-2, such as a family member, sexual partner, or through occupational contact. Neonatal infection is transmitted via exposure to active lesions during vaginal birth.

Risk Factors

- Unprotected sex (ano-genital herpes)
- Medical occupations (e.g., dentists, dental technicians, nurses, and respiratory care unit personnel)
- Vaginal birth (neonatal herpes)
- Wrestling (herpes gladiatorum)
- Compromised immune system

Signs and Symptoms

The clinical manifestations and the clinical course depend on the following: anatomic site of the lesions, age at first episode of infection, subtype of the virus, and immune status of the patient. Initial episodes of HSV-1 or HSV-2 can be severe and are often accompanied by systemic signs and symptoms.

- Oral-facial infections—gingivostomatitis (inflammation of the gums and oral mucosa), pharyngitis, fever, facial neuralgia, malaise, myalgias, loss of appetite, irritability, cervical adenopathy, and lesions of the lip, face, gingiva, tongue, and hard and soft palate
- Genital infections—fever, headache, malaise, myalgias, pain, itching, dysuria, vaginal and urethral discharge, inguinal lymphadenopathy, and lesions of the external genitalia, cervix, and urethra. Perianal and anal infections may occur after anal intercourse.
- Neonatal infection (usually disseminated disease)—fever, hypothermia, progressive jaundice, hepato-splenomegaly, vesicular skin lesions, loss of appetite, vomiting, lethargy, respiratory distress, cyanosis, circulatory collapse, and death (if untreated). Neurologic sequelae are common.
- Eye infections (herpes keratitis)—pain, blurred vision, conjunctivitis, edema, corneal lesions, and blindness. (In the United States, HSV is the most common cause of corneal blindness.)
- Infection in immunocompromised persons (usually disseminated disease)—widespread dermal, mucosal, and visceral disease (including pneumonia), long-lasting localized lesions
- Herpetic whitlow (primary or recurrent HSV infection of the finger or hand)—edema, erythema, tenderness, vesicular or pustular lesions, fever, and axillary lymphadenopathy (often from occupational exposure, e.g., dentists)

DIFFERENTIAL DIAGNOSIS

- Tonsillitis
- Viral encephalitis (or other viral infections)
- Dermatitis
- Vulvovaginitis
- Impetigo
- Conjunctivitis
- Bacterial meningitis
- Bacterial pneumonia

DIAGNOSIS
Physical Examination

Because HSV has been isolated from many visceral and mucocutaneous sites, there is considerable variability in the clinical manifestations and the course of infection. Primary infections tend to be more severe and of longer duration. Recurrent infections are common because HSV remains latent in the nerve cells of the ganglia or cranial nerve until a trigger causes reactivation after the primary infection.

Laboratory Tests

- Tissue cultures—to show characteristic multinucleated giant cells
- Antigen detection—for group and type discrimination
- Polymerase chain reaction (PCR)—especially for CNS infections
- Serologic assays, especially tissue-specific assays (e.g., complement fixation, passive hemagglutination, indirect immunofluorescence, radioimmunoassay, complement-mediated cytolysis, antibody-dependent cellular cytolysis)—to type isolates

Pathological Findings

Entry of HSV infection is at mucosal surfaces or breaks in the skin, but disseminated infections may also involve visceral organs and the central nervous system. After the primary infection, HSV infection is maintained by the nerve ganglion cells in a latent state. Reactivation results in the normal pattern of gene expression, replication, and release of HSV. HSV can be shed even if the infection is subclinical.

Imaging

Magnetic resonance imaging (MRI) and computed tomography (CT)—to locate involved areas of HSV encephalitis

Other Diagnostic Procedures

- Electroencephalography (EEG) to locate involved areas of HSV encephalitis.
- Staining of scrapings with Wright, Giemsa, or Papanicolaou stains—to diagnose skin lesions and to view intranuclear inclusions
- Immunoblotting techniques
- Cell-mediated immunity assay

TREATMENT OPTIONS
Treatment Strategy

Limited skin lesions can be treated with over-the-counter preparations. Antiviral chemotherapy with acyclovir can successfully treat HSV infections.

Drug Therapies

Lower dosages of antivirals listed below are for recurrent infections, and higher dosages are for primary infections.

- Intravenous acyclovir (45 to 60 mg/kg/day for 21 days)—for neonatal herpes

- Intravenous acyclovir (10 mg/kg/day every eight hours for 10 to 14 days)—for HSV encephalitis
- Oral acyclovir (200 to 400 mg three to five times/day)—for mucocutaneous herpes, oral acyclovir (200 to 400 mg tid for 10 days), oral valacyclovir (500 to 1,000 mg bid), and oral famciclovir (125 to 250 mg tid for 5 to 10 days)—for genital lesions
- Oral famciclovir (500 mg bid) and acyclovir (400 mg bid)—to reduce frequency and severity of recurrences
- Ganciclovir—effective against both HSV-1 and HSV-2 but generally too toxic for practical use
- Idoxuridine, trifluridine (one drop 1% solution every two hours), topical vidarabine, acyclovir, and interferon—for herpetic keratitis
- Intravenous foscarnet (40 mg/kg every eight hours for 10 to 24 days)—for acyclovir-resistant HSV

Complementary and Alternative Therapies

Enhancing the immune system and inhibiting the herpes virus may be achieved through nutritional and herbal support.

NUTRITION

- Avoid alcohol, caffeine, refined foods, sugars, saturated fats, and high arginine-containing foods (seeds, grains, nuts, nut butters, and chocolate). Arginine promotes HSV replication.
- Increase intake of high lysine-containing foods (fish, chicken, eggs, potatoes, and dairy products) during active herpes infection. Lysine inhibits HSV replication.
- Vitamin C (1,000 mg tid) and acidophilus (one capsule with meals) may reduce the duration of outbreaks.
- Beta-carotene (50,000 to 100,000 IU/day) inhibits viral activity.
- Zinc (30 mg/day) inhibits viral replication.
- L-Lysine (500 to 1,000mg/day for prevention; 2,000 mg bid to qid during an outbreak) may reduce duration and frequency of outbreaks.
- Thymus extract can help strengthen the immune system.
- Selenium (250 mcg/day) may reduce duration and frequency of outbreaks.
- Vitamin A (200,000 IU/day for 3 days at onset of outbreak) can be helpful to decrease length and severity of symptoms. Contraindicated for pregnant women and those with liver disease.

HERBS

Herbs are generally a safe way to strengthen and tone the body's systems. As with any therapy, it is important to ascertain a diagnosis before pursuing treatment. Herbs may be used as dried extracts (capsules, powders, teas), glycerites (glycerine extracts), or tinctures (alcohol extracts). Unless otherwise indicated, teas should be made with one teaspoon herb per cup of hot water. Steep covered 5 to 10 minutes for leaf or flowers, and 10 to 20 minutes for roots. Drink 2 to 4 cups/day. Tinctures may be used singly or in combination as noted.

Topical cream applications of concentrated extracts of lemon balm *(Melissa officinalis)* and/or glycyrrhizic acid (from licorice root) can provide symptomatic relief and reduce severity and duration of outbreak. They may be applied to both oral and genital lesions. For best results, apply at first sign of outbreak.

Internal treatment supports anti-viral activity and immune function. For acute infection, combine equal parts of the following herbs in a tincture (30 to 60 drops tid to qid) or a tea (three to four cups/day). Coneflower *(Echinacea purpura),* licorice root *(Glycyrrhiza glabra),* lemon balm, yarrow *(Achillea millefolium),* chamomile *(Matricaria recutita),* and

St. John's wort *(Hypericum perforatum).* Licorice is contraindicated in hypertension. For recurrent infections, substitute lomatium *(Lomatium dissectum)* and astragalus *(Astragalus membranosus)* for yarrow and chamomile, and use the new formula in tincture form, 30 drops tid. These herbs have a deep-acting, immune-stimulating effect. Lemon balm *(Melissa officianalis)* can be used topically or internally for prevention and treatment of HSV.

HOMEOPATHY

An experienced homeopath should assess individual constitutional types and severity of disease to select the correct remedy and potency. For acute prescribing use three to five pellets of a 12X to 30C remedy every one to four hours until acute symptoms resolve.

- *Apis mellifica* when lesions are swollen, stinging, and burning; relieved by cold applications.
- *Graphites* for genital herpes on inner thigh with tremendous itching.
- *Petroleum* for genital herpes that spread to anus and thighs.

PHYSICAL MEDICINE

Ice packs applied to oral lesions or to the sacral area for genital lesions may help reduce pain and inflammation. Stress reduction techniques, such as meditation, yoga, or tai chi, improve immune function and help to reduce frequency of outbreaks.

ACUPUNCTURE

Boosting the immune system, pain relief, and balancing normal physiology are ways in which acupuncture may be helpful.

MASSAGE

Therapeutic massage helps to reduce the effects of stress which may exacerbate HSV.

Patient Monitoring

Patients with primary infections must be counseled about infectivity, recurrences, asymptomatic shedding of virus, pregnancy, and sex. Identifying triggers (e.g, ultraviolet light) can help to reduce recurrences if steps are taken to avoid them (e.g, sunscreen). Avoiding contact with infectious lesions (e.g., condoms, gloves) can help prevent primary infections.

OTHER CONSIDERATIONS

Prevention

Sex should be avoided during outbreaks as condoms do not completely prevent herpes infections. Virus may be transmitted even when no lesions are visible. Cesarean section is advised for pregnant women genitally infected with either HSV-1 or HSV-2 as some recurrences may be asymptomatic. Avoid sunburn or use sunscreen to reduce the risk of recurrent herpes of the lips.

Complications/Sequelae

- Herpes keratitis is associated with encephalitis and blindness.
- Genital herpes increases a woman's risk of cervical cancer.
- Infection with herpes at the time of delivery can result in serious, life-threatening infection in the infant.
- A primary infection during pregnancy may result in spontaneous abortion or life-threatening infection in the fetus.
- Oral-facial herpes has been implicated as the etiologic agent in Bell's palsy and erythema multiforme
- Primary infections can be associated with herpes encephalitis and aseptic meningitis.

Prognosis

Most herpes infections resolve without sequelae except for infections in neonates and immunocompromised persons. Frequent recurrences should be expected.

Pregnancy

Primary HSV infection in the third trimester of pregnancy can be associated with high mortality and mobidity. Cesarean section is indicated if active genital lesions are present. If an infant becomes infected during delivery, neonatal herpes ensues, often resulting in disseminated infection; neurologic deficits and death are common without antiviral treatment.

Nutritional support is indicated in pregnancy. Topical herbal applications may provide symptomatic relief and decrease duration and severity of outbreaks.

REFERENCES

Balch JF, Balch PA. *Prescription for Nutritional Healing.* 2nd ed. Garden City Park, NY: Avery Publishing; 1997:317–319.

Bartram T. *Encyclopedia of Herbal Medicine.* Dorset, England: Grace Publishers; 1995:226–227.

Fauci AS, Braunwald E, Isselbacher KJ et al, eds. *Harrison's Principles of Internal Medicine.* 14th ed. New York, NY: McGraw-Hill; 1998:1080–1086.

Holmes KK, Mardh PA, Sparling PF. *Sexually Transmitted Diseases.* 2nd ed. New York, NY: McGraw-Hill; 1995:391–408.

Krugman S, Katz SL, Gershon AA, et al. *Infectious Diseases of Children.* St. Louis, Mo: Mosby-Year Book; 1992:175–188.

Lad VD. *The Complete Book of Ayurvedic Home Remedies.* New York, NY: Harmony Books; 1998:200–201.

Mandell GL, Douglas RG Jr, Bennett JE. *Principles and Practice of Infectious Diseases.* 3rd ed. New York, NY: Churchill Livingstone; 1990:1144–1151.

Milman N, Scheibel J, Jessen O, et al. Lysine prophylaxis in recurrent herpes simplex labialis: a double-bline, controlled crossover study. *Acta Derm Venereol.* 1980;60:85–87.

Morrison R. *Desktop Guide to Keynotes and Confirmatory Symptoms.* Albany, Calif: Hahnemann Clinic Publishing; 1993:29, 171, 172, 289.

Murray MT, Pizzorno JE. *Encyclopedia of Natural Medicine.* 2nd ed. Rocklin, Calif: Prima Publishing; 1998:360, 520–524.

Thein DJ, Hurt WC. Lysine as a prophylactic agent in the treatment of recurrent herpes simplex labialis. *Oral Surg Oral Med Oral Pathol.* 1984;58:659–666.

Tyler VE: *Herbs of Choice: The Therapeutic Use of Phytomedicinals.* New York, NY: PharmaceuticalProducts Press; 1994:162–166.

Werbach, M. *Nutritional Influences on Illness.* New Canaan, Conn: Keats Publishing; 1988:213–215.

Wöbling RH, Leonhardt K. Local therapy of herpes simplex with dried extract from *w* 1994;1:25–31.

■ HERPES ZOSTER (VARICELLA-ZOSTER) VIRUS

OVERVIEW

Definition

Varicella–zoster virus (VZV) is the etiologic agent for two diseases: varicella (chickenpox) and herpes zoster (shingles). Chickenpox is a very common contagious disease that mostly affects children 2 to 10 years of age and is usually benign; however, chickenpox in adults or immunocompromised persons can have visceral complications and can be fatal (15%). Second attacks of varicella may occur, but these attacks are usually mild and more common in immunocompromised persons. Herpes zoster is caused by a reactivation of the latent VZV and most frequently affects immunocompromised individuals and older people (>50 years of age).

Etiology

- Exposure to VZV at school, at home, or in the hospital
- Depression of cellular immunity to VZV leads to herpes zoster

Risk Factors

- Infected family member or close contact with an infected person
- Immunosuppression (e.g., with cancer, chemotherapy, radiation, immunosuppressive medication, lymphoma)
- Surgery or insult to the spinal cord
- Lack of vaccination

Signs and Symptoms

The typical rash of chickenpox is characterized by maculopapules, vesicles, and scabs in various stages of development on the trunk, scalp, face, and extremities. The typical rash of herpes zoster is unilateral with a dermatomal distribution; lesions begin as maculopapules, then progress to vesicles and scabs on the face (trigeminal ganglia), trunk (thoracic ganglia), shoulders and neck (cervical ganglia), and lower extremities (lumbar or sacral ganglia).

- Varicella: low-grade fever, malaise (fatigue), headache, loss of appetite, rash, and pruritus
- Zoster: rash with dermatomal distribution (T3 to L3), tingling and itching progressing to severe pain, zoster ophthalmicus (if the ophthalmic branch of the trigeminal nerve is involved), erythematous maculopapular rash, acute neuritis, postherpetic neuralgia

DIFFERENTIAL DIAGNOSIS

Chickenpox has a characteristic rash with lesions in all different stages of development and a history of recent exposure. In contrast, herpes zoster may be very difficult to diagnose without serologic testing in the prodromal stage. Appropriate differential diagnosis of herpes zoster must exclude:

- Disseminated herpes simplex virus
- Rickettsialpox
- Impetigo
- Disseminated coxsackievirus infection
- Dermatitis herpetiformis and eczema herpeticum
- Stevens–Johnson syndrome

DIAGNOSIS

Physical Examination

Chickenpox can be easily recognized clinically by the following.

- Maculopapular rash along with fever; mild constitutional symptoms
- Progression of macules to papules, vesicles, and pustules, which eventually crust
- Crops of lesions in all phases of development
- White shallow ulcers in the mouth

Herpes zoster usually presents with the following.

- Unilateral rash within a dermatome
- Maculopapules that progress to vesicles and eventually crust
- Moderate to severe neuralgia

Laboratory Tests

- Restriction endonuclease analysis—to determine the molecular identity of the VZV
- In situ hybridization and polymerase chain reaction (PCR)—to detect viral DNA in vesicular fluid
- Fluorescent antibody to membrane antigen (FAMA)—to detect VZV antibodies and immune status
- Latex agglutination (LA) test—to make a serologic diagnosis
- Enzyme-linked immunosorbent assay (ELISA)—to make a serologic diagnosis and to determine immune status
- Radioimmunoassay (RIA)—to determine immune status

Pathological Findings

- Ballooning degeneration of epidermal cells
- Multinucleated giant cells on Tzanck smear
- Eosinophilic intranuclear inclusions
- Invasion (of lesions) by polymorphonuclear leukocytes
- Hemorrhage, edema, and lymphocytic infiltration in ganglia during herpes zoster virus infection

Other Diagnostic Procedures

- Biopsy for immunofluorescence testing

TREATMENT OPTIONS

Treatment Strategy

Shorten the duration of the current infection and make the patient as comfortable as possible. Because chickenpox is benign in most children, there are no recommendations for treatment other than over-the-counter lotions to relieve itching. However, a vaccine is available for healthy children, and postexposure prophylaxis is recommended for high-risk groups.

- For immunocompetent children who have never been infected—live attenuated varicella vaccine
- For immunocompromised children, adults, or children with AIDS—varicella–zoster immune globulin (VZIG) or intravenous zoster immune plasma (ZIP) (given within 96 hours of exposure to be effective)

Drug Therapies

- Acetaminophen—for fever (aspirin is contraindicated in children)
- Acyclovir (800 mg five times/day for five to seven days, for adolescents and adults with chickenpox; 800 mg five times/day for 7 to 10 days, for patients with herpes zoster; 10 to 12.5 mg/kg intravenously every eight hours for seven days—for varicella in immunocompromised patients; 800 mg orally qid, for varicella in a woman in the third trimester of pregnancy)
- Valacyclovir (1 g tid for 7 to 10 days)—to accelerate healing of herpes zoster
- Prednisone (60 mg/day for seven days, then 30 mg/day for seven days, then 15 mg/day for seven days)—for pain relief of herpes zoster in normal host (to be taken with acyclovir)
- Antipruritic drugs—usually topical agents
- Capsaicin cream (from cayenne pepper), amitriptyline hydrochloride, and fluphenazine hydrochloride—for pain relief of herpes zoster or post-herpetic neuralgia

Complementary and Alternative Therapies
May be helpful in reducing the duration and severity of the disease.

NUTRITION
- Avoid foods that inhibit immune activity and stimulate inflammation, such as saturated fats, refined foods, sugars, and juice.
- Beta-carotene (50,000 to 100,000 IU/day), zinc (30 to 50 mg/day), vitamin C (1,000 to 1,500 mg tid to qid), vitamin E (400 to 800 IU/day) promote immune function and healing of the lesions.
- Calcium (1,000 to 1,500 mg/day), Magnesium (200 mg bid to tid), and B complex (50 to 100 mg/day) protect nerve integrity.
- Additional B_{12} (500 to 1,000 mcg) may be required, especially with post-herpetic neuralgia.
- Vitamin A (200,000 to 300,000 IU/day for 3 days, then 100,000 to 150,000 IU/day for 3 days, then 50,000 IU/day for three days) helps decrease severity and length of symptoms. Contraindicated in pregnancy and liver disease.

HERBS
Herbs are generally a safe way to strengthen and tone the body's systems. Ascertain a diagnosis first. Herbs may be used as dried extracts (capsules, powders, teas), glycerites (glycerine extracts), or tinctures (alcohol extracts). Unless otherwise indicated, teas should be made with 1 tsp. herb per cup of hot water. Steep covered 5 to 10 minutes for leaf or flowers, and 10 to 20 minutes for roots. Drink 2 to 4 cups/day. Tinctures may be used singly or in combination as noted.
- Topical cream applications of concentrated extract of glycyrrhizic acid (from licorice root) can provide symptomatic relief. A poultice made from powdered slippery elm (Ulmus fulva), comfrey (Symphytum officinalis), and goldenseal root (Hydrastis canadensis) is soothing, aids healing, and reduces the likelihood of secondary infection.
- Internal treatment supports anti-viral activity and immune function. For acute infection, combine equal parts of the following herbs in a tincture (30 to 60 drops tid to qid) or a tea (3 to 4 cups/day). Coneflower (Echinacea purpura), licorice root (Glycyrrhiza glabra), burdock root (Arctium lappa), lemon balm (Melissa officinalis), chamomile (Matricaria recutita), and St. John's wort (Hypericum perforatum). Licorice is contraindicated in hypertension.
- For pain relief and post-herpetic neuralgia combine equal parts tincture of Jamaican dogwood (Piscidia erythrina), wild lettuce (Lactuca virosa), valerian (Valeriana officinalis), marigold (Calendula officinalis), and St. John's wort with 1/2 part yellow jasmine (Gelsemium sempiverens). Take 30 to 60 drops tid to qid.

HOMEOPATHY
An experienced homeopath should select the correct remedy and potency. For acute prescribing use 3 to 5 pellets of a 12X to 30C remedy every one to four hours until acute symptoms resolve.
- Lachesis for herpes zoster across left side of back with flushes of heat
- Mezereum for herpes zoster of the face with headaches and facial neuralgias
- Petroleum for herpes zoster with intense itching that is worse at night

PHYSICAL MEDICINE
Tepid oatmeal baths may provide relief from itching and burning. Use Aveeno, as commercially available, or place one cup of oats in a sock and let soak in tub. Squeeze the sock to release the soothing oat milk. Prepare a tea from peppermint leaf (Mentha piperita), cool and place in a spray bottle. Spray on lesions for temporary pain relief.

ACUPUNCTURE
Immune function may be stimulated with acupuncture treatments, decreasing the duration and intensity of herpes zoster and post-herpetic neuralgia.

Patient Monitoring
During an outbreak of either varicella or herpes zoster, patients should be monitored for secondary bacterial infections. VZV lies dormant for many years after initial presentation as chickenpox. No further treatment is necessary unless the virus is reactivated as shingles.

OTHER CONSIDERATIONS
Prevention
Varicella is uncomplicated in most children, usually conferring lifelong immunity. A vaccine is now available for healthy children who have never been exposed to varicella. However, rigid isolation and prophylaxis is recommended for high-risk groups such as immunocompromised children, and adults.

Complications/Sequelae
Central nervous system (CNS) involvement of chickenpox, including benign cerebellar ataxia, aseptic meningitis, encephalitis, transverse myelitis, Guillain–Barré syndrome, and Reye's syndrome, is usually benign. Varicella pneumonia can be serious and is more common in adults. Aspirin should not be given to manage elevated temperatures in children because of the association with Reye's syndrome. Severe varicella infections are seen in children treated with cancer chemotherapy or corticosteroids and children with AIDS. CNS involvement of herpes zoster includes meningoencephalitis, granulomatous angiitis (rare), transverse myelitis.

Prognosis
Most cases resolve in two to three weeks. Immunity usually results after one episode. Severe and often fatal infections may occur in newborn infants and patients receiving corticosteroids, cancer chemotherapy, or radiation. VZV resistance to acyclovir has been reported in HIV-positive patients.

Pregnancy
High doses of vitamins are contraindicated. Topical applications may be used for symptomatic relief.

REFERENCES
Fauci AS, Braunwald E, Isselbacher KJ et al, eds. Harrison's Principles of Internal Medicine. 14th ed. New York, NY: McGraw-Hill; 1998:1086–1088.
Krugman S, Katz SL, Gershon AA, et al. Infectious Diseases of Children. St. Louis, Mo: Mosby-Year Book; 1992:587–609.
Mandell GL, Douglas RG Jr, Bennett JE. Principles and Practice of Infectious Diseases. 3rd ed. New York, NY: Churchill Livingstone; 1995:1153–1158, 2237–2240.
Morrison R. Desktop Guide to Keynotes and Confirmatory Symptoms. Albany, Calif: Hahnemann Clinic Publishing; 1993:218, 249, 289.

■ HIV AND AIDS
OVERVIEW
Definition
In the early 1980s, Kaposi's sarcoma, pneumocystis carinii pneumonia (PCP), and other conditions becoming prevalent in homosexual men in United States cities were recognized as the result of a profound acquired immunodeficiency. This acquired immune deficiency syndrome, or AIDS, was soon understood to be a worldwide health problem. AIDS is caused by the human immunodeficiency virus (HIV), which attacks CD4 T lymphocytes. The infection results in cell death and impaired immune response. HIV most directly affects the central nervous, gastrointestinal, and pulmonary systems. A massive research effort has produced better treatments, resulting in longer survival and improved quality of life. But there is still no vaccine or cure for AIDS.

Etiology
- Infection by HIV, a member of the lentivirus group of retroviruses. Seventy percent of transmission is through sexual contact. Parenteral transmission is mainly among intravenous drug users. Blood transfusions and blood products caused many infections, especially among hemophiliacs, but screening procedures have nearly eliminated this risk.
- Transmission to and from health care workers is also rare, due to increased precautions.
- Children, comprising fewer than 1% of cases, generally acquire the infection perinatally.

Risk Factors
- Unprotected sex
- Anal intercourse
- Multiple sex partners
- Intravenous drug use
- Occupational needlestick or other contact with infectious body fluids
- Exposure to contaminated blood products
- Children born to HIV-infected mothers

Signs and Symptoms
- Chronic infections
- Fever
- Weight loss
- Night sweats
- Skin lesions or rashes
- Oral candidiasis (thrush)
- Persistent lymphadenopathy
- Shortness of breath, cough, and/or chest pain
- Diarrhea, abdominal pain, and/or vomiting
- Blurred vision
- Headache
- Depression
- Dementia
- Herpes
- Kaposi Sarcoma
- Malignancies

DIFFERENTIAL DIAGNOSIS
- Candidiasis
- Cholecystitis
- Gastroenteritis
- Herpes zoster
- Idiopathic thrombocytopenic purpura
- Meningitis
- Pancreatitis
- Pneumonia (pneumocystis carinii)
- Syphilis
- Tuberculosis

DIAGNOSIS
Physical Examination
Evaluate for oral candidiasis, "cottage cheese and ketchup" appearance of retina, adenopathy, skin abnormalities, respiratory symptoms, abdominal tenderness, dementia.

Laboratory Tests
Complete blood work-up, including testing for HIV RNA levels. CD4 count below 200/mm3 indicates increased susceptibility to opportunistic infections. Arterial blood gas, for suspected pneumocystis carinii pneumonia (PCP). Stool sample for culture, ova and parasites, Cryptosporidium.

Imaging
Chest X ray for PCP, tuberculosis. Head CT if neurological symptoms are present.

Other Diagnostic Procedures
A blood test is all that is required to establish a diagnosis of HIV infection. Other procedures are intended to evaluate the progression toward AIDS and diagnose any opportunistic infections. Cerebrospinal fluid analysis if neurological symptoms are present or meningitis is suspected.

TREATMENT OPTIONS
Treatment Strategy
Antiretroviral treatments attempt to slow progression of HIV infection to AIDS, while antibiotics and other therapies are used against opportunistic infections and other complications as they arise. Alternative treatments may be used to support the immune system, help in coping with disease symptoms and side effects from conventional treatments, and improve quality of life. Any delay in onset of severe illness, as well as maintenance of the patient's general condition and avoidance of "wasting syndrome," may buy time for better treatments to be developed.

Drug Therapies
Appropriate treatment depends on the stage of the infection and complicating conditions. Antiretrovirals, such as Zidovudine, 200 mg orally tid, or Lamivudine, 150 mg orally bid, are generally prescribed, together with protease inhibitors such as Indinavir, 800 mg orally tid. These medications have significant side effects, and when to begin administering them to asymptomatic patients is a matter for careful consideration. When prescribing for complications, interactions and contraindications must be carefully considered, as HIV/AIDS patients may have a number of medical problems at any one time and are usually taking multiple medications. Compliance with the prescribed regimen is important to avoid encouraging resistant viral strains.

For pneumocystis carinii pneumonia: Antibiotics, trimethoprim/sulfamethoxazole being the first choice and pentamidine a good alternative. Prednisone if PaO2 is less than 70, but prednisone is contraindicated with systemic fungal infection.

For cryptococcal meningitis: amphotericin B, with flucytosine

For oral candidiasis: clotrimazole

For toxoplasmosis: pyrimethamine; synergistic with sulfanomides

For cytomegalovirus: ganciclovir; interacts with zidovudine

Complementary and Alternative Therapies

These may be effective at slowing the progression from HIV to AIDS. In addition, they can be used as an adjunctive therapy or by themselves to treat some opportunistic infections. See the related conditions. A combination of nutrition and herbal treatment may be effective. Homeopathy can be effective to treat symptoms. Training in biofeedback, guided imagery, and hypnosis have been shown to result in decreased fever, fatigue, pain, headache, nausea and insomnia, and increased resilience.

NUTRITION

A good quality multivitamin is important for health maintenance. Megadoses of some nutrients should be avoided, unless specifically indicated. For example, doses of zinc greater than 30 mg, unless during an acute infection, can decrease immune functioning.

- Multivitamin: two to six capsules/day (Some vitamin formulas may be more difficult to absorb; check doses, as multivitamin doses may vary from brand to brand.)
- Vitamin C (1 to 2 g/day), beta-carotene (150,000 to 300,000 IU/day), and zinc (30 mg/day): optimizes immune function
- N-acetyl cysteine (1,500 to 2,000 mg/day): increases glutathione and is protective of the lungs
- Selenium (100 to 400 mcg/day): important antioxidant, may actually have antiviral effects
- Vitamin E (400 to 800 IU/day): antioxidant, may also slow bone marrow suppression from AZT
- Vitamin B complex (50 to 100 mg/day): depleted in stress
- Vitamin B_{12} (1,000 mcg IM): one injection a month to counter effects of medications, two times a week for peripheral neuropathy
- Magnesium (500 to 750 mg/day): important in protein biosynthesis. Decrease dose if diarrhea develops.
- Coenzyme Q10 (10 mg/day): may improve T cell/suppresser ratios
- L-glutamine (30 to 40 g in five doses of 6 to 8 g each for at least 7 to 10 days): primary fuel for the cells lining the gastrointestinal tract; helps restore muscles during wasting. Serum levels are not an adequate reflection of body status.
- L-carnitine (2,000 mg/day): with wasting or high serum triglycerides
- Consider gluten or other food allergies, which can lead to diarrhea and other malabsorption problems; food sensitivities and allergies increase (e.g., lactose intolerance) with the use of antiretrovirals. Hypoallergenic protein supplementation may help slow wasting.

HERBS

Herbs are generally a safe way to strengthen and tone the body's systems. As with any therapy, it is important to ascertain a diagnosis before pursuing treatment. Herbs may be used as dried extracts (capsules, powders, teas), glycerites (glycerine extracts), or tinctures (alcohol extracts). Unless otherwise indicated, teas should be made with 1 tsp. herb per cup of hot water. Steep covered 5 to 10 minutes for leaf or flowers, and 10 to 20 minutes for roots. Drink 2 to 4 cups/day. Tinctures may be used singly or in combination as noted.

- To stimulate immune function and provide antiviral support: Licorice (*Glycyrrhiza glabra*), 1/4 to 1/2 solid extract twice a day, inhibits HIV replication in vitro; helps regenerate liver cells; not used if hypertensive. St. John's wort (*Hypericum perforatum*), at 250 mg tid, inhibits binding and entry of HIV into host cells and elevates mood. Huang qi (*Astragalus membranaceus*), 250 to 500 mg powdered solid extract,

inhibits HIV-1 replication and stimulates the appetite. Use one to two of these herbs.

- To stimulate digestion and prevent diarrhea, take one to three of the following herbs, which stimulate the appetite (15 to 60 drops tid with meals): gentian (*Gentiana lutea*) tonic, historically used as an antiparasitic, to be avoided with ulcers; dandelion (*Taraxacum officinale*) cholagogue, historically used for liver problems; goldenseal (*Hydrastis canadensis*) anti-inflammatory, mild laxative, do not exceed recommended dose for long-term use
- Garlic (*Allium sativum*) is a strong antioxidant, enhances natural killer cell activity in AIDS patients, and lowers lipids; historic use in digestive disorders
- Siberian ginseng (*Eleutherococcus sentecosus*), 30 to 60 drops tid or one cup tea tid: increases T cell, NK cell, and cytotoxic killer cell function; regulates the adrenal glands and enhances endurance
- Milk thistle (*Silybum marianum*): supportive treatment for toxic liver damage, especially important with medications used in HIV/AIDS
- Acidophilus (two to five million organisms tid): beneficial gut bacteria that are depleted in chronic antibiotic use

HOMEOPATHY

An experienced homeopath should assess individual constitutional types and severity of disease to select the correct remedy and potency. For acute treatment, see the appropriate condition.

PHYSICAL MEDICINE

- Weight training may be helpful in maintaining muscle mass and a sense of well-being.
- Hyperthermia. Immersion in hot water (103° to 105° F) to raise core body temperature, increases CD4 counts; should only be done with supervision. This may be too depleting in debilitated or hypotensive patients.

ACUPUNCTURE

May be very helpful to treat infections, stimulate immune system, and increase general sense of well-being

MASSAGE

Massages have been shown to enhance the immune system and decrease anxiety.

PATIENT MONITORING

Patients must be seen regularly to evaluate disease progression and monitor for complications. CD4 counts should be taken every three months.

OTHER CONSIDERATIONS

Prevention

Safe-sex practice or abstinence would prevent most cases of AIDS. Avoid bodily fluids of HIV carriers. Needle-exchange programs have the potential for reducing cases among intravenous drug users. Health care workers should continue to take universal precautions.

Complications/Sequelae

It is the nature of immune system failure that complications are common and severe. While 70% to 80% of patients recover fully from pneumocystis carinii pneumonia, respiratory failure is a possibility. Other complications may include hydrocephalus from cryptococcal meningitis and blindness from cytomegalovirus, numerous opportunistic infections, kaposi sarcoma, and malignancies.

Prognosis

HIV has a long latency period; the median time for progression to AIDS is 11 years. AIDS itself seems to be uniformly lethal, generally in one to two years. Those time spans are beginning to increase as treatments improve.

Pregnancy

Zidovudine administered to pregnant AIDS patients is the only therapy yet known to reduce the likelihood of transmission to the child. A decision must be made, based on the patient's condition, whether to postpone treatment until after the first trimester to reduce the risk to the fetus. Likewise the possible teratogenic effects of other medications must be weighed against the advisability of postponing more aggressive combination treatment for the mother.

REFERENCES

Auerbach J, Oleson T, Solomon G. A behavioral medicine intervention as an adjunctive treatment for HIV-related illness. *Psychology and Health.* 1992;6:325–334.

Blumenthal M, ed. *The Complete German Commission E Monographs.* Boston, Mass: Integrative Medicine Communications; 1998:119–120, 134, 169–170.

Dubin J. *HIV Infection and AIDS.* Emergency Medicine Online. 1998. Accessed at www.emedicine.com/emerg/topic253.htm on February 13, 1999.

Dworkin BM. Selenium deficiency in HIV infection and the acquired immunodeficiency syndrome (AIDS). *Chem Biol Interact.* 1994;91:181–186.

Fawzi WW, Mbise RL, Hertzmark E, et al. A randomized trial of vitamin A supplements in relation to mortality among human immunodeficiency virus-infected and uninfected children in Tanzania. *Pediatr Infect Dis J.* 1999;18:127–133.

Gruenwald J, Brendler T, Jaenicke C et al, eds. *PDR for Herbal Medicines.* Montvale, NJ: Medical Economics Company; 1998:626–627, 866–867, 903–904, 1138–1139, 1174–1175.

Guidelines for the use of antiretroviral agents in HIV-infected adults and adolescents. U.S. Department of Health and Human Services. December 1, 1998.

Hamilton Nunnelley EM. *Biochemistry of Nutrition: A Desk Reference.* New York, NY: West Publishing Company; 1987:183–184.

Hanna L. Complementary and alternative medicine: exploring options and making decisions. *Bulletin of Experimental Treatments for AIDS.* January 1998.

Hayashi K, Hayashi T, Kojima I. A natural sulfated polysaccharide, calcium spirulan, isolated from Spirulina platensis: in vitro and ex vivo evaluation of anti-herpes simplex virus and anti-human immunodeficiency virus activities. *AIDS Res Hum Retroviruses.* 1996;12:1463–1471.

Lissoni, P, Vigore L, Rescaldani R, et al. Neuroimmunotherapy with low-dose subcutaneous interleukin-2 plus melatonin in AIDS patients with CD4 cell number below 200/mm3: a biological phase-II study. J Biol Regul Homeost Agents. 1995;9:155–158.

Nerad JL, Gorbach SL, et al. Nutritional aspects of HIV infection. *Infect Dis Clin North Am.* 1994;8:499–515.

Noyer CM, Simon D, Borczuk A, Brandt LJ, Lee MJ, Nehra V. A double-blind placebo-controlled pilot study of glutamine therapy for abnormal intestintal permeability in patients with AIDS. *Am J Gastroenterol.* 1998;93:972–975.

Patarca R, Fletcher MA. Massage therapy is associated with enhancement of the immune system's cytotoxic capacity. *Int J Neurosci.* February 1996;84:205–217.

Remacha AF, Cadafalch J. Cobalamin deficiency in patients infected with the human immunodeficiency virus. *Semin Hematol.* 1999;36:75–87.

■ HYPERCHOLESTEROLEMIA

OVERVIEW
Definition
Hypercholesterolemia, or hyperlipidemia—abnormally high levels of fats (cholesterol, triglycerides, or both) in the blood—may be present without symptoms and yet put the patient at risk for generalized atherosclerosis, coronary artery disease or carotid artery disease. The risk of having a heart attack or stroke increases as a person's total cholesterol level increases. Total cholesterol level is ideally about 140 to 200 milligrams of cholesterol per deciliter of blood (mg/dL) or less. Moderate risk is 200 to 240 mg/dL; high risk is 240 mg/dL or higher.

Cholesterol and triglyceride levels are highest in people with hereditary hyperlipidemia, sometimes regardless of their diet and exercise level. Hereditary hyperlipidemia, or hyperlipoproteinemia, is a condition that interferes with the body's ability to metabolize and eliminate fats. Each of the five main types of hyperlipoproteinemia produces a different profile and risks.

- Type I hyperlipoproteinemia (familiar hyperchylomicronemia) is a rare disorder, present at birth. Patients have recurrent bouts of abdominal pain and an enlarged liver and spleen, and develop xanthomas on their skin.
- Type II hyperlipoproteinemia (familiar hypercholesterolemia) results in accelerated atherosclerosis and early death, usually from a heart attack. Patients have a high level of LDL cholesterol, and xanthomas grow in the tendons and skin.
- Type III hyperlipoproteinemia leads to high levels of VLDL cholesterol and triglycerides. Atherosclerosis often blocks arteries and reduces blood flow to the legs by middle age.
- Type IV hyperlipoproteinemia is common and affects several members of a family. A high level of triglycerides may increase a person's risk of developing atherosclerosis.
- Type V hyperlipoproteinemia is uncommon. The body can't metabolize and eliminate excess triglycerides. Although hereditary, it can result from alcohol abuse, poorly controlled diabetes, kidney failure, or eating after a period of starvation.

Etiology
High fat levels:
- A diet high in saturated fat and cholesterol
- Cirrhosis of the liver
- Poorly controlled diabetes
- Underactive thyroid gland
- Overactive pituitary gland
- Kidney failure
- Porphyria
- Heredity

High triglyceride levels:
- Excess calories in diet
- Acute and chronic alcohol abuse
- Severe uncontrolled diabetes
- Kidney failure
- Certain drugs (estrogens, oral contraceptives, corticosteroids, and to some extent thiazide diuretics)
- Elevated serum insulin

Risk Factors
- Obesity
- Diet rich in saturated fat
- Sedentary lifestyle
- Stress

- Hereditary hyperlipidemia
- Hyperhomocysteinemia

Signs and Symptoms
High fat levels may cause few, if any, symptoms. Diagnosis is usually made through blood tests. Severe symptoms may include:
- Fat deposits that form growths, or xanthomas, in the tendons and skin
- Extremely high levels of triglycerides (800 mg/dL and higher), which may cause enlargement of the liver and spleen and symptoms of pancreatitis, such as severe abdominal pain

DIFFERENTIAL DIAGNOSIS
- Hypothyroidism
- Obstructed liver disease
- Nephrotic syndrome
- Diabetes

DIAGNOSIS
Physical Examination
See "Signs and Symptoms" above.

Laboratory Tests
A blood sample determines total cholesterol. A sample used to measure HDL cholesterol, LDL cholesterol, and triglycerides is most effective after 12 hours of fasting. The following results represent the ideal range:
- Total cholesterol: 120 to 200 mg/dL
- Chylomicrons: None (after 12 hours of fasting)
- Very low-density lipoproteins (VLDL): 1 to 30 mg/dL
- Low-density lipoproteins (LDL): 60 to 160 mg/dL
- High-density lipoproteins (HDL): 35 to 65 mg/dL
- LDL to HDL ratio: less than 3.5
- Triglycerides: 10 to 160 mg/dL

Other Diagnostic Procedures
- Clinical observation of suspected hypercholesterolemia or a routine health screening will provide laboratory confirmation of elevated cholesterol triglycerides.
- Serum or urinary homocysteine levels

TREATMENT OPTIONS
Treatment Strategy
- Diet should be low in cholesterol and saturated fat to reduce LDL cholesterol level.
- Exercise to reduce LDL cholesterol level and increase HDL cholesterol level.
- Drinking a small amount of alcohol on a regular basis may raise HDL cholesterol level and lower LDL cholesterol level, but more than two drinks daily could have the opposite effect.
- Maintain an appropriate weight.
- Stop smoking.
- Avoid caffeine (may increase cholesterol levels).
- Consider a lipid-lowering drug for high cholesterol levels if behavioral intervention trial is unsuccessful.
- When cholesterol levels are very high and don't respond to usual treatments, specific blood tests are in order to identify the exact cause of the condition and to treat it appropriately.

Drug Therapies
- Bile acid sequestrants: cholestyramine/cholestipol—used to treat elevated LDL by promoting bile acid excretion and increasing LDL receptors in liver. One to six packets per day. Common side effects include

bloating, constipation, and elevated triglycerides.
- Nicotinic acid—used to treat elevated LDL and VLDL by decreasing VLDL synthesis. 500 mg to 3 gm/day to tid can cause cutaneous flushing, GI upset (which usually resolve over a few weeks), and elevated glucose, uric acid, and liver function tests
- HMG CoA reductase inhibitors (statins): Pravastatin, Simvastatin, Atorvastatin, Fluvastatin, and Lovastatin treat elevated LDL. 20 to 80 mg/day, single or divided dose. These drugs inhibit cholesterol synthesis and upregulate LDL receptors in the liver. Side effects include myositis (muscle inflammation), arthralgias (joint pains), GI upset, and elevated liver function tests.
- Fibric acid derivatives: gemfibrozil—used to treat elevated triglycerides and elevated remnants by stimulating lipoprotein lipase (an enzyme that breaks down lipids in lipoproteins). May decrease VLDL synthesis. Side effects include myositis (muscle inflammation), GI upset, gallstones, and elevated liver function tests.

Complementary and Alternative Therapies
The digestion, metabolism, and utilization of fats, as well as minimizing the effects of hypercholesterolemia, are areas in which alternative therapies can be very effective. Begin with dietary suggestions and nutritional support, as needed. Herbs can be used to facilitate the metabolism of cholesterol.

NUTRITION
- Avoid saturated fats which contribute to cholesterol synthesis and contribute to oxidative stress.
- Vegetable proteins have been shown to lower cholesterol levels, while animal and milk proteins have been shown to raise them. Thus a vegetarian or semi-vegetarian diet has been shown to be efficacious in lowering cholesterol.
- Increase foods high in omega-3 oils which can help decrease cholesterol (cold water fish, nuts, and seeds).
- Reduce consumption of sugar and simple carbohydrates. The digestion of these foods causes a rise in serum insulin which can lead to an increase in lipid production.
- Include foods that help reduce cholesterol, such as those high in water-soluble fiber—legumes, grains, and fruits containing pectin.
- Increase foods that support the liver, such as beets, carrots, yams, artichokes, dark bitter greens, and lemons.
- Consider digestive enzymes in cases where poor fat digestion is a factor.
- Omega-3 fatty acids (1,000 to 1,500 mg bid to tid) decrease synthesis, increase breakdown of triglycerides, and lower total cholesterol levels. Found in fish oils capsules (EPA's cicosapentaenoic acid) and flax seed.
- Niacin reduces total cholesterol while increasing the levels of the protective lipoprotein HDL. The amount of niacin needed to achieve these results is very high. Inositol hexa-niacinate (IHN) 500 mg tid causes no short-term reactions, and is safe for the liver.
- Selenium (200 mcg/day) is needed for normal lipid metabolism.
- L-Taurine (200 mg/day) conjugates cholesterol and facilitates its excretion.
- Vitamin C (1,000 mg tid) and vitamin E (400 to 800 IU/day) decrease oxidative stress and are needed for cholesterol metabolism.
- B complex, especially vitamin B_{12} (1,000 mcg/day), folic acid (400 to 800 mcg/day), betaine (1,000 mg/day), and vitamin B_6 (50 to 100 mg/day), are essential to methionine metabolism. The addition of these vitamins will reduce high levels of homocysteine.
- Coenzyme Q10 (50 to 100 mg/day) is an antioxidant and reduces oxidative damage to the circulatory system.

- Chromium (200 mcg one to three times a day) helps to stabilize glucose levels and reduce lipid oxidation secondary to diabetes.
- Magnesium (200 mg bid to tid) is needed for many metabolic pathways and has blood pressure lowering effects.
- Panthenine (500 mg tid) is a form of pantethenic acid that has shown effectiveness in reducing serum cholesterol.

HERBS
Herbs are generally a safe way to strengthen and tone the body's systems. As with any therapy, it is important to ascertain a diagnosis before pursuing treatment. Herbs may be used as dried extracts (capsules, powders, teas), glycerites, or tinctures (alcohol extracts). Unless otherwise indicated, teas should be made with one teaspoon herb per cup of hot water. Steep covered 10 to 20 minutes and drink two to four cups/day. Tinctures may be used singly or in combination as noted.
- Garlic (*Allium sativum*) has the effect of reducing cholesterol. It is most effective when included in the diet in the raw form, or taken in capsules.
- Herbs that support the liver, and promote bile production and excretion may be taken singly or in combination. Herbs to consider include milk thistle (*Silybum marianum*), dandelion root (*Taraxacum officinale*), burdock root (*Arctium lappa*), blue flag (*Iris versicolor*), greater celandine (*Chelidonium majus*), and blue vervain (*Verbena hastata*). Greater celandine should be taken with caution (no more than 2 ml/day) as it can lead to bilary colic. Tinctures (15 to 20 drops/dose), or infusions (one heaping tsp./dose), are best taken 10 to 20 minutes before meals.
- Hawthorn berries (*Crataegus oxyanthoides*) help to lower high blood pressure, promote cholesterol metabolism, and suppress cholesterol synthesis, as well as strengthening connective tissue and cardiac muscle. Dried extracts are taken 200 mg bid to tid, or tincture 30 drops tid.
- Ginger (*Zingiber officinalis*) has been shown to lower cholesterol levels.
- Alfalfa (*Medicago sativa*) has been shown to lower cholesterol levels.

HOMEOPATHY
An experienced homeopath should assess individual constitutional types and severity of disease to select the correct remedy and potency. For acute prescribing use 3 to 5 pellets of a 12X to 30C remedy every 1 to 4 hours until acute symptoms resolve. Constitutional homeopathy is useful as a supportive therapy.

ACUPUNCTURE
Acupuncture can assist with improving liver/gallbladder function, and in strengthening the cardiovascular system.

Patient Monitoring
Avoiding high-fat foods can help reduce cholesterol, and some foods actually have a cholesterol-lowering effect (see "Nutrition").

OTHER CONSIDERATIONS
Prevention

Lifestyle changes (quitting smoking, eating a low-fat diet, exercising, and reducing stress) are recommended first. If these actions aren't adequate, then lipid-lowering drugs can be prescribed.

Complications/Sequelae
- Atherosclerosis
- Coronary heart disease

Prognosis

Maintaining an appropriate weight, eating a low-fat diet, and exercising can have a significant impact on the patient's cholesterol level and long-term prognosis.

REFERENCES

Auer W, Eiber A, Hertkorn E, et al. Hypertension and hyperlipidaemia: garlic helps in mild cases. *Br J Clin Pract.* 1990;44:3–9.

Barrie SA, Wright JV, Pizzorno JE. Effects of garlic on platelet aggregation, serum lipids and blood pressure in humans. *J Orthomelec.* 1987;2:15–21.

Bordia A. Effect of garlic on blood lipids in patients with coronary heart disease. *Am J Clin Nutr.* 1981;34:2100–2103.

Bordia A, Bansal HC, Arora SK, et al. Effect of the essential oils of garlic and onion on alimentary hyperlipemia. *Atherosclerosis.* 1975;21:15–19.

Jain AK, Vargas R, et al. Can garlic reduce levels of serum lipids? A controlled clinical study. *Am J Med.* 1993;94:632–635.

Johns Hopkins Health Information. Accessed at http://www.intelihealth.com on January 25, 1999.

Murray MT, Pizzorno JE. *The Encyclopedia of Natural Medicine.* 2nd ed. Rocklin, Calif: Prima Publishing; 1998.

Silagy C, Neil A. Garlic as a lipid lowering agent-a meta-analysis. *JR Coll Physicians Lond.* 1994;28:39–45.

Steiner M, Khan AH, Holbert D, Lin RI. A double-blind crossover study in moderately hypercholesterolemic men that compared the effect of aged garlic extract and placebo administration on blood lipids. *Am J Clin Nutr.* 1996;64:866–870.

Vorberg G, Scneider B. Therapy with garlic: Results of a placebo-controlled, double-blind study. *Br J Clin Pract.* 1990;7–11.

Warshafsky S, Kramer RS, Sivak SL. Effect of garlic on total serum cholesterol: a meta-analysis. *Ann Intern Med.* 1993;119:599–605.

Werbach, M. *Nutritional Influences on Illness.* New Canaan, Conn: Keats Publishing; 1988.

Yamamoto M. Serum HDL-cholesterol increasing and fatty liver improving actions of *Panax ginseng* in high cholesterol diet-fed rats with clinical affect on hyperlipidemia in man. *Am J Chin Med.* 1983;1:96–101.

■ HYPERKALEMIA

OVERVIEW

Definition

Hyperkalemia is an excess of serum potassium. Most potassium in the body (98%) is found within cells. Small changes in extracellular potassium levels can disturb the cellular membrane potential, with profound effects on the cardiovascular and neuromuscular systems. Excess potassium is ordinarily excreted in the urine, and hyperkalemia is most often a result of renal insufficiency. It may also be precipitated by conditions that cause the release of potassium from the cells into the bloodstream, such as tissue trauma. Untreated, hyperkalemia may be associated with up to 67% mortality, mainly due to the effect of the potassium imbalance on cardiac function.

Etiology

- Renal insufficiency
- Acidosis (e.g., diabetic ketoacidosis)
- Increased potassium intake
- Hypoaldosteronism (Addison's disease)
- Rhabdomyolysis
- Hemolysis (sickle-cell disease, venipuncture, blood transfusions, burns, tumor lysis)
- Side effect of some medications

Risk Factors

- Renal failure (acute or chronic)
- Trauma, especially crush injuries or burns
- Diet high in potassium (bananas, oranges, tomatoes, high protein diets, salt substitutes)
- Use of medications such as potassium supplements, potassium-sparing diuretics, digoxin, nonsteroidal anti-inflammatory drugs, cyclosporine, succinylcholine, heparin, ACE inhibitors, and beta-blockers

Signs and Symptoms

- Fatigue
- Weakness
- Paresthesia
- Paralysis
- Palpitations
- Difficulty breathing

DIFFERENTIAL DIAGNOSIS

- Pseudohyperkalemia—e.g., from hemolysis during phlebotomy, erythrocyte fragility disorders
- Laboratory error—False high potassium reading may occur in patients with high platelet or white cell count.
- Other neurologic syndromes
- Heart disease/congestive heart failure

DIAGNOSIS

Physical Examination

Assess for weakness and paresthesia. Check for evidence of dialysis sites and signs of trauma. Deep tendon reflexes or motor strength may be decreased. Pulse may be slow or irregular.

Laboratory Tests

- Potassium level—upper limit of normal is 5 to 5.5 mEq/liter
- Digoxin level
- Calcium level—hypocalcemia exacerbates cardiac effects
- Glucose level—if patient has diabetes
- BUN and creatinine—to evaluate renal status
- Arterial blood gas—if acidosis suspected

Other Diagnostic Procedures

Assess patient's overall condition and stability. Perform blood workup and monitor cardiac and renal function.

Electrocardiography should always be performed and may reveal the following anomalies, usually in order of progression. Note that life-threatening cardiac arrhythmias can occur without warning at almost any level of hyperkalemia.

- Peaked T-waves, shortened QT interval, ST-segment depression
- Widening of QRS complex, increases in PR interval, P-wave flattening
- P-wave disappearance, QRS widening to sine wave
- Ventricular fibrillation, asystole

TREATMENT OPTIONS

Treatment Strategy

Hyperkalemia is a life-threatening condition, and treatment must be prompt and aggressive. Patients presenting in the emergency room should be evaluated as to cardiac status and held under continuous electrocardiographic monitoring with frequent checks of vital signs. If renal failure is detected, admit patients to the ICU and consult a nephrologist. Treatment is aimed at stabilizing cardiac function, promoting movement of potassium from the extracellular environment to the cells, and encouraging excretion of excess potassium. Once the acute condition is stabilized, the root cause of the hyperkalemia should be determined and treated. Dialysis may be indicated if more conservative treatments fail.

Drug Therapies

- Calcium—Works quickly to stabilize membrane resting potential, ameliorating cardiac and neuromuscular effects. However, calcium does not lower potassium level and its effects last only about one hour, so other treatment must be started as well. Give 10 ml of 10% calcium gluconate solution IV over two minutes, or 5 ml of 10% calcium chloride solution IV over two minutes. Contraindicated in hypercalcemic patients.
- Insulin—Promotes potassium shift intracellularly. In normoglycemic patients, 10 units IV with 1 ampule D 50 to prevent hypoglycemia
- Sodium bicarbonate—Promotes potassium shift intracellularly; 1 mEq/kg, up to 50 to 100 mEq, slow IV or continuous drip. Caution required in patients with renal failure due to high sodium and fluid load.
- Beta agonists—Promote potassium shift intracellularly; 2.5 mg albuterol mixed with saline via high flow nebulizer every 20 minutes as tolerated. Safety in pregnancy is not established. Monitor for tachycardia and nervousness.
- Diuretics—Cause potassium excretion from kidneys but effects may be slow and inconsistent; furosemide (Lasix) 40 mg IV push. Dose may need to be doubled for patients with renal failure. Safety in pregnancy is not established. Contraindicated in hypovolemic patients.
- Binding resins—Promote potassium/sodium exchange in gastrointestinal system; sodium polystyrene sulfonate (Kayexalate) 15 to 30 g (4 to 8 tsp) in 50 to 100 ml of 20% sorbitol orally every 3 to 4 hours, or retention enema 50 g in 200 ml of 20% sorbitol for 30 to 60 minutes every four hours. Sorbitol contraindicated in post-op patients; may cause colonic necrosis. Caution required in patients with renal failure due to sodium load. Safety in pregnancy is not established.

Complementary and Alternative Therapies

Hyperkalemia is an acute, life-threatening condition requiring immediate and aggressive medical intervention. Alternative therapies may be appropriate for concurrent support and in treatment of the underlying cause once the patient has been stabilized.

NUTRITION

- Avoid alcohol, caffeine, refined foods, sugar, and saturated fats (meat proteins and dairy products). In addition, eliminate high potassium foods, such as bananas, from the diet.
- Increase water intake, as dehydration can exacerbate hyperkalemia
- Eat small amounts of protein and favor vegetable proteins and fish over chicken and red meats.
- Small, frequent meals can help prevent hypoglycemia. Insulin release potentiates intracellular potassium shift.
- Magnesium (200 mg bid to tid) is essential for the sodium-potassium pump. It also has vasodilatory effects and may help stabilize cardiac arrhythmias.

HERBS

Herbs are generally a safe way to strengthen and tone the body's systems. As with any therapy, it is important to ascertain a diagnosis before pursuing treatment. Herbs may be used as dried extracts (capsules, powders, teas), glycerites (glycerine extracts), or tinctures (alcohol extracts). Unless otherwise indicated, teas should be made with one teaspoon herb per cup of hot water. Steep covered 5 to 10 minutes for leaf or flowers, and 10 to 20 minutes for roots. Drink 2 to 4 cups/day. Tinctures may be used singly or in combination as noted.

Of primary concern is the effect of hyperkalemia on the heart. While most kidney tonics are rich in potassium and should be avoided, some cardiac glycosides and flavonoids have a neutral effect on potassium levels and are protective of cardiac function.

- Hawthorn (*Crataegus oxyacantha*) increases cardiac output without increasing cardiac load. It has a mild vasodilatory effect, helps to stabilize cardiac arrhythmias, and also supports liver function. Compromised liver function and poor fat digestion can exacerbate hyperkalemia. Drink 3 to 4 cups of tea/day. Hawthorn is a relatively safe herb and may be used long-term.
- Lily of the valley (*Convalleria majalis*) increases cardiac output and has a regulating effect on heart rhythm. It is a secondary diuretic which relieves edema and has a neutral to slightly lowering effect on sodium and potassium. This herb has toxic side effects and should not be used without physician supervision.

HOMEOPATHY

An experienced homeopath should assess individual constitutional types and severity of disease to select the correct remedy and potency.

PHYSICAL MEDICINE

Contrast hydrotherapy. Alternating hot and cold applications brings nutrients to the site and diffuses metabolic waste from inflammation. The overall effect is decreased inflammation, pain relief, and enhanced healing. Use the applications over the kidneys. Alternate 3 minutes hot with 1 minute cold. Repeat 3 times. This is 1 set. Do 2 to 3 sets/day.

ACUPUNCTURE

Acupuncture may be helpful in supporting normal kidney function and minimizing the effects of hyperkalemia.

MASSAGE

Swedish massage may help to stimulate the kidneys; whether this is appropriate for a particular patient depends on his or her condition and the underlying cause of the hyperkalemia.

Patient Monitoring

Continue cardiac monitoring; track serum potassium levels while patient remains in hospital. Measure urine output and potassium excretion levels. Repeat potassium tests 2 to 3 days after discharge. Monitor for renal insufficiency.

OTHER CONSIDERATIONS

Prevention

Patients should be advised to avoid foods high in potassium. Medications should be reviewed to avoid those which predispose to hyperkalemia. If the problem was precipitated by noncompliance with a dialysis schedule, encourage the patient to make this a priority.

Complications/Sequelae

Severe hyperkalemia is itself a life-threatening emergency that can lead to cardiac and/or respiratory arrest. Over-correction of the potassium level must also be guarded against.

Prognosis

Many of the therapies for hyperkalemia discussed above begin to work in about half an hour. However, they address only the immediate ion balance and not the root cause of the hyperkalemia. The prognosis depends on treating for such conditions as renal failure or diabetic ketoacidosis.

Pregnancy

Hyperkalemia in pregnancy is a medical emergency.

REFERENCES

Blumenthal M, ed. *The Complete German Commission E Monographs*. Boston, Mass: Integrative Medicine Communications; 1998:162.

Lee HS, Yu YC, Kim ST, Kim KS. Effects of moxibustion on blood pressure and renal function in spontaneously hypertensive rats. *Am J Chin Med*. 1997;25: 21–26.

Wheeless CR. Management of Hyperkalemia. *Wheeless' Textbook of Orthopaedics*. 1996. Accessed at http://wheeless.belgianorthoweb.be/oo3/24.htm on 2/17/99.

Zwanger M. *Hyperkalemia*. Emergency Medicine Online Text. 1998. Accessed at http://www.emedicine.com/emerg/topic261.htm on 2/13/99.

■ HYPERTENSION

OVERVIEW
Definition

Hypertension is an average or sustained systolic blood pressure over 140 mm Hg and/or a diastolic blood pressure over 90 mm Hg. Hypertension has an overall incidence of 20%, with onset usually occurring after age 20. The prevalence rises with age to over 50% over age 65. Ninety-five to 99% of hypertensive individuals have essential hypertension. Persons with hypertension are three to four times more likely to experience a major cardiovascular event (e.g., myocardial infarction, cerebrovascular accident, congestive heart failure).

Categories of hypertension (measured in mm Hg):

Stage 1 (mild)	Systolic BP 140 to 159	Diastolic BP 90 to 99
Stage 2 (moderate)	Systolic BP 160 to 179	Diastolic BP 100 to 109
Stage 3 (severe)	Systolic BP 180 to 209	Diastolic BP 110 to 119
Stage 4 (very severe)	Systolic BP >210	Diastolic BP >120

Etiology

- Essential, or primary, hypertension has no identifiable cause.
- Secondary hypertension may be caused by renal, endocrine, and vascular conditions; coarctation of the aorta, certain neurological conditions, acute stress, and chronic heavy alcohol use. Use of oral contraceptives, decongestants, and antidepressants may also cause secondary hypertension.

Risk Factors

Hypertension is more common in African Americans at all ages and in persons from lower socioeconomic groups. Individual risk factors include the following.

- Family history
- Alcohol use
- High sodium intake
- Stress
- Sedentary lifestyle
- Obesity
- High sugar intake

Signs and Symptoms

Essential hypertension has no symptoms except in extreme cases or after cardiovascular complications result. Extremely high blood pressures may cause headaches.

Severe hypertension or hypertensive crisis (usually secondary hypertension) with end-organ damage may produce headache, nausea and vomiting, seizure, retinopathy, and other symptoms.

DIFFERENTIAL DIAGNOSIS

Tests to determine possible causes are performed only if a secondary cause is suspected.

DIAGNOSIS
Physical Examination

Hypertension is diagnosed through blood pressure measurements. Guidelines include controlling the patient's posture when taking the blood pressure; restricting the use of caffeine, nicotine, and other stimulants before taking the blood pressure; using the appropriate size cuff; and taking at least three readings at least one week apart.

Diagnostic procedures focus on screening for causes and risk factors, assessing potential end-organ damage from sustained hypertension.

The history should include past blood pressure levels, family history, past conditions, diet (especially salt and cholesterol intake), exercise, current medications, alcohol and tobacco use, and stressors.

Physical examination should include the following.

- Blood pressure taken on right and left arms, both sitting and standing
- Heart rate and rhythm
- Peripheral and femoral pulses
- Fundoscopy
- Weight
- Complete family and patient history

Laboratory Tests

- Complete blood count
- Calcium level
- Creatinine level
- Potassium level
- Sodium level
- Fasting glucose and insulin levels
- Cholesterol levels
- Uric acid level
- Urinalysis

Pathological Findings

There are pathological findings only if organ damage has begun to occur from sustained hypertension; see "Complications."

Imaging

Only required for differential diagnosis or if end-organ damage is suspected:

- Chest X ray
- Ultrasonography
- IVP and renal arteriogram
- Provocative renal nuclear scan
- Digital subtraction arteriography
- Angiogram

Other Diagnostic Procedures

Only required for differential diagnosis or if end-organ damage is suspected:

- Plasma catecholamines
- Urinary metanephrines
- Plasma renin
- Electroencephalography

TREATMENT OPTIONS
Treatment Strategy

The goal of treatment is to lower the risk of future cardiovascular damage by lowering the blood pressure to below 140 mm Hg (systolic) and 90 mm Hg (diastolic). In stage 3 or 4 hypertension, significant partial reduction is acceptable.

Nonpharmacological therapies may be used with or without drug therapy. Nondrug therapies are generally used with stage 1 hypertension and should be evaluated over the course of 6 to 12 months. Drug treatment is usually required for more severe hypertension and usually provides control within 1 to 3 months.

Lifestyle modifications that lower blood pressure include the following.

- Weight reduction
- Sodium restriction
- Discontinuation or restriction of alcohol
- Discontinuation of caffeine

- Exercise
- Patient education about the importance of lowering blood pressure
- Biofeedback and relaxation techniques

Drug Therapies

Each case should be considered individually, yet drug therapy is recommended for patients with sustained systolic pressure over 160 mm Hg or diastolic pressure over 100 mm Hg. Traditionally, therapy with a diuretic or beta-blocker is tried first. The dosage may be modified or an additional drug from another class may be added. Ten percent of patients may require three drugs.

- Diuretics—e.g., hydrochlorothiazide (Hydrodiuril; 12.5 to 50 mg/day); side effects include decreased level of potassium and increased cholesterol and glucose levels; contraindicated in patients with gout and diabetes
- Potassium-sparing agents—spironolactone (Aldactazide; 25 to 100 mg/day); side effects include hyperkalemia and gynecomastia

Adrenergic inhibitors include the following.

- Alpha-blockers—doxazosin (Cardura; 1 to 20 mg/day); side effects include postural hypotension and lassitude
- Beta-blockers—acebutolol (Sectral; 200 to 800 mg/day); side effects include congestive heart failure, bronchospasm, masking of hypoglycemia induced by insulin, depression, insomnia, fatigue; contraindicated relatively in heart failure, airway disease, heart block, diabetes, and peripheral vascular disease
- Alpha/beta blockers—labetalol (Normodyne; 200 to 1,200 mg/day in two doses); side effects include postural hypotension and beta-blocker side effects
- Centrally acting sympatholytics—methyldopa (Aldomet; 500 to 3,000 mg/day in two doses); side effects include hepatic disorders, sedation, dry mouth
- Peripherally acting sympatholytics—reserpine (Serpasil; 0.05 to 0.25 mg/day); side effects include sedation and depression
- Calcium-channel blockers—verapamil (Isoptin; 90 to 480 mg/day); side effects include constipation, nausea, headache, conduction defects; use with caution in heart failure or block
- Dihydropyridines—amlodipine (Norvase; 2.5 to 10 mg/day); side effects include flushing, headache, ankle edema
- Direct vasodilators—hydralazine (Apresoline; 50 to 400 mg/day in two doses); side effects include headache, tachycardia, lupus syndrome
- Angiotensin-converting enzyme (ACE) inhibitors—benazepril (Lotensin; 5 to 40 mg/day); side effects include cough, rash, loss of taste; use with caution in renovascular disease

Complementary and Alternative Therapies

Mind-body techniques (such as biofeedback, yoga, meditation, and stress management), nutritional and herbal support may be effective in improving hypertension and concurrent pathologies.

NUTRITION

- Avoid caffeine and decrease intake of refined foods, sugar, and saturated fats (meats and dairy products). Some kinds of hypertension respond to a reduction of salt intake.
- Eliminate food allergens as these may exacerbate hypertension. Increase dietary fiber, vegetables and vegetable proteins, and essential fatty acids (cold-water fish, nuts, and seeds).
- MaxEPA, flax oil, or evening primrose oil (1,000 to 1,500 mg one to two times/day) lowers cholesterol and mildly reduces hypertension.
- Magnesium (200 mg bid to tid) induces mild vasodilation to decrease blood pressure.
- Zinc (30 mg/day) may help reduce blood pressure that is associated with high levels of cadmium (usually secondary to cigarette smoking).
- Coenzyme Q10 (50 to 100 mg one to two times/day) is protective to the cardiovascular system.
- B complex (50 to 100 mg/day) with additional folic acid (800 mcg/day), B₁₂ (1,200 mcg/day), and Betaine (1,000 mg/day) may increase resistance of stress and lower blood pressure that is secondary to homocysteinemia.
- Vitamin E (400 IU/day) reduces platelet aggregation.
- Some patients are sensitive to grains. A trial of limiting grain-based foods in the diet should be implemented to assess the effect on blood pressure.

HERBS

Herbs are generally a safe way to strengthen and tone the body's systems. As with any therapy, it is important to ascertain a diagnosis before pursuing treatment. Herbs may be used as dried extracts (capsules, powders, teas), glycerites (glycerine extracts), or tinctures (alcohol extracts). Unless otherwise indicated, teas should be made with one teaspoon herb per cup of hot water. Steep covered 5 to 10 minutes for leaf or flowers, and 10 to 20 minutes for roots. Drink two to four cups/day. Tinctures may be used singly or in combination as noted.

Hawthorn (*Crataegus oxyacantha*), linden flowers (*Tilia cordata*), passionflower (*Passiflora incarnata*), valerian (*Valeriana officinalis*), and cramp bark (*Viburnum opulus*) may be safely used long-term. These herbs relax and strengthen the cardiovascular system while moderately reducing blood pressure. Combine equal parts in a tincture, 20 to 30 drops tid or qid. Hawthorn may be taken as a dried extract, 250mg tid.

Dandelion leaf (*Taraxecum officinalis*) has a diuretic effect and spares potassium. Drink three to four cups/day.

The following herbs that have a stronger hypotensive effect and may have toxic side effects. These herbs must be used under the supervision of a qualified practitioner. Lily of the valley (*Convallaria majalis*), night-blooming cereus (*Cactus grandifloris*), mistletoe (*Viscum album*), motherwort (*Leonorus cardiaca*), and Indian tobacco (*Lobelia inflata*). Combine 3 to 4 of these herbs with equal parts of cramp bark and valerian and take 30 to 60 drops tid.

HOMEOPATHY

An experienced homeopath should assess individual constitutional types and severity of disease to select the correct remedy and potency.

ACUPUNCTURE

Acupuncture may be helpful in reducing blood pressure, alleviating stress, and addressing concurrent pathologies.

MASSAGE

Therapeutic massage may be effective in reducing the effects of stress and inducing relaxation and lowered blood pressure.

Patient Monitoring

Since patient compliance is poor with antihypertensive medications, with up to 20% of patients discontinuing the drug, patient education and follow-up are critical. Even after blood pressure is stabilized, changes in the medical regimen will be required for some patients for months and years. Schedule follow-up visits every three to six months.

OTHER CONSIDERATIONS

Prevention

Individuals with high normal or stage 1 hypertension may be able to prevent hypertension with a low-sodium diet, exercise, relaxation techniques, weight reduction, alcohol avoidance, and smoking cessation.

Complications/Sequelae

The complications of untreated hypertension include the following.

- Stroke
- Aortic aneurysm
- Myocardial infarction
- Congestive heart failure
- Cardiac enlargement
- Left ventricular hypertrophy
- Renal insufficiency
- Cerebral thrombosis or embolization

Prognosis

Controlled hypertension results in greatly diminished risks of complications and a generally good prognosis.

Pregnancy

Mild elevation of blood pressure can be normal in pregnancy, however, pregnancy-induced hypertension can progress rapidly to life-threatening sequelae. Blood pressure should be monitored frequently during pregnancy. Hawthorn, linden flowers, passionflower, valerian, and cramp bark may be used safely in pregnancy after the first trimester. Further intervention must be under the supervision of a physician.

REFERENCES

Barker LR, Burton JR et al, eds. *Principles of Ambulatory Medicine.* 4th ed. Baltimore, Md: Williams & Wilkins; 1995:803–843.

Bartram T. *Encyclopedia of Herbal Medicine.* Dorset, England: Grace Publishers; 1995:240.

Dambro MR. *Griffith's 5 Minute Clinical Consult 1999.* Baltimore, Md: Lippincott Williams & Wilkins; 1999.

Detre Z, Jellinek H, Miskulin R. Studies on vascular permeability in hypertension. *Clin Physiol Bichem.* 1986;4:143–149.

Golik A, Zaidenstein R, Dishi V, et al. Effects of captopril and enalapril on zinc metabolism in hypertensive patients. *J Am Coll Nutri.* 1998;17:75–78.

Kwan CY. Vascular effects of selected antihypertensive drugs derived from traditional medicinal herbs. *Clin Exp Pharmacol Physiol.* 1995;(suppl 1):S297–S299. Review.

Liva R. Naturopathic specific condition review: hypertension. Protocol Journal of Botanical Medicine. 1995;1:222.

Murray MT. *The Healing Power of Herbs.* Rocklin, Calif: Prima Publishing; 1991:90–96, 107–112.

Murray MT, Pizzorno JE. *Encyclopedia of Natural Medicine.* 2nd ed. Rocklin, Calif.:Prima Publishing; 1998.

Stein JH, ed. *Internal Medicine.* 4th ed. St. Louis, Mo: Mosby-Year Book; 1994:302–323.

Werbach M. *Nutritional Influences on Illness.* New Canaan, Conn: Keats Publishing; 1988:227–240.

The fifth report of the joint national committee on detection, evaluation, and treatment of high blood pressure. *Arch Intern Med.* 1993;153:154.

■ HYPERTHYROIDISM

OVERVIEW
Definition

Hyperthyroidism occurs when the thyroid gland produces excessive amounts of thyroid hormone. The condition can take three different forms. Graves' disease appears as a goiter in the neck along with eye and skin changes.Graves' disease is an autoimmune condition. It stems from an antibody that stimulates the thyroid to produce excessive amounts of thyroid hormones. In the process, the antibody overwhelms the usual thyroid-stimulating hormone. The stimulation causes the thyroid to grow, creating a goiter in the neck. In Graves' ophthalmopathy, the extraoccular muscles show edema, increased connective tissue fatty infiltration, and infiltration by lymphocytes. In toxic nodular goiter, one or more nodules in the thyroid, which are benign thyroid tumor, produce an excess of thyroid hormone. Secondary hyperthyroidism occurs when the pituitary gland stimulates the thyroid to overproduce thyroid hormones.

The ailment varies in severity. Most cases can be treated effectively with medication. Surgery may be necessary if conservative treatment fails. Left untreated, hyperthyroidism is potentially fatal. One complication, thyroid storm, is a life-threatening emergency that requires immediate treatment. It manifests itself as sudden, extreme overactivity of the thyroid gland, produces fever, weakness, loss of muscle, restlessness, mood swings, confusion, altered consciousness, and an enlarged liver with mild jaundice.

Estimates suggest that at least two million Americans, and possibly double that number, suffer from some degree of hyperthyroidism. Thyroid problems affect four times as many women as men, and more elderly individuals than younger people. All types of hyperthyroidism cause the body's cells to burn fuel so rapidly that they waste much of it in the form of heat.

Etiology

While several different factors trigger hyperthyroidism, stress is thought to play a role in the onset of the disease. The disease appears most often in individuals between the ages of 20 and 40.

Risk Factors

- Age between 20 and 40 years
- Stress
- Pregnancy
- In newborns, a mother with Graves' disease
- Intestinal dysbiosis
- Antibiotic overusage
- Family history

Signs and Symptoms

- Tachycardia
- Tachyarrythmia/palpitations
- Bruit over thyroid gland
- Hypertension
- Swelling at the base of the neck
- Moist skin and increased perspiration
- Shakiness and tremor
- Nervousness
- Confusion
- Increased appetite accompanied by weight loss
- Difficulty sleeping
- Swollen, reddened, and bulging eyes
- Constant stare (infrequent blinking, lid lag)
- Sensitivity of eyes to light

- Occasionally, raised, thickened skin over shins, dorsum of feet, back, hands, or even face
- In thyroid storm: fever, very rapid pulse, agitation, and possibly delirium
- Altered menses

DIFFERENTIAL DIAGNOSIS

- Depression
- Anxiety
- Hyperactivity
- Neurologic disease with resultant tremor
- Heart disease
- Drugs

DIAGNOSIS
Physical Examination

Patient is typically restless and anxious. Look for a slight tremor when patient sticks out tongue and extends the fingers. Examination of the thyroid gland while the patient swallows will yield evidence of enlargement. Auscultation may exhibit a bruit.

Laboratory Tests

Serum thyroxine (T_4) assay on free T_4 and the thyroid-hormone-binding ratio give accurate assessments of the state of the thyroid. If necessary, test also for an increase in the concentration of thyroxine and a decrease in that of thyroid-stimulating hormone. Serum triiodothyronine (T_3) assay also helps to differentiate between Graves' disease, toxic nodular goiter, T_3 toxicosis, and secondary hyperthyroidism.

Other Diagnostic Procedures

- Perform a radioactive iodine uptake test.
- Radioactive iodine uptake tests indicate the source of the overstimulation that results in the disease.
- Thyroid ultrasound

TREATMENT OPTIONS
Treatment Strategy

Three basic forms of treatment are available for the various manifestations of hyperthyroidism: thyroid depressive drugs, radioactive iodine, and surgery. Surgery is now the therapy of last resort.

Drug Therapies

Although the thyroid gland needs a small amount of iodine to function properly, a large amount of this element prevents the gland from releasing excess thyroid hormone. Thus, a one-time dose of radioactive iodine in liquid form has become the most popular method of treatment. The dose depends on the size of the thyroid and the findings of the radioactive iodine uptake test. The health care provider must assess the effect of the initial dose after 2 to 3 months. Depending on the result, he or she should plan follow-up visits every 6 to 12 weeks. Can cause hypothyroidism and is contraindicated in pregnancy.

Alternatively, prescribe thyroid depressive drugs in tablet form. Propylthiouracil and methimazole, the drugs most commonly used, decrease production of thyroid hormone. Oral doses should start high; adjust the doses downward according to the results of blood tests for the thyroid hormone. Typical starter doses usually bring hyperthyroidism under control within 6 to 12 weeks. Larger doses can control the condition faster, but may increase risk of adverse effects, such as allergic reactions, nausea, loss of taste and, rarely, depressed synthesis of blood cells in the bone marrow.

Beta-blocking drugs such as propranolol help to control some of the symptoms of hyperthyroidism, particularly in a thyroid storm. They slow heart rates, reduce tremors, and control anxiety. However, they do not control abnormal thyroid function.

Surgical Procedures

Suggest surgery for patients who have very large goiters, cannot receive radioactive iodine, do not tolerate other drugs, or do not benefit from medical treatment. The surgery involves removal of parts or most of the thyroid gland; and permanently controls hyperthyroidism in more than 90% of patients. However, it can lead to hypothyroidism in some patients, who must take replacement thyroid hormone from then on.

Complementary and Alternative Therapies

May minimize symptoms of mild thyroid dysfunction. Moderate to severe cases may need concurrent treatment with conventional therapies.

NUTRITION

Foods that depress the thyroid and should be included in the diet are broccoli, cabbage, brussel sprouts, cauliflower, kale, spinach, turnips, soy, beans, and mustard greens. Sorghum, flaxseed, cassava, and pulses contain cyanogenic glycosides which depress thyroid function. Avoid refined foods, dairy products, wheat, caffeine, and alcohol. Food allergies play a role in any autoimmune disease and should be assessed if that is suspected.

- Essential fatty acids are anti-inflammatory and help to modulate immune function. Take 1,000 to 1,500 mg tid.
- Bromelain (250 to 500 mg tid between meals) is a proteolytic enzyme that reduces inflammation.
- Vitamin C (1,000 mg tid to qid) supports immune function and decreases inflammation.
- Calcium (1,000 mg/day) and magnesium (200 to 600 mg/day) are co-factors for many metabolic processes.
- Vitamin E (400 IU bid) can help protect the heart during periods of tachycardia.
- Coenzyme Q10 (50 mg bid) can help protect the heart during periods of tachycardia.
- Lithium has anti-thyroid properties. Doses of as little as 20 mg per day of elemental lithium may augment other anti-thyroid treatments.

HERBS

Herbs are generally a safe way to strengthen and tone the body's systems. Ascertain a diagnosis before pursuing treatment. Herbs may be used as dried extracts (capsules, powders, teas), glycerites (glycerine extracts), or tinctures (alcohol extracts). Unless otherwise indicated, teas should be made with 1 tsp. herb per cup of hot water. Steep covered 5 to 10 minutes for leaf or flowers, and 10 to 20 minutes for roots. Drink 2 to 4 cups/day. Tinctures may be used singly or in combination as noted.

- Bugleweed (Lycopus virginica) and lemon balm (Melissa officinalis) help to normalize the over-active thyroid. Motherwort (Leonorus cardiaca) may relieve heart palpitations and Passionflower (Passiflora incarnata) reduces anxiety. Combine two parts of Bugleweed with one part each of lemon balm, motherwort, and passionflower and take in tincture form, 30 to 60 drops tid to qid.
- Quercetin (250 to 500 mg tid) is an anti-inflammatory.

- Turmeric (Curcuma longa) potentiates bromelain and should be taken between meals, 500 mg tid.
- Milk thistle (Silibum Marianum) helps the liver to provide proper binding proteins to sequester thyroid hormone. 300 to 600 mg tid.
- Hawthorne berry (Cratagus Oxycantha) helps to protect the heart during periods of tachycardia. 1/4 tsp. of the solid extract, or 1,000 mg of the herb, tid.
- Lemon balm (Mellissa officinalis) inhibits the binding of TSH and thyroid-stimulating antibodies to TSH receptors.
- Immune suppressing herbs such as Stephania tetranda and Hemidesmus indicus help break the circle of cellular damage in chronic inflammation.
- Anti-inflammatory herbs such as licorice (Glycyrrhiza glabra) and Rehmania glutinosa are systemic anti-inflammatories and support the adrenals as well.

HOMEOPATHIC REMEDIES

An experienced homeopath should assess individual constitutional types, severity of disease, and select the correct remedy and potency.

PHYSICAL MEDICINE

Ice packs to the throat will help to decrease inflammation. Castor oil packs to the throat will also reduce inflammation. Apply oil directly to skin, cover with a clean soft cloth (e.g., flannel) and plastic wrap. Leave in place for 30 to 60 minutes. For best results use three consecutive days in one week.

ACUPUNCTURE

Acupuncture may help correct hormonal imbalances and addressing underlying deficiencies/excesses involved in hyperthyroidism.

MASSAGE

Therapeutic massage may relieve stress and increase sense of well-being.

Patient Monitoring

Monitor patients during/after treatment. Watch for signs of hypothyroidism.

OTHER CONSIDERATIONS
Complications/Sequelae

Liquid radioactive iodine may have long-term effects on mortality. Patients who experience severe weight loss/muscle wasting after treatment should follow a diet that provides supplemental calories and protein.

Pregnancy

Thyroid testing during pregnancy may have variable and unreliable results. Mild pathology may not be detected until after pregnancy. A thyroid storm is a rare complication in pregnancy and may be life-threatening. Thyroid treatment in pregnancy should be supervised by a physician.

REFERENCES
Bartram T. *Encyclopedia of Herbal Medicine.* Dorset, England: Grace Publishers; 1995:422.
Berkow R. *Merck Manual.* 16th ed. Whitehorse Station, NJ: The Merck Publishing Group; 1992.
Blumenthal M, ed. *The Complete German Commission E Monographs.* Boston, Mass: Integrative Medicine Communications; 1998:432.
Hoffman D. *The New Holistic Herbal.* New York, NY: Barnes & Noble Books; 1995:95.

■ HYPOGLYCEMIA

OVERVIEW
Definition
Hypoglycemia is characterized by an inadequate concentration of glucose in circulating blood (low blood sugar). Beta cells in the pancreas secrete the hormone insulin after meals in response to an increase in plasma glucose concentrations. Insulin, in turn, lowers plasma glucose concentrations by increasing the rate at which glucose is taken up by cells. A deficiency of plasma glucose (e.g., after exercise, during pregnancy) because of increased glucose utilization causes the alpha cells of the pancreas to secrete the hormone glucagon. Glucagon, in turn, stimulates the release of glucose that is stored in the liver as glycogen to make up for the deficit. These glucoregulatory mechanisms can become overworked by lifestyle factors such as stress or poor diet, or by disease, or as a result of genetic predisposition.

Hypoglycemia is typically divided into two categories: fasting (postabsorptive) hypoglycemia and reactive (postprandial) hypoglycemia. Fasting hypoglycemia is associated with medications (e.g., sulfonylureas) and serious disease states (e.g., critical organ failure, various cancers, prolonged starvation). Reactive hypoglycemia is associated with postprandial hypoglycemia that becomes symptomatic several hours after a meal, and often with exercise. It is usually not associated with a serious preexisting disorder.

Etiology
Reactive causes include:
- Fasting hypoglycemia
- Prolonged starvation
- Postprandial hypoglycemia, especially with exercise
- Gastric surgery

Fasting (postabsortive) causes include:
- Drugs (e.g., insulin, sulfonylureas, alcohol)
- Organ failure (e.g., renal, cardiac, or hepatic failure)
- Hormone deficiencies (e.g., growth hormone, cortisol)
- Endogenous hyperinsulinism (e.g., insulinoma)
- Non-beta cell tumors (e.g., fibrosarcoma, mesothelioma)
- Congenital enzyme abnormalities (e.g., glycogen storage disease type 1)

Risk Factors
- Diabetes (especially insulin excess and impaired glucose counter-regulation)
- Excessive use of alcohol, tobacco, coffee, or caffeine-containing drinks
- Treatment for diabetes (e.g., sulfonylureas)
- Cancer
- Poor diet (e.g., excessive intake of simple carbohydrates and/or inadequate protein intake)
- Congenital enzyme abnormalities
- Severe illness (e.g., organ failure, sepsis)

Signs and Symptoms
Clinical manifestations of low glucose levels are nonspecific but can range from mild (subtle impairment) to severe and life-threatening (coma, death). Because glucose is critical for proper brain function, low levels manifest in the brain first.
- Headache
- Depression, anxiety
- Palpitations
- Bizarre behavior, mental confusion
- Blurred vision, vertigo
- Excessive sweating
- Tremulousness, incoordination
- Slurred speech
- Seizures (common in children but rare in adults)
- Fatigue
- Coma
- Irritability

DIFFERENTIAL DIAGNOSIS
- Diabetes
- Depression
- Premenstrual syndrome and menopause
- Central nervous system tumors or abnormalities
- Psychiatric disturbances
- Dumping syndrome

DIAGNOSIS
Physical Examination
Hypoglycemia is most often suspected on the basis of the history or the presenting symptoms which may include irritability, confusion, tremulousness, diaphoresis, and tachycardia. Screening laboratory tests are essential. The diagnosis of hypoglycemia is based on Whipple's triad: symptoms of hypoglycemia, low plasma glucose concentrations, relief of symptoms when normal plasma glucose levels are restored.

Laboratory Tests
- Blood and plasma glucose
- Serum insulin, calcium, phosphate, uric acid, lipids, creatinine
- Liver tests
- Insulin antibodies
- Plasma and urine corticosteroids

Pathological Findings
- Fasting plasma glucose levels of 60 to 105 mg/dL are normal.
- Fasting plasma glucose levels of 45 to 60 mg/dL suggest hypoglycemia.
- Fasting plasma glucose levels less than 45 mg/dL indicate severe hypoglycemia
- Fasting plasma glucose levels over 140 mg/dL indicate diabetes.

Imaging
Computed tomography (CT) scans are used to diagnose non-beta cell tumors, insulinomas, or other tumors that may be responsible for hypoglycemia.

Other Diagnostic Procedures
- Glucose tolerance test (GTT [fasting])
- Glucose-insulin tolerance test (G-ITT)
- Hypoglycemic index (e.g., calculation of the fall in blood glucose 90 minutes before the nadir divided by the value of the nadir; a hypoglycemic index > 0.8 indicates reactive hypoglycemia)
- Symptom assessment
- C-peptide suppression test
- Glucose infusion test
- Measurement of counter-regulatory hormone concentrations

TREATMENT OPTIONS
Treatment Strategy
Fasting hypoglycemia can be a medical emergency because of the adverse effects of prolonged low blood sugar on the brain, whereas reactive hypoglycemia is usually self-limited and rarely produces dangerous symptoms. However, it is imperative to establish the existence of hypoglycemia and to

distinguish between the two hypoglycemic states. Plasma glucose concentrations must be raised to normal levels as quickly as possible. Clinical improvement should be expected in less than 10 minutes. If there is no improvement after 15 minutes, the initial treatment should be repeated.

Drug Therapies

- Oral administration of glucose if the patient is awake enough to swallow (10 to 20 g carbohydrate)
- Intravenous administration of glucose for patients unable to swallow (25 ml of 50% glucose solution)
- Subcutaneous or intramuscular injection of glucagon (1 mg) is an alternative to the above treatments, but patients must also eat because the effect of glucagon is short.
- Intravenous mannitol (40 g as a 20% solution over 20 minutes) and glucocorticoids (dexamethasone, 10 mg) may be used to treat a delayed recovery (e.g., patient who remains in a coma after glucose levels return to normal).

Complementary and Alternative Therapies

Alternative therapies may also be useful in regulating blood sugar in the short term.

NUTRITION

- Small frequent meals, preferably five to six a day, high in protein and complex carbohydrates.
- Minimize simple carbohydrates including sugar, refined foods, juices, and fruit.
- Eliminate caffeine, alcohol, and tobacco.

Some patients with normal lab values may respond well to dietary changes.

Vitamins and minerals essential to normal glucose regulation include:

- Chromium picolinate—100 to 200 mcg tid with meals
- Magnesium—200 mg bid to tid
- Vanadyl sulfate—10 to 20 mg/day
- Zinc—15 to 30 mg/day
- B complex—50 to 100 mg/day
- Niacinamide—500 mg/day
- Pyridoxine (B_6)—100 mg/day
- Pantothenic acid (B_5)—250 mg/day
- Vitamin C—1,000 mg bid to tid
- Vitamin E—400 IU/day

HERBS

Herbs are generally a safe way to strengthen and tone the body's systems. As with any therapy, it is important to ascertain a diagnosis before pursuing treatment. Herbs may be used as dried extracts (capsules, powders, teas), glycerites, or tinctures (alcohol extracts). Unless otherwise indicated, teas should be made with 1 tsp. herb per cup of hot water. Steep covered 10 to 20 minutes and drink 2 to 4 cups/day. Tinctures may be used singly or in combination as noted.

- Siberian ginseng *(Eleuthrococcus senticosus)* provides adrenal support. Use tincture 20 drops bid, or dried extract 100 mg tid for two to three weeks, with a one week rest before resuming.
- A tincture of equal parts of licorice root *(Glycyrrhiza glabra)*, gotu kola *(Centella asiatica)*, Siberian ginseng, and ginger root *(Zingiber*

officinale), 10 to 15 drops tid, may be used in combination to strengthen the adrenals and alleviate hypoglycemic symptoms.

HOMEOPATHY

An experienced homeopath should assess individual constitutional types and severity of disease to select the correct remedy and potency. Constitutional homeopathy can provide overall support, but the underlying cause must be addressed.

ACUPUNCTURE

May be beneficial in decreasing stress and increasing coping skills.

Patient Monitoring

If a hypoglycemic mechanism is obvious and treatable (or self-limited), then no further diagnostic workup is necessary. If a hypoglycemic mechanism is not apparent, further studies are necessary to determine the cause.

OTHER CONSIDERATIONS
Prevention

Diet is one of the most important factors in avoiding hypoglycemic episodes. The diet of choice for hypoglycemia should be low in simple carbohydrates and high in protein and complex carbohydrates. Refined and simple sugars, alcohol, coffee, tobacco, and caffeine-containing soft drinks should be avoided. Avoid fasting, and favor more frequent smaller meals over fewer larger meals. Regular moderate exercise may improve glucose metabolism by increasing insulin sensitivity and glucose tolerance.

Complications/Sequelae

Untreated post-absorptive hypoglycemia can result in coma, brain damage or death.

Prognosis

Patients with reactive hypoglycemia can expect no long-term ill effects because there is no underlying pathology. However, the prognosis for patients with fasting hypoglycemia depends largely on the underlying disease causing the hypoglycemia, which may be progressive and sometimes fatal.

Pregnancy

Pregnancy may be a predisposing factor in reactive hypoglycemia and adult-onset diabetes.

REFERENCES

Anderson RA, Polansky MM, Bryden NA, Bhathena SJ, Canary JJ. Effects of supplemental chromium on patients with symptoms of reactive hypoglycemia. *Metabolism.* 1987;36:351–355.

Branch WT Jr. *Office Practice of Medicine.* 3rd ed. Philadelphia, Pa: WB Saunders; 1994:574–575.

Fauci AS, Braunwald E, Isselbacher KJ, et al: *Harrison's Principles of Internal Medicine.* 14th ed. New York, NY: McGraw-Hill; 1998:2069–2071.

Mowry DB. *The Scientific Validation of Herbal Medicine.* New Canaan, Conn: Keats Publishing; 1986:25.

Tyler VE. *Herbs of Choice: The Therapeutic Use of Phytomedicinals.* New York, NY: Pharmaceutical Products Press; 1994:141.

Wilson JD, Foster DW. Williams *Textbook of Endocrinology.* 8th ed. Philadelphia, Pa: WB Saunders; 1992:1232–1248.

Wyngaarden JB, Smith LH Jr. *Cecil Textbook of Medicine.* 17th ed. Philadelphia, Pa: WB Saunders; 1985:1342–1348.

■ HYPOTHYROIDISM

OVERVIEW
Definition
Hypothyroidism occurs when the thyroid gland produces too little thyroid hormone, when there is decreased conversion from T_4 to T_3, when there is an overproduction of reverse T_3 (Wilson's syndrome), or when the body is not efficiently using thyroid hormone. It can take several forms.

- In Hashimoto's thyroiditis, the most common type, the gland shrinks and loses its function.
- Post-therapeutic hypothyroidism may follow overzealous treatment for hyperthyroidism (excess production of thyroid hormone). Medical and surgical treatments for hyperthyroidism can leave patients' thyroids incapable of producing enough thyroid hormone.
- Goitrous hypothyroidism results from an extreme shortage of iodine in the diet. Almost unknown in the United States since the introduction of iodized salt, it produces a goiter in the neck.

Other types of hypothyroidism can stem from inherited enzymatic deficiencies or the failure of other glands in the body. According to some estimates, as many as 11 million Americans suffer some degree of hypothyroidism. However, the majority of those cases go undiagnosed.

Hypothyroidism can occur in either sex at any age, although middle-aged women are most commonly affected. Note that infants, adolescents, and adults show different sets of symptoms. The disease has a wide variety of symptoms, and they often reveal themselves slowly and subtly. Untreated, hypothyroidism can cause anemia, a low body temperature, heart failure and, ultimately, a condition known as myxedema coma. This type of coma, triggered by exposure to cold, infection, or drugs such as sedatives, is potentially fatal. It leads to a slowdown in breathing, seizures, and a reduction in the flow of blood to the brain. Myxedema coma is extremely rare in warm climates, but not uncommon in cold regions.

Etiology
- In Hashimoto's thyroiditis, often called primary hypothyroidism, an autoimmune response occurs in which antibodies in the blood destroy tissues in the thyroid gland. As a result, the thyroid decreases in size and reduces its production of thyroid hormones.
- Post-therapeutic hypothyroidism results from the treatment of hyperthyroidism with radioactive iodine or surgical removal of part or all of the thyroid gland. The treatment can leave the patient's thyroid unable to produce sufficient amounts of thyroid hormone.
- Goitrous hypothyroidism is caused by a lack of iodine in the diet, a problem in some developing countries (The thyroid requires a steady supply of iodine to operate correctly).

Risk Factors
- Treatment for hyperthyroidism
- Chronic lack of iodine in the diet
- Inherited enzymatic defects
- For women, reaching middle age

Signs and Symptoms
- Slow pulse
- Lethargy
- Hoarse voice
- Slowed speech
- Puffy face
- Loss of eyebrows from the sides
- Drooping eyelids
- Intolerance to cold
- Weight gain
- Constipation
- Dry, scaly, thick, coarse hair
- Raised, thickened skin over the shins
- Carpal tunnel syndrome
- Confusion
- Depression
- In children, growth retardation, delayed teething, and mental deficiency
- Dementia
- Headaches
- Menstrual cramps or other menstrual disorders

DIFFERENTIAL DIAGNOSIS
- Euthyroid sick syndrome
- Depression
- Alzheimer's disease or other types of dementia
- Carpal tunnel syndrome

DIAGNOSIS
Physical Examination
Patients typically report muscle aches and the inability to stay warm in cool or cold temperatures. Tests of reflexes indicate brisk contraction and slow relaxation times. As symptoms progress, patients show puffy faces, dry, thickened skin, hoarseness, and hearing loss. The palms and soles have slightly orange hues, evidence of carotene deposits. The heart is enlarged.

Laboratory Tests
Blood tests may show decreased levels of thyroid hormone, increased thyroid-stimulating hormone, and the presence of auto-antibodies, differentiating between primary and secondary hypothyroidism. Patients with primary hypothyroidism, for example, will not respond to radioactive iodine uptake tests, while most of those with secondary hypothyroidism will show a brisk response. Blood tests can also indicate the presence of anemia, a symptom of untreated hypothyroidism. Hypercholesterolemia may be found with hypothyroidism.

Other Diagnostic Procedures
When necessary, perform two radioactive iodine uptake tests four days apart.

TREATMENT OPTIONS
Treatment Strategy
Providers can prescribe several thyroid hormones as replacement therapy. Typically, condition improves within two to three weeks of the start of daily hormone therapy, and all symptoms disappear within a few months. However, patients must continue this treatment for the rest of their lives.

Drug Therapies
Health care providers must initially choose between synthetic preparations of the human thyroid hormone and dried forms of animal thyroid hormone. Providers generally prefer synthetic versions of thyroxine, liothyronine, or combinations of the two. They typically prescribe 100 to 125 mcg of the medication daily, to be taken orally. Evidence suggests that patients absorb about 90% to 95% of the dose.

Key to effective treatment is calibration of the medication. Particularly in older patients, treatment should start with small doses of thyroid hormone. Providers then gradually increase the dose until the individual's blood level of thyroid-stimulating hormone returns to normal. With appropriate calibration of doses, the patient will reach this stage about eight weeks after the start of daily therapy.

Specialists recommend that providers not prescribe liothyronine alone over long periods. It tends to cause chemical hyperthyroidism for at least several hours per day, thereby exposing the patient to above normal cardiac risks. Since myxedema coma represents an emergency situation, providers should administer replacement hormones intravenously.

Complementary and Alternative Therapies
Thyroid function can be effectively supported with nutrition and herbs, although concurrent treatment with conventional medicine may be necessary in moderate to severe cases.

NUTRITION
Avoid foods that suppress thyroid function, including broccoli, cabbage, brussel sprouts, cauliflower, kale, spinach, turnips, soybeans, peanuts, linseed, pinenuts, millet, cassava, and mustard greens. Avoid refined foods, dairy products, wheat, caffeine, and alcohol.

- Essential fatty acids (1,000 to 1,500 mg bid) are necessary for hormone production. It may be wise to avoid flaxseed oil due to high levels of cyanogenic glycosides. A better choice for omega 3 oils for the hypothyroid patient would be cold water fish oils or borage oil.
- Vitamin C (1,000 mg tid to qid), vitamin A (10,000 to 25,000 IU/day), B complex [50 to 100 mg/day, augmented with vitamins B_2 (riboflavin, 15 mg), B_3 (niacin, 25 to 50 mg), and B_6 (pyridoxine, 25 to 50 mg)], selenium (200 mcg/day), iodine (300 mcg/day), vitamin E (400 IU/day), and zinc (30 mg/day) are necessary for thyroid hormone production.
- L-tyrosine (500 mg bid-tid) also supports normal thyroid function. In a small percentage of patients it may cause caffeine-like symptoms. Patients with insomnia should avoid taking L-tyrosine in the evening. (May rarely exacerbate hypertension.)
- Calcium (1,000 mg/day) and magnesium (200 to 600 mg/day) are co-factors for many metabolic processes.

HERBS
Herbs are generally a safe way to strengthen and tone the body's systems. Ascertain a diagnosis before pursuing treatment. Herbs may be used as dried extracts (capsules, powders, teas), glycerites (glycerine extracts), or tinctures (alcohol extracts). Unless otherwise indicated, teas should be made with 1 tsp. herb per cup of hot water. Steep covered 5 to 10 minutes for leaf or flowers, and 10 to 20 minutes for roots. Drink 2 to 4 cups/day.

A combination that would support thyroid function includes herbs rich in minerals. Combine equal parts of the following herbs for a tea (3 to 4 cups/day) or tincture (20 to 30 drops tid). Horsetail (*Equisetum arvense*), oatstraw (*Avena sativa*), alfalfa (*Medicago sativa*), and gotu kola (*Centella asiatica*).

Seaweeds such as kelp (*Alaria esculenta*), bladderwrack (*Fucus vesiculosis*), Irish moss (*Chondrus crispus*) may be taken as foods or in capsule form due to their salty and unfamiliar taste. Many patients would not tolerate the seaweed taste in a tea beverage.

Coleus foreskohlii (1 to 2 ml tid) stimulates thyroid function with an increase in thyroid hormone production. Also, herbs such as guggul (*Commiphora guggul*—25 mg of guggulsterones tid) and hawthorne (*Crataegus oxyacantha*—500 mg bid) are taken to counteract hypercholesterolemia which often attends hypothyroidism.

HOMEOPATHY
For patients that do not want to take whole tissue glandulars, homeopathic glandulars are available for hypothyroidism.

PHYSICAL MEDICINE
Contrast hydrotherapy to the neck and throat may stimulate thyroid function. Alternating hot and cold applications brings nutrients to the site and diffuses metabolic waste from inflammation. The overall effect is decreased inflammation, pain relief, and enhanced healing. Alternate three minutes hot with one minute cold. Repeat three times. This is one set. Do two to three sets/day.

Exercise helps sensitize thyroid gland to hormones and improves its function. Stress reduction techniques such as yoga, meditation, or tai chi help to lower cortisol levels. High cortisol levels may decrease T_3/reverse T_3 ratios.

ACUPUNCTURE
Acupuncture may be helpful in correcting hormonal imbalances and addressing underlying deficiencies involved in hypothyroidism.

MASSAGE
Therapeutic massage may be useful in relieving stress, improving circulation, and increasing the overall sense of well-being.

Patient Monitoring
Monitor patients carefully during and after any treatment.

OTHER CONSIDERATIONS
Prevention
A diet using small amounts of iodized salt may help prevent goitrous hypothyroidism.

Complications/Sequelae
Watch out for brief swings into hyperthyroidism with certain treatments.

Prognosis
Expect to see beneficial effects of hormone replacement therapy within two to three weeks of starting the course of treatment. Symptoms should disappear within a few months, by which time patients will have settled into a maintenance dose of hormone.

Pregnancy
Thyroid testing during pregnancy may have variable and unreliable results. Mild pathology may not be detected until after pregnancy. Thyroid treatment in pregnancy should be done with the supervision of a physician.

REFERENCES
Bartram T. *Encyclopedia of Herbal Medicine.* Dorset, England: Grace Publishers; 1995:304.
Berkow R. *Merck Manual.* 16th ed. Whitehorse Station, NJ: The Merck Publishing Group; 1992.
Murray MT, Pizzorno JE. *Encyclopedia of Natural Medicine.* Rocklin, Calif: Prima Publishing; 1998:386–390.

■ INFANTILE COLIC

OVERVIEW
Definition
Colic is a state of excessive crying seen in infants, typically during the late afternoon or early evening. From 15% to 20% of infants develop colic, and it seems to be more common in firstborns and in boys than in later-born infants and in girls. Colic is not a disease or syndrome caused by bacteria or viruses. It is seen in otherwise healthy infants and can begin as early as 2 weeks of age. It is self-limited, only rarely lasting until the infant is 6 months old.

Etiology
No cause has been proven for this disorder, but theories include those listed below.

- Stage in the development of an immature central nervous system or digestive system
- Response to emotional and family stress—need for comfort
- Reflection of differences in infant temperament and physiology
- Intolerance to foods in mother's diet, specifically, dairy products, caffeine, or gassy foods
- Introducing food into infant's diet too early

Risk Factors
- In breast-fed infants, a maternal diet that includes dairy products, caffeine, or gassy foods
- In bottle-fed infants, cow's milk formula or iron-fortified formula intolerance
- Overstimulation or understimulation of infant
- Caregiver smoking
- Antibiotics given at birth or to mother during labor

Signs and Symptoms
- Inconsolable crying that lasts more than three hours for three or more days a week in a healthy infant 2 weeks to 3 months of age
- Crying accompanied by vigorous kicking, pulling the legs up tightly to the body, and making tight fists
- May have swollen or distended stomach, burp, or pass gas often
- Infant appears to be in pain
- Arched back and clenched fists
- Frequent spitting up after feeding

DIFFERENTIAL DIAGNOSIS
- Bladder infection
- Ear infection
- Kidney infection
- Gastrointestinal reflux
- Severe constipation
- Intussusception
- Volvulus
- Testicular torsion
- Occult fracture

DIAGNOSIS
Physical Examination
Infant appears healthy, eats well, and is gaining weight, with no fever or diarrhea. Cradle cap and dry skin often occur with colic, in which case suspect food intolerance.

Laboratory Tests
In the absence of poor feeding, diarrhea, weight loss, fever, black, green, or bloody stools in an infant less than 2 months old, or the persistence of crying beyond 6 months of age, no laboratory tests are needed.

Other Diagnostic Procedures
- Make sure the infant is properly fed, burped, comfortably clothed, and has a clean diaper.
- Evaluate the history of crying offered by the caregiver.

TREATMENT OPTIONS
Treatment Strategy
Because there is no identified cause, treatment involves finding what is effective from among the items listed below, and supporting the parents.

- For a breast-fed infant, decrease the time between nursing sessions (nurse on demand) and have the mother eliminate dairy products, caffeine, and all foods that give the mother gas (sensitive foods may include citrus, spicy foods, and soy).
- For a bottle-fed infant, change to a formula that is not based on cow's milk. May need hypoallergenic formula.
- Do not offer solid foods to the infant before 6 months of age.
- Instruct parents to try holding the infant close, offering a pacifier, rocking, rubbing the back, giving infant a warm bath, taking a car ride, playing music, or placing the infant in an infant swing to ease the crying. Try these various strategies until one works.
- Remind parents that this condition should last only a few months. Encourage them to take breaks if the crying becomes unbearable, join a support group, or call the pediatrician if they fear they will harm the baby.
- Review with parents different methods of burping.

Drug Therapies
No drugs are currently recommended, although simethicone may be helpful.

Complementary and Alternative Therapies
Eliminating gas-producing foods and using supportive herbal or homeopathic therapies can help reduce or eliminate infantile colic. Reducing stimuli and placing the infant in a dim, quiet room may help to calm the baby.

NUTRITION
Follow dietary changes as noted in "Treatment Strategy" above. Acidophilus (especially *Bifidus* spp.) can be given to both the breastfeeding mother and infant. Use 1 capsule with meals tid for adult; 1 capsule/day for infant (break capsule open and administer powder in divided doses throughout the day). This will help to normalize bowel flora.

HERBS
Herbs are generally a safe way to strengthen and tone the body's systems. As with any therapy, it is important to ascertain a diagnosis before pursuing treatment. Herbs may be used as dried extracts (capsules, powders, teas), glycerites (glycerine extracts), or tinctures (alcohol extracts). Unless otherwise indicated, teas should be made with 1 tsp. herb per cup of hot water. Steep covered 5 to 10 minutes for leaf or flowers, and 10 to 20 minutes for roots. Drink 2 to 4 cups/day. Tinctures may be used singly or in combination as noted.

A tea made from fennel seed *(Foeniculum vulgare)* or anise seed *(Pimpinella anisum)* may be administered directly to the infant (1 tsp. before and after feedings) or drunk by the breastfeeding mother (1 cup three to six times/day). Both fennel and anise act as gastrointestinal relaxants and help to expel gas.

Other herbs that have relaxing effects and help reduce colic are lemon balm *(Melissa officinalis)*, catnip *(Nepeta cateria)*, peppermint *(Mentha piperita)*, spearmint *(Mentha spicata)*, and linden flower *(Tilia cordata)*. These may be added to the above tea as needed.

HOMEOPATHY

An experienced homeopath should assess individual constitutional types and severity of disease to select the correct remedy and potency. For acute prescribing use 3 to 5 pellets of a 12X to 30C remedy every one to four hours until acute symptoms resolve. For infants, dissolve about 5 pellets in $1/4$ cup of water and give 1 tsp. every four hours.
- *Carbo vegetalis* for flatulent colic and burping.
- *Chamomilla* for colic with irritability that is relieved by constant holding and walking.
- *Magnesia phosphoricum* for colic that is better when bending double.

Combination remedies for colic, as commercially available, may be used as needed.

PHYSICAL MEDICINE

Warm baths may help to relax and soothe colicky infants. Add 3 to 4 drops of essential oil of lavender or lemon balm to enhance the benefit.

MASSAGE

Clockwise abdominal massage may help to relieve spasm and expel gas. Use 3 to 5 drops of tincture of catnip *(Nepeta cateria)* in 1 to 2 tsp. of almond or olive oil to enhance effectiveness. Apply warmth.

Patient Monitoring

Additional diagnostic producers may be required if the following symptoms develop:
- Colic persists or recurs daily: may be ear, bladder, or kidney infection;

formula may need to be changed or further foods eliminated from nursing mother's diet.
- An infant less than 2 months old develops black or blood stools, vomiting, diarrhea, or fever.

OTHER CONSIDERATIONS
Prevention

Colic may occur less often if one can:
- Nurse infant on demand (typically, every two to four hours) or use a non-iron-fortified formula for bottle-fed infant.
- Respond to the infant's cries quickly.
- Cultivate a support network of family/friends to help.
- Not smoke.
- Elevate infant's head during and after feedings.

Complications/Sequelae

Infants generally outgrow colic with no subsequent problems. Parents should be cautioned not to shake the infant, which can produce the potentially fatal shaken infant syndrome.

Prognosis

Colic usually responds to one or more treatments and typically resolves before the infant is 6 months of age. Colicky babies, however, often grow up to have other allergy-related conditions, such as otitis media, asthma, and digestive problems.

REFERENCES

Ayllon T. *Stopping Baby's Colic.* New York, NY: Putnam; 1989.

Boericke W. *Materia Medica.* 9th ed. Santa Rosa, Calif: Boericke and Tafel; 1927:151.

Jones S. *Crying Baby, Sleepless Nights: Why Your Baby Is Crying and What You Can Do About It.* Boston, Mass. The Harvard Common Press; 1992.

Kemper KJ. *The Holistic Pediatrician.* New York, NY: HarperPerennial; 1996.

Kruzel T. *The Homeopathic Emergency Guide.* Berkeley, Calif: North Atlantic Books; 1992:126–128.

Schiff D, Shelov P, eds. *American Academy of Pediatrics: The Official, Complete Home Reference Guide to Your Child's Symptoms, Birth Through Adolescence.* New York, NY: Villard Books; 1997.

Wilen J, Wilen L. *Folk Remedies That Work.* New York, NY. HarperPerennial; 1996.

■ INFLUENZA

OVERVIEW
Definition
Influenza, or "flu," is a viral infection of the respiratory tract. Its symptoms are usually systemic and more severe than those of other viral respiratory infections such as the common cold. Regional and local influenza epidemics lasting three to six weeks occur almost every winter. While most cases run their course in one to two weeks, life-threatening complications such as pneumonia are possible, especially in the elderly and in patients with chronic illnesses. Between 20,000 and 40,000 people die of influenza in the United States annually, and pandemics occurring a few times a century may kill many more.

Etiology
There are three main types of orthomyxoviruses that cause influenza.

- Influenza A: Responsible for near-annual epidemics of disease with relatively severe symptoms. Mutates by gradual antigenic drift and also by occasional abrupt protein changes (antigenic shift) which can cause pandemics, as occurred most recently in 1918 ("Spanish flu"), 1957 ("Asian flu") and 1968 ("Hong Kong flu").
- Influenza B: Near-annual outbreaks, but usually less serious than type A influenza. Mutates by antigenic drift only.
- Influenza C: Causes mild illness, or is asymptomatic. Not responsible for epidemics. Antigenically stable.

The viruses are mainly spread via aerosols of respiratory secretions released through sneezing and coughing.

Risk Factors
- Age (highest risk in school-age children and the elderly)
- Health-care provider
- Residence in a nursing home or other chronic care facility
- Chronic cardiovascular or pulmonary disorders (including asthma)
- Compromised immune system

Signs and Symptoms
- Sudden onset of fever (101 to 104°F)
- Chills
- Headache
- Muscle aches
- Fatigue
- Nonproductive cough
- Sore throat
- Sneezing, rhinorrhea and/or nasal obstruction
- Loss of appetite
- Nausea, vomiting, or diarrhea, especially in children

DIFFERENTIAL DIAGNOSIS
- Common cold
- Pharyngitis
- Laryngitis
- Herpes esophagitis
- Bronchitis
- Pneumonia

DIAGNOSIS
Physical Examination
Patients appear ill, febrile, and coughing. They may not exhibit all the classical symptoms, but evidence of upper respiratory infection is generally apparent. Lungs are usually clear.

Laboratory Tests
Viral testing of throat swabs or washings.

Imaging
Chest X rays should be taken if complicating pneumonia is suspected.

Other Diagnostic Procedures
Diagnosis may often be made by symptoms alone, particularly when an epidemic is underway.

TREATMENT OPTIONS
Treatment Strategy
Specific antiviral therapies are available for influenza. Medications are given to relieve symptoms until the antivirals take effect. Complementary therapies can be part of this process. Antibiotics are not effective against the viruses that cause influenza; however, some health care providers choose to administer them to patients particularly vulnerable to complicating bacterial pneumonia. Rest and fluids are recommended.

Drug Therapies
Antiviral drugs amantadine (Symadine, Symmetrel), 100 mg bid for 10 days, or rimantadine (Flumadine) administered within 48 hours of illness onset. Effective against influenza A only. Relieve symptoms with OTC acetaminophen, ibuprofen, cough suppressant, and decongestant. Never give aspirin to children or teenagers with a viral illness because of the risk of Reye's syndrome.

Complementary and Alternative Therapies
A combination of herbs and nutrition may be quite effective at relieving symptoms and speeding healing. The backbone of treatment is rest and fluids. The correct homeopathic treatment can be helpful in relieving symptoms.

NUTRITION
- Vitamin C (1,000 mg tid to qid), vitamin A (25,000 IU/day) or beta-carotene (200,000 IU/day), and zinc (25 to 90 mg/day) are nutrients that optimize immune system functioning. High doses of vitamin A are contraindicated in women who are or may become pregnant in the next three months. High doses of vitamin A and zinc should not be used for longer than two to six weeks. Some practitioners recommend 300,000 IU of vitamin A for three days, then 150,000 IU for three days. The World Health Organization recommends a similar protocol for treating measles in developing countries.
- Decrease sugar consumption. Sugar decreases lymphocyte and neutrophil activity.

HERBS
Herbs are generally a safe way to strengthen and tone the body's systems. As with any therapy, it is important to ascertain a diagnosis before pursuing treatment. Herbs may be used as dried extracts (capsules, powders, teas), glycerites (glycerine extracts), or tinctures (alcohol extracts). Unless otherwise indicated, teas should be made with 1 tsp. herb per cup of hot water. Steep covered 5 to 10 minutes for leaf or flowers, and 10 to 20 minutes for roots. Drink 2 to 4 cups/day. Tinctures may be used singly or in combination as noted.

- Coneflower *(Echinacea angustifolia)*—immune modulating
- Goldenseal *(Hydrastis canadensis)*—immune modulating, antimicrobial, bitter, astringent
- Licorice *(Glycyrrhiza glabra)*—antiviral, anticolic, soothing to mucous membranes
- Yarrow *(Achillea millefolium)*—antibacterial, astringent, antispas-

modic, especially with fever

- Elder *(Sambucus canadensis)*—diaphoretic, anticatarrhal, especially for lungs
- St. John's wort *(Hypericum perforatum)*—antiviral, pain relief, anti-depressant
- Mix a combination of coneflower and goldenseal with two to four of the other herbs listed. Drink 3 to 6 cups tea/day, or take 30 to 60 drops tincture three to six times/day.
- Garlic/ginger tea (2 to 3 cloves of garlic and 2 to 3 slices of fresh ginger) drunk as a tea keeps the lungs clear and acts as anti-microbial. May be used in addition to above herbs.

HOMEOPATHY

An experienced homeopath should assess individual constitutional types and severity of disease to select the correct remedy and potency. For acute prescribing use 3 to 5 pellets of a 12X to 30C remedy every one to four hours until acute symptoms resolve.

- Combination remedy of *Aconite, Gelsemium, Eucalyptus, Ipecacuanha, Phosphorus, Bryonia,* and *Eupatorium perfoliatum* (trade name Oscillococcinum) can be very effective.
- *Gelsemium* for influenza that leaves the patient weak and forgetful, especially with diarrhea
- *Eupatorium perfoliatum* for influenza with deep achiness, especially with sneezing and coughing
- *Nux vomica* for influenza with violent vomiting and irritability

ACUPUNCTURE

May be helpful at alleviating symptoms and speeding healing. Usually very helpful in decreasing length and severity of symptoms.

Patient Monitoring

Elderly patients, or those who have underlying renal insufficiency, seizure disorders, or psychosis, should be carefully monitored while on antiviral drugs, as there have been occasional cases of seizures, hallucinations, and delirium, particularly with high doses.

OTHER CONSIDERATIONS
Prevention

Each year a killed-virus vaccine is prepared based on expectations (based on antigenic and gene sequence changes) of the virus types that will be circulating that winter. The vaccines are 70% to 90% effective if administered before the flu season (December through March in the United States). Side effects have generally been minor, with the exception of an increased rate of Guillain-Barré syndrome accompanying the 1976 swine flu vaccination. Influenza viruses for the vaccines are grown in chick embryos, so the vaccines should not be administered to patients with chicken or egg allergies. Antibodies to a particular viral strain are long-lasting; however, the mutation rate is such that a new vaccination is advisable each year. Antiviral drugs may be administered to those for whom the vaccine is contraindicated, or who did not get immunized with enough time before an outbreak for antibodies to develop. They are 50% to 80% effective for prevention of type A influenza only.

Complications/Sequelae

The most common complication of influenza, occurring frequently in elderly patients and others with impaired immune systems, is bacterial pneumonia. This results from viral damage to the lungs' defenses, allowing proliferation of *Pneumococci, Staphylococci,* or *Haemophilus influenzae* bacteria. Occasionally, actual viral invasion of the alveoli may result in interstitial pneumonia, a serious disease with high mortality from lung hemorrhage and edema. Patients with underlying cardiac or pulmonary disease are at higher risk for this complication. Bronchitis and asthma may be exacerbated by influenza. Non-respiratory complications may include pericarditis, myocarditis, myositis, rhabdomyolysis, and Reye's syndrome (particularly in children). Following influenza, fatigue may be present for two weeks.

Prognosis

In uncomplicated influenza the symptoms generally last one to five days, but they can last up to two weeks.

Pregnancy

Studies suggest that pregnancy may increase the risk of serious influenza complications due to decreased lung capacity, increases in heart rate and oxygen consumption, and immunologic changes. The CDC has recommended vaccination for women who will be in the second or third trimester of pregnancy during the flu season. No adverse fetal effects are known.

REFERENCES

Baron S. *Medical Microbiology.* University of Texas Medical Branch; 1996:58. Available at http://129.109.112.248/microbook/ch058.htm.

Blumenthal M, ed. *The Complete German Commission E Monographs.* Boston, Mass: Integrative Medicine Communications; 1998:446.

Bräunig B, Dorn M, Knick E. *Echinacea purpurea radix* for strengthening the immune response in flu-like infections. *Z Phytotherapie.* 1992;13:7–13.

Dorn M. Mitigation of flu-like effects by means of a plant immunostimulant. *Natur und Ganzheitsmedizin.* 1989; 2:314–319.

Gruenwald J, Brendler T, Jaenicke C et al, eds. *PDR for Herbal Medicines.* Montvale, NJ: Medical Economics Company; 1998:604–605.

Hoffman D. *The New Holistic Herbal.* New York, NY: Barnes & Noble Books; 1995: 191.

Influenza. Centers for Disease Control and Prevention. Accessed at www.cdc.gov/nci-dod/diseases/flu/fluinfo.htm on February 13, 1999.

Kennedy M. Influenza viral infections: presentation, prevention and treatment. *Nurse Pract.* September 1998.

Kruzel T. *The Homeopathic Emergency Guide.* Berkeley, Calif: North Atlantic Books; 1992:190–196.

Murray MT, Pizzorno JE. *Encyclopedia of Natural Medicine.* Rocklin, Calif: Prima Publishing; 1998:66–68.

Ody P. *The Complete Medicinal Herbal.* New York, NY: DK Publishing; 1993.

Roettger B. Homeopathy as an effective treatment for colds and flus. *Nutrition Science News Magazine.* August 1995.

Savtsova ZD, Zalesskii VN, Orlovskii AA. The immunocorrective effect of laser reflexotherapy in experimental influenza infection [in Russian]. *Zh Mikrobiol Epidemiol Immunobiol.* January 1990:75–80.

Scaglione, et al. Efficacy and safety of the standardized ginseng extract G115 for potentiating vaccination against common cold and/or influenza syndrome. *Drugs Exp Clin Res.* 1996;22:65–72.

Tan D. Treatment of fever due to exopathic wind-cold by rapid acupuncture. *J Tradit Chin Med.* 1992;12:267–271.

Wagner H. Herbal immunostimulants for the prophylaxis and therapy of colds and influenza. *Eur J Herbal Med.* 1997;3(1).

■ INSECT BITES AND STINGS

OVERVIEW
Definition
Biting and stinging insects may cause allergic reactions. Stinging insects include apids (honeybees, bumblebees), vespids (yellow jackets, hornets, wasps), and formicids (fire and harvester ants). Biting insects include *Triatoma* (kissing bugs, conenose bugs), *Culicidae* (mosquitoes), *Tabanidae* (horseflies, deerflies), spiders (black widow, brown recluse), and others (bedbugs, black flies). There are more allergic reactions to stinging insects (0.4% to 4% of the United States population) than to biting insects. Approximately 40 stings each year are fatal.

Risk Factors
- Increased risk of systemic reaction if previous sting resulted in urticaria or airway obstruction
- Males—2:1 predominance
- Age—elderly (death more common) and children (for frequency of stings but not for fatal reactions)

Signs and Symptoms
Stinging insects:
- Large local reactions—pinprick sensation, red papule or wheal, site of bite is warm and tender, edema, possible ulceration or necrosis
- Systemic toxic reactions—shortness of breath, vomiting, diarrhea, fever, muscle spasms, dizziness, loss of consciousness
- Systemic reactions (anaphylaxis)—generalized urticaria, pruritus, erythema, angioedema (e.g., of lips or periorbital area), laryngoedema, asthma, abdominal cramps, diarrhea, hypotension secondary to anaphylactic shock, possible respiratory or cardiovascular failure

Biting insects:
- Urticarial or pruritic papules, pruritic wheals
- Arthus reaction and systemic symptoms; anaphylactic reactions (rare)
- Lesions, crusting, and infection from excoriation
- Myiasis (cutaneous, intestinal, or atrial larvae infestation)
- Systemic infections: Lyme disease, rocky mountain fever, plague, malaria, dengue fever, etc.

DIFFERENTIAL DIAGNOSIS
- Lyme disease
- Coronary and respiratory diseases
- Anaphylaxis from another source (e.g., insulin, latex, etc.)

DIAGNOSIS
Physical Examination
Check patient for papules or wheals that spread. Evaluate presence of a systemic reaction (e.g., difficulty breathing, nausea, diarrhea, fever, muscle spasms). Evaluate lesions for infection from scratching. Assess patients who have traveled to Central or South America/Africa for myiasis.

Laboratory Tests
- CBC. Sed Rate. Lyme titer.
- Skin tests (using Hymenoptera venoms) determine venom-specific immunoglobulin E (IgE) antibodies.
- Radioallergosorbent test (RAST) determines clinical sensitivity.
- Immunoglobulin G (IgG) levels—low venom-specific levels are associated with treatment failure in yellow jacket and mixed vespid immunotherapy.

Pathological Findings
Toxic reactions:
- Nonimmunologic

- Cutaneous reactions mediated by IgE or IgG antibodies
- Leukocyte histamine release

Systemic reactions:
- Endogenous vasoactive materials released as a result of allergen-IgE interaction with mast cell and basophil surfaces
- Elevated IgE in 80% of patients with positive skin tests

Other Diagnostic Procedures
- Systemic reactions only—pure venom skin test determines sensitivity but cannot discriminate local from systemic reactions.

TREATMENT OPTIONS
Treatment Strategy
Local reactions usually do not require treatment unless they are severe. Anaphylaxis is a medical emergency. For large local reactions (most resolve in three to seven days with no treatment):
- Remove stinger and cleanse wound.
- Apply ice pack or cool compresses.
- Apply paste of one tsp. meat tenderizer mixed with one tsp. water to stinger site.

For systemic reactions:
- Recline, elevating lower extremities.
- Venous tourniquet decreases systemic absorption.
- Maintain airway and give oxygen.

Drug Therapies
- Antihistamines and analgesics can be taken for pruritus and swelling.
- Topical steroids and systemic glucocorticoids are commonly used but with poor scientific evidence.
- Antibiotics if infection is suspected.

For systemic reactions:
- Aqueous epinephrine (1:1,000, 0.3 to 0.5 ml; 0.01 ml per kg for children)—repeat dosage every 15 to 20 minutes as necessary.
- Intravenous epinephrine (1:100,000) can be administered in an acute care facility for anaphylactic shock.
- Nebulized epinephrine can help alleviate upper-airway edema.
- Parenteral antihistamines (e.g., diphenhydramine hydrochloride [Benadryl], 5 mg per kg each 24 hours in divided doses) increase systemic vascular resistance, elevate diastolic pressure, decrease itching; higher doses for patients not responding to epinephrine.

Complementary and Alternative Therapies
High doses of bioflavonoids and vitamins may reduce severity and duration of reactions from insect bites as well as reducing recurrent reactions. Homeopathic remedies can provide relief.

NUTRITION
- B complex (50 to 100 mg/day), especially B_1 (50 to 100 mg one to two times/day) and B_{12} (1,000 mcg/day) can be used in prevention as a mosquito repellant.
- Vitamin C helps to stabilize mast cells and reduce histamine release. For severe reactions take 1,000 mg every two hours to bowel tolerance (i.e., loose stools) which may be over 10,000 mg/day. After acute episode, take 1,000 mg tid to qid.
- Bromelain (250 to 500 mg qid between meals) is a proteolytic enzyme that has anti-inflammatory effects. (also found in commercial meat tenderizer preparations). Combined with saliva and applied to the sting or bite they help to break down the proteins in the venom.

HERBS
Herbs are generally a safe way to strengthen and tone the body's systems.

Ascertain a diagnosis before pursuing treatment. Herbs may be used as dried extracts (capsules, powders, teas), glycerites (glycerine extracts), or tinctures (alcohol extracts). Unless otherwise indicated, teas should be made with 1 tsp. herb per cup of hot water. Steep covered 5 to 10 minutes for leaf or flowers, and 10 to 20 minutes for roots. Drink 2 to 4 cups/day. Tinctures may be used singly or in combination as noted.

- Licorice root *(Glycyrrhiza glabra)* supports the immune system and reduces inflammation. Take 500 to 1,000 mg every three to four hours during acute reaction; contraindicated in hypertension.
- Quercetin is a bioflavonoid that has powerful anti-inflammatory effects. Take 500 to 800mg bid for severe reactions. For mild to moderate reactions, take 500 mg qid. People with extreme sensitivities to onions may not tolerate quercetin.
- Turmeric *(Curcuma longa)* is an anti-inflammatory that potentiates the effects of bromelain. Take 250 to 500 mg qid with bromelain.
- Herbs that increase immune function, enhance peripheral and lymphatic circulation, and help to restore dermal integrity may be helpful in reducing the severity and duration of the allergic response. Combine equal parts of coneflower *(Echinacea purpura)*, cleavers *(Galium aparine)*, oat straw *(Avena sativa)*, red clover *(Trifolium pratense)*, elder *(Sambucus canadensis)*, and marigold *(Calendula officinalis)*. This is best used as a tea, 4 to 6 cups/day, to increase hydration. Tincture may be used as well (30 to 60 drops qid).
- Poultice of raw grated potato or plantain leaves *(Plantago major)* may soothe itching, relieve swelling, and enhance healing.
- Make a strong tea from peppermint *(Mentha piperita)* using 1 heaping tsp./cup. Place in spray bottle and chill. Spray on stings and bites to relieve itching.
- Witch hazel mixed with a few drops of lavender oil can be used as a cooling compress.
- Bug repellent herbs include lavender, citronella, eucalyptus, and pennyroyal. Mix 15 drops of each essential oil with 1 oz. of food-grade oil (e.g., almond or olive). May need frequent application, tid to qid.

HOMEOPATHY

An experienced homeopath should assess individual constitutional types and severity of disease to select the correct remedy and potency. For acute prescribing use 3 to 5 pellets of a 12X to 30C remedy every one to four hours until acute symptoms resolve.

- *Aconite* for acute swelling with anxiety and fear.
- *Apis mellifica* for stinging pains with rapid swelling that feels better with cold applications. Patient is fatigued and apathetic.
- *Belladonna* for rapid, intense swelling with redness and heat. Patient is thirstless and calm.
- *Ledum* for puncture wounds, especially with coldness surrounding injury.
- Topical homeopathic preparations containing *Ledum, Arnica, Calendula, Hypericum,* and/or *Urtica* may provide symptomatic relief. Do not apply over broken skin.

Patient Monitoring

Because biphasic anaphylactic episodes can occur, patients with significant hypotension or bronchospasm should be observed for 8 to 12 hours or admitted. Referral to an allergist is warranted with anaphylaxis.

OTHER CONSIDERATIONS
Prevention

- Venom immunotherapy for patients with systemic reactions reduces anaphylaxis risk to 1% to 2% if sting occurs during therapy; increase usual maintenance dose of 100 mcg to 200 mcg when treatment fails; risks include systemic reactions (observe patient for at least 20 minutes); treatment usually ends after three years (five years in severe cases) in spite of continued positive venom skin tests.
- Emergency insect stinging kits (EpiPen, Epi-EZ-Pen, Ana-Kit) have both epinephrine (1.6 to 4.8 mg) and antihistamines (e.g., diphenhydramine [Benadryl], 25 to 50 mg).
- Diethyltoluamide (deet) repels only biting insects; use concentration above 75%; toxic if ingested and may damage synthetic clothing.
- Citronella is an effective, nontoxic plant source; reapply frequently.
- Wear a Medic Alert bracelet if susceptible to systemic reactions.
- Keep bites clean, refrain from scratching to prevent secondary infection.
- Do not use scented hair oils or perfumes.
- Wear shoes and long pants, and no floral-patterned or dark clothing.

Complications/Sequelae

- Secondary infection from scratching and poor hygiene
- Excessive epinephrine—can cause hypertension and arrhythmia, especially with coexisting heart disease
- Reaction to venom immunotherapy (12% of patients)
- Encephalitis, vasculitis, renal failure, nephrotic syndrome
- Multiple stings can cause systemic toxic reaction in nonallergic patients and may be fatal.
- Biting insects may transfer disease (e.g., mosquitoes/malaria).

Prognosis

- 50% of patients have recurrent allergic reactions.
- Immunologic tests cannot predict subsequent urticarial reactions.
- Spontaneous remission is highest in children under age 16.

Pregnancy

Large doses of vitamins and bioflavonoids are contraindicated in pregnancy. Small doses of vitamin C (500 to 1000 mg tid) may provide relief. Topical preparations, excluding essential oils, are safe.

REFERENCES

Habif TP. *Clinical Dermatology.* 3rd ed. St. Louis, Mo: Mosby-Year Book; 1996.
Kruzel T. *The Homeopathic Emergency Guide.* Berkeley, Calif: North Atlantic Books; 1992:198–200.
Middleton E, ed. *Allergy: Principles and Practice.* 5th ed. St. Louis, Mo: Mosby-Year Book; 1998.
Rakel RE, ed. *Conn's Current Therapy.* 50th ed. Philadelphia, Pa: WB Saunders; 1998.

■ INSOMNIA

OVERVIEW
Definition
Insomnia is a disorder or a symptom of another condition, not a disease. It is the persistent inability or difficulty with falling or staying asleep. It frequently impairs daytime functioning. At some time during the year, approximately one-third of adults suffer from some form of insomnia.

Etiology
Insomnia may have distinct underlying physical and/or mental causes, or it may have no discernable cause. In idiopathic insomnia (up to 50% of all insomnia cases), the patient's polysomnogram is usually normal. Transient situational insomnia is caused by work or school stress or family illness. Other causes of insomnia include the following:

- Substance abuse—caffeine, alcohol, recreational drugs, long-term sedative use, stimulants, decongestants, bronchodilators
- Disruption of circadian rhythms—shift work/travel across time zones
- Menopause—prevalent in 30% to 40% of menopausal women
- Elderly—normal decrease in depth, length, continuity of sleep
- Medical illness—gastro-esophageal reflux disease (GERD), fibromyalgia, hyperthyroidism, dementia, arthritis, and other painful conditions

Risk Factors
- Age—elderly are more affected
- Night-time occupation
- Travel crossing time zones
- Substance abuse, including caffeine
- Asthmatics—use of bronchodilators

Signs and Symptoms
- Impaired sleep onset
- Impaired sleep maintenance (e.g., frequent waking)
- Early-morning waking
- Subjective sense of unsatisfying sleep
- Daytime drowsiness and impaired functioning
- Anticipatory anxiety

DIFFERENTIAL DIAGNOSIS
- Psychiatric—character disorder, depression, anxiety, psychosis
- Medical causes—thyroid disorders, gastric and peptic ulcers, chronic pain, cardiopulmonary dysfunction, urinary frequency, Parkinson's disease, and dementia
- Sleep apnea syndrome
- Narcolepsy
- Nocturnal myoclonus

DIAGNOSIS
Physical Examination
Surgical and medical history and physical examination are essential diagnostic tools, as the patient may not appear tired.

Laboratory Tests
Tests rule out differential diagnosis or underlying causes (e.g., toxic screen test for substance abuse, thyroid-stimulating hormone test for hyperthyroidism).

Pathological Findings
- Rapid-eye-movement (REM) sleep and non-rapid-eye-movement (NREM) sleep changes from its normal pattern in people with sleep disorders but rarely for those with idiopathic insomnia.

Other Diagnostic Procedures
Polysomnogram can determine biologic causes; includes electroencephalogram, electrocardiogram, respiration, electro-oculogram (eye movement), electromyogram (muscle tone), and blood oxygen saturation.

TREATMENT OPTIONS
Treatment Strategy
Identify initiating stressor(s), rule out underlying illnesses, and develop a strategy to help the patient cope with and alleviate the symptoms. Comorbidity must be determined and treated first to avoid inaccurate or even harmful treatment (e.g., benzodiazepine for a patient with sleep apnea). Also recommend:

- Maintain good sleep hygiene.
- Keep a regular sleep/wake schedule.
- Exercise early in the day, not in the evening.
- Do not nap. However, some people who become overtired may actually sleep better if they take a nap.
- Set up optimal conditions for sleep and have relaxing bedtime rituals.

Drug Therapies
For idiopathic insomnia:

- Pharmacologic—sedative hypnotic compounds reduce sleep latency and increase continuity.
- Benzodiazepine (BZD) class (triazolam .125 mg/day, clonazepam 0.5 mg/day, or flurazepam 15 mg/day with anxiety); use lowest dose with elderly; side effects—daytime sleepiness, ataxia, addiction; do not use with alcohol or for sleep apnea; withdraw slowly.
- Tricyclic antidepressants (Elavil)—amitriptyline (10 to 100 mg at bedtime)

Complementary and Alternative Therapies
Herbs may be effective for treating both short term and chronic insomnia. Nutrition can be an important adjunctive treatment. Mind/body treatments, such as yoga, psychotherapy, and relaxation methods may be helpful.

NUTRITION
- Calcium/magnesium: regulate relaxation, especially with muscle tension and physical restlessness, 500/250 Ca/Mg bid
- B-complex: B vitamins are depleted under stress: they may be stimulating in certain individuals, so take in the morning.
- 5-HTP is a form of tryptophan now available which is particularly helpful for difficulty staying asleep. 5-HTP increases seratonin levels. Dose is 50 mg before bed. 5-HTP will help within one week if it will be helpful at all. Dietary sources of tryptophan include turkey, eggs, fish, dairy products, bananas, and walnuts. (Tryptophan as a supplement was removed from the market after a contaminant caused severe side effects.)
- Melatonin: manufactured in the pineal gland, from tryptophan, is responsible for appropriate circadian rhythms and is used to prevent jet lag. Dose is 1 to 3 mg before bed. Note that a lower dose may be effective when a higher dose is not.
- Niacinamide: muscle relaxant, gentle tranquilizing effects. Dose is 70 to 280 mg/day, either in divided doses during the day (anxiolytic), or at bed time.

HERBS
Herbs are generally a safe way to strengthen and tone the body's systems. As with any therapy, it is important to ascertain a diagnosis before pursuing treatment. Herbs may be used as dried extracts (capsules, powders, teas), glycerites (glycerine extracts), or tinctures (alcohol extracts). Unless otherwise indicated, teas should be made with 1 tsp. herb per cup of hot

water. Steep covered 5 to 10 minutes for leaf or flowers, and 10 to 20 minutes for roots. Drink 2 to 4 cups/day. Tinctures may be used singly or in combination as noted. The herbs are listed in order of increasing strength; use the gentlest herb that is effective.

- Chamomile *(Chamomilla recutita):* mild sedative, calms gastric upset. One cup of chamomile tea before bed is often all that is needed for mild insomnia. In a few patients, chamomile may cause gastric upset.
- Lemon balm *(Melissa officinalis)* alone, or in combination with catnip *(Nepeta cataria):* nervous sleeping disorders and mild digestive complaints; one cup tea or 30 to 60 drops tincture one to three times a day.
- Passionflower *(Passiflora incarnata):* the aerial parts of passionflower are a very effective herbal remedy for insomnia taken 2 to 4 ml one half hour before bedtime.
- Valerian *(Valeriana officinalis):* sedative, anodyne, bitter. Side effects of too high a dose may be nausea and/or grogginess. Traditionally used in combination with passionflower and hops *(Lupuli strobulus)* for treatment of acute stress. Persons with depression should avoid hops. Dose is equal parts herb at 1 cup one to three times a day, or tincture 30 to 60 drops one to three times a day.
- Kava kava *(Piper methisticum):* spasmolytic, anxiolytic, sedative; very effective for short term management of stress and insomnia. Should not be used for more than three months without medical supervision. Dose is 15 to 30 drops ($^1/_2$ to 1 ml) tincture one to three times a day, or $^1/_4$ to $^1/_2$ ml of concentrated liquid extract three times a day.
- St. John's wort *(Hypericum perforatum):* for insomnia with anxious depression; dose is 15 to 60 drops ($^1/_2$ to 2 ml) tid, or 250 mg tid of herb or herb extract for depression. Side effects may include skin rash, photosensitivity, and gastric upset. It may take four to six weeks to become effective.
- Jamaican dogwood *(Piscidia piscipula):* Jamaican dogwood is a powerful remedy for insomnia, particularly when the sleeplessness is due to nervous tension and pain. Taken 1 to 2 ml just before bedtime, Jamaican dogwood is arguably the strongest herbal anodyne for sleeplessness. Jamaican dogwood combines well with passionflower, valerian, kava, and St. John's wort.
- Essential oils (three to five drops added to a bath) may be effective as part of a bedtime ritual. Commonly used herbs are lavender *(Lavendula officinalis),* rosemary *(Rosemarinus officinalis),* and chamomile *(Chamomilla recutita).*

HOMEOPATHY

An experienced homeopath should assess individual constitutional types and severity of disease to select the correct remedy and potency. For acute prescribing use 3 to 5 pellets of a 12X to 30C remedy every one to four hours until acute symptoms resolve.

- *Arsenicum alba* for insomnia caused by anxiety (especially about their health), especially in perfectionists who develop panic attacks
- *Nux vomica* for insomnia from over use of stimulants, caffeine, drugs or tobacco, especially in competitive, aggressive people
- *Coffea cruda* for insomnia from a racing mind, especially if the stress is adjusting to a positive event.
- *Ignatia imara* for insomnia (or excessive sleeping) after grief

ACUPUNCTURE

May be effective at treating both insomnia and some of its underlying causes.

MASSAGE

May be beneficial for its systemic relaxing properties.

Patient Monitoring

Chronic insomnia and exhaustion increases risks for accidents and the likelihood of comorbid conditions.

OTHER CONSIDERATIONS

Prevention

Establishing good sleep habits is the best method to avoid insomnia when there is no comorbidity or complicating factors. A healthy diet and regular exercise also help to prevent insomnia and alleviate stress. Alcohol disrupts the quality of sleep and regular use before bed should be avoided.

Complications/Sequelae

- BZDs can cause oversedation if used for substance abuse or sleep apnea patients.
- Elderly patients need special attention with insomnia treatment. Education about the need for less sleep is important. Pain medication needs to be adequate to permit good sleep. However, caution in not oversedating is important to avoid falls and other complications.

Prognosis

Without comorbidity, or with successful treatment of comorbid condition, most patients recover within a few weeks or after the stressful event has been resolved. Chronic insomnia with sedative dependence can take years to overcome.

Pregnancy

Insomnia usually occurs in the later months of pregnancy when the mother's size and need to urinate disrupt sleep. The best treatment is naps during the day.

REFERENCES

Blumenthal M, ed. *The Complete German Commission E Monographs.* Boston, Mass: Integrative Medicine Communications; 1998:422, 431.

Bravo SQ, et al. Polysomnographic and subjective findings in insomniacs under treatment with placebo and valerian extract (LI 156). Proceedings of the Second International Congress on Phytomedicine, Munich. *Eur J Clin Pharmacol.* 1996;50:552.

DreBring H. Insomnia: Are valerian/balm combinations of equal value to Benzodiazepine? *Therapiewoche.* 1992;42:726.

Emser W. Phytotherapy of insomnia—a critical overview. *Pharmacopsychiatry.* 1993;26:150.

Fauci AS, Braunwald E, Isselbacher KJ et al, eds. *Harrison's Principles of Internal Medicine.* 14th ed. New York, NY: McGraw-Hill; 1998.

Goroll, Allan H, ed. *Primary Care Medicine.* 3rd ed. Philadelphia, Pa: Lippincott-Raven; 1995.

Rakel RE, ed. *Conn's Current Therapy.* 50th ed. Philadelphia, Pa: WB Saunders; 1998.

■ INTESTINAL PARASITES

OVERVIEW
Definition
The two major classes of intestinal parasites are helminths and protozoa. Helminths are multicellular worms (with the exceptions of *Strongyloides* and *Hymenolepis nana*) with complex life cycles. Helminths cannot multiply in the host and will eventually clear up without reinfection. Protozoa are single-cell organisms capable of multiplying within the host. There is usually a direct fecal–oral transmission, with direct person-to-person transmission uncommon. Intestinal parasites affect 5% to 30% of the U.S. population, dependent on geographic and socioeconomic factors. Less than 10% of parasitologic reports routinely identify helminths.

Etiology
- Helminth pathogens include cestodes (tapeworms), trematodes (flukes), hookworms, and various nematodes (roundworms).
- Protozoan pathogens include *Entamoeba histolytica* (amebiasis), *Giardia lamblia* (giardiasis), *Cryptosporidium, Isospora belli, Enterocytozoon bieneusi* (microsporidiosis), and free-living amebas and blood/tissue protozoa (e.g., *Plasmodium* [malaria]).

Risk Factors
- Demographics—endemic areas
- International travel
- Poor sanitation (food and water)
- Poor personal hygiene
- Age—children at a higher risk
- Child and institutional care facilities
- Acquired immunodeficiency syndrome (AIDS)

Signs and Symptoms
Symptoms vary depending upon the intestinal parasite and may include the following.
- Malodorous diarrhea
- Midepigastric pain/tenderness
- Nausea/vomiting
- Fatigue
- Gas/bloating
- Weight loss
- Dysentery (e.g., amebiasis)
- Passing a worm
- Perirectal or vulvar rash/pruritus

DIFFERENTIAL DIAGNOSIS
- Food poisoning/bacterial
- Pyogenic abscesses diarrhea (e.g., *E. coli*)
- Typhoid
- Inflammatory bowel disease
- Hemorrhoids
- Peptic ulcer
- Influenza

DIAGNOSIS
Physical Examination
The patient may appear anorexic. There may be abdominal bloating and/or tenderness to palpation. Increased bowel sounds are often present with auscultation. Perirectal or vulvar rash or rectal prolapse may be visible.

Laboratory Tests
Tests for some intestinal parasites should be based on an assessment of the risk profile for the patient.
- Fecal testing—identifies ova, larvae, or adult helminths and trophozoites or cysts of protozoa. Collect sample before use of anti-diarrheal agents, antibiotics, or barium for X ray to avoid detection problems. Prompt examination or use of preservative is necessary; three (five for pinworm) samples required for accurate detection. Complete exam includes use of wet mounts, permanent stains (for laboratory's records), and concentration techniques.
- Serological testing—reliable tests available for only a few parasitic diseases (e.g. ameba).
- Eosinophilia—associated with degree of mucosal invasion
- Biopsy of tissue to detect helminths in tissue or parasites in mucosa

Pathological Findings
- Gross or occult blood with amebic colitis
- Ulceration and inflammation of bowel, rarely a lesion
- Trophozoites invade tissue, most parasites do not

Imaging
Rarely required for diagnosis. X ray with barium, ultrasound, or CT are sometimes used to diagnose amebomas, liver abscesses, and colitis.

Other Diagnostic Procedures
- String test—samples duodenal contents (e.g., for *Giardia lamblia, Cryptosporidium, Strongyloides*), rarely used
- "Scotch tape" test—identifies pinworm ova on perianal skin.
- Sigmoidoscopy—may show muco-purulent colitis and ulceration.
- Endoscopy of upper intestinal tract—can extract fluid or tissue for biopsy, impression smear, and microscopic examination; usually for *Giardia lamblia* and *Strongyloides*

TREATMENT OPTIONS
Treatment Strategy
Medication, diet, and patient education for personal hygiene and to avoid reinfection. Some of the most effective drugs with the least side effects are not available in this country (e.g., Tinidazole for giardia or amebiasis) or are available only from the Centers for Disease Control (e.g., Ivermectin for various nematodes).

Drug Therapies
Symptomatic treatment—initiate after drug therapy has begun. Drug therapy for helminths, selected examples (adult dosages):
- Albendazole—for various roundworms and tapeworms; 400 mg once, three days in severe cases; for pinworms repeat dose after two weeks. Used with glucocorticoids for neurocysticercosis (prevents complications from dying cysticerci) 15 mg/kg/day in three doses, 8 to 28 days.
- Mebendazole—for various roundworms; 100 mg bid for three days, longer periods for echinococcosis (tapeworm). Mild side effects (e.g., diarrhea) except with long administration.
- Pyrantel pamoate—for various roundworms; 11 mg/kg of body weight up to one g, once, but several times for hookworm. Available over-the-counter for pinworms; is well-tolerated.
- Praziquantel—for most flukes and tapeworms; 40 mg/kg/day in 2 doses once, to 75 mg/kg/day in 3 doses for 2 days. Mild side effects—headache, dizziness, nausea, abdominal pain. Use with glucocorticoids for neurocysticercosis; 50 mg/kg/day in 3 doses for 15 days.

Drug therapy for protozoa, selected examples (adult dosages):

- Metronidazole (Flagyl)—250 mg tid for five days commonly used for giardia, but not FDA approved for this use; use for *B. hominis* concurrently eradicates giardia. Use 750 mg tid for 10 days for liver abscesses and cysts of *E. histolytica,* follow with iodoquinol for severe amebiasis and abscesses, *B. coli, Trichomonas vaginalis;* avoid all alcohol, disulfiram-like reaction can occur. Side effects—nausea, metallic taste, dry mouth, headache, and rarely encephalopathy, pancreatitis, ataxia, seizures, and peripheral neuropathy.
- Trimethoprim/sulfamethoxazole—for *Isospora belli;* 160/800 mg qid for 10 days, then bid for three weeks. Side effects—self-limited diarrhea (severe with AIDS), possible liver, skin, or bone marrow toxicity from sulfamethoxazole.
- Chloroquine—oral therapy for malaria; 600 mg base then 300 mg base at 6, 24, and 48 hours.

Complementary and Alternative Therapies
Identification of the organism is imperative before initiating any therapy. The following nutritional guidelines will help to inhibit organism growth. Many of the herbs suggested have toxic side effects and should only be used under the supervision of a qualified practitioner. It is important to maintain good bowel elimination during treatment.

NUTRITION
- Avoid simple carbohydrates such as refined foods, fruits, juices, dairy products (contain lactose sugar), and all sugars.
- Eliminate caffeine and alcohol.
- Increase intake of raw garlic, pumpkin seeds, pomegranates, beets, and carrots, all of which have vermifuge properties. Ensure adequate intake of water and dietary fiber to promote good bowel elimination.
- Digestive enzymes will help to normalize digestion and restore the local environment to its normal state which is inhospitable to parasites. Papain taken 30 minutes before and after meals helps to kill worms. Acidophilus supplements will help normalize bowel flora.
- Vitamin C (1,000 mg tid to qid), zinc (20 to 30 mg/day), and beta carotene (100,000 IU/day) support the immune system.

HERBS
Ascertain a diagnosis before pursuing treatment. Herbs may be used as dried extracts (capsules, powders, teas), glycerites (glycerine extracts), or tinctures (alcohol extracts). Unless otherwise indicated, teas should be made with 1 tsp. herb per cup of hot water. Steep covered 5 to 10 minutes for leaf or flowers, and 10 to 20 minutes for roots. Drink 2 to 4 cups/day. Tinctures may be used singly or in combination as noted.

The following herbs are listed according to increasing strength and toxicity. Use only under the supervision of a qualified practitioner. The most gentle herb that is effective should be used for treatment.

Vermifuges include the following.
- Garlic *(Allium sativum)* 1 clove tid.
- Thyme *(Thymus vulgaris)* or oregano *(Oreganum vulgare)* oil, 1 to 2 enteric-coated capsules tid to qid.
- Wormwood *(Artemisia absinthum)* may be used as a tea (3 cups/day) or tincture (1 to 2 tsp. tid).
- Quassia *(Picrasma excelsor)* is specifically for threadworms. Prepare a cold infusion tea (1 heaping tbsp. soaked in 1 qt. of water overnight) and drink throughout the day.
- Black walnut *(Juglans nigra)* may be used as a tea (3 cups/day) or tincture (30 drops tid to qid).

- Male fern *(Dryopteris filix-mas)* is specific for tapeworm. Large doses are extremely poisonous and may induce toxic liver damage.
- Tansy *(Tanacetum vulgare)* may be used in combination with wormwood for treatment of roundworm and threadworm. Drink 1 cup of tea one to two times/day, or use tincture at 30 to 60 drops bid to tid. Large doses of this herb can be highly toxic.

Anti-parasitic herbs include the following. Use together in a tea (1 cup tid) or tincture (30 to 60 drops tid).
- Barberry *(Berberis vulgaris)*
- Oregon grape *(Berberis aquafolium)*
- Goldenseal *(Hydrastis canadensis)*
- Wormseed *(Chenopodium ambrosoides)*

Topical applications for roundworm include oils of garlic (use with a carrier oil such as olive oil to avoid skin irritation), thyme, or lavender.

HOMEOPATHY
An experienced homeopath should assess individual constitutional types and severity of disease to select the correct remedy and potency. For acute prescribing use 3 to 5 pellets of a 12X to 30C remedy every one to four hours until acute symptoms resolve.
Cina is specific for pinworms; with restless agitation and itching rectum
Rumex crispus for marked itching immediately on uncovering or undressing
Spigellia for worm infestations with piercing and sharp pains

MASSAGE
May help stimulate bowel function and elimination.

Patient Monitoring
The patient must receive adequate hydration and diet. Patient education prevents transmission or reinfection. Retesting must take into account the lifecycle of the parasite (usually three to four weeks for protozoa and five to six weeks for helminth) and the likelihood of reinfection.

OTHER CONSIDERATIONS
Prevention
The best prevention is good community sanitation and personal hygiene.

Complications/Sequelae
Complications occur more frequently in the elderly, AIDS patients, or immunocompromised patients. Complications involving the central nervous system may be severe.

Prognosis
The course and prognosis vary with the specific intestinal parasite.

Pregnancy
Treatment for intestinal parasites during pregnancy should be closely followed by a qualified practitioner.

REFERENCES
Fauci AS, Braunwald E, Isselbacher KJ et al, eds. *Harrison's Principles of Internal Medicine.* 14th ed. New York, NY: McGraw-Hill; 1998.
Morrison R. *Desktop Guide to Keynotes and Confirmatory Symptoms.* Albany, Calif: Hahnemann Clinic Publishing; 1993:128, 329, 353.
Rakel RE, ed. *Conn's Current Therapy.* 50th ed. Philadelphia, Pa: WB Saunders; 1998.

■ IRRITABLE BOWEL SYNDROME

OVERVIEW

Definition

Irritable bowel syndrome presents itself as a variety of lower abdominal symptoms, including pain, cramping, gassiness, and either or both diarrhea and constipation. Symptoms often appear after eating or during stress and result from abnormal motility. Because the gastrointestinal tract is particularly sensitive to stimuli, the effect of stress, diet, drugs, hormones, and minor irritants can aggravate its tendency to contract abnormally.

The syndrome generally takes two forms. Spastic colon, often triggered by eating a meal, produces periods of constipation, diarrhea, or both, along with abdominal pain. Painless diarrhea comes on urgently, generally during or after a meal, or on waking after a night's sleep.

IBS often starts in young adulthood. Between 10% and 20% of the population has symptoms of the syndrome at some time. It accounts for half of all gastrointestinal referrals, and is a major cause of lost work or school time. It affects twice as many women as men. Some women show more symptoms during menstruation.

Etiology

No underlying anatomic or definitive etiologic cause has emerged. The symptoms result from abnormal motility, and the contractions become disorganized, harsh, or spasmodic. The erratic propulsion that results can cause sudden, explosive elimination of stools, or can delay any elimination. Chronic stress or depression often trigger attacks. Eating in general can cause immediate need for a bowel movement. Specific foods such as high-fat meals, wheat, dairy products, and citrus fruits, as well as drinks containing caffeine or alcohol, can aggravate the condition.

Risk Factors

- Stress
- Depression
- In some cases, eating specific foods, including wheat, dairy products, or citrus fruits
- In some cases, alcohol or caffeine
- Familial predisposition

Signs and Symptoms

- Crampy pain in the lower abdomen
- Bloating
- Gassiness
- Changes in bowel habits
- Diarrhea or constipation, or both alternately
- Need for bowel movement immediately on waking or after eating
- Relief of pain after bowel movement
- Feeling of incomplete emptying after bowel movement
- Mucus in feces

DIFFERENTIAL DIAGNOSIS

- Inflammatory bowel diseases (ulcerative colitis or Crohn's disease)
- Diverticulosis
- Duodenal ulcer
- Lactose intolerance
- Biliary tract disease
- Abuse of cathartics
- Amebiasis, giardiasis, or other parasitic disease
- *Campylobacter* enteritis
- Allergic gastroenteropathy
- Colonic polyps
- Colonic neoplasms
- Ischemic enteropathy (in patients over age 60)
- Ovarian neoplasms and cysts
- Uterine fibroids
- Hyperthyroidism
- Infections
- Diabetes mellitus

DIAGNOSIS

Physical Examination

Patients with either form of IBS usually appear in good health. Palpation of the abdomen may show tenderness. Rectal examination often indicates a rectum that is empty or contains hard, firm feces. A pelvic examination of women serves to eliminate alternative diagnoses.

Laboratory Tests

- A stool sample—preferably a three-day slide series—can reveal the presence of blood, ova, parasites or bacteria.
- Biochemical profiling, including serum amylase, and urinalysis, also serves to narrow the diagnosis—ESR, CBC.

Imaging

Abdominal ultrasound, a barium enema X ray, X rays of the small bowel or the upper gastrointestinal tract, and colonoscopy can also help to rule out organic causes of IBS-like symptoms

Other Diagnostic Procedures

Sigmoidoscopy, particularly with a flexible instrument, shows the state of the colon up to 60 centimeters, the area in which 65% to 70% of colonic neoplasms and polyps are found. In cases of IBS, this procedure often triggers spasm and pain, but shows no abnormalities.

TREATMENT OPTIONS

Treatment Strategy

Sympathetic understanding plays a major role in treatment. Explain the nature of the condition, and assure the patient that he or she has no major underlying organic disease. Outline the extreme sensitivity of the patient's bowels to stimuli such as stress, food, drugs, and hormones. Remember that no two IBS patients are alike. Encourage patients to avoid, wherever possible, stressful situations that may trigger episodes of IBS.

Drug Therapies

- Oral doses of antispasmodic agents such as hyoscyamine (Anaspaz, Cytospaz, Levsin) or dicyclomine (Bentyl, Bemote, Di-Spaz) can reduce the pain of spasm. They should be taken 30 to 60 minutes before meals. Oral doses of amitriptyline, taken 30 to 60 minutes before meals, reduce depression and bowel spasms.
- Bulk-producing agents (psyllium, as in Metamucil) or antiflatulents (simethicone, as in Mylicon) as symptoms indicate
- Lactose capsules for lactose intolerance, as indicated
- Patients with diarrhea should take loperamide (as in Imodium) before meals, as needed.

Complementary and Alternative Therapies

Irritable bowel syndrome is a multi-factoral condition that can often be successfully treated with alternative therapies. Most important are proper eating habits, stress reduction, and gastrointestinal support. Incorporating nutritional supplements may help reduce the effects of stress. Intestinal support can include fiber, acidophilus, peppermint oil capsules, or a tea of fennel or ginger. Chronic IBS may also respond to digestive enzymes and a supportive tincture. Stress reduction techniques through biofeedback, hypnosis, or counseling can help patients to deal with stress.

NUTRITION

- Removal of known food allergens or food irritants is imperative. The most common food allergens are dairy, wheat, corn, peanuts, citrus, soy, eggs, fish, and tomatoes. An elimination/challenge trial may be helpful in uncovering sensitivities. Remove all suspected allergens from the diet for two weeks. Add in one food every three days and wait for reaction which may include digestive upset, headache, fatigue, flushing, or worsening of symptoms.
- Fiber supplementation helps reduce abdominal pain, cramping, and gas. Supplements include psyllium, flax meal, slippery elm (*Ulmus rubra*) powder, marshmallow root (*Althea officinalis*) powder.
- Digestive enzymes taken 20 minutes before meals can help enhance digestion and normalize bowel function.
- One teaspoon of raw bran with each meal, supplemented by extra fluids, provides fiber reliably.
- Pro-flora supplements such as acidophilus and lactobacillus species taken bid to tid can help to re-balance normal bowel flora and reduce gas and bloating.
- Magnesium 200 mg bid to tid and B-complex (50 to 100 mg/day) with extra B$_5$ (pantothenic acid; 100 mg/day) may help to reduce the effects of stress.
- Low-fat diets may relieve abdominal pain following meals. Patients with spasm and constipation often benefit from dietary fiber supplementation.

HERBS

Ascertain a diagnosis before pursuing treatment. Herbs may be used as dried extracts (capsules, powders, teas), glycerites (glycerine extracts), or tinctures (alcohol extracts). Unless otherwise indicated, teas should be made with 1 teaspoon herb per cup of hot water. Steep covered 5 to 10 minutes for leaf or flowers, and 10 to 20 minutes for roots. Drink 2 to 4 cups/day. Tinctures may be used singly or in combination as noted.

- Enteric-coated peppermint oil (*Mentha piperita*): one to two capsules (0.2 ml peppermint oil/capsule) tid after meals. Peppermint oil is a potent spasmolytic that reduces bowel irritability.
- A tea of fennel seed (*Foeniculum vulgare*) or ginger root (*Zingiber officinalis*) taken after meals promotes elimination of intestinal gas and good digestion.
- A tincture of equal parts of the following herbs may be taken before meals (30 drops tid): Valerian (*Valeriana officinalis*), passionflower (*Passiflora incarnata*), anise seed (*Pimpinella anisum*) extract, meadowsweet (*Filependula ulmaria*), wild yam (*Dioscorea villosa*), and milk thistle (*Silybum marianum*). Combined, they enhance digestion, relieve spasm, and reduce inflammation.

HOMEOPATHY

An experienced homeopath should assess individual constitutional types and severity of disease to select the correct remedy and potency.

PHYSICAL MEDICINE

- Electric heating pads, hot water bottles, and long hot baths can relieve painful spasms and cramping in the abdomen.
- Regular exercise, such as walking, can reduce stress, and encourages bowel movements in constipated individuals.
- Castor oil pack. Used externally, castor oil is a powerful anti-inflammatory. Apply oil directly to skin, cover with a clean soft cloth (e.g., flannel) and plastic wrap. Place a heat source (hot water bottle or heating pad) over the pack and let sit for 30 to 60 minutes. For best results, use for three consecutive days.
- Abdominal breathing helps to induce the relaxation response and may aid normal physiological functioning (e.g., digestion). Chewing food thoroughly enhances digestion. Enzyme release begins in the mouth.

ACUPUNCTURE

Acupuncture can be useful in reducing frequency and duration of IBS episodes as well as providing overall support to gastrointestinal function.

MASSAGE

Therapeutic massage may be beneficial in reducing the effects of stress and increasing the overall sense of well-being.

Patient Monitoring

Insist on regular follow-up visits, to ensure that symptoms remain under control, and to detect any possible organic diseases of the gastrointestinal tract. Make patients aware that they may suffer episodes of abdominal symptoms related to psychologic stress and depression.

OTHER CONSIDERATIONS
Prevention

Best to develop pattern of regular exercise, to reduce stress and aid GI motility. A diet generally higher in fiber and lower in fat.

Complications/Sequelae

Depression or anxiety associated with unresolved symptoms.

Prognosis

Recurrences throughout life, particularly at times of high stress or relaxed preventative measures.

Pregnancy

Pregnancy may exacerbate symptoms of IBS. Treatment must be supervised by an experienced practitioner.

REFERENCES
Berkow R, ed. *Merck Manual of Diagnosis and Therapy.* 16th ed. Rahway, NJ: The Merck Publishing Group; 1992.

Dambro MR. *Griffith's Five-Minute Clinical Consult.* New York, NY: Lippincott, Williams and Wilkins; 1998.

Koch TR. Peppermint oil and irritable bowel syndrome [In Process Citation]. *Am J Gastroenterol.* 1998;93:2304–2305.

Liu JH, Chen GH, Yeh HZ, Huang CK, Poon SK. Enteric-coated peppermint-oil capsules in the treatment of irritable bowel syndrome: a prospective, randomized trial. *J Gastroenterol.* 1997;32:765–768.

Murray MT, Pizzorno JE. *Encyclopedia of Natural Medicine.* Rocklin, Calif: Prima Publishing; 1998:396–400.

Pittler MH, Ernst E. Peppermint oil for irritable bowel syndrome: a critical review and metaanalysis. *Am J Gastroenterol.* 1998;93:1131–1135.

■ LARYNGITIS

OVERVIEW

Definition

Laryngitis is an irritation and swelling of the larynx and the surrounding area. It can cause a patient's voice to become hoarse, and possibly to disappear altogether. The condition can take both acute and chronic forms, although the symptoms and treatment are often the same for both types. Acute laryngitis is most common in late fall, winter, and early spring. In general, it resolves within one or two weeks, with or without treatment. The chronic form is often associated with external factors such as smoking and regular exposure to industrial fumes and other allergens. The most common cause in pediatric cases is acute infection, whereas laryngitis in adults tends to have a chronic, non-infectious cause.

Etiology

Both acute and chronic laryngitis are usually caused by a viral infection—influenza A, B, parainfluenza, adenovirus, rhinovirus. They can occasionally result from a bacterial infection—*Streptococcus*. Excessive use of the voice, esophageal reflux, irritations, trauma, allergies to inhaled substances, and autoimmune reactions can also lead to the condition. Laryngitis often accompanies colds, and also appears during the course of a variety of other ailments, including bronchitis, pneumonia, influenza, pertussis, measles, and diphtheria.

Risk Factors

- Presence of upper respiratory tract infection
- Chronic bronchitis, rhinitus, sinusitis
- Smoking
- Allergy to and exposure to pollen, dust, and allergens in the workplace
- Alcoholism, or excessive drinking
- Overuse or abuse of voice

Signs and Symptoms

- Unnatural change in the voice
- Hoarseness
- Aphonia
- Tickling, scratchiness, and rawness in the throat
- A constant urge to clear the throat
- Fever, malaise, dysphagia may occur in more severe cases
- Difficulty breathing if the larynx is swollen
- Inflammation of the larynx's lining

DIFFERENTIAL DIAGNOSIS

- Gastroesophageal reflux disease
- Diphtheria
- Laryngeal cancer
- Throat cancer
- Vocal chord polyps
- Vocal chord nodules
- Croup
- Thyroid disease

DIAGNOSIS

Physical Examination

Examination of the throat may or may not reveal redness, suggesting the possibility of strep throat. Indirect examination of the larynx may reveal a mild to marked swelling of the organ's mucous membrane. This examination can help to differentiate between laryngitis and diphtheria.

Laboratory Tests

A throat culture will indicate the presence of strep throat or other bacterial infection.

Other Diagnostic Procedures

- Ask patient to describe symptoms completely
- Evaluate the throat and larynx by examination. Fiberoptic or indirect laryngoscopy
- Virus or bacterial culture

TREATMENT OPTIONS

Treatment Strategy

If a bacterial infection has caused the laryngitis, appropriate antibiotics should be prescribed. Laryngitis that results from viral causes has no specific treatment. It can benefit from any one of a variety of relatively unaggressive methodologies, depending on the extent of the condition. Treatment of accompanying acute or chronic bronchitis can improve the laryngitis.

Advise patients to rest their voices for about a week, either by not speaking or by whispering. Patients should also be warned to avoid irritants, such as smoke, cold air, and alcohol. Advise patients to get plenty of rest, increase fluid intake, and consider additional humidification. Such passive treatment presents particular difficulties for children.

Drug Therapies

Antibiotics clear up the bacterial form of laryngitis: 250 mg penicillin or 250 mg erythromycin for 10 to 12 days. Typical medications include broad-spectrum antibiotics such as amoxicillin and tetracycline, taken orally. Antihistamines and inhaled steroids should be prescribed to treat allergies related to laryngitis

Complementary and Alternative Therapies

Alternative treatments may be effective in cases of acute, chronic, or recurrent laryngitis. Use nutritional support along with lozenges, teas, and an appropriate gargle combination.

NUTRITION

- Zinc lozenges (as commercially available): Boosts the immune system and relieves soreness.
- Vitamin C (1,000 mg tid to qid): needed for proper immune function and to strengthen mucous membranes
- B-complex (50 to 100 mg/day): Enhances immune function, especially during stress.

HERBS

Herbs are generally a safe way to strengthen and tone the body's systems. As with any therapy, it is important to ascertain a diagnosis before pursuing treatment. Herbs may be used as dried extracts (capsules, powders, teas), glycerites (glycerine extracts), or tinctures (alcohol extracts). Unless otherwise indicated, teas should be made with 1 tsp. herb per cup of hot water. Steep covered 5 to 10 minutes for leaf or flowers, and 10 to 20 minutes for roots. Drink 2 to 4 cups/day. Tinctures may be used singly or in combination as noted.

- Slippery elm (*Ulmus rubra*) soothes irritated tissues and promotes healing.
- Licorice (*Glycyrrhiza glabra*) has antiviral properties and is soothing to the throat. Licorice is contraindicated in hypertension.

Gargles: Use 5 drops of each tincture listed below in $\frac{1}{4}$ cup of water. Gargle and swallow four to six times a day.

- Laryngitis gargle: Coneflower *(Echinacea purpurea)*, sage *(Salvia officinalis)*, and marigold *(Calendula officinalis)* are soothing and anti-inflammatory herbs.
- Anti-microbial gargle: Coneflower, goldenseal *(Hydrastis canadensis)*, and myrrh *(Commiphora molmol)* are anti-bacterial and immune-stimulating herbs.
- Pain relief gargle: Propolis, peppermint *(Mentha piperita)*, and ginger *(Zingiber officinalis)* are antimicrobial and anodyne herbs.

HOMEOPATHY

An experienced homeopath should assess individual constitutional types and severity of disease to select the correct remedy and potency. For acute prescribing use 3 to 5 pellets of a 12X to 30C remedy every one to four hours until acute symptoms resolve.

- *Aconite* for laryngitis that comes on after a shock
- *Spongia tosta* for laryngitis from coughing
- *Phosphorus* for hoarseness that is painless or with burning pains
- *Arum* for laryngitis from over-use
- *Causticum* for hoarseness that comes with every cold and is relieved with cold drinks

ACUPUNCTURE

Acupuncture may be helpful in enhancing immune function.

MASSAGE

Therapeutic massage is helpful in reducing the effects of stress.

OTHER CONSIDERATIONS

Prevention

Avoid abusing or overusing the voice, environmental irritants, and smoking.

Complications/Sequelae

Chronic hoarseness

Prognosis

Laryngitis usually resolves within one to two weeks. Children typically take one week to recover their voices.

Pregnancy

Caution with antibiotics. Goldenseal *(Hydrastis canadensis)* should be used with caution in pregnancy.

REFERENCES

Berkow R, ed. *Merck Manual of Diagnosis and Therapy.* 16th ed. Rahway, NJ: Merck Research Laboratories; 1992.

Berkow R, Beers MH, Fletcher AJ, eds. *Merck Manual, Home Edition.* Rahway, NJ: Merck & Co; 1997.

Ballenger JJ, Snow JB, eds. *Otorhinolaryngology.* 15th ed. Philadelphia, Pa: Williams and Wilkins; 1996;30:535–555.

Hoffman D. *The New Holistic Herbal.* New York, NY: Barnes & Noble Books; 1995: 47.

Larson DE, ed. *Mayo Clinic Family Health Book.* 2nd ed. New York, NY: William Morrow and Company; 1996.

■ LOW BACK PAIN

OVERVIEW

Definition

Low back pain, which affects 60% to 80% of the adult population at one time or another, is sharp or diffuse pain and often is accompanied by inflexibility and tenderness at the lumbar region. Usually caused by mechanical stress injuries or overload, the pain frequently radiates and affects the buttocks and legs as well. The majority of low back problems are acute or episodic, resulting from sharp or consistent strain. Less frequently, low back pain is a symptom of more serious injury, spinal deterioration, or disease. Back pain can interfere, to a greater or lesser degree, with the patient's ability to engage in work, recreation, and other normal activities.

Etiology

- The most common cause of low back problems is relatively minor trauma or injury to the supporting muscles, the surrounding soft tissue (tendons, ligaments, or joint capsules) or spinal disks of the lumbar region. Generally, repeated twisting or lifting of heavy objects triggers the injury.
- After significant back strain or injury, a prolapsed or herniated disk is the type of serious low back injury most frequently seen. An incomplete tear in the annulus fibrosus of the intervertebral disk can cause a bulge that then irritates the lower lumbar roots. Some ruptures cause intervertebral fluids to leak, which can induce inflammation.
- Compression fractures at the lower part of the spine occur relatively frequently in older women with osteoporosis. A sudden stress or shock can cause one or more of the vertebrae to collapse on one side, producing a wedge-like distortion, throwing the muscles into spasm, and compressing the nerve root.
- Other causes of low back pain include a number of degenerative and mechanical conditions, most commonly lumbar degenerative disk disease (chronic low back pain) which develops over time as the intervertebral disks wear down and lose elasticity; spondylosis (degenerative spondylolisthesis, arthritis of the spine), which occurs when overuse, injury, or aging causes the intervertebral disks to thin and the spaces between the disks to narrow; and spinal or lumbar stenosis, which develops as the spinal canal narrows, causing crowding around the spinal cord and nerve roots, and buckling of intervertebral disk and interlaminar ligaments.
- Low back pain can be caused by sciatica (lumbar radiculopathy), irritation of the fifth lumbar or first sacral nerve root usually as a result of a herniated disk; and by sacrolitus, an inflammatory condition usually associated with certain inflammatory bowel diseases and rheumatic disorders. Other seemingly unrelated conditions can produce low back pain, including ovarian cyst, nephrolithiasis, pancreatitis, ulcers, infection (usually indicated by fever, chills, and sweats), or metastatic cancers (usually indicated by night sweats and severe night pain).
- A psychological component may be involved in many back problems.

Risk Factors

Men and older people are particularly prone to lower back problems, as are people who regularly lift, twist, bend, and operate vibrating equipment. Trauma, infection, heredity, a history of intermittent sciatica, poor overall fitness, and smoking seem to increase a person's risk for developing degenerative back conditions. In addition, people who suffer from depression or have such personality disorders as hysteria and hypochondriasis have higher incidences of lower back problems. For reasons that are not altogether clear, those who are not particularly satisfied with their work or are paid poorly seem to suffer more lower back injuries or chronic back problems.

Signs and Symptoms

- Tenderness, pain, and stiffness in the lower back
- Pain that radiates into the buttocks or legs
- Difficulty standing erect or in one position for an extended time
- Discomfort while sitting
- Weakness and leg fatigue while walking

DIFFERENTIAL DIAGNOSIS

Since low back pain can be a symptom of other conditions, careful diagnosis is important to determine if the pain is caused by structural abnormalities or inflammatory process, or is referred by organic disease and conditions, and develop a treatment plan.

- Lumbar degenerative disk disease (chronic low back pain)
- Spondylosis (degenerative spondylolisthesis)
- Spinal or lumbar stenosis
- Sciatica (lumbar radiculopathy)
- Spinal fracture
- Herniated nucleus pulposus or ruptured intervertebral disk
- Sacroilitis
- Ovarian cyst
- Nephrolithiasis
- Pancreatitis
- Ulcers
- Osteomyelitis
- Infection
- Metastatic tumors, myeloma, lymphoma
- Depression
- Osteoporosis with compression fractures
- Spinal tuberculosis
- Fibromyalgia
- Ulcerative colitis
- Reiter's syndrome
- Psoriatic arthritis
- Enteric arthritis
- Prostate or testicular problems

DIAGNOSIS

Physical Examination

Patients who have acute or episodic back sprain typically experience diffuse tenderness in the low back or sacroiliac region, normal reflexes, and normal motor strength. Range of motion testing may elicit complaints of pain. With chronic back pain, reports of stiffness, especially when rising from a seated position, are more common.

As the patient sits and raises a straightened leg, a midline bulge of the intervertebral disk coupled with mild bilateral discomfort may indicate a ruptured disk. With the patient prone, observe for pain with hip extension. Patient may also have difficulty standing erect, electing to assume a stooped posture.

Diminished knee and/or ankle reflexes may indicate stenosis. As the patient stands with the spine extended (leaning backwards), the pain may become immediately more severe. In some cases, neurologic examinations reveal loss of normal nerve function as evidenced in weakness, loss of sensation, or loss of reflexes. The patient may present with a history of bowel and bladder dysfunction.

Laboratory Tests

Alkaline phosphatase to rule out bone tumor. CBC, ANA, sed rate rheumatoid factor to rule out rheumatoid arthritis, infection, and osteomyelitis.

Pathological Findings

Blood tests that reveal elevated erythrocyte sedimentation rate or WBC suggest infection.

Imaging

Plain radiographs are usually not helpful in determining back sprain. However, X rays may be recommended to rule out more serious conditions. For example, if the patient complains of pain at rest or at night, or history of trauma, AO and lateral radiographs are indicated to rule out infection or tumor. Although a prolapsed or bulging disk may not be evident in routine X rays, it may be seen on an MRI or CT scan.

AP and lateral radiographs may show age-appropriate changes in the case of degenerative disk disease, such as anterior osteophytes and reduced height of the intervertebral disk. There may also be a "vacuum sign" with apparent air (nitrogen) in the disk space.

In stenosis, radiographs may reveal degeneration, marked narrowing of the intervertebral disk, and degenerative scoliosis. End plate changes around the disk space and marginal osteophyte formation around the facet joints may also be evident.

Other Diagnostic Procedures

If the pain does not subside and functioning does not return after a few days of bed rest and limited activity, further tests and specific imaging may be necessary to rule out long-term chronic or degenerative back problems. In some cases, strength testing on a treadmill will reveal weakness in toe or heel walking, or in large toe dorsiflexion. This may indicate stenosis. Testing for sensation with pinprick, temperature, and light touch test may be helpful in making an accurate diagnosis.

TREATMENT OPTIONS

Treatment Strategy

For most low back problems, one to two days of bed rest and 10 days of NSAIDs or other non-narcotic pain-relieving medication is all that is needed until the inflammation and muscle spasm subsides. For chronic back pain, managing pain and minimizing disability over time becomes the focus of treatment. Physical therapy and manipulation are beneficial in muscle spasm and in correcting biomechanical dysfunction.

Drug Therapies

NSAIDs or other non-narcotic pain medications such as aspirin or acetaminophen are usually sufficient to manage the pain. Muscle relaxants in the first week or two may also be advisable.

For chronic back pain, a continuous course of NSAIDs may be necessary. Occasional low-dose, rapidly tapered oral steroids, or an epidural steroid injection, may be used to reduce inflammation. While steroids can produce dramatic results, they have little lasting benefit and tend to become less effective over time.

Other therapies—Physical therapy and spinal manipulation may be helpful in the first three to four weeks following an episode of low back pain. Once the acute pain has diminished, exercises, aerobic conditionings, and strengthening can help prevent long-term back problems. Proper posture is essential.

If other treatments are not effective in relieving pain and restoring function, surgery may be recommended. For example, in the case of a prolapsed or herniated disk, surgery may be necessary to remove part or all of a disk to prevent long-term nerve damage. Newer procedures, including percuta-neous discectomy, laser discectomy, and endoscopic discectomy use a large needle or tube inserted through the skin to remove the disks. For severe cases of lumbar stenosis, a laminectomy may be recommended to stabilize the spinal column.

Complementary and Alternative Therapies

Alternative therapies can be effective for easing muscle tension, correcting spinal imbalances, relieving discomfort, and averting long-term back problems by improving muscle and joint health. Relaxation techniques, biofeedback, supervised exercises, and gentle exercises such as Tai Chi, Chi Kung, and yoga may be quite helpful to prevent reoccurrence. Electromyographic (EMG) biofeedback can help, specifically when chronic pain is related to muscle spasms.

NUTRITION

- B-complex: B_1 (50 to 100 mg), B_2 (50 mg), B_3 (25 mg); B_5 (100 mg); B_6 (50 to 100 mg), B_{12} (100 to 1,000 mcg), folate (400 mcg/day) are reduced when in stress/pain
- Anti-oxidants: vitamin E (400 IU/day), vitamin C (1,000 to 3,000 mg/day)
- Calcium (1,500 to 2,000 mg) and magnesium (700 to 1,000 mg) to regulate muscle contraction and ease spasm
- Bromelain (250 to 500 mg tid away from food) anti-inflammatory, works especially well with turmeric

HERBS

Ascertain a diagnosis before pursuing treatment. Herbs may be used as dried extracts (capsules, powders, teas), glycerites (glycerine extracts), or tinctures (alcohol extracts). Unless otherwise indicated, teas should be made with 1 tsp. herb per cup of hot water. Steep covered 5 to 10 minutes for leaf or flowers, and 10 to 20 minutes for roots. Drink 2 to 4 cups/day. Tinctures may be used singly or in combination as noted. Mix three to six of the following herbs (1 cup tea or 30 to 60 drops of tincture three to six times/day).

Relaxants: Black haw (*Viburnum prunifolium*) spasmolytic; petasites (*Petasites hybridus*) acute muscle spasm, not for long-term use; valerian (*Valeriana officinalis*) antispasmodic, especially with sleeplessness; wild yam (*Dioscorea villosa*) antispasmodic, especially with joint pains and long-term stress; turmeric (*Curcuma longa*) anti-inflammatory, especially with digestive problems; Jamaican dogwood (*Piscidea piscipula*) spasmolytic

Pain relief: White willow bark (Salix alba) anti-inflammatory and analgesic; devil's claw (Harpagophytum procumbens) analgesic, anti-inflammatory, especially with joint problems; St. John's wort (Hypericum perforatum) anti-inflammatory, especially with neuralgia and/or anxiety

Circulatory stimulants may be added if there is decreased circulation or congestion in the area: rosemary leaves (Rosemariana officinalis), especially with digestive problems; gingko (Ginkgo biloba), especially with poor circulation

Topical treatment may be quite helpful for acute problems. Mix one to two drops of essential oil or 5 to 10 drops of tincture into 1 tbsp. vegetable oil, and rub into the affected area: St. John's wort for nerve pain; leopard's bane (Arnica montana) anti-inflammatory, external use only; lobelia (Lobelia inflata) anti-spasmodic

HOMEOPATHY

An experienced homeopath should assess individual constitutional types and severity of disease to select the correct remedy and potency. For acute prescribing use 3 to 5 pellets of a 12X to 30C remedy every one to four hours until acute symptoms resolve.

- *Aesculus* for dull pain with muscle weakness and increased circulation to affected area
- *Arnica montana* especially with a bruised feeling and/or pain as a result of trauma
- *Colocynthis* for weakness in the small of the back with sudden severe cramping
- *Gnaphalium* for sciatica that alternates with numbness, especially if sitting makes it better
- *Lycopodium* for burning pain, especially with gas and/or bloating
- *Rhus toxicodendron* for stiffness and pain in the small of the back that is worse in the morning; may have restlessness

PHYSICAL MEDICINE

- Chiropractic or osteopathic manipulation can help to release muscle spasm, improve flexibility, and increase parasympathetic response to induce pain relief. For chronic back pain, postural treatments such as the Alexander Technique or Hellerwork may also be suitable. Electromyographic (EMG) biofeedback may be helpful when chronic pain is related to muscle spasms.
- Contrast hydrotherapy. Alternating hot and cold applications brings nutrients to the site and diffuses metabolic waste from inflammation. The overall effect is decreased inflammation, pain relief, and enhanced healing. If possible, immerse the part being treated. Alternate three minutes hot with one minute cold. Repeat three times. This is one set. Do two to three sets/day. This is useful in both acute and chronic back problems.
- Castor oil pack. Used externally, castor oil is a powerful anti-inflammatory. Apply oil directly to skin, cover with a clean soft cloth (e.g. flannel) and plastic wrap. Place a heat source (hot water bottle or heating pad) over the pack and let sit for 30 to 60 minutes. For best results, use for three consecutive days. This can be very helpful in chronic back problems, especially with ligament involvement.

ACUPUNCTURE

May help to relieve spasm and pain and increase circulation to the affected area, thus decreasing pain and inflammation.

MASSAGE

Massage may be helpful both acutely and to prevent chronic problems. Reflexology can be taught to patients for self-treatment.

Patient Monitoring

Follow closely for treatment compliance in initial acute phase and then for following weeks of therapy.

OTHER CONSIDERATIONS

Prevention

Appropriate physical activity and exercise will help strengthen back and torso muscles. Maintaining a healthy weight and good posture lowers risk of developing recurrent back strain or chronic back pain. Learning to bend and lift appropriately, sleeping on a firm mattress, sitting in steady and supporting chairs, and wearing good supportive shoes that fit well are important factors in averting and minimizing lower back problems.

Complications/Sequelae

People with low back problems may experience mild to marked functional impairment, specifically in walking, and pain while carrying out the simplest of tasks. In addition, they may have trouble sleeping and difficulty concentrating. Severe symptoms may limit vocational and recreational activities and affect mood and sexual interest. While depression is usually not the cause of chronic low back pain, it may complicate treatment, hindering eventual recovery.

Prognosis

Eighty five percent of all patients with back pain improve within one month. For those whose symptoms persist for more than six months, the risk for long-term disability is considerable.

Pregnancy

Pregnant women are at increased risk for back problems due to body changes and hormonal relaxation of the ligaments and tendons. Physical medicine techniques, proper body mechanics, and exercise are the safest treatments. Some women actually experience relief of chronic back pain in pregnancy.

REFERENCES

Balch JF, Balch PA. *Prescription for Nutritional Healing.* 2nd ed. Garden City Park, NY: Avery Publishing Group; 1997:149–150.

Bartram T. *Encyclopedia of Herbal Medicine.* Dorset, England: Grace Publishers; 1995:238–239, 277–278.

Blumenthal M, ed. *The Complete German Commission E Monographs.* Boston, Mass: Integrative Medicine Communications; 1998:81–82, 136–137, 183, 197, 222–223, 226–227, 230–231.

Gruenwald J, Brendler T, Jaenicke C et al, eds. *PDR for Herbal Medicines.* Montvale, NJ: Medical Economics Company; 1998:662–663, 786–787, 871–872,

Kitade T, Odahara Y, Shinohara S, et al. Studies on the enhanced effect of acupuncture analgesia and acupuncture anesthesia by D-phenylalanine (2nd report): schedule of administration and clinical effects in low back pain and tooth extraction. *Acupunct Electrother Res.* 1990;15:121–135.

Kruzel T. *The Homeopathic Emergency Guide.* Berkeley, Calif: North Atlantic Books; 1992:30–38.

Morrison R. *Desktop Guide to Keynotes and Confirmatory Symptoms.* Albany, Calif: Hahnemann Clinic Publishing; 1993:36–39, 59–61.

Mowrey D. *The Scientific Validation of Herbal Medicine.* New Canaan, Conn: Keats Publishing; 1986:223–227.

Murray MT, Pizzorno JE. *Encyclopedia of Natural Medicine.* Rocklin, Calif: Prima Publishing; 1998:338.

Snider RK, ed. *Essentials of Musculoskeletal Care.* Rosemont, Ill: American Academy of Orthopaedic Surgeons; 1997.

Werbach M. *Nutritional Influences on Illness.* New Canaan, Conn: Keats Publishing Inc.; 1987:1987: 342-345.

■ MENOPAUSE

OVERVIEW
Definition

Menopause is the cessation of regular menstrual cycles, a normal physiological and biological event (unless from oophorectomy) that occurs in women at an average age of 51. Today, 50 million women in the United States have reached menopause. The experience of menopause varies enormously between individuals and among cultural groups. While up to 80% of American women experience hot flashes within a collection of symptoms, a study of Mayan Indians found that no women experienced hot flashes. Although women's life expectancy has greatly increased over time, the average age of menopause onset remains constant. Most women will spend one-third of their life postmenopausal.

Etiology

- Ovarian failure
- Depletion of oocytes
- Depletion of functional gonadotropin-sensitive ovarian follicles—reduces and eventually eliminates estradiol production, resulting in cessation of menses
- Estrone—predominate postmenopausal estrogen is one-third as potent as estradiol
- Hysterectomy and certain medical treatments for endometriosis and cancer

Risk Factors

- Premature ovarian failure—menopause before age 40; karyotypic abnormalities and autoimmune disorders need to be ruled out
- Age
- Smoking—hastens follicular depletion

Signs and Symptoms

- Amenorrhea—the cessation of uterine bleeding for more than one year is clinically determined to be menopause; average duration is four years from early menstrual changes to complete cessation of menses
- Vasomotor symptoms—including hot flashes (flushing of face, neck, and upper trunk; may be accompanied by palpitations, dizziness, headaches); night sweats (with subsequent depression and irritability from insomnia); cold hands and feet
- Vaginal atrophy—dryness may result in postcoital bleeding; vulvar pruritus
- Urinary tract atrophy—increased frequency, burning, nocturia, incontinence
- Mood symptoms—depression, irritability, tension; usually correlate with sleep disturbances
- Facial hirsutism (from androgens) and wrinkles (from lack of estrogen)
- Osteoporosis—bone fractures possible; risk increases with premature menopause
- Coronary heart disease (CHD)—twice as many women die from CHD than cancer. Marked increase in susceptibility after menopause.

DIFFERENTIAL DIAGNOSIS

- Pregnancy—perimenopausal women may neglect to use contraception
- Endometrial cancer
- Excessive exercise—causing cessation of menses
- Uterine leiomyoma
- Hypothalamic dysfunction
- Mood and anxiety disorders

DIAGNOSIS
Physical Examination

Unless there is premature menopause or concurrent illness, the patient appears normal. The uterus may be smaller on bimanual examination.

Laboratory Tests

- Follicle-stimulating hormone (FSH)—values rise in response to estrogen decline; ≥ 40 mIU/mL is diagnostic of menopause; may fluctuate daily until postmenopause; diagnoses premature ovarian failure; helps rule out differential diagnosis
- Estradiol-17 beta decreases from 120 pg/mL to below 20 pg/mL; estrone becomes the main circulating estrogen; eventually, estradiol results only from estrone conversion
- Estrone—production decreases from 80 to 300 mg/day to 40 mg/day
- Androstenedione (primary androgen)—decreases from 1,500 to 800 mg/mL; testosterone levels decline far less than estrogen
- Luteinizing hormone (LH)—maximum increase two to three years postmenopause; abnormal pulse frequency and amplitude patterns; levels drop below FSH levels

Pathological Findings

- Follicular atresia
- Thinning of vaginal epithelium
- Lack of estrogen decreases bone density and intestinal calcium absorption
- Arteriosclerosis
- Osteoporosis

Imaging

May be done for osteoporosis detection

Other Diagnostic Procedures

Menopause is defined as a 12-month cessation of menses, usually with history of vasomotor complications. FSH measurement is rarely used solely for diagnosis. Commonly used procedures are endometrial sampling, Pap smears, and regular pelvic exams. Endometrial biopsy for differential diagnosis

TREATMENT OPTIONS
Treatment Strategy

Estrogen replacement therapy can help prevent osteoporosis and coronary artery disease. Serious side effects of hormone replacement therapy warrant careful individual evaluation and consideration of alternatives. Supplementation with calcium and other micronutrients and regular exercise help prevent these conditions.

Drug Therapies

- Estrogen—relieves hot flashes and vaginal atrophy and retards osteoporotic bone loss and fractures. Studies point toward possible CHD and Alzheimer's disease prevention. Use the lowest effective dose. Continuous administration avoids uterine bleeding. Estrogen use increases risk of breast cancer, uterine (endometrial) cancer, thromboembolism, pulmonary embolus, and gallbladder disease. Side effects include bloating, nausea, adult-onset asthma, and breast tenderness.
- Conjugated equine estrogens (e.g., Premarin 0.625 mg/day, or 1.25 mg/day with severe vasomotor symptoms)—most commonly used form; can cause metabolic changes in the liver; contraindicated with obesity, smoking, hypertension or cholesterol, varicose veins
- Estradiol—most easily metabolized delivering estrogen directly into the blood stream; available in transdermal patch (e.g., Estraderm,

1.0 mg/day of estradiol, 0.05 mg/day of transcutaneous estrogen)

- Vaginal creams—for urogenital atrophy, four to six weeks for initial effect, then twice weekly
- Progesterone—may potentiate estrogen, allowing for lower estrogen dosage (e.g., medroxyprogesterone, 2.5 to 10 mg/day); eliminates uterine cancer caused by estrogen therapy; may slow osteoporosis but does not prevent CHD or urogenital atrophy; side effects—bloating, depression, breast tenderness
- Methyltestosterone—increases libido; may decrease osteoporosis of the spine; 1.25 to 5.0 mg/day; side effect—facial hirsutism
- Alendronate—equally effective treatment for osteoporosis prevention
- Lipid-lowering drugs and aspirin—alternative treatment for CHD
- Estriol—weaker form of estrogen; best used in combination with 10% each estrone and estradiol (e.g., Tri-estrogen 2.5 to 5 mg/day, therapeutically equivalent to 0.625 to 1.25 mg/day conjugated estrogen); add progesterone for women with intact uterus; early studies show fewer adverse effects than other estrogens
- Estrogel—rubbed on abdomen and absorbed into the body; commonly used in France

Complementary and Alternative Therapies

Alternative therapies may be effective alone or in conjunction with standard treatment. Alternative medicine has much to offer for improving cardiovascular health and preventing osteoporosis. Relaxation techniques, stress management, yoga, and meditation can help with perimenopausal symptoms. Weight-bearing and aerobic exercise are crucial for cardiovascular health and osteoporosis prevention. Exercise increases endorphin release, aiding pain relief and mood elevation. Walking, swimming, and biking are less stressful on the joints.

NUTRITION

- Soy (25 to 50 mg soy/day) contains soy isoflavones (phytoestrogens); studies suggest relief of hot flashes and vaginal atrophy, and increased protection from osteoporosis and breast cancer.
- Vitamin E (400 to 1,600 IU/day) can balance vasomotor instability, decrease hot flashes, and is cardioprotective. High doses may be contraindicated in hypertension.
- Calcium/magnesium (1,000/500 mg/day for women taking estrogen and 1,500/750 mg/day for those who are not) is best absorbed with meals and sufficient gastric juices. Citrate or citramate forms may be the most absorbable forms.
- Avoiding smoking, alcohol, caffeine, and spicy foods may help decrease hot flashes.
- A combination of Vitamin C (1,200 mg), hesperidin (900 mg), and hesperidin methyl chalcone (900 mg) relieves hot flashes in a majority of women.
- Gamma-oryzanol (from rice bran oil) 300 mg/day gives partial or total relief of hot flashes in over 80 percent of users.

HERBS

Herbs are generally a safe way to strengthen and tone the body's systems. As with any therapy, it is important to ascertain a diagnosis before pursuing treatment. Herbs may be used as dried extracts (capsules, powders, teas), glycerites (glycerine extracts), or tinctures (alcohol extracts). Unless otherwise indicated, teas should be made with 1 tsp. herb per cup of hot water. Steep covered 5 to 10 minutes for leaf or flowers, and 10 to 20 minutes for roots. Drink 2 to 4 cups/day. Tinctures may be used singly or in combination as noted.

- Black cohosh (Cimicifuga racemosa) relieves vasomotor symptoms and depression; Remifemin is the most tested extract of black cohosh.

Toxicology studies show long-term use to be safe; side effect may be mild stomach upset; historic use in climacteric depression; 2 mg/day

- Chaste tree (Vitex agnes-castus) for irregular menstrual cycles; normalizes pituitary function; may take up to six months for full therapeutic effect
- Angelica (Angelica archangelica) relieves vasomotor symptoms
- Licorice (Glycyrrhiza glabra) is an estrogen-balancing herb, especially with chronic stress (regulates cortisol); not for use with hypertension; 250 mg tid, 30 to 60 drops tincture tid, or 1 cup of tea tid
- Ginkgo (Ginkgo biloba) improves memory and peripheral circulation, to treat depression and prevent Alzheimer's disease; may take up to 12 weeks for full effect; 120 mg bid to tid

HOMEOPATHY

An experienced homeopath should assess individual constitutional types and severity of disease to select the correct remedy and potency. For acute prescribing, use 3 to 5 pellets of a 12X to 30C remedy every one to four hours until acute symptoms resolve.

- Mulimen—German combination remedy (chasteberry, black cohosh, St. John's wort, cuttlefish ink) shown effective for hot flashes in 1992 study
- Ferrum phosphoricum, Graphites, Lycopodium—for symptoms occurring during sexual intercourse
- Amyl nitrosum, Lachesis, Sulphur—for hot flashes

PHYSICAL MEDICINE

Kegel exercises increase pelvic muscle tone, which helps to prevent incontinence and bladder or uterine prolapse.

ACUPUNCTURE

Acupuncture enhances endorphin release and stimulates kidney function. May also help to balance hormones and relieve vasomotor symptoms.

MASSAGE

Massage increases circulation and promotes general relaxation. Use water-soluble nonestrogen lubricants, vegetable oil, or vitamin E oil for vaginal atrophy.

Patient Monitoring

Women should have an annual Pap smear and mammography.

OTHER CONSIDERATIONS
Prevention

Menopause is not a disease but a natural process of aging. Certain symptoms may be prevented and more serious complications avoided with appropriate treatment.

Complications/Sequelae

Possible complications from estrogen use include the following.

- Breast cancer—no correlation with <5 years use
- Endometrial cancer—eliminated by concurrent progesterone use
- Thromboembolism—30 in 100,000 risk
- Pulmonary embolus
- Pancreatitis—use of transdermal patch obviates most of the risk
- Gallbladder disease—twice as prevalent
- Adult-onset asthma—twice as prevalent

Complications possibly prevented from estrogen use include the following.

- Decrease in vasomotor symptoms
- Osteoporosis—slows progression, reducing fractures 30% to 50%

- CHD—observational studies indicate decreased CHD; not confirmed by randomized clinical trials
- Alzheimer's disease—effects on central nervous system may decrease risk; unproven

Prognosis

All symptoms of menopause will progress more slowly and risks for several diseases can be reduced if managed appropriately.

REFERENCES

Bartram T. Encyclopedia of Herbal Medicine. Dorset, England: Grace Publishers; 1995:291–292.

Blumenthal M, ed. The Complete German Commission E Monographs. Boston, Mass: Integrative Medicine Communications; 1998:108, 466.

Devine A, Dick IM, Heal SJ, et al. A 4-year follow-up study of the effects of calcium supplementation on bone density in elderly postmenopausal women. Osteoporosis Int. 1997;7:23–28.

Gruenwald J, Brendler T, Jaenicke C et al, eds. PDR for Herbal Medicines. Montvale, NJ: Medical Economics Company; 1998:647–648, 871–872.

Kistner RW, ed. Kistner's Gynecology: Principles and Practice. 6th ed. St. Louis, Mo: Mosby-Year Book; 1995.

Murray MT. The Healing Power of Herbs: The Enlightened Person's Guide to the Wonders of Medicinal Plants. Rocklin, Calif: Prima Publishing; 1995:163–164.

Murray MT, Pizzorno JE. Encyclopedia of Natural Medicine. Rocklin, Calif: Prima Publishing; 1998.

Thys-Jacobs S, Starkey P, Bernstein D, Tian J. Calcium carbonate and the premenstrual syndrome: effects on premenstrual and menstrual symptoms. Premenstrual Syndrome Study Group. Am J Obstet Gynecol. 1998;179:444–452.

Villa ML, Packer E, Cheema M, et al. Effects of aluminum hydroxide on the parathyroid-vitamin D axis of postmenopausal women. J Clin Endocrinol Metab. 1991;73:1256–1261.

Vorberg G. Treatment of menopause symptoms—Successful hormone-free therapy with Remifemin®. ZFA. 1984;60:626–629.

Weiss RF. Herbal Medicines. Beaconsfield, England: Beaconsfield Publishers; 1998:317–319.

■ MOTION SICKNESS

OVERVIEW

Definition

Motion sickness is discomfort that occurs during travel in a moving vehicle such as a car, boat, or airplane. It represents a normal response to sensory conflict and changes in motion patterns.

Etiology

Motion sickness occurs when vestibular system input conflicts with visual cues, e.g., when the body senses rolling motions which are not visually apparent from inside a ship's cabin, or conversely during a "virtual reality" simulation when the eyes perceive movement that is not experienced by the body. Asymmetry can occur between right and left otolith mass.

Risk Factors

- Exposure to motion stimuli
- Youth and/or inexperience with the form of motion
- Predisposition to nausea or vomiting
- Fear or anxiety
- Exposure to unpleasant odors
- Poor ventilation
- Zero gravity
- Asian descent
- Female gender

Signs and Symptoms

- Dizziness
- Pallor
- Cold sweating
- Hypersalivation
- Nausea
- Vomiting
- Fatigue
- Headache
- Malaise

DIFFERENTIAL DIAGNOSIS

- Migraine
- Vestibular disease
- Metabolic disorders
- Vertigo
- Viral illness

DIAGNOSIS

Patient rarely arrives at a physician's office actually suffering from motion sickness; more often a health care provider will be asked for advice and preventatives after an episode and/or in anticipation of future travel.

Physical Examination

Patient may appear pale and/or weak, complain of nausea, and possibly have an elevated heart rate.

Laboratory Tests

Laboratory tests are not necessary to establish a diagnosis of motion sickness. However, in clinical studies, elevated salivary cortisol is sometimes used as an index.

Other Diagnostic Procedures

Question patient about the precipitating event and course and duration of symptoms to establish a diagnosis of motion sickness.

TREATMENT OPTIONS

Treatment Strategy

Motion sickness is not in itself dangerous, but may become dangerous if it occurs during the operation of machinery or during driving. Removing or minimizing exposure to the stimuli will help to alleviate the symptoms. Avoid fixation on moving objects.

Drug Therapies

For the short term, suggest OTC antihistamines:

- Cyclizene (Marezine): 50 mg 30 to 60 minutes before travel and every four to six hours as necessary. For children ages 6 to 11, 25 mg every six to eight hours. Not recommended for children younger than 6.
- Dimenhydrinate (Dramamine): 50 to 100 mg every four to six hours. For children ages 6 to 11, 25 to 50 mg every six to eight hours. For children ages 2 to 5, 12.5 to 25 mg every six to eight hours.
- Meclizine (Bonine, Antivert, Dramamine II): 25 to 50 mg once daily. Not recommended for patients younger than 12.

Antihistamines are effective for both prevention and treatment. These products are contraindicated in patients with breathing problems, glaucoma, or an enlarged prostate causing difficulties in urination. Antihistamines often cause drowsiness and should not be used while driving. The drowsiness effect is most pronounced with dimenhydrinate.

For the longer term, scopolamine patch placed behind the ear six to eight hours before travel will last up to three days. Side effects may include dry mouth, drowsiness, blurred vision, and disorientation. Scopolamine is not effective if administered after the onset of symptoms and may interact with alcohol, antihistamines, and antidepressants.

Phenytoin, amphetamine, and other norepinephrine-releasing agents (e.g., 25 mg promethazine in combination with 25 mg ephedrine one hour before travel) can be effective if not contraindicated.

Complementary and Alternative Therapies

Digestive herbs and/or homeopathic remedies may be helpful in preventing and relieving motion sickness. As with most therapies, alternative therapies for motion sickness are best used before the onset of symptoms.

NUTRITION

Avoid alcohol and caffeine. If there is concurrent respiratory involvement, eliminate pro-inflammatory and mucus promoting foods such as dairy products, fruit, and sugar. Ginger root *(Zingiber officinalis)* sliced and chewed may prevent the onset of motion sickness. Encapsulated ginger, crystallized ginger or ginger snaps may also be effective. Ginger may be as effective as Dramamine if taken one hour before needed. Sips of lemon water may help relieve nausea from motion sickness.

HERBS

Herbs are generally a safe way to strengthen and tone the body's systems. As with any therapy, it is important to ascertain a diagnosis before pursuing treatment. Herbs may be used as dried extracts (capsules, powders, teas), glycerites (glycerine extracts), or tinctures (alcohol extracts). Unless otherwise indicated, teas should be made with one teaspoon herb per cup of hot water. Steep covered 5 to 10 minutes for leaf or flowers, and 10 to 20 minutes for roots. Drink 2 to 4 cups/day. Tinctures may be used singly or in combination as noted.

Ginger root *(Zingiber officinalis)* in a tea (frequent small sips) or tincture (30 drops in 1/2 cup of water as needed). May add peppermint

(Mentha piperita) and/or chamomile *(Matricaria recutita)* if there is vomiting.

Black horehound *(Ballota nigra)* may help relieve nausea secondary to inner ear problems. May be used as tea (one cup tid) or tincture (30 drops tid).

HOMEOPATHY

An experienced homeopath should assess individual constitutional types and severity of disease to select the correct remedy and potency. For acute prescribing use three to five pellets of a 12X to 30C remedy every one to four hours until acute symptoms resolve.

- *Cocculus* for motion sickness and vertigo from watching moving objects.
- *Petroleum* for motion sickness with cold sensation in the abdomen.
- *Tabacum* for unrelenting nausea with cold sweat.

ACUPUNCTURE

P6 acupressure may reduce symptoms of sea sickness. Use "Sea Bands" as commercially available, as these may be very effective.

MASSAGE

Massage or other relaxation techniques may help control motion sickness.

Patient Monitoring

Patients should be instructed to report any unusual side effects resulting from medication for motion sickness.

OTHER CONSIDERATIONS

Prevention

Patients should avoid reading while in a moving vehicle, preferably keeping their eyes on the scene outside. Driving or piloting the vehicle provides protection from motion sickness, since it necessarily involves constant observation of the outside environment. For children, an elevated car seat allowing a view out the window is helpful. Patients should get as much fresh air as possible, avoid twisting the neck, and avoid eating or drinking heavily before travel. If possible, select a seat or cabin where the vehicle's motion is least perceptible, such as near the waterline of a boat or in the center of a plane. Diaphragmatic breathing may help prevent motion sickness.

Complications/Sequelae

Motion sickness has no long-term complications.

Prognosis

The symptoms generally disappear quickly after travel is concluded. Patients often acclimate during a trip of several days or after repeated exposures to the same type of experience.

Pregnancy

Ginger should be used with caution in the first trimester of pregnancy.

REFERENCES

Blumenthal M, ed. *The Complete German Commission E Monographs.* Boston, Mass: Integrative Medicine Communications; 1998:429.

Dobie TG, May JG. The effectiveness of a motion sickness counselling programme. *Br J Clin Psychol.* 1995;34 (part 2):301–311.

Gresty MA, Grunwald EA. Medical perspective of motion sickness. Proceedings of the International Workshop on Motion Sickness: Medical and Human Factors; May 1997; Marbella, Spain.

Helling K, Hausmann S, Flottmann T, Scherer H. Individual differences in susceptibility to motion sickness [in German]. *HNO.* 1997;45:210–215.

Hoffman D. *The New Holistic Herbal.* New York, NY: Barnes & Noble Books; 1995:181.

Hu S, Stritzel R, Chandler A, Stern RM. P6 acupressure reduces symptoms of vection-induced motion sickness. *Aviat Space Environ Med.* 1995;66:631–634.

Jozsvai EE, Pigeau RA. The effect of autogenic training and biofeedback on motion sickness tolerance. *Aviat Space Environ Med.* 1996;67:963–968.

Morrison R. *Desktop Guide to Keynotes and Confirmatory Symptoms.* Albany, Calif: Hahnemann Clinic Publishing; 1993:133, 288, 379.

Pray WS. Motion sickness: a sensory conflict. *U.S. Pharmacist.* March 1998.

Ramsey A. Virtual reality induced symptoms and effects: a psychophysiological prespective. Proceedings of the International Workshop on Motion Sickness: Medical and Human Factors. Marbella, Spain, May 1997.

Stern RM, Hu S, Uijtdehaage SH, Muth ER, Xu LH, Koch KL. Asian hypersusceptibility to motion sickness. *Hum Hered.* 1996;46:7–14.

■ MYOCARDIAL INFARCTION

OVERVIEW
Definition
Myocardial infarction (MI) is the result of continuous and/or complete reduction in blood flow to a portion of the myocardium, thus producing some degree of myocardial death and necrosis. Oxygen deprivation results from blockage of coronary arteries supplying blood to the myocardium typically brought on by atherosclerotic plaque. Total coronary artery occlusion results in acute MI with Q wave formation (non Q wave infarctions have greatly narrowed infarct-related artery without total obstruction). Introduction of coronary care units in the 1960s and recent practices of urgent reperfusion and advances in pharmacologic interventions have decreased mortality rates from 30% to 40%, to 15% to 20% of admissions.

Etiology
- Atherosclerosis, resulting in narrowed or occluded arteries
- Thrombosis, the immediate cause, caught within artherosclerotic plaque
- Coronary vasomotor spasm
- Coronary artery embolism
- Congenital anomalies
- Arteritis
- Trauma

Risk Factors
- Smoking
- High fat diet, excess body weight
- Family history of early MI
- Diabetes
- Second generation oral contraceptives
- Hostile, aggressive personality (Type A)
- Hypertension
- Hypercholesterolemia
- Males and postmenopausal females
- Cocaine or amphetamine abuse

Signs and Symptoms
- Pain, heaviness, tightness, burning—in chest (substernal), back, left arm, jaw, neck
- Dyspnea
- Dizziness, weakness
- Nausea, vomiting
- Anxiety
- Arrhythmia
- Hypotension, hypertension

DIFFERENTIAL DIAGNOSIS
- Pulmonary embolism
- Unstable angina
- Esophagitis, or esophageal spasm
- Myocarditis
- Cholecystitis
- Pericarditis
- Aortic dissection
- Hiatal hernia
- Chest wall pains
- Pneumothorax
- Gastroenteritis/P.U.D.

DIAGNOSIS
Physical Examination
- "Crushing" chest pain, S4 gallop, ectopic impulse, systolic murmurs
- Crackles—indicate elevated left ventricle (LV) filling pressure
- Hypotension, elevated jugular venous pulse, clear lung auscultation—indicate right ventricular infarction
- S3 gallop—indicates systolic dysfunction

Laboratory Tests
- Serum cardiac enzymes increase as myocardial necrosis evolves
- MB fraction of creatine kinase (CK-MB)—rises within six hours, peaks within 24 hours, and declines within 72 hours of MI; gold standard for diagnosis
- Lactate dehydrogenase (LDH)—rises after 24 hours, peaks three to six days and returns to normal in a week to 10 days; increases diagnostic specificity
- Troponin T (cTnT) and cardiac-specific troponin I (cTnI)—better sensitivity and specificity than CK-MB. Serum levels increase 3 to 12 hours after MI, peak at 24 to 48 hours, and return to baseline in 5 to 14 days.

Pathological Findings
- Atherosclerotic plaque leads to platelet–fibrin thrombosis, resulting in coronary artery occlusion
- Myocardium becomes ischemic, resulting in transmural spread of necrosis
- Depth of plaque fissure, extent of atherosclerotic stenosis, thrombogenic plaque constituents—determine magnitude of thrombosis

Imaging
- Chest X ray to differentiate pneumothorax
- CT/MRI or aortography to differentiate aortic dissection
- Noninvasive radionuclide imaging—shows perfusion; e.g., technetium 99m sestamibi; for nondiagnostic ECGs, persistent chest pain

Other Diagnostic Procedures
- Electrocardiogram (ECG)—diagnoses ventricular dysrhythmias and monitors sinus tachycardia (ST)-segment changes
- History of symptoms; physical examination
- Test cardiac enzyme levels
- ST elevation—at least 1 mm in two contiguous precordial leads or in inferior limb leads; appears early in MI
- Hyperacute T waves invert as ST segments return to normal
- Q waves often appear with ST elevation
- Left bundle branch block (LBBB)—Q waves in V5 and V6 with 7 mm ST elevation
- Echocardiagram
- Two-dimensional—determines ventricular function, wall and valvular abnormalities
- Doppler—diagnoses mitral regurgitation or ventricular septal rupture
- Angiography—diagnoses coronary occlusion and wall abnormalities for chest pain or nondiagnostic ECG

TREATMENT OPTIONS
Treatment Strategy
- Immediate management of the patient aims to identify need for reperfusion, relieve pain, provide oxygen, and prevent or treat complications of MI.

- Rapid reperfusion can reduce infarct size, preserve ventricular function, stop transmural spread of necrosis, increase electrical stability, and reduce morbidity and mortality. There are three main methods of reperfusion: thrombolytic therapy, percutaneous transluminal coronary angioplasty (PTCA) and other mechanical reperfusion, and surgery.
- Treatment for all patients includes analgesics, nitroglycerin, anticoagulants, antiplatelet therapy, beta-andronergic antagonists, and oxygen supplementation.

Drug Therapies

Thrombolytic therapy. Ninety percent of patients with acute MI have complete occlusion of the infarct-related artery.

- Perform within 60 to 90 minutes, little benefit after 12 hours
- Restores artery patency

Thrombolytic drugs include:

- Streptokinase (SK)—70 minutes to lysis; half-life 20 minutes; coronary patency: 55% at 90 minutes, 85% at 24 hours; antigenic; 1.5 million units intravenously in 30 to 60 minutes, slower if blood pressure falls
- Tissue plasminogen activator (Alteplase, rt-PA)—45 minutes to lysis; half-life six minutes; coronary patency: 75% at 90 minutes, 85% at 24 hours; nonantigenic; 100 mg IV in 90 minutes; 15 mg bolus, then 0.75 mg/kg over 30 minutes, then 0.50 mg/kg over 60 minutes
- Anisoylated plasminogens streptokinase activator complex (Anistreplase APSAC)—more expensive but longer fibrinolytic activity than streptokinase; 30 mg IV in five minutes
- Reteplase (r-PA) is similar to alteplase, 10 units as a two minute bolus, repeated after 30 minutes
- Aspirin—antiplatelet affect; 169 to 320 mg then 85 mg for maintenance, consider contraindications
- Heparin—improves coronary patency, controversial; best results with t-PA; 1,000 units/hour for 8 to 72 hours
- Contraindications for thrombolytic therapy—severe bleeding, hypertension, liver or renal disease, pregnancy, recent surgery, stroke

Surgical Procedures

PTCA—mechanical reperfusion

- Percutaneous transluminal coronary angioplasty (PTCA)—Superior treatment; can re-establish arterial blood flow in 90% of patients without some of the risks associated with fibrinolytic agents. Few facilities can perform expeditiously.
- Intra-aortic balloon counterpulsation—maintains perfusion; for hypotension, ventricular rupture, mitral regurgitation; PTCA adjunct, CABG adjunct; temporizing method prior to PTCA, CABG or to allow heart to recover
- Intracoronary stenting—stabilizes dissection during PTCA

Coronary artery bypass surgery (CABG)—for free wall and acute septal rupture, mitral regurgitation, refractory cardiogenic shock. To be utilized when the disease is too extensive for mechanical repurfusion.

General Measures

- Analgesia—morphine sulfate 4 to 8 mg doses; intravenous morphine 2 to 4 mg, can be repeated every 5 to 10 minutes
- Nitroglycerin—for recurrent ischemia, congestive heart failure (CHF), hypertension. 0.4 mg sublingual, can be given every five minutes in the absence of hypotension. Good response should be followed by IV nitroglycerin at 10 mcg/minute
- Antiplatelet therapy with aspirin. 325 mg chewed to enhance absorption

- Anticoagulants—for thromboembolic complications. Heparin IV bolus of 80 units/kg followed by infusion of 18 units/kg/hour
- Oxygen—2 to 4 L per minute by nasal cannula
- Angiotensin-converting enzyme (ACE) inhibitors—reduce ventricular dilation and remodeling; monitor renal function and hypotension, Captopril 6.25 mg orally, titrate to 25 to 50 mg orally tid over 24 to 48 hours
- Beta blockers—reduce cardiac rupture, reinfarction, ventricular fibrillation. Metoprolol 5 mg, repeated every five minutes to a total of 15 mg, then switch to oral metoprolol or atenolol

Complementary and Alternative Therapies

Alternative therapies are most appropriate to prevent the first MI, minimize damage from an MI, and reduce the risk of a future MI, once the patient has been properly diagnosed and stabilized. There are no substitutes for immediate and appropriate medical care with a presentation of chest pain and/or suspected MI. See related subjects under angina, hypertension, and atherosclerosis.

NUTRITION

- L-carnitine (9 g/day IV for five days, then 6 g/day orally for 12 months) was studied within 24 hours of onset of chest pain and was found to decrease left ventricular dilation.
- Diet: In another study, a diet high in antioxidants (vitamin C, vitamin E, and beta-carotene), soluble dietary fiber, and one that replaces fat with oils showed reduced plasma lipid peroxide and lactate dehydrogenase cardiac enzyme levels. This may reduce myocardial necrosis and reperfusion injury.
- Bromelain (400 to 800 mg/day) has been used for thrombolysis and may help dissolve plaque.

HERBS

Herbs should not be used in lieu of immediate medical attention. Herbs can be used as general heart tonics and specifically applied to treating conditions associated with MI, such as atherosclerosis, congestive heart failure, hypercholesterolemia, hypertension, and hypertriglyceridemia.

HOMEOPATHY

Homeopathy should not be used in lieu of immediate medical attention. An experienced homeopath should assess individual constitutional types and severity of disease to select the correct remedy and potency of heart tonics.

PHYSICAL MEDICINE

Beneficial for rehabilitation.

ACUPUNCTURE

Useful for pain and rehabilitation.

MASSAGE

Beneficial for rehabilitation.

Patient Monitoring

Immediate:

- Electrocardiogram—2- to 3-lead bedside
- Cardiac rate and rhythm
- Look for complications

OTHER CONSIDERATIONS
Prevention

Regular exercise, stress reduction, weight management, and avoidance or management of risk factors

Complications/Sequelae

Electrical:

- Sinus bradycardia
- Ventricular or sinus tachycardia
- Atrial fibrillation

Mechanical:

- Rupture of free wall, interventricular septum, or papillary muscle
- Mitral regurgitation
- Hypertension
- LV failure/CHF
- Acute pericarditis
- Dressler's syndrome
- Cardiac arrest/sudden death
- Anxiety, depression

Prognosis

Killip subgroups:

- Class I—no evidence of pulmonary congestion or shock (mortality < 5%)
- Class II—mild pulmonary congestion, isolated S3 gallop (mortality 10%)
- Class III—pulmonary edema, LV dysfunction, mitral regurgitation, S3 gallop, severe CHF (mortality 30%)
- Class IV—systemic hypoperfusion, hypotension, cardiogenic shock (80% mortality)

REFERENCES

Iliceto S, Scrutinio D, Bruzzi P, et al. Effects of L-carnitine administration on left ventricular remodeling after acute anterior myocardial infarction: the L-Carnitine Ecocardiografia Digitalizzata Infarto Miocardico (CEDIM) Trial. *J Am Coll Cardiol.* August 1995;26:380.

Kruzel T. *The Homeopathic Emergency Guide.* Berkeley, Calif: North Atlantic Books; 1992:58–60.

Murray MT. *The Healing Power of Herbs: The Enlightened Person's Guide to the Wonders of Medicinal Plants.* Rocklin, Calif: Prima Publishing; 1998:184.

Rakel RE, ed. *Conn's Current Therapy.* 50th ed. Philadelphia, Pa: WB Saunders; 1998.

Singh RB, Niaz MA, Agarwal P, Begom R, Rastogi SS. Effect of antioxidant-rich foods on plasma ascorbic acid, cardiac enzyme, and lipid peroxide levels in patients hospitalized with acute myocardial infarction. *J Am Diet Assoc.* July 1995;95:775–780.

Singh RB, Singh NK, Niaz MA, Sharma JP. Effect of treatment with magnesium and potassium on mortality and reinfarction rate of patients with suspected acute myocardial infarction. *Int J Clin Pharmacol Thera.* 1996;34:219–225.

Washington Manual of Medical Therapeautics. 29th ed. Philadelphia, Pa: Lippincott-Raven Publishers; 1998.

■ OBESITY

OVERVIEW
Definition
Overweight is defined as a body-mass index (BMI) over 25 and obesity as a BMI over 30 (BMI is defined as the weight in kilograms divided by the square of the height in meters). A BMI over 25 is associated with increased health risks. Historically, obesity was defined as a body weight greater than 20% above a desirable weight as defined by the Metropolitan Life Insurance Company tables of weights and heights. However, the BMI is the current standard. Approximately 33% of Americans 20 to 75 years of age are overweight, and of these, approximately one-third are severely obese. For both men and women, the prevalence of overweight increases with age.

Etiology
While there is no single underlying etiology of simple obesity, excessive weight reflects an imbalance between energy input and energy output. However, genetic and environmental factors may also play a role; for example, total body fat stores and the total number of fat cells are determined genetically and can make an individual susceptible to obesity. In addition, there are a number of rare congenital syndromes in which all affected individuals are obese, such as Prader–Willi syndrome, Cushing's syndrome, Alström's syndrome, Laurence-Moon-Biedl syndrome, Cohen's syndrome, and Carpenter's syndrome.

- Genetic predisposition
- Insulinoma
- Hypothalamic disorders
- Overeating
- High-fat diet
- Decreased physical activity
- Prescription medications (e.g., steroids, phenothiazines, tricyclic antidepressants, antiepileptics, anti- hypertensives)
- Psychological factors (e.g., disturbance in body image, reaction to separation or death)

Risk Factors
- Familial predisposition
- Sedentary lifestyle
- High-fat diet

Signs and Symptoms
BMI over 25 to 30

DIFFERENTIAL DIAGNOSIS
- Cushing's disease—characterized by weight gain in the face, thorax, and abdomen, but sparing the buttocks and extremities
- Hypothyroidism (60% of patients have only a modest weight gain)
- Hypothalamic tumors (e.g., craniopharyngiomas)
- Stein–Leventhal syndrome (in women)—characterized by obesity, hirsutism, and infertility
- Klinefelter's syndrome (in men)—characterized by increased adipose tissue and reduced muscle mass

DIAGNOSIS
Physical Examination
After determining the level of obesity in an individual patient, it is essential to determine whether complications such as diabetes, hypertriglyceridemia, and hypertension exist. It is also important to assess an obese patient's willingness and motivation to lose weight. Many obese patients are content being "overweight" and do not view 30 or 50 extra pounds as a problem. In addition, careful assessment of any previous history of weight loss; fac-

tors related to the onset of obesity; details of the patient's current eating habits; emotional well-being; and the patient's weight-losing goals is essential to the success of any treatment program.

Laboratory Tests
- Fasting serum glucose
- Thyroid function tests
- Serum cholesterol and triglycerides

Pathological Findings
Android (male) fat distribution is characterized by fat distributed above the waist. Upper body fat distribution appears to occur by hypertrophy of adipocytes. There is a higher morbidity and mortality associated with upper body than lower body fat distribution. Gynecoid (female) fat distribution is characterized by fat distributed in the lower body such as the buttocks, hips, and thighs. Lower body fat distribution appears to occur by hyperplasia (i.e., differentiation of new fat cells). Because it is easier to reduce the size of fat cells than the number of them, people with a lower body fat distribution often have a harder time losing weight.

- Hyperplasia of adipocytes: Even if weight is lost, the number of fat cells is fixed.
- Hypertrophy of adipocytes: Cell size will return to normal with weight loss.

Imaging
- Generally not necessary for diagnosis
- Dual energy X-ray absorptiometry—to analyze body fat
- Magnetic resonance imaging and computed tomography—to measure regional fat distribution

Other Diagnostic Procedures
- Waist measure—above 35" in women or 40" in men is abnormal
- Waist:hip ratio—to measure abdominal girth (> 0.85 in women and >1.0 in men is abnormal)
- Body-mass index (BMI)—to measure level of obesity (BMI of 20 to 25 is considered normal)
- Weight and height tables from Metropolitan Life Insurance Company—to indicate the weight at which longevity is highest (does not distinguish between obesity and overweight)
- Skinfold thickness measured by skin calipers (triceps, biceps, subscapular, suprailiac)—to estimate total body fat
- Underwater weighing—to calculate fat-free mass and body fat.
- Measure total body water (fixed fat-free mass (FFM) equals water mass/0.73), which is subtracted from total body weight to obtain total body fat.

TREATMENT OPTIONS
Treatment Strategy
Lifelong lifestyle changes (e.g., exercise, behavior modification) and diet modification are necessary to control weight in obese patients. Many obese patients may have consumed more calories than they metabolized in their weight-gaining phase but currently may be eating enough merely to maintain weight gained previously. Health care providers must assess the risks associated with obesity on an individual basis, using the BMI and fat distribution as well as co-morbidities as guides for treatment. Risk assessment may be critical to the process of setting goals and providing motivation. No drug treatment has been shown to be safe and effective for long-term weight loss. Surgical therapies for morbid obesity include gastric bypass (Roux-en-Y procedure), or stapling and liposuction for moderate fat redistribution.

OBESITY
··

CONDITIONS

It is important to enroll family members, especially spouses, in any lifestyle and diet changes that will affect the interactions of the relationship. Family activities such as shopping, cooking, and eating out all have an impact on diet and caloric intake.

Drug Therapies

- Diuretics—for temporary use to reduce water retention; does not reduce adipose tissue stores
- Ephedrine (20 to 60 mg/day) plus caffeine (200 to 600 mg/day)—to transiently increase the basal metabolic rate. (These over-the-counter drugs should not be taken by patients with heart disease, high blood pressure, thyroid disease, diabetes, or an enlarged prostate.)

Complementary and Alternative Therapies

The main thrust of alternative therapy is increasing basal body metabolism and addressing the behavioral component. The bottom line is to expend more calories than are consumed. Most obese people have tried many diets and are frustrated with their lack of success. Alternative therapies can help stabilize blood sugars, promote a custom tailored exercise plan, and treat emotional well being. Mind/body techniques can be helpful, especially in reframing the goal of weight loss to the goal of health. Individual treatment plans addressing family history, personal health risks, and past successes can be important information in designing a plan. It is interesting to note that rates of both obesity and eating disorders are rising rapidly in the United States.

Behavior modification (e.g., keeping a food journal, eating a diet low in total and saturated fats, beginning an exercise program, counseling to change eating and exercise habits) can be effective. Special emphasis should be placed on what has and has not been successful in the past.

NUTRITION

- Protein: While the standard weight loss diet is low protein, high complex carbohydrates, some people will do better with a high protein, low carbohydrate diet. Regular meals that contain protein are important for blood sugar stabilization. In either diet, it is important to use many foods that the patient enjoys. Liberal consumption of oat bran or garlic helps lower lipids slightly. Anecdotally, some people lose weight by eating protein at breakfast, which decreases afternoon or pre-dinner gorging and cravings for sweets.
- Fluid: Six to eight glasses daily of non-sugared, caffeine-free drinks flush toxins, and increase a sense of satiety.
- Fiber: Increasing dietary fiber (e.g., fruits, vegetables, psyllium, chitin, guar gum, glucomannan, gum karaya, and pectin) promotes weight loss by enhancing blood sugar control, reducing the number of calories that are absorbed, and increasing satiety.
- Allergies: Many people find that avoiding allergenic foods (wheat, dairy, soy, eggs, and citrus) allows for diuresis and improved digestion. Other allergic foods may be discovered by using an IgG Elisa food allergy test.
- Multiple vitamin to address any dietary imbalances
- Chromium picolinate (200 to 500 mcg/one to two times per day): claimed to preferentially burn fat, proven to increase insulin sensitivity, stabilize blood sugars. Helpful in those patients with sugar cravings.
- Vitamin C (3,000 to 6,000 mg/day) speeds up metabolism, acts as an anti-inflammatory, and is needed for cholesterol metabolism.
- Essential fatty acids (primrose oil, 2 to 4 g/day; flaxseed oil, 1 to 3 tbsp/day): One study showed reduction in appetite and some weight loss without dieting. Fat cravings may be exacerbated by a fatty acid deficiency.

- Lecithin, choline, methionine: (1 g/day of each) aids proper fat metabolism and decreases fat cravings
- Thiamine: (2.5 mg/day) plays a role in fatty-acid metabolism and may decrease ketone formation, increased ketones may play a role in excessive hunger; in order to avoid imbalance, supplement with a B-complex: B_1 (50 to 100 mg), B_2 (50 mg), B_3 (25 mg), B_5 (100 mg), B_6 (50 to 100 mg), B_{12} (100 to 1,000 mcg), folate (400 mcg/day)
- Kelp (1,000 to 2,000 mg/day, equivalent to 250 to 500 mcg of iodine per day) may aid in weight loss, as it provides nutrients for thyroid functioning.
- L-glutamine (1,000 mg tid) may blunt carbohydrate craving.
- Coenzyme Q10 is important in fatty-acid metabolism, may help break down fat into energy
- 5-Hydroxytryptophan (5-HTP; 100 to 300 mg/day) to reduce food intake by promoting satiety. Acts as an anti-depressant, especially with sleep disturbances
- Fasting: For patients who don't have diabetes, fasting or juice fasting one day a week is helpful to reset the appetite control system.

HERBS

Herbs are generally a safe way to strengthen and tone the body's systems. As with any therapy, it is important to ascertain a diagnosis before pursuing treatment. Herbs may be used as dried extracts (capsules, powders, teas), glycerites (glycerine extracts), or tinctures (alcohol extracts). Unless otherwise indicated, teas should be made with 1 tsp. herb per cup of hot water. Steep covered 5 to 10 minutes for leaf or flowers, and 10 to 20 minutes for roots. Drink 2 to 4 cups/day. Tinctures may be used singly or in combination as noted.

Ma Huang (*Ephedra sinica*) is used to stimulate the sympathetic nervous system in order to burn more fat. It is a constituent of most OTC weight loss products (1 cup tea or 30 drops tincture/day in the morning). Reacts with cardiac glycosides (arrhythmias), MAO-inhibitors (potentiates sympathomimetic effects), and secale alkaloids (hypertension). Patients need to be warned of the side effects and only use ephedra short term (if at all).

A combination of four to six of the following herbs can be taken tid before meals (1 cup tea or 30 drops tincture).

- Peppermint (*Mentha piperita*) carminative, spasmolytic, historically to reduce appetite
- Bladder wrack (*Fucus vesiculosus*) historic use in obesity
- Parsley (*Petroselinum crispum*) diuretic, historic use in gastrointestinal conditions
- Dandelion (*Taraxacum officinale*) diuretic, dyspepsia
- Hawthorne (*Cretaegus oxyacantha*) reduces peripheral vascular resistance, historically a sedative
- St. John's wort (*Hypericum perforatum*) anti-depressant, historically with nerve pain
- Valerian (*Valeriana officinalis*) bitter spasmolytic, sedative
- Milk thistle (*Silybum marianum*) dyspepsia, specifically for liver and gallbladder
- Lavender (*Lavendula officinalis*) carminative, spasmolytic, relaxant
- Gentian (*Gentiana lutea*) carminative, digestive stimulation

HOMEOPATHY

Homeopathic remedies may be of help in treating obesity, but the constitutional remedy for the specific individual should be prescribed by an experienced practitioner.

PHYSICAL MEDICINE

Daily exercise program: exercise is critical to maintaining weight loss. While 20 minutes of aerobic execise a day is ideal, as little as 10 minutes/day can help stabilize blood sugar and thereby reduce cravings. Gentle exercise (walking, yoga, swimming, biking) can increase cardiovascular health without undue stress on joints.

ACUPUNCTURE

Acupuncture can be used to help balance the body's metabolism, stabilize blood sugar, correct digestive disorders, control certain eating disorders, aid in elimination and relieve stress, anxiety and depression that may lead to overeating.

MASSAGE

May be beneficial. By decreasing stress, cortisol is decreased, which will help to stabilize blood sugar and help prevent or treat diabetes.

Patient Monitoring

A good provider–patient relationship is an essential ingredient for a successful treatment program. All obese patients must be monitored for the medical and psychological complications of obesity.

OTHER CONSIDERATIONS

Prevention

Lifestyle changes are the key to successful weight loss in obese patients. Regular exercise and a long-term low-calorie diet can help to raise the basal metabolic rate (the rate at which calories are burned) and reset the set point (the weight the body tries to maintain by regulating the amount of food and calories consumed).

Complications/Sequelae

There is a known increase in morbidity (and mortality) associated with many of the complications of obesity.

- Type II diabetes mellitus (adult-onset diabetes)—rare in individuals with a BMI <22
- Hypertension (blood pressure >160/95 mm Hg)— especially in patients 20% over ideal weight
- Coronary artery disease
- Hypercholesterolemia
- Hypertriglyceridemia as a result of increased insulin resistance and hyperinsulinemia
- Congestive heart failure and sudden death as a result of increased blood volume, stroke volume, cardiac output, and left ventricular end-diastolic volume
- Respiratory problems (e.g., pickwickian syndrome, pulmonary hypertension)
- Circulatory problems, such as varicose veins and venous stasis, which predisposes patients to venous thromboembolic disease
- Endometrial and postmenopausal breast cancer in women, prostate cancer in men, and colorectal cancer in men and women

- Gallbladder disease as a result of increased secretion of biliary cholesterol
- Obstructive sleep apnea as a result of fat accumulation in the tracheopharyngeal area
- Arthritis as a result of excess stress on joints especially of the lower extremities
- Skin problems, such as acanthosis nigricans

Prognosis

Eating and exercise habits are hard to change. Most obese patients have long histories of unsuccessful attempts to lose weight. Approximately 10% to 60% of patients who attempt diet therapy are able to lose at least 20 pounds; however, only between 10% and 20% of patients are able to maintain their weight loss over time. Patients should be told that losing 15 to 20 pounds is often responsible for a 10% to 25% decrease in health risks associated with obesity.

Pregnancy

The complications of obesity can complicate pregnancy, resulting in increased risk for the fetus. Pregnancies in obese women should be considered high risk.

- Gestational diabetes
- Hypertension
- Preeclampsia
- Abnormally large infants resulting in difficult deliveries
- Increase rate of cesarean sections with complications
- Increased incidence of fetal distress and meconium staining

REFERENCES

Balch JF, Balch PA. *Prescription for Nutritional Healing.* 2nd ed. Garden City Park, NY: Avery Publishing; 1997:406–412.

Bartram T. *Encyclopedia of Herbal Medicine.* Dorset, England: Grace Publishers; 1995:315.

Blumenthal M, ed. *The Complete German Commission E Monographs.* Boston, Mass: Integrative Medicine Communications; 1998:125–126, 169–170, 179–181.

Branch Jr WT. *Office Practice of Medicine.* 3rd ed. Philadelphia, Pa: WB Saunders; 1994:1053–1065.

Cangiano C, Ceci F, Cascino A, et al. Eating behavior and adherence to dietary prescriptions in obese adult subjects treated with 5-hydroxytryptophan. *J Clin Nutr.* 1992;56:863–867.

Fauci AS, Braunwald E, Isselbacher KJ, et al., eds. *Harrison's Principles of Internal Medicine.* 14th ed. New York, NY: McGraw-Hill; 1998:454–462.

Gruenwald J, Brendler T, Jaenicke C et al, eds. *PDR for Herbal Medicines.* Montvale, NJ: Medical Economics Company; 1998:779–780, 1022–1024, 1138–1139.

Mowrey DB. *The Scientific Validation of Herbal Medicine.* New Canaan, Conn: Keats Publishing; 1986:277–282.

Murray MT, Pizzorno JE. *Encyclopedia of Natural Medicine.* 2nd ed. Rocklin, Calif: Prima Publishing; 1998:437–446, 680–694.

Nestel PJ, et al. Arterial compliance in obese subjects is improved with dietary plant n-3 fatty acid from flaxseed oil despite increased LDL oxidizability. *Arterioscler Thromb Vasc Biol.* 1997;17:1163–1170.

Uusitupa M. New aspects in the management of obesity: operation and the impact of lipase inhibitors. *Curr Opin Lipidol.* 1999;10:3–7.

Wyngaarden JB, Smith LH Jr, Bennett, JC. *Cecil Textbook of Medicine.* 19th ed. Philadelphia, Pa: WB Saunders; 1992:1162–1169.

■ OSTEOARTHRITIS

OVERVIEW
Definition
Osteoarthritis is characterized by degenerative joint changes that cause pain, tenderness, limited range of motion, crepitus, and inflammation. As many as 90% of individuals over age 40 show degenerative changes radiographically, although not all of these individuals have symptoms. Osteoarthritis is the most common form of arthritis and most frequently affects the articular cartilage and subchondral bones of the hands, knees, hips, and spine. Osteoarthritis is characterized as primary if there is no apparent predisposing cause or secondary if it is associated with an underlying medical condition. Primary osteoarthritis can be localized to one or two joints or generalized to three or more joints. Osteoarthritis affects men and women nearly equally; however, under age 45 men are affected more frequently, and over age 55 women are affected more frequently. Approximately 40 million Americans have osteoarthritis.

Etiology
Primary osteoarthritis appears to be caused by the cumulative effects of repetitive occupational or recreational joint use (with professions such as baseball pitchers, ballet dancers, dock workers), which leads to a destruction of the cartilage when individuals are in their 50s and 60s. Degenerative changes are usually age-related, but may also occur as a result of fractures and other mechanical abnormalities.

There may also be a genetic predisposition. Secondary osteoarthritis is associated with an underlying medical condition (e.g., Wilson's disease, acromegaly, hemochromatosis, hypoparathyroidism), which can often be treated, resulting in a resolution of the osteoarthritis.

Risk Factors
- Increasing age
- Genetic predisposition
- Obesity
- Major trauma
- History of inflammatory joint disease
- Metabolic disorders (e.g., hemochromatosis, acromegaly, calcium pyrophosphate deposition disease [CPPD])
- Congenital bone and joint disorders
- Certain occupations (e.g., baseball players, ballet dancers, dock workers)

Signs and Symptoms
- Morning stiffness or stiffness after inactivity for less than 15 minutes
- Joint pain, worsened by movement and improved with rest (in severe cases, constant pain)
- Soft tissue swelling
- Bony crepitus (crackling noise with movement)
- Bony hypertrophy causing gross deformities (e.g., Heberden's nodules of distal interphalangeal joints)
- Limited range of motion
- Subluxation (incomplete or partial dislocation)

DIFFERENTIAL DIAGNOSIS
- Rheumatoid arthritis
- Septic arthritis
- Claudication
- Bursitis
- Neuropathy
- Osteoporosis
- Metastatic bone disease
- Gout

DIAGNOSIS
Physical Examination
The patient often presents with pain that is localized to one or more joints, especially after exercise or movement. Bony hypertrophy (enlargement) and inflammation (redness, warmth) often accompany the pain. Loss of function and pain at rest usually indicate severe disease. Observe the patient for the extent of deformity and disability.

Laboratory Tests
Most laboratory values are normal, but they are helpful in ruling out other forms of arthritis and possible underlying precipitating causes (e.g., metabolic disorders associated with secondary osteoarthritis).
- Complete blood count (mononuclear cells usually predominate)
- Erythrocyte sedimentation rate (ESR)
- Urinalysis
- Chemistry panel
- Synovial fluid analysis to rule out CPPD, gout, septic arthritis

Pathological Findings
- Irregular loss of cartilage, especially in weight-bearing joints
- Joint space narrowing
- Synovial inflammation (synovitis)
- Bony sclerosis (eburnation)
- Bone cysts
- Increased number of osteophytes (spurs) at joint margins, the radiologic hallmark of osteoarthritis
- Periarticular muscle wasting
- Areas of cartilagenous repair, but inferior repair tissue
- Gross deformity, loose bodies, and subluxation

Imaging
Magnetic resonance imaging (MRI) has replaced computed tomography (CT) scans and myelography for diagnosis and evaluation of osteoarthritis of the spine. MRI is not particularly helpful in evaluating peripheral osteoarthritis.
- X rays—to detect joint space narrowing as cartilage is lost, bony sclerosis, bony cysts, osteophytosis
- Arthroscopy—to diagnose osteoarthritis
- Myelography—to evaluate patients preoperatively

Other Diagnostic Procedures
Radiographic evidence of osteoarthritis is not always symptomatic; the diagnosis is based on clinical findings, history, and radiographic features. Pain and disability may be associated with atrophy of the muscles around the joints; this is especially true of the knee.

TREATMENT OPTIONS
Treatment Strategy
The goals of treatment are individualized to reduce pain, minimize disability, and maintain range of motion and mobility. Many patients with osteoarthritis are not able to perform even the simple activities of daily living (ADLs), such as bathing and dressing. Patients should be told that therapy is palliative not curative.

Drug Therapies
- Aspirin—as needed for inflammation and analgesia, within tolerance
- Acetaminophen (4,000 mg/day)—to reduce pain
- Nonsteroidal anti-inflammatory drugs (NSAIDs)—ibuprofen (Motrin), 1,200 mg/day, and naproxen (Naprosyn), 1,000 mg/day—to reduce pain and inflammation. Approximately 30% of peptic ulcer disease cases in the elderly (over age 65) can be attributed to NSAID use;

in addition, there is some evidence linking NSAIDs with acceleration of the progression of osteoarthritis because they appear to inhibit cartilage repair. However, this is controversial.

- Tramadol (50 to 300 mg/day)—a weak opioid for refractory pain control
- Intra-articular or periarticular glucocorticoids—for symptomatic relief. Oral corticosteroids are contraindicated.
- Capsaicin cream—to reduce pain by depleting nerve endings of substance P

Complementary and Alternative Therapies

The etiology and pathogenesis of osteoarthritis are diverse and somewhat unpredictable. Alternative therapies can help improve joint function and decrease inflammation by providing nutritional, herbal, and lifestyle support.

Exercise that combines muscle strengthening and aerobic conditioning can help improve joint stability and function. Weight loss is essential for overweight patients. Proper body mechanics and rest, when indicated, are important considerations.

NUTRITION

- Reduce pro-inflammatory foods such as refined foods, sugar, saturated fats (meat and dairy products), and omega-6 fatty acids.
- Omega-3 fatty acids reduce inflammation. Increase cold-water fish, nuts, and seeds or supplement with essential fatty acids (such as fish oil, 1,000 to 1,500 mg bid).
- Increase whole grains, vegetables, and legumes.
- Vitamin C (1,000 mg tid to qid) to support the growth and integrity of the cartilage.
- Vitamin E (400 to 800 IU/day) inhibits breakdown of cartilage and stimulates new cartilage formation.
- Vitamin A (5,000 IU/day) or beta-carotene (50,000 IU/day), zinc (20 to 30 mg/day), and selenium (200 mcg/day) are antioxidants that protect cartilage and reduce oxidative damage secondary to inflammation.
- Boron (3 mg/day) helps slow joint degeneration.
- Glucosamine sulfate (500 mg tid) promotes cartilage synthesis and repair of damaged joints. The overall effect is one of increased joint integrity and significant pain relief. Glucosamine sulfate has, in at least some studies, been shown to be more effective than ibuprofen at relieving pain as well as being better tolerated than ibuprofen or other NSAIDs.
- S-Adenosylmethionine (SAM) (1,200 mg/day for 21 days, then tapered to 200 mg/day). SAM stimulates production of cartilage and is a mild analgesic and anti-inflammatory agent. It has only recently become available in the United States.
- Niacinamide (500 to 1,000 mg tid) increases joint mobility and reduces pain. High doses of niacinamide require that liver function tests and serum glucose be monitored periodically.

HERBS

Herbs are generally a safe way to strengthen and tone the body's systems. As with any therapy, it is important to ascertain a diagnosis before pursuing treatment. Herbs may be used as dried extracts (capsules, powders, teas), glycerites (glycerine extracts), or tinctures (alcohol extracts). Unless otherwise indicated, teas should be made with 1 tsp. herb per cup of hot water. Steep covered 5 to 10 minutes for leaf or flowers, and 10 to 20 minutes for roots. Drink 2 to 4 cups/day. Tinctures may be used singly or in combination as noted.

- Hawthorn (*Crataegus oxyacantha*) and bilberry (*Vaccinium myr-*

tillus) are high in flavonoids, especially anthocyanidins and proanthocyanidins, which enhance the integrity of connective tissue. Take 100 to 200 mg dried extract bid to tid.
- Devil's claw (*Harpagophytum procumbens*), yucca (*Yucca bacata*), turmeric (*Curcuma longa*), black cohosh (*Cimicifuga racemosa*), ginger root (*Zingiber officinalis*), boswellia (*Boswellia serrata*), teasel root (*Dipsacus asper*), and meadowsweet (*Filependula ulmaria*) may be combined in equal parts as tea (1 cup tid) or tincture (30 to 60 drops tid) to reduce inflammation and relieve pain.

HOMEOPATHY

An experienced homeopath should assess individual constitutional types and severity of disease to select the correct remedy and potency. For acute prescribing use 3 to 5 pellets of a 12X to 30C remedy every one to four hours until acute symptoms resolve.

- *Arnica montana* for arthritis with sore, stiff joints that are worse in damp, cold weather.
- *Bryonia alba* for arthritic pain that is worse with movement and cold, and is better with heat.
- *Pulsatilla* for wandering arthritis that is worse on initiating movement but is relieved by continued movement. The pain feels worse with heat and better with cold applications.
- *Rhus toxicodendron* for arthritis that is worse on waking in the morning, worse in damp and cold weather or before storms, and worse with exertion. The pains feel better with heat, dry weather, and motion.

PHYSICAL MEDICINE

Contrast hydrotherapy. Alternating hot and cold applications brings nutrients to the site and diffuses metabolic waste from inflammation. The overall effect is decreased inflammation, pain relief, and enhanced healing. If possible, immerse the part being treated. Alternate three minutes hot with one minute cold and repeat three times. This is one set. Do two to three sets/day.

Castor oil pack. Used externally, castor oil is a powerful anti-inflammatory. Apply oil directly to skin, cover with a clean soft cloth (e.g., flannel) and plastic wrap. Place a heat source (hot water bottle or heating pad) over the pack and let sit for 30 to 60 minutes. For best results use three consecutive days.

ACUPUNCTURE

Acupuncture can do much in the way of pain relief, reducing inflammation, and strengthening overall health.

MASSAGE

Therapeutic massage may be beneficial in enhancing joint mobility, increasing circulation, and alleviating pain.

Patient Monitoring

The disability caused by osteoarthritis varies according to the site of the disease; for example, disease of the interphalangeal joints does not cause the limitation of function or pain that is caused by osteoarthritis in a weight-bearing joint. Joint deterioration is not inevitable but appears to be associated with aging and obesity. Although radiographic features of osteoarthritis may progress with age, the progression appears to be gradual, and treatment in some cases appears to slow progression. Patients should be told that while there is no cure, the disability experienced by patients with rheumatoid arthritis is uncommon in patients with osteoarthritis.

Patients should be monitored for the harmful effects of the NSAIDs, such as gastro-intestinal bleeding. Patients should be instructed to examine their stools for changes in color, and have stools monitored periodically for occult blood. In addition, patients should be monitored for renal failure by checking blood urea nitrogen and creatinine levels.

OTHER CONSIDERATIONS
Prevention
Since osteoarthritis appears to be exacerbated by obesity, patients can expect a more benign course if they lose weight.

Complications/Sequelae
GI bleeding and decreased renal function with NSAID and aspirin use

Prognosis
Expect a progressive course to the condition. Joint effusions and joint enlargement occur later in the course of the condition. Most advanced stages include full cartilage loss.

Pregnancy
Most women who become pregnant are normally too young to have primary osteoarthritis; however, if they have an underlying condition with which osteoarthritis is associated (secondary osteoarthritis), they should consult their health care provider concerning the safety of the palliative medications.

REFERENCES
Fauci AS, Braunwald E, Isselbacher KJ et al, eds. *Harrison's Principles of Internal Medicine.* 14th ed. New York, NY: McGraw-Hill, 1998:1935–1941.

Kelly WN. *Textbook of Internal Medicine.* 3rd ed. Philadelphia, Pa: Lippincott-Raven; 1997:1121–1124.

Koopman WJ. *Arthritis and Allied Conditions: A Textbook of Rheumatology.* 13th ed. Baltimore, Md:Williams & Wilkins; 1997:1985–2006.

Lockie A, Geddes N. *The Complete Guide to Homeopathy.* New York, NY: DK Publishing, 1995:154–155.

Morrison R. *Desktop Guide to Keynotes and Confirmatory Symptoms.* Albany, Calif: Hahnemann Clinic Publishing; 1993:38,74,314,326.

Murray MT. *Encyclopedia of Nutritional Supplements.* Rocklin, Calif: Prima Publishing; 1996:336–342, 365–373, 475

Murray MT, Pizzorno JE. *Encyclopedia of Natural Medicine.* 2nd ed. Rocklin, Calif: Prima Health; 1998:695–705.

■ OSTEOMYELITIS

OVERVIEW
Definition
Osteomyelitis is an infection of the bone, caused usually by bacteria but occasionally by fungi. Several forms of osteomyelitis exist. Hematogenous osteomyelitis, which occurs most often in children, generally develops in bones with a good blood supply and rich marrow. Vertebral osteomyelitis begins as a gradually developing back pain. Posttraumatic osteomyelitis commonly occurs in patients with infected prostheses.

Once established in the bone, the infections can spread outward to the adjacent soft tissue, where it causes abscesses. Antibiotics are first line treatment. Unsuccessful treatment can result in chronic osteomyelitis. While often symptom-free for long periods, this condition causes bone pain, recurring infections, and constant or intermittent drainage of pus through the skin. The drainage creates sinus tracts between the bone and the skin. It affects children more than adults.

Etiology
The infection is most commonly *Staphylococcus aureus* but consider other microorganisms such as *Mycobacterium tuberculosis*. It starts in soft tissue adjacent to bone or enters the body from external sources. It reaches the bone via several routes (including the bloodstream, open wounds, surgery on bones) and causes the bone marrow to swell. As it presses against the bone's rigid outer wall, the marrow compresses blood vessels, reducing the supply of blood to the bone or cutting it off entirely. Without treatment, parts of the bone may die. Prosthetic devices may be source of irritation.

Risk Factors
- Open bone fracture
- Bone surgery
- Attachment of metal to a bone
- Kidney dialysis
- Intravenous use of illegal drugs
- Implanted prosthesis
- Foot ulcers
- Diabetes
- Trauma

Signs and Symptoms
Symptoms can be acute or chronic, depending on etiology.
- Intense pain and a sensation of heat at the site of the affected bone
- Tenderness and swelling
- Persistent back pain, unrelieved by rest, heat, or analgesics
- Abscesses in tissue surrounding the painful bone
- Fever, in some cases
- Fatigue, irritability, malaise
- Inflammation, generally localized with or without drainage

DIFFERENTIAL DIAGNOSIS
- Infectious arthritis
- Charcot's joint (neuropathic joint disease)
- Bone tumors
- Cellulitis
- Other systemic infection
- Gout
- Other sources of localized inflammation

DIAGNOSIS
Physical Examination
Patient typically looks sick, particularly children. They report tenderness when palpated above the affected area of the bone. Fever is not necessarily an indictor of osteomyelitis; patients may show minimal fever or no fever. Check patient's TB status. Consider old chest X rays and family history.

Laboratory Tests
Samples of blood, pus, joint fluid and, if necessary, the bone itself serve to diagnose the infection and to identify the bacteria or fungi responsible.
- An elevated white blood cell count typifies osteomyelitis in children, but rarely in adults.
- ESR is typically high in both children and adults, particularly in cases of vertebral osteomyelitis.
- Blood cultures indicate the pathogen that caused infection, most commonly *S. aureus*. Fungal and tubercular infections are almost impossible to diagnose without cultures.

Pathological Findings
Pyogenic bacteria

Imaging
Radionuclide bone scans that use technetium phosphate give positive indications of the condition, but they are less useful when osteomyelitis stems from infected prostheses, because the technetium phosphate accumulates in fracture sites, new bone, overlying areas of cellulitis, and aseptic loosened areas of the prostheses. In these cases, conventional X rays reveal changes. Computed tomography can help define the amount of bone destruction and indicate the presence of complications of the infection, such as abscesses. Magnetic resonance imaging serves to distinguish infection in soft tissue alone from that in the bone.

Other Diagnostic Procedures
- Palpate areas of apparent infection for signs of warmth and tenderness.
- Carry out blood tests for white blood cell count and ESR.
- Perform blood culture to identify cause of infection.
- Biopsy the bone, where necessary, by needle aspiration or open surgery.
- Needle biopsy of the infected bone itself, or open surgical biopsy, is generally required to diagnose vertebral osteomyelitis. Aspiration applies to the intervertebral disk space that appears infected.

TREATMENT OPTIONS
Treatment Strategy
A three-week course of antibiotics forms the first line of treatment of osteomyelitis. Choice of antibiotic depends on identification of the infectious agent. Bed rest should frequently accompany the treatment. Surgery is necessary when detection and treatment of the infection occur too late to halt its spread.

Extended bed rest and immobilization of the affected bones are recommended in conjunction with antibiotics or antimicrobials.

Drug Therapies
Courses of antibiotics lasting several weeks should clear up infections identified early. If diagnostic techniques identify the nature of the infection precisely, antibiotic specific to that infection should be prescribed. Antimicrobials recommended for chronic osteomyelitis and forms of the condition caused by fractures or infections in sites adjacent to the bone.

Oxacillin and nafcillin, effective against *S. aureus*, the most common source of infection, should be given intravenously to children when tests do not reveal a precise cause of infection. Start intravenously; change to oral administration within days. For children, intravenous administration should start as soon as the patient is diagnosed and hospitalized.

In cases of osteomyelitis that result from foot ulcers or diabetes, medical treatment should include such antimicrobial agents as cefoxitin, cefotetan, or a combination of aminoglycoside and clindamycin.

Surgical Procedures

Surgery may be necessary when osteomyelitis is identified late. Surgery is an option more often in cases of chronic osteomyelitis, osteomyelitis caused by fractures and infections in soft tissue contiguous to the bone, and that originating in foot ulcers. Surgery can drain abscesses adjacent to the infected bone and remove all dead tissue and bone. Antimicrobial or antibiotic therapy should follow all cases of surgery.

Infected prostheses should be surgically removed, following several weeks of antibiotic treatment, to permit a new prostheses to be implanted at the same time.

Complementary and Alternative Therapies

Osteomyelitis requires immediate medical attention. Alternative therapies can be used concurrently to stimulate the immune system and optimize recovery.

NUTRITION

For overall immune support and to enhance healing, use the following.
- Vitamin C (1,000 mg tid to qid)
- Zinc (30 to 50 mg/day for 1 month, then reduce to 25 mg/day)
- Vitamin E (400 to 800 IU/day)
- Vitamin A (10,000 to 15,000 IU/day) (avoid in pregnancy or women considering becoming pregnant)
- Acidophilus (1 to 3 capsules/day, or 1 to 5 million organisms/day)— to prevent antibiotic-induced diarrhea and yeast infections

HERBS

Ascertain a diagnosis before pursuing treatment. Herbs may be used as dried extracts (capsules, powders, teas), glycerites, or tinctures (alcohol extracts). Unless otherwise indicated, teas should be made with 1 tsp. herb per cup of hot water. Steep covered 10 to 60 minutes and drink 2 to 4 cups/day. Tinctures may be used singly or in combination.

Use one or more herbs from each category. Make a tincture using equal parts. Take 15 to 20 drops tid to qid.
- Immune support: coneflower *(Echinacea angustifolia)*, lomatium *(Lomatium dissectum)*, astragalus *(Astragalus membranaceus)*
- Anti-microbials: goldenseal *(Hydrastis canadensis)*, barberry *(Berberis vulgaris)*, garlic *(Allium sativum)*
- Analgesics: valerian *(Valeriana officianalis)*, St. John's wort *(Hypericum)*
- For improved circulation: ginkgo biloba *(Ginkgo folium)* 120 mg bid

Alteratives are traditionally known as blood cleansers. Use the following herbs in combination as an infusion. Drink 2 to 3 cups a day.
- Red clover *(Trifolium pratense)*, burdock root *(Arctium lappa)*, yellow dock *(Rumex crispus)*, yarrow *(Achillea millefolium)*, cleavers *(Galium aparine)*, and licorice root *(Glycyrrhiza glabra)*. Licorice is contraindicated in hypertension.

Topical applications aid abscess healing: Make a paste from the powders of goldenseal root *(Hydrastis canadensis)* and slippery elm *(Ulmus fulva)*. Apply as needed.

HOMEOPATHY

An experienced homeopath should assess individual constitutional types and severity of disease to select the correct remedy and potency. For acute prescribing use 3 to 5 pellets of a 12X to 30C remedy every one to four hours until acute symptoms resolve.
- *Arnica* for use after trauma or injury, especially with bruising or a bruised, "beat up" feeling
- *Ledum* for puncture wounds that lead to abscesses, especially if they feel better with cold applications
- *Silica* for enlarged, suppurating glands or abscesses, especially in depleted individuals

ACUPUNCTURE

May help stimulate immune response, reducing inflammation, pain, edema, and fever.

Patient Monitoring

Careful monitoring is essential during antibiotic and antimicrobial treatments. Look for rapid responses—24 to 48 hours—to the administration of antibiotics and antimicrobials.

OTHER CONSIDERATIONS

Prevention

Avoid strenuous activity or weight-bearing exercise until healed.

Complications/Sequelae

Patients who do not receive treatment soon after the onset of infection and those with immune deficiency may develop chronic osteomyelitis. Infections that spread from foot ulcers to bones in the foot often involve several types of bacteria and are difficult to cure by antibiotics alone. Abcess may occur. Cure may require removal of the infected bone. Massage is contraindicated in osteomyelitis due to concerns of spreading infection.

Prognosis

Most patients respond well with no long-term problems. Chronic osteomyelitis can be quiescent for months to years.

REFERENCES

Berkow R, ed. *Merck Manual of Diagnosis and Therapy.* 16th ed. Rahway, NJ: Merck Research Laboratories; 1992.

Dambro MR. *Griffith's Five-Minute Clinical Consult.* New York, NY: Lippincott, Williams and Wilkins; 1998.

Larson DE, ed. *Mayo Clinic Family Health Book.* 2nd ed. New York, NY: William Morrow and Company; 1996.

■ OSTEOPOROSIS

OVERVIEW

Definition

Osteoporosis is a progressive skeletal disease characterized by a reduction of bone mass, which can cause bone fractures and deformity. Osteoporosis affects over 25 million people each year—80% of them are women. Osteoporosis may be secondary to chronic liver or kidney disease, arthritis, or malabsorption diseases, or caused by prolonged use of corticosteroids. Rare forms include idiopathic or juvenile osteoporosis. Most common is postmenopausal osteoporosis, where accelerated bone resorption is the result of reduced estrogen, and involutional osteoporosis, characterized by the imbalance of bone resorption and formation.

Etiology

Most osteoporosis is caused by increasing bone resorption that is due to decreased estrogen and progesterone production following menopause. Additionally, women lose about 15% to 30% of their bone mass on average between the age of 30 and menopause. Decreased testosterone in aging men accelerates osteoporosis as well. Other causes include the following.

- Glucocorticoid and heparin use
- Juvenile osteoporosis—a rare disorder affecting children ages 8 to 14; self-limited, usually resolves in four to five years
- Renal failure
- Hyperthyroidism
- Hyperparathyroidism
- Hyperadrenalism
- Upper intestinal surgery
- Calcium, magnesium, and micronutrient deficiencies
- Low vitamin D intake and/or insufficient sunlight exposure
- Cushing's syndrome
- Anorexia nervosa
- Chronic heparin therapy
- Hypogonadism
- Exogenous glucocorticoid administration
- Thyrotoxicosis
- Hyperprolactinemia
- Low calcium absorption (low gastric acidity)
- Long term diuretic or antibiotic use

Risk Factors

- Women
- Age—25% of women at age 60 and 50% of women at age 75 have vertebral fractures
- Caucasians, Asians more prone to the condition
- Thin women with history of amenorrhea and low body fat
- Smokers; regular alcohol or caffeine drinkers; people whose diets are high in phosphates or low in calcium
- Family history
- Depression—effects hypothalamic–pituitary axis
- Sedentary lifestyle or prolonged immobilization
- Nulliparous women
- Heavy metal toxicity
- Chronic broad-spectrum antibiotic use (destroys normal intestinal flora, leading to malabsorption of nutrients and decreased vitamin K production)

Signs and Symptoms

- Periodontal disease—an early warning sign
- Loss of height
- Hunched back/spinal deformity
- Back pain
- Fracture without trauma

DIFFERENTIAL DIAGNOSIS

- Malignancies (e.g., multiple myeloma, lytic metastatic carcinoma)
- Osteomalacia
- Paget's disease
- Skeletal hyperparathyroidism

DIAGNOSIS

Physical Examination

The patient with more established disease may have deformities (e.g., dorsal spine, wrist) and typically appears hunched. Distribution of weight changes in women with thickening in the waist and upper back and thinning of the hips and breasts. Periodic measurements demonstrate loss of height.

Laboratory Tests

- Urinary test—indicates breakdown of bone products
- Tests identify secondary osteoporosis or underlying illnesses but are normal with primary osteoporosis (e.g., serum calcium, phosphate, creatinine, or thyroid)
- Serum assays of bone-specific alkaline, phosphatase, osteocalcin, and C-terminal procollagen peptides help monitor effectiveness of therapy
- Thyroid function usually normal in primary forms of osteoporosis

Pathological Findings

- Decrease in cortical bone thickness and in the size and number of trabeculae of the cancellous bone
- Biochemical indices of bone absorption are usually increased
- Lack of estrogen decreases bone density, sensitivity of bone to parathyroid hormone (PTH), intestinal calcium absorption, and increases calcitonin and osteoclastic bone resorption
- Decrease in 1,25-dihydroxy vitamin D (calcitriol, the active form of vitamin D) causes lower calcium absorption and hypercalciuria

Imaging

Radiographic screening for bone loss may determine the need for treatment. Early changes of intervertebral space and accentuation of cortical plates, and late changes plate fractures and intervertebral compression and deformity will be seen on X ray. Current bone density does not predict future bone density.

- Quantitative digital radiography
- Single-photon absorptiometry of the forearm
- Dual-photon absorptiometry of the 2nd to 4th lumbar vertebrae
- Quantitative computerized tomography and dual energy X ray absorptiometry—measure cortical and trabecular bone and total body bone mineral density levels

Other Diagnostic Procedures

Risk factors are not diagnostic. Physical evidence may be present, and most compelling. The most reliable diagnostic tools are imaging techniques.

TREATMENT OPTIONS

Treatment Strategy

A variety of pharmacological, hormonal, and phytomedicinal treatments slow the effects of osteoporosis. Imaging must be repeated to insure adequate treatment is being given. Diet and exercise, with caution as to any increased mechanical stresses, may be essential to maximize treatment plans.

Drug Therapies

- Estrogen—slows bone loss and fractures by decreasing resorption, increasing intestinal calcium absorption, and lowering renal calcium excretion. It cannot increase bone growth. Bone loss resumes when treatment is stopped. Many practitioners advocate treating with the lowest dosage possible. Estrogen use may be correlated with an increased risk of breast cancer and uterine cancer, abnormal blood clotting, and gall bladder disease.
- Conjugated equine estrogens (e.g., Premarin 0.625 mg/day)—most commonly used form; can cause metabolic changes in the liver; contraindicated with obesity, smokers, high blood pressure or cholesterol, varicose veins
- Estradiol—most easily metabolized delivering estrogen directly into the blood stream; available in transdermal patch (e.g., Estraderm, 1.0 mg/day of estradiol, 0.05 mg/day of transcutaneous estrogen)
- Progesterone—enhances bone formation; may potentiate estrogen, allowing for lower estrogen dosage (e.g., medroxyprogesterone, 2.5 to 5 mg/day; progesterone, 0.625 mg, such as Provera); eliminates uterine cancer caused by estrogen therapy
- Calcium—1,000 mg/day for postmenopausal women on estrogen and 1,500 mg/day for those not on estrogen; preserves cortical bone mass, no effect on trabecular; taken early in life aids prevention; better absorption if taken with meals; no known adverse effects up to 2,500 mg/day
- Bisphosphonates (e.g., alendronate 10 mg/day)—alternative to estrogen; increases bone density and reduces fractures (take upon rising with eight ounces water; do not lie down or eat for 1/2 hour); side effects: esophagitis, especially with overdose, abdominal pain, heartburn, nausea
- Selective Estrogen Receptor Modulators (SERMS)—estrogen-like effects with reduced breast cancer risk (e.g., raloxifene, 60 mg/day); side effects: hot flashes or blood clotting (uncommon)
- Vitamin D—increases intestinal absorption of calcium and osteoblast activity (800 IU/day); take with calcium

Complementary and Alternative Therapies

Nutritional and herbal support, in particular, can slow bone loss and enhance absorption of essential vitamins and minerals. Weight-bearing exercise and stress management should be part of any program.

NUTRITION

- Eliminate refined foods, alcohol, caffeine, tobacco, sugar, phosphorous (carbonated drinks and dairy products), aluminum-containing antacids, and high amounts of sodium chloride (table salt) and animal proteins. Sea salt, soy sauce, tamari, or kelp granules are preferable to table salt because they contain many other trace minerals.
- Increase intake of complex carbohydrates, essential fatty acids (cold-water fish, nuts, and seeds), legumes, and soy. Soy, although is has less calcium than dairy, contains calcium that is more readily absorbed. Isoflavones found in soy may inhibit bone resorption and increase bone building activity. Studies suggest 30 to 50mg/day of soy to optimize bone mass.
- Dark berries (blueberries, blackberries, cherries, and raspberries) contain anthocyanidins which help to stabilize collagen found in bone matrix.
- Mineral-rich foods, especially non-dairy sources of calcium, should be increased. Although dairy is a good source of calcium, it also contains high amounts of phosphorus which inhibits calcium absorption and increases urinary calcium excretion. Non-dairy sources of calcium, although lower in actual calcium content, may provide more bioavailable calcium. Particularly beneficial are almonds, black-strap molasses, dark leafy greens, sardines, sea vegetables, soy, tahini, prunes, and apricots.
- Calcium citrate or aspartate (1,000 to 1,500 mg/day) are the preferred forms of calcium. Calcium requires sufficient stomach acid (HCl) for adequate digestion and this is often low in the elderly. Calcium carbonate buffers stomach acid and may not be the best form. Oyster shell calcium may contain heavy metals or other contaminants and is poorly digested.
- Magnesium (200 mg bid to tid) enhances calcium uptake, is necessary for hormone production, and is cardioprotective. Magnesium may actually increase bone density and may be a more important factor than calcium.
- Vitamin K (100 to 500 mcg/day) is needed to produce osteocalcin, a protein found in bone tissue that increases calcium uptake. Vitamin K is produced by intestinal flora that may become depleted after antibiotic use. Foods high in vitamin K include dark leafy greens. Vitamin K may interfere with coumadin.
- Boron (0.5 to 3 mg/day) is needed for calcium absorption. Women at high risk for breast cancer should use boron with caution as some studies suggest that it increases estrogen metabolism.
- Manganese (5 to 20 mg/day) is a trace mineral that is often low in osteoporosis. It helps produce the collagen matrix onto which calcium is laid down.
- Zinc (10 to 30 mg/day) is needed for normal bone growth. Copper (1 to 2 mg/day) is often low in osteoporosis and is needed with long-term zinc supplementation.
- Chromium (200 to 600 mcg/day) should be used in patients with unstable blood sugars. Poor glucose regulation is associated with increased bone loss.
- Essential fatty acids (1,000 mg bid) are necessary for hormone production.
- B-complex (50 to 100 mg/day) reduces the effects of stress. Elevated cortisol levels from stress increase bone loss. Folic acid (1 to 5 mg/day), B_6 (100 mg/day), and B_{12} (1,000 mcg/day) should be taken for hyperhomocysteinemia which interferes with collagen crosslinking.

HERBS

Herbs are generally a safe way to strengthen and tone the body's systems. As with any therapy, it is important to ascertain a diagnosis before pursuing treatment. Herbs may be used as dried extracts (capsules, powders, teas), glycerites (glycerine extracts), or tinctures (alcohol extracts). Unless otherwise indicated, teas should be made with 1 tsp. herb per cup of hot water. Steep covered 5 to 10 minutes for leaf or flowers, and 10 to 20 minutes for roots. Drink 2 to 4 cups/day. Tinctures may be used singly or in combination as noted.

- Some herbs have phyto-estrogen/progesterone properties. These can be used to support hormone levels which may minimize bone loss. Natural progesterone may be more effective at increasing bone density than synthetic progestins. It is important to note that natural progesterone may not be strong enough to offset the risk of uterine cancer posed by conventional estrogen replacement therapy. Other herbs can be used in osteoporosis to provide minerals and enhance digestion. Liver support is also recommended to help with metabolizing hormones and normalizing ratios. Chaste tree *(Vitex agnus-cactus)* and black cohosh *(Cimicifuga racemosa)* help to normalize pituitary function. Chaste tree must be taken long term (12 to 18 months) for maximum effectiveness. Standardized black cohosh is commercially available as Remifemin (one tablet bid) through Enzymatic Therapies. Use only under physician supervision with hormone therapy. Re-evaluate after six months of use.

- Black cohosh, licorice *(Glycyrrhiza glabra)*, and squaw vine (Mitchella repens) help to balance estrogen levels. Licorice is contraindicated in hypertension.
- Chaste tree, wild yam *(Dioscorea villosa)*, and lady's mantle *(Alchemilla vulgaris)* help to balance progesterone levels.
- Tea brewed from nettles is high in calcium.
- Kelp *(Nereocystis luetkeana)*, bladderwrack *(Fucus vesiculosis)*, oatstraw *(Avena sativa)*, nettles *(Urtica diocia)*, and horsetail *(Equisetum arvense)* are rich in minerals and may also help support a sluggish thyroid.
- Milk thistle *(Silybum marianum)*, dandelion root *(Taraxacum officinalis)*, vervain *(Verbena hastata)*, and blue flag *(Iris versicolor)* support the liver and may help restore hormone ratios. Taken together as a tea before meals, they are slightly bitter and enhance digestion.
- Topical applications of natural progesterone may vary in the amount of active hormone they contain. Usually composed of wild yam, the natural progesterone sterols are converted in the laboratory to make them bioavailable. Progesterone levels should be checked periodically with natural progesterone use. Natural estrogen, an 80-10-10 mixture of estriol, estradiol, and estrone also works well as a substitute for premarin in doses of 2.5 to 10 mg/day. It may have less cancerogenic activity for the uterus and breast.

HOMEOPATHY
An experienced homeopath should assess individual constitutional types and severity of disease to select the correct remedy and potency. For acute prescribing use three to five pellets of a 12X to 30C remedy every one to four hours until acute symptoms resolve. A combination of homeopathic tissue salts such as *Calcarea carbonicum, Calcarea fluoricum,* and *Silica* may be helpful. Take as directed.

ACUPUNCTURE
Acupuncture may be helpful in treating concurrent pathologies such as hormone imbalances and poor blood sugar control.

MASSAGE
Therapeutic massage may be beneficial in enhancing circulation and increasing overall sense of well-being.

Patient Monitoring
Patients with identified osteoporosis, after stabilization, are seen yearly to assess and adjust therapy as necessary.

OTHER CONSIDERATIONS
Fluoride treatments increase cancellous bone at the expense of cortical bone (i.e., increases both bone density and bone fragility).

Prevention
Thirty percent of women will not be identified with osteoporosis without bone density tests, allowing initiation of treatment. Prevention of bone fracture is key to osteoporosis treatment. Weight bearing exercise before onset with proper diet and increased calcium and vitamin D, as well as many factors listed under "Drug Therapies" are actually preventive measures. Osteoporosis is thought to be a teenagers' disease as this is when its onset takes root. Adequate calcium/magnesium intake and proper nutrition, coupled with weight-bearing exercise throughout childhood and adulthood are the primary preventative measures for osteoporosis.

Complications/Sequelae
Fractures, the most common complication, are a significant cause of debility and death (e.g., 25% within a year of a hip fracture). Acute and chronic pain can be disabling, and result in associated depression and anxiety.

Prognosis
Osteoporosis will progress more rapidly without estrogen treatment but will progress regardless. Nearly 1.5 million fractures result each year, often causing chronic care status or death. In most patients, stabilization of skeletal manifestations and reduced pain should be predicted with aggressive therapy.

Pregnancy
The etiology is unknown for osteoporosis appearing during or just after pregnancy.

REFERENCES
Chapuy MC, Arlot ME, Duboeuf F, et al. Vitamin D_3 and calcium to prevent hip fractures in elderly women. *N Engl J Med.* 1992;327:1637–1642.

Chesney RW. Vitamin D. Can an upper limit be defined? *J Nutr.* 1989;119:1825–1828.

Fauci AS, Braunwald E, Isselbacher KJ et al, eds. *Harrison's Principles of Internal Medicine.* 14th ed. New York, NY: McGraw-Hill; 1998.

Feskanich D, Weber P, Willett WC, Rockett H, Booth SL, Colditz GA. Vitamin K intake and hip fractures in women: a prospective study. *Am J Clin Nutr.* 1999;69:74–79.

Gaby AR. *Preventing and Reversing Osteoporosis: Every Woman's Essential Guide.* Rocklin, Calif: Prima Publishing; 1995.

Goroll AH, ed. *Primary Care Medicine.* 3rd ed. Philadelphia, Pa: Lippincott-Raven; 1995.

Werbach M. *Nutritional Influences on Illness.* New Canaan, Conn: Keats Publishing; 1988:331–340.

■ OTITIS MEDIA

OVERVIEW

Definition

Otitis media is an infection with inflammation of the middle ear, common in infants and children under the age of 7, due to their immature immune systems and short, relatively horizontal, easily blocked eustachian tubes. Fluid may persist in the middle ear for weeks or months, causing at least some temporary hearing loss at an important time for language and cognitive development. Acute otitis media (AOM) is usually accompanied by a viral upper respiratory infection. Otitis media with effusion (OME) refers to the presence of fluid in the middle ear. It is generally asymptomatic and is often diagnosed during well-child examinations.

Etiology

Blockage and swelling of eustachian tubes resulting from one or more of the causes listed below.

- Respiratory infection
- Allergies
- Tobacco smoke or other environmental irritants
- Infection and/or hypertrophy of the adenoids
- Sudden increase in pressure such as during an airplane descent
- Drinking while lying on the back
- Excess mucus and saliva produced during teething

The bacteria that cause most cases of acute otitis media are *Streptococcus pneumoniae* (25% to 35% of cases), *Haemophilus influenzae* (20% to 25%), *Moraxella catarrhalis* (10% to 15%), *S. pyogenes*—Group A (2% to 3%) and *Staphylococcus aureus* (1%). Some of the remaining cases are caused by viral infections. For OME, the most common causes are *H. influenzae* (15%), *M. catarrhalis* (10%), *S. pneumoniae* (7% and rising), and *S. aureus* (3%). Otitis media is not contagious in itself, but may be precipitated in multiple children by a contagious respiratory infection.

Risk Factors

- Youth
- Male gender
- Winter
- Bottle feeding, especially lying on the back
- Pacifier use
- Group day care
- Allergies
- Exposure to tobacco smoke
- Sibling(s) prone to ear infections
- Enlarged adenoids or chronic sinusitis
- Native American or Inuit background
- Down syndrome
- Craniofacial anomalies
- Compromised immune system
- Children who have their first episode before 6 months of age are more likely to repeat

Signs and Symptoms

- Pain in the ear, usually worse at night; crying, irritability, disrupted sleep
- Feeling of "fullness," sometimes manifested in an infant as head-shaking
- Difficulty hearing
- Fever
- Vomiting and diarrhea
- Bulging eardrum

An episode of AOM may be followed by several weeks of OME.

DIFFERENTIAL DIAGNOSIS

- Otitis externa
- "Ear-pulling" due to itching or teething

DIAGNOSIS

Physical Examination

Otoscopic examination reveals a red, opaque, bulging eardrum in AOM. Spontaneous perforation may occur. In OME, clear or yellow fluid may be seen through a translucent eardrum. A retracted eardrum (short arm of the malleus is prominent, long arm of the malleus appears shortened) indicates a partial vacuum in the eustachian tube, inhibiting drainage. Alternatively, an eardrum distended by fluid or fixed air pressure from a blocked eustachian tube obscures the malleus. Pneumatic otoscopy may reveal decreased mobility of the eardrum, indicating fluid or fixed air pressure in the middle ear.

Laboratory Tests

Tympanocentesis (needle aspiration) may be employed to identify the bacteria involved in the infection, but this painful and invasive test should be done only when (1) the child is seriously ill or has not responded to standard antibiotic treatment and (2) precise identification of the disease-causing organism is essential.

Imaging

Otomicroscope for detailed visualization if necessary. If AOM is complicated by mastoiditis, computed tomography (CT) should be used to detect intracranial complications such as epidural abscess.

Other Diagnostic Procedures

Take patient history with special attention to recent respiratory infections or other causative factors. Examine eardrums using a pneumatic otoscope. Take temperature in both ears. A difference of more than 0.5° C is suggestive of AOM in the warmer ear.

A tympanometer (a soft rubber probe with an airtight seal) is placed in the ear canal, emits a sound, and measures its reflection, thus calculating the amount of the sound that is transmitted to the middle ear. This transmission is lower than normal in the fluid-filled ear.

An audiometer or other formal hearing test may be employed to discern any hearing loss, especially as a complication of chronic infection.

TREATMENT OPTIONS

Treatment Strategy

Many acute otitis media cases are self-limiting. However, delaying treatment requires follow-up visits for monitoring, and complications can be significant. Therefore, antibiotics are standard treatment.

Drug Therapies

AOM: First-line treatment is amoxicillin (Amoxil, 500 mg orally qid for 7 to 10 days), or azithromycin (Zithromax) if penicillin allergy is present. Second-line treatment is amoxicillin-clavulanate (Augmentin, 500 mg orally qid for 7 to 10 days) or cefuroxime axetil (Ceftin, 500 mg orally bid for 7 to 10 days). Parents should be reminded of the importance of completing the course. Combine with pain relief measures such as acetaminophen and/or ibuprofen.

OME: Begin with observation alone, or with antibiotics. Administer a hearing test if the condition is not resolved within 6 to 12 weeks. Guidelines advise treating with either antibiotics or myringotomy with tympanostomy tube insertion if fluid and a 20-dB hearing loss are present after 12 weeks.

Tube insertion is recommended if OME is still present four to six months after initial diagnosis.

Complementary and Alternative Therapies

A large percentage of otitis media are self-limiting. Nutritional support, herbs, and homeopathic remedies are gentle ways to reduce recurrences and alleviate pain and acute infection.

Otitis media with effusion (OME) has a strong association with allergies. Suspect an allergic component if the child's first otitis occured before the age of 6 months, at or near the introduction of solid food or formula, or infections are recurrent and/or accompanied by eczema, asthma, or other atopic conditions. The following guidelines pertain to both AOM and OME unless otherwise indicated.

NUTRITION

Eliminate all food allergens from the diet. The most common allergenic foods are dairy, soy, citrus, peanuts, wheat, fish, eggs, corn, and tomatoes. An elimination/challenge trial may be helpful in uncovering sensitivities. Remove suspected allergens from the diet for two weeks. Re-introduce foods at the rate of one food every three days. Watch for reactions which may include gastrointestinal upset, mood changes, flushing, and exacerbation of symptoms. A rotation diet, in which the same food is not eaten more than once every four days, may be helpful in recurrent OME.

Essential fatty acids are anti-inflammatory and support immune function. Children should be supplemented with cod liver oil or other fish oils (1/2 to 1 tsp./day). Vitamin C (100 to 250 mg bid to tid) enhances immunity and decreases inflammation. Vitamin C from rose hips or palmitate is citrus-free and hypoallergenic.

HERBS

Herbs are generally a safe way to strengthen and tone the body's systems. As with any therapy, it is important to ascertain a diagnosis before pursuing treatment. Herbs may be used as dried extracts (capsules, powders, teas), glycerites (glycerine extracts), or tinctures (alcohol extracts). Unless otherwise indicated, teas should be made with one teaspoon herb per cup of hot water. Steep covered 5 to 10 minutes for leaf or flowers, and 10 to 20 minutes for roots. Drink two to four cups/day. Tinctures may be used singly or in combination as noted.

Herbal eardrops may be effective at reducing infection, pain, and fluid accumulation. Note: Eardrops are contraindicated if perforation of the tympanic membrane is suspected. An ear oil from mullein flower (*Verbascum thapsus*) and garlic (*Allium sativum*) has pain reduction and antimicrobial effects. For otitis with pain, include one of the following oils: St. John's wort (*Hypericum perforatum*), Indian tobacco (*Lobelia inflata*), or monkshood (*Aconitum napellus*). Place three to five drops in ear bid to qid. Note that monkshood is toxic if taken internally.

Internal treatment should include one or more of the following:
- Coneflower (*Echinacea angustifolia, purpurea,* and *pallida*) may be taken as tincture or glycerite, 20 drops tid to qid. For chronic otitis, consider the following herbs that support the lymphatics and mucus membranes. Eyebright (*Euphrasia officinalis*), cleavers (*Galium aparine*), marigold (*Calendula officinalis*), and elderberry (*Sambucus canadensis*) may be combined in a tea (two to four ounces tid), tincture (10 to 20 drops tid), or glycerite (20 drops tid).

HOMEOPATHY

An experienced homeopath should assess individual constitutional types and severity of disease to select the correct remedy and potency. For acute prescribing use three to five pellets of a 12X to 30C remedy every one to four hours until acute symptoms resolve.
- *Aconite* for otitis that comes on suddenly after exposure to cold or wind; child has bright red ears and high fever
- *Belladonna* for sudden onset of otitis with great sensitivity and pain
- *Chamomilla* for otitis with intense irritability, especially with teething

PHYSICAL MEDICINE

A hot pack applied to ear and side of neck may relieve pain. Blanche one-half of an onion, wrap in cheesecloth and apply hot to ear. The sulphur bonds in the onion will be soothing. May also use a hot water bottle or a sock filled with raw rice and heated.

Craniosacral therapy may be effective in enhancing lymph flow.

MASSAGE

Gentle massaging of the neck may assist lymph flow.

Patient Monitoring

Patient should return if AOM does not improve within 48 to 72 hours. Recheck within two to four weeks to ensure that infection has cleared and determine extent, if any, of effusion. Children with OME should be rechecked every four to six weeks until the fluid resolves, with special attention to detecting any retraction pocket ("pouch") in the eardrum that could lead to accumulation of dead skin cells (cholesteatoma). Tubes should be checked two to three weeks after insertion and every six months thereafter.

OTHER CONSIDERATIONS

Prevention

Reduction of environmental factors such as exposure to tobacco smoke and respiratory infections. Breast feeding reduces incidence of AOM. Xylitol-sweetened chewing gum helps prevent ear infections by inhibiting *Streptococcus.* Prophylactic antibiotics may be prescribed for children who are particularly prone to otitis media. Adenoidectomy has a modest benefit in reducing the frequency of recurrent ear infections in patients for whom more conservative measures have not been successful. The *S. pneumonial* vaccine is becoming increasingly important, but current versions are not particularly effective before 2 years of age; a preparation effective in children as young as 3 months old is under investigation. The *H. influenzae* (Hib) vaccine does not protect against the "nontypeable" *Haemophilus* species that causes ear infections. Conservative introduction of solid foods as child is weaning may help prevent otitis and allergic conditions. If there is a strong family history of allergies or atopic conditions and/or if the child's immunity has been compromised in infancy, delay the introduction of highly allergenic foods until 1 year or older.

Complications/Sequelae
- Hearing loss, usually temporary
- Failure of perforation in eardrum to close, requiring repair
- Chronic purulent otitis media from external bacteria entering via perforation
- External eczematoid otitis, from drainage via perforation
- Facial paralysis from pressure on nerve
- Ossicular discontinuity, requiring surgical correction
- Cholesterol granuloma, requiring surgical removal

- Labyrinthitis, requiring early treatment to preserve hearing
- Mastoiditis
- Meningitis
- Brain abscess or empyema
- Cholesteatoma, a dangerous complication that can result in bone and tissue destruction

Serious complications have become less common with the use of antibiotics. However, physicians must be on guard for resistant organisms.

Prognosis

Symptoms of AOM should improve within 48 to 72 hours. It tends to resolve quickest in older children, during the summer, in mild cases, and in children without significant prior history of ear infections. OME that does not resolve within a few months with conservative treatment should be treated more aggressively.

REFERENCES

Bitnun A, Allen UD. Medical therapy of otitis media: use, abuse, efficacy and morbidity. *J Otolaryngol.* 1998;27(suppl 2):26–36.

Bizakis JG, Velegrakis GA, Papadakis CE, Karampekios SK, Helidonis ES. The silent epidural abscess as a complication of acute otitis media in children. *Int J Pediatr Otorhinolaryngol.* 1998;45:163–166.

Cohen R, Levy C, Boucherat M, Langue J, de la Rocque F. A multicenter, randomized, double-blind trial of 5 versus 10 days of antibiotic therapy for acute otitis media in young children. *J Pediatr.* 1998;133:634–639.

Gehanno P, Nguyen L, Barry B, et al. Eradication by ceftriaxone of streptococcus pneumoniae isolates with increased resistance to penicillin in cases of acute otitis media. *Antimicrob Agents Chemother.* 1999;43:16–20.

Kruzel T. *The Homeopathic Emergency Guide.* Berkeley, Calif: North Atlantic Books; 1992:243–245.

Reichenberg-Ullman J, Ullman R. Healing otitis media through homeopathy. 1996. Available at www.healthy.net/library/articles/rbullman/ottis.htm.

Uhari M, Kontiokari T, Koskela M, Niemela M. Xylitol chewing gum in prevention of acute otitis media: double-blind randomised trials. *Br Med J.* 1996;313:1180–1184.

Wright E.D, Pearl AJ, Manoukian JJ. Laterally hypertrophic adenoids as a contributing factor in otitis media. *Int J Pediatr Otorhinolaryngol.* 1998;45:207–214.

■ PARKINSON'S DISEASE
OVERVIEW
Definition

Parkinson's disease is a chronic, progressive disorder of the central nervous system (CNS) characterized by gait difficulty, postural instability, rigidity, and tremor due to the loss of dopaminergic neurons in the substantia nigra, which leads to dopamine depletion. Parkinson's disease is the most common form of parkinsonism and is classified as idiopathic or primary. Rate of occurrence is higher in later life (age 50 and above; average age of onset, 60); 5% to 10% of patients are under the age of 40, and 5% of all patients have a familial history of the disease. The disease affects men and women equally. The other major subtypes of parkinsonism are listed below.

- Postencephalitic parkinsonism
- Drug-induced parkinsonism
- Striatonigral degeneration
- Arteriosclerotic parkinsonism
- Toxin-induced parkinsonism
- Parkinsonism-dementia complex of Guam

Etiology

A combination of oxidative damage, environmental toxins, genetic predisposition, and accelerated aging have been identified as the most likely etiologic factors. True etiology is unknown.

Risk Factors

- Environmental factors or toxicants (such as pesticides and viruses)
- Family history of parkinsonism (due to a mutant alpha synuclein gene)
- Endogenous neurochemicals (free radicals)
- Normal age-related wearing away of dopamine-producing neurons

Signs and Symptoms

- Tremor, most present unilaterally; increases with stress and improves with rest
- Rigidity
- Bradykinesia; creates gait disturbance and postural abnormalities
- Poor balance
- Walking problems
- Blepharospasm

Secondary symptoms may include the following.

- Memory loss
- Sleep disturbances
- Stooped posture
- Ocular abnormalities
- Constipation or incontinence through dysautonomia
- Dementia in 20% of patients
- Speech, breathing, and swallowing problems

DIFFERENTIAL DIAGNOSIS

- Essential (benign, familial) tremor
- Shy–Drager syndrome (multiple system atrophy)
- Progressive supranuclear palsy
- Wilson's disease
- Huntington's disease
- Hallervorden–Spatz syndrome
- Alzheimer's disease
- Creutzfeldt–Jakob disease
- Depression
- Diffuse Lewy body disease
- Olivopontocerebellar atrophy
- Post-traumatic encephalopathy

DIAGNOSIS
Physical Examination

Patient exhibits consistent presence of tremors and one or more of the other physical symptoms, including relatively immobile face with widened palpebral fissures, infrequent blinking, and fixity of facial expression; seborrhea of the scalp and face is common.

Laboratory Tests

There are no objective tests for Parkinson's disease.

Pathological Findings

The presence of Lewy bodies are considered the hallmark of the disease but can be identified only at autopsy.

Imaging

Neuroimaging techniques hold promise in providing markers for the disease. PET can quantify activity of the dopamine system by measuring activity of the dopamine transporter (DAT). MRI can be used to rule out a mass lesion in the brain, multiple but clinically silent cerebral infarcts, or normal pressure hydrocephalus.

Other Diagnostic Procedures

- As this is a neurodegenerative disease that is treatable, a therapeutic response to levodopa should confirm the diagnosis.
- Clinician interview and observation assesses symptoms and degree of severity. A careful patient history, such as the Schwab and English Activities of Daily Living Scale, can be used to confirm diagnosis and severity of symptoms.
- Evaluate for substance abuse and other medical conditions.

Several standardized instruments can help in assessment and determination of appropriate treatment.

- Activities of Daily Living (ADL) Scale
- NYU Parkinson Disease Disability Scale
- Hoehn and Yahr Scale
- Columbia University Scale
- Cornell-UCLA Scale
- Webster Scale
- University of British Columbia Scale

TREATMENT OPTIONS
Treatment Strategy

Depending on the type, number, and severity of symptoms, treatment options include the following.

- Pharmacotherapy
- Surgery (e.g., cryothalamotomy and pallidotomy)
- Exercise to improve mobility and physical, occupational, or speech therapy as required

Drug Therapies

- Levodopa (L-3,4-dihydroxyphenylalanine; 25/100 mg increased gradually to 25/250 mg; tid for both), a dopamine precursor, is transformed into dopamine by nerve cells; most effective for bradykinesia and rigidity; side effects include severe nausea and vomiting, low blood pressure, involuntary movements, restlessness.
- Carbidopa is used in combination with levodopa; available in combined form as Sinemet (25/100 or 50/200 mg); prevents levodopa from being metabolized until it reaches the brain; allows for smaller doses of levodopa and reduces levodopa's side effects.
- Selegiline (deprenyl) inhibits enzyme monoamine oxidase B (MAO-B), which metabolizes dopamine in the brain; prolongs response to levodopa by protecting dopamine-producing neurons from toxic effect;

side effects include nausea, orthostatic hypotension, insomnia; contraindicated for patients taking fluoxetine and meperidine.

- Anticholinergics such as benztropine (Cogentin; 0.5 to 2 mg tid) and biperiden (Akineton; 1 to 3 mg qid) block action of acetylcholine; used when symptoms are mild and before Sinemet; side effects include dry mouth, constipation, urinary retention, hallucinations, memory loss, blurred vision, and confusion.
- Amantadine (110 mg bid) potentiates the release of endogenous dopamine; side effects include restlessness, confusion, skin rashes, edema, disturbances of cardiac rhythm); may be combined with anticholinergics
- Dopamine antagonists such as bromocriptine (Parlodel; 2.5 to 10 mg tid) and pergolide (Permax; 1 mg tid) activate dopamine receptors; taken alone or with Sinemet.
- Catechol-O-methyltransferase (COMT) inhibitors such as tolcapone (Tasmar) increase availability of levodopa in the brain; can be taken with levodopa

Complementary and Alternative Therapies

CAM therapies do not take the place of pharmaceutical treatment. They may, however, provide some relief of symptoms and slow the progression of the disease. The primary focus is decreasing oxidation. Hair analysis may be useful to determine if there is heavy metal toxicity.

NUTRITION

- Essential fatty acids are anti-inflammatory. Dietary manipulation includes reducing animal fats and increasing fish. A mix of omega-6 (evening primrose, black currant, borage, pumpkin seed) and omega-3 (flax seed and fish oils) may be most optimum (2 tbsp. oil/day or 1,000 to 1,500 mg bid).
- Anti-oxidants vitamin C (1,000 mg tid), vitamin E (400 to 800 IU/day), and the trace mineral selenium (200 mcg) may slow progression of Parkinson's, and are often found in a complex together. Other antioxidants that are often recommended are alpha-lipoic acid, grape seed extract, and pycnogenol.
- Vitamin B_6 (10 to 100 mg/day) may help with symptom control, but should be given with zinc (30 mg/day) to counteract B_6's ability to interfere with l-dopa metabolism.
- A vitamin B complex is helpful.
- Manganese: Excessive exposure increases the risk of Parkinson's.
- Amino acids: Low protein diets may help control tremors. However, D-tyrosine (100 mg/kg/day) increases dopamine turnover. Patients with Parkinson's may be deficient (since the major source is meats, dairy, and eggs), and supplementation may be beneficial.
- Glutathione: antioxidant, found in low levels in patients with Parkinson's. (200 mg bid)
- Choline increases brain function; thus, various forms are recommended including lecithin, phosphatidyl choline, and DMAE. (Dimethylaminoethanol), which stimulates the production of choline.
- Neurotransmitters made from amino acids such as glutamic acid and GABA (Gamma-aminobutyricacid) often are used in treating Parkinson's.

HERBS

Herbs are generally a safe way to strengthen and tone the body's systems. As with any therapy, it is important to ascertain a diagnosis before pursuing treatment. Herbs may be used as dried extracts (capsules, powders, teas), glycerites (glycerine extracts), or tinctures (alcohol extracts). Unless otherwise indicated, teas should be made with 1 tsp. herb per cup of hot water. Steep covered 5 to 10 minutes for leaf or flowers, and 10 to 20 minutes for roots. Drink 2 to 4 cups/day. Tinctures may be used singly or in combination as noted.

- Gotu kola *(Centella asiatica):* traditionally used as a CNS stimulant, with historic use in Parkinson's. One cup tea bid, or 30 to 60 drops tincture bid
- Ginkgo *(Ginkgo biloba):* circulatory stimulant, increases cerebral vascular sufficiency and antioxidant (as a supplement 120 mg/day)
- Hawthorn *(Crataegus oxyacanthus):* circulatory stimulant, antioxidant (2 to 5 g/day)
- Herbs specific to the liver such as milk thistle, globe artichoke, and bupleurum provide liver support and reduce free radical damage.
- Nervine herbs such as St. John's wort, skullcap, oats, and lemon balm help support the structure of the nervous system.

HOMEOPATHY

An experienced homeopath should assess individual constitutional types and severity of disease to select the correct remedy and potency. For acute prescribing use 3 to 5 pellets of a 12X to 30C remedy every one to four hours until acute symptoms resolve. For chronic prescribing use 30C 5 pellets once or twice daily.

- *Argentum nitricum* for ataxia, trembling, awkwardness, painless paralysis
- *Causticum* for Parkinson's with restless legs at night, contractures, especially when patient prefers wet, rainy weather
- *Mercurius vivus* for Parkinson's that is worse at night, especially with panic attacks
- *Plumbum metallicum* for Parkinson's, especially with a history of arteriosclerosis
- *Zincum metallicum* for Parkinson's with great restless, especially with depression

PHYSICAL MEDICINE

Chelation therapy with I.V. EDTA may be effective if the Parkinson's is due to heavy metal toxicity or environmental toxins.

ACUPUNCTURE

May be helpful, particularly for the tremor associated.

MASSAGE

May help with increasing circulation, decreasing muscle spasm, and increasing the overall sense of well-being.

Patient Monitoring

Patients receiving pharmacological therapy must be closely monitored for drug effectiveness, side effects, and adjustments. Concomitant medical conditions and their pharmacological therapies may influence the treatment of Parkinson's; these conditions include glaucoma, heart disease, high blood pressure, and stomach/intestinal diseases. Psychotherapy can help reduce anxiety and depression; however, medications for anxiety and depression may worsen symptoms of Parkinson's disease in some patients.

OTHER CONSIDERATIONS

Prevention

There are no known ways to prevent or avoid Parkinson's disease. Early use of selegiline may delay progression of symptoms. Avoid drugs known to cause tardive dyskinesia.

Complications/Sequelae

Patients over 60 may have increased side effects from certain pharmacological interventions such as anticholinergic drugs, including hallucinations, confusion, and psychosis.

Prognosis

Parkinson's disease is irreversible and progressive. Choosing the proper pharmacotherapies can improve symptoms, especially in the early to mid stages.

REFERENCES

Bartram T. *Encyclopedia of Herbal Medicine*. Dorset, England: Grace Publishers; 1995:328–329.

Blumenthal M, ed. *The Complete German Commission E Monographs*. Boston, Mass: Integrative Medicine Communications; 1998:138.

Fauci AS, Braunwald E, Isselbacher KJ et al, eds. *Harrison's Principles of Internal Medicine*. 14th ed. New York, NY: McGraw-Hill; 1998.

Morrison R. *Desktop Guide to Keynotes and Confirmatory Symptoms*. Albany, Calif: Hahnemann Clinic Publishing; 1993:32–33, 111–113, 244–247, 303–304, 401–403.

National Institutes of Health. Accessed at www.ninds.nih.gov/healinfo/disorder/parkinso/pdhtr.htm on January 16, 1999.

Parkinson's Disease Foundation. Accessed at www.pdf.org/ on January 16, 1999.

Perry TL, Godin DV, Dansen S. Parkinson's disease: a disorder due to nigral glutathione deficiency. *Neurosci Lett*. 1982;33:305–310.

Thierney LM Jr, McPhee SJ, Papadakis MA. *Current Medical Diagnosis & Treatment 1999*. 38th ed. Stamford, Conn: Appleton & Lange; 1999.

Werbach, M. *Nutritional Influences on Illness*. New Canaan, Conn: Keats Publishing; 1988:346–349.

■ PEPTIC ULCER

OVERVIEW

Definition

Peptic ulcers are lesions of the mucosal lining of the stomach and the duodenum which penetrate the muscularis mucosae, and are called gastric ulcers (GU) and duodenal ulcers (DU), respectively. They may also affect the distal esophagus as a result of chronic gastrointestinal reflux. Duodenal ulcers are the most common. Often a chronic disorder, peptic ulcers affect about 10% of the population. They are declining in Western countries as a whole but are increasing in the elderly population. Recent work in understanding the pathogenesis of acid-peptic disease, and the role of *Helicobacter pylori (H. pylori)* have resulted in refined and more effective treatments.

Etiology

- *H. pylori* damages gastric mucosa; implicated in 90% of duodenal and 70% to 80% of gastric ulcers; unknown concurrent pathogenic factors are present as only 15% to 20% of those infected with *H. pylori* will actually develop ulcers
- Nonsteroidal anti-inflammatory drug (NSAID) ingestion causes overproduction of gastric acid unrelated to the presence of *H. plyori*. It causes up to 25 % of GUs. Acid and pepsin are corrosive agents that overpower the gastroduodenal's defense system's ability to protect the epithelium with adequate mucin and to regenerate the lining quickly.
- Zollinger–Ellison syndrome—gastric-acid stimulating pancreatic islet cell tumors; causes steatorrhea-type diarrhea and gastric acid hypersecretion.
- Rarely, gastrinoma.

Risk Factors

- Age (elderly)
- Smokers are twice as likely to develop and more likely to die from ulcer, possibly from decreased pancreatic bicarbonate secretion, diminishing mucosal defense.
- Genetics or higher rate of familial *H. pylori* infection
- Blood type O
- Chronic stress may exacerbate but not cause ulcers. Acute stress in life-threatening and surgical emergencies can cause ulcers.
- Increased risk with chronic pulmonary disease, renal transplants, chronic renal failure, alcoholism, systemic mastocytosis, and hyperparathyroidism
- NSAID, alcohol, and caffeine use are loosely associated.

Signs and Symptoms

DUs:

- Epigastric pain (often burning or gnawing) occurs after eating and lasts from one to three hours; relieved by milk and antacids; episodic with periods of remission.
- Increased pain, vomiting of blood, tarry or red stools, and significant weight loss are indications of perforation, gastric outlet obstruction, or hemorrhaging.

GUs:

- Epigastric pain (gnawing, burning) is sometimes relieved by food or antacids and sometimes not.
- Vomiting and nausea (without obstruction)
- Antral gastritis from *Helicobacter pylori*
- Nonsteroidal anti-inflammatory drug (NSAID)–induced ulcers—sometimes painless

DIFFERENTIAL DIAGNOSIS

- Non-ulcer dyspepsia
- Crohn's disease
- Ulcerative colitis
- Gastric carcinomas
- Gastritis
- Pancreatitis
- Gall bladder disease

DIAGNOSIS

Physical Examination

- Epigastric tenderness in the midline or slightly to the right of the midline
- Hyperactive bowel sounds upon auscultation
- Rigid, board-like abdomen and surrounding tenderness

Laboratory Tests

All antral biopsy specimen tests are accurate for detection of *H. pylori*. Serological tests are accurate for patients previously untreated for *H. pylori*.

- Serum antibodies to IgG and IgA are elevated with *H. pylori*; enzyme-linked immunosorbent assay (ELISA) test is commonly used.
- Giemsa and Warthin-Starry stains identify *H. pylori*.
- Rapid urease test—antral mucosal biopsy specimens identify *H. pylori* with 90.2% sensitivity and 100% specificity.

Pathological Findings

- Increase in gastric acid secretion after *H. pylori* infection, returning to normal within a year
- Basal levels and serum gastric levels from eating are increased
- Somatostatin deficiency

Imaging

- Barium radiographic examination is commonly used for initial diagnosis.

Other Diagnostic Procedures

- Diagnosis for ulcers typically begins with barium radiographic or endoscopic examination.
- Urea breath test identifies *H. pylori* with 100% specificity and sensitivity.
- Establish location of ulcer, as gastric ulcers develop into malignancies in up to 5% of cases, requiring absolute diagnosis and documented resolution.
- Endoscopy is more accurate than X ray, detects greater detail, deformities, and hemorrhaging, and is better for carcinoma detection.

TREATMENT OPTIONS

Treatment Strategy

The treatment approach as determined by the National Institutes of Health (NIH) Consensus Development Conference advocates the eradication of *H. pylori* with concurrent use of antisecretory agents for first occurrences and recurrence. Unless recurrent bleeding is life threatening, maintenance with antisecretory agents may not be warranted. Gastric ulcers generally take longer and are more difficult to heal than duodenal ulcers.

Drug Therapies

- For *H. pylori* "triple therapy" is considered most efficacious, but variations of the regimen are commonly used. *H. pylori* that is resistant to antibiotics, especially to the macrolides and imidazoles (e.g., metronidazole), is problematic worldwide. Side effects of triple therapy include diarrhea and pseudomembranous colitis. Two-week treatment may be combined with H_2-receptor antagonists and proton-pump inhibitors:

- Amoxicillin 500 mg qid OR tetracycline 500 mg bid
- Bismuth subsalicylate (Pepto-Bismol) 2 tablets qid
- Metronidazole 250 mg tid
- H_2-receptor antagonists (e.g., cimetidine 400 mg bid, ranitidine 150 mg bid) inhibit gastric acid secretion; serious side effects are infrequent (e.g., reversible hepatitis with ranitidine).
- Proton-pump inhibitors (e.g., omeprazole 20 mg/day, lansoprazole 30 mg/day) decrease gastric acid secretion.
- Antacids are used for relief of symptoms and to aid healing of ulcers.
- Sucralfate (1,000 mg qid) acts to protect the ulcer crater with an adherent coating; acts only locally (not absorbed); used for up to two months.
- Colloidal bismuth compounds (e.g., bismuth subcitrate 240 mg bid, bismuth subsalicylate 500 mg qid) can eradicate *H. pylori* and are also antacids. They increase gastric mucosal secretion of prostaglandins, bicarbonate, and glycoprotein mucus.
- Surgery is indicated for perforation, gastric outlet obstruction, hemorrhaging, and patients who do not respond to medical treatments. To be considered in the aggressive treatment of GU if other therapies fail.

Complementary and Alternative Therapies
Nutritional and herbal support help to heal gastric mucosa, fight infection, and reduce recurrence. In addition, mind-body techniques such as meditation, progressive muscle relaxation, tai chi, yoga, and stress management may alleviate symptoms and enhance healing.

NUTRITION
- Avoid dairy, caffeine, alcohol, and sugar. Coffee, even decaffeinated, should be eliminated because of irritating oils.
- Eliminate any known food allergens. Food allergies can be tested for using an IGG ELISA food allergy panel, or by an elimination diet.
- Include sulphur-containing foods such as garlic, onions, broccoli, cabbage, brussel sprouts, and cauliflower in the diet. Sulphur is a precursor to glutathione that provides antioxidant protection to the gastric mucosa. N-acetyl cysteine (200 mg bid) is also a precursor to glutathione.
- Bananas contain potassium and plantain, both of which yield benefits.
- Acidophilus (one capsule with meals) can help normalize bowel flora and inhibit *H. pylori*.
- Essential fatty acids (1,000 to 1,500 mg bid to tid) reduce inflammation and inhibit the growth of *H. pylori*.
- Vitamin C (1,000 mg tid) decreases nitrosamines which are linked to stomach cancer and inhibits *H. pylori*.
- Zinc (30 to 50 mg/day) enhances healing.
- Vitamin E (400 IU/day) enhances healing and provides antioxidant protection.
- Vitamin A (50,000 IU/day for two weeks followed by 10,000 to 25,000 IU/day) for longer term maintenance.
- Glutamine (500 to 3,000 mg tid) promotes healing of ulcers. Cabbage juice (1 quart/day) is high in glutamine, although it may initially be irritating.

HERBS
Herbs are generally a safe way to strengthen and tone the body's systems. As with any therapy, it is important to ascertain a diagnosis before pursuing treatment. Herbs may be used as dried extracts (capsules, powders, teas), glycerites (glycerine extracts), or tinctures (alcohol extracts). Unless otherwise indicated, teas should be made with 1 tsp. herb per cup of hot water. Steep covered 5 to 10 minutes for leaf or flowers, and 10 to 20 minutes for roots. Drink 2 to 4 cups/day. Tinctures may be used singly or in combination as noted.

- DGL (deglycyrrhizinated licorice), 250 mg qid 15 to 20 minutes before meals and one to two hours after last meal, increases local circulation and facilitates healing of the gastric mucosa. This preparation has most of the hypertensive factor of licorice root removed and is therefore safe to take long-term and in cases of hypertension.
- Quercetin (250 to 500 mg before meals) or catechin (500 to 1,000 mg before meals) are bioflavonoids that reduce gastric inflammation and reactions to irritants and allergies.
- Powders of slippery elm (*Ulmus rubra*) and marshmallow root (*Althea officinalis*) may be taken singly or together, one tsp. bid to tid to decrease inflammation and encourage healing.
- A soothing carminative tea taken before meals can reduce spasm and normalize digestion. Combine equal parts of three to six of the following herbs in a tea and sip before meals. Chamomile (*Matricaria recutita*), lemon balm (*Melissa officinalis*), catnip (*Nepeta cateria*), passionflower (*Passiflora incarnata*), meadowsweet (*Filependula ulmaria*), peppermint (*Mentha piperita*), and valerian (*Valeriana officinalis*).

For *H. pylori*:
- Bismuth subcitrate (120 mg qid for eight weeks) may be helpful in eradicating *H. pylori* and reducing recurrence of peptic ulcer disease. It is poorly absorbed, which decreases the likelihood of side effects; however, it is associated with neurotoxicity if used long-term. Combining it with barberry (*Berberis vulgaris*), goldenseal (*Hydrastis canadensis*), and/or Oregon grape (*Berberis aquifolium*) may potentiate its antimicrobial effects. Take one or more in tincture form, 30 to 60 drops tid.

HOMEOPATHY
An experienced homeopath should assess individual constitutional types and severity of disease to select the correct remedy and potency. For acute prescribing use 3 to 5 pellets of a 12X to 30C remedy every one to four hours until acute symptoms resolve.
- *Argentum nitricum* for abdominal distention with belching and violent splinter-like pains that radiate across abdomen. May crave sweets.
- *Arsenicum album* for ulcers with intense burning pains and nausea. Patient cannot bear the sight or smell of food and is thirsty but only drinks in small sips.
- *Lycopodium* for bloating after eating with burning that lasts for hours. Patient is hungry soon after eating and wakes hungry and irritable in the morning.

ACUPUNCTURE
Acupuncture may be helpful in reducing the effects of stress and improving overall digestive function.

MASSAGE
Therapeutic massage can alleviate stress and increase sense of well-being.

Patient Monitoring
- Patient compliance with triple therapy is often problematic.
- GUs that do not heal in two to three months are potentially signs of malignancy, requiring endoscopic examination.

OTHER CONSIDERATIONS
Prevention
- Smoking increases the risk of developing ulcers and delays ulcer healing.
- Eliminate food allergies or foods that continually produce dyspeptic symptoms.

- Eat a fiber-rich diet.
- If symptomatic, avoid milk and caffeine, as they stimulate gastric acid secretion.
- Limit use of NSAIDs, aspirin, and cortisone drugs.
- Alcohol damages the gastric mucosal barrier.

Complications/Sequelae
- Increased pain, vomiting of blood, tarry or red stools, and significant weight loss are indications of perforation, gastric outlet obstruction, or hemorrhaging, usually requiring surgery.
- 2% to 5% of suspected GUs are actually ulcerated adenocarcinomas, or GUs that will develop into malignancies.

Prognosis
- Mortality rates for ulcers complicated by perforation, gastric outlet obstruction, or hemorrhaging can be as high as 23%, especially in the elderly.
- DUs—60% recur in a year, 80% to 90% within two years; but only 5% to 15% recur after treatment that eradicates *H. pylori*

Pregnancy
- Amoxicillin—preferred drug
- Tetracycline—U.S. FDA rating D, drug to be avoided during pregnancy; positive evidence of fetal risk for pregnancy and lactation
- Bismuth compounds—no FDA rating but has warnings; high doses and prolonged use contraindicated
- Metronidazole—contraindicated in first trimester; with caution after first trimester; carcinogenic and adverse effects for lactation
- Nutritional guidelines and herbal support are safe in pregnancy. The effects of high doses of bioflavonoids in pregnancy are unknown. Do not use bismuth subcitrate in pregnancy.

REFERENCES
Blumenthal M, ed. *The Complete German Commission E Monographs*. Boston, Mass: Integrative Medicine Communications; 1998:427, 432.
Fauci AS, Braunwald E, Isselbacher KJ et al, eds. *Harrison's Principles of Internal Medicine*. 14th ed. New York, NY: McGraw-Hill; 1998.
Kruzel T. *The Homeopathic Emergency Guide*. Berkeley, Calif: North Atlantic Books; 1992:134–137.
Murray M, Pizzorno JE. *Encyclopedia of Natural Medicine*. 2nd ed. Rocklin, Calif: Prima Publishing; 1998:522–523.
Sabiston DC, ed. *Textbook of Surgery*. 15th ed. Philadelphia, Pa: WB Saunders; 1998.

■ PERICARDITIS

OVERVIEW

Definition

Pericarditis encompasses all the numerous disorders of the pericardium. The pericarditis disease processes fall into three categories:

- Acute pericarditis: inflammation of the pericardium (sometimes with effusion) with numerous etiologies
- Pericardial effusion or pericardial tamponade: increased intrapericardial pressure from effusion of the pericardia causing hemodynamic compromise
- Constrictive pericarditis or chronic pericardial disease: pericardium thickening and fibrosis, usually resulting from chronic inflammation

Pericardial effusion and constrictive pericarditis can occur together (effusive-constrictive pericarditis). The condition is common in adolescents and young adults, with males affected more than females. Pericarditis and pericardial effusion are common manifestations of AIDS. Pericarditis is common in end-stage renal failure.

Etiology

Acute pericarditis and pericardial effusion are idiopathic, or include:

- Viral—coxsackie, echo, adenovirus, Epstein-Barr, measles, mumps, influenza, infectious mononucleosis, poliomyelitis, varicella, hepatitis B, cytomegalovirus
- Bacterial—haemophilus (notably children), staphylococcus, streptococcus, pneumococcus, salmonella, meningococcus, Lyme disease, legionella, mycoplasma
- Fungal—candida, histoplasmosis, Aspergillus, Nocardia
- Parasitic—protozoal
- Drug-induced—procainamide, hydralazine, anticoagulant, nicotinic acid, bleomycin, phenytoin, minoxidil, mesalamine
- Neoplastic (especially common in patients older than 50)—breast, lung, lymphoma, leukemia, melanoma, mesothelioma
- Mycobacterium tuberculosis
- Connective tissue disease—systemic lupus erythematosus, rheumatoid arthritis, rheumatic fever, scleroderma, polyarteritis (nodosa), acute rheumatic fever
- Acquired immunodeficiency syndrome (AIDS)
- Cardiac trauma or rupture
- Metabolic disease—hemodialysis, uremia, myxedema, cholesterol pericarditis, chylopericardium
- Radiation
- Myocardial infarction
- Dressler's syndrome
- Aortic dissection
- Sarcoidosis
- Pancreatitis
- Inflammatory bowel disease
- Amyloidosis

Constrictive pericarditis results from pericardial thickening and fibrosis, either long after acute bacterial, fungal, viral, neoplastic, or uremic pericarditis or from chronic inflammation.

Risk Factors

- Chest trauma
- Exposure to viral, bacterial, fungal or parasitic pathogens

Signs and Symptoms

Acute pericarditis:

- Chest pain (often sudden, usually sharp, generally retrosternal with radiation to the trapezial ridge)
- Pain intensified by lying down, coughing, and deep breathing, eased by sitting up and leaning forward
- Breathing splinted
- Fever, malaise, flushing
- Myalgia
- Odynophagia
- Anorexia
- Anxiety

Pericardial effusion:

- Dyspnea
- Cyanosis
- Relative hypotension
- Tachycardia
- Altering consciousness

Constrictive pericarditis:

- Dyspnea
- Distension of jugular veins
- Peripheral edema
- Pulmonary congestion
- Fatigue
- Abdominal swelling
- Acute myocardial infarction
- Pneumonia
- Pulmonary emboli
- Aortic dissection
- Pneumothorax
- Cholecystitis
- Pancreatitis

DIAGNOSIS

Physical Examination

See Signs and Symptoms

Laboratory Tests

Acute pericarditis:

- Blood count and cultures
- Viral and fungal serologies
- Antistreptolysin-O (ASO) titer
- Cold agglutinins
- Heterophile test
- Thyroid function test
- Blood urea nitrogen (BUN)
- Creatinine
- Connective tissue disease screens
- Pericardial effusion: pericardial fluid analysis
- Will see leukocytosis with increased erythrocyte sedimentation rate (ESR)
- Possible elevated creatine kinase (CK)
- Possible elevated lactate dehydrogenase (LDH)
- Possible elevated serum glutamic-oxaloacetic (SGOT)

Pathological Findings

- Acute inflammation of pericardium

Imaging

- Chest X ray: small pleural effusion with transient infiltrates
- Chest CT scan or MRI: calcified or thickened pericardium

Other Diagnostic Procedures

If pericardial effusion is suspected, explore the patient history for viral and flulike illnesses, trauma, and chronic hemodialysis.

• Electrocardiogram
• Echocardiogram
• Right heart catheterization
• Pericardiocentesis
• Pericardial biopsy

TREATMENT OPTIONS

Treatment Strategy

Outpatient treatment is possible, but hospitalization is often appropriate until the etiology or possible complications are known, to rule out myocardial infarction and to watch for cardiac tamponade. Patients with acute significant pericardial effusion should be hospitalized.

Drug Therapies

For idiopathic causes, aspirin and nonsteroidal anti-inflammatory therapy are generally suitable. Corticosteroids may be prescribed for short-term use. Avoid anticoagulants (hemopericardium risk).

• Aspirin—650 mg every four hours for two weeks; standard contraindications, precautions, and interactions
• Ibuprofen—400 to 600 mg every six hours for two weeks
• Indomethacin—25 to 50 mg every six to eight hours for two weeks
• Colchicine—0.6 to 1.2 mg/day
• Azathioprine, prednisone—60 mg/day for two to three days (if other drugs are ineffective)

Surgery may be needed for purulent pericarditis, uremia, and neoplasm etiologies, ineffective drug therapy, chronic acute pericarditis. Pericardial drainage may be needed with cardiac tamponade and hypotension.

Complementary and Alternative Therapies

Alternative therapies may have benefit as supportive treatments for some of the causes of pericarditis. Homeopathics could be tried in addition to drug therapies. The relief from symptoms can be quite dramatic.

NUTRITION

• Vitamin C (1,000 mg tid) may help stabilize mast cells and decrease inflammation. It also aids in fighting infection, and is an anti-oxidant. Vitamin C is depleted in infections and inflammatory conditions.
• Coenzyme Q10 (50 mg bid) is an important anti-oxidant; it may help prevent heart muscle damage and speed recovery.
• Consider sodium restriction for patients with constrictive pericarditis.
• If pericarditis is of viral origin supplement with vitamin A (300,000 IU/day for 3 days).
• Flax oil (3 g bid) decreases inflammation of pericardium.
• Avoid saturated fats, alcohol, and sugars, which can lead to increased inflammation and lowered immune function.
• Consume at least 5 servings of fruits and vegetables per day. These foods are anti-inflammatory and protect the heart.

HERBS

Herbs are generally a safe way to strengthen and tone the body's systems. As with any therapy, it is important to ascertain a diagnosis before pursuing treatment. Herbs may be used as dried extracts (capsules, powders, teas), glycerites (glycerine extracts), or tinctures (alcohol extracts). Unless otherwise indicated, teas should be made with 1 tsp. herb per cup of hot water. Steep covered 5 to 10 minutes for leaf or flowers, and 10 to 20 minutes for roots. Drink 2 to 4 cups/day. Tinctures may be used singly or in combination as noted.

• Hawthorn (Crataegus oxyacantha) decreases capillary permeability, stabilizes collagen, anti-oxidant, increases cardiac contractility, anti-

atherosclerotic, anti-hypertensive (mild ACE inhibitor) with very low toxicity. Dose is 60 drops tincture tid, 1 tsp. berries steeped for 10 minutes in hot water, or 100 to 250 mg tid as a supplement.
• Linden (Tilia cordata) is used for hypertension with nervous tension, may be useful adjunctive treatment where there is anxiety. Dose is one tsp. dried blossoms/cup hot water tid or 60 drops tincture tid.
• Blue monkshood (Aconitum napellus) has been described as an herbal remedy for pericarditis without significant effusion. CAUTION: As this herb can be highly toxic, even fatal, it is not recommended unless prescribed by an experienced health care provider.
• If pericarditis is of viral origin recommend echinacea 500 mg or 60 drops of tincture 6 to 8 times per day.

HOMEOPATHY

An experienced homeopath should assess individual constitutional types and severity of disease to select the correct remedy and potency. For acute prescribing use 3 to 5 pellets of a 12X to 30C remedy every one to four hours until acute symptoms resolve.

• Aconite for sudden, sharp pains accompanied by anxiety (especially fear of dying) and restlessness
• Spongia tosta for the sensation that the chest will explode, anxiety, faintness, sweating; patient may be flushed
• Cactus grandiflorus for the feeling that there is a band around the chest or a great weight on the chest; palpitations; feels better in the open air and worse at night

ACUPUNCTURE

Can be very helpful in decreasing inflammation, enhancing immune response, and regulating cardiac function.

Patient Monitoring

Re-evaluate symptoms and cardiac status in two weeks. Consider follow-up chest X ray and electrocardiogram after four weeks. Follow-up advised with recurrence of symptoms.

OTHER CONSIDERATIONS

Prevention

If patient is overweight, weight loss is recommended.

Complications/Sequelae

• Pericardial tamponade
• Noncompressive effusion
• Right-side heart failure

Prognosis

Course depends on cause and complications, although pericarditis generally is self-limiting, and symptoms and inflammation resolve in two to four weeks. A small percentage of acute pericarditis patients experience recurrence within months. Constrictive pericarditis is gradually progressive.

REFERENCES

Andreoli TE, Bennett JC, Carpenter CCJ. Cecil Essentials of Medicine. 3rd ed. Philadelphia, Pa: WB Saunders; 1993:110–114.
Dambro MR. Griffith's 5-Minute Clinical Consult–1999. Baltimore, Md: Lippincott Williams & Wilkins; 1999:792–793.
Fleming T, Gruenwald J, Brendler T, Jaenicke C, eds. PDR for Herbal Medicines. Montvale, NJ: Medical Economics Company; 1998:606–608.
Stein JK, ed. Internal Medicine. 4th ed. St. Louis, Mo: Mosby-Year Book; 1994:248–252.
Stoller JK, Ahmad M, Longworth DL, eds. The Cleveland Clinic Intensive Review of Internal Medicine. Baltimore, Md: Williams & Wilkins; 1998:759–760.

■ PERTUSSIS
OVERVIEW
Definition
Pertussis is a disease reported since the 1500s. Pertussis, meaning intense or violent cough, is a highly communicable, bacterial infection of the respiratory system. The gasping inspiratory sounds, heard mostly in young children, give it its common name, whooping cough. Patients are contagious for three weeks, with an incubation period of one to two weeks. Before a vaccine for pertussis was developed in 1948, it was the leading cause of death from communicable disease for children under age 14 in the United States. Worldwide reduction in the use of the vaccine in recent years has caused an increase in incidence of pertussis.

Etiology
Bordetella pertussis and *B. parapertussis,* small gram-negative coccobacilli, are the infectious organisms that produce pertussis in humans. Aerosol droplets are usually spread from the cough of infected patients. The bordetella organism adheres to the cilia of the epithelial cells lining the mucosa of the respiratory tract, producing the pertussis toxin, causing local tissue reaction, and eventually systemic illness.

Risk Factors
- Lack of immunization to pertussis
- Exposure to infected person(s)

Signs and Symptoms
After an incubation period of 5 to 20 days, there are three phases (catarrhal, paroxysmal, and convalescent) each with its own signs and symptoms.
Catarrhal phase (one to two weeks):
- Upper respiratory tract infection; often indistinguishable from the common cold but increasingly severe
- Low-grade fever
- Rhinitis
- Anorexia

Paroxysmal phase (one to four weeks):
- Cough increases (2 to 50 episodes a day) and fever subsides
- Sudden, forceful inspirations (whooping sound)
- Paroxysms of cough include bulging eyes, tongue protrusion, lacrimation, cyanosis.
- Vomiting (thick secretions), choking, and/or apnea follow paroxysms.
- Patient may not appear ill between paroxysms; infants often exhausted and may lose consciousness

Convalescent phase (two weeks to several months):
- Residual cough
- Older children and adults with previous vaccine or illness have nonspecific bronchitis-like symptoms, usually without the characteristic whooping sound.

DIFFERENTIAL DIAGNOSIS
- Acute upper respiratory infections
- Pneumonias
- Bronchiolitis
- Cystic fibrosis
- Tuberculosis
- Foreign bodies in respiratory tract
- Chronic obstructive pulmonary disease
- Leukemia

DIAGNOSIS
Physical Examination
The patient initially presents with cold-like symptoms. Paroxysms may occur following a slight startle. Often a child who appears well begins to flail and gasp as the face reddens, eyes water, and the inspiratory whoop may be heard. Adults describe feelings of strangulation and bursting headache before air again enters the lungs.

Laboratory Tests
- Pertussis organisms are cultured from respiratory tract secretions (highly specific, but not sensitive) or nasopharyngeal secretions (more sensitive); negative cultures occur with patients taking antibiotics or with previous vaccination.
- Direct fluorescein-conjugated antibody (DFA) staining of nasopharyngeal secretions effectively identifies *B. pertussis;* may give false negatives and positives; only reliable in experienced laboratories.
- Serologic tests (now commercially available) show that IgM and IgA are elevated with infection.

Pathological Findings
- Lymphocytosis is stimulated by pertussis toxin.
- White blood count is elevated (15,000 to 60,000).
- Pertussis toxin causes leukocyte dysfunction, insulin secretion, and histamine sensitivity.
- Local epithelial damage results from tracheal cytotoxin, dermonecrotic factor, and adenylate cyclase.

Imaging
Chest X ray may be clear or show mild infiltrates.

Other Diagnostic Procedures
Available laboratory tests are generally used for research and patients with severe complications. Pertussis should be suspected for severe cough (longer than two weeks) with post-tussive vomiting, leukolymphocytosis, inspiratory whoop, and known exposure. A lack of immunization is not a good indicator of possible pertussis, as a large percentage of immunized people contract pertussis.

TREATMENT OPTIONS
Treatment Strategy
Treatment is largely to control symptoms and prevent spread. Quarantine for four weeks. Parenteral fluid and nutrition, oxygen supplementation, and mechanical ventilation may be required.

Drug Therapies
- Antibiotics—usually erythromycin (40 to 50 mg/kg/day, with a maximum dose of 2 kg, in four divided doses for 14 days) reduces transmission and is effective even for infants. Unless given in the catarrhal phase, antibiotics do not reduce the severity or length of illness.
- Corticosteroids (e.g., betamethasone, 0.075 mg/kg/day) may reduce severity and length of paroxysms, especially for infants.
- Albuterol (0.3 to 0.5 mg/kg/day) reduces the severity of cough paroxysms.
- Immediate resuscitation from loss of consciousness is essential to avoid anoxic brain damage and death.
- Suctioning of secretions, oxygen administration, parenteral fluids and electrolytes are used for infants and protracted illness.
- Mist by tent may benefit infants.
- Do not use cough suppressants.

Complementary and Alternative Therapies

Pertussis is more serious in children under the age of 2 and in the elderly. For those people with healthy immune systems, pertussis can be treated with nutrition, herbs, and homeopathy with excellent results. Alternative therapies require intensive nursing on the part of the caretaker.

NUTRITION

Note: Doses given are for children. Adults should double the amounts.
- Eliminate mucus-forming foods such as dairy, bananas, wheat, and meat products.
- Encourage small, frequent meals of vegetable broths, steamed vegetables, and fresh fruit (especially pineapple and grapes) and vegetable juices. Add therapeutic foods to broths, including onions, garlic, ginger, leeks, turnips, carrots, and leafy greens.
- Vitamin C (200 to 500 mg tid), zinc (10 to 15 mg/day), and beta-carotene (10,000 to 25,000 IU/day) support the immune system.

HERBS

Herbs are generally a safe way to strengthen and tone the body's systems. As with any therapy, it is important to ascertain a diagnosis before pursuing treatment. Herbs may be used as dried extracts (capsules, powders, teas), glycerites (glycerine extracts), or tinctures (alcohol extracts). Unless otherwise indicated, teas should be made with 1 tsp. herb per cup of hot water. Steep covered 5 to 10 minutes for leaf or flowers, and 10 to 20 minutes for roots. Drink 2 to 4 cups/day. Tinctures may be used singly or in combination as noted.

Respiratory and immune-stimulating herbs are used in a variety of modalities. For best results use both internal and external treatment.

Catarrhal stage: Use immune-stimulants, expectorants, and antiseptics to facilitate expectoration, enhance immunity, and reduce severity of infection. Choose two herbs from each of the first three categories. Combine in equal parts in a tea ($^1/_2$ cup every three to four hours), a tincture or glycerite (30 drops every three to four hours).

Paroxysmal stage: In addition to the above formula, add anti-spasmodic herbs to ease cough. Combine 2 parts of catnip with two to four of the other anti-spasmodic herbs in a tincture or glycerite (20 drops every one to two hours).

Immune-stimulating herbs:
- Coneflower (*Echinacea purpurea*)
- Usnea lichen (*Usnea spp.*)
- Garlic (*Allium sativum*)
- Astragalus (*Astragalus membranaceus*)

Expectorants:
- Licorice root (*Glycyrrhiza glabra*)
- Elecampane (*Inula helenium*)
- Mullein (*Verbascum thapsus*)

Antiseptics:
- Thyme (*Thymus vulgaris*)
- Hyssop (*Hyssopus officinalis*)
- Anise seed (*Pimpinella anisum*)

Antispasmodics:
- Indian tobacco (*Lobelia inflata*)—should not be more than $^1/_4$ of a combination.
- Catnip (*Nepeta cateria*)
- Chamomile (*Matricaria recutita*)
- Cramp bark (*Viburnum opulus*)
- Valerian (*Valeriana officinalis*)

Garlic (*Allium sativum*) and ginger root (*Zingiber officinalis*) can be made into a syrup and given throughout the course of illness. Combine 10 to 12 cloves of sliced garlic with 10 to 12 slices of fresh ginger root. Using 2 cups of raw sugar, layer ginger, garlic, and sugar in a glass jar. Let sit in cool place for two days. Strain and store in amber jar. Give $^1/_2$ to 1 tsp. tid. Garlic and ginger can also be combined in a tea. Using 2 to 3 cloves of garlic and 2 to 3 slices of ginger, simmer in 1 cup of water for 10 to 15 minutes. Drink $^1/_2$ cup tid to qid. May add honey and lemon for flavor.

HOMEOPATHY

An experienced homeopath should assess individual constitutional types and severity of disease to select the correct remedy and potency. For acute prescribing use 3 to 5 pellets of a 12X to 30C remedy every one to four hours until acute symptoms resolve.
- *Aconite* for sudden onset of cough and great thirst for cold drinks
- *Belladonna* for sudden onset, high fever with flushed face and irritability
- *Drosera* for cough that is aggravated by tickle in the throat or on lying down. Paroxysms of coughing may be so severe that the patient cannot catch his or her breath
- *Bryonia alba* for cough that is dry and painful and is aggravated by eating and any motion
- *Arnica montana* for painful cough with nosebleed. Child may cry in anticipation of cough
- *Antimonium tartaricum* for rattling cough and weakness that prevents expectoration
- *Ipecacuanha* for persistent nausea with paroxysmal cough leading to or ending in gagging or vomiting

PHYSICAL MEDICINE
- Chest rubs. Use 3 to 6 drops of essential oil (camphor, thyme, eucalyptus, rosemary) with 1 tbsp. food grade oil (almond, flax, or olive). Rub on chest to increase circulation and ease spasm.
- Castor oil pack. Used externally, castor oil is a powerful anti-inflammatory and may help prevent consolidation in pertussis. Apply oil directly to chest, cover with a clean soft cloth (e.g., flannel) and plastic wrap. Place a heat source (hot water bottle or heating pad) over the pack and let sit for 30 to 60 minutes. For best results use three consecutive days in one week. Use daily during acute infection. Can add three to six drops of essential oil (see chest rub) to enhance the benefit.
- Herbal steams. Place 3 to 6 drops of essential oil (see chest rub) in a humidifier or a warm bath. This will help thin mucus and open respiratory passages.
- Contrast hydrotherapy. Alternating hot and cold applications to the chest and/or back increases circulation to the chest, brings nutrients to the lungs, and diffuses metabolic waste from inflammation. The overall effect is decreased inflammation, pain relief, and enhanced healing. Alternate three minutes hot with one minute cold. Repeat three times. This is one set. Do two to three sets/day.
- Warming sock treatment. Before bed, place cold, damp socks on warmed feet and cover with dry wool socks. Let child sleep with the wet socks on overnight. This will stimulate immune function, decrease congestion, and may allow more restful sleep.
- Tapotement and postural drainage may also help prevent consolidation and decrease duration of illness.

ACUPUNCTURE

Both acupuncture and acupressure are used for children. May enhance immunity and decrease duration and severity of infection.

MASSAGE

See chest rubs under physical medicine. Foot massage has an overall relaxing effect and can help induce relaxation and sleep in an anxious child.

Patient Monitoring

Patients who have serious complications, severe paroxysms, or are under one year of age should be hospitalized.

OTHER CONSIDERATIONS

Prevention

Vaccination (0.5 mL, intramuscularly)

- 80% to 90% effective but lasts only up to 12 years (disease is less severe and often undiagnosed in older child and adult); studies show observer bias in efficacy of vaccine
- Typically given with diphtheria and tetanus

The following whole-cell (DTP) side effects have led to reduction in use.

- Inoculation site soreness
- Fever
- Persistent (more than three hours) crying
- Seizures
- Encephalopathy

Acellular (DTaP)—rare, infrequent side effects similar to DTP

- Patient should be isolated for seven days.
- Antibiotic (erythromycin) prescribed to nonimmunized, exposed person may prevent pertussis.

Complications/Sequelae

- Death in infants (more common in infants under 6 months of age)
- Pneumonia—low-grade fever after the catarrhal phase is indicative of secondary infection (10% of infants)

- Otitis media
- Seizures
- Coma
- Encephalopathy (1%)

Interathoracic and intraabdominal pressure during paroxysms can cause the following.

- Umbilical and inguinal hernias
- Subconjuctival, scleral, and cerebral hemorrhages
- Hemoptysis
- Rectal prolapse
- Periorbital edema
- Subcutaneous emphysema
- Pneumothorax or pneumomediastinum

Prognosis

Without complications, complete recovery can be expected.

Pregnancy

Pertussis is generally uncomplicated in healthy adults. Nutritional support and homeopathics are safe in pregnancy. Herbal treatment should be under the supervision of a qualified practitioner.

REFERENCES

Bartram T. *Encyclopedia of Herbal Medicine.* Dorset, England: Grace Publishers; 1995:452–453.

Behrman RE, Kliegman R, eds. *Nelson Textbook of Pediatrics.* 15th ed. Philadelphia, Pa: WB Saunders; 1996.

Blumenthal M, ed. *The Complete German Commission E Monographs.* Boston, Mass: Integrative Medicine Communications; 1998:432.

Bove M. *An Encyclopedia of Natural Healing for Children and Infants.* New Canaan, Conn: Keats Publishing; 1996:205–208.

Rakel RE, ed. *Conn's Current Therapy.* 50th ed. Philadelphia, Pa: WB Saunders; 1998.

Rosen P, Barkin R, eds. *Emergency Medicine: Concepts and Clinical Practice.* 4th ed. St. Louis, Mo: Mosby-Year Book; 1996.

Scott J. *Natural Medicine for Children.* London, England: Gaia Books Ltd; 1990:133–134.

■ PHARYNGITIS
OVERVIEW
Definition
Pharyngitis is an inflammation of the throat, caused by a virus or, less frequently, bacteria. Both types of infection lead to the same symptoms, which include a sore throat, pain when swallowing, and occasionally breathing difficulty. Among viral infections, pharyngitis can occur in association with the common cold, influenza, and infectious mononucleosis. Bacterial infections responsible for the condition include beta-streptococcus, *Mycoplasma pneumoniae,* and those involved in sexually transmitted diseases such as gonorrhea. About one in five patients with a streptococcal infection have pharyngitis. Symptoms differ little between viral and bacterial pharyngitis, although they may be more marked in the bacterial form. Differentiation between the two requires a throat culture. Chronic pharyngitis can result from continual exposure to infection or irritants. Many cases of acute viral pharyngitis subside without any treatment beyond rest. Bacterial forms generally require antibiotics, once the bacterium has been identified. In rare cases, untreated bacterial pharyngitis can lead to rheumatic fever, glomerulonephritis, otitis media, mastoiditis, pneumonia, or meningitis.

Etiology
Acute pharyngitis stems from a viral infection, such as a common cold, or a bacterial infection, such as Group A beta-hemolytic streptococcus. The viral form often accompanies such disorders as the common cold, influenza, and infectious mononucleosis. Continuing infection of the sinuses, lungs, or mouth can lead to chronic pharyngitis. So can constant irritation of the pharynx that results from smoking, breathing heavily polluted air, or consuming too much alcohol over a long duration.

Risk Factors
- Presence of an upper respiratory viral infection
- Bacteria such as beta-hemolytic streptococcus, *Staphylococcus aureus, Candida albicans, Mycoplasma pneumoniae,* or *Chlamydia pneumoniae*
- Sexually transmitted diseases, such as gonorrhea
- Continuing infection of the sinuses, lungs, or mouth
- Long-term tobacco smoking
- Long exposure to throat irritants (for example, in the workplace)
- Overuse of alcohol
- Fatigue

Signs and Symptoms
- Sore throat
- Pain when swallowing
- In rare cases, difficulty breathing
- Inflammation of the pharyngeal mucous membrane
- A whitish membrane or exudate of pus covering the pharyngeal mucous membrane
- Fever, headache, chills
- Enlarged lymph nodes in the neck
- Enlarged tonsils, tonsillar exudates

DIFFERENTIAL DIAGNOSIS
- Infectious mononucleosis
- Adenovirus infection
- Respiratory infection
- Polio
- Scarlet fever
- Leukopenia
- Lymphoma

DIAGNOSIS
Physical Examination
Patients generally exhibit fever. Lack of fever to mild fever suggests a viral infection, while mild to moderate fever indicates bacterial pharyngitis. Examination of the throat reveals mild to severe inflammation and redness, often accompanied by a whitish membrane. A discharge of pus suggests bacterial rather than viral infection. Normal-sized or slightly enlarged lymph nodes suggest viral infection, while slightly to moderately enlarged lymph nodes increase the likelihood of a bacterial cause. In children, lymph nodes can become very enlarged with both viral and bacterial infection.

Laboratory Tests
An elevated white blood count typifies both viral and bacterial pharyngitis. A throat culture proves negative in the case of the viral form, and positive for streptococcus or other bacteria in the case of bacterial infection.

Pathological Findings
Identifiable on culture.

Other Diagnostic Procedures
- Ask patient to describe symptoms completely.
- Evaluate the throat by examination, seeking extent of inflammation and presence of a whitish membrane and pus.
- Check for enlarged lymph nodes in the patient's neck.
- Screen for gonoccal infection.

TREATMENT OPTIONS
Treatment Strategy
Once strong suspicion or positive confirmation that a bacterial infection has caused the pharyngitis, prescribe appropriate antibiotics. Pharyngitis that stems from a viral cause has no specific treatment beyond bed rest and simple forms of self-treatment, such as gargling and aspirin. Advise the patient to get plenty of rest.

Drug Therapies
Penicillin VK 250 mg tid, taken orally for 6 to 10 days, remains the drug of choice against Group A streptococcal pharyngitis, primarily to prevent rheumatic fever. As an alternative, intravenous penicillin G benzathine, or a first-generation cephalosporin. For patients allergic to penicillin, erythromycin 300 to 400 mg tid makes a suitable substitute.

Suggest over-the-counter analgesics such as aspirin or an aspirin substitute to relieve the pain of the sore throat. Take caution in prescribing aspirin for patients under 18. Patients can relieve discomfort with throat lozenges and by gargling with half a teaspoon of salt in a glass of warm water several times daily. A soft or liquid diet including warm broths also helps to avoid irritating the throat.

Complementary and Alternative Therapies
Established strep infection should be treated with antibiotics. Alternative treatments can be effective in cases of acute, chronic, or recurrent pharyngitis. Begin with nutritional support at the first sign of a sore throat. Use the tincture and/or the tea throughout the course of infection. For mild or non-infectious pharyngitis, licorice or slippery elm in lozenges or teas to soothe irritation may be all that is needed.

NUTRITION
- Zinc (30 mg/day or lozenges) boosts the immune system and relieves soreness.
- Vitamin C (1,000 mg tid to qid) is needed, as bowel tolerates, for

proper immune function and to strengthen mucous membranes.

- Beta-carotene (50,000 to 100,000 IU/day) restores integrity of mucous membranes and supports immunity.

HERBS

Herbs are generally a safe way to strengthen and tone the body's systems. As with any therapy, it is important to ascertain a diagnosis before pursuing treatment. Herbs may be used as dried extracts (capsules, powders, teas), glycerites (glycerine extracts), or tinctures (alcohol extracts). Unless otherwise indicated, teas should be made with 1 tsp. herb per cup of hot water. Steep covered 5 to 10 minutes for leaf or flowers, and 10 to 20 minutes for roots. Drink 2 to 4 cups/day. Tinctures may be used singly or in combination as noted. Note: Lozenges (as commercially available) should be used as directed.

- Slippery elm *(Ulmus rubra):* Soothes irritated tissues and promotes healing. Use as lozenge or tea.
- Licorice *(Glycyrrhiza glabra):* Anti-viral properties and soothing to the throat. Use as lozenge or tea. Licorice is contraindicated in hypertension.
- Garlic/Ginger tea *(Allium sativum/Zingiber officinalis):* Anti-microbial and warming herbs. Use two cloves of garlic and two to three slices of fresh ginger root. Simmer in one cup of water for 10 minutes. Drink warm. May add lemon and honey for flavor.
- Tincture of two parts coneflower *(Echinacea purpurea),* two parts goldenseal *(Hydrastis canadensis),* and one part propolis, should be taken every three to four hours. Place 30 drops in 1/4 cup water. Gargle and swallow.

HOMEOPATHY

An experienced homeopath should assess individual constitutional types and severity of disease to select the correct remedy and potency. For acute prescribing use 3 to 5 pellets of a 12X to 30C remedy every one to four hours until acute symptoms resolve.

- *Apis* for red, swollen throat with burning pains. Patient is thirstless and feels better with cold drinks.
- *Belladonna* for bright red throat and tongue that feels worse on the right side. Patient is thirsty.
- *Lycopodium* for dryness of throat; pain begins on right side and goes to left. Pain is relieved with hot drinks.

PHYSICAL MEDICINE

Chiropractic treatment may be a helpful adjunct, especially in children.

ACUPUNCTURE

Acupuncture may be helpful in improving immune function.

MASSAGE

Patients with chronic pharyngitis may respond to therapeutic massage and other mind-body therapies that reduce the effects of stress and increase the overall sense of well-being.

OTHER CONSIDERATIONS

Prevention

Avoid contact with infected persons.

Complications/Sequelae

- Rheumatic fever
- Systemic infection
- Otitis media
- Septicemia
- Rhinitis
- Sinusitis

Prognosis

Acute pharyngitis usually remits within a week to ten days. Ensure that patients prescribed antibiotics complete their course of treatment. Patients with chronic pharyngitis caused by irritants should stop smoking or drinking alcohol, and avoid exposure to heavily polluted air.

Pregnancy

Use caution with antibiotic therapy. Goldenseal *(Hydrastis canadensis)* is contraindicated in pregnancy.

REFERENCES

Berkow R, ed. *Merck Manual.* 16th ed. Rahway, NJ: Merck Research Laboratories; 1992.

Larson DE, ed. *Mayo Clinic Family Health Book.* 2nd ed. New York, NY: William Morrow and Company; 1996.

Lewis WH, Elvin-Lewis MPF. *Medical Botany/Plants Affecting Man's Health.* New York, NY: John Wiley & Sons; 1977.

Morrison R. *Desktop Guide to Keynotes and Confirmatory Symptoms.* Albany, Calif: Hahnemann Clinic Publishing; 1993:5, 28.

■ PREECLAMPSIA

OVERVIEW

Definition

Preeclampsia involves the development of hypertension accompanied by protein in the urine and edema in women, and occurs between the 20th week of pregnancy and the first week after delivery. Early-stage preeclampsia produces few clinical signs, but symptoms progressively appear. Left untreated, it can develop into eclampsia, a potentially fatal ailment that produces seizures, bleeding, or liver or kidney problems in the woman and threatens the life of her unborn child. Preeclampsia develops in about 5% of pregnant women. That proportion has fallen in recent years, presumably because of improved prenatal care. The mothers of 26 in every 1,000 live-born infants will have had the condition, which may develop into the second leading cause of maternal mortality. The condition, sometimes called toxemia, is more common in first pregnancies and in women who already have hypertension or vascular disease. Babies of women with preeclampsia may weigh less than those born to women without preeclampsia, and are four to five times more likely than others to experience problems soon after birth. About one woman in 200 with preeclampsia develops eclampsia.

Eclampsia also may be associated with a bleeding problem called disseminated intravascular coagulation, in which the body's blood clotting products are depleted. A group of symptoms called HELLP (hemolysis, elevated liver function tests and low platelets) may also occur.

Etiology

The cause for preeclampsia or eclampsia is unknown. Despite the nickname toxemia, no one has isolated any toxic substance in pregnant women's blood that can cause the symptoms. Potential causes include genetic, dietary, vascular, and neurological factors.

Risk Factors

- First pregnancy
- Teenage pregnancy
- Pregnancy over the age of 40
- Multiple pregnancies, multiple fetuses
- Preeclampsia in prior pregnancy
- History of hypertension
- History of diabetes
- History of kidney disease
- African-American patient

Signs and Symptoms

Preeclampsia:

- Blood pressure of more than 140/90 mm of Hg
- Increase of 30 mm Hg systolic or 15 mm Hg diastolic, when blood pressure is under 140/90
- Excessive weight gain of more than five pounds per week
- Very sudden weight gain over one or two days
- Edema, particularly of the hands and face on arising
- Protein in the urine
- Reduction of amount of urine

Eclampsia:

- Pain in the upper right side of the abdomen
- Disturbances to vision, such as seeing flashing lights

DIFFERENTIAL DIAGNOSIS

- Chronic hypertension
- Pregnancy-induced hypertension
- Pregnancy-worsened hypertension
- Kidney disease
- Lupus or autoimmune diseases
- Strenuous jobs that require a hectic pace or heavy lifting

DIAGNOSIS

Physical Examination

Measure blood pressure. Look for edema in the hands and face, and particularly around the eyes, caused by fluid retention. Pitting edema in lower extremities. Check reflexes for hyperreflexia.

Laboratory Tests

- A 24-hour urine indicates the level of protein and amount of urine.
- Obtain routine laboratory tests, including CBC with platelets, urinalysis, electrolyte levels, uric acid concentration, prothrombin time, and partial thromboplastic time.
- Obtain levels of BUN and creatinine, to rule out unsuspected kidney disease.
- Obtain liver function tests to rule out liver involvement.

Pathological Findings

Fibrin in kidneys and liver.

Other Diagnostic Procedures

A 24-hour urine test to measure protein. Assess lab results for differentiating diagnosis.

TREATMENT OPTIONS

Treatment Strategy

The type of treatment depends on the severity of preeclampsia. Patients with a blood pressure of 150/110 mm, with marked edema, or high levels of protein in the urine have severe preeclampsia, and require hospitalization and vigorous therapy. The initial goal of treatment is to prevent development of eclampsia or the HELLP (hemolysis, elevated liver enzymes, and low platelet count) syndrome, which poses great risk of maternal or fetal/neonatal morbidity and mortality.

Having stabilized the hospitalized patient, the provider should aim to deliver the fetus as soon as possible. Delivery may represent the best form of treatment for severe preeclampsia, yet a balanced treatment plan should consider the severity of preeclampsia, the gestational age of the fetus, and the assessment of maternal and fetal well being. For patients near term, the provider can induce labor or perform a Caesarean section. In pregnancies that are less than 28 weeks, in which the fetus has low chances of surviving delivery, many providers try to forestall labor. However, prolonging such pregnancies with worsening symptoms causes maternal complications and death of the fetus in 87% of cases. Providers often recommend induction of labor in pregnancies less than 24 weeks with severe preeclampsia, despite the minimal likelihood of a viable fetus. For pregnancies of 24 to 28 weeks, conservative management with constant monitoring of mother and fetus is generally the therapy of choice.

In cases of mild preeclampsia, prescribe bed rest and advise the patient to lie on her left side, to increase her output of urine and lessen intravascular dehydration. She should also drink more water than usual. Check blood pressure and urinary protein every two days. Ensuring fetal well being includes fetal heart tones and a non-stress test. Fetal growth should be monitored by ultrasound every few weeks. If the mother's condition does not improve, she should be hospitalized, stabilized, and prepared for delivery. If possible, close monitoring should continue after delivery, as one in four cases of eclampsia occurs at this stage—normally within two to four days of delivery. Examine patients every two weeks for the first two months after delivery.

Drug Therapies

For hospitalized patients with mild preeclampsia, fluids and intravenous magnesium sulfate usually reduce blood pressure to normal levels. Loading dose of 4 g IV in 200 ml saline over 20 to 30 minutes, maintenance dose then 1 to 2 g/hour IV. Toxicity therapy for above is calcium gluconate, one g over two to three minutes. If intravenous magnesium
sulfate does not reduce blood pressure within four to six hours, use an intravenous infusion of hydralazine.

Avoid driving the blood pressure below 130/80 in cases of severe preeclampsia, which would decrease perfusions of the uterus so severely as to endanger the fetus. If the patient's urine output does not increase, a solution of furosemide, given intravenously, produces diuresis.

Complementary and Alternative Therapies

Preeclampsia can appear and progress rapidly. It is imperative that the patient be underqualified medical care. Alternative therapies can be used preventatively or concurrently with medical treatment.

NUTRITION

- Omega-3 oils (1,000 mg tid) are highly beneficial in pregnancy, and help reduce inflammation.
- Increasing protein intake may help minimize preeclampsia.
- Magnesium 200 mg bid to tid, has mild vasodilatory effects and helps reduce high blood pressure.

HERBS

Herbs are generally a safe way to strengthen and tone the body's systems. As with any therapy, it is important to ascertain a diagnosis before pursuing treatment. Herbs may be used as dried extracts (capsules, powders, teas), glycerites, or tinctures (alcohol extracts). Unless otherwise indicated, teas should be made with one teaspoon herb per cup of hot water. Steep covered 10 to 20 minutes and drink two to four cups/day. Tinctures may be used singly or in combination as noted.

Herbs that can be used to treat mild hypertension in pregnancy include the following. Passion flower *(Passiflora incarnata)*, hawthorn berries *(Crataegus oxyanthoides)*, cramp bark *(Viburnum opulus)*, milk thistle *(Silybum marianum)*, and Indian tobacco *(Lobelia inflata)*. Use equal parts of each in a tincture, 20 drops tid to qid.

ACUPUNCTURE

May be helpful in lowering blood pressure and generally improving circulation.

Patient Monitoring

Hospitalized patients require ongoing assessment after delivery. Examine patient at least every two weeks for the first two months after delivery. Blood pressure may remain high for up to eight weeks after delivery.

OTHER CONSIDERATIONS

Patients should remove rings as soon as fingers begin to swell.

Complications/Sequelae

Eclampsia remains a threat after delivery, usually within four days.

Prognosis

Preeclampsia is a condition to be aggressively and continually managed. Patients hospitalized should be closely followed, depending on the severity of the preeclampsia and the absence or presence of any complications.

REFERENCES

Berkow R, ed. *Merck Manual of Diagnosis and Therapy.* 16th edition. Rahway, NJ: The Merck Publishing Group; 1992.

Berkow R, Beers MH, Fletcher AJ, eds. *Merck Manual, Home Edition.* Rahway, NJ: Merck & Co; 1997.

Klonoff-Cohen HS, Cross JL, Pieper CF. Job stress and preeclampsia. *Epidemiol.* 1996;7:245–249.

Larson DE, ed. *Mayo Clinic Family Health Book.* 2nd ed. New York, NY: William Morrow and Company; 1996.

Murray M. *Encyclopedia of Nutritional Supplements.* Rocklin, Calif: Prima Health; 1996.

Scalzo R. *Naturopathic Handbook of Herbal Formulas.* Durango, Colo: 2nd ed. Kivaki Press; 1994.

■ PRIMARY PULMONARY HYPERTENSION

OVERVIEW

Definition

Pulmonary hypertension can appear as a single disease entity (primary) or in conjunction with another cardiopulmonary disease (secondary). It is characterized by increased pulmonary artery pressure and pulmonary vascular resistance. Three subtypes include thrombotic, plexogenic, and veno-occlusive.

Etiology

Many cases of pulmonary hypertension are idiopathic or primary, especially in young women. However, many diseases of the heart or respiratory system can also cause pulmonary hypertension. All cause narrowing of the pulmonary blood vessels, increasing resistance to blood flow through the lungs. To maintain pulmonary blood flow, pulmonary arterial pressure increases. Possible causes include the following.

- Congenital heart disease (e.g., atrial and ventricular septal defects; patent ductus arteriosus)
- Mitral stenosis or regurgitation
- Chronic obstructive pulmonary disease (e.g., emphysema)
- Interstitial lung disease
- Obesity and the hypoventilation syndrome
- Pulmonary thromboembolism
- Dexfenfluramine and other diet drugs

Risk Factors

- Autoimmune disorders (e.g., systemic lupus erythematosus, rheumatoid arthritis)
- Morbid obesity, especially accompanied by sleep apnea, or hypoventilation syndrome
- Interstitial lung disease
- Family history of pulmonary hypertension (7% of cases)
- Human immunodeficiency virus
- Collagen vascular diseases
- Cocaine use
- Male gender

Signs and Symptoms

All of the signs and symptoms are nonspecific, suggesting other more common respiratory diseases. Pulmonary hypertension presents initially as dyspnea on exertion; over time, however, the dyspnea occurs even at rest.

- Exertional dyspnea, often the only presenting symptom
- Excessive fatigue
- Exertional syncope or near syncope
- Cough
- Pleuritic chest pain
- Peripheral edema
- Hemoptysis
- Palpitations

Closer examination reveals the following signs.

- Loud P2
- Right ventricular lift
- Murmur of tricuspid or pulmonic insufficiency
- Right ventricular S4

DIFFERENTIAL DIAGNOSIS

- Chronic obstructive pulmonary disease (COPD)
- Thromboembolic disease
- Pulmonary veno-occlusive disease
- Coronary artery disease
- Psychogenic dyspnea

DIAGNOSIS

Physical Examination

Classic findings include a reduced carotid pulse, increased jugular venous pressure, an accentuated second heart sound (S2), right-sided third and fourth heart sounds, tricuspid regurgitation, and right ventricular lift. There may be peripheral cyanosis and edema. The right ventricle and central pulmonary arteries are enlarged on chest X ray. The EKG and the echocardiogram reveal right ventricular hypertrophy. Hypoxia and hypercapnia are almost always present.

Pathological Findings

Under normal circumstances the pulmonary vascular system is a high-flow, low-pressure, and low-resistance system, even during exercise. In pulmonary hypertension there is a decrease in the cross-sectional area of pulmonary blood vessels because of vasoconstriction, obstruction, or obliteration. Pulmonary arterial pressure and vascular resistance increase with increased flow and eventually even with rest, leading to right ventricular hypertrophy and deficient cardiac output. Ohter findings: remodeling of pulmonary vasculature from chronic high flow (pressure), obliteration of the pulmonary vasculature, vasoconstriction from interstitial lung disease, microthrombotic lesions in small pulmonary arteries.

Imaging

- High-resolution computed tomography (CT)
- Echo-Doppler (shows right ventricular enlargement)
- Chest x-ray (shows enlarged central pulmonary arteries)
- Pulmonary angiography

Other Diagnostic Procedures

- Open lung biopsy
- Balloon septostomy
- Ventilation and perfusion lung scanning
- ECG to detect right ventricular hypertrophy

These studies are used to exclude secondary causes of pulmonary hypertension.

- Pulmonary function tests (e.g., spirometry, gas exchange analysis)
- Chest X ray
- Two-dimensional M-mode, Doppler, and transesophageal echocardiography
- Arterial blood gases
- Doppler or transesophageal echocardiography
- Pulmonary artery catheterization
- Sleep studies

TREATMENT OPTIONS

Treatment Strategy

Treatment is entirely dependent on the cause. With secondary pulmonary hypertension, the underlying disease must be treated. Hypoxia and hypercapnia can be treated palliatively with supplemental oxygen, and vasodilators and anticoagulants as needed. Patients must be counseled to avoid unnecessary physical stress because pulmonary vascular resistance increases dramatically with exercise. Withdrawal of appetite suppressant drugs sometimes, but not always, may lead to stabilization or resolution of pulmonary hypertension.

Drug Therapies

- Supplemental oxygen for hypoxemic patients
- Vasodilator therapy: adenosine, 50 mcg/kg/min, in increasing doses until symptoms of pulmonary reactivity occur; prostacyclin, two ng/kg/min, every 30 minutes until side effects occur; nitric oxide may be effective in a subset of patients with primary pulmonary hyperten-

sion, via inhalation of 5 to 10 parts/million, until no longer effective

- Calcium-channel blockers, e.g., nifedipine, 120 to 240 mg/day or diltiazem, 540 to 900 mg/day, to improve survival. Treatment should not be given, however, without direct measurements of pulmonary artery pressures. As yet there is no clear role for such therapies in secondary pulmonary hypertension.
- Anticoagulants (e.g., warfarin)—if the primary disease is thromboembolic pulmonary disease
- Diuretics—for right ventricular failure

Complementary and Alternative Therapies

Use to enhance respiratory function and strengthen cardiovascular and pulmonary circulation.

NUTRITION

- Coenzyme Q10 (100 mg bid) supports cardiac function, is an antioxidant, and oxygenates tissues.
- L-Carnitine (500 mg tid) improves endurance and is needed for efficient cardiac function.
- Magnesium aspartate (200 mg bid to tid) increases efficiency of cardiac muscle and decreases vascular resistance.
- Potassium aspartate (20 mg/day) improves heart contractility.
- Vitamin E (400 IU/day) is an antioxidant and is cardioprotective.
- Vitamin C (1,000 to 1,500 mg tid) is an antioxidant, improves vascular integrity, and stimulates immune function.
- Taurine (500 mg bid) enhances the efficiency of cardiac function.
- Selenium (200 mcg/day) is a cardioprotective antioxidant.
- Choline (250 to 500 mg/day) and Inositol (150 to 200 mg/day) are part of the phospholipid membrane and positively effect parasympathetic activity and vasodilation.

HERBS

Herbs are generally a safe way to strengthen and tone the body's systems. Ascertain a diagnosis first. Herbs may be used as dried extracts (capsules, powders, teas), glycerites (glycerine extracts), or tinctures (alcohol extracts). Unless otherwise indicated, teas should be made with 1 teaspoon herb per cup of hot water. Steep covered 5 to 10 minutes for leaf or flowers, and 10 to 20 minutes for roots. Drink 2 to 4 cups/day. Tinctures may be used singly or in combination as noted.

The following herbs tonify the respiratory system, improve vascular tone, lower blood pressure, and increase the efficiency of cardiac function. Combine them in equal parts in tincture form and take 30 drops tid to qid.

- Hawthorn (Crataegus oxyacantha) increases cardiac output without increasing cardiac load. Strengthens the integrity of vasculature and has mild vasodilation activity.
- Garlic (Allium sativum) enhances expectoration, is hypotensive, immune-stimulating, and anti-atherosclerotic.
- Rosemary (Rosemarinus officinalis) strengthens cardiac function, is anti-atherosclerotic, antispasmodic, and improves circulation to the lungs.
- Linden flowers (Tilia cordata) is an antispasmodic, hypotensive, anti-atherosclerotic, respiratory relaxant, and expectorant. Also stimulates immune function.
- Ginkgo (Ginkgo biloba) improves peripheral blood flow and decreases platelet aggregation.
- Indian tobacco (Lobelia inflata) stimulates respiratory function, is anti-spasmodic, and hypotensive. Used in high doses this herb can have toxic side effects. Using small amounts in a formula (one-fourth or less) will minimize the risk of toxicity.

HOMEOPATHY

An experienced homeopath should assess individual constitutional types and severity of disease to select the correct remedy and potency.

PHYSICAL MEDICINE

Castor oil pack. Apply oil directly to chest, cover with a clean soft cloth (e.g. flannel) and plastic wrap. Place a heat source (hot water bottle or heating pad) over the pack and let sit for 30 to 60 minutes. Use for three consecutive days.

Contrast hydrotherapy. Alternating hot and cold applications to the chest brings nutrients to the lungs and diffuses metabolic waste from inflammation. The overall effect is decreased inflammation, pain relief, and enhanced healing. Alternate three minutes hot with one minute cold and repeat three times. This is one set. Do two to three sets/day. For debilitated patients use cool and warm applications.

Steams. Using three to six drops of essential oils in a humidifier, vaporizer, atomizer, or warm bath will stimulate respiration and circulation. Consider eucalyptus, rosemary, thyme, and/or lavender. This treatment will also minimize risk of secondary infection due to COPD or interstitial lung disease.

ACUPUNCTURE

May support treatment of symptoms through an increase in circulation.

Patient Monitoring

Primary pulmonary hypertension is a relatively rare disease that most often affects women in their 30s and 40s; however, it is seen at all ages from infancy to over 60 years of age.

OTHER CONSIDERATIONS
Prevention

Pulmonary hypertension has been associated with exogenous agents, collagen vascular diseases, autoimmune disorders, and HIV. Weight control, avoiding diet drugs, and smoking cessation all play a part in prevention.

Complications/Sequelae

Cor pulmonale, or hypertrophy of the right ventricle, is inevitable. Other complications include thromboembolism, heart failure, and sudden death.

Prognosis

Patients with primary pulmonary hypertension generally live only three to five years from the time of the diagnosis. Patients usually die a sudden death from heart failure. While the prognosis is generally poor, survival depends on the severity of the pulmonary hypertension and the degree of right ventricular hypertrophy.

Pregnancy

Pregnancy is contraindicated with pulmonary hypertension because it is extremely dangerous for both the mother and the child.

REFERENCES

Bartram T. *Encyclopedia of Herbal Medicine*. Dorset, England: Grace Publishers; 1995:195, 270, 276, 376.

Bordow RA, Moser KM. *Manual of Clinical Problems in Pulmonary Medicine*. 4th ed. Boston, Mass: Little, Brown; 1996:304–311,353,424, 431–434.

Fauci AS, Braunwald, E, Isselbacher KJ et al, eds. *Harrison's Principles of Internal Medicine*. 14th ed. New York, NY: McGraw-Hill; 1998:1466–1468.

Fishman AP, Elias JA, Fishman JA, et al. *Fishman's Pulmonary Diseases and Disorders*. 3rd ed. New York, NY: McGraw-Hill; l998: 1261–1296.

Hinshaw HC, Murray JF. *Disease of the Chest*. 4th ed. Philadelphia, Pa: WB Saunders; 1980:684–697.

Woodley M, Whelan A. *Washington Manual of Therapeutics*. 27th ed. Boston, Mass: Little, Brown; 1992:211–212.

■ PROSTATITIS

OVERVIEW

Definition

Prostatitis is characterized by irritative voiding symptoms and perineal or suprapubic discomfort. It may be the most common genitourinary ailment in men younger than age 50, resulting in an estimated 2 million visits to physicians each year. The bacterial form of prostatitis most often occurs in men ages 70 and older. The four subtypes are:

- Acute bacterial prostatitis—the least common form; often associated with bacteriuria; usually caused by enteric gram-negative bacilli
- Chronic bacterial prostatitis—a relatively uncommon disorder sometimes associated with an underlying defect in the prostate
- Nonbacterial prostatitis—the most common form; causes unknown
- Prostatodynia—symptoms similar to nonbacterial prostatitis; no objective findings, such as the presence of infection-fighting cells

Etiology

Infection by a bacterial pathogen is the most common factor in the etiology of prostatitis; the etiology of nonbacterial prostatitis and prostatodynia is unknown.

Risk Factors

- Recent urinary tract infection
- Prior sexually transmitted disease, such as gonorrhea or chlamydia.
- Smoking
- Excess alcohol consumption

Signs and Symptoms

Signs and symptoms may vary depending on subtype; some patients are asymptomatic. Common symptoms include:

- Recurrent urinary tract infections
- Urinary frequency and urgency
- Dysuria
- Nocturia
- Fever
- Chills
- Generalized malaise
- Bladder outlet obstruction
- Painful ejaculation, bloody semen, or sexual dysfunction
- Pain localized to lower back (sacral), pelvis, or perineum

DIFFERENTIAL DIAGNOSIS

- Chronic urethritis
- Cystitis
- Anal disease

DIAGNOSIS

Physical Examination

Although often not definitive, a physical examination may find the prostate tender, swollen, and indurate; may be warm to palpitating finger in rectum; hardness and nodules may indicate a malignancy.

Laboratory Tests

Urine and blood cultures to detect infection or cancerous cells. In the case of nonbacterial prostatitis, cultures are negative but increased numbers of leukocytes are seen on prostatic secretions.

Pathological Findings

Enteric gram-negative organisms are the most commonly found bacterial pathogens in prostatitis; gram-negative organisms (e.g., *Enterococcus)* are sometimes associated with acute and chronic forms.

Imaging

In most cases, imaging tests are not required. However, pelvic radiographs and transrectal ultrasound may help detect prostatic calculi.

Other Diagnostic Procedures

- Clinician interview and physical examination: Take medical history and conduct prostate exam.
- Conduct a cytoscopic examination of the urethra, prostate, and bladder in cases of nonbacterial prostatitis to rule out interstitial cystitis.

TREATMENT OPTIONS

Treatment Strategy

Antibiotics are the treatment of choice, either intravenously or orally. Symptomatic relief is achieved with pain relievers, stool softeners, anti-inflammatory agents, and hot sitz baths. Periodic prostatic massage may also relieve symptoms, but an acutely inflamed prostate gland should not be massaged until antibacterial agent has established adequate blood levels. Surgery (transurethral resection or drainage) is indicated if calculi are detected or fever and pain persist; side effects of resection include retrograde ejaculation and some cases of impotence or incontinence.

Drug Therapies

Several antibiotics are recommended for treating prostatitis, depending on the subtype. They include:

- Ampicillin and aminoglycoside (parenteral) is recommended initially until organisms' sensitivities are determined in acute bacterial prostatitis; oral antibiotics such as trimethoprim-sulfamethoxazole or quinolones are then used to complete a fou- to six-week regimen.
- Trimethoprim-sulfamethoxazole is associated with successful cure rates in chronic prostatitis; also effective are carbenicillin, erythromycin, cephalexin, and quinolones; therapy duration is controversial but usually lasts from 6 to 12 weeks.
- Erythromycin (250 mg qid) is recommended for nonbacterial prostatitis to treat ureaplasma, mycoplasma, or chlamydia; recommended duration is 14 days to be continued for four to six weeks if response is favorable; oxybutynin (5 mg orally tid), propantheline (15 mg orally tid), and diazepam (2 mg orally tid) are also recommended treatments.

Complementary and Alternative Therapies

Various therapies can be effective during acute infection. With chronic or nonbacterial prostatitis, these therapies may have much to offer. A combination of herbs and nutrition can be effective. Homeopathy may offer significant symptomatic relief.

NUTRITION

- Vitamin C (1,000 mg tid to qid)
- Zinc (60 mg/day) has been shown to reduce the size of the prostate.
- Selenium (200 mcg/day) is an antioxidant concentrated in the prostate.
- Essential fatty acids (1,000 to 1,500 mg one to two times/day) are anti-inflammatory; for optimum prostaglandin concentrations.
- Pumpkin seeds have been used historically to help maintain a healthy prostate.
- Diet: Avoid simple sugars, alcohol (especially beer), and coffee; consume plenty of water (48 oz. per day).

HERBS

Herbs are generally a safe way to strengthen and tone the body's systems. As with any therapy, it is important to ascertain a diagnosis before pursuing treatment. Herbs may be used as dried extracts (capsules, powders, teas), glycerites (glycerine extracts), or tinctures (alcohol extracts). Unless otherwise indicated, teas should be made with 1 tsp. herb per cup of hot water. Steep covered 5 to 10 minutes for leaf or flowers, or 10 to 20 minutes for roots. Drink 2 to 4 cups/day. Tinctures may be used singly or in combination as noted.

Saw palmetto *(Serenoa repens):* Studies show this could possibly be as effective as prescribed antimicrobial therapy. Dose of 160 mg bid is difficult to achieve in tea or tincture; extract standardized for 85% to 95% of fatty acids and sterols is recommended.

Cernilton, a flower pollen extract (500 to 1,000 mg bid to tid), has been used extensively in Europe to treat prostatitis due to inflammation or infection. It also has a contractile effect on the bladder and relaxes the urethra.
- Bearberry *(Arctostaphylos uva-ursi):* diuretic, urinary antiseptic
- Goldenseal *(Hydrastis canadensis):* diuretic, antiseptic, antimicrobial
- Coneflower *(Echinacea purpurea):* improves immune function
- Corn silk *(Zea mays):* diuretic, soothing demulcent

Take a combination of the above herbs, 1 cup tea or 60 drops tincture tid.

HOMEOPATHY
An experienced homeopath should assess individual constitutional types and severity of disease to select the correct remedy and potency. For acute prescribing, use 3 to 5 pellets of a 12X to 30C remedy every one to four hours until acute symptoms resolve.
- *Chimaphila umbellata* for retention of urine with an enlarged prostate
- *Pulsatilla* for pain after urination, especially with involuntary urination
- *Pareira* for painful urination, especially with painful urging or pain in the bladder
- *Lycopodium* for painful urination with reddish sediment in the urine, especially with impotence
- *Thuja* for urethritis, prostatitis, specifically if there is a forked stream of urine or genital condyloma

PHYSICAL MEDICINE
Kegel exercises increase pelvic circulation and improve muscle tone.

ACUPUNCTURE
May improve urinary flow and decrease edema and inflammation of prostatic tissues.

MASSAGE
May help reduce symptoms, especially with chronic or recurring prostatitis. Focus may be on the lower abdominal area, lower back, and around the sacrum.

OTHER CONSIDERATIONS
Men should have a yearly prostate examination after age 40, even if they have no symptoms of prostate problems.

Prevention
Warm sitz baths, increased water consumption, and avoidance of prolonged bicycle riding, horseback riding, and other exercises that irritate the region below the prostate may help prevent recurrence. Sexual activity may reduce the chances of prostatitis and reduce the likelihood of recurrence by easing fluid congestion in the prostate. However, sexual intercourse during infection may further irritate prostate and hinder recovery.

Complications/Sequelae
Infection may spread to testicles and epididymis. Chronic form may cause destruction of gland, bladder neck scarring, and stricture formation. Impotence may develop in some cases.

Prognosis
Antimicrobial therapy is usually effective, and recurrence is variable. Chronic prostatitis is more difficult to cure; suppressive antibiotic therapy may be used to prevent symptoms and recurrent urinary tract infections. Recurrent symptoms are common in nonbacterial prostatitis; serious sequelae do not usually result.

REFERENCES
Bartram T. *Encyclopedia of Herbal Medicine.* Dorset, England: Grace Publishers; 1995:52, 128, 203.
Berkow R, ed. *The Merck Manual of Diagnosis and Therapy.* 16th ed. Rahway, NJ: The Merck Publishing Group; 1992.
Blumenthal M, ed. *The Complete German Commission E Monographs.* Boston, Mass: Integrative Medicine Communications; 1998:75, 201.
Buck AC, Rees RWM, Ebeling L. Treatment of chronic prostatitis and prostadynia with pollen extract. *Br J Urol.* 1989;64:496–499.
Conn RB, Borere WZ, Snyder JW, eds. *Current Diagnosis 9.* Philadelphia, Pa: WB Saunders; 1996.
Driscoll CE, Bope ET, Smith CW JR, Carter BL, eds. *The Family Practice Desk Reference.* 3rd ed. St. Louis, Mo: Mosby-Year Book; 1996.
Gruenwald J, Brendler T et al, eds. *PDR for Herbal Medicines.* Montvale, NJ: Medical Economics Company; 1998:817, 1,229.
Morrison R. *Desktop Guide to Keynotes and Confirmatory Symptoms.* Albany, Calif: Hahnemann Clinic Publishing; 1993:119, 228–231, 341, 388–389.
Murray MT, Pizzorno JE. *Encyclopedia of Natural Medicine.* Rocklin, Calif: Prima Publishing; 1998:480–486.
Thierney Jr LM, McPhee SJ, Papadakis MA, eds. *Current Medical Diagnosis & Treatment 1999.* 38th ed. Stamford, Conn: Appleton & Lange; 1999.
Werbach, M. *Nutritional Influences on Illness.* New Canaan, Conn: Keats Publishing; 1988:82–84.

■ PSORIASIS

OVERVIEW

Definition

Chronic papulosquamous dermatological disorder presenting as raised, reddish pink lesions covered with silvery, opaque scales and well-defined borders. Lesions occur predominantly on the scalp, elbows, knees, groin, and sacrum, although not limited to these areas. May appear as a few spots or involve large areas. Increased ratio of cyclic GMP over cyclic AMP within the dermis stimulates a high cell production rate. Newly generated cells rise to the skin's surface within days, accumulating in thick, crusty patches. The condition afflicts more than six million people in the U.S. of both sexes, all ages, is negatively affected by emotional stress, is not contagious, and has genetic traits. (Patients with Crohn's disease have a seven-fold risk increase; chromosome 16 is implicated in both disorders.) Severe cases can be physically painful and emotionally traumatic due to its unsightly appearance. Approximately 10% of psoriasis sufferers develop psoriatic arthritis, a phenomenon unique among skin disorders. Although there is no cure, symptoms can be managed in most instances. The disease may take one of several forms:

- Chronic, plaque-type (most common)
- Guttate
- Psoriatic erythroderma
- Pustular
- Flexural
- Ostraceous

Etiology

Specific etiology uncertain; several factors are implicated:

- Immune system dysfunction (HLA antigen involvement)
- Genetic traits (Portions of chromosomes 16, 17, 20, 6)

Trigger events:

- Emotional stress
- Skin injuries/sunburn
- Streptococcal infection (symptoms sometimes first appear two weeks after strep throat)
- Certain drugs (chloroquine, gold, lithium, beta-blockers)
- Acidic foods

Risk Factors

- Familial/genetic predisposition
- Race (incidence highest among Caucasians)
- Immune system diseases (including AIDS)
- Obesity
- Alcoholism
- Streptococcal infections elsewhere in the body
- Skin damage
- Rheumatoid arthritis

Signs and Symptoms

Symptoms wax and wane. Manifestations include:

- Raised skin lesions, deep pink with red borders and silvery surface scales; may be cracked and painful
- Blisters oozing aseptic pus (pustular or guttate type—occurs only on palms or plantars)
- Pitted, discolored, and possibly thickened fingernails and/or toenails; may be separated from underlying skin
- Itching in some cases
- Joint pain (psoriatic arthritis) in some cases
- New lesions may appear following injuries to the skin.

DIFFERENTIAL DIAGNOSIS

- Eczema
- Dermatitis
- Other skin disorders
- Squamous cell carcinoma
- Cutaneous lupus erythematosus
- Intertrigo or candidiasis

DIAGNOSIS

Physical Examination

Unsightly raised dermal lesions deep pink or red in color with white or silvery scales; pustules on palms and plantars; pitted, discolored nails.

Laboratory Tests

- Elevated cGMP relative to cAMP
- Decreased dermal keratohyalin
- Increased intracellular calcium and calmodulin levels
- Low zinc/high copper levels
- Possible B_{12}, folate, and iron deficiencies
- Possible anemia

Pathological Findings

- Dermal surface lesions due to abnormally rapid cell growth, deposit, and accumulation
- Abnormal microvasculature dermal permeability

Other Diagnostic Procedures

- Skin biopsy, if necessary

TREATMENT OPTIONS

Treatment Strategy

Identifying cause of onset in relation to emotional trauma, skin injury, viral/bacterial infection, diet, weight gain may help define treatment options. Although blood tests will not confirm diagnosis, laboratory tests for levels of cCMP/cAMP, HLA antigens, and levels of calcium, zinc, and certain drugs may also help determine mode of treatment, which includes:

- Topical medications
- Systemic drugs
- Light therapy—solar and ultraviolet radiation
- Dietary modification—avoid triggers, lose weight
- Vitamin/mineral supplementation
- Exercise
- Elimination therapy (certain medications and acidic foods)

Drug Therapies

Reduce epidermal proliferation rate and/or halt the inflammatory process. Topical Creams and Lotions:

- Corticosteroids: Reduce inflammation/irritation (use only to begin treatment; prolonged use causes skin thinning, pigment changes, and suppresses the immune system, causing vengeful flare-ups upon cessation.)
- Petroleum jelly: Softens skin and retains moisture
- Salicylic acid ointments: Promote scale shedding
- Capsaicin ointment: Prevents blood vessel development in affected areas; blocks inflammatory skin chemicals; should be used with care, and never on open wounds or sores as it would be very painful
- Calcitriol (or calcipotriene) ointment (vitamin D3 analogue): May be as effective as corticosteroids with fewer side effects.
- Coal tar ointments/shampoos: Ease discomfort, improve effectiveness of UV light therapy (may cause folliculitis; increased squamous cell carcinoma risk)

- Etretinate: Good response with few side effects (for severe cases unresponsive to other treatments)
- Anthralin: Applied for 30 to 60 minutes only to affected area (irritates healthy skin; stains last several weeks)

Ultraviolet light: Natural sunlight in short increments (sunburn detrimental)

- PUVA: Artificial long-wave light therapy in combination with oral psoralen (photosynthesizing agent), effective in recalcitrant cases (significant carcinogenic risk in long-term treatments)
- UVB: Artificial short-wave light therapy in combination with topical medications such as coal tar (no significant increase in carcinogenic risk factor)
- Liquid nitrogen: freeze moderate-sized lesions

Systemic/Oral drugs (in difficult cases):

- Methotrexate: anti-cancer drug (long-term use causes hepatic, renal, hematologic toxicity; nausea; vomiting; diarrhea; significant risk of squamous cell and increased risk of metastatic carcinoma)
- Psoralen: With UVB therapy; least toxic oral medication
- Tegison (vitamin A analogue): inhibits rapid skin cell growth, particularly with UV therapy (numerous side effects)
- NSAIDs: for pain/inflammation of psoriatic arthritis

Complementary and Alternative Therapies

Therapies are aimed at detoxifying the entire body and regulating cAMP/gAMP ratios. Patients often benefit from mind/body therapies and stress management. Exercise increases cAMP and improves overall health. Proper hydration aids in elimination. Herbs and nutrition may be helpful by themselves or as adjunctive therapy.

NUTRITION

- Limit alcohol, refined foods, simple sugars, and saturated fats found in meat and dairy as these foods tend to exacerbate this condition. Avoid acidic foods (pineapple, oranges, coffee, tomato) and any allergic foods (wheat, citrus, milk, corn, eggs are the most common).
- Essential fatty acids: omega-3 and omega-6 (oily fish, flax seed oil, 1,000 mg bid)
- Vitamins: B_{12} (100 to 1,000 mcg) may need to be intramuscular injections, folate (400 mcg/day), vitamin E (400 to 800 IU/day)
- Minerals: found to be low in patients with psoriasis; zinc (30 mg/day), selenium (200 mcg/day)
- Quercetin: 500 mg tid before meals, decreases cAMP, decreases gut inflammation
- Digestive enzymes facilitate proper protein digestion and should be taken with each meal. This is particularly important as incomplete protein digestion inhibits the formation of cAMP, thus contributing to the cell proliferation which characterizes psoriasis.

HERBS

Herbs are generally a safe way to strengthen and tone the body's systems. As with any therapy, it is important to ascertain a diagnosis before pursuing treatment. Herbs may be used as dried extracts (capsules, powders, teas), glycerites (glycerine extracts), or tinctures (alcohol extracts). Unless otherwise indicated, teas should be made with 1 tsp. herb per cup of hot water. Steep covered 5 to 10 minutes for leaf or flowers, and 10 to 20 minutes for roots. Drink 2 to 4 cups/day. Tinctures may be used singly or in combination as noted.

- Topical creams may alleviate discomfort. Chickweed (Stellaria media) relieves itching and marigold (Calendula officinalis) speeds healing of open lesions.
- Milk thistle (Silybum marianum) decreases cAMP breakdown, liver protectant

- Yellow dock (Rumex crispus), red clover (Trifolium pratense), and burdock (Arctium lappa) are alteratives.
- Sarsaparilla (Smilax sarsaparilla) binds endotoxins, shown in studies to be effective in psoriasis
- Mix equal parts of the above herbs and use 1 cup tea tid or 30 to 60 drops tincture tid. This is especially effective if sipped or take 5 to 15 minutes before meals to stimulate digestion. Coleus (Coleus forskohlii) (tincture, 1 ml tid) increases cAMP, and has been used historically for psoriasis.

HOMEOPATHY

In homeopathic philosophy, treating a skin condition is not beneficial. Constitutional treatment by a homeopathic prescriber who will address the whole person may help. Homeopathic treatment of skin problems can result in an initial worsening of any skin condition before resolution.

PHYSICAL MEDICINE

Sunlight/ultraviolet light is a beneficial treatment for those with psoriasis. Exposure to the sun or UVB for half an hour daily is a helpful treatment.

Patient Monitoring

Follow-up is important in severe cases, particularly when treatment includes corticosteroids.

OTHER CONSIDERATIONS

Prevention

Prevention may not be possible, but avoid triggering drugs (lithium, NSAIDs, salicylates, white willow (Salix alba), penicillin, and others). Treatment aims at avoiding flare-ups and lengthening periods of remission. A stressful even often precedes the initial episode, thus stress management techniques often help with successful treatment.

Complications/Sequelae

- Secondary infections
- Arthritis
- Serious bowel involvement
- Exfoliate erythrodermatitis
- Rebound after corticosteroids

Prognosis

Aggressive control and treatment usually beget a benign course.

Pregnancy

Oral medications and topical creams absorbed into the bloodstream can be damaging to the fetus. Use caution when treating psoriasis.

REFERENCES

Blumenthal M, ed. The Complete German Commission E Monographs. Boston, Mass: Integrative Medicine Communications; 1998:169–170.

The Editors of Time-Life Books. The Medical Advisor. Alexandria, Va: Time-Life Books; 1996.

Ergil KV. Medicines from the Earth: Protocols for Botanical Healing. Harvard, Mass: Gaia Herbal Research Institute; 1996:207–211.

Gruenwald J, Brendler T et al, eds. PDR for Herbal Medicines. Montvale, NJ: Medical Economics Company; 1998:903–904, 114, 1157.

Syed TA, et al. Management of psoriasis with aloe vera extract in a hydrophilic cream: a placebo-controlled, double-blind study. Trop Med Int Health. 1996;1:505–509.

Walker JP, Brown EH. The Alternative Pharmacy. Paramus, NJ: Prentice Hall Press; 1998.

Werbach MR. Nutritional Influences on Illness. New Canaan, Conn: Keats Publishing Inc; 1988:370–373.

■ PULMONARY EDEMA

OVERVIEW

Definition

Pulmonary edema is characterized by the abnormal accumulation of pulmonary interstitial or alveolar fluid. Pulmonary edema due to heart disease increases in adults over age 40; the incidence rate due to non-cardiogenic causes is approximately 150,000 cases each year. The two primary subtypes are:

- Cardiogenic pulmonary edema—associated with congestive heart failure or other heart disease
- Noncardiogenic pulmonary edema—associated with a number of clinical conditions (e.g., acute severe asthma, lymphatic blockade, lymphangitis carcinomatosis, iatrogenic fluid overload, drug intoxication)

Other forms of pulmonary edema in which the exact mechanisms have not been fully explained include:

- Narcotic-overdose pulmonary edema
- High-altitude pulmonary edema
- Neurogenic pulmonary edema

Etiology

Causes are cardiogenic or noncardiogenic. The biological factors in the etiology of pulmonary edema include altered capillary permeability (e.g., from infections or inhaled toxins), increased pulmonary venous pressure (e.g., from left ventricle failure, mitral stenosis, or pulmonary venous disease), and decreased plasma oncotic pressure (e.g., hypoalbuminemia).

A variety of noncardiogenic factors can also cause pulmonary edema, including shock, drug overdose (e.g., from heroin), high altitude, transfusion reactions, CNS trauma, the Hanta virus, multiple trauma, eclampsia, and oxygen toxicity.

Risk Factors

- Hypertension
- Diabetes
- Coronary or valvular heart disease
- Obesity
- Smoking

Signs and Symptoms

- Dyspnea
- Tightness in chest
- Angina
- Rales
- Rhonchi
- Cyanosis
- Diaphoresis
- Pink, frothy sputum
- Anxiety
- Lower extremity edema

DIFFERENTIAL DIAGNOSIS

Differentiate cardiogenic from noncardiogenic causes:

- Pneumonia
- Asthma
- COPD exacerbation
- Hyperventilation syndrome

DIAGNOSIS

Physical Examination

Signs of pulmonary edema include tachypnea, tachycardia, and elevated blood pressure. A fever may indicate concurrent infection. Other physical presentations include cyanosis, diaphoresis, retractions, wheezing, rales, cough with pink and frothy sputum, S_3 gallop or murmur (may indicate valvular disease), peripheral edema, and bruits. The Swan-Ganz catheter may be used to obtain pulmonary vascular pressure and differentiate between cardiogenic and noncardiogenic forms.

Laboratory Tests

A variety of laboratory tests can help in detecting underlying etiology but are not considered specific for pulmonary edema.

- Blood tests, including CBC with differential, electrolyte, BUN, creatinine, and serum protein concentrations
- Urinalysis and microscopic examination of urine to detect proteinuria

Pathological Findings

- Imbalance of Starling forces
- Decreased plasma oncotic pressure
- Increased negativity of interstitial pressure
- Altered alveolar-capillary membrane permeability
- Lymphatic insufficiency

Imaging

- Echocardiogram to determine underlying cause, such as valvular disease or cardiomyopathy
- Chest X ray to reveal interstitial edema and pulmonary vasculature shadows (Clinical presentations may not appear on chest X rays for up to 12 hours; may also take up to four days to clear after clinical improvement.)

Other Diagnostic Procedures

Acute pulmonary edema is a life-threatening medical emergency. As a result, treatment may have to begin before making a complete diagnosis. The primary goal after initial treatment is to distinguish between cardiogenic and noncardiogenic forms. Diagnostic measures include taking a detailed medical history, including past history of cardiac and pulmonary disease, hypertension, shortness of breath, orthopnea, dyspnea on exertion, faintness, chest pain, recent weight gain, general edema, recent infection, and exposure to toxic inhalants or smoke. Diagnosis of pulmonary edema resulting from chronic forms of heart failure should focus on identifying underlying cardiac disorder (e.g., arrhythmia or infection). Tests include:

- Arterial blood gas
- ECG
- Pulmonary function

TREATMENT OPTIONS

Treatment Strategy

Depending on the cause of pulmonary edema, several general measures are recommended for immediate stabilization and long-term prevention against recurrent episodes.

- Administration of 100% oxygen (to achieve arterial PO_2 greater than 60 mm Hg) via nasal cannula or mask. Maintain patient in sitting position with legs dangling (facilitates respiration and reduces venous return) or elevate head of bed 30 degrees.
- Mechanical ventilation

- Rotating tourniquet applied to extremities
- Pharmacotherapy
- Surgery (indicated in rare cases, including valvular heart disease or ventricular septum rupture after myocardial infarction)

Drug Therapies

- Morphine (2 to 5 mg) as needed to reduce congestion and anxiety
- Diuretics, such as furosemide (40 to 80 mg) or ethacrynic acid (40 to 100 mg), given intravenously to reduce circulating blood volume
- Vasodilators, such as IV nitroglycerin (10 to 20 mcg/min increased by 10 to 20 mcg/min every five minutes until effective) or sodium nitroprusside administered intravenously (10 mcg/min litrated to goal of systolic blood pressure of 100 to 110 mm Hg) to decrease afterload and left ventricular work
- Digoxin can be administered orally (usual loading dose is 1 mg in 3 to 4 doses/24 hours, intravenously or orally) to achieve serum levels of 1.00 to 1.5 ng/ml; prior to administration, check for previous digoxin use and adverse reactions; also check for history of renal, pulmonary, liver, or thyroid disease; some medications used by patient might affect digoxin.
- Dobutamine (2.5 to 15 mcg/kg/min) or dopamine (2 to 20 mcg/kg/min) for inotropic support
- Aminophylline (theophylline ethylenediamine) (240 to 480 mg intravenously) to diminish bronchoconstriction, increase renal blood flow and sodium excretion, and augment myocardial contractility

Complementary and Alternative Therapies

Pulmonary edema is most often a sign of advanced pathology. Alternative therapies may be helpful in strengthening the cardiopulmonary system and reducing the severity of the disease.

NUTRITION

- Increase dietary potassium and magnesium with diuretic use (e.g., bananas, apricots, nuts, seeds, dandelion leaves *[Taraxacum officinalis],* and green leafy vegetables).
- Coenzyme Q10 (100 mg bid) supports cardiac function, is an antioxidant, and oxygenates tissues.
- L-Carnitine (500 mg tid) improves endurance and is needed for efficient cardiac function.
- Magnesium aspartate (200 mg bid to tid) increases efficiency of cardiac muscle and decreases vascular resistance. In addition, magnesium and calcium (1,000 mg/day) influence intra- and inter-cellular fluid exchange and may be depleted with diuretic use.
- Potassium aspartate (20 mg/day) improves heart contractility and should be supplemented with diuretic use.
- Vitamin E (400 IU/day) is an antioxidant and is cardioprotective.
- Vitamin C (1,000 to 1,500 mg tid) is an antioxidant, improves vascular integrity, and stimulates immune function.
- Taurine (500 mg bid) enhances the efficiency of cardiac function and may increase diuresis.
- Raw heart concentrate (100 to 200 mg/day) provides essential nutrients to the heart.
- Selenium (200 mcg/day) is an antioxidant that protects both heart and lung tissues.
- Choline (250 to 500 mg/day) and Inositol (150 to 200 mg/day) are part of the phospholipid membrane and positively effect parasympathetic activity and vasodilation.

HERBS

Herbs are generally a safe way to strengthen and tone the body's systems. As with any therapy, it is important to ascertain a diagnosis before pursuing treatment. Herbs may be used as dried extracts (capsules, powders, teas), glycerites (glycerine extracts), or tinctures (alcohol extracts). Unless otherwise indicated, teas should be made with 1 teaspoon herb per cup of hot water. Steep covered 5 to 10 minutes for leaf or flowers, and 10 to 20 minutes for roots. Drink 2 to 4 cups/day. Tinctures may be used singly or in combination as noted.

The goals of herbal therapy are to enhance the function of the cardiopulmonary systems, improve vascular tone, and increase diuresis. A general diuretic should contain herbs that support circulation and lymphatic drainage. They are best administered in a tea (4 to 6 cups/day), although a tincture may be used (30 to 60 drops qid). Combine three of these herbs with equal parts of two to three additional herbs from the following categories, according to the underlying cause. Cleavers *(Gallium aparine),* yarrow *(Achillea millefolium),* oatstraw *(Avena sativa),* elder *(Sambucus canadensis),* red clover *(Trifolium pratense),* fresh parsley *(Petroselenium crispus),* and dandelion leaf *(Taraxacum officinalis).*

Non-cardiogenic pulmonary edema:
- Garlic *(Allium sativum)* enhances expectoration, is hypotensive, and immune-stimulating. (Garlic can also be taken as capsules, 1,000 to 4,000 mg/day.)
- Rosemary *(Rosemarianus officinalis)* strengthens cardiac function, is anti-spasmodic, and improves circulation to the lungs.
- Linden flowers *(Tilia cordata)* is an anti-spasmodic, hypotensive, anti-atherosclerotic, respiratory relaxant, and expectorant. Also stimulates immune function.
- Indian tobacco *(Lobelia inflata)* stimulates respiratory function, is anti-spasmodic, and hypotensive. At high doses this herb has toxic side effects. Used as part of a formula (.25 or less) minimizes risk of toxicity. You may substitute mullcin *(Verbascum thapsus),* which also stimulates respiratory function.
- Thyme leaf *(Thymus vulgaris)* enhances expectoration, tonifies respiratory system, and increases circulation.

For cardiogenic pulmonary edema:
- Hawthorn *(Crataegus oxyacantha)* increases cardiac output without increasing cardiac load. Strengthens the integrity of vasculature and has mild vasodilation propeties.
- Motherwort *(Leonorus cardiaca)* has anti-spasmodic properties, relieves heart palpitations, and enhances cardiac function.
- Rosemary *(Rosemarianus officinalis)* strengthens vasculature and is an antispasmodic heart tonic.

The following herbs may be very effective in pulmonary edema with cardiac involvement. Because of their potential side effects they should only be used under physician supervision. All three increase cardiac output without increasing cardiac load, have diuretic properties, and have regulating effects on heart rhythm.
- Lily of the valley *(Convalleria majalis)*
- Night blooming cereus *(Cactus grandiflorus)*
- Broom *(Sarothamnus scoparius)*

HOMEOPATHY

An experienced homeopath should assess individual constitutional types and severity of disease to select the correct remedy and potency.

PHYSICAL MEDICINE

Contrast hydrotherapy. Alternating hot and cold applications brings nutrients to the site and diffuses metabolic waste from inflammation. The overall effect is decreased inflammation, pain relief, and enhanced healing. Using this technique with hand and/or foot baths may help to improve circulation and lymphatic drainage. If possible, immerse the part being treated (as with an extremity). Alternate 3 minutes hot with 1 minute cold. Repeat three times. This is one set. Do two to three sets/day.

Castor oil pack. Used externally, castor oil is a powerful anti-inflammatory. Apply oil directly to chest, cover with a clean soft cloth (e.g. flannel) and plastic wrap. Place a heat source (hot water bottle or heating pad) over the pack and let sit for 30 to 60 minutes. For best results use three consecutive days. Add four to six drops of essential oils, such as eucalyptus, lavender, rosemary, and thyme, to increase benefit.

Postural drainage may be helpful in relieving pulmonary congestion. Tapotement can help prevent consolidation.

ACUPUNCTURE
Acupuncture may improve cardio-pulmonary function and provide support in the treatment of underlying cause.

MASSAGE
Therapeutic massage can assist with increasing circulation and lymphatic drainage.

Patient Monitoring
Once immediate treatment for the acute stage of pulmonary edema is completed, a careful search for underlying cause should be initiated. Strategic measures are needed for long-range stabilization, which may include surgery.

OTHER CONSIDERATIONS
Prevention
Prompt treatment of cardiac disorders can reduce risk. Dietary approaches, such as a low-salt diet and maintaining an ideal weight, and smoking cessation are recommended to prevent heart disease.

Complications/Sequelae
Pulmonary edema can be fatal. It is sometimes misdiagnosed as asthma.

Prognosis
Highly dependent on etiology. Mortality is 50% to 60% for noncardiogenic pulmonary edema and higher for cardiogenic shock. Following acute phase, pulmonary edema is often manageable through medications and treatment of underlying disease.

Pregnancy
Conventional treatments are indicated as this may be life-threatening.

REFERENCES
Bartram T. *Encyclopedia of Herbal Medicine*. Dorset, England: Grace Publishers; 1995:73, 80, 155, 156.

Blumenthal M, ed. *The Complete German Commission E Monographs*. Boston, Mass: Integrative Medicine Communications; 1998:423, 425.

Dambro MR, ed. *Griffith's 5 Minute Clinical Consult*. Baltimore, Md: Williams & Wilkins; 1998.

Fauci AS, Braunwald E, Isselbacher KJ et al, eds. *Harrison's Principles of Internal Medicine*. 14th ed. New York, NY: McGraw-Hill; 1998.

Thierney LM Jr, McPhee SJ, Papadakis MA, eds. *Current Medical Diagnosis & Treatment 1999*. 38th ed. Stamford, Conn: Appleton & Lange; 1999.

■ RAYNAUD'S PHENOMENON

OVERVIEW

Definition

According to the U.S. National Heart, Lung, and Blood Institute, Raynaud's phenomenon is characterized by episodic vasospastic attacks resulting in digital ischemia. Fingers are most often affected, rarely toes. Sudden spasmodic contractions of arterioles occur when patient is exposed to cold or becomes stressed; episodes are intermittent and may last minutes or hours. Approximately 5% to 10% of the United States population is affected, with women being affected five times more often than men. It occurs usually between the ages of 20 to 40 in women and later in life for men. An estimated 80% to 90% of women with scleroderma have Raynaud's phenomenon. The two major subtypes are:

- Raynaud's disease or syndrome (primary/idiopathic), in which cases persist for more than two to three years without evidence of an associated disease. Progressive disease—spasms become more frequent and more severe.
- Secondary Raynaud's phenomenon, a less common form resulting from underlying disease, such as connective tissue disease. Increased morbidity and poorer prognosis.

Etiology

Biologic factors (e.g., abnormalities in the adrenergic receptor); psychodynamic influences (e.g., stress); underlying disease (e.g., systemic lupus erythematosus)

Risk Factors

- Cigarette smoking
- Age in women (onset primarily between the ages of 20 and 40)
- Occupation (using vibrating tools like chainsaws and jackhammers)
- Pharmaceuticals (including ergot preparations) methysergide, beta-adrenergic receptor antagonists, chemotherapeutic agents such as bleomycin, vinblastine, cisplatin; and some over-the-counter cold medications and prescription narcotics
- Existing autoimmune or connective tissue disorder
- Electric shock injury
- Previous frostbite
- Repeated physical stress (such as that resulting from typing or piano playing)
- Primary pulmonary hypertension
- Exposure to cold

Signs and Symptoms

- Changes in skin color in the fingers or toes and sometimes in the nose, legs, or earlobes (may occur in three phases: pallor, cyanosis, rubor)
- Throbbing, tingling, numbness, and pain
- Atrophy of the terminal fat pads
- Gangerous ulcers near fingertips

DIFFERENTIAL DIAGNOSIS

- Rheumatoid arthritis
- Systemic sclerosis (including more localized CREST)
- Systemic lupus erythematosus
- Mixed connective tissue disease
- Thromboangiitis
- Thoracic outlet compression syndrome
- Carpal tunnel syndrome
- Acrocyanosis
- Cryoglobulinemia
- Reflex sympathetic dystrophy

DIAGNOSIS

Physical Examination

White-blue-red sequence of changes in digits after exposure to cold or emotional disturbance; secondary form may present pitting scars and ulcers of the skin or gangrene in fingers or toes.

Laboratory Tests

A variety of laboratory tests may reveal abnormalities, but they are not considered diagnostic alone.
These include:

- Nail fold capillaroscopy, to distinguish between primary and secondary forms
- Antinuclear antibody test (ANA), to assess for antibodies due to connective tissue disease or other autoimmune disorder
- Erythrocyte sedimentation rate (ESR), to measure inflammation

Pathological Findings

Appears to result from an exaggeration of normal physiological responses involving vasculature constriction. May include episodic digital ischemia secondary to exaggerated reflex sympathetic vasoconstriction; enhanced digital vascular responsiveness to cold or normal sympathetic stimuli; normal reflex sympathetic vasoconstriction superimposed on local digital vascular disease; enhanced adrenergic neuroeffector activity.

Other Diagnostic Procedures

- Clinician interview—assess symptoms and degree of severity; detailed medical history and patient report essential since attacks are intermittent; if psychological in origin, patient may have an attack due to stress when being examined
- Evaluate for medical conditions, stress, possible pharmacological side effects
- The Allen test (radial/ulnar arteries) may help distinguish between occlusion vs. vasospasm. The Taylor-Pelmear scale system is used to classify vibration-induced disease. Provocative exposure to cold.

TREATMENT OPTIONS

Treatment Strategy

The primary goal is to reduce frequency and severity of episodes, prevent tissue damage, and treat underlying disease if present. Conservative non-drug and self-help measures (e.g., dressing warmly and avoiding the cold, smoking cessation) are used for mild and infrequent episodes. For severe cases, options include:

- Pharmacotherapy
- Sympathectomy (if symptoms are progressive)

Drug Therapies

- Calcium channel blockers (vasodilators) such as nifedipine (sustained-release, 10 to 30 mg tid) and diltiazem (30 to 90 mg tid) may benefit severe cases, especially with presence of peripheral vasoconstriction without significant organic vascular disease; side effects include headache, dizziness, flushing, palpitations, dyspepsia, pruritus, and edema.
- Adrenergic blocking agents such as resperine (0.25 to 0.5 mg tid) may increase nutritional blood flow to digits; side effects include hypotension, nasal stuffiness, lethargy, and depression.
- Postsynaptic alpha-adrenergic antagonist such as prazosin (1 to 5 mg tid)
- Doxazosin and terazosin
- Sympatholytic agents, including methyldopa, guanethidine, and phenoxybenzamine
- Prostoglandins to inhibit platelet aggregation; side effects include voiding and/or diarrhea and hypertension

- Angiotensin-converting enzyme inhibitors such as captopril reduce peripheral resistance, sympathetic nervous system activity reduction, and norepinephrine release due to angiotensin suppression.
- Serotonin S2 antagonist (Ketanserin) antagonizes serotonin S2 and blocks 1adrenergic receptors to inhibit vasoconstriction and platelet aggregation stimulated by serotonin; not available in the United States.
- Nitroglycerine relaxes smooth muscle, dilates veins, lowers oxygen need in the myocardial tissues, inhibits platelet aggregation.

Complementary and Alternative Therapies

Raynaud's is a poorly understood syndrome that may be helped with alternative therapies that improve circulation and support general health. Begin with nutritional support and circulatory stimulants.

Biofeedback may allow patient to bring digit temperature under voluntary control. Autogenic training has been found to be an effective technique for Raynaud's phenomenon.

NUTRITION

- Vitamin E (400 to 800 IU/day) improves circulation and inhibits platelet aggregation.
- Vitamin C (1,000 mg bid to tid) supports connective tissue and reduces inflammation.
- B-complex (50 to 100 mg/day) reduces the effects of stress.
- Coenzyme Q10 (100 mg bid) enhances tissue oxygenation.
- Calcium (1,500 mg/day) and Magnesium (200 mg tid) relieve spasm.
- Omega-3 oils (1,500 mg bid to tid) are anti-inflammatory and inhibit platelet aggregation.
- Zinc (30 to 50 mg/day) is required for normal immune function.

HERBS

Herbs are generally a safe way to strengthen and tone the body's systems. As with any therapy, it is important to ascertain a diagnosis before pursuing treatment. Herbs may be used as dried extracts (capsules, powders, teas), glycerites, or tinctures (alcohol extracts). Unless otherwise indicated, teas should be made with one teaspoon herb per cup of hot water. Steep covered 10 to 20 minutes and drink two to four cups/day. Tinctures may be used singly or in combination as noted.

The following herbs are circulatory stimulants with other properties as well. Use one or more tinctures in combination, 20 to 30 drops bid.

- Hawthorn berries (Crataegus oxyanthoides)—enhances vascular integrity, and has mild vasodilatory effects
- Ginkgo (Ginkgo biloba)—120 to 160 mg/day for dried extracts, inhibits platelet aggregation
- Rosemary (Rosemariana officinalis)—is a gentle relaxant
- Ginger root (Zingiber officinalis)—is a mild anodyne
- Prickly ash bark (Xanthoxylum clava-herculis)—enhances lymph activity and vascular integrity

HOMEOPATHY

An experienced homeopath should assess individual constitutional types and severity of disease to select the correct remedy and potency.

ACUPUNCTURE

Acupuncture may be useful as an adjunctive therapy to increase circulation and reduce vasospasm.

MASSAGE

Therapeutic massage or bath using essential oils may help ease symptoms. A basic formula includes six drops of a blend of nutmeg (Myristica fragrans), 15 drops, lavender (Lavandula angustifolia), 5 drops, and geranium, 10 drops, for bath; add two tbsp. vegetable oil for massage; other essential oils used in massage include cypress (Cupressus sempervirens), neroli (Citrus aurantium), lemon (Citrus limon), or rose (Rosa gallica) in 2 tsp. base oil.

Patient Monitoring

All patients should avoid or quit smoking since nicotine is a vasoconstrictor.

OTHER CONSIDERATIONS
Prevention

Patient should protect himself or herself from exposure to cold and guard against cuts and other injury to affected areas. Exercise, such as raising arms above head and whirling them vigorously, may help circulation. Biofeedback may help patient prevent or stop attacks.

Complications/Sequelae

Dry gangrene is a serious but rare complication. Other complications include ulceration of affected parts and deformities of fingers/fingernails or toes/toenails.

Prognosis

Progressive course, yet management techniques are successful in 40% to 60% of symptoms of Raynaud's phenomenon patients. Mild cases of vibration-induced disease should recover if causal activity is avoided. .

Pregnancy

Some medications used to treat Raynaud's phenomenon may affect the growing fetus.

REFERENCES

Balch JF, Balch PA. *Prescription for Nutritional Healing.* 2nd ed. Garden City Park, NY: Avery Publishing Group; 1997.

Batchelder HJ. Allopathic specific condition review: Raynaud's disease. *The Protocol Journal of Botanical Medicine.* 1996;2:134–137.

Fauci AS, Braunwald E, Isselbacher KJ et al, eds. *Harrison's Principles of Internal Medicine.* 14th ed. New York, NY: McGraw-Hill; 1998.

Mitchell W, Batchelder HJ. Naturopathic specific condition review: Raynaud's disease. *The Protocol Journal of Botanical Medicine.* 1996;2:138–140.

Thierney LM Jr, McPhee SJ, Papadakis MA, eds. *Current Medical Diagnosis & Treatment 1999.* 38th ed. Stamford, Conn: Appleton & Lange; 1999.

■ REITER'S SYNDROME

OVERVIEW

Definition

Reiter's syndrome is a reactive arthritis, either sexually transmitted (*Chlamydia trachomatis* or *Ureaplasma urealyticum*) or follows enteric bacterial infection (dysenteric) and classically has a triad of symptoms: arthritis, conjunctivitis, and urethritis. Mouth and skin ulcerations are now recognized as a fourth feature. Only a third of patients present with the triad, making Reiter's syndrome difficult to diagnose. Differing clinical manifestations depend on gender, genetics, and race.

Etiology

The syndrome has arthritic features appearing one to three weeks after the triggering infection. Infectious agents have been found in affected joints, but etiology of joint involvement is unknown. Microbial antigens within the synovium suggest possible continuing infection or that the arthritis is caused by the persistence of antigens.

- HLA-B27 gene—20% of people with the gene get Reiter's; about 80% of people with Reiter's are HLA-B27+

Dysentery triggers:

- Salmonella—6.4% to 6.9% develop Reiter's; 60% are HLA-B27$^+$ or have B27 cross-reactive antigens
- Shigella—0.2% to 2% develop Reiter's; most are HLA-B27$^+$
- Campylobacter—occasionally
- Yersinia—predominately in Scandinavia; 60% to 80% are HLA-B27

Sexually transmitted disease triggers (1% to 3% following nongonococcal infections):

- Chlamydia—50% of Reiter's patients have antibodies to *C. trachomatis;* 50% are HLA-B27$^+$; a T-cell-mediated, chlamydial antigen-specific immune response is being researched.
- Reiter's is not in itself a sexually transmitted disease.

Risk Factors

- Sexual intercourse with chlamydia-infected partner
- White males ages 20 to 40
- HLA-B27 gene and associated infective pathogens
- Food poisoning, bacterial dysentery

Signs and Symptoms

Not every symptom type occurs for each patient.

- Arthritic disorders—pain, swelling, stiffness, redness
- Spondyloarthropathy—joints of the spine and sacroiliac
- Small joints of the fingers and toes (digital periostitis; "sausage digits"), wrists, feet (plantar fascitis), or ankles (Achilles tendinitis)
- Conjunctivitis—affects 40%; usually brief, mild
- Keratitis, corneal ulceration, scleritis
- Iritis—affects 5%; scarring and permanent damage can occur; pain and light sensitivity
- Urethritis—affects 33%; burning during urination may not occur; pus drainage from penis
- Prostatitis—prostate tender on palpation
- Circinate balanitis—affects 33% of men; shallow ulcerations on the shaft or glans of the penis; painless
- Keratoderma blennorrhagica—papulosquamous eruptions on soles, palms, and glans penis; purulent with thick keratotic outer layer
- Mouth—inflammation of hard and soft palate; often painless
- Costochondritis—inflammation of the breastbone cartilage
- Anorexia or weight loss, malaise, morning stiffness, fever

DIFFERENTIAL DIAGNOSIS

- Ankylosing spondylitis
- Crohn's disease associated arthritis
- Inflammatory bowel disease associated arthritis
- Ulcerative colitis
- Psoriatic arthritis
- Lyme disease
- Gonococcal bacterial arthritis

DIAGNOSIS

Physical Examination

Patient may have fever, severe pain, and weight loss during acute phase.

Laboratory Tests

- Serological test—antecedents for Yersinia or Chlamydia support diagnosis
- Inflammation—indicated by erythrocyte sedimentation rate and C-reactive protein levels
- Synovial fluid—>2,000 cells/ml, mostly polymorphonuclear leukocytes
- Urinalysis or urine culture—determines bacterial infection

Pathological Findings

- Synovial/joint inflammation—cellular infiltration of polymorphonuclear leukocytes, lymphocytes, and plasma cells; heterotopic bone formation
- Enthesitis—inflammation and erosion where the tendons and muscles insert into the bone
- Mucocutaneous lesions—thickening of the horny layer, acanthosis, parakeratosis
- Intestines—acute and chronic lesions, inflammation of the colon and terminal portion of the ileum

Imaging

- X-rays—reveal spurs, calcifications, periosteal thickening, joint and articular margin erosion, sacroiliitis; enthesitis appears as erosions and reactive new bone formation; abnormalities in 70% of chronic patients
- Scintigraphy—more sensitive in sacroiliac and enthesitis detection
- Computerized tomography—assesses sacroiliac and spondylitic involvement

Other Diagnostic Procedures

Diagnosis of Reiter's is difficult. History of infecting agent helps, but can occur without trigger. Exclusion of other diagnoses, the presence of spine and sacroiliac arthritis, and appearance of non-joint symptoms, especially urethritis, determines correct diagnosis. Skin lesions typical of Reiter's permit a more definitive diagnosis. The HLA-B27 genetic marker is not diagnostic but helps confirm diagnosis.

TREATMENT OPTIONS

Treatment Strategy

Treatment focuses on symptom management. Specialists for each discrete symptom are usually needed, as each symptom may require a different strategy. Physical and occupational therapy may help patients improve muscle tone, maintain mobility, alleviate gait disturbances, and learn to perform tasks with less stress on joints.

Drug Therapies

- Nonsteroidal anti-inflammatory drugs (NSAIDS)—Indomethacin (2 to 3 mg/kg/day, especially effective in 75 mg bid slow-release); side effects include gastrointestinal irritation, bleeding, ulceration, headaches, dizziness

- Corticosteroids—oral or local injection into joint; decreases inflammation and controls pain
- Sulfasalazine—experimental, promising sulfa-based drug for peripheral arthritis; 2 to 3 g/day; well-tolerated; monitor blood counts with long-term use for bone marrow suppression
- Methotrexate—orally or by injection for chronic arthritis; 7.5 to 15 mg/week; experimental; blood and liver tests for bone marrow and liver toxicity, respectively; contraindicated with acquired immunodeficiency syndrome (AIDS)

Complementary and Alternative Therapies

Alternative therapies may be effective at alleviating symptoms. Treatment strategy is very similar to rheumatoid arthritis, with specific nutrients and herbs for the eyes and lower urinary tract.

NUTRITION

- Glucosamine sulfate (500 mg tid—higher doses required for obese patients or those taking diuretics): stimulates cartilage growth and may be as effective for pain relief as NSAIDs without the side effects. May take one to three months to see relief. Anecdotal cases find cartilage regeneration.
- Avoid nightshade family (tomatoes, potatoes, eggplant, peppers, tobacco); decrease saturated fats and alcohol (inflammatory); increase oily fish, nuts, and flaxseed (anti-inflammatory); increase fruits and vegetables (bioflavonoids); and avoid any allergenic foods.
- Antioxidants: Vitamin C (1,000 to 3,000 mg/day), vitamin E (400 to 800 IU/day), beta-carotene (25,000 IU/day), selenium (200 mcg/day)
- Essential fatty acids (2 tbsps. oil/day or 1,000 to 1,500 mg bid): a mix of omega-6 (evening primrose) and omega-3 (flaxseed).
- Minerals: zinc (45 mg/day), copper (1 mg/day), bromelain (500 mg tid)—anti-inflammatory

HERBS

Ascertain a diagnosis before pursuing treatment. Herbs may be used as dried extracts (capsules, powders, teas), glycerites (glycerine extracts), or tinctures (alcohol extracts). Unless otherwise indicated, teas should be made with 1 tsp. herb per cup of hot water. Steep covered 5 to 10 minutes for leaf or flowers, and 10 to 20 minutes for roots. Drink 2 to 4 cups/day. Tinctures may be used singly or in combination as noted.

Turmeric (Curcuma longa)—anti-inflammatory: 400 mg tid is equally effective as phenybutazone 300 mg/day for duration of morning stiffness, walking time, and joint swelling, with greater safety and tolerability, works especially well with bromelain.

For urethritis:

- Juniper (Juniperus communis): diuretic historically used for inflammatory conditions of the lower urinary tract, avoid with kidney disease
- Uva ursi (Arctostaphylos uva-ursi): antibacterial and anti-inflammatory for lower urinary tract, for acute use only

- Horsetail (Equisetum arvense): soothing diuretic with historic use for rheumatic disease
- Licorice (Glycyrrhiza glabra): anti-inflammatory, soothing, not for use with hypertension
- Meadowsweet (Filipendula ulmaria): anti-inflammatory with historic use as a diuretic and for rheumatism

Mix three to four of these herbs in equal amounts and use 1 tsp. of mixture. Drink 1 cup tea tid or 30 drops tincture tid, daily during acute flare-up, and two weeks of the month as a preventive.
For iritis:

- Horsetail, licorice, meadowsweet (see above)
- Eyebright (Euphrasia officinalis) and bilberry (Vaccinium myrtillus): historically used for inflammation of the eyes; drink 30 to 60 drops tincture tid, 1 cup tea tid, and use tea to make compresses for acute relief.

ACUPUNCTURE

As with other forms of arthritis, acupuncture may be effective at stimulating the immune system, and reducing inflammation.

Patient Monitoring

Patients are sometimes hospitalized during the acute phase. Prolonged follow-up is necessary to confirm diagnosis, treat changing symptoms, and avoid further complications.

OTHER CONSIDERATIONS
Complications/Sequelae

- Blindness
- Aortic root necrosis

Prognosis

Initial attacks last three to six months. Syndrome manifests within 10 to 30 days of infection. Mean duration is 19 weeks. Fifty percent of people with one to two attacks have no further symptoms. Most people with a third attack develop chronic Reiter's syndrome. The intensity of attacks tends to maintain a consistent pattern, but few (15%) patients have permanent joint damage. Patients maintain near-normal lifestyles with physical/occupational modifications.

Pregnancy

Drugs must be evaluated for safety during pregnancy.

REFERENCES

Bartram T. *Encyclopedia of Herbal Medicine.* Dorset, England: Grace Publishers; 1995:368–369.

Gruenwald J, Brendler T, Jaenicke C et al, eds. *PDR for Herbal Medicines.* Montvale, NJ: Medical Economics Company; 1998.

Koopman WJ, ed. *Arthritis and Allied Conditions.* 13th ed. Baltimore, Md: Lippincott, Williams & Wilkins; 1996.

Murray MT, Pizzorno JE. *Encyclopedia of Natural Medicine.* 2nd ed. Rocklin, Calif: Prima Publishing; 1998.

Weiss RF. *Herbal Medicines.* Beaconsfield, England: Beaconsfield Publishers; 1998:339.

■ RHEUMATOID ARTHRITIS
OVERVIEW
Definition
Rheumatoid arthritis (RA) is a chronic systemic inflammatory autoimmune disease. Main characteristics include symmetrical synovitis and joint erosion; extra-articular manifestations affect the lungs, eyes, heart, and blood vessels. RA affects approximately 1% of the population, striking women in a 3:1 ratio to men. The usual age of onset lies between 30 and 60, but the disease can strike at any age. Symptom severity and disease progression vary widely between individuals. Onset may be rapid or insidious.

Etiology
The etiology of RA remains elusive, but a genetic link involving the major histocompatibility complex class II antigens has been identified. Medical researchers suspect that environmental factors in conjunction with genetic predisposition may trigger RA.

Risk Factors
- Genetic predisposition
- Environmental factors may include bacterial or viral infection and hormonal status
- Psychological stress (possible)
- Female gender
- Typically ages 30 to 60, although RA occurs at all ages

Signs and Symptoms
- Malaise, low-grade fever, weight loss, and stiffness in and about joints following inactivity
- Morning stiffness lasts for more than one hour
- Arthritis of more than three joints; specifically, proximal interphalangeal, metacarpophalangeal, wrist, elbow, knee, ankle, and metatarsophalangeal joints
- At least one affected hand joint; specifically, wrist, metacarpophalangeal, or proximal interphalangeal joint
- Extra-articular symptoms such as rheumatoid nodules, pleural effusion, pericarditis, lymphadenopathy, splenomegaly with leukopenia, vasculitis, normochromic, normocytic anemia, and elevated ESR.

DIFFERENTIAL DIAGNOSIS
- Ankylosing spondylitis and seronegative spondyloarthropathy
- Diffuse connective tissue disease, including systemic lupus erythematosus, scleroderma, dermatomytosis/polymyositis, vasculitis, and mixed connective tissue disease
- Other forms of arthritis, including infectious arthritis, reactive arthritis, and osteoarthritis
- Glucocorticoid withdrawal syndrome
- Gout, pseudogout
- Calcium pyrophosphate dihydrate deposition disease
- Chronic fatigue syndrome
- Fibromyalgia
- HIV infection
- Intermittent hydrarthrosis
- Lyme disease
- Malignancy, occult malignancy
- Parkinson's disease (with regard to swan neck deformities of the hands)
- Polymyalgia rheumatica and giant cell arteritis

DIAGNOSIS
Physical Examination
The patient experiences joint stiffness, tenderness, and pain; the affected joints are swollen and may be warm to the touch. Approximately 20% of patients present with subcutaneous nodules located over bony prominences or within bursas or tendon sheaths. Some patients exhibit splenomegaly and lymph node enlargement; low-grade fever, anorexia, weight loss, fatigue, and weakness are more common. In advanced cases, symptoms include skin and muscle atrophy; dryness of the eyes, mouth, and other mucous membranes; and physical deformities.

Laboratory Tests
Blood tests reveal several abnormalities:
- Rheumatoid factor (IgM antibody directed against IgG) present in 80% of cases
- Antinuclear antibodies present in 25% of cases
- Elevated erythrocyte sedimentation rate
- Elevated levels of gamma globulins (typically IgM and IgG)
- Platelet count may elevate due to inflammation
- Moderate hypochromic normocytic anemia
- Leukopenia (frequent with splenomegaly)

Arthrocentesis may reveal:
- Straw-colored joint fluid that is slightly cloudy and contains flecks of fibrin
- White blood cell counts at 5,000 to 25,000 per mm (>85% polymorphonuclear leukocytes)
- IgG may approach serum levels
- Depressed glucose level (may be less than 25 mg/dL)

Pathological Findings
- Synovitis
- Pannus formation (i.e., thickening of synovium)
- Cartilage breakdown
- Bone erosion

Imaging
In later stages of the disease, x-rays can reveal joint space narrowing and joint destruction.

Other Diagnostic Procedures
- Patient's report of symptoms
- Physician assessment of physical symptoms
- Results of laboratory tests
- American College of Rheumatology criteria (five of the following seven, with numbers 1 through 4 continuous for at least six weeks): (1) Morning stiffness greater than one hour; (2) Arthritis in at least three joint groups with soft tissue swelling or fluid; (3) Swelling involving at least one of the following joint groups: ploximal interpalangeal, metacarpophalangeal, or wrists; (4) Symmetrical joint swelling; (5) Subcutaneous nodules; (6) Positive rhematoid factor test; (7) Radiographic changes consistent with RA

TREATMENT OPTIONS
Treatment Strategy
Treatment is typically aimed at relieving symptoms, preventing joint degradation, and preserving joint function. Traditional treatment involves a conservative approach using nonpharmacologic therapy and nonsteroidal anti-inflammatory drugs for up to a year before resorting to aggressive therapies. However, as substantial joint destruction can occur within two years of developing RA, the current recommendation is to treat RA earlier and more aggressively. Other general treatment strategies include the following.
- Whole-body rest to reduce systemic inflammatory response and combat RA-associated fatigue

- Articular rest such as joint relaxation techniques, assistive devices, and splints
- Heat and cold treatment
- Exercise to preserve joint motion, strength, endurance
- Surgery (e.g., carpal tunnel release, resection of metatarsal heads, total hip or total knee arthroplasty) to address joint destruction, deformation, or refractory pain

Drug Therapies

Nonsteroidal anti-inflammatory drugs (NSAIDs) such as aspirin, ibuprofen, ketoprofen, naproxen, tolmetin, diclofenac, and diflunisal reduce pain and inflammation. Gastrointestinal side effects are common and may include ulcers and bleeding. The recently FDA-approved celecoxib selectively inhibits cyclo-oxgenase-2 and has a reduced risk of gastrointestinal side effects. Many more "COX-2" drugs are expected to be approved shortly.

Disease-modifying anti-rheumatoid drugs (DMARDs) include gold salts (injectable or oral), antimalarials (e.g., hydroxychloroquine), penicillamine, and sulfasalazine. DMARDs also include immunosuppressive drugs such as methotrexate, azathioprine, and cyclophosphamide. Beneficial effects may not be apparent for weeks or months. Most DMARDs have serious side effects including gastrointestinal symptoms, thrombocytopenia, myelosuppression, proteinuria, and hepatotoxicity.

Costicosteroids (glucocorticoids) have both anti-inflammatory and immuno-suppressive effects. Drugs such as prednisone (5 to 15 mg predinsone or equivalent daily, for short-term use) and methylprednisolone relieve symptoms quickly and may be given orally or by injection. Side effects include osteoporosis, mood changes, fluid retention and weight gain, and hypertension.

Some patients do not respond to individual DMARDs and better results may be achieved through drug combination. For example, a combination of methotrexate, hydroxychloroquine, and sulfasalazine may be more effective than methotrexate alone.

Experimental therapy options include the following.
- Zileuton, a 5-lipoxygenase inhibitor, is under FDA review for treatment of mild synovitis
- Oral Type II collagen
- Minocycline
- Recombinant human interleukin-1 receptor antagonist
- Antibodies to TNF-α
- Anti-CD4 monoclonal antibodies
- Cyclosporine
- Mycophenolate mofetil

Complementary and Alternative Therapies

The goal of therapy is to decrease inflammation and preserve joint function. Because some, but not all, cases of RA respond to dietary changes, a trial should be informative and may be helpful. Proper nutrition is often a mainstay of complimentary therapies. Herbs may be helpful for decreasing the severity and frequency of attacks. Treatment is long term.

NUTRITION
- The most common allergic foods are wheat, corn, and dairy. Elimination/challenge diets may identify whether these foods constitute a problem. Avoid foods completely for two weeks, then reintroduce the foods one at a time, every three days, and note symptoms. Citrus, chocolate, alcohol, red meat, flour products, spices, and carbonated drinks may also aggravate RA.
- A vegetarian diet high in antioxidants may provide relief from the symptoms. This diet has high amounts of flavanoids (green tea, blueberry, elderberry) and low amounts of saturated fats.
- A small percentage of people respond dramatically to a diet free of nightshades. They include peppers, eggplant, tomatoes and white potatoes. A month-long trial is recommended.
- Selenium levels are low in people who have RA. One clinical study demonstrated that selenium combined with vitamin E reduces RA symptoms. Dose is 50 to 75 mcg/day of selenium and 400 to 800 IU of vitamin E.
- Zinc (45 mg/day) and manganese (45 mg/day) have both been found to be low in RA.
- Omega-3 fatty acids suppress the production of inflammatory compounds produced by white blood cells. Dose is 1,000 to 1,500 IU/day.
- Bromelain is a proteolytic enzyme that when taken away from food is an anti-inflammatory (when taken with meals, it acts as a digestive enzyme). Dose is 2,000 to 2,500 mg bid.
- Quercetin stabilizes mast cells, found in increased numbers in the synovial membranes of affected joints. Dose is 250 to 500 mg tid away from food.

HERBS
Herbs are generally a safe way to strengthen and tone the body's systems. As with any therapy, it is important to ascertain a diagnosis before pursuing treatment. Herbs may be used as teas, dried extracts (capsules, powders), glycerites (glycerine extracts), or tinctures (alcohol extracts). Unless otherwise indicated, teas should be made with 1 tsp. herb per cup of hot water. Steep covered 5 to 10 minutes for leaf or flowers, and 10 to 20 minutes for roots. Drink 2 to 4 cups/day. Tinctures may be used singly or in combination as noted.
- Devil's Claw *(Harpagophytum procumbens):* analgesic, anti-inflammatory
- Ginseng *(Panax ginseng):* adaptogen (tonic for long-term stress), specific for chronic disease or condition and the effects of suppressive medications
- Ginger *(Zingiber officinale):* antispasmodic, digestive stimulant, anti-inflammatory
- Valerian *(Valeriana officinalis):* sedative, anodyne, antispasmodic, bitter. Helpful for pain control, especially if pain causes sleep disturbances.
- Blue flag *(Iris versicolor):* cholagogue (stimulates liver to process effects of inflammation)
- Wild yam *(Dioscorea villosa):* antispasmodic, bitter, specific for RA, adaptogen
- Horsetail *(Equisitum arvense):* diuretic, stabilizes connective tissue
- Devil's claw and three to five of the above herbs can be mixed as either tincture 30 to 60 drops tid, or 1 cup tea tid.

Other herbs to consider to reduce excessive immune response include gana derma, maitake mushroom *(Grifold frondosa),* and turmeric. Other anti-inflammatory herbs to consider include boswelia, sarsparilla *(Smilax* species), gotu kola *(Centella asiatica),* and ashwaganda (winter cherry).

HOMEOPATHY
An experienced homeopath should assess individual constitutional types and severity of disease to select the correct remedy and potency. For acute prescribing use 3 to 5 pellets of a 12X to 30C remedy every one to four hours until acute symptoms resolve.
- *Rhus toxicodendron* for arthritis that feels worse in the morning, in damp, cold weather and/or before a storm, and feels better with heat, dry weather, and upon moving the joints
- *Bryonia alba* for arthritis that feels better with pressure, feels worse

with any movement, and/or cold weather, but also feels worse with getting overheated
- *Ruta graveolens* for arthritic pains that feel worse after exertion, feel better after resting, especially with a history of strains/sprains to the joints
- *Calcarea carbonica* for arthritis that is associated with weakness and cold clammy extremities that feel worse in the cold

ACUPUNCTURE
May be helpful at decreasing pain, improving joint function, and delaying disease process.

MASSAGE
May be helpful in relieving symptoms and increasing mobility.

Patient Monitoring
- Side effects of pharmacologic treatment
- Osteoporosis prevention
- Periodic blood tests and X rays

OTHER CONSIDERATIONS
Complications/Sequelae
- Joint infection
- Cardiopulmonary complications
- Systemic vasculitis
- Gastrointestinal complications
- Amyloidosis
- Joint erosion or destruction
- Skin vasculitis

Prognosis
RA varies widely among individuals. Approximately 15% to 20% of cases have an intermittent course with periods of partial to complete remission. Flare-ups may involve more joints than were initially affected, but remission periods often last longer than flare-ups. A further 10% of cases have periods of long clinical remission. The majority of cases (65% to 70%) are progressive; the rate of progression can be slow or rapid.

Early age of onset, high rheumatoid factor titer, and elevated erythrocyte sedimentation rate correspond to a poor prognosis. Involvement of more than 20 to 30 joints and presence of extra-articular symptoms also correspond with a poor outcome. Women generally have a poorer outcome than men. Individuals experiencing unrelieved symptoms for two or more years are at increased risk of premature death due to infection, heart disease, respiratory failure, renal failure, and gastrointestinal disease.

Pregnancy
- Seventy-five percent of female RA patients experience symptom remission with pregnancy.
- Most DMARDs must be paired with effective contraception.

REFERENCES
American College of Rheumatology, Clinical Guidelines Committee. Guidelines for rheumatoid arthritis management. *Arthritis Rheum.* 1996;39:713–722.

Blumenthal M, ed. *The Complete German Commission E Monographs.* Boston, Mass: Integrative Medicine Communications; 1998:121, 135, 150–151, 138, 226–227.

Gruenwald J, Brendler T, Jaenicke C et al, eds. *PDR for Herbal Medicines.* Montvale, NJ: Medical Economics Company; 1998:810.

Kelley WN, Harris ED, Sledge CB, eds. *Textbook of Rheumatology.* 5th ed. Philadelphia, Pa: WB Saunders Company; 1997: chap 55.

Mazzetti I, Grigolo B, Borzai RM, Meliconi R, Facchini A. Serum copper/zinc superoxide dismutase levels in patients with rheumatoid arthritis. *J Clin Lab Res.* 1996;26(4):245–249.

Morrison R. *Desktop Guide to Keynotes and Confirmatory Symptoms.* Albany, Calif: Hahnemann Clinic Publishing; 1993:73–75, 85–86, 226, 329–330.

Mulherrin DM, Thurnham DI, Situnayake RD. Glutathione reductase activity, riboflavin status, and disease activity in rheumatoid arthritis. *Ann Rheum Dis.* 1996;55:837–840.

Murray MT, Pizzorno JE. *Encyclopedia of Natural Medicine.* Rocklin, Calif: Prima Publishing; 1998:492–501.

Tierney Jr LM, McPhee SJ, Papadakis MA, eds. *Current Medical Diagnosis & Treatment, 1999.* Stamford, Conn: Appleton & Lange; 1999.

Weisman MH, Weinblatt ME, eds. *Treatment of the Rheumatic Diseases: Companion to the Textbook of Rheumatology.* Philadelphia, Pa: WB Saunders Company; 1995: chap 3.

Wylie G, et al. A comparative study of Tenidap, a cytokine-modulating anti-rheumatic drug, and diclofenac in rheumatoid arthritis: a 24 week analysis of a 1-year clinical trial. *Br J Rheumatol.* 1995;34:554–563.

Zurier RB, Rossetti RG, Jacobson EW, et al. Gamma-linolenic acid treatment of rheumatoid arthritis. A randomized, placebo-controlled trial. *Arthritis Rheum.* 1996;39:1808–1817.

■ ROSEOLA

OVERVIEW

Definition

Roseola infantum (exanthem subitum or sixth disease) is a nonspecific febrile disease with an incubation period of one to two weeks, usually followed by skin rash. Ninety percent of cases (B variant) occur in the first two years of life, with a prevalence of 30% for children in the United States. Five percent (A variant) occur in adult patients with the acquired immunodeficiency syndrome (AIDS) or lymphoproliferative disease.

- As much as ninety percent of all people older than age two are seropositive for one or both variants.
- Immune response includes presence of antibodies, T-cell reactivity, and cytokines.

Etiology

Roseola is most often caused by the human herpesvirus 6 (HHV-6). The virus was isolated in 1986 from the peripheral blood mononuclear cells of AIDS and lymphoproliferative patients. As much as 80 to 90% of adults are seropositive for HHV-6. As maternal antibodies to roseola decrease, infants first become susceptible. It is still unknown how the disease is acquired but may be from viral shedding in saliva. The incubation period is 5 to 15 days. As many as 7% of cases may be caused by other rare pathogens or enteroviruses.

Risk Factors

- Age—under age three
- AIDS or other immunocompromised patients (e.g., transplant recipients)—the virus becomes pathogenic when reactivated in these patients.
- Males and females are equally likely to acquire roseola.

Signs and Symptoms

- Fever—sudden onset of high fever (103° to 106°F), usually lasting three to four days; child usually remains alert and active. Fever subsides promptly with appearance of rash.
- Rash—usually appears as fever resolves and lasts for three to four days; may be measles-like (macular, coalescent) or rubella-like (papular); discrete, nonpruritic, rose-colored lesions are two to three mm in diameter; usually appears first on trunk and spreads to neck and extremities but spares face
- Seizures—relatively rare, appearing at height of fever; resolves when fever subsides; may occur without rash
- Bulging anterior fontanelle
- Respiratory symptoms, inflamed tympanic membranes, and diarrhea occur in about half of the cases.

DIFFERENTIAL DIAGNOSIS

- Bacterial pneumonia
- Measles
- Rubella
- Drug reactions
- Entero- or adenoviral diseases
- Sepsis
- Urinary tract infection
- Meningitis
- Fifth disease
- Otitis media

DIAGNOSIS

Physical Examination

Patient may be either listless or normally active with high fever. Nonpruritic, rose-colored lesions usually appear as fever resolves.

Laboratory Tests

- Complete blood count during primary infection—white cell count averages 8,000/mm^3, leukopenia with relative lymphocytosis
- Serologic tests show serum IgM and IgG antibodies to HHV-6; must exclude human cytomegalovirus
- Increase in neutrophils and an infrequent elevated number of monocytes
- With rare cases of encephalopathy, DNA may be found in the cerebrospinal fluid.
- Viral cell culture (or culture on tissue from affected organs) is done primarily for research purposes or for clinical management in post-primary infections

Pathological Findings

- Viral latency is supported by viral nucleic acid in both peripheral blood mononuclear cells and saliva in seropositive adults and children.
- Enlarged spleen—occurs but is uncommon

Other Diagnostic Procedures

Diagnosis is by exclusion of other diseases and by observation of the pattern of fever and rash. Roseola can be suspected when it is known to be in the community.

TREATMENT OPTIONS

Treatment Strategy

There is no cure for roseola. Most cases are self-limiting and benign. Cool baths reduce temperature and lightweight bed clothes can lessen the effects of the condition.

Drug Therapies

- Antipyretics (e.g., acetaminophen 10 to 15 mg/kg every four hours, maximum 2.6 g/day)—lower fever, analgesic properties ease discomfort; caution with aspirin for children as Reye's syndrome may develop.
- High fluid intake prevents dehydration.
- Sedatives (e.g., diazepam [Valium]) may reduce chance of seizures in children prone to convulsions.
- Phenobarbital is sometimes given for seizures.

Complementary and Alternative Therapies

The main focus is on managing the symptoms and on preventing febrile seizures (brought on by a rapid rise in the temperature or too high a temperature). The correct homeopathic remedy can be very effective. Herbal teas are diaphoretic, anti-pyretic and calming. Adult doses are listed, unless otherwise specified. The formula to determine the child's dose is (age of child/20) x adult dose = child dose. Adult doses may given to the mother for breastfeeding babies.

NUTRITION

Immune stimulating: vitamin C (1,000 mg tid), zinc (30 to 60 mg/day) and beta-carotene (250,000 IU/day).

HERBS

Herbs are generally a safe way to strengthen and tone the body's systems. As with any therapy, it is important to ascertain a diagnosis before pursuing treatment. Herbs may be used as dried extracts (capsules, powders, teas), glycerites (glycerine extracts), or tinctures (alcohol extracts). Unless otherwise indicated, teas should be made with one teaspoon herb per cup of hot water. Steep covered 5 to 10 minutes for leaf or flowers, and 10 to 20 minutes for roots. Drink 2 to 4 cups/day. Tinctures may be used singly or in combination as noted.

- Catnip *(Nepeta cataria)* is an anti-pyretic, sedative, spasmolytic.
- Peppermint *(Mentha piperita)* is a carminative, spasmolytic, historic use for colds and fevers
- Elder *(Sambuccus nigra)* to disperse fever; calming
- Fennel *(Foeniculum vulgare)* for dyspepsia; decreases upper respiratory catarrh, calming
- Yarrow *(Achillea millifolium)* for loss of appetite, to disperse a fever
- Chamomile *(Matricaria recutita)* stimulates immune system, relaxing (to allow for sleep)

Mix four to six of the above and drink as a tea, 1 cup tid to qid or tincture, 60 drops tid to qid. In addition, a strong tea (2 tbsp. herb) can be made and added to a bath to prevent fever from going too high or rising too rapidly in children susceptible to febrile seizures.

Garlic/ginger tea (one to three cloves garlic and one to three slices of fresh ginger) may be drunk to stimulate the immune system and prevent upper respiratory infections. Lemon and a sweetener may be added for flavor. Avoid honey in children less than 2 years old.

HOMEOPATHY

An experienced homeopath should assess individual constitutional types and severity of disease to select the correct remedy and potency. For acute prescribing use three to five pellets of a 12X to 30C remedy every one to four hours until acute symptoms resolve.

- *Aconitum nappellus* for rapid onset of a high fever, especially with restless anxiety
- *Belladonna* for high fever where the face and/or body are burning hot to the touch, especially with irritability and sensitivity to noise or light, or with a history of febrile seizures
- *Chamomilla* for fever with one cheek red and the other pale, with hypersensitivity and irritability
- *Pulsatilla* for fever, child is thirstless, clingy and wants to be held all the time

PHYSICAL MEDICINE

Warming socks. Put cotton socks wet with cold water and wrung out on the feet. Put wool socks on top of the cotton socks and go to bed. This treatment, while uncomfortable at first, will help disperse a fever and allow for a good night's sleep.

Wet sheet wrap. To bring down a fever, wrap the child in a cotton sheet that is wet with cold water and wrung out. Next wrap the child in another blanket. Especially in infants, this will disperse a fever and allow a restful sleep.

ACUPUNCTURE

Acupressure for children may be quite calming and help release the fever.

MASSAGE

Gentle massage may relieve discomfort. A foot massage may help to disperse the fever and relax the child. Some children will not want to be touched.

Patient Monitoring

There is no need for patient monitoring once the disease has been correctly diagnosed and the roseola rash appears. However, children with previous febrile seizures should be closely monitored.

OTHER CONSIDERATIONS

Prevention

Avoiding crowded environments, such as daycare centers, and infected children is the only prevention. There is no vaccine.

Complications/Sequelae

- Febrile seizures
- Mononucleosis
- Encephalitis (rare)
- Meningitis
- Hepatitis

Prognosis

In the absence of complications, the prognosis is good for children with roseola.

REFERENCES

Behrman RE, Kliegman RM, Nelson WE, Arvin AM, eds. *Nelson Textbook of Pediatrics.* 15th ed. Philadelphia, Pa: WB Saunders; 1996.

Bove M. *An Encyclopedia of Natural Healing for Children and Infants.* Stamford, Conn: Keats Publishing; 1996:174–176.

Fauci AS, Braunwald E, Isselbacher KJ et al, eds. *Harrison's Principles of Internal Medicine.* 14th ed. New York, NY: McGraw-Hill; 1998.

Morrison R. *Desktop Guide to Keynotes and Confirmatory Symptoms.* Albany, Calif: Hahnemann Clinic Publishing; 1993:3–6, 58–62, 115–117, 310–315.

■ SEIZURE DISORDERS

OVERVIEW

Definition

Seizures are a temporary neurologic event that results from abnormal, hyper-synchronous discharges from neurons in the central nervous system (CNS). Seizures can be variously characterized according to behavioral and electroencephalographic (EEG) changes. Recurrent seizures from one of many chronic processes are considered epilepsy; however, a single seizure or recurrent seizures from a correctable cause (e.g., febrile seizures) are not considered epilepsy.

The International League Against Epilepsy published a Classification of Epileptic Seizures in 1981 in which all seizures were classified according to clinical features and EEG changes. The three major categories of seizures are: partial, generalized, and unclassified.

Partial (or focal) seizures can be isolated to certain areas of the cerebral cortex and are further classified as simple-partial seizures (consciousness is preserved), complex-partial seizures (consciousness is lost), or partial seizures with secondary generalization.

Generalized seizures usually involve both cerebral hemispheres and are further classified as absence seizures (petit mal—brief loss of consciousness), generalized tonic-clonic seizures (grand mal—tonic contractions followed by unresponsiveness), atonic seizures (transient loss of muscle tone), andmyoclonic seizures (transient muscle contractions).

Unclassified epileptic seizures include neonatal seizures, West syndrome (infantile spasms), Lennox-Gastaut syndrome, juvenile myoclonic epilepsy, and reflex epilepsy (e.g., seizures resulting from certain stimuli such as a flickering light).

Etiology

- CNS infection (e.g., bacterial meningitis, encephalitis)
- Drug toxicity or withdrawal (e.g., alcohol or illicit drug use)
- Genetic mutations (e.g., myoclonic epilepsy with ragged red fibers [MERRF])
- Head trauma
- Electrolyte or metabolic derangements
- Drugs that lower the seizure threshold
- High fevers
- Brain abnormalities (e.g., tumors, stroke)
- Hypoglycemia and hypocalcemia

Risk Factors

- History of febrile seizures
- Family history of seizures
- History of stroke
- Alzheimer's disease

Signs and Symptoms

The physical presentations a seizue are varied in duration, severity, and characteristics. Signs may include the following.

- Prodrome of generalized seizures (aura), including lethargy, depression, irritability, myoclonic jerks of limbs, abdominal pains, pale complexion, headache, constipation, or diarrhea
- Loss of consciousness
- Total or partial body muscle spasm (tonic contractions)
- Apnea (cessation of breathing)
- Cyanosis (bluish coloring) of skin and mucus membranes

- Dilated pupils that are unreactive to light
- Bowel or bladder incontinence
- Increased pulse and blood pressure
- Increased salivation and sweating
- Deep coma, postictal confusion, and deep sleep

Repeated seizures over a long period of time may result in:

- Absentmindedness
- Automatisms (e.g., lip smacking, chewing, fumbling)
- Declining school or work performance
- Loss of postural muscle tone

DIFFERENTIAL DIAGNOSIS

- Stokes-Adams attack
- Transient ischemic attack
- Syncope
- Hysterical (psychogenic) seizures
- Metabolic disturbances (e.g., delirium tremens)
- Migraine syndromes
- Sleep disorders (e.g., narcolepsy)
- Movement disorders (e.g., tics)

DIAGNOSIS

Physical Examination

Initially, providers must attend to the seizure patient's respiratory and cardiovascular status and vital signs. After the patient is stable, a detailed history must be taken from family member, witnesses, and the patient (if possible) to determine definitively whether the patient actually experienced a seizure. Precipitating events (e.g., head trauma) and risk factors (e.g., family history of seizures) must be considered. The presence or absence of "auras," which are experienced by up to 60% of seizure patients, automatisms, myoclonus, postures (i.e., whether or not the patient fell), continence (loss of bowel function), and postictal confusion must be noted. These signs can help to differentiate the type of seizure experienced.

Laboratory Tests

Laboratory values are often normal in seizure patients.

- Complete blood count to diagnose metabolic disorders and as a baseline before treatment
- Urine and blood toxicologic screens to determine any underlying drug use
- Serum electrolytes and liver function tests for baseline values before beginning treatment

Pathological Findings

In many cases, the brains of patients with generalized seizures appear normal; however, some seizure disorders have definable lesions: harartomas, vascular abnormalities, areas of neuronal loss, fibrosis, scars, and tumors. In addition, traumatic (e.g., cortical contusions) or hypoxic (e.g., degeneration of Purkinje cells) effects can result from the seizures themselves.

Imaging

- Magnetic resonance imaging (MRI) to diagnose cerebral lesions (e.g., tumors, vascular malformations)
- Computed tomography (CT) to diagnose CNS infection and cerebral lesions when MRI is not available
- Positron emission tomography (PET) to localize epileptogenic areas in cases refractory to medical treatment
- Single photon emission computed tomography (SPECT) to localize epileptogenic areas in cases refractory to medical treatment

Other Diagnostic Procedures

- An electroencephalogram (EEG) is the primary diagnostic tool used to categorize seizures. The epileptiform abnormalities (spikes and waves) on the EEG are recorded in 60% to 90% of patients.
- Lumbar puncture—to diagnose meningitis, encephalitis, and human immunodeficiency virus
- Closed-circuit television EEG (CCTV/EEG) for long-term monitoring in a hospital setting to localize epileptogenic foci for resective surgery
- Ambulatory EEG for long-term monitoring at home, school, or work to localize epileptogenic foci for resective surgery

TREATMENT OPTIONS

Treatment Strategy

Treating the seizure patient can be challenging. It includes diagnosing and treating any underlying condition (e.g., surgical removal of cerebral lesions, focal brain resection, temporal lobectomy, lesionectomy, hemispherectomy) that may be causing the seizure activity. Precipitating events (e.g., lack of sleep, alcohol ingestion) should be identified and then avoided. The goal of therapy is to stop the seizure without adverse side effects, to prevent recurrences, and to help patients readjust to their home life and work environment.

Drug Therapies

Ideally, patients should take only one medication. However, many patients need several medications for complete seizure control. Approximately 30% to 70% of seizure patients will have a second seizure within 1 year. Side effects from seizure medication are experienced by over 50% of patients. These include gastrointestinal complaints, gingival hypertrophy, weight gain or loss, hair loss or hirsutism, coarsening of facial features (especially children), drowsiness, impaired memory and concentration, depression, mood swings, insomnia, dizziness, tremor, headache, ataxia, dermatitis, hepatotoxicity, bone marrow suppression, aplastic anemia, thrombocytopenia, lymphyadenopathy, and osteomalacia.

- Carbamazepine (Tegretol), 600 to 1,800 mg/day for tonic-clonic and focal-onset seizures
- Phenytoin (Dilantin), 300 to 500 mg/day for tonic-clonic and focal-onset seizures
- Valproic acid (Depakote), 750 to 2,000 mg/day for tonic-clonic, absence, myoclonic, and focal-onset seizures
- Phenobarbital (Luminol), 60 to 180 mg/day for tonic-clonic and focal-onset seizures
- Primidone (Mysoline), 750 to 1,250 mg/day for tonic-clonic and focal-onset seizures
- Lamotrigine (Lamictal), 150 to 500 mg/day for focal-onset seizures and Lennox-Gastaut syndrome
- Gabapentin (Neurontin), 900 to 2,400 mg/day for focal-onset seizures
- Ethosuximide (Zarontin), 750 to 1,500 mg/day for absence seizures
- Clonazepam (Klonopin), 1 to 12 mg/day for absence and myoclonal seizures
- Felbamate (Felbatol), 2400 to 3,600 mg/day for focal-onset seizures and Lennox-Gastaut syndrome

Complementary and Alternative Therapies

Some mild cases of seizures may be controlled by alternative therapies, specifically nutrition, the cornerstone of alternative treatment. Herbal treatment may be helpful if low blood sugar and/or stress are initiating factors. Precautions regarding sudden cessation of drugs must be adhered to as there are currently no adequate replacements to drug therapies and/or surgical interventions.

NUTRITION

- A ketogenic diet (high fat, low protein, low carbohydrate) produces ketones in the blood stream, which may help control the frequency of seizures, especially if low blood sugar, or skipping eals, is a trigger. Some studies have shown a connection with food allergies and seizures in children. Avoid alcohol, caffeine, and aspartame.
- Taurine: (500 mg tid) neuroinhibitory amino acid that inhibited experimentally induced seizures
- Folic acid: (400 mcg/day) depleted during seizures and in some persons with seizures, although higher doses than 400 mcg may actually precipitate some seizures. Should take with B_{12}
- B_{12}: (100 to 200 mcg/day)
- B_6: (20 to 50 mg/kg) especially in children may help control seizures; depleted in dilantin therapy. However, B_6 may inhibit dilantin's effects.
- Magnesium: 500 to 750 mg/day (should be in a 1:1 ratio in people taking calcium) for normal muscle and neuronal function
- Manganese: (5 to 15 mg/day) depleted in epileptics, especially in children
- Zinc: (30 mg/day) may be depleted by some medications, some concern that excess zinc may disrupt zinc/copper ratios and increase seizures, especially without sufficient taurine
- Dimethyl glycine: (100 mg bid) anecdotal evidence for decreasing medication requirements

HERBS

Herbs are generally a safe way to strengthen and tone the body's systems. As with any therapy, it is important to ascertain a diagnosis before pursuing treatment. Herbs may be used as dried extracts (capsules, powders, teas), glycerites (glycerine extracts), or tinctures (alcohol extracts). Unless otherwise indicated, teas should be made with 1 tsp. of herb per cup of hot water. Steep covered 5 to 10 minutes for leaf or flowers, and 10 to 20 minutes for roots. Drink 2 to 4 cups/day. Tinctures may be used singly or in combination as noted.

- Passionflower (*Passiflora incarnata*): to both prevent and treat seizures, may be effective without side effects, especially where stress is a precipitating factor. Dose is 30 drops tid to qid.
- Skullcap (*Scutellaria lateriflora*): anti-spasmodic and calmative herb, with historic use for epilepsy
- Valerian (*Valeriana officinalis*): spasmolytic, sedative, historically used for epilepsy, large doses may cause lethargy or gastrointestinal upset that resolve with discontinuation
- The above herbs may be used singly or in combination at 1 cup tea tid or 30 to 60 drops tincture tid. In addition, use milk thistle (*Silybum marianum*) to protect the liver from ill effects of some medications (70 to 210 mg tid).

HOMEOPATHY

An experienced homeopath should assess individual constitutional types and severity of disease to select the correct remedy and potency. For acute prescribing use 3 to 5 pellets of a 12X to 30C remedy every one to four hours until acute symptoms resolve. If symptoms persist consult with an experienced homeopath.

- *Artemesia vulgaris* for convulsions after exertion and/or visual stimulation
- *Oenanthe* for violent seizures, especially exacerbated menstrually or after a head injury
- *Bufo* for convulsions accompanied by delayed development
- *Cicuta* for violent seizures with arching of the back, especially with a long postictal drowsiness and/or after head injury
- *Cuprum metallicum* for seizures with mental dullness and/or difficulty breathing

- *Causticum* for seizures during menses or after a fright or receiving bad news
- *Belladonna* as general remedy, especially for convulsions followed by nausea

PHYSICAL MEDICINE
Chiropractic, osteopathic, or naturopathic manipulation may be quite helpful, especially in children with seizures or seizures appearing after a head trauma.

ACUPUNCTURE
Acupuncture may be helpful with specific acupressure points that have been used to stop seizures.

Patient Monitoring
Because of the toxicity of the antiepileptic therapy, patients must be monitored closely for myriad side effects, the most serious of which include hepatotoxicity, bone marrow suppression, aplastic anemia, thrombocytopenia, lymphyadenopathy, hirsutism, osteomalacia, and ataxia. In addition, determining the correct dosage or drug combinations is an inexact science at present; thus, patients must be monitored closely for many months until seizures are under control and side effects are tolerable. Starting and stopping antiepileptic medications must be done slowly, often by overlapping drugs for several weeks. Monitoring should continue regularly to ensure patient compliance with the drug schedule.

OTHER CONSIDERATIONS
Prevention
Some patients can identify events that seem to trigger seizures such as alcohol, lack of sleep, stress, and, in certain individuals, visual or auditory stimuli (e.g., video games, music). Thus, these situations must be avoided. Also, strict compliance with the drug schedule is mandatory to ensure therapeutic blood levels. Dangerous activities such as swimming, operating equipment, working at heights, and driving are contraindicated initially, and perhaps forever, depending on the seriousness of the seizure disorder and the success of treatment.

Complications/Sequelae
- The diagnosis of a seizure disorder can drastically alter a person's outlook and restrict their productivity; in addition, patients may face occupational discrimination and loss of independence if they are unable to drive. Depression or other psychological disturbances may result.
- Serious injuries are often sustained with the first seizure and in seizure disorders that are refractory to treatment. Head injuries and broken bones are common sequelae.

- The long-term effects of antiepileptic drugs on the growth and development of children is unknown.
- Generalized status epilepticus is characterized by a series of grand mal seizures without regaining consciousness. This must be treated as a medical emergency as irreversible neurologic sequelae are common.
- Absence status is characterized by absence seizures that may last for hours. This may be labeled inattention or daydreaming by young schoolchildren who may fall behind developmentally if the seizure disorder is not diagnosed.

Prognosis
Approximately 60% of adults who have successful therapeutic treatments and are seizure-free for two to five years can stop taking their medication. The exact point at which a drug-free trial should occur is unknown, but often providers make a first attempt after two years. Seizures that are refractory to drug therapy (20%) may respond successfully to surgery if they fit the criterion for a good surgical candidate. The diagnosis of a seizure disorder can drastically alter a person's outlook and restrict their productivity.

Pregnancy
While it is not uncommon for women with a seizure disorder to have a normal pregnancy and delivery, there may be changes in the frequency of the seizures, which can have a teratogenic effect. Also, women who experience grand mal seizures while pregnant are more likely to experience premature labor, spontaneous abortion, toxemia, and placental abruptio and hypoxia. In addition, infants of women who are taking antiepileptic drugs have malformations two to three times as often as healthy women. These malformations include cleft lip and palate, cardiac abnormalities, anencephaly, and neural tube defects.

REFERENCES
Adams RD, Victor M, Ropper AH. *Principles of Neurology.* 6th ed. New York, NY: McGraw-Hill; 1997:313–341.

Bartram T. *Encyclopedia of Herbal Medicine.* Dorset, England: Grace Publishers; 1995:170–171.

Fauci AS, Braunwald E, Isselbacher KJ et al, eds. *Harrison's Principles of Internal Medicine.* 14th ed. New York, NY: McGraw-Hill Book Company; 1998:2311–2325.

Gruenwald J, Brendler T, Jaenicke C et al, eds. *PDR for Herbal Medicines.* Montvale, NJ: Medical Economics Company; 1998:1128, 1135, 1204, 1219.

Morrison R. *Desktop Guide to Keynotes and Confirmatory Symptoms.* Albany, Calif: Hahnemann Clinic Publishing; 1993:46,76,111–114,124,146–147,276.

Murray MT. *Encyclopedia of Nutritional Supplements.* Rocklin, Calif: Prima Publishing; 1996:84.

Murray MT. *The Healing Power of Herbs.* 2nd ed. Rocklin, Calif: Prima Publishing; 1995:40,91.

Rowland LP. *Merritt's Textbook of Neurology.* 9th ed. Media, Pa: Williams & Wilkins; 1995:845–868.

Werback MR. *Nutritional Influences on Illness.* New Canaan, Conn: Keats Publishing, Inc; 1987:189–193.

■ SEXUAL DYSFUNCTION
OVERVIEW
Broadly defined, sexual dysfunction is the general inability to enjoy sexual intercourse. Sexual disorders include sexual desire (libido) problems, disorders in the psychophysiologic processes of the sexual response cycle (desire, excitement, orgasm, resolution), and pain with sexual intercourse. Sexual dysfunctions are classified as primary (lifelong) or secondary (acquired after normal sexual functioning) and may be generalized (not limited to certain situations, partners, or stimulation) or situational.

Definition
This large group of vasocongestive and orgasmic disorders affects both males and females and may affect more than half of all couples at some time. The major subtypes are:
- Male erectile disorder (impotence)—the inability to attain or maintain an erection for sexual intercourse
- Ejaculation disturbances—primarily premature ejaculation in men
- Vaginismus—spasm of the vagina preventing penetration and sometimes causing pain during coitus
- Sexual aversion disorder—the inhibition of sexual arousal and excitement
- Orgasmic disorders—delayed or absent orgasm in either males or females who otherwise have normal sexual desires and arousal
- Dyspareunia (sexual pain disorders)
- Sexual dysfunction due to general medical condition
- Substance-induced sexual dysfunction

Etiology
Psychological influences (e.g., anger, fear, guilt, depression, and anxiety); interpersonal issues (e.g., marital discord and boredom); alcohol and drug use; certain medications; neurologic insult and/or biological causes can be factors in the etiology of sexual dysfunction.

Risk Factors
- Medical comorbidity (e.g., diabetes, pelvic cancer, genitourinary disorders, urethral strictures, genital infections,endocrine and hormonal disorders)
- Pharmacological (e.g., antihypertensive, antipsychotic, and antidepressant medications)
- Alcohol or drug abuse
- Cigarette smoking (atherosclerosis of the penile artery may account for nearly 50% of impotence cases in men over 50)
- Depression, anxiety, or issues of self esteem
- Age 65 and over in men
- Stressful life events
- Vascular surgery
- Previous sexual trauma
- Cultural pressures and expectations
- Fatigue

Signs and Symptoms
Dependent on the disorder:
- Premature or retarded ejaculation in men
- Inability to maintain an erection
- Pain during intercourse
- Lack or loss of sexual desire
- Difficulty achieving orgasm
- Anxiety and/or depression
- Inadequate vaginal lubrication in women

DIFFERENTIAL DIAGNOSIS
- Sexual dysfunction due to a general medical condition
- Substance-induced sexual dysfunction
- Sexual dysfunction due to combined factors (i.e., psychological and general medical condition)
- Sexual dysfunction not otherwise specified
- Personality disorder
- Relational problem
- Pseudo-dysparenia

DIAGNOSIS
Physical Examination
Varies depending on the type of sexual dysfunction. Examples of physical presentations include:
- Involuntary spasm in the perineal muscles surrounding the distal third of the vagina (vaginismus)
- Structural abnormalities of the penis, such as genital infections, Peyronie's disease, and lesions (dyspareunia and male erection disorder)
- Infectious vaginitis and atrophic vaginitis (female sexual arousal disorder)
- Scars, vulvar inflammation, clitoral inflammation or adhesions, and dermatitis (female dyspareunia)

Laboratory Tests
Specific laboratory tests are available to aid diagnosis of sexual dysfunctions resulting from underlying medical conditions; these are usually not considered diagnostic alone. Blood tests, such as serum-free testosterone, luteinizing hormone (if low testosterone level), and serum prolactin tests can help detect hormonal problems and distinguish between psychological and organic causes for sexual dysfunctions like impotence and sexual aversion disorders.

Imaging
CTs and MRIs are helpful for differential diagnosis (e.g., evaluating the sella turcica for pituitary tumors).
Duplex ultrasound can ascertain blood flow in cavernous arteries (erectile dysfunction).

Other Diagnostic Procedures
- Clinician interview—assess symptoms and degree of severity; may include routine sexual history, modified sexological examination (e.g., sensitivity of vulva to touch); gather information on ethnic, cultural, religious, and social background, which may impact a patient's sexual desires, expectations, and attitudes
- Evaluate for concurrent substance abuse, medical conditions, psychiatric conditions
- Nocturnal penile tumescence measurements taken during REM sleep help to differentiate between psychological and organic causes.

TREATMENT OPTIONS
Treatment Strategy
Depending on the type, severity, and duration of the sexual dysfunction, one or more of the following are recommended.
- Psychotherapy and sex therapy, especially interpersonal therapy
- Behavioral therapy (e.g., dysfunctions like premature ejaculation and vaginismus may stem from conditioned responses)
- Pharmacotherapy, and adjusting/alleviating existing medications
- Surgery of penile venous system for severe cases in which venous leakage occurs; NIH recommends procedure be performed in investigational setting at medical centers

- Penile prostheses
- Vacuum/constrictive devices for erectile dysfunction

Drug Therapies

- Sildenafil citrate (Viagra)—enhances natural response to sexual stimulation in men by blocking effect of enzyme that breaks down cyclic guanosine monophosphate (cGMP); complications include serious cardiovascular event (e.g., myocardial infarction and sudden cardiac death), primarily in patients with preexisting risk factors; other side effects include anxiety, priapism, and temporary vision loss or decreased vision; contraindicated for patients taking nitrates
- Tricyclics or MAOIs—for treating panic states leading to sexual aversion disorder
- Testosterone—for treating low androgen levels in erectile dysfunction and impotence (200 mg IM/every two weeks for three to four months)
- Vasodilators—such as papaverine, phentolamine, or prostaglandin E1 used alone or in combination and administered via penile injections for erectile dysfunction; may cause priapism and transient hypertension
- Nefazodone (Serzone) and other antidepressants—may help decrease psychological side effects of sexual dysfunction; contraindicated for use with MAOIs or in pregnant women
- Dibucaine (1%) or lidocaine (1%)—ointment applied externally for vulval distress

Complementary and Alternative Therapies

Sexual dysfunction that is secondary to decreased peripheral circulation, hormonal imbalance, or depression and/or anxiety may be reduced with the use of alternative therapies. Mind-body techniques such as meditation, progressive muscle relaxation, yoga, tai chi, and stress management may be helpful in relieving anxiety around sexual performance.

NUTRITION

- Vitamin C (1,000 mg tid) to support vascular integrity.
- Vitamin E (400 IU/day), B$_6$ (50 to 100 mg/day), and zinc (30 mg/day) to support hormone production.
- Magnesium (200 mg bid) supports hormone production and is a vasodilator.
- B-complex (50 to 100 mg/day) helps to reduce the effects of stress and may improve symptoms of depression and/or anxiety.

HERBS

Herbs are generally a safe way to strengthen and tone the body's systems. As with any therapy, it is important to ascertain a diagnosis before pursuing treatment. Herbs may be used as dried extracts (capsules, powders, teas), glycerites (glycerine extracts), or tinctures (alcohol extracts). Unless otherwise indicated, teas should be made with one teaspoon herb per cup of hot water. Steep covered 5 to 10 minutes for leaf or flowers, and 10 to 20 minutes for roots. Drink two to four cups/day. Tinctures may be used singly or in combination as noted.

Consider the following herbs for sexual dysfunction related to vascular insufficiency.

- Ginkgo (Ginkgo biloba, 50 to 100 mg/day) increases peripheral circulation and may improve sexual function related to arterial insufficiency. Long-term treatment (six months or more) may be required for best results. Ginkgo should be used cautiously with other blood-thinning agents (e.g. coumadin).
- Hawthorn (Crataegus oxyacantha), rosemary (Rosemarinus officinalis), ginger root (Zingiber officinalis), and Prickly ash bark (Xanthoxylum clava-herculis) are circulatory stimulants.

Use singly or in combination, 3 cups of tea/day or 20 to 30 drops tincture tid.

- Yohimbe bark (Pausinystalia yohimbe) is used for sexual dysfunction, however, because of its side effects it should not be used without physician supervision.

Consider these herbs for sexual dysfunction secondary to hormonal imbalance.

- Chaste tree (Vitex agnus-cactus) helps to normalize pituitary function but must be taken long term (12 to 18 months) for maximum effectiveness. Use only under physician supervision with hormone therapy.
- Saw palmetto (Serenoa repens) may reduce excessive androgen production.
- Damiana (Turnera diffusa) may support testosterone levels. It is also tonifying to the central nervous system and may help alleviate anxiety and depression in conjunction with sexual dysfunction.
- Milk thistle (Silybum marianum), dandelion root (Taraxacum officinale), and vervain (Verbena hastata) support the liver and may help restore hormone ratios. Use equal parts in a tea (1 cup before meals), or tincture (15 to 20 drops before meals).

For sexual dysfunction associated with depression or anxiety, consider the following.
St. John's wort (Hypericum perforatum), kava kava (Piper methysticum), skullcap (Scutellaria laterifolia), lemon balm (Melissa officinalis), passionflower (Passiflora incarnata), and gotu kola (Centella asiatica). Combine equal parts in a tea (one cup bid) or tincture (20 to 30 drops bid). It may take up to six weeks to see best results.

HOMEOPATHY

An experienced homeopath should assess individual constitutional types and severity of disease to select the correct remedy and potency.

PHYSICAL MEDICINE

Contrast sitz baths may relieve symptoms and promote circulation, relieving pelvic vascular congestion. You will need two basins that can be comfortably sat in. Fill one basin with hot water, one with cold water. Sit in hot water for three minutes, then in cold water for one minute. Repeat this three times to complete one set. Do one to two sets per day three to four days per week.

MASSAGE

Therapeutic massage may be beneficial in reducing the effects of stress and increasing overall sense of well-being.

Patient Monitoring

Sexual dysfunctions tend to be chronic and episodic and require long-term monitoring.

OTHER CONSIDERATIONS
Prevention

In cases that are primarily psychological in nature, continued psychological, behavioral, and interpersonal therapy decreases chances of a relapse. Men should avoid smoking to help prevent vascular problems associated with erectile dysfunction.

Complications/Sequelae

Drug side effects (e.g., androgen replacement therapy may have significant health risks for men with normal testosterone levels, especially in cases of unrecognized prostate cancer)
Sexual dysfunctions can adversely affect other areas of social functioning.

Prognosis

Sexual disorders are usually recurrent and chronic; a spontaneous remission occurs in 15% to 30% of patients with acquired erectile dysfunction; increased sexual experience often leads to control of premature ejaculation in males.

Pregnancy

Fluctuations in libido may be normal during and after pregnancy and should not be treated.

REFERENCES

American Psychiatric Association. *Diagnostic and Statistical Manual of Mental Disorders.* 4th ed. Washington, DC: American Psychiatric Association; 1994.

Blumenthal M, ed. *The Complete German Commission E Monographs.* Boston, Mass: Integrative Medicine Communications; 1998:383.

Conn RB, Borer WZ, Snyder JW. *Current Diagnosis* (No. 9). Philadelphia, Pa: WB Saunders; 1996:9.

Hoffman D. *The New Holistic Herbal.* New York, NY: Barnes & Noble Books; 1995:195.

Murray MT. *The Healing Power of Herbs: The Enlightened Person's Guide to the Wonders of Medicinal Plants.* Rocklin, Calif: Prima Publishing; 1995:127, 149–150.

Scalzo R. *Naturopathic Handbook of Herbal Formulas.* Durango, Colo: 2nd ed. Kivaki Press; 1994:66.

Tierney LM, McPhee SJ, Papadakis, MA, eds. *Current Medical Diagnosis & Treatment 1999.* Stamford, Conn: Appleton & Lange; 1999.

■ SINUSITIS

OVERVIEW

Definition

Sinusitis is an inflammation and infection of the paranasal sinuses that causes impaired sinus mucociliary clearance. It affects approximately 31 million adults and children in the United States. Sinusitis has many similar characteristics to rhinitis, and can also be called rhinosinusitis.

Etiology

Sinusitis is most often caused by an upper respiratory tract infection or through bacterial infection (*S. pneumoniae, H. influenzae*, or by fungal or viral entities). This is followed by allergic rhinitis, dental infection, or manipulation, and trauma to the sinuses. Disease of the anterior ethmoid-middle meatal complex (ostiomeatal complex) is the most frequent local cause of chronic sinusitis.

Risk Factors

- Upper respiratory infections
- Allergic rhinitis
- Immunodeficiency, Kartagener's syndrome, and cystic fibrosis
- Nosocomial sinusitis from foreign nasal bodies
- Nasal polyps, nasal septal deviation, and spurs
- Anatomic abnormalities that narrow the ostiomeatal channels
- Cold air, cigarette smoke, decongestants, and metal vapors

Signs and Symptoms

- Inflammation and edema of nasal mucosa, purulent sinonasal secretion (yellow or green), or postnasal drip
- Headache, pain, sinus tenderness, or toothache
- Cough or pharyngitis
- Fever, in half of patients
- Loss of smell
- General malaise

DIFFERENTIAL DIAGNOSIS

- Upper respiratory tract infection (common cold)
- Tension and vascular headaches
- Meningitis
- Brain and epidural abscesses
- Viral, allergic, or vasomotor rhinitis
- Tumors or cysts

DIAGNOSIS

Physical Examination

Physical findings may include tenderness, purulent sinonasal obstruction and secretion, and postnasal drip. Look for three of the following findings: maxillary toothache, colored nasal discharge, poor response to nasal decongestants, abnormal sinus transillumination, purulent secretions

Laboratory Tests

- Culture and biopsy for chronic and fungal sinusitis
- Microscopic examination shows sheets of polymorphonuclear neutrophils as well as bacteria
- Skin test to determine underlying allergy
- Blood test to reveal immunoglobulin serum levels and antibody response to specific antigens (i.e., allergies)
- Nasopharyngeal culture

Pathological Findings

- Bacterial titers exceeding 1,000 CFU per ml, primarily *Streptococcus pneumoniae, H. influenzae*, and *Branhamella (Moraxella)*

catarrhalis for acute sinusitis
- Anaerobes of the *Bacteroides, Fusobacterium, Streptococcus, Veillonella*, and *Corynebacterium* species as well as anaerobic gram-positive cocci for chronic sinusitis (some studies show this to be inaccurate with anaerobes found in as few as 7.6% of cases)
- Gram-negative bacteria, such as *Pseudomonas aeruginosa, Klebsiella pneumoniae*, and *Enterobacter* species for nosocomial sinusitis
- Normal ciliated epithelium replaced by stratified squamous epithelium in chronic sinusitis
- Goblet cell hyperplasia, mononuclear cell infiltration, and basement membrane thickening
- Edema, inflammation, and thickened mucosa

Imaging

- Computed tomography (CT)—shows the ostiomeatal complex as well as other sinuses; evaluates disease, anatomic obstructions, fine bony structure, and soft-tissue complications; diagnoses fungal sinusitis
- Conventional sinus radiograph—diagnoses maxillary and frontal sinus disease; poor for ostiomeatal complex
- Flexible fiberoptic rhinoscopy—reveals purulent drainage in sinus ostia
- Transillumination—maxillary and frontal sinuses; often inaccurate

Other Diagnostic Procedures

- Endoscopy exam—differentiates between purulence and allergic mucosal thickening; reveals ostiomeatal disease
- Irrigation of the maxillary antrum—distinguishes between purulence and allergic mucosal thickening; identifies tumors

TREATMENT OPTIONS

Treatment Strategy

Nonsurgical treatment includes antibiotics, decongestants, avoiding allergens, steam or mist inhalation for drainage and symptom relief, and hydration to thin secretions. Surgical treatment for restoration of ventilation and mucociliary functioning is attempted when nonsurgical measures have failed.

Drug Therapies

- Antibiotics—For first cases of sinusitis, amoxicillin (500 mg tid) is generally used. With penicillin resistance and treatment failure, use broad-spectrum antibiotics such as cefuroxime (Ceftin, 250 to 500 mg bid), cefaclor (Ceclor, 500 mg bid), amoxicillin/clavulanic acid (Augmentin, 500 mg bid), clarithromycin (Biaxin, 250 to 500 mg bid), or an azithromycin (Zithromax) pack for patients allergic to penicillins. Antibiotics are taken for 10 to 14 days in acute cases and for up to six weeks in chronic cases.
- Decongestants—Oral decongestants, such as pseudoephedrine (60 mg tid to qid), cause urinary retention in older male patients; monitor their use with hypertensive patients. Nasal sprays, such as oxymetazoline (Afrin, tid), should be used for three to five days only; there is a risk of tachyphylaxis and rebound if used longer.
- Nasal steroid spray for allergic/chronic sinusitis (e.g., triamcinolone)

Surgical therapies include functional endoscopic surgery (FESS)—to remove diseased tissue (reduced comorbidity and damage to normal anatomy compared to external surgery); external surgery—for osteomyelitis, orbital or intracranial complications, and failure of FESS

Complementary and Alternative Therapies

A combination of physical medicine and herbal or homeopathic treatment is often effective for treating both acute and chronic rhinosinusitis.

NUTRITION

- Vitamin C (1,000 mg tid), zinc (30 to 60 mg/day), beta-carotene (15,000 IU/day) to support immunity.
- Bromelain (500 mg tid between meals) and Quercetin (500 mg tid between meals) are anti-inflammatory
- Avoid mucous-producing foods, such as dairy products, bananas and any known allergens. Drink plenty of fluids. Decrease sugar intake.

HERBS

Ascertain a diagnosis before pursuing treatment. Herbs may be used as dried extracts (capsules, powders, teas), glycerites (glycerine extracts), or tinctures (alcohol extracts). Unless otherwise indicated, teas should be made with 1 tsp. herb per cup of hot water. Steep covered 5 to 10 minutes for leaf or flowers, and 10 to 20 minutes for roots. Drink 2 to 4 cups/day. Tinctures may be used singly or in combination as noted.

- Wild indigo *(Baptesia tinctoria)*—specific for upper respiratory and sinus infections, increases phagocytosis
- Eyebright *(Euphrasia officinalis)*—anticatarrhal, specific for sinus
- Licorice *(Glycyrrhiza glabra)*—antiviral, soothing, especially with exhaustion and/or heartburn, avoid with hypertension
- Coneflower *(Echinacea purpurea)*—stimulates the immune system
- Goldenseal *(Hydrastis canadensis)*—antiviral, antibacterial, digestive tonic

A combination of all of the above herbs, equal parts, may be very effective. 1 cup tea or 30 to 60 drops tincture every two to four hours. May add:

- Jamaican dogwood *(Piscidia piscipula)* or St. John's wort *(Hypericum perforatum),* in equal parts, may be added for pain relief.
- Garlic/Ginger tea—two to three cloves of garlic *(Allium sativum)* and two to three slices of fresh ginger *(Zingiber officinalis).* Steep 5 to 15 minutes and drink, breathing in the steam. Stimulates immune system and stimulates drainage, prevents sinus problems from extending into lungs.
- Essential oils for bath or steam. For a steam, place two to five drops in a pot, bring to a simmer and hold head over the pot. For a bath, add 5 to 10 drops of oil to the bath. Eucalyptus, lavender, and thyme are specific for upper-respiratory infections. Lavender and rosemary are also calming. These essential oils have antiseptic properties.

HOMEOPATHY

An experienced homeopath should assess individual constitutional types and severity of disease to select the correct remedy and potency. For acute prescribing use 3 to 5 pellets of a 12X to 30C remedy every one to four hours until acute symptoms resolve.

- *Arsenicum album* for sinusitis with watery, excoriating discharge
- *Kali bichromicum* for sinusitis with thick "gluey" discharge, postnasal drip, especially with ulceration
- *Pulsatilla* for thick, bland, greenish discharge, especially if patient is weepy and is not thirsty
- *Nux vomica* for sinusitis with coryza, and a stopped up feeling, especially if patient is impatient and/or angry

PHYSICAL MEDICINE

- Contrast hydrotherapy. Alternating hot and cold applications brings nutrients to the site and diffuses metabolic waste from inflammation. Use washcloths over the sinus area. Alternate three minutes hot with one minute cold. Repeat three times. Do two to three sets/day.
- Nasal lavage to shrink membranes/increase drainage. Mix salt and water to taste like tears. Rinse each nostril by holding head over sink and letting water run from upper nostril to lower nostril. Keep nostrils lower than throat to prevent salt water draining into back of throat.
- Cranio-sacral therapy (osteopathic/chiropractic) can be very effective at decreasing the frequency of infections/headaches.

ACUPUNCTURE

May be helpful for both acute and chronic sinusitis.

Patient Monitoring

Patients not responding to therapy should see an otolaryngologist.

OTHER CONSIDERATIONS

Fungal sinusitis should be suspected for patients who do not respond to antibiotic therapy and for immunocompromised patients.

Prevention

Avoid known allergens, cold air, cigarette smoke, topical drugs, swimming, and metal vapors, and follow a diet that reduces mucus production.

Complications/Sequelae

Orbital infection from acute ethmoid sinusitis requires hospitalization, surgical drainage, and intravenous culture-specific antibiotics.

- Osteomyelitis of the frontal bones (Pott's puffy tumor), especially in children
- Intracranial spread of infection results in meningitis, subdural empyema, and abscesses; male adolescents are most at risk.
- Sphenoid sinusitis—Delayed diagnosis is associated with serious morbidity and mortality.
- Otitis media—frequently present with children
- Abscess—extradural, subdural, brain,or retrobulbar

Prognosis

An acute sinus infection lasts no longer than 8 weeks; a chronic sinus infection lasts for at least 4 weeks after initiation of treatment.

Pregnancy

Tetracycline is contraindicated in pregnancy.

REFERENCES

Barkin R, Rosen P, eds. *Emergency Medicine: Concepts and Clinical Practice.* 4th ed. St. Louis, Mo: Mosby-Year Book; 1996.

Blumenthal M, ed. *The Complete German Commission E Monographs.* Boston, Mass: Integrative Medicine Communications; 1998:122–123.

Gruenwald J, Brendler T, et. al, eds. *PDR for Herbal Medicines.* Montvale, NJ: Medical Economics Company; 1998:684–685.

Kruzel T. *The Homeopathic Emergency Guide.* Berkeley, Calif: North Atlantic Books; 1992:286–290.

Middleton E, ed. Allergy: *Principles and Practice.* 5th ed. St. Louis, Mo: Mosby-Year Book; 1998.

Rakel RE. *Conn's Current Therapy.* 50th ed. Philadelphia, Pa: WB Saunders; 1998.

■ SLEEP APNEA

OVERVIEW

Definition

Sleep apnea is a disorder that involves repeated episodes of upper airway occlusion and transient respiratory arrest during sleep. Types include obstructive (caused by upper airway obstruction, seen in up to 4% of adults), central (caused by CNS's failure to initiate respirations during sleep, termed "Ondine's curse"), and mixed. Apneas have significant adverse cardiovascular effects, create sleep disruptions that cause daytime exhaustion, and are associated with increased mortality.

Etiology

In obstructive apnea, the upper airway is narrowed or obstructed by blocked nasal passages, large tonsils or adenoids, large tongue, short lower jaw, or fatty tissue resulting from obesity. In central apnea, the CNS respiratory control stops working during sleep, possibly an inherited neurologic problem, acquired neuromuscular disorder, or triggered by obstructive apnea.

Risk Factors

- Obesity (67% of patients)
- Insensitive breathing reflex
- Incoordination of breathing muscles
- Male gender (three times more common among men)
- Middle age (can occur at any age, but worsens as patients grow older)
- Drugs such as alcohol, sedatives, hypnotics, short-acting beta blockers
- Prematurity in infants
- Allergies
- Nasal obstruction

Signs and Symptoms

- Loud, irregular snoring punctuated by quiet periods when patient is not breathing for more than 10 seconds; episodes can occur up to 100 times or more per hour
- Excessive daytime sleepiness and fatigue
- Morning headaches, sore throat, dry mouth, cough
- Personality or behavior change (depression, moodiness, irritability)
- Change in alertness, memory
- Impotence
- Hypertension (in 20% to 30% of hypertensive patients)

DIFFERENTIAL DIAGNOSIS

- Narcolepsy
- Insomnia
- Other sleep disorder (periodic leg movement, restless leg syndrome)
- Hypothyroidism
- Temporal Lobe Epilepsy
- Laryngospasm

DIAGNOSIS

Physical Examination

Daytime sleepiness and/or a partner's report of snoring usually prompt treatment. Check weight and blood pressure. May try overnight oximetry during sleep at home to evaluate O_2 levels. If significant pattern of low O_2 levels, refer to a sleep clinic.

Laboratory Tests

- Thyroid hormone levels for hypothyroidism.
- Allergy panel.
- Albumin levels for true hypocalcemia.

Other Diagnostic Procedures

- Refer to otolaryngologist to rule out anatomic or inflammatory causes.
- Epworth Sleepiness Scale to evaluate degree of daytime sleepiness. (Eliminate caffeine before taking test.)
- Refer to sleep clinic.
- Portable or ambulatory monitoring. Sleep test done in-home; appropriate only if symptoms are obvious and severe and patient requires urgent treatment but cannot come to sleep clinic.
- Multiple Sleep Latency Test. Performed day after all-night sleep study to assess level of daytime sleepiness and rule out other causes.
- Definitive test is polysomnography, all-night observation in a sleep clinic, where the apneic episodes can be detected.

TREATMENT OPTIONS

Treatment Strategy

- Lose weight.
- Decrease or eliminate use of alcohol, antihistamines, tranquilizers, and short-acting beta-blockers.
- Treat allergies and upper respiratory infections.
- Develop regular sleep habits and sleep for sufficient periods.
- Avoid supine posture; sleep sitting up or on side.
- Humidify air at night.
- Gargle with salt (without swallowing) to shrink tonsils.
- Eliminate smoking or other irritants.
- Raise the head of the bed.
- CPAP (continuous positive airway pressure) device for moderate to severe cases
- Surgery for moderate to severe cases (tonsillectomy, nasal surgery, uvulopalatopharyngoplasty)

Drug Therapies

Drugs for treating central apnea include the following.

- Acetazolamide. Results promising.
- Clomipramine. Side effects (e.g., impotence) limit use. Patient may develop tolerance in 6 to 12 months.
- Doxapram. Experimental; side effects are hyperactivity, irregular heart rhythm, increased blood pressure, nausea and diarrhea, urinary retention; not for use in those with cardiac problems.
- Aminophylline, theophylline, almitrine, naloxone, medroxyprogesterone, tryptophan. No appreciable improvement; serious side effects.
- Oxygen. Not consistently effective.

Drugs for treating obstructive apnea include the following.

- Medroxyprogesterone. Somewhat effective; side effects are fluid retention, nausea, depression, excess hair growth, breast tenderness; not for use in patients with blood-clotting disorders, liver disease, breast or genital cancer, or pregnant women.
- Protriptyline. Used rarely; side effects are decreased REM sleep, dry mouth, constipation, urinary hesitancy or frequency, impotence, confusion (elderly); not for use if arrhythmias, very high blood pressure, glaucoma, or prostate disease are present.

Surgical Procedures

Devices for treating central apnea include the following.

- Diaphragmatic pacemaker. Requires delicate surgery with risk of developing obstructive apnea and injuring phrenic nerves; not practical for most patients.
- Continuous positive airway pressure (CPAP) ventilator. Keeps airway open to eliminate apneic spells; can be uncomfortable and reduce quality of sleep.
- Negative pressure ventilator (cuirass). Requires tight fit and careful adjustment of rate; can be uncomfortable and reduce quality of sleep.

Devices for treating obstructive apnea include the following.

- CPAP ventilator. Excellent results; pressure settings 5 to 20 cm H_2O; side effects are discomfort or claustrophobia wearing mask, inconvenience, nasal congestion, sneezing.
- Tongue-retaining device. Pulls tongue forward; use generally limited to non-obese patients with no nasal obstruction.
- Jaw retainers. Custom-fitted to pull jaw forward; still experimental; side effects are excess saliva, exacerbation of TMJ or dental problems.
- Internal dilators or external nose strips. Available over-the-counter; effectiveness unproven.

Surgery options include the following.

- Nasal surgery. By itself not usually effective; may be needed to allow use of CPAP.
- Uvulopalatopharyngoplasty (UPPP). Smooths and removes excess tissue from soft palate and throat; effectiveness greater than 20%, with success depending on body weight control. Outpatient in healthy uncomplicated cases; one to two days in hospital for others. Risk from anesthesia; results include pain, difficulty swallowing.
- Laser-assisted uvulopalatoplasty (LAUP). Treats snoring, but leaves apnea potential.
- Maxillofacial surgery. Effectiveness not proven; risks include difficulty healing, inconvenience, added orthodontics, possible need for reoperation, effect of general anesthestic on breathing, pneumonia, difficulty swallowing, 50% to 75% failure rate in five years.

Complementary and Alternative Therapies

Alternative therapies may be useful in treating the allergic component of this condition. Homeopathy and nutrition could be most likely to have a positive affect. While many supplements are touted as good for weight loss, none have proven to be as effective as decreasing caloric input and increasing exercise.

NUTRITION

- Diet: clinical trial of eliminating mucous producing foods (dairy and bananas) for two weeks, reintroducing them and noticing any difference
- Essential fatty acids (EFAs) moderate inflammatory response, decrease allergic response; EFAs are found to be low in obese individuals
- Chromium helps regulate insulin and decrease insulin resistance, may not be effective at burning fat preferentially, but effective at stabilizing blood sugar and decreasing sugar cravings

HOMEOPATHY

An experienced homeopath should assess individual constitutional types and severity of disease to select the correct remedy and potency. For acute prescribing use three to five pellets of a 12X to 30C remedy every one to four hours until acute symptoms resolve.

- *Grindelia* for sleep apnea with advanced cardiac or respiratory illness, patient starts from sleep with a sensation of suffocation
- *Lachesis* for sleep apnea, especially if the patient also has frequent nightmares; patient is unable to sleep on their right side, and is very loquacious
- *Sambucus nigra* for difficulty breathing at night; patient may actually jump up out of bed with a feeling of suffocation, especially with nasal obstruction or asthma

- *Spongia tosta* for patients with a sense of suffocation that may wake them, constriction, tickling or dryness of the throat, a harsh, dry cough
- *Digitalis* used homeopathically helps sleep apnea in persons who have a slow heartbeat that may be accompanied by palpitations, and fear of dying from heart problems
- *Opium* for sleep apnea with loud snoring; heavy sleep that is difficult to disturb, especially if associated with narcolepsy
- *Sulphur* for sleep apnea with insomnia and nightmares, especially with skin rashes that become worse with heat

Patient Monitoring

- Refer for nutritional counseling or supervised exercise program for weight loss and maintenance.
- Follow-up with sleep clinic or home health care products supplier if using CPAP device.
- Refer to psychological counseling for personality/behavioral problems.
- Suggest support group, such as AWAKE or American Sleep Apnea Association (ASAA).

OTHER CONSIDERATIONS

Prevention

Weight loss is key in preventing continuance or recurrence of obstructive apnea.

Complications/Sequelae

- Nocturnal sudden death (2,000 to 3,000/year in U.S.)
- Chronic heart enlargement or arrhythmias
- Psychological and memory problems
- Marital discord
- Pulmonary hypertension

Prognosis

With treatment, patients are able to lead normal lives. Untreated, or if treatment is discontinued, significant health issues and even premature death can result.

Pregnancy

- Nasal congestion that produces snoring is common in pregnancy but should not be confused with apnea.
- Apnea may cause fetal distress because of low oxygen supply in the blood; early recognition and treatment are required.

REFERENCES

Caldwell JP. *Sleep: Everything You Need to Know.* Buffalo, NY: Firefly Books; 1997.

Dunkell S. *Goodbye Insomnia, Hello Sleep.* New York, NY: Carol Publishing Group; 1994

Lipman DS. *Snoring From A to ZZZZ: Proven Cures for the Night's Worst Nuisance.* Portland, Ore: Spencer Press; 1996.

Morrison R. *Desktop Guide to Keynotes and Confirmatory Symptoms.* Albany, Calif: Hahnemann Clinic Publishing; 1993.

Pascualy RA, Soest SW. *Snoring and Sleep Apnea: Personal and Family Guide to Diagnosis and Treatment.* 2nd ed. New York, NY: Demos Vermande; 1996.

Smolley LA, Bruce DF. *Breathe Right Now: A Comprehensive Guide to Understanding and Treating the Most Common Breathing Disorders.* New York, NY: WW Norton & Co; 1998.

■ SPRAINS AND STRAINS
OVERVIEW
Definition
A sprain is an injury to a ligament or to the site of its attachment to bone, most often the ankle, knee, elbow, or wrist, which usually results in painful swelling.

- Grade 1—least severe type of sprain; minimal or mild pain, swelling, and disability. Edema, tenderness, and function loss is minimal to mild. Joint is stable. The ligament or muscle has less than 20% of its fibers damaged.
- Grade 2—moderate pain, swelling, and disability; moderate edema, tenderness and functional loss. Unstable joint, but flexion of the ligament will result in a solid endpoint. Twenty to 70% tissue fibers damaged.
- Grade 3—severe symptoms in all six categories. Joint is unstable, and flexion of the ligament results in an absent or mushy endpoint. Over 70% of the tissue fibers are damaged, or ligament or muscle is completely ruptured.

A strain is a tear or other injury to muscle tissue or tendon, commonly occurring in the muscles that support the neck, thigh, groin, and ankle.

Etiology
Sprain—extrinsic load (i.e., twisting) to a joint, which causes the ligaments to deform past their elastic limit. The extent to which the bones depart from their normal alignment will determine the severity of the injury to the tendon.

Strain—tension on a muscle that is stronger than the tensile capacity of its weakest structural element. Usually occurs during activities that require muscle activation and stretching simultaneously.

Risk Factors
- Poor conditioning
- Ill-fitting sports equipment
- Inadequate warm-up before activity

Signs and Symptoms
- Pain
- Stiffness
- Swelling
- Joint instability

DIFFERENTIAL DIAGNOSIS
First, differentiation must be made between a sprain and a strain.
Sprains:
- Strain
- Avulsion fracture
- Hairline fracture
- Contusion
- Ecchymosis
- Tendon rupture (especially Achilles)
- Hematoma
- Septic joint
- Inflammatory arthropathies
- Tendinitis

Strains:
- Underlying tumor involving the muscle or its attachment
- Infectious and inflammatory muscle syndromes
- Sprain
- Contusion

- Tendinitis
- Fracture

DIAGNOSIS
Physical Examination
Pain and swelling in the affected area, usually acute within the first 48 hours of the injury

Pathological Findings
Damage to the muscle, tendon, or ligament, depending on the severity and grade of the injury

Imaging
X rays may be indicated when the patient suffers from a grade 2 or grade 3 sprain, or is experiencing pain over a bone. The attached ligament can pull a piece of bone off during the injury, resulting in an avulsion fracture. X rays are not useful for strains. Although rarely necessary, a magnetic resonance image (MRI) will reveal complete tears of the ligament, as edema and bleeding and muscle-tendon pathology (achilles or rotator cuff tear).

Appropriate stress films show ligament instability.

Other Diagnostic Procedures
Determine degree of injury for sprains (see Overview), and extent of pain/tenderness in strains.

TREATMENT OPTIONS
Treatment Strategy
Over several days following injury, RICE treatment—rest, ice, compression (tape, etc.), and elevation of the affected joint.

Ice reduces pain, bleeding, and inflammation. It may also reduce secondary damage to other parts of the joint. However, the overall clinical benefit is not known. Bleeding and inflammation may play an important role in the healing process. Wrap the affected area in elastic bandage in more severe cases. Cast may be required to stabilize grade 3 injuries.

Activity that involves the affected area should be limited for an average of seven days.

Physical therapy—Grade 1 injury: strapping/taping or orthotic for two to three weeks. Grade 2: weight-bearing brace/orthotic/cast for four to eight weeks. Grade 3: weight-bearing cast for three to six weeks followed by orthotic or strapping for three to six weeks. Surgery may be indicated. All to be followed by appropriate exercise regimen for return of function.

Drug Therapies
Pain relief through analysis may allow the patient to mobilize the affected area and resume activity. When injuries are more severe or chronic, however, continued use of analgesics may lead to aggravation of the condition. Analgesics should not be used to mask pain so that activity can be resumed without proper immobilization. Reduction in the inflammatory response can also hasten the mobilization of the injured area, but the role of inflammation in healing is unknown and interference could theoretically slow tissue repair. Muscle spasms often accompany sprains and strains and can interfere with rehabilitation.

Over-the-counter pain relievers and anti-inflammatory agents usually help; however, product label dosage recommendations may be inadequate for moderate to severe injuries.
- Aspirin—325 mg, one to two tablets every four hours

- Naproxin—210 mg, two to three tablets every 8 to 12 hours
- Ibuprofen—200 mg, two to three tablets every four to six hours
- Analgesic balms
- Acetaminophen—325 mg, one to two tablets every four hours

Complementary and Alternative Therapies

Specific nutrients and herbs may help restore the integrity of connective tissue, reduce inflammation, and provide pain relief.

NUTRITION

- Vitamin C (1,000 to 1,500 mg tid) to reduce inflammation and support connective tissue.
- Bromelain (250 to 500 mg tid between meals) is a proteolytic enzyme that helps to reduce inflammation.
- Beta carotene (50,000 IU/day) is needed for collagen synthesis.
- Zinc (15 to 30 mg/day) supports immune function and healing.
- Vitamin E (400 IU/day) has antioxidant effects.
- Adequate protein intake is important.

HERBS

Herbs are generally a safe way to strengthen and tone the body's systems. As with any therapy, it is important to ascertain a diagnosis before pursuing treatment. Herbs may be used as dried extracts (capsules, powders, teas), glycerites (glycerine extracts), or tinctures (alcohol extracts). Unless otherwise indicated, teas should be made with 1 tsp. herb per cup of hot water. Steep covered 5 to 10 minutes for leaf or flowers, and 10 to 20 minutes for roots. Drink 2 to 4 cups/day. Tinctures may be used singly or in combination as noted.

Bioflavanoids, a constituent found in dark berries and some plants, have anti-inflammatory properties and strengthen connective tissue by promoting collagen synthesis. The following are bioflavanoids that may be taken in dried extract form as noted.

- Quercetin: 250 to 500mg tid
  - Hawthorn (Crataegus oxyacantha): 500 mg tid
- Turmeric (Curcuma longa) potentiates the effect of bromelain. Take 250 to 500 mg each of turmeric and bromelain, tid between meals.

The following combination of antispasmodic, analgesic, and circulatory stimulants may help to relieve congestion and provide pain relief. Black cohosh (Cimicifuga racemosa), cramp bark (Viburnum opulus), Jamaican dogwood (Piscidia erythrina), feverfew (Tanacetum parthenium), poke root (Phytolacca americana), and valerian (Valeriana officinalis). Combine equal parts in a tea (1 cup tid to qid), or tincture (15 drops every 15 minutes to acute relief, up to eight doses; or 20 to 30 drops qid).

HOMEOPATHY

An experienced homeopath should assess individual constitutional types and severity of disease to select the correct remedy and potency. For acute prescribing use 3 to 5 pellets of a 12X to 30C remedy every one to four hours until acute symptoms resolve.

- Arnica montana for acute injury with bruised sensation and sensitivity to pressure
- Rhus toxicodendron for sprains and strains with great restlessness
- Ruta graveolens for stiffness and pain from injury or chronic overuse

Topical homeopathic creams containing Leopard's Bane (Arnica montana) and/or St. John's wort (Hypericum perforatum) may provide pain relief. Do not apply over broken skin.

Arnica oil may be applied topically for pain relief, provided the skin is not broken.

PHYSICAL MEDICINE

Castor oil pack. Used externally, castor oil is a powerful anti-inflammatory, especially helpful for chronic or severe injury. Apply oil directly to skin, cover with a clean soft cloth (e.g., flannel) and plastic wrap. Place a heat source (hot water bottle or heating pad) over the pack and let sit for 30 to 60 minutes. For best results, use for three consecutive days.

ACUPUNCTURE

Acupuncture may provide pain relief and increase local circulation.

MASSAGE

Therapeutic massage is effective at increasing circulation and may relieve spasm in surrounding muscle groups.

Patient Monitoring

Monitor for recurring sprains and strains. Once a muscle or tendon is injured, it is susceptible to re-injury, especially if patient returns to full activity too soon.

OTHER CONSIDERATIONS

Prevention

Basic physical fitness and strength training are important preventive measures.

Warm-up exercises increase energy output and increase the temperature of muscles, improve coordination between the brain and muscles, reducing uncontrolled muscle movements.

Warm-ups should begin with stretching movements of the large muscle groups that are to be exercised more heavily. Jogging and exercise bikes are good initial exercises, to be followed by exercises more specific to the activity to be pursued. Lastly, the warm-up routine should include event-specific movements, such as throwing a football or swinging a racket. Warm-ups should last 15 or 20 minutes.

Half of all athletic injuries are due to inappropriate training or inadequate warm-up, and most of these errors result from a failure to follow the principle of slow progression. Sudden increases in intensity or duration of an activity often lead to over-use injuries such as sprains and strains.

Preventive training can take the form of muscle training, mobility and flexibility training (flexibility of the joint is limited by tight connective tissue), coordination and propioceptic training, and sport-specific training that reinforces good technique in recurring, stress-inducing movements.

Improper technique often causes excess load on joints, so correction of technique can prevent sprains and strains. Another method for reducing load is to decrease the speed of the activity.

Patient should not return to full activity until the affected joint has returned to 90% strength and flexibility.

Complications/Sequelae

- Strains: recurrent strains and complete muscle tears
- More chronic pain and joint instability
- Recurrent sprains
- Complete tear of muscle or tendon

- Stress fracture
- Degenerative arthritis from chronic joint instability

Prognosis

Inflammation occurs for up to 72 hours, followed by gradual reduction of swelling.

Recovery time is as follows: grade 1, 4 to 6 weeks; grade 2, 2 to 3 months; grade 3, 4 to 6 months. Patient may return to high-impact activity when range of motion, strength, and function of the injured joint is nearly equal to the uninjured side.

Pregnancy

High doses of vitamin C are contraindicated in pregnancy. Bromelain, quercetin, and turmeric should be used with caution.

REFERENCES

Balch JF, Balch PA. *Prescription for Nutritional Healing.* Garden City Park, NY: Avery Publishing Group; 1997.

Birrer RB, ed. *Sports Medicine for the Primary Care Physician.* Boca Raton, Fla: CRC Press; 1994.

Blumenthal M, ed. *The Complete German Commission E Monographs.* Boston, Mass: Integrative Medicine Communications; 1998:429.

Brown DJ. *Herbal Prescriptions for Better Health.* Rocklin, Calif: Prima Health; 1996.

Kibler WB, Herring S, Press J, Lee P. *Functional Rehabilitation of Sports and Musculoskeletal Injuries.* Gaithersburg, Md: Aspen Publishers; 1998.

Morrison R. *Desktop Guide to Keynotes and Confirmatory Symptoms.* Albany, Calif: Hahnemann Clinic Publishing; 1993:38, 326, 330.

Null G. *The Clinician's Handbook of Natural Healing.* New York, NY: Kensington Publishing Corp; 1997.

Olshevsky M, Noy S, Zwang M, Burger R. *Manual of Natural Therapy.* New York, NY: Facts on File; 1989.

Strauss RH, ed. *Sports Medicine.* Philadelphia, Pa: WB Saunders Company; 1991.

Ullmann D. *The Consumer's Guide to Homeopathy.* New York, NY: G. P. Putnam's Sons; 1995.

Zachazewski JE, Magee DJ, Quillen WS. *Athletic Injuries and Rehabilitation.* Philadelphia, Pa: WB Saunders Company; 1996.

■ TENDINITIS

OVERVIEW

Definition

Tendinitis is the painful inflammation of a tendon and its attachments to bone. It is most often the result of the stress from a particular occupation (e.g., drywall hangers, musicians, painters) or sport (e.g., baseball, basketball, tennis, swimming). Acute tendinitis may heal within a few days or weeks, but it may also become chronic if it is not treated acutely. Pain may initially be only a dull ache with movement of the affected limb; however, with time, if untreated, it may become severe, allowing only limited movement and causing disability. The areas most commonly affected by tendinitis are the shoulder (e.g., bicipital tendinitis, supraspinatus tendinitis, rotator cuff tendinitis, or impingement syndrome), elbow (e.g., lateral epicondylitis [tennis elbow] or medial epicondylitis [golfer's elbow], wrist and thumb (e.g., stenosing tenosynovitis [de Quervain's disease]), knee (e.g., patellar tendinitis [jumper's knee]), and ankle (e.g., Achilles and peroneal tendinitis).

Calcific tendinitis, which occurs when calcium deposits in a joint, is not usually preceded by an identified trauma. There is much disagreement over the cause of this type of tendinitis. Although some investigators hypothesize that it results from chronic tendinitis, it appears to be associated with chronic diseases, such as diabetes mellitus. Calcific tendinitis presents as an acute inflammatory reaction, often resembling gout, that is often bilateral (e.g., in both shoulders), progressing to a pattern of exacerbations and remissions.

Etiology

- Sports, with over- or undertraining or poor technique
- Trauma
- Infections (e.g., gonococcal disease)
- Inflammatory conditions (e.g., Reiter's syndrome, ankylosing spondylitis)
- Ill-fitting shoes (Achilles tendinitis)
- Falling
- Carrying or lifting heavy objects

Risk Factors

- Participation in sports activities
- Occupations involving repetitive activities
- Poor ergonomic positioning with office activities
- Alcoholism, because of an inadequate neurologic function
- Diabetes, because of an inadequate vascular supply

Signs and Symptoms

- Edema (usually minimal)
- Localized tenderness
- Pain, which may or may not be present at rest but is always triggered or exacerbated by movement of the affected limb
- Warmth and redness
- Crepitus (crackling)

DIFFERENTIAL DIAGNOSIS

It is often difficult to distinguish between tendinitis and bursitis. Bursitis is the inflammation of the small fluid-filled sacs (bursa) located between tendons and bones, which cushion tissues from friction. Bursitis is usually characterized by a dull, persistent ache, while tendinitis typically causes sharp pain on movement. The two conditions often coexist.

- Bursitis—inflammation of the bursa (fluid-filled sacs)
- Polyarthritis—arthritis in many joints
- Vasculitis—inflammation of the blood vessels
- Periosteitis—inflammation of the periosteum (connective tissue that covers bone)
- Fibrositis—inflammation of muscle sheaths and fascial layers
- Polymyalgia rheumatica—severe pain and stiffness in proximal muscle groups
- Diseases of the muscles, bones, or spine (e.g., Reiter's syndrome, gout, rheumatoid arthritis)
- Malingering
- Fibromyalgia
- Carpal tunnel syndrome

DIAGNOSIS

Physical Examination

Pain at the point of inflammation is usually worsened by movement, but there may also be pain at rest. The patient may exhibit crepitus when moving the affected joint and complain of numbness and tingling. Range of motion may be normal or limited because of the pain. Severe swelling is uncommon and may indicate arthritis.

Pathological Findings

- Shoulder: impingement of supraspinatus tendon between acromion and greater tuberosity of the humerus, fibrosis and thickening, tear of the rotator cuff, degenerative bony changes (e.g., bony spurs, sclerosis, cyst formation)
- Knee: calcifications, fibrosis of the tendon, degenerative changes, necrotic areas
- Elbow: small tears (microtears) of the tendon of the extensor carpi radialis brevis, inflammation of tendinous sheath over extensor carpi radialis and extensor communis, granulation tissue, degenerative changes
- Wrist and thumb: inflammation of abductor pollicis longus and extensor pollicis brevis tendons, proliferation of fibrous tissue
- Foot: thickening of the Achilles tendon, adhesions between the tendon and tendon sheath

Imaging

- Computed tomography, to evaluate intra-articular abnormalities
- Magnetic resonance imaging, to diagnose tendinitis, tears, or tumors

Other Diagnostic Procedures

- Individual tests, chosen for their specificity, sensitivity, and cost-benefit profile
- X rays, which are often normal in the early stages
- Arthroscopy, to diagnose arthritis, calcific tendinitis, osteonecrosis, and cancer and to treat any abnormalities found
- Arthrography, to establish the correct diagnosis
- Ultrasonography, to diagnose intra-articular abnormalities
- Electromyography, to rule out neurologic problems
- Nerve conduction velocity studies

TREATMENT OPTIONS

Treatment Strategy

In all cases of tendinitis, treatment depends on the severity of the symptoms. Conservative treatment is attempted initially, progressing to surgery if needed. Health care providers will prescribe ice, analgesia, rest, temporary immobilization, massage, steroid injections, light exercise, physical therapy, and finally surgery for refractory cases.

Drug Therapies

- Nonsteroidal anti-inflammatory drugs (NSAIDS): indocin (25 to 50 mg tid) and ibuprofen (200 to 600 mg bid to tid)

- Injection of lidocaine and corticosteroids (1 to 3 mL 1% lidocaine, 1 to 3 mL 0.5% bupivacaine, and 10 to 30 mg triamcinolone). Only three or four injections spaced three weeks apart should be given. Steroid injections directly into weight-bearing tendons are contraindicated because there is a risk of tendon rupture. Injections should be into the tendon sheath or bursa.
- Colchicine (for calcific tendinitis only)

Complementary and Alternative Therapies

A combination of essential fatty acids (EFAs), castor oil packs, and homeopathic treatment is often sufficient for simple tendinitis. Other therapies may be added as needed.

- Ice, especially after the initial injury, to increase circulation to inflamed tissues and decrease pain caused by congestion
- Rest
- Massage or chiropractic for improved circulation
- Temporary immobilization (e.g., slings, splints, crutches) of the affected limb. The shoulder should not be immobilized for a long period of time because further loss of range of motion (frozen shoulder) may occur from adhesions, capsular tightening, and muscle shortening.
- Flexibility and strengthening exercises after acute phase has passed
- Physical therapy (e.g., range of motion exercises)
- Ultrasonography (phonophoresis with 10% lidocaine cream or arnica gel)—high-frequency sound to heat an area and increase the blood supply
- Transcutaneous electrical nerve stimulation (TENS)—electricity used to control pain
- Proper occupational ergonomics (i.e., stop repetitive or offending activity)

NUTRITION

- Vitamin C (500 to 1,000 mg tid) to aid in healing, increase immune function, and reduce inflammation
- Calcium (1,500 mg/day) and magnesium (750 mg/day) to aid healing of connective tissues and muscles
- Vitamin A (15,000 IU/day) to increase immune function and tissue healing
- Vitamin E (400 to 800 mg/day) to reduce inflammation
- Bromelain: 250 to 750 mg tid between meals to reduce inflammation and prevent swelling after trauma or surgery
- Essential fatty acids (EFAs) (1,000 to 15,000 IU one to three times/day, anti-inflammatory)

HERBS

Herbs are generally a safe way to strengthen and tone the body's systems. As with any therapy, it is important to ascertain a diagnosis before pursuing treatment. Herbs may be used as dried extracts (capsules, powders, teas), glycerites (glycerine extracts), or tinctures (alcohol extracts). Unless otherwise indicated, teas should be made with 1 tsp. herb per cup of hot water. Steep covered 5 to 10 minutes for leaf or flowers, and 10 to 20 minutes for roots. Drink 2 to 4 cups/day. Tinctures may be used singly or in combination as noted.

- Bioflavonoids (500 to 1,000 mg tid) to reduce inflammation and maintain healthy collagen
- Curcumin, yellow pigment of tumeric (Curcuma longa)— (200 to 400 mg tid) between meals to reduce inflammation; serves as an antioxidant
- Willow (Salix alba) bark tea (2 to 3 tsp. per 1 cup of boiling water tid) for analgesic effect (Caution: If allergic to aspirin, do not take aspirin-like herbs.)
- Licorice (Glycyrrhiza glabra)—3 cups tea/day to reduce inflamma-

tion (Caution: Long-term use is associated with headaches, water retention, potassium loss, high blood pressure, and lethargy.)
- Comfrey (Symphytum officinale)—1 tsp. per 1 cup boiling water qid to aid healing and for pain relief. Use as the water in contrast hydrotherapy.

HOMEOPATHY

An experienced homeopath should assess individual constitutional types and severity of disease to select the correct remedy and potency. For acute prescribing, use 3 to 5 pellets of a 12X to 30C remedy every 1 to 4 hours until acute symptoms resolve.

Externally:
Homeopathic treatments for tendinitis include creams or gels. *Arnica* cream by itself or in combination with *Calendula officinalis, Hamamelis virgineana, Aconitum napellus,* and *Belladonna,* applied three to six times/day, speeds healing and decreases discomfort.
- For acute injuries, start with *Arnica,*.

Internally:
- *Bryonia* for pains that are worse with the slightest motion or when jarred. The pain feels worse with cold and better with heat.
- *Phytolacca* for tendinitis where the pain is focused at the insertion of the tendons and that feels worse with heat
- *Rhus toxicodendron* for tendinitis with restlessness that is worse in the morning
- *Rhododendron* for tendinitis that gets worse with barometric pressure changes

PHYSICAL MEDICINE

- Orthotics or heel lift and shoe correction (Achilles tendinitis)
- Elbow strap and small (2 lb.) weights (tennis elbow)
- Contrast hydrotherapy. Alternating hot and cold applications brings nutrients to the site and diffuses metabolic waste from inflammation. The overall effect is decreased inflammation, pain relief, and enhanced healing. After first 24 to 48 hours, soak affected part for three minutes in hot water, then 30 seconds in cold water.

MASSAGE

May be helpful for pain relief and improving range of motion.

Patient Monitoring

Tendinitis often presents in three stages: Stage 1, a dull ache precipitated by strenuous activity and resolving with rest; stage 2, pain precipitated by minor movements (e.g., dressing); and stage 3, constant pain. Patients should be seen every three to four weeks until the tendinitis resolves.

OTHER CONSIDERATIONS

Prevention

Proper stretching and warm-up exercises can be preventive measures for athletes at risk for tendinitis. Braces are used for forearms, knees, and ankles to give added stability and support to reduce recurrences. For occupational injuries, job ergonomics must be reviewed and modified to prevent recurrences.

Complications/Sequelae

- Tendon rupture
- After surgery, some patients do not attain their preinjury functional level.
- Degenerative changes are often seen in patients over 40 with chronic tendinitis.
- After steroid injection, there may be atrophy of the soft tissues surrounding a joint or iatrogenic infections. In addition, steroids

may weaken the collagen structure of tendons, potentiating the risk for tendon rupture.

Prognosis

Although most case of tendinitis resolve within a few days to weeks of treatment, recurrences are common, particularly with athletes and individuals in occupations that require overhead or repetitive motions.

Pregnancy

- Stenosing tenosynovitis (de Quervain's disease) is common in pregnancy, but usually resolves spontaneously without treatment.
- A health care provider should be consulted for the proper dosage of vitamin A.

REFERENCES

Balch JF, Balch PA. *Prescription for Nutritional Healing.* 2nd ed. Garden City Park, NY: Avery Publishing; 1997:174–175.

Duke JA. *The Green Pharmacy.* Emmaus, Pa: Rodale Press; 1997:106–109.

Kelly WN, Harris Jr ED, Ruddy S, Sledge CB. *Textbook of Rheumatology.* 5th ed. Philadelphia, Pa:WB Saunders Company; 1997:372–373, 386, 422–429, 462–463, 486, 558–559, 598–599, 603–606, 642.

Koopman WJ. *Arthritis and Allied Conditions: A Textbook of Rheumatology.* 13th ed. Baltimore, Md:Williams & Wilkins; 1997:44,1769–1771, 1795, 1894–1896.

Millar AP. *Sports Injuries and Their Management.* Sydney, Australia: Maclennan & Petty; 1994:10–14, 84–85, 101–103, 111–112,118–119, 8830–8831.

Morrison R. *Desktop Guide to Keynotes and Confirmatory Symptoms.* Albany, Calif: Hahnemann Clinic Publishing; 1993:72–74, 298.

Murray MT, Pizzorno JE. Encyclopedia of Natural Medicine. 2nd ed. Rocklin, Calif: Prima Publishing; 1998:805–809.

Noble J. *Textbook of General Medicine and Primary Care.* Boston, Mass: Little, Brown; 1987:228–229, 288–290, 293–296.

Vinger PF, Hoener EF, eds. *Sports Injuries: The Unthwarted Epidemic.* Boston, Mass: John Wright; 1982:227, 255.

■ THYROIDITIS

OVERVIEW

Definition

Thyroiditis is an inflammatory condition of the thyroid gland. Patient may present with clinical features of hyperthyroidism or hypothyroidism. There are several types, both common (Hashimoto's, subacute, silent) and rare (suppurative, Riedel's). These vary by cause, course, and histopathology:

- Hashimoto's (struma lymphomatosa, lymphadenoid goiter, chronic lymphocytic thyroiditis): is an autoimmune disorder closely related to Graves' disease, with a familial tendency; it is the most common cause of hypothyroidism in patients not previously treated for overactive thyroid.
- Subacute (de Quervain's thyroiditis, granulomatous thyroiditis, giant cell thyroiditis): self-limited inflammation; a prodromal upper respiratory infection is common.
- Silent (acute lymphocytic thyroiditis): related to Hashimoto's; self-limited, usually occurring in young to middle-aged women; hyper- or hypothyroidism may spontaneously resolve.
- Suppurative: rare disorder usually occurring in the course of a systemic infection.
- Riedel's (chronic fibrous thyroiditis, Riedel's struma, wood thyroiditis, ligneous thyroiditis, invasive thyroiditis): rarest form; found most frequently among middle-aged women; may cause both hypothyroidism and hypoparathyroidism.

Etiology

Hashimoto's is an immune disorder, with lymphocytes gradually replacing thyroid tissue; gland enlarges, and hypothyroidism slowly develops. Subacute is most likely a viral infection, with leaked thyroid hormone causing transient thyrotoxicosis, followed by hypothyroidism. The trigger for silent thyroiditis is unknown, but may involve an autoimmune mechanism. The suppurative form is caused by pyogenic organisms. Riedel's is caused by multifocal systemic fibrosis syndrome.

Risk Factors

- Prodromal upper respiratory tract infection (subacute)
- Pregnancy
- Graves' disease (Hashimoto's)
- Positive family history or preceding autoimmune diseases or conditions

Signs and Symptoms

Hashimoto's:

- Firm, symmetrically enlarged, lobulated gland not tender on palpation; few pressure symptoms
- Progressive worsening of hypothyroid symptoms—cool, dry skin, slow pulse rate (<60 bpm), swelling around eyes, hoarseness, slow reflexes

Subacute:

- Acute, painful enlargement of thyroid; pain possibly radiating to ears or jaw
- Dysphagia
- Malaise and low-grade fever

Silent:

- Mild hyperthyroid symptoms—rapid heartbeat, slight nervousness, hyperactivity, weight loss (5 to 10 lbs.), increased perspiration
- Thyroid moderately enlarged and firm but not tender or painful

Suppurative:

- Severe pain, tenderness, redness, fluctuation in thyroid area

Riedel's:

- Thyroid asymmetrically enlarged, stony, adheres to neck structures
- Signs of compression and invasion—dysphagia, dyspnea, hoarseness

DIFFERENTIAL DIAGNOSIS

- Graves' disease
- Goiter
- Carcinoma
- Thyrotoxicosis
- Sore throat
- Dental problems
- Ear infection

DIAGNOSIS

Physical Examination

With Hashimoto's, the gland is firm, symmetrically enlarged, not tender on palpation, with few pressure symptoms. With subacute, the gland is acutely painful, with pain radiating to the ears and jaw. If no pain is present, silent form is likely. Suppurative produces severe pain and redness. With Riedel's, the enlarged gland is asymmetric and hard.

Laboratory Tests

- TSH and serum T4 and T3 levels: Hashimoto's—T4, 5 mcg/100 ml, TSH >5.0 mcU/ml; subacute—suppressed TSH (<0.1 mcU/ml), elevated serum or free T4; silent—increased T4 and decreased TSH
- Radioiodine uptake: very low to zero in hyperthyroid phase of subacute; high in chronic forms; low in Riedel's
- Thyroid antibody test: high titers in Hashimoto's; possible in other types
- Erythrocyte sedimentation rate: elevated in subacute; markedly elevated in silent
- Biopsy: only if antibodies not detected and no apparent cause for symptoms; see giant cells in silent thyroiditis

Pathological Findings

Lymphocyte infiltration, fibrosis, atrophy (lymphocyte), mononuclear cell infiltrate, giant cells (granulomatous)

Imaging

Thyroid radiodine scan (granulomatous)

TREATMENT OPTIONS

Treatment Strategy

The course of each type of thyroiditis generally involves three phases: hyperthyroid phase, hypothyroid phase, and return to euthyroid status. Treatment is symptomatic and individualized to type and phase.

Drug Therapies

Hashimoto's:

- Levothyroxine: 0.1 to 0.15 mg daily if hypothyroidism or large goiter present

Subacute:

- Aspirin: two tablets three to four times daily as needed to relieve pain and inflammation
- Steroids (such as prednisone or dexamethasone): at lowest dose that relieves pain; gives relief in 24 hours, but continue four to six weeks after pain is gone; severe cases only
- Propranolol: 10 to 40 mg every six hours for thyrotoxic symptoms
- Thyroxine: 0.05 to 0.1 mg/daily for hypothyroidism symptoms

Silent:

- Short-term beta-blockers: as needed for hyperthyroid symptoms
- Levothyroxine: as needed for hypothyroid symptoms

Suppurative:

- Antibiotics and surgical drainage: as needed for marked fluctuation

Riedel's:
- Partial thyroidectomy: to relieve pressure

Complementary and Alternative Therapies
Concurrent therapy with medications may be necessary.

NUTRITION
- Foods that depress the thyroid are broccoli, cabbage, brussel sprouts, cauliflower, kale, spinach, turnips, soy, beans, and mustard greens. These foods should be included in the diet for hyperthyroid conditions and avoided for hypothryroid conditions.
- Avoid refined foods, sugar, dairy products, wheat, caffeine, and alcohol.
- Essential fatty acids are anti-inflammatory and necessary for hormone production. Take 1,000 to 1,500 flaxseed oil mg tid.
- Calcium (1,000 mg/day) and magnesium (200 to 600 mg/day) are cofactors for many metabolic processes.

For hyperthyroid conditions:
- Bromelain (250 to 500mg tid between meals) is a proteolytic enzyme that reduces inflammation.
- Vitamin C (1,000 mg tid to qid) supports immune function and decreases inflammation.

For hypothyroid conditions:
- Vitamin C (1,000 mg tid to qid), vitamin A (10,000 to 25,000 IU/day), B-complex (50 to 100 mg/day), selenium (200 mcg/day), iodine (300 mcg/day), vitamin E (400 IU/day), and zinc (30 mg/day) are necessary for thyroid hormone production.
- L-tyrosine (100 mg bid) also supports normal thyroid function. May exacerbate hypertension.

HERBS
Ascertain a diagnosis before pursuing treatment. Herbs may be used as dried extracts (capsules, powders, teas), glycerites (glycerine extracts), or tinctures (alcohol extracts). Unless otherwise indicated, teas should be made with one teaspoon herb per cup of hot water. Steep covered 5 to 10 minutes for leaf or flowers, and 10 to 20 minutes for roots. Drink two to four cups/day. Tinctures may be used singly or in combination as noted.

For hyperthyroid conditions:
- Bugleweed (*Lycopus virginica*) and lemon balm (*Melissa officinalis*) help to normalize the over-active thyroid.
- Motherwort (*Leonorus cardiaca*) relieves heart palpitations and passionflower (*Passiflora incarnata*) reduces anxiety. Combine two parts of bugleweed with one part each of lemon balm, motherwort, and passionflower in a tincture, 30 to 60 drops tid to qid.
- Quercetin (250 to 500 mg tid) is an anti-inflammatory.
- Turmeric (*Curcuma longa*) potentiates bromelain and should be taken between meals, 500 mg tid.
- Ginkgo biloba (*Gingko folium*) 80 to 120 mg bid.

For hypothyroid conditions:
- A combination that would support thyroid function includes herbs rich in minerals. Combine the following for a tea (3 to 4 cups/day) or tincture (20 to 30 drops tid). Horsetail (*Equisetum arvense*), oatstraw (*Avena sativa*), alfalfa (*Medicago sativa*), gotu kola (*Centella asiatica*), and bladderwrack (*Fucus vesiculosis*)

HOMEOPATHY
An experienced homeopath should assess individual constitutional types and severity of disease, to select the correct remedy and potency.

PHYSICAL MEDICINE
For hyperthyroid conditions: ice packs to the throat for inflammation. For hypothyroid conditions: contrast hydrotherapy to the neck and throat may stimulate thyroid function. Alternating hot and cold applications brings nutrients to the site and diffuses metabolic waste from inflammation. The overall effect is decreased inflammation, pain relief, and enhanced healing. Alternate three minutes hot with one minute cold and repeat three times. This is one set. Do two to three sets/day. In addition, exercise sensitizes thyroid gland to hormones and improves its function.

ACUPUNCTURE
Acupuncture may be helpful in correcting hormonal imbalances and addressing underlying deficiencies and excesses involved in thyroiditis.

Patient Monitoring
- Hashimoto's is associated with other autoimmune diseases (Addison's disease, pernicious anemia, etc.), so monitor the patient for these.
- Because Hashimoto's can progress to hypothyroidism, schedule yearly checkups and begin treatment promptly.
- Repeat thyroid function tests 3 to 12 months in lymphocytic thyroiditis, and every three to six weeks in granulomatous thyroiditis, until euthyroid.

OTHER CONSIDERATIONS
Complications/Sequelae
- High doses of glucocorticoids can cause stomach ulcers, bone loss.
- Hypothyroidism my develop after silent or Hashimoto's thyroiditis.

Prognosis
Some degree of compromise or disability is expected for 6 to 12 months: hyperthyroid phase, 1 to 3 months; hypothyroid phase, 3 to 6 months, then gradual return to euthyroid.

Pregnancy
Thyroid testing during pregnancy may have variable and unreliable results. Mild pathology may not be detected until after pregnancy.

REFERENCES
Blumenthal M, ed. *The Complete German Commission E Monographs.* Boston, Mass: Integrative Medicine Communications; 1998:432.

The Burton Goldberg Group, compilers. *Alternative Medicine: The Definitive Guide.* Tiburon, Calif: Future Medicine Publishing Inc; 1997.

Ferri FF. *Ferri's Clinical Advisor: Instant Diagnosis and Treatment.* St Louis, Mo: Mosby-Year Book;1999.

Hoffman D. *The New Holistic Herbal.* New York, NY: Barnes & Noble Books; 1995:95.

Murray MT, Pizzorno JE. *Encyclopedia of Natural Medicine.* Rocklin, Calif: Prima Publishing; 1998:386–390.

Noble J, ed. *Textbook of Primary Care Medicine.* 2nd ed. St Louis, Mo: Mosby-Year Book; 1996.

Tierney Jr LM, McPhee SJ, Papadakis MA, eds. *Current Medical Diagnosis and Treatment.* Norwalk, Conn: Appleton & Lange; 1994.

■ ULCERATIVE COLITIS

OVERVIEW

Definition

Ulcerative colitis (UC) is a chronic nonspecific inflammatory bowel disease (IBD) involving the mucosa and submucosa of the colon. It involves the rectum and is characterized by ulceration, bloody diarrhea and rectal bleeding. Disease severity depends on degree and extent of inflammation and proximal colonic involvement. UC may present at all ages, but onset peaks between 15 and 30 years with a secondary onset peak between 60 and 70; it is a serious, relapsing-remitting disease with significant morbidity and mortality affecting at least 50 per 100,000 people in the United States. Higher incidence in Jewish population. Familial incidence is established; 10% to 20% of UC patients have at least one family member affected with IBD. Medical management controls symptoms in most cases, but colectomy is necessary in about 25% of those affected.

Etiology

Unknown. Infectious, genetic, immunologic, and psychological causes likely.

Risk Factors

- Jewish ethnicity (Ashkenazi Jews in particular)
- Positive family history
- A diet high in margarine or chemically modified fat (diet of combined western foods)
- Psychological disturbances

Signs and Symptoms

UC typically manifests as bloody diarrhea interspersed with asymptomatic intervals. Onset may be acute and fulminant, but more often is insidious, with progressively severe urgency to defecate, mild abdominal cramps, and blood and mucus in stools. Symptoms may include violent diarrhea, high fever, malaise, abdominal tenderness or pain, anemia, anorexia, weight loss, and arthralgias. In UC confined to the rectosigmoid area, stool may be normal or hard and dry, with mucus discharged between or accompanying bowel movements. Stool abnormality increases with proximal involvement, with up to 20 bowel movements a day, diffuse cramping, distressing tenesmus, passage of pus, nocturnal sweats, pain, and diarrhea.

DIFFERENTIAL DIAGNOSIS

- Crohn's disease
- Hemorrhoids
- Viral, bacterial, and parasitic infections; "Gay bowel" syndrome
- Diverticulitis
- Irritable bowel syndrome
- Radiation proctitis
- Drug- or toxin-induced enterocolitis
- Vasculitis of the intestinal tract
- Colonic carcinoma
- Tuberculosis
- Diarrhea associated with infection
- Diarrhea associated with antibiotics

DIAGNOSIS

Physical Examination

Patients with mild or moderate disease usually look well and exhibit few abnormal signs; bowl sounds and rectal exam (apart from blood) are often normal. Those with severe disease may also look deceptively well, but usually exhibit tachycardia, tender colon, and systemic complications. Diagnosis is made on the basis of history, absence of fecal pathogens, and endoscopic and histological appearances of the colon.
■ Mild inflammatory changes include the following.

- Loss of normal vascular pattern
- Fine granularity of mucosa
- Pinpoint hemorrhage to mucosal swabbing
- Exudation of mucopus

Progressive inflammatory changes include the following.

- Coarse granularity and pinpoint ulceration
- Confluent hemorrhage
- Confluent mucopus progressing to gross ulcerations
- Spontaneous hemorrhage
- Exudation of pus
- Pseudopolyps
- Epithelial dysplasia

Acute disease stage includes the following.

- Loss of haustrations
- Thickening of smooth muscle of colon
- "Lead pipe" appearance of colon
- Occasional colonic stricture

Laboratory Tests

- Nonspecific
- Iron deficiency anemia
- Leukocytosis
- Hypoalbuminemia
- Elevated ESR
- Electrolyte imbalance

Pathological Findings

Endoscopic appearance of mucosa ranges from normal-appearing to complete denudation; UC is characterized by an even "micro-carpet" of tiny ulcers. Sigmoidoscopic appearance is rarely normal even during asymptomatic intervals. Pathologic changes include:

- Degeneration of reticulin fibers beneath mucosal epithelium
- Occlusion of subepithelial capillaries
- Infiltration of lamina propria with plasma cells, eosinophils, lymphocytes, mast cells, and polymorphonuclear leukocytes
- Crypt abscesses, epithelial necrosis, and mucosal ulceration

Imaging

- Radiography (plain view of abdomen)
- Air contrast barium enema
- Ultrasonography and CT may help determine extent of disease and complications

Other Diagnostic Procedures

- Stool samples
- Rectal exam
- Endoscopy with biopsy
- Presence of IL-1ra allele 2 gene is marker for disease severity
- State-Trait Anxiety Inventory (Form Y); Sacks' sentence completion tests (psychological influences)

TREATMENT OPTIONS

Treatment Strategy

The goal of treatment is to control inflammation, prevent complications, and replace nutritional and blood losses. Severe cases may require hospitalization; perforations and hemorrhage may occur without warning. Control of active disease with drug therapy depends upon extent and severity of mucosal ulceration. Most widely used are steroids and 5-aminosalicylic acid (5-ASA) drugs. Corticosteroids can induce remissions but do not prevent relapses. When indicated, total proctocolectomy with ileoanal pull through and pouch is the preferred surgical procedure. Indications

for surgery include:
- Severe inflammation unresponsive to medical therapy
- Chronic active disease
- Cancer prophylaxis
- Growth retardation in children

Drug Therapies

Sulfasalazine is the treatment of choice for flare-ups, chronic treatment, and to reduce frequency of relapse (1 to 4 g/day). Diarrhea may be treated cautiously with diphenoxylate, loperamide, or opiates. Use of antidiarrheal agents in severe disease could precipitate toxic megacolon. Toxic megacolon requires immediate surgery if no improvement within 24 hours after hospitalization

- Ulcerative proctitis and proctosigmoiditis may be treated topically with corticosteroid or mesalamine enema, foam, or suppository; oral prednisone if refractory (20 to 60 mg/day); osmotic purgation to relieve constipation
- Parenteral or oral corticosteroids (prednisone 20 to 60 mg/day) for more severe flare-ups; patients with chronic activity (10% to 15%) require continuous low-dose corticosteroids
- Immunomodulators such as 6-mercaptopurine and azathioprine reduce need for corticosteroids
- Oral prednisone (20 to 60 mg/day) or parenteral corticosteroids and sulfasalazine (one g bid or tid) and parenteral ACTH are useful in severe active disease; iron and parenteral hyperalimentation if indicated; antibiotics in toxic megacolon
- A new class of topically-acting corticosteroids (budesonide, fluticasone, beclomethasone dipropionate, prednisolone-21-methasulphobenzoate, tixocortol pivalate) is an alternative in treating active UC
- Cyclosporine may induce remission
- Nicotine patches may induce remission but are not helpful in maintaining remission

Complementary and Alternative Therapies

Nutritional and herbal support, mind-body techniques, and physical aids can help reduce the frequency and severity of ulcerative colitis as well as improve the integrity of intestinal mucosa and correct nutritional deficiencies. Stress reduction techniques through biofeedback, hypnosis, or counseling can help patients to deal productively with stress. Other mind-body therapies such as: yoga, tai chi, meditation, psychotherapy; stress management such as yoga, deep breathing, stretching, regular exercise (walking), meditation, prayer, visualization, and hypnotherapy; and support groups such as the Crohn's-Colitis Foundation of America (CCFA) may also be helpful.

NUTRITION
- Decrease refined foods, sugars, and saturated fats.
- Eliminate all food allergens from the diet. The most common allergenic foods are dairy, soy, citrus, peanuts, wheat, fish, eggs, corn, and tomatoes. An elimination/challenge trial may be helpful in uncovering sensitivities. Remove suspected allergens from the diet for two weeks. Re-introduce foods at the rate of one food every three days. Watch for reactions which may include gastrointestinal upset, mood changes, headaches, flushing, and exacerbation of symptoms.
- A rotation diet, in which the same food is not eaten more than once every four days, may be helpful in reducing symptoms.
- Specific foods that may exacerbate ulcerative colitis are dairy, Brassica vegetables (cabbage, brussel sprouts, broccoli, cauliflower, and kale) and gluten-containing grains (wheat, oats, barley, triticale, rye).
- Fiber supplementation can help reduce abdominal pain, cramping, and gas. These supplements include psyllium, flax meal, slippery elm (*Ulmus fulva*) powder, and marshmallow root (*Althea officinalis*)

powder. There may be increased bloating and gas initially but this should resolve within 7 to 10 days.
- Pro-flora supplements taken bid to tid can help to re-balance normal bowel flora and reduce gas and bloating.
- Essential fatty acids may be protective of intestinal mucosa. Max-EPA or fish oil (3 to 4 g, up to 18 g/day).
- Bromelain (250 to 500 mg between meals) is a proteolytic enzyme that reduces inflammation.
- Minimum 48 oz of water/day
- Eliminate caffeine and alcohol

IBD is associated with low levels of the following nutrients due to poor absorption, competitive inhibition from medications, or increased requirement.
- Biotin (300 mcg/day)
- Beta-carotene (50,000 IU/day)
- Vitamin A (50,000 IU/day for one month, then 10,000 IU/day)
- Vitamin C (1,000 mg tid)
- Vitamin D (100 to 200 IU/day) is associated with secondary hyperparathyroidism and osteomalacia, possibly due to poor calcium absorption and utilization.
- Vitamin K (10 mg/day) may help normalize prothrombin levels and decrease bleeding.
- B vitamins, specifically thiamine (100 to 250mg/day), pantothenic acid (100 mg/day), riboflavin (50 mg/day), B12 (1,000 mcg/day), and folic acid (800 mcg/day). Folic acid may be depleted with sulfasalazine use, which is a competitive inhibitor with folic acid.
- Magnesium (200 mg bid to tid) is associated with weakness, hypotension, and tetany.
- Calcium (1,000 mg/day)
- Zinc (100mg bid for one month, then 20 to 30 mg/day)
- Elemental iron (30 mg bid), especially with chronic blood loss. Glycinate form is least constipating and 30% more absorbable than ferrous sulphate.
- Selenium (200 mcg/day) protects against oxidative damage.

HERBS
Ascertain a diagnosis before pursuing treatment. Herbs may be used as dried extracts (capsules, powders, teas), glycerites (glycerine extracts), or tinctures (alcohol extracts). Unless otherwise indicated, teas should be made with 1 tsp. herb per cup of hot water. Steep covered 5 to 10 minutes for leaf or flowers, and 10 to 20 minutes for roots. Drink 2 to 4 cups/day. Tinctures may be used singly or in combination as noted. The goal of herbal therapy is to relieve spasm, reduce inflammation, and encourage healing of the intestinal mucosa.
- Enteric-coated peppermint oil: one to two capsules (0.2ml peppermint oil/capsule) tid after meals. Peppermint oil *(Mentha piperita)* is a potent spasmolytic that reduces bowel irritability.
- A tincture of equal parts of the following herbs may be taken before meals (20 to 30 drops tid): Cramp bark *(Viburnum opulus)*, passionflower *(Passiflora incarnata)*, meadowsweet *(Filependula ulmaria)*, wild yam *(Dioscorea villosa)*, valerian *(Valeriana officinalis)*, and lemon balm *(Melissa officinalis)*. Combined, they enhance digestion and relieve spasm.
- For acute exacerbation with bleeding, use equal parts of the following herbs in a tincture (30 drops qid): Coneflower *(Echinacea purpurea)*, goldenseal *(Hydrastis canadensis)*, and geranium *(Geranium maculatum)*
- Licorice root *(Glycyrrhiza glabra)* and marshmallow root *(Althea officinalis)* are soothing and promote healing of gastrointestinal mucosa. Make a tea of licorice root by steeping 1 tsp. in one cup

of hot water for 20 minutes. Drink 3 cups/day. (Contraindicated in hypertension.) For marshmallow root tea, soak 1 heaping tbsp. of root in one quart of cold water overnight. Strain and drink throughout the day.

- Quercetin (250 to 500 mg before meals) may help reduce reactions to food sensitivities.

HOMEOPATHY

An experienced homeopath should assess individual constitutional types and severity of disease to select the correct remedy and potency. For acute prescribing use 3 to 5 pellets of a 12X to 30C remedy every one to four hours until acute symptoms resolve.

- *Arsenicum album* for intense cramping and burning, with scanty dark blood in stool. Patient is restless, chilly, and anxious about their health.
- *China* for extreme bloating and gurgling in abdomen; bloody stools and exhaustion.
- *Phosphorus* for painless diarrhea with prostration and thirst for cold drinks.
- *Sulphur* for morning diarrhea that drives patient out of bed.
- *Mercurius vivus* for IBD associated with canker sores and metallic taste.

PHYSICAL MEDICINE

Castor oil pack. Used externally, castor oil is a powerful anti-inflammatory. Apply oil directly to skin, cover with a clean soft cloth (e.g. flannel) and plastic wrap. Place a heat source (hot water bottle or heating pad) over the pack and let sit for 30 to 60 minutes. For best results, use for three consecutive days.

ACUPUNCTURE

Ulcerative colitis may respond to acupuncture which can help alleviate spasm and normalize digestive function.

Patient Monitoring

Regularly scheduled appointments to evaluate disease activity, and psychological well-being. The extreme variability and high incidence of relapse and morbidity predispose patients to anxiety and depression.

OTHER CONSIDERATIONS

Prevention

Severely ill patients must be monitored closely for peritonitis, perforation, and toxic megacolon; long-term patients for epithelial dysplasia and cancer. Annual liver tests and cholangiography for cholestasis are recommended. Laboratory parameters measured serially during treatment are useful indicators of disease activity.

Complications/Sequelae

Local:
- Hemorrhage
- Perforations
- Peritonitis
- Strictures
- Perianal abscesses
- Rectovaginal fistulas
- Pseudopolyposis
- Toxic megacolon
- Carcinomatous changes
- Colon cancer

Systemic:
- Peripheral arthropathy
- Ankylosing spondylitis
- Erythema nodosum
- Pyoderma gangrenosum
- Episcleritis
- Aphthous ulceration of the mouth
- Fatty liver
- Primary sclerosing cholangitis
- Cholangiocarcinoma
- Growth retardation in children
- Depression and anxiety

Prognosis

The typically relapsing-remitting course of UC depends upon severity of initial attack, extent of proximal colonic involvement, and response to medical treatment. There is no cure excepting colectomy. Left-sided and ulcerative proctitis have the most favorable prognosis. Drug treatment is effective for about 70% to 80% of patients; surgery becomes necessary in the remaining 20% to 30%. About 45% of patients are symptom-free at any given time; most suffer at least one relapse in any 10-year period. About 5% succumb to fulminant UC or require immediate colectomy; a smaller percentage have a single attack without recurrence; and about 15% experience continuous symptoms refractory to medication and rarely achieve full remission. In the 25% of patients with ulcerative proctitis (disease localized to the rectum), 10% to 30% experience late proximal spread. UC in children affects the entire colon in 50% of cases. The prognosis is affected by the extent and the severity of the disease, and by the physical condition of the patient.

Pregnancy

Maintenance treatment should be continued, with pregnancy timed to inactive phase of disease and relapses treated aggressively with corticosteroids. Corticosteroids and sulfasalazine are safe and nonteratogenic; immunosuppressive agents are not recommended. Goldenseal, geranium, and quercetin are contraindicated in pregnancy. In addition, high doses of vitamins should be avoided.

REFERENCES

Berkow R, ed. *The Merck Manual of Diagnosis and Therapy.* 16th ed. Rahway, NJ: Merck Research Laboratories; 1992.

Blumenthal M, ed. *The Complete German Commission E Monographs.* Boston, Mass: Integrative Medicine Communications; 1998:427–428, 432.

Greenfield, S.M. et al. A randomized controlled study of evening primrose oil and fish oil in ulcerative colitis. *Aliment Pharmacol Ther.* 1993;7:159–166.

Roediger WE, Moore J, Babidge W. Colonic sulfide in pathogenesis and treatment of ulcerative colitis. *Dig Dis Sci.* 1997;42:1571–1579.

Weatherall DJ, Ledingham JGG, Warrell DA, eds. *Oxford Textbook of Medicine.* 3rd ed. New York, NY: Oxford University Press; 1996.

Werbach, M. *Nutritional Influences on Illness.* New Canaan, Conn: Keats Publishing; 1988:424–427.

Wyngaarden JB, Smith LH, Bennett JC, eds. *Cecil Textbook of Medicine.* Philadelphia, Pa: WB Saunders; 1992.

■ URETHRITIS
OVERVIEW
Definition
Urethritis is infection and inflammation of the urethral lining caused by bacterial infections, and may involve the bladder, prostate, and reproductive organs. Urethritis can affect males and females of all ages; however, females are at higher risk due to proximity of urethral opening to anus and vagina, increasing the likelihood of bacterial contamination.

Sexually transmitted pathogens *Chlamydia trachomatis, Neisseria gonorrhoeae* (co-infection common), and herpes simplex are primary causes of urethritis, particularly in men; however, often no infection can be documented. Vaginitis triggered by *Candida albicans* or *Trichomonas vaginalis,* and bacterial vaginosis, are also contributing causes for women. In bacteria-negative cultures, urethritis and vaginitis account for most urinary disorders in women.

Of the organisms which cause nongonococcal urethritis (NGU), chlamydia is the most common and most serious, with 75% of infected women and 50% of infected men remaining asymptomatic. Left untreated, it can lead to permanent damage of reproductive organs in both men and women. Implications tend to be more severe in women due to the internal nature of the infection, which often goes without notice until complications arise.

Etiology
- Bacteria and other organisms entering the urethra, including *Chlamydia trachomatis, Neisseria gonorrhoeae, Ureaplasma urealyticum, Mycoplasma hominis, Candida albicans, Trichomonas vaginalis,* and herpes viruses
- Bruising during sexual intercourse (women)
- Infection reaching the urethra via venous system from prostate gland or through the penis opening; in older men, classical urinary tract pathogens are a more common cause than STDs
- Bacterial infection following course of antibiotics
- Reiter's syndrome

Risk Factors
- Unprotected sex
- History of sexually transmitted diseases
- Multiple sex partners, or sexual relations with individual who has multiple sex partners
- Urinary catheter or instrumentation
- Bacteria-resistant drugs
- Prior history of kidney stones, prostatitis, epididymitis, genital injury
- Reiter's syndrome, which has a genetic predisposition
- Increased caffeine intake

Signs and Symptoms
In both sexes but particularly women, the disease may be asymptomatic.
In men:
- Burning during urination
- Purulent or whitish-mucus urethral discharge
- Burning or itching around the penile opening
In women:
- Painful urination and/or unusual vaginal discharge
- Cervicitis
- Salpingitis
- Pelvic inflammatory disease

DIFFERENTIAL DIAGNOSIS
- Reiter's syndrome
- Gonorrhea
- Allergic reactions
- Other urinary tract infections

DIAGNOSIS
Physical Examination
- Watery and thin discharge *(C. trachomatis)*
- Purulent discharge *(N. gonorrhoeae)*
- Inflammation of penile opening

Laboratory Tests
- Presence of white blood cells in urine specimen
- Gram stain of urethral discharge which shows >4 WBCs per HPF
- Intracellular gram-negative diplococci strongly suggests gonorrhea
- Absence of gram-negative cocci strongly suggests NGU (gram stains are less than 100% sensitive for chlamydial infections)
- Syphillis and HIV serology to rule out other STDs

Pathological Findings
- Unusual urethral/vaginal discharge in 50 to 75% of cases
- In males, possible inflammation and irritation at penis opening
- Urethral strictures

Other Diagnostic Procedures
- Thorough medical and sexual history, including date of symptom onset and prior history of STDs
- Genital examination
- Evaluation of laboratory evidence for infection *(C. trachomatis* requires specimen of intracellular and urethral cellular material; collect specimen with calcium alginate swab inserted two to three cm into urethra)
- Evaluation of sexual partners may aid diagnosis in asymptomatic disease

C. trachomatis:
- Immunofluorescent testing
- Enzyme-linked immunoassay
- DNA probing of cervical samples

TREATMENT OPTIONS
Treatment Strategy
- Therapy must often be administered presumptively.
- Antimicrobial therapy directed against etiologies.
- Chlamydial disease may persist even after successful treatment of gonococcal component.
- Impress upon patient importance of treatment compliance.
- All sex partners should be treated.
- Sexual abstinence recommended until treatment regimen is completed, as disease can remain active even after symptoms have disappeared.

Drug Therapies
Urethritis:
- Tetracycline (500 mg qid for seven days)
- Erythromycin (500 mg qid for seven days; preferred in pregnancy)

N. gonorrhoeae:
- Ceftriaxone (250 mg IM once a day)
- Ofloxacin (400 mg once a day)
- Ciprofloxacin (500 mg once a day)

C. trachomatis:
- Doxycycline (100 mg bid for 10 days)
- Ofloxacin (300 mg orally bid for 10 days)

Trichomonas urethritis/vaginitis:

- Metronidazole (2 g orally once a day; contraindicated in pregnancy)
- Clindamycin (300 mg orally bid for seven days)

Herpes simplex:
- Acyclovir (400 mg orally tid for 10 days)
- Famciclovir (250 to 500 mg orally bid for 10 days)
- Valacyclovir (1,000 mg orally bid for 10 days)

Persistent/recurrent disease:
- Retreatment with antimicrobials

Complementary and Alternative Therapies

Nutrition, herbs, and homeopathic remedies are useful in fighting infection, relieving pain, and tonifying the urinary system.

NUTRITION

- Eliminate any known food allergens. Food allergies can be tested for using an IgG ELISA food allergy panel, or by an elimination diet.
- Eliminate refined foods, fruit juices, caffeine, alcohol, and sugar, which may compromise immune function and irritate the urinary tract.
- Cranberries and blueberries contain substances that inhibit the adhesion of bacteria to the urinary tract.
- Vitamin C (1,000 mg tid) stimulates immune system and acidifies urine, which inhibits bacterial growth.
- Beta-carotene (25,000 to 50,000 IU/day) is necessary for immune function and mucous membrane integrity.
- Zinc (30 to 50 mg/day) supports immune function.

HERBS

Herbs are generally a safe way to strengthen and tone the body's systems. As with any therapy, it is important to ascertain a diagnosis before pursuing treatment. Herbs may be used as dried extracts (capsules, powders, teas), glycerites (glycerine extracts), or tinctures (alcohol extracts). Unless otherwise indicated, teas should be made with 1 tsp. herb per cup of hot water. Steep covered 5 to 10 minutes for leaf or flowers, and 10 to 20 minutes for roots. Drink 2 to 4 cups/day. Tinctures may be used singly or in combination as noted.

Herbal therapy should be instituted at the first sign of symptoms and continued for three days beyond resolution of symptoms. Treatment of infectious urethritis is best accomplished through teas because of the flushing action of the additional fluid intake. Combine two herbs from each of the following categories and drink 4 to 6 cups/day.

Urinary antiseptics are antimicrobial and include the following.
- Uva ursi (*Arctostaphylos uva ursi*)
- Buchu (*Agathosma betulina*)
- Thyme leaf (*Thymus vulgaris*)
- Pipsissewa (*Chimaphila umbellata*)

Urinary astringents tone and heal the urinary tract and include the following.
- Horsetail (*Equisetum arvense*)
- Plantain (*Plantago major*)
- Cleavers (*Galium aparine*)

Urinary demulcents soothe the inflamed urinary tract and include the following.
- Corn silk (*Zea mays*)
- Couch grass (*Agropyron repens*)
- Marshmallow root (*Althea officinalis*) is best used alone in a cold infusion. Soak one heaping tbsp. of marshmallow root in one quart of cold water overnight. Strain and drink during the day in addition to the other urinary tea.

For advanced or recurrent infections, prepare a tincture of equal parts of goldenseal (*Hydrastis canadensis*) and coneflower (*Echinacea purpurea*). Take 30 drops four to six times/day in addition to the urinary tea.

For non-infectious urethritis or for urethritis with severe pain and spasm, add kava kava (*Piper methysticum*) to any of the above formulas. A peri-wash may be helpful in reducing pain with urination. Place 1 tsp. of the coneflower/goldenseal tincture in an eight-ounce peri bottle. Fill with water. Rinse off after each urination.

HOMEOPATHY

An experienced homeopath should assess individual constitutional types and severity of disease to select the correct remedy and potency. For acute prescribing use 3 to 5 pellets of a 12X to 30C remedy every one to four hours until acute symptoms resolve.
- *Staphysagria* for urinary infections associated with sexual intercourse
- *Apis mellifica* for stinging pains that are exacerbated by warmth
- *Cantharis* for intolerable urging with "scalding" urine
- *Sarsaparilla* for needing to stand to urinate, with burning after urination

ACUPUNCTURE

May be helpful in enhancing immune function.

Patient Monitoring

- Recurrent or persistent symptoms require careful re-evaluation and retreatment with antimicrobials when urethral discharge tests positive or demonstrates increased numbers of polymorphonuclear leukocytes.
- Monitor general condition/medications.
- Encourage patient self-care.
- Monitor closely for treatment compliance, particularly for STD-related urethritis.

OTHER CONSIDERATIONS

Treat patient's sexual partner(s) if STD-related.

Prevention

- Wipe from front to back following bowel movement, wash genitalia with soapy water, shower rather than bath (for women only).
- Drink eight glasses of water daily.
- Protected sex with latex condom when outside of a monogamous relationship

Complications/Sequelae

- When left untreated, gonococcal urethritis—common in men—may cause urethral stricture with increased risk of periurethral abscess; may perforate the peritoneal scrotum, causing urethral fistula.
- Untreated chlamydia increases risk of acquisition/transmission of HIV, causes pelvic inflammatory disease (PID) in women, and—in men—affects the testicles, which leads to complications and possible infertility.
- Infection spread to ureters/kidneys

Prognosis

- When associated with low-grade infection and treated appropriately, seldom produces long-term illness; however, recurrence is common.
- STDs or NGU can be effectively treated with antibiotic medication. When asymptomatic or left untreated, complications—including infertility—may result, and disease transmission to sex partners is inevitable.

Pregnancy

NGU:
- Permanent damage to reproductive organs/infertility in both sexes.
- Difficulties during pregnancy, premature delivery, low birth weight.

- Ear, eye, and lung infections in newborns. (Resultant neonatal conjunctivitis can permanently damage eyesight.)
- Nutritional guidelines are safe to follow in pregnancy. Herbal therapies should be used only with physician supervision.
- Avoid tetracyclines.

REFERENCES

Bartram T. *Encyclopedia of Herbal Medicine.* Dorset, England: Grace Publishers; 1995:436–437.

Berkow R, Beers MH. *The Merck Manual of Diagnosis and Therapy.* Rahway, NJ: Merck and Company; 1992.

Blumenthal M, ed. *The Complete German Commission E Monographs.* Boston, Mass: Integrative Medicine Communications; 1998:432.

Bowie WR. Approach to men with urethritis and urologic complications of sexually transmitted diseases. *Med Clin North Am.* 1990;74:1543–1557. Accessed at www.thriveonline.com.

Hoffman D. *The New Holistic Herbal.* New York, NY: Barnes & Noble Books; 1995:109–110.

Kruzel T. *The Homeopathic Emergency Guide.* Berkeley, Calif: North Atlantic Books; 1992:98–102.

Shealy CN. *The Illustrated Encyclopedia of Healing Remedies.* Boston, Mass: Element Books Limited; 1998.

Tierney LM, et al, eds. *Current Medical Diagnosis & Treatment 1999.* 38th ed. Stamford, Conn: Appleton & Lange; 1999.

Virtual Hospital: University of Iowa Family Practice Handbook. 3rd ed. Available at www.vh.org.

■ URINARY INCONTINENCE

OVERVIEW

Definition

Urinary incontinence (inability to control urination or the involuntary loss of urine from the bladder) afflicts more than 13 million people in the United States of both sexes and all age groups. Incidence is higher in the elderly and two-fold greater in women. Exercise and behavioral therapies have a high degree of success; medication and surgery are effective in a select group over the short-term. Many drugs have unwanted and/or serious side effects: Surgery should be considered only when other treatment options fail. Diagnostic categories are:

- Stress incontinence (SUI): Most common form among women primarily due to pregnancy, childbirth, menopause. Weakened pelvic floor muscles fail to support bladder and resultant pressure interferes with muscles that close the urethra. Leakage occurs with physical stress (e.g., coughing, sneezing).
- Urge (or reflex) incontinence (UI): Leakage accompanied by sudden unexplained need to urinate (e.g., when touching water). May be due to nerve damage (e.g., from Alzheimer's disease, stroke, brain tumor, injury, surgery).
- Overflow incontinence (OI): Rare in women. Bladder overextension due to blocked urethra or inability of bladder muscles to expel urine. Caused by neurological damage (e.g., from diabetes), tumors, urinary stones, enlarged prostate.
- Mixed incontinence (MI): SUI/UI in combination.
- Functional incontinence (FI): Impaired cognitive abilities and/or restricted movement (e.g., confined to a wheelchair) prevents timely access to toilet.
- Transient incontinence (TI): Triggered by medication, UTIs, restricted mobility, stool impaction.

Etiology

- Neurological damage/disorders (dementia, spinal cord injury, multiple sclerosis, stroke)
- Low estrogen levels in women
- Physical changes (from pregnancy or enlarged prostate, stool impaction, tumor)
- Medications
- Urinary tract infections (UTIs)
- Weak urethral sphincter
- Weak pelvic floor muscle

Risk Factors

- Overweight
- Hysterectomy before age 45
- At least one live birth
- Labor exceeding 24 hours
- Prostate disease or hypertrophy in males
- Physical problems associated with age/debility
- Neurologic damage or disorders

Signs and Symptoms

- Involuntary urination
- Perineal irritation
- Frequent and unusual urinary urge

DIFFERENTIAL DIAGNOSIS

- Vaginal discharge in women
- UTIs
- Urethral discharge in men
- Medication effects (diuretics)

DIAGNOSIS

Physical Examination

- Urine leakage
- Findings specific to risk factors

Laboratory Tests

Urinalysis to determine urinary tract/bladder infection, urinary stones, diabetes, glomerular disease, tumor.

Pathological Findings

- Urethral sphincter incompetence
- Prostatic hypertrophy
- Bladder tumor
- UTI

Imaging

- Pelvic ultrasound
- Renal ultrasound
- Transrectal ultrasound (prostate)

Other Diagnostic Procedures

- Physical examination
- Neurological assessment
- Medical history
- Interview for pattern of voiding/leakage, straining/discomfort associated with urination
- Test for stress incontinence (e.g., vigorous coughing to detect urine loss)
- Urodynamics
- Voidin cystourethrogram

TREATMENT OPTIONS

Treatment Strategy

Along with the drug therapies and surgical procedures listed below, the following may be necessary.

- Catheters
- Urethral plugs
- Condom catheters
- Absorbent pads, undergarments, diapers

Drug Therapies

- Antibiotics: For UTIs or sexually transmitted diseases
- Anticholinergics: For UI, reduce detrusor muscle contractions/increase urethral resistance (imipramine [Tofranil] 10 to 25 mg up to tid; oxybutinin [Ditropan] 2.5 to 5 mg up to tid; hyoscyamine [Cystospaz], hyoscyamine sulfate [Levsin/Levsinex, Cystospaz-M], and flavoxate [Urispas] all 100 to 200 mg tid or qid). High instance of undesirable/intolerable side effects
- Antimuscarinic/ganglionic-blockers: Propantheline (Pro-Banthine) 15 to 30 mg every four to six hours. High incidence of side effects including confusion, agitation, coronary artery disease, especially in the elderly.
- Cholinergics: For underactive detrusor, bethanechol (Duvoid, Myotonachol, Urecholine); contraindicated with asthma, bradycardia, Parkinson's disease. Can produce intolerable sweating/excessive salivation
- Sympathomimetics: For SUI, phenylpropanolamine (found in Ornade) 25 to 100 mg bid; or pseudoephedrine (found in Sudafed) 15 to 30 mg tid; caution with hypertension, angina, hyperthyroidism, diabetes
- Hormones: SUI in women, increase urethral resistance (conjugated estrogens [Premarin] 1.25 to 2.5 mg/day in cream; .3 to .625 mg/day

orally with Estradiol [Estrace]); increased risk of endometrial cancer, particularly with unopposed estrogen

Surgical Procedures

Success rate higher in younger patients; effectiveness deteriorates over time; long-term success rate estimated at 75% to 90% for five years.

- Artificial sphincter: Inflatable cuff surrounding bladder neck activated by mechanism implanted in scrotum or labia.
- Supportive devices: String secured to the bladder and attached to muscle, bone, or ligament; in severe SUI, a wide sling elevates bladder.

Complementary and Alternative Therapies

The main thrust of alternative therapies is Kegel exercises, biofeedback, and preventing any exacerbating conditions. Underlying conditions (e.g., malnutrition, dementia, prostatitis, and UTIs) need to be addressed. Yoga may be beneficial. Habit training (establishing toilet times to increase regularity of voiding) may also help treat this condition.

NUTRITION

- Eliminate caffeine, alcohol, sweetener substitutes, simple sugars.
- Cranberries and blueberries contain substances which inhibit the adhesion of bacteria to bladder tissue. This may be useful in preventing infections which can exacerbate incontinence. Also helps to deodorize urine.
- Vitamin C (1,000 mg tid) acidifies urine which inhibits bacterial growth.
- Beta-carotene (25,000t to 50,000 IU/day) is necessary for immune function and mucous membrane integrity.
- Zinc (30 mg/day) supports immune function, often deficient in the elderly.
- Calcium (1,000 mg/day) and magnesium (500 mg/day) together may help to improve sphincter control.

HERBS

Herbs are generally a safe way to strengthen and tone the body's systems. As with any therapy, it is important to ascertain a diagnosis before pursuing treatment. Herbs may be used as dried extracts (capsules, powders, teas), glycerites (glycerine extracts), or tinctures (alcohol extracts). Unless otherwise indicated, teas should be made with 1 teaspoon herb per cup of hot water. Steep covered 5 to 10 minutes for leaf or flowers, and 10 to 20 minutes for roots. Drink 2 to 4 cups/day. Tinctures may be used singly or in combination as noted.

Urinary astringents have been used historically for sphincter tone and connective tissue integrity. Demulcents soothe irritated tissue and may decrease spasm of the bladder.

These urinary astringents tone and heal the urinary tract and can be taken long term at 1 cup/day or 30 drops tincture/day.

- Horsetail *(Equisetum arvense)* also helps with connective tissue integrity
- Plantain *(Plantago major)* is an astringent and demulcent

Marshmallow root *(Althea officinalis)* is a urinary demulcent, best used alone in a cold infusion. Soak 1 heaping tbsp. of marshmallow root in 1 quart of cold water overnight. Strain and drink during the day in addition to other teas.

HOMEOPATHY

An experienced homeopath should assess individual constitutional types and severity of disease to select the correct remedy and potency. For acute prescribing use three to five pellets of a 12X to 30C remedy every one to four hours until acute symptoms resolve.

- *Causticum* for SUI, especially with retention from holding the urine and frequent urges to urinate
- *Natrum muriaticum* for SUI, vaginal dryness, painful coition, especially with a history of grief
- *Pareira* for retention of urine from an enlarged prostate
- *Sepia* for SUI with sudden urging, especially with prolapsed uterus and vaginitis
- *Zincum* for SUI, urinary retention from prostate problems, unable to urinate standing, must sit

ACUPUNCTURE

May be of help, depending on cause.

Patient Monitoring

Compliance with behavioral techniques is essential and may require close monitoring and reinforcement. Physician must be alert to and monitor side effects of medications, or for infections following implants/surgery.

OTHER CONSIDERATIONS

Early treatment is most beneficial; embarrassment often causes delay in seeking help.

Prevention

- Pelvic muscle strengthening (Kegel) exercises during and after pregnancy
- Maintenance of healthy prostate in men; maintenance of healthy pelvis in women
- Maintenance of optimal body weight for height/age

Complications/Sequelae

- Drugs: Considerable risk of unwanted, intolerable and/or serious side effects; contraindication with other medications
- Surgery: Possible complications
- Catheters: UTIs

Prognosis

Most cases can be vastly improved with appropriate management; effectiveness may deteriorate with age.

Pregnancy

Pregnancy increases risk of incontinence; effect of drugs upon fetus must be determined before administered during pregnancy.

REFERENCES

Bartram T. *Encyclopedia of Herbal Medicine.* Dorset, England: Grace Publishers; 1995:247.

Blumenthal M, ed. *The Complete German Commission E Monographs.* Boston, Mass: Integrative Medicine Communications; 1998:432.

Dambro MR. *Griffith's 5 Minute Clinical Consult:* Baltimore, Md: Williams & Wilkins; 1998.

Fauci AS, Braunwald, E, Isselbacher KJ et al, eds. *Harrison's Principles of Internal Medicine.* 14th ed. New York, NY: McGraw-Hill; 1998:1466–1468.

Morrison R. *Desktop Guide to Keynotes and Confirmatory Symptoms.* Albany, Calif: Hahnemann Clinic Publishing; 1993:111–113, 258–261, 286, 402.

Olshevsky M, Noy S, Zwang M, et al. *Manual of Natural Therapy.* New York, NY: Facts on File Inc; 1989.

Thom DH, Van den Eeden SK, Brown JS. Evaluation of parturition and other reproductive variable as risk factors for urinary incontinence. *Obstet Gynecol.* 1997;90:983–989.

Ullman D. *The Consumer's Guide to Homeopathy.* New York, NY: The Putnam Publishing Group; 1995.

■ URINARY TRACT INFECTION IN WOMEN
OVERVIEW
Definition
Urinary tract infection is a bacterial infection with, or causing, inflammation of urothelium. It occurs predominantly in women ages 14 to 61. Isolated UTIs occur in 25% to 30% of all women; recurrent UTIs occur in 60%, 95% of which are due to exogenous reinfection.

Etiology
- Gram-negative bacteria causes UTIs, including *Escherichia coli, Enterobacter sp, Klebsiella sp,* and *Proteus mirabilis,* and, less commonly, *Pseudomonas aeruginosa, Serratia marcescens,* and *Trichomonas vaginalis* protozoa.

Risk Factors
- Changes in sexual activity: partner, frequency, intensity
- Diabetes mellitus
- Pregnancy
- Use of irritant chemicals (detergents, spermicides)
- Use of irritant contraceptive devices (e.g., diaphragm)
- Use of oral contraceptives
- Heavy antibiotic use, eliminating "barrier" micro-organisms
- Urinary tract abnormality or obstruction (tumor, calculi, stricture, inability to empty bladder completely)
- Previous UTIs less than 6 months apart
- Catheterization, hospitalization, chronic antimicrobial therapy, immuno-suppressants, and corticosteroids; may trigger UTIs

Signs and Symptoms
- Painful urination, with a burning sensation, frequency, and urgency
- Blood or pus in urine
- Pain or cramping in the lower abdomen
- Chills, fever (fever may be the only symptom in infants and children)
- Strong-smelling urine

DIFFERENTIAL DIAGNOSIS
- Vaginitis
- Pyelonephritis (Up to one-third of UTI patients with mild lower UTI symptoms may have acute uncomplicated pyelonephritis.)
- Urethritis
- Sexually transmitted disease
- Hematuria due to another condition, such as a tumor, calculi, Tb, or, rarely, parasitic disease (malaria)
- Intraperitoneal disease

DIAGNOSIS
Physical Examination
- Enlarged, tender kidney upon palpation
- Abdominal rigidity upon palpation
- Costovertebral tenderness upon palpation
- Urinary symptoms: frequency, urgency, pain (only occurs in one-third of patients with lower UTI)

Laboratory Tests
- Urinalysis with macro/micro examination
- Suprapubic needle aspiration culture if unable to obtain clean catch: bacterial count is greater than 102 CFU/ml
- Urine culture to differentiate urethritis (bacterial colony greatest in urethral culture) and UTI (bacterial colony greater than or equal to 10^5 CFU/ml)

- Vaginal culture to differentiate vaginitis (bacterial colony greatest in vaginal culture)

Pathological Findings
In recurrent UTIs, periurethral flora culture, indicating prolonged coliform bacterial colonization, confirm virulence over normal host defenses (urine, urine flow, urinary tract mucosa, urinary tract bacterial inhibitors)

Imaging
Recurrent or infant UTIs:
- Plain film x-ray, ultrasound, endoscopic imaging, or VCUG
- Intravenous pyelogram (IVP)

Other Diagnostic Procedures
Urine culture (indications: pregnancy, history of UTI, diabetes mellitus, age over 65, immunosuppression, urologic abnormality, gross hematuria, unresolved or recurrent UTI symptoms, UTI symptoms for three or more days, fever, chills, flank pain, and recent—within the previous two weeks—antimicrobial therapy, hospital or nursing home stay, increase in sexual activity, or urethral catheter) Types:
- Vaginal—swab vaginal introitus with sterile cotton applicator; place in 5 ml saline or standard transport broth
- Urethral—void, 5 to 10 ml
- Midstream—void, 200 ml midstream
- Suprapubic needle aspiration of the bladder

TREATMENT OPTIONS
Treatment Strategy
Antibiotics eliminate bacteria and prevent progression of infection to kidneys. NSAIDs, urinary antiseptics, herbal, and homeopathic treatments are considered for symptomatic relief.

Drug Therapies
General considerations: patient compliance, type of infection (isolated vs. recurrent; uncomplicated vs. complicated, cost, strength, dose, side effects, efficacy, and length (7 to 10 vs. 1 to 3 days) of treatment. Commonly used for UTI:
- Amoxicillin: 250 to 500 mg every eight hours
- Fluoroquinolone (Ciprofloxacin): 250 mg every 12 hours
- Trimethoprim/Sulfamethoxazole (TMP/SMX): 160 mg trimethoprim/ 800 mg sulfamethoxazole every 12 hours

Also used:
- Ampicillin: 250 to 500 mg qid
- Cotrimoxazole: 160 to 800 mg every 12 hours
- Nitrofurantoin: 40 to 100 mg every six hours

Used in severe UTI, with sepsis:
- Aminoglycosides (gentamicin sulfate, kanamycin sulfate): single intramuscular dose of 5 mg/kg gentamicin, or 0.5 g gentamicin parenterally every eight hours.

Complementary and Alternative Therapies
Nutrition, herbs, and homeopathic remedies may be useful in fighting infection, relieving pain, and tonifying the urinary system.

NUTRITION
- Eliminate refined foods, fruit juices, caffeine, alcohol, and sugar which may compromise immune function. Cranberries and blueberries contain substances which inhibit adhesion of bacteria to bladder tissue.
- Vitamin C (1,000 mg tid) acidifies urine, inhibits bacterial growth.
- Beta-carotene (25,000 to 50,000 IU/day) is necessary for immune

function and mucous membrane integrity.
- Zinc (30 to 50 mg/day) supports immune function.

HERBS

Ascertain a diagnosis before pursuing treatment. Herbs may be used as dried extracts (capsules, powders, teas), glycerites (glycerine extracts), or tinctures (alcohol extracts). Unless otherwise indicated, teas should be made with 1 tsp. herb per cup of hot water. Steep covered 5 to 10 minutes for leaf or flowers, and 10 to 20 minutes for roots. Drink 2 to 4 cups/day. Tinctures may be used singly or in combination as noted.

Herbal therapy should be instituted at the first sign of symptoms and continued for three days beyond resolution of symptoms. Treatment of UTI's is best accomplished through teas because of the flushing action of the additional fluid intake. Combine two herbs from each of the following categories and drink 4 to 6 cups/day.
- Urinary antiseptics are antimicrobial: uva ursi (*Arctostaphylos uva ursi*), buchu (*Agathosma betulina*), thyme leaf (*Thymus vulgaris*), Pipsissewa (*Chimaphila umbellata*)
- Urinary astringents tone and heal the urinary tract: horsetail (*Equisetum arvense*), plantain (*Plantago major*)
- Urinary demulcents soothe the inflamed urinary tract: Corn silk (*Zea mays*), couch grass (*Agropyron repens*)

Marshmallow root (*Althea officinalis*) is best used alone in a cold infusion. Soak 1 heaping tbsp. of marshmallow root in 1 quart of cold water overnight. Strain and drink during the day in addition to the other tea.

For advanced or recurrent infections prepare a tincture of equal parts of goldenseal (*Hydrastis canadensis*) and coneflower (*Echinacea purpurea*). Take 30 drops four to six times/day.

HOMEOPATHY

An experienced homeopath should assess individual constitutional types and severity of disease to select the correct remedy and potency. For acute prescribing use 3 to 5 pellets of a 12X to 30C remedy every one to four hours until acute symptoms resolve.
- *Staphysagria* for UTI's associated with sexual intercourse
- *Apis mellifica* for stinging pains that are exacerbated by warmth
- *Cantharis* for intolerable urging with "scalding" urine
- *Sarsaparilla* for burning after urination

Patient Monitoring

For chronic UTIs, perform follow-up urinalysis. For isolated UTIs, no follow-up necessary unless pain persists.

OTHER CONSIDERATIONS

Prevention
- Drink unsweetened cranberry juice, or take cranberry juice extract.
- Urinate before and after sexual intercourse.
- Recheck diaphragm fit.

- Drink plenty of fluids, such as water and herb teas. Avoid sweetened fruit juices and other sweetened drinks.
- Avoid sexual activity until infection is resolved.

Complications/Sequelae
- Pyelonephritis
- Renal abscess
- Gram-negative sepsis

Prognosis

Antibiotics stop symptoms of uncomplicated, isolated UTIs within 24 to 48 hours and destroy bacteria with indicated duration of treatment. Herbal remedies treat UTIs while homeopathic remedies relieve the symptoms.

Pregnancy

Risk factors for complications include the following.
- Untreated bacteriuria (develops into pyelonephritis 20% to 40% of the time)
- Undetected UTI

Treatment during pregnancy includes the following.
- Routine urinalysis during first trimester
- Antibiotics for positive cultures
- Prophylaxis if recurrent UTIs during pregnancy
- Hospitalization for acute pyelonephritis

REFERENCES

Avorn J, Monane M, Gurwitz JH, Glynn RJ, Choodnovskiy I, Lipsitz LA. Reduction of bacteriuria and pyuria after ingestion of cranberry juice. *JAMA.* 1994; 271:751–754.

Berkow R, ed. *The Merck Manual.* 16th ed. Rahway, NJ: Merck and Company Inc; 1992.

Blumenthal M, ed. *The Complete Commission E Monographs, American Botanical Council.* Boston, Mass: Integrative Medicine Communications; 1998:432.

Engel JD, Schaeffer AJ. Evaluation of and antimicrobial therapy for recurrent urinary tract infections in women. *Urol Clin N Am.* 1998;25: 685–701.

Goodman-Gilman A, Rall T, Nies A, Palmer T. *The Pharmacological Basis of Therapeutics.* 8th ed. New York, NY: Pergamon Press; 1990.

Howell A, Vorsa N, Der Marderosian A, Foo Lai Yeap. Inhibition of the adherence of P-fimbriated Escherichia cola to uroepithelia-cell surfaces by proanthocyanidin extracts in cranberries. *N Engl J Med.* 1998;339:1085–1086. Letter.

Kruzel T. *The Homeopathic Emergency Guide.* Berkeley, Calif: North Atlantic Books; 1992:98–102.

Murray M, Pizzorno J. *Encyclopedia of Natural Medicine.* Rocklin, Calif: Prima Publishing; 1990.

Ofek I, Goldhar J, Zafriri D, Lis H, Adar R, Sharon N. Anti-Escherichia coli adhesion activity of cranberry and blueberry juices. *N Engl J Med.* 1991;324:1599. Letter.

Schmidt DR, Sobota AE. An examination of the anti-adherence activity of cranberry juice on urinary and nonurinary bacterial isolates. *Microbios.* 1988;55:173–181.

Schultz V, Hansel R, Tyler VE. *Rational Phytotherapy: A Physician's Guide to Herbal Medicine.* New York, NY: Springer; 1997.

Sobel JD. Pathogenesis of urinary tract infection: role of host defenses. *Infect Dis Clin of North Am.* 1997;11:531–549.

Sobota AE. Inhibition of bacterial adherence by cranberry juice: potential use for the treatment of urinary tract infections. *J Urol.* 1984;131:1013–1016.

Ullman D. *The Consumer's Guide to Homeopathy.* Tarcher/Putnam; 1996.

Werbach M, Murray M. *Botanical Influences on Illness: A Sourcebook of Clinical Research.* Tarzania, Calif: Third Line Press; 1994.

Zafriri D, Ofek I, Adar R, Pocino M, Sharon N. Inhibitory activity of cranberry juice on adherence of type 1 and type P fimbriated Escherichia coli to eucaryotic cells. *Antimicrob Agents Chemother.* 1989;33:92–98.

■ UROLITHIASIS
OVERVIEW
Definition
Also called nephrolithiasis or kidney stones, urolithiasis is the presence of calculi in the urinary tract. The male-to-female incidence ratio is 4:1, with 240,000 to 720,000 Americans affected yearly. Eighty percent of calculi are composed of calcium (either oxalate or phosphate), with others composed of struvite, uric acid, or cystine.

Etiology
Type of stone indicates cause.
- Calcium type I—increased small bowel absorption of calcium unrelated to intake
- Calcium type II—increased dietary calcium intake
- Calcium type III—increased vitamin D synthesis (secondary to renal phosphate loss)
- Calcium oxalate—Idiopathic in origin, or through primary intestinal disorders, chronic diarrhea with inflammatory bowel disease or steatorrhea
- Struvite (magnesium ammonium phosphate)—mainly in women and can be large, stag's horn shape; secondary to infection with urease-producing organisms (*Proteus, Pseudomonas, Providencia,* and less commonly *Klebsiella*)
- Uric acid—metabolic defects or dietary excess of uric acid; bowel disease or chemotherapy
- Cystine—secondary to chronic diarrhea, type I renal tubular acidosis, chronic hydrochlorothiazide treatment, idiopathic

Risk Factors
- Excess intake of calcium, oxalate, or purines in predisposed individuals
- Inadequate fluid intake
- Sedentary occupation
- Area of high humidity, elevated temperatures (summer)
- Hyperparathyroidism
- Renal tubule defects (renal tubule acidosis)
- Bowel disease
- Ileal bypass for obesity
- Genetics—cystinuria is an autosomal recessive disorder and homozygous type has markedly increased cystine excretion;
- Excessive intake of certain vitamins and minerals
- Gout
- Use of certain diuretics

Signs and Symptoms
May be asymptomatic, but the following are usually seen.
- Sudden onset of severe flank pain
- Nausea and vomiting
- Patient in constant motion in attempt to lessen the pain
- Pain referred to testes or labium as the stone moves
- Fever and chills (infection)
- Pain radiating anteriorly over the abdomen

DIFFERENTIAL DIAGNOSIS
- Urinary tract infection
- Pyelonephritis
- Diverticulitis
- Pelvic inflammatory disease
- Ovarian pathology
- Drug addiction
- Appendicitis
- Small bowel obstruction
- Ectopic pregnancy
- Cadmium toxicity

DIAGNOSIS
Physical Examination
Patient is in extreme pain and constantly moving. Pain occurs episodically as the stone moves down the ureter and may be referred. Severity of symptoms does not reflect stone size. Patient may be asymptomatic, with stone found incidentally on plain film.

Laboratory Tests
- Urinalysis—Possibly microscopic or gross hematuria, but absence does not exclude stones. Exclude infection.
- Urine pH—Persistent urinary pH <5.0 indicates uric acid or cystine stone; persistent urinary pH >7.5 indicates struvite stone
- Urine culture and sensitivity tests
- Serum chemistries for calcium, electrolytes, phosphate, and uric acid
- 24-hour urine collection for calcium, uric acid, phosphate, oxalate, citrate excretion (recurrent cases only) and to collect stones for analysis

Pathological Findings
Analysis of stone to determine type—assume 80% are calcium, 20% struvite, 5% uric acid, 5% cystine.

Imaging
- Plain abdominal film and renal ultrasound—radiopaque stones
- Ultrasound with a full bladder—to confirm stone in the ureterovesical junction
- Intravenous urography—to confirm diagnosis
- Intravenous pyelogram—to determine size and location of stone and degree of obstruction
- Unenhanced helical CT scan—rim sign or halo of the calculus

Other Diagnostic Procedures
Metabolic evaluation for recurrent stone formation:
- 24-hour urine collection to check volume, urinary pH, calcium, uric acid, oxalate, and citrate excretion
- Second collection on restricted calcium (400 mg/day), sodium (100 mEq/day), and oxalate diet
- Serum parathyroid hormone and calcium load tests at third visit

TREATMENT OPTIONS
Treatment Strategy
Usually conservative management eventually results in stone passage. Treatment depends on type of stone, ability or inability to pass, and presence of complications. All patients should drink at least six to eight glasses of water daily plus one at bedtime and one during the night. For calcium type II stones, follow a low-calcium diet, restrict sodium to 1 g/kg daily, and increase bran intake.

Surgical Procedures
Surgery is recommended for patients with severe pain unresponsive to medications, serious bleeding, and persistent fever, nausea, or significant urinary obstruction. If no medical treatment is provided after surgery, stones recur in 50% of patients within five years.
- Extracorporeal shock wave lithotripsy (ESWL)— outpatient procedure that shatters stones under 2 cm and without complications
- Urethroscopy for stones in lower third of ureter
- Percutaneous nephrolithotomy when in upper two-thirds of ureter and greater than 2 cm in size

Drug Therapies

- Narcotics—as needed to control acute severe pain
- Allopurinol—for uric acid calculi; 100 to 300 mg/day to control hyperuricemia
- Potassium citrate—for uric acid calculi; 100 mEq tablets bid to raise urinary pH
- HCTZ—for calcium type I stones; 25 to 50 mg/day.
- Cellulose phosphate—for calcium type I stones; 10 g/day to decrease bowel absorption
- Orthophosphates—for calcium type III stones; to inhibit vitamin B synthesis

Complementary and Alternative Therapies

Symptomatic urolithiasis requires medical attention. Alternative therapies aid in preventing recurrent episodes and increasing the overall vitality of the urogenital system. Start with nutritional guidelines for prevention of recurrence. Herbs and homeopathics can be used for acute pain relief and long-term tonification of the urinary tract.

NUTRITION

- Reduce intake of sugar, refined foods, animal products (meats and dairy), caffeine, alcohol, soft drinks, and salt.
- Increase intake of water, fiber, vegetables, whole grains, and vegetable proteins.
- Minimize oxalate-containing foods such as spinach, rhubarb, beets, nuts, chocolate, black tea, wheat bran, strawberries, and beans.
- Include foods rich in magnesium and low in calcium, such as barley, bran, corn, rye, oats, soy, brown rice, avocado, banana, and potato.
- Magnesium citrate (200 to 400 mg/day)—may increase the solubility of calcium oxalate and calcium phosphate.
- Pyridoxine (B_6, 10 to 100 mg/day)—is essential for the metabolism of oxalic acid.
- Folic acid (5 mg/day)—for uric acid stones.

HERBS

Herbs are generally a safe way to strengthen and tone the body's systems. As with any therapy, it is important to ascertain a diagnosis before pursuing treatment. Herbs may be used as dried extracts (capsules, powders, teas), glycerites, or tinctures (alcohol extracts). Unless otherwise indicated, teas should be made with 1 teaspoon herb per cup of hot water. Steep covered 10 to 20 minutes and drink 2 to 4 cups/day. Tinctures may be used singly or in combination as noted.

- For acute pain relief, combine tinctures of wild yam (*Dioscorea villosa*), cramp bark (*Viburnum opulus*), kava (*Piper methysticum*), and Jamaican dogwood (*Piscidia erythrina*). Take 15 drops every 15 minutes for up to 8 doses.
- Drink an infusion of equal parts of gravel root (*Eupratorium*), corn silk (*Zea mays*), Pipsissewa (*Chimaphila umbellata*), and kava (*Piper methysticum*) 1 tsp./cup, 3 to 4 cups/day.

HOMEOPATHY

An experienced homeopath should assess individual constitutional types and severity of disease to select the correct remedy and potency. For acute prescribing use 3 to 5 pellets of a 12X to 30C remedy every one to four hours until acute symptoms resolve.

Remedies that may be considered for acute pain relief include the following.

- *Berberis*—for sharp, stitching pains that radiate to groin.
- *Colocynthis*—for restlessness with pains that feel better bending forward.
- *Ocimum*—for nausea and vomiting from the pain.

PHYSICAL MEDICINE

Castor oil pack. Used externally, castor oil is a powerful anti-inflammatory. Apply oil directly to skin, cover with a clean soft cloth (e.g. flannel) and plastic wrap. Place a heat source (hot water bottle or heating pad) over the pack and let sit for 30 to 60 minutes. For best results, use for three consecutive days.

Patient Monitoring

Fifty percent of patients pass the stone within 48 hours. For complications or recurrences, refer patient to a urologist. Admit patients to the hospital when they have persistent vomiting, suspected urinary tract infection, pain unresponsive to oral analgesics, or obstructing calculus with a solitary kidney.

OTHER CONSIDERATIONS

Prevention

Maintain proper hydration and dietary restrictions to avoid future development of stones. Determine and treat underlying cause. Alkalinize urine (maintain pH >7.5 with cautious use of penicillamine) in patients with recurrent cystine stones.

Complications/Sequelae

Urinary tract infection and obstruction can result in extensive kidney damage.

Prognosis

Annual rate of recurrence after first stone is 3%, after second stone 6%. This condition is painful but usually produces no permanent damage. Majority of patients will pass the stone within 48 to 72 hours of onset of symptoms.

Pregnancy

Do not perform ESWL on women of childbearing age who have a stone in the lower ureter; the effect on the ovary is not known. Rule out ectopic pregnancy and/or ruptured ovarian cyst.

REFERENCES

Ferri FF. *Ferri's Clinical Advisor: Instant Diagnosis and Treatment.* St Louis, Mo: Mosby-Year Book; 1999.

Tierney LM Jr, McPhee SJ, Papadakis MA, eds. *Current Medical Diagnosis and Treatment 1994.* Norwalk, Conn: Appleton & Lange; 1994.

Grases F, et al. Urolithiasis and phytotherapy. *Int Urol Nephrol.* 1994;26:507–511.

Larson DE, ed. *Mayo Clinic Family Health Book.* 2nd ed. New York, NY: William Morrow and Company; 1996.

Scalzo R. *Naturopathic Handbook of Herbal Formulas.* Durango, Colo: 2nd ed. Kivaki Press; 1994.

The Burton Goldberg Group, compilers. *Alternative medicine: The Definitive Guide.* Tiburon, Calif: Future Medicine Publishing; 1997.

■ VAGINITIS

OVERVIEW

Definition

Vaginitis is the inflammation of the femal vagina, of which there are various types. Some are caused by an increase in abnormal organisms (e.g., trichomonads) and others by an increase in normal flora (e.g., Candida, *Gardnerella vaginalis, anaerobes*). Candidiasis in the vaginal tract is called vulvovaginitis and is the most common cause of vaginal discharge in women. The Candida yeast-like fungus causes approximately 40% of all vaginitis, and about 75% of women get Candida vaginitis at some time.

Etiology

Candida vaginitis is primarily caused by *Candida albicans* but may be caused by *C. tropicalis* or *C. glabrata*. Yeast is a part of the normal flora of the vaginal tract in nearly one third of women; infection occurs when there are changes in host resistance or bacterial flora. A small amount of vaginal discharge is normal at midcycle and should not be confused with vaginitis.

Risk Factors

- Antibiotic therapy—especially with broad spectrum types
- Pregnancy—from increased heat and moisture and hormonal shifts
- Diabetes
- Corticosteroid use
- Immunosuppressive drugs and conditions
- Human immunodeficiency virus (HIV) infection—frequent candidiasis can be an early sign of HIV in women
- Anemia
- Hypothyroidism
- Oral contraception—controversial, predominately for recurrence
- Being overweight
- High sugar intake
- Use of panty hose, constrictive clothing, or underwear that is not cotton

Signs and Symptoms

- Vaginal and vulvar pruritus (proportional to the number of organisms)
- Thin, creamy, or curd-like vaginal discharge; more copious during pregnancy; nonodorous
- Red, swollen, painful vaginal mucous membranes and external genitalia
- Satellite lesions (tender, red, discrete pustules that spread to thighs and anus)

DIFFERENTIAL DIAGNOSIS

- Trichomoniasis
- *Gardnerella vaginalis*
- Anaerobes
- Vaginal foreign bodies (retained tampons)
- Allergic reaction to douching or vaginal contraception
- Gonorrhea (especially in prepubertal girls)
- Contact dermatitis/vaginitis, including latex in condoms

DIAGNOSIS

Physical Examination

- Vagina may appear hyperemic, bright red, with dry, white, and curd-like plaques or may have no erythema
- Vulva may have fissures, edema, and erythema
- Discharge appears creamy or curd-like

Laboratory Tests

- Microscopic wet mount scraping of vaginal plaque, discharge, or vulva scraping mixed with 10% potassium hydroxide (KOH) shows yeast, spores, and/or pseudohyphae; 50% to 70% accuracy rate.

- Gram stain is more sensitive; identifies both mycelial and blastospore forms.
- pH
- Wet prep for trichomonas.

For recurrent infections (vaginal pH <4.5):
- Culture's findings on Nickerson's or Sabouraud's media
- Glucose tolerance test rules out diabetes
- HIV testing
- Possibly obtain endocervical swabs for chlamydia and gonorrhea detection assays

Pathological Findings

- Pustule lesion dissects horizontally under the stratum corneum and peels it away; may appear like hyperplastic indurated plaques, atrophic inflamed plaques, or a leukoplakic area
- Accumulation of scale and inflammatory cells
- The pH of discharge is normal

TREATMENT OPTIONS

Treatment Strategy

Topical treatment is initiated before systemic, but patient preference may influence choice. Length of treatment and dose are both typically increased for chronic infection. Patients should avoid excessive exertion and sweating, keep vaginal area as dry as possible during infection, avoid sexual relations until symptoms clear, take showers instead of baths, and use unscented soap. Use proper hygiene when cleansing after bowel movement by wiping from front to back. Wear cotton underwear and avoid pantyhose and tight-fitting pants.

Drug Therapies

Topical and oral therapies are considered to be almost equally effective.

- Topical therapies—may initially cause burning from inflammation: polyenes (nystatin)—one tablet bid for two weeks placed high in the vagina with applicator; 70% to 80% effective; no systemic side effects; azole derivatives such as imidazole (e.g., miconazole, butoconazole) and triazole (e.g., fluconazole, terconazole)—intravaginal cream one to five days, also may be used externally for satellite lesions; 85% to 90% effective; no systemic side effects.
- Oral therapies: fluconazole—75% to 92% effective; 150 mg once; often considered the treatment of choice; contraindicated for pregnancy; appears to help HIV infected women; ketoconazole—83% effective, but higher rate of recurrence with cessation of short- and long-term therapy; 400 mg/day for five days, or for two weeks with recurrent infection; oral nystatin helps reduce intestinal colonization.

Complementary and Alternative Therapies

With the exception of pelvic inflammatory disease, gonoccocal, and chlamydia infections, alternative therapies for acute and chronic vaginitis can be effective for treating both symptoms and causes. Begin with a douche and an acidophilus supplement. For chronic or recurrent vaginitis, also incorporate vitamins, minerals, and herbs into the treatment plan.

Topical Applications: Use only one of the following douches at one time. Do not douche during menstrual flow. For first time or acute infection try the vinegar douche or boric acid capsules. For chronic vaginitis, use the herbal combination douche. For recurrent vaginitis, use the Betadine douche. Discontinue douching immediately if there is pain or exacerbation of symptoms.

- White vinegar: 1 to 2 tbsp. white vinegar to 1 pint of water. Douche daily for 10 to 14 days.
- Boric acid: One capsule (600 mg) inserted daily for 10 to 14 days.

May cause irritation or problems from systemic absorption.

- Herbal combination: Mix equal parts of oregano leaf (*Origanum vulgare*), goldenseal root (*Hydrastic canadensis*), and coneflower (*Echinacea purpura*). Steep 1 heaping tbsp. of herbal mixture in one pint of water. Cool and douche daily for 10 to 14 days.
- Povidone iodine (Betadine): Douche with one part iodine to 100 parts water twice daily for 10 to 14 days. Prolonged use can suppress thyroid function.

NUTRITION

- Avoid simple and refined sugars (breads, pasta, baked goods, sweets), dairy products, alcoholic beverages, peanuts, fresh or dried fruit, fruit juice, and all known food allergens. Eat whole foods with plenty of protein, fresh vegetables, and grains.
- Lactobacillus acidophilus re-establishes normal flora in the body and prevents the over-growth of Candida. Take one capsule orally bid to tid, and insert one capsule into the vagina nightly (not to exceed 14 nights).
- Vitamin A (10,000 IU/day) or beta-carotene (50,000 IU/day) enhances the integrity of the vaginal mucosa. Required for proper immune functioning. Avoid high doses of vitamin A in pregnant patients or those who plan to get pregnant within three months.
- Zinc (30 mg/day) and vitamin E (400 to 800 IU/day) are essential for immune function.
- Vitamin C (1,000 mg tid to qid) optimizes immunity and helps to restore the integrity of vaginal mucosa.

HERBS

Ascertain a diagnosis before pursuing treatment. Herbs may be used as dried extracts (capsules, powders, teas), glycerites (glycerine extracts), or tinctures (alcohol extracts). Unless otherwise indicated, teas should be made with 1 tsp. herb per cup of hot water. Steep covered 5 to 10 minutes for leaf or flowers, and 10 to 20 minutes for roots. Drink 2 to 4 cups/day. Tinctures may be used singly or in combination as noted.

- Pau d'arco tea has antifungal effects. Drink 2 to 4 cups/day.
- Garlic (*Allium sativum*) has antimicrobial, antifungal, and immune stimulating properties. Prepare a tea with two cloves of garlic. Drink 2 to 4 cups/day. May add lemon and honey for flavor.

HOMEOPATHY

An experienced homeopath should assess individual constitutional types and severity of disease to select the correct remedy and potency. For acute prescribing use 3 to 5 pellets of a 12X to 30C remedy every one to four hours until acute symptoms resolve.

- *Calcarea carbonica* for intense itching with thick white or yellowish discharge that is worse before menses.
- *Borax* for burning pains with egg-white colored discharge that occurs midcycle.
- *Sepia* for burning pains with milky white discharge and pressure in vaginal area. Depression and irritability is usually present.
- *Graphites* for backache with thin white discharge that is worse in the morning and when walking.

- *Arsenicum album* for burning, offensive discharge in a patient who is easily chilled.
- Homeopathic combinations are also available as creams to apply intravaginally.

ACUPUNCTURE

Acupuncture may relieve pelvic congestion and improve immune function.

Patient Monitoring

Patients should be educated about the various risks for infection. Strict diabetic control is essential for diabetic patients. There is no specific follow-up unless infection persists. Repeat pelvic examination and a culture is then warranted. Treating the partner will minimize the possibility of reinfection.

OTHER CONSIDERATIONS

Prevention

- Avoid risks (see above).
- Avoid sweating, overheating. and sexual relations until symptoms clear.
- Use unscented soap, take showers instead of baths, and proper hygiene.

Complications/Sequelae

- Chronic Candida vaginitis—no definitive cure
- Often a result of persistent yeast in vagina, not recurrent infection
- Use oral and topical therapies together in higher doses for two to three weeks; maintenance therapy with azoles.
- Additional risk factors include oral contraception, vaginal douching, increased frequency of sexual intercourse
- Fifteen percent of men have symptomatic balanitis and should be treated to prevent recurrent female infection.
- Antifungal therapy or acidophilus supplementation is started prophylactically with known antibiotic-associated Candida vaginitis.
- HIV infection and diabetes predispose patients to chronic infections.
- Secondary bacterial infections

Prognosis

Some cases of Candida vaginitis resolve spontaneously while others progress or become chronic. Recurrence is common. Chronic cases should be evaluated for systemic infections.

Pregnancy

Treatment should only be conducted under the supervision of a physician.

REFERENCES

Dambro MR. *Griffith's 5-Minute Clinical Consult–1999*. Baltimore, Md: Lippincott Williams & Wilkins; 1999:358–361.

Fauci AS, Braunwald E, Isselbacher KJ et al, eds. *Harrison's Principles of Internal Medicine*. 14th ed. New York, NY: McGraw-Hill; 1998.

Habif TP. *Clinical Dermatology*. 3rd ed. St. Louis, Mo: Mosby-Year Book; 1996.

Morrison R. *Desktop Guide to Keynotes and Confirmatory Symptoms*. Albany, Calif: Hahnemann Clinic Publishing; 1993:43, 69, 85, 171, 346.

Murray MT, Pizzorno JE. *Encyclopedia of Natural Medicine*. 2nd ed. Rocklin, Calif: Prima Publishing; 1998:530–535.

■ WARTS

OVERVIEW

Definition

Warts (verrucae) are small, benign, usually painless, and sometimes self-limiting growths on the skin caused by human papillomaviruses (HPV).

- Common warts *(Verrucae vulgares)*
- Flat warts *(Verrucae planae)*
- Genital warts *(Condylomata acuminata)*
- Plantar warts *(Verruca plantaris)*

Although prevalence is highest in children and lowest in the elderly, warts affect all age groups. Genital warts are contagious; common, flat, and plantar warts generally are not. All warts can spread from one part of the body to another. Warts can disappear without treatment, and reappear.

Etiology

Human papillomaviruses (HPV)

Risk Factors

- Contact with affected persons or shed skin with HPV (particularly for genital warts)
- Trauma
- Immunosuppressive diseases (e.g., AIDS) and drugs
- Atopic dermatitis
- Communal facilities (locker rooms)

Signs and Symptoms

General characteristics:
- Appear singularly, clustered
- Sometimes painful

Common warts:
- Round and asymmetric
- Can grow from tiny (1 mm), smooth, flesh-tone papules to large (5 to 10 mm), thick, rough plaques
- May form mosaics (1 to 3 cm in diameter)
- Found anywhere, but generally on the hands

Flat warts:
- Small (1 to 3 mm) papules with flat tops
- Usually flesh-tone or pink
- Sometimes itchy
- Generally found on the face and back of hands

Genital warts (venereal warts):
- Tiny flat papules that grow to resemble common warts
- Generally found on external genitalia, pubic, and perineal regions
- May be found intravaginally and in the anal canal

Plantar warts:
- Rough, thickened, scarcely elevated papules
- Sometimes exhibiting black dots, indicating thrombosed capillaries
- Often quite tender, possible leg/back pain from disrupted posture
- Found on the sole of the foot, sometimes completely covering the heel or plantar region

DIFFERENTIAL DIAGNOSIS

- Corns or clavi
- Scar tissue
- Skin tags
- Molluscum contagiosum
- Moles
- Condyloma lata
- Calluses
- Seborrheic keratoses
- Skin cancer

DIAGNOSIS

Physical Examination

General clinical characteristics of warts include:
- Disturbed skin lines
- Tiny black dots (thrombosed capillaries)
- Previous trauma to sites (e.g., fingers, nails, knees, face, scalp)

Other Diagnostic Procedures

- Warts usually can be diagnosed by location, appearance, and, if necessary, paring or debridement.
- Genital warts: Check intravaginally and in the anal canal.
- Plantar warts: To confirm diagnosis (vs. corns or clavi), pare lesion and look for characteristic black dots (thrombosed capillaries).
- Electron microscopy
- Immunohystochemistry
- Nucleic acid hybridization

TREATMENT OPTIONS

Treatment Strategy

Although asymptomatic warts can be ignored (with some risk of spreading), treatment may be desirable because warts can be embarrassing and disfiguring.

A number of treatments are available, including drug therapy (usually the initial therapy), cryosurgery (minimal scarring), electrosurgery, laser vaporization, curette and desiccation (scarring possible), and excision (scarring possible). Actual treatment depends on the location, type, and severity of warts. Because warts are benign, avoid treatments that could be harmful or could result in scarring.

Advise patients not to self-treat warts on mucous membranes or genitals and to be aware of scarring when treating warts on the face. Also, advise patients to keep warts covered during treatment.

Drug Therapies

Common, flat, and plantar warts: 12% to 40% salicylic acid, sometimes paired with lactic acid, qid (OTC). To optimize treatment, review guidelines with patients:
- Soak wart in warm water or bathe before treatment.
- Dry wart area.
- Apply medication per manufacturer's instructions.
- Keep area dry during treatment.

Some practitioners advise filing (pumice stone) before application.

Less common drugs include trichloroacetic acid or cantharidin (common warts), tretinoin (retinoic acid, Retin-A) (flat warts, notably on the face), benzoyl peroxide, bleomycin (intradermal injection), and cimetidine.

Genital warts: physician-applied podophyllin 25% in tincture of benzoin weekly or patient-applied podofilox 0.5 bid three days/rest four days, repeat up to four cycles. U.S. FDA-approved intralesional interferon alfa-n3 can be effective for persistent and recurring external genital warts. Covering warts for a week at a time with waterproof tape can cure warts by preventing viral growth. Plantar warts sometimes respond to hot-water soaks, 113°F water for 30 to 45 minutes, two to three times/week for six to eight weeks.

Complementary and Alternative Therapies

Nutritional and herbal support may enhance immune function and minimize recurrence of HPV. Some cases of HPV may respond to alternative therapies alone.

NUTRITION

- Eliminate caffeine, alcohol, refined foods, and sugar.
- Avoid saturated fats, which increase inflammation (animal protein and dairy products).
- Increase whole grains, fresh vegetables, fruits, legumes, and essential fatty acids (nuts, seeds, and cold-water fish).
- Vitamin C (1,000 to 1,500 mg tid), beta-carotene (100,000 IU/day), vitamin E (400 IU/day), and zinc (15 to 30 mg/day) support immune function. Vitamin E may also be used topically to treat warts.
- B complex (50 to 100 mg/day) helps to reduce the effects of stress which can weaken the immune system. Folic acid (800 mcg/day) is especially recommended for cervical HPV.
- Selenium (200 mcg/day) has antioxidant activity and supports immune function.

HERBS

Herbs are generally a safe way to strengthen and tone the body's systems. As with any therapy, it is important to ascertain a diagnosis before pursuing treatment. Herbs may be used as dried extracts (capsules, powders, teas), glycerites (glycerine extracts), or tinctures (alcohol extracts). Unless otherwise indicated, teas should be made with 1 tsp. of herb per cup of hot water. Steep covered 5 to 10 minutes for leaf or flowers, and 10 to 20 minutes for roots. Drink 2 to 4 cups/day. Tinctures may be used singly or in combination as noted.

Anti-viral herbs that support the immune system. Combine tinctures of 1 part of goldenseal (Hydrastis canadensis) with 2 parts each of the following: lomatium (Lomatium dissectum), licorice root (Glycyrrhiza labra), coneflower (Echinacea purpurea), osha (Ligusticum porteri), thuja leaf (Thuja occidentalis). Take 30 drops bid.

Topical applications are most effective for eradicating warts. Discontinue any topical application if irritation should develop in the surrounding skin.

For plantar, flat, and common warts use one or more of the following applications. The application may need to be repeated nightly for up to three weeks. Wart will turn black as it begins to die.

- Peel patch. Cut a piece of banana peel and place over wart before going to bed. Tape in place.
- Raw garlic patch. Cover wart and surrounding skin with a thin layer of castor or olive oil. Apply a thin slice of fresh garlic; tape in place.

To maximize benefit, place 2 to 4 drops of tincture of thuja or greater celandine (Chelidonium majus) on the wart before application.

For genital HPV, paint the warts with vitamin A or beta-carotene once or twice daily. Add 3 to 4 drops each of thuja, echinacea, and lomatium for best results. Cervical involvement may need to be treated under the supervision of a physician. A retention douche with 1 tsp. each of thuja, echinacea, and lomatium in 2 cups of water may be helpful in resolving superficial warts.

HOMEOPATHY

Thuja is the classic remedy for warts, although by no means the only remedy that expresses warts. For the greatest benefit, an experienced homeopath should assess individual constitutional types and severity of disease to select the correct remedy and potency.

ACUPUNCTURE

May be helpful in stimulating immune system.

Patient Monitoring

Monitor patients with diabetes or poor circulation for infections.

OTHER CONSIDERATIONS

Prevention

- Avoid contact with warts, particularly genital warts.
- Cover warts during treatment and avoid wound fluid.
- Use footwear in public areas.
- Do not scratch, pick, or bite warts.
- Do not share towels and washcloths with affected persons.

Complications/Sequelae

All warts: auto inoculation; scars
Common warts: nail deformity
Plantar warts: chronic pain from plantar wart removal
Genital warts: intraepithelial neoplasms

Prognosis

Although some warts will disappear without treatment, usually within 6 to 24 months, resolution without remission cannot be guaranteed.

With treatment, resolution for common, flat, and plantar warts can be six weeks or more; for genital warts, 20 weeks or more. If treatments are unsuccessful, first consider cryosurgery (multiple treatments may be needed) and then consider electrosurgery, laser vaporization, curette and desiccation, or excision.

Pregnancy

High doses of vitamins and herbs are contraindicated in pregnancy. Topical applications are safe. Pregnant women should not use podophyllin.

REFERENCES

Barker LR, et al, eds. *Principles of Ambulatory Medicine.* 4th ed. Baltimore, Md: Williams and Wilkins; 1995:1467–1469.

Berkow R, Beers MH. *The Merck Manual of Medical Information.* Whitehouse Station, NJ: Merck Research Laboratories; 1997:984–985.

Brodell RT. *Infect* Med. SCP Communications, Inc.; 1996:13:56–60, 66.

Dambro MR. *Griffith's 5-Minute Clinical Consult–1999.* Baltimore, Md: Lippincott Williams and Wilkins; 1999:1166–1169.

Duke JA. *The Green Pharmacy.* Emmaus, Pa: Rodale Press; 1997: 452–455.

Ewald GA, McKenzie CR, eds. *Manual of Medical Therapeutics.* 28th ed. Boston, Mass: Little, Brown and Company; 1995:20–21.

Lockie A, Deddes N. *The Complete Guide to Homeopathy.* New York, NY: DK Publishing Inc; 1995:187, 189, 227.

Ody P. *The Complete Medicinal Herbal.* New York, NY: DK Publishing Inc; 1993:160–161.

Pray WS. *Nonprescription Product Therapeutics.* Baltimore, Md: Lippincott Willliams & Wilkins, in press.

Scalzo R. *Naturopathic Handbook of Herbal Formulas.* 2nd ed. Durango, Colo: Kivaki Press; 1994:73.

Walker LP, Brown EH. *The Alternative Pharmacy.* Paramus, NJ: Prentice Hall Press; 1998:353–354.

HERBS

Aloe
Barberry
Bilberry
Black Cohosh
Burdock
Cat's Claw
Cayenne
Celery Seed
Chamomile, German
Chamomile, Roman
Comfrey
Devil's Claw
Echinacea
Eucalyptus
Evening Primrose
Feverfew
Flaxseed
Garlic
Ginger
Ginkgo Biloba
Ginseng, American
Ginseng, Asian
Ginseng, Siberian
Goldenseal
Grape Seed Extract
Green Tea
Hawthorn
Kava Kava
Lemon Balm
Licorice
Milk Thistle
Pau D'Arco
Peppermint
Saw Palmetto
St. John's Wort
Stinging Nettle
Valerian

■ ALOE

Aloe vera/Aloe barbadensis/Aloe ferox (Botanical)
Liliaceae (Plant Family)
Aloe barbadensis/capensis (Pharmacopeial)

OVERVIEW

Aloe vera has a long history of use as a medicinal plant, with written record going back to 1750 BC. The plant has a wide variety of uses because different parts of the plant have different medicinal properties. The mucilaginous gel that is most widely associated with aloe vera comes from the inner part of the leaf. It is separated from the pericyclic tubules, specialized cells that are under the epidermis of the leaf. Those cells have a bitter yellow latex or juice that is dried to form a pharmaceutical product called aloe latex. Aloe gel is used for wound healing, both internally and externally. It greatly speeds the healing of many skin injuries, including ulcerations, burns, frostbite, and abrasions. Aloe latex is a powerful cathartic and is used for constipation. Because it can cause painful cramping, it is not used as often as gentler herbal laxatives. Lower doses of aloe latex can be effective in preventing kidney stone formation or reducing their size. Lower doses can also be effective as a stool softener, which is particularly helpful in the case of hemorrhoids.

Aloe gel is now found in many commercial skin-care products, shampoos, and conditioners. But some studies have shown that it does not retain its healing ability when stored. There is now a stabilized form of the gel that may be able to be stored and still retain the healing action, but fresh aloe gel from the leaves is still the best option.

Aloe gel may also be taken internally, often in a liquid form called aloe juice. In this form, aloe can help heal peptic ulcers by inhibiting stomach acids that irritate ulcers. Aloe juice also improves digestion by destroying many bacteria that cause infection.

Recent studies have shown that aloe juice has important HIV-fighting properties. Its antiviral ability attacks the virus itself, but more important, it greatly enhances the action of AZT. A polysaccharide constituent of aloe, acetylated mannose, worked synergistically with AZT in vitro to inhibit HIV replication, and researchers believe the supplemental use of acetylated mannose may reduce required AZT dosage by as much as 90%.

MACRO DESCRIPTION

A perennial plant; yellow flowers; tough, fleshy leaves grow up to 20 inches long, 5 inches across, up to 30 per plant; grows to 4 feet. Grown in most tropical and subtropical locations, including Caribbean, southern United States, Latin America, and the Middle East.

PART USED/PHARMACEUTICAL DESIGNATIONS

• Leaves

CONSTITUENTS/COMPOSITION

Anthraquinones, aloins, anthranoids, aglycones, polysaccharides (including glycoproteins and mucopolysaccharides), and prostaglandins

COMMERCIAL PREPARATIONS

Aloe gel is best fresh from an aloe plant. Slit a leaf lengthwise and remove gel. Aloe gel is also available commercially in stabilized form. Aloe latex is available as a powder or in 500 mg capsules for use as a laxative. Aloe juice is available in liquid form.

MEDICINAL USES/INDICATIONS

• Aloe was historically used to treat burns.

• Traditional herbal actions: antibacterial, antifungal, anesthetic, antipyretic, antipruritic; moisturizer, vasodilator, anti-inflammatory, anthelmintic, cathartic, stomachic, demulcent, emmenagogue, laxative combined with carminative, vulnerary

• Clinical applications: burns (due to radiation, sunburn, and other causes), headaches, dry skin, rashes (due to dermatitis, poison ivy, or insect bites), kidney stones, hemorrhoids, hives, HIV, constipation, wound healing, peptic ulcers, immune system enhancement, diabetes, asthma

PHARMACOLOGY

Aloe vera contains vitamins C and E and zinc, which are all important for wound healing. Glycoproteins in aloe gel inhibit and break down bradykinin, a mediator of pain and inflammation. Aloe gel also inhibits thromboxane, which also causes inflammation. Aloe gel stimulates fibroblast and connective tissue formation, a healing action that most other anti-inflammatories don't have. The polysaccharides in aloe seem to stimulate skin growth and repair as well. Aloe also increases blood flow to burned tissue, which helps it heal.

Aloe gel has been particularly effective in healing diabetic leg ulcers because along with its other wound healing capabilities, it also lowers blood sugar.

Aloe gel's antibacterial and antifungal ability compares favorably with that of silver sulfadiazine, an antiseptic used regularly in treatment of extensive burns. Aloe vera extract has been shown to kill *Pseudomonas aeruginosa, Klebsiella pneumoniae, Serratia marcescens, Citrobacter species, Enterobacter cloacae, Streptococcus pyogenes, Streptococcus agalactiae, Staphylococcus aureus, Escherichia coli, Streptococcus faecalis,* and *Candida albicans.*

Aloe's active cathartic component is aloin. In small doses, it gives tone to intestinal muscle. In larger doses, it becomes a strong purgative, increasing colonic secretions and peristaltic contractions in the large intestine. It is harsher on the system than other anthraquinone laxatives, such as cascara and senna. The anthraquinones in aloe latex prevent kidney stone formation by binding calcium in the urinary tract and reducing the growth rate of urinary calcium crystals.

Aloe juice heals peptic ulcers by inhibiting pepsin when the stomach is empty, releasing it only to digest food. It inhibits the release of hydrochloric acid by preventing the binding of histamine to parietal cells. It also heals and prevents other irritants from reaching the ulcer. Aloe juice aids the digestive process by increasing gastric pH, reducing yeast infections, and improving water retention.

Acemannan, an antiviral compound of aloe juice, is a powerful immune system stimulant. It enhances macrophage activity, the function of T cells and interferon production. Acemannan has been effective for treatment of HIV, influenza, and measles. It has a direct antiviral effect on HIV by inhibiting glycosylation of viral glycoproteins. Even more promising, it enhances the action of AZT. Studies show that acemannan, combined with suboptimal noncytotoxic concentrations of AZT, acts synergistically to inhibit replication of HIV and herpes simplex virus type 1.

DOSAGE RANGES AND DURATION OF ADMINISTRATION

- The dosage for dry aloe extract is very small (50 to 200 mg).
- For general use: dosage of gel or juice 2 tbsp. tid (the standardized aloe product measure to hydroxyanthracene derivatives is not widely available in the USA)
- For prevention of kidney stones: 2 to 3 tbsp. daily
- For laxative purposes: 500 to 1,000 mg daily (care should be taken that laxative doses of aloe are accompanied by carminative herbs to prevent griping)
- For burns or wound healing, topically: aloe vera gel applied liberally (fresh gel from aloe plant is best)
- For hemorrhoids, as a stool softener: dry aloe extract, 0.05 to 0.2 g
- For HIV: 800 to 1,600 mg of acemannan a day (equivalent to .5 to 1 liter of aloe vera juice, although amount of acemannan may vary in different products)
- For constipation: 20 to 30 mg hydroxyanthracene derivatives per day, calculated as anydrous aloin

SIDE EFFECTS/TOXICOLOGY

Aloe gel is safe for external use, unless it causes a rare allergic reaction. Discontinue use if it irritates the skin. It is not useful for treatment of deep, vertical wounds (e.g., cesarean incision). Aloe latex may cause severe intestinal cramps or diarrhea.

WARNINGS/PRECAUTIONS/CONTRAINDICATIONS

Pregnant or nursing mothers should not ingest aloe latex. It may cause uterine contractions and trigger miscarriage. Contraindicated for gastrointestinal illness, intestinal obstruction, appendicitis, and abdominal pain of unknown origin. May aggravate ulcers, hemorrhoids, diverticulosis, diverticulitis, colitis, and irritable bowel syndrome. If taken over a long time, can cause dependence or disturbance of electrolyte balance. May cause urine to turn a harmless red color. Should not be used for children under 12.

INTERACTIONS

Chronic use of aloe latex could cause potassium deficiency, which could interfere with cardiac glycoside and antiarrhythmic drugs. Potential for potassium deficiency is increased if used with thiazide diuretics, licorice, or corticosteroids.

REGULATORY AND COMPENDIAL STATUS

German Commission E approves aloe latex for chronic constipation, with certain reservations.

REFERENCES

Blitz JJ, et al. Aloe vera gel in peptic ulcer therapy: preliminary report. *J Am Osteopath Assoc.* 1963;62:731–735.

Blumenthal M, ed. *The Complete German Commission E Monographs.* Boston, Mass: Integrative Medicine Communications. 1998.

Castleman M. *The Healing Herbs.* New York, NY: Bantam Books. 1991.

Danhof I. Potential benefits from orally-injested internal aloe vera gel. International Aloe Science Council Tenth Annual Aloe Scientific Semina; 1991; Irving, Texas.

Duke J. *The Green Pharmacy.* Emmaus, Penn: Rodale Press. 1997.

Fahim MS, Wang M. Zinc acetate and lyophilized *Aloe barbadensis* as vaginal contraceptive. *Contraception.* 1996;53:231–236.

Fulton JE Jr. The stimulation of postdermabrasion wound healing with stabilized aloe vera gel-polyethylene oxide dressing. *J Dermatol Surg Onco.* 1990;16:460.

Grindlay D, Reynolds T. The aloe vera phenomenon: a review of the properties and modern uses of the leaf parenchyma gel. *J Ethnopharmacol.* 1986;16:117–151.

Gruenwald J, Brendler T, Jaenicke C et al, eds. *PDR for Herbal Medicines.* Montvale, NJ: Medical Economics Company. 1998.

Heggers J, et al. Beneficial effects of aloe in wound healing. *Phytother Res.* 1993;7:S48–S52.

Murray M, Pizzorno J. *Encyclopedia of Natural Medicine.* Rocklin, Calif: Prima Publishing. 1991.

Murray M. *Healing Power of Herbs.* Rocklin, Calif: Prima Publishing. 1995.

Newall C, et al. *Herbal Medicines.* London, England: Pharmaceutical Press. 1996.

Plemmons JM, et al. Evaluation of acemannan in the treatment of aphthous stomatitis. *Wounds.* 1994;6.

Saoo K, et al. Antiviral activity of aloe extracts against cytomegalovirus. *Phytother Res.* 1996;10:348–350.

Schmidt JM, Greenspoon JS. Aloe vera dermal wound gel is associated with a delay in wound healing. *Ostet Gynecol.* 1991;78(1).

Shida, T. et al. 1985. Effect of aloe extract on peripheral phagocytosis in adult bronchial asthma. Planta Med 51.

Schmidt JM, Greenspoon JS. Aloe vera dermal wound gel is associated with a delay in wound healing. *Ostet Gynecol.* 1991;78(1).

Syed TA, et al. Management of psoriasis with aloe vera extract in a hydrophilic cream: a placebo-controlled, double-blind study. *Trop Med Int Health.* 1996;1:505–509.

Tyler V. *The Honest Herbal.* New York, NY: Pharmaceutical Products Press. 1993.

Vazquez B, et al. Anti-inflammatory activity of extracts from aloe vera gel. *J Ethnopharmacol.* 1996;55:69–75.

■ BARBERRY/BARBERRY BARK/BARBERRY ROOT/BARBERRY ROOT BARK

Berberis vulgaris (Botanical)
Berberidaceae (Plant Family)
Berberis vulgaris/Berberidis cortex/Berberidis radix/Berberidis radicis cortex (Pharmacopeial)

OVERVIEW

In traditional folk medicine, barberry soothes sore throats, treats diarrhea or constipation, and eases inflammation and infection of the urinary, gastrointestinal, and respiratory tracts. It may reduce the discomfort of arthritis and rheumatism, soothe psoriasis, and treat chronic yeast infections. These uses reflect barberry's reputation as an herbal antibiotic.

Sought after as an alternative to goldenseal (a once-endangered botanical regarded as "king" of herbal antibiotics by some individuals), barberry and other herbs with similar constituents (e.g. berberine) and actions are termed mucous membrane tonics and adaptogens by herbalists. Mucous membrane tonics regulate the flow of mucous; they may increase or decrease mucous secretion. Adaptogens also allow immune factors already present within the body to stimulate antibacterial responses during illness.

The study of barberry's isoquinoline alkaloid constituents has overshadowed study of the plant as a whole. These constituents are potentially therapeutic, with bactericidal, smooth muscle, and cardiovascular effects.

Barberry was used in ancient Egypt to prevent the plague, during the middle ages in Europe as a purgative and antiseptic, and by Native Americans as tea to stimulate the appetite. It has other uses as well; the yellow color of the root and inner bark provide a semi-colorfast clothing dye, and the berries can be made into jam or sugared for cake decorations.

MACRO DESCRIPTION

Deciduous shrub grows to nine feet. Branches, gray, bear thorns. Leaves alternate or in rosette formation, can be various colors, spiny teeth, four to five leaves per branch. Flowers, bright yellow, in $2^1/_2$ inch racemes, bloom April to June. The berries are red and grow in drooping bunches. Inner bark is yellow.

The bark of the stem and root, and the root itself, are used medicinally. Traditionally, the berries were also used as a tonic in tea, but they do not contain isoquinoline alkaloids and are more closely associated with culinary use. Barberry grows in the northeastern United States, particularly in New England, and is native to Europe.

PART USED/PHARMACEUTICAL DESIGNATIONS

- Roots
- Berry
- Root bark
- Stem bark

CONSTITUENTS/COMPOSITION

Isoquinoline alkaloids berberine, berbamine, oxyacanthine, jatrorrhizine, columbamine, palmatine, magnoflorine; also, resin, tannins

COMMERCIAL PREPARATIONS

Crude bark for tea or powdered in capsules; aqueous alcohol or alcohol extracts available as 1:5 tinctures or standardized fluid extracts (standardized to 8% to 12 % isoquinoline alkaloids); ointment

MEDICINAL USES/INDICATIONS

- Traditional: Berry as tea, diuretic, expectorant, laxative, appetite stimulant; root bark and bark as tea, anti-inflammatory, diaphoretic, astringent, antiseptic, laxative, bitter tonic, alterative (blood purifier), cholagogue (liver stimulant that promotes bile excretion)
- Conditions: chronic diarrhea, dysentery, indigestion, eye ailments, mouth sores, jaundice, hepatitis, fever, hemorrhage, arthritis, rheumatism, low back pain, stomach bacterial infections, *H. pylori*
- Clinical applications (listed as "unapproved" in German Commission E monograph): Inflammation/infection of the kidneys and urinary, bronchial, and gastrointestinal tracts; liver, spleen, and circulatory disorders; spasms; and chronic candidiasis

PHARMACOLOGY

Herbalists provide much of the information available on the usage and effects of whole barberry rootbark and bark preparations. While these sources often corroborate empirical results of barberry use, scientific study tends to focus on determining the scope and application of the bactericidal activity of the isoquinoline alkaloid constituents. At least one study demonstrated superior anti-inflammatory actions of whole barberry extract, compared to single constituents. By using tissue or bacterial cultures and single alkaloid preparations, researchers have determined antimicrobial, bactericidal, anti-inflammatory, immune-stimulant, hypotensive, antifibrillatory, antiarrhythmic, sedative, anticonvulsant and smooth muscle effects.

Berberine has in vitro antibacterial activity. Actions against *Staphylococcus, spp., Streptomyces, spp., Chlamydia, spp., Corynebacterium diphtheria, Escherichia coli, Salmonella typhi,Vibrio cholerae, Diplococcus pneumoniae, Pseudomonas, spp., Shigella dysenteriae, Entamoeba histolytica, Trichomonoas vaginalis, Neisseria gonorrhoeae, N. menengitidis, Treponema palidum, Giardia lamblia, Leishmania donovani,* and *Candida albicans* may be due to adhesion blockage of the streptococci to host cells through the depletion of lipoteichoic acid and fibronectin. In other studies berberine raised blood flow to the spleen; reduced fever, possibly by altering interferon response to microorganisms; stimulated bile secretion; altered bilirubin levels; inhibited brain tumor cells in rats; and was superior to sulfacetaminde against *Chlamydia trachomatis*.

In vitro studies demonstrate that oxyacanthine dilates blood vessels, modulates adrenaline, and is bactericidal to *Bacillus subtilis, Colpidium colpoda*. Palmatine is antiarrhythmic, adrenocorticotrophic, analgesic, and bactericidal. Jatrorrhizine is sedating, hypotensive, and fungicidal. In animal studies, one experiment showed a berbamine-induced immune response in mice with influenza.

These actions have not been scientifically demonstrated to occur in the human body. Berberine absorption in the small intestine is poor, and large doses obtained through excess intake of berberine-containing plant preparations cause negative side effects on the stomach and small intestines. However, because it is excreted through the urine, it may have antibiotic actions specific to that area of the body. This remains to be proven, but concurs with traditional use.

DOSAGE RANGES AND DURATION OF ADMINISTRATION

For throat, urinary, gastrointestinal, respiratory inflammation or infection, including chronic candidiasis, any of the following can be taken for five to seven days.

- Tea: 2 to 4 g steeped dried root tid

- Tincture (1:5): 3 to 6 ml tid
- Dry extracts: 250 to 500 mg tid

For skin disorders: 10% extract of barberry in ointment, applied topically tid

SIDE EFFECTS/TOXICOLOGY

American Herbal Products Association safety rating: 2b. Safe with appropriate use, but do not use during pregnancy. Due to a lack of scientific documentation of barberry's purported therapeutic uses, the German Commission E monograph lists barberry as an unapproved herb.

Barberry root and root bark preparations have not caused any of the toxic effects noted with excessive or lethal doses of berberine. (At doses higher than 0.5 g, berberine causes lethargy, nose bleeds, difficulty breathing, skin and eye irritation, kidney irritation, nausea, vomiting, diarrhea. Small doses stimulate respiratory system, large doses lead to respiratory paralysis. Lethal doses cause hemorrhagic nephritis.)

WARNINGS/CONTRAINDICATIONS/PRECAUTIONS

Over-consumption of berberine-containing plant medicines may irritate mucous membranes, particularly in the stomach. Do not use during pregnancy.

INTERACTIONS

Excess berberine intake may interfere with B vitamin assimilation.

REGULATORY AND COMPENDIAL STATUS

In the United States, barberry is a dietary supplement; in Germany the Commission E does not approve therapeutic use due to lack of scientific documentation of effects.

REFERENCES

Amin AH, Subbaiah, TV, Abbasi KM. Berberine sulfate: antimicrobial activity, bioassay, and mode of action. *Can J Microbiol.* 1969;15:1067–1076.

Bergner P. Goldenseal and the common cold; goldenseal substitutes. *Medical Herbalism: A Journal for the Clinical Practitioner.* Winter 1996–1997;8:1.

Blumenthal M, ed. *The Complete German Commission E Monographs.* Boston, Mass: Integrative Medicine Communications; 1998.

Foster S, Duke JA. *A Field Guide to Medicinal Plants: Eastern and Central North America.* Boston, Mass: Houghton Mifflin; 1990.

Harborn, J, Baxter H. *Phytochemical Dictionary: A Handbook of Bioactive Compounds from Plants.* Washington DC: Taylor & Francis; 1993.

Ivanovska N, Philipov S. Study on the antiinflammatory action of *Berberis vulgaris* root extract, alkaloid fractions, and pure alkaloids. *Int J Immunopharmacol.* 1996;18:552–561.

Kowalchik C,Hylton W, eds. *Rodale's Illustrated Encyclopedia of Herbs.* Emmaus Pa: Rodale Press; 1998.

Leung A, Foster S. *Encyclopedia of Common Natural Ingredients Used in Food, Drugs, and Cosmetics.* 2nd ed. New York, NY: John Wiley & Sons; 1996.

McGuffin M, Hobbs C, Upton R, Goldberg A. *American Herbal Products Associations's Botanical Safety Handbook.* Boca Raton, Fla: CRC Press; 1996.

Muller K, et al. The antipsoriatic Mahonia aquifolium and its active constituents; I. Pro- and antioxidant properties and inhibition of 5-lipoxygenase. *Planta Med.* 1994;60:421–424.

Murray M. *The Healing Power of Herbs: the Enlightened Person's Guide to the Wonders of Medicinal Plants.* Rocklin, Calif: Prima Publishing; 1995.

Murray M, Pizzorno J. *Encyclopedia of Natural Medicine.* 2nd ed. Rocklin, Calif: Prima Publishing; 1998:310.

Shamsa F, et al. Antihistaminic and anticholinergic activity of barberry fruit *(Berberis vulgaris)* in the guinea-pig ileum. *J Ethnopharmacol.* 1999;64:161–166.

Sotnikova R, et al. Relaxant properties of some aporphine alkaloids from Mahonia aquifolium. *Methods Find Exp Clin Pharmacol.* 1997;19:589–597.

Sun D, Courtney HS, Beachey EH. Berberine sulfate blocks adherence of Streptococcus pyogenes to epithelial cells, fibronectin, and hexadecane. *Antimicrob Agents Chemother.* 1988;32:1370–1374.

■ BILBERRY
Vaccinium myrtillus (Botanical)
Ericaceae (Plant Family)
Myrtilli fructus/Myrtilli folium (Pharmacopeial)

OVERVIEW
In World War II British pilots noticed that eating bilberries or bilberry preserves before flying nightly bombing raids improved their vision. Since then, studies have shown that bilberry contains more than 15 different anthocyanosides, flavonoid compounds that not only improve visual acuity, but are important for the treatment of many eye disorders, including cataracts, macular degeneration, diabetic retinopathy, and night blindness. A botanical relative of blueberry, cranberry, and huckleberry, the anthocyanosides in bilberry are also known for their ability to stabilize collagen, rebuild capillaries, inhibit platelet aggregation, reduce hyperglycemia, relax smooth muscle, and increase gastric mucus. Dried bilberry fruit is rich in tannins and pectin, making it an effective treatment for diarrhea, both historically and in modern day European usage.

Bilberry extract contains the highest percentage of anthocyanidin content (25% compared to 0.1% to 0.25% in fresh fruit), making it the most effective means of treatment. This extract improves the delivery of oxygen and blood to the eyes, the maintenance of which is necessary to prevent cataracts and macular degeneration. The extract is also a powerful antioxidant, preventing free radical damage that can cause cataracts and macular degeneration and lead to cancer and heart disease. Bilberry extract's ability to stabilize and strengthen collagen protects the integrity of the eye tissue against glaucoma. The anthocyanosides also strengthen the area of the retina that controls vision and the adaptation between dark and light, improving poor night vision and poor day vision in particular.

The ability of bilberry extract to strengthen capillaries not only protects the eye from the hemorrhaging associated with diabetic retinopathy, but also makes it an important aid for other vascular disorders as well. Because this strengthening power is combined with the ability to reduce platelet aggregation, the extract may help prevent ischemic stroke without risking hemorrhagic stroke. It is also very effective for varicose veins and hemorrhoids and helps reduce the risk of artherosclerosis. As an antioxidant, bilberry is able to raise the levels of intracellular vitamin C, which increases the protection to the capillary walls, improving circulation. The collagen stabilizing, antioxidant, and anti-inflammatory properties of the extract make it very helpful for treatment of arthritis.

Bilberry leaves have been used historically to treat diabetes mellitus by lowering blood glucose levels, an ability that may be related to their chromium content. Use of bilberry extract to prevent and improve diabetic retinopathy is documented. These uses are not approved, however, by the German Commission E, which refers to a lack of documented evidence for bilberry leaves' efficacy.

Anthocyanosides help protect against ulcers by stimulating mucus flow that protects the stomach lining from digestive acids. Their ability to relax smooth muscle is thought to relieve dysmenorrhea as well.

MACRO DESCRIPTION
Deciduous shrub, grows to 16 inches. Stems are multibranched and erect; leaves are pointed and oval; flowers are small, pink, and white; berries are round and purple-black when ripe. Native to Europe, Asia, and North America. Flowers from April through June. Fruit collected July through September.

PART USED/PHARMACEUTICAL DESIGNATIONS
- Fruit

CONSTITUENTS/COMPOSITION
Catechins, invertose, flavonone glycosides, and anthocyanosides (particularly glycosides of malvidin, cyanidin, and delphinidin).

COMMERCIAL PREPARATIONS
Fresh or dried berries; tea made from dried leaves or dried berries; bilberry extract (standardized for 25% anthocyanidin)

MEDICINAL USES/INDICATIONS
Traditional herbal actions: antioxidant, stimulates gastric mucus, breaks down plaque deposits on arterial walls, strengthens capillary walls and causes new capillary formation, vasodilator, reduces platelet aggregation, astringent, antidiarrheal, muscle relaxant, membrane and collagen stabilizing, anti-inflammatory, vascular tonic

Clinical applications: eye disorders (poor night and day vision, cataracts, glaucoma, diabetic retinopathy, macular degeneration), ulcers, ischemic stroke, angina, diarrhea, dysmenorrhea, circulation, rheumatoid arthritis, varicose veins, hemorrhoids, circulation problems, vascular disorders, diabetes, capillary fragility

PHARMACOLOGY
Research on the pharmacology of the bilberry has focused primarily on its anthocyanoside content. Anthocyanosides strengthen and protect collagen by reinforcing its natural matrix, preventing free radical damage, and inhibiting cleavage caused by inflammation and the release of compounds that cause inflammation (e.g., histamine). This protects tissue from secondary damage from inflammation and aids the regeneration of new tissue after injury.

Anthocyanosides build and strengthen capillaries by increasing intracellular vitamin C levels and decreasing capillary permeability. This aids the circulation of blood to connective tissue in the body, promoting healing after injury or damage from inflammation. Stronger capillaries prevent hemorrhage, such as the eye damage caused by diabetic retinopathy. Anthocyanosides also improve circulation in the larger arteries and veins, reducing platelet aggregation, which aids in the treatment of vascular disorders, such as varicose veins, hemorrhoids, and atherosclerosis. As well as improving circulation and blood flow in the eyes, anthocyanosides also increase the regeneration of rhodopsin in the retina. This purple pigment is crucial to the optimal functioning of the rods, cells that are important for night vision and light adaptation.

The tannins in dried bilberry are effective for treating nonspecific, acute diarrhea. Tannins act as astringents, reducing intestinal inflammation by thickening the surface protein layer of the mucous membrane. This slows the secretion process and protects against resorption of toxins. Germany's Commission E has officially recognized and positively evaluated bilberry fruit, but not bilberry leaf, for nonprescription and clinical applications.

DOSAGE RANGES AND DURATION OF ADMINISTRATION
- For eye conditions and circulation: standardized bilberry extract (with 25% anthocyanidin) in encapsulated form, dose of 480

mg/day in two to three divided dosages. After improvement, maintenance dose of 240 mg/day for prevention.

- For dysmenorrhea or ulcer prevention: 20 to 40 mg extract tid, $^1/_2$ cup of fresh bilberries (difficult to acquire in the U.S.), or tincture (1: 5) 2 to 4 ml tid.
- For diarrhea: 5 to 10 g crushed dried bilberry in cold water, brought to a boil for 10 minutes, then strained.
- For diabetes mellitus: Pour boiling water over 1 g (approximately $1^1/_2$ tsp.) bilberry leaf, and strain after 10 to 15 minutes. Do not continue use for long duration.

SIDE EFFECTS/TOXICOLOGY

There are no side effects or toxicity associated with bilberry fruit or extract. Prolonged overuse of bilberry leaf may result in severe hydroquinone poisoning, which, with continued chronic use, could be fatal.

WARNINGS/CONTRAINDICATIONS/PRECAUTIONS

There are no known contraindications for bilberry fruit or extract. Its use is not contraindicated during pregnancy or lactation. Prolonged overuse of bilberry leaves could result in chronic intoxication or death.

REGULATORY AND COMPENDIAL STATUS

In Germany, Commission E has approved the use of bilberry fruit and extract for treatment of diarrhea and inflammation of the mouth.

Commission E has not approved therapeutic use of bilberry leaves, because efficacy has not been documented.

REFERENCES

Blumenthal M, ed. *The Complete German Commission E Monographs.* Boston, Mass: Integrative Medicine Communications; 1998.

Bomser J, et al. In vitro anti-cancer activity of fruit extracts from *Vaccinium* species. *Planta Med.* 1996;62:212–216.

Brown D. *Herbal Prescriptions for Better Health.* Rocklin, Calif: Prima Publishing; 1996.

Detre Z, Jellinek H, Miskulin R. Studies on vascular permeability in hypertension. *Clin Physiol Bichem.* 1986;4:143–149.

Duke J. *The Green Pharmacy.* Emmaus, Pa: Rodale Press; 1997.

Gruenwald J, Brendler T, Jaenicke C et al, eds. *PDR for Herbal Medicines.* Montvale, NJ: Medical Economics Company Inc; 1998.

Havsteen B. Flavonoids, a class of natural products of high pharmacological potency. *Biochem Pharmacol.* 1983;32:1141–1148.

Morazzoni P, Bombardelli E. *Vaccinium myrtillus L. Fitoterapia.* 1996;LXVII:3–29.

Murray M. *The Healing Power of Herbs.* Rocklin, Calif: Prima Publishing; 1995.

Orsucci, PL. et al. Treatment of diabetic retinopthy with anthocyanosides: a preliminary report. *Clin Oc.* 1983;5:377.

Perossini M, et al. Diabetic and Hypertensive retinopathy therapy with Vaccinium myrtillus anthocyanosides (Tegens): Double blind placebo controlled clinical trial. *Annali di Ottalmaologia e Clinica Ocaulistica.* 1987;CXII.

Schulz V et al. *Rational Phytotherapy.* Berlin, Germany: Springer-Verlag; 1998.

Tyler V. *Herbs of Choice.* New York, NY: Haworth Press Inc; 1994.

■ BLACK COHOSH
Cimicifuga racemosa (Botanical)
Ranunculaceae (Plant Family)
Cimicifugae racemosae rhizoma (Pharmacopeial)

OVERVIEW

Black cohosh *(Cimicifuga racemosa)* is a native American plant whose roots may provide a safe alternative to synthetic hormones in treating menopause and other female reproductive symptoms. The botanical has been widely used for more than 40 years in Europe and is approved by the German Commission E for premenstrual discomfort, dysmenorrhea, and menopausal symptoms. Black cohosh is sometimes called "black snake-root," "bugbane," "bugwort," or "squawroot."

Although physicians widely recommend hormone replacement therapy (HRT) for menopause, only 10% to 20% of menopausal women take it. Only half of patients who receive prescriptions for HRT have them filled and fewer than 40% of those who start HRT are still taking it a year later. The primary reason women avoid HRT is fear of breast cancer. While shying away from conventional hormone treatment, Americans are embracing alternative therapies. One in three uses botanicals, herbals, or other alternative treatments at some time.

In a German study involving 629 female patients, black cohosh improved physical and psychological menopausal symptoms in more than 80% of the subjects within six to eight weeks. The botanical was well tolerated, with only 7% of patients reporting mild, transient stomach upset. A double-blind study of 60 patients showed that black cohosh relieved menopausal depression and anxiety better than both conjugated estrogens and diazepam (Valium). Patients taking black cohosh also exhibited greater increases in the number of superficial cells in the vaginal lining. The number of daily hot flashes dropped from an average of five to fewer than one in the black cohosh group. The estrogen group reported a decrease from 5 to 3.5. More than 80% of the women taking black cohosh also reported improvements in tinnitus, heart palpitations, vertigo, and headaches.

Another significant benefit black cohosh offers over synthetic estrogen is that it does not stimulate the growth of estrogen-dependent, breast cancer cells. In vitro studies suggest it may actually inhibit growth of these cells. Studies of Remifemin brand black cohosh have shown that it enhances the effects of tamoxifen in preventing a recurrence of breast cancer.

Black cohosh relieves menopausal symptoms by suppressing the secretion of luteinizing hormone (LH) and lessening its ability to bind with receptors in the hypothalamus. Sudden bursts of LH cause hot flashes, heart palpitations, headaches, and thinning of the vaginal lining. Unlike synthetic estrogens, it does not affect follicle-stimulating hormone or prolactin release.

Although most studies have focused on black cohosh's effect on symptoms of menopause, it is also used to treat other ailments including arthritic inflammation, mild hypertension, respiratory congestion, rheumatoid arthritis, sciatica, osteoarthritis, tinnitus, muscular and neurological pain, and nervous conditions.

MACRO DESCRIPTION

Black cohosh is a member of the buttercup family. It is a hardy perennial that grows in the shady woodlands of the United States and Canada. It grows up to five feet tall, and has a stout black rhizome and straight, dark brown roots. Small white flowers sprout from long, feathery racemes in June and July. The rhizome and roots are harvested in the fall.

PART USED/PHARMACEUTICAL DESIGNATIONS
- Roots
- Rhizome

CONSTITUENTS/COMPOSITION

Cimicifugin (macrotin) and isoflavone formononetin. Triterpene glycosides (principally the xylosides actein, cimicifugoside, and 27-deoxyacteine), also are present in black cohosh. Other constituents are aromatic acids (including ferulic, isoferulic, and salicylic acids) tannins, resin, fatty acids, sugars, and starch.

COMMERCIAL PREPARATIONS

The unrefined dried roots and rhizome of black cohosh are odorless and have a bitter, acrid taste. Black cohosh is available over the counter in drugstores and health-food stores in several forms. The most familiar are capsules and tablets. The botanical also is available as a liquid tincture that can be mixed in water and as a dried root that's simmered in water to make a drink similar to tea. Several natural menopause treatments are made from a combination of black cohosh and other botanicals.

MEDICINAL USES/INDICATIONS

Black cohosh was traditionally used as an emmenagogue, anti-spasmodic, ulcerative (blood purifier), sedative, and nervine tonic. Clinical applications include the following.

- Relieves symptoms of premenstrual syndrome and painful menstruation
- Diminishes physical effects of menopause including hot flashes, heart palpitations, tinnitus, vertigo, and headaches. Tinnitus may respond best to a combination of black cohosh and the botanical Ginkgo biloba
- Eases menopause's psychological effects including depression, nervousness, and irritability
- Increases the number of superficial cells in the vaginal lining, which diminishes dryness and discomfort
- Reduces inflammation associated with arthritis and rheumatism.
- Slightly lowers arterial blood pressure by decreasing constriction of peripheral blood vessels
- Acts as an expectorant by increasing blood flow to the lungs and thinning respiratory mucus

It is unknown whether black cohosh mimics synthetic estrogen's tendency to lessen the risk of osteoporosis and heart disease.

PHARMACOLOGY

Black cohosh's estrogenic activity is associated with cimicifugin (macrotin) and the isoflavone formononetin. The botanical's antihypertensive effect is associated with actein. Ferulic and isoferulic acids give black cohosh its anti-inflammatory properties.

DOSAGE RANGES AND DURATION OF ADMINISTRATION

The recommended dose is 40 mg per day of the crude drug. The following doses should be taken tid.
- Powdered root or as tea: 1 to 2 g
- Fluid extract (1:1): 4 ml (1 tsp.)
- Solid (dry powdered) extract (4:1): 250 to 500 ml
The following dose should be taken bid.

- Remifemin brand tablets of equivalent (containing one mg of 27-deoxyacteine per tablet): two tablets. The German Commission E had recommended administration be limited to six months. The recommendation was made before recent toxicology studies on rats, which suggest black cohosh is safe for long-term use. The U.S. FDA regulates black cohosh as a dietary supplement, providing no guidelines for dosage or duration.

SIDE EFFECTS/TOXICOLOGY

- Rats given approximately nine times the therapeutic daily dose of two mg of 27-deoxyacteine for six months displayed no teratogenic, mutagenic, or carcinogenic effects.
- Mild gastrointestinal symptoms are the most common side effects. They include nausea, vomiting, diarrhea, and abdominal pain. Other side effects include dizziness, visual dimness, headaches, tremors, joint pain, and bradycardia.
- Although the six-month rat study attempted to replicate long-term human effects, long-term human studies have not been done.

WARNINGS/CONTRAINDICATIONS/PRECAUTIONS

Black cohosh is contraindicated in pregnancy, particularly during the first two trimesters because overdose may lead to premature birth. However, the botanical is often used late in pregnancy to stimulate labor. No data is available to support the use of black cohosh in women who are breastfeeding. The Germany Commission E lists no contraindications in the use of black cohosh. The botanical is appropriate for patients not suited for HRT including those with a history of breast cancer, unexplained uterine bleeding, liver and gallbladder disease, pancreatitis, endometriosis, uterine fibroids, and fibrocystic breast disease. Do not confuse black cohosh with blue cohosh, a botanical with similar properties, but less data on safety and efficacy.

INTERACTIONS

Black cohosh taken with oral contraceptives or synthetic estrogen may intensify the side effects of those drugs.

REGULATORY AND COMPENDIAL STATUS

Black cohosh has been approved by the German Commission E for the treatment of premenstrual discomfort, dysmenorrhea, and menopause discomforts.

REFERENCES

Beuscher N. *Cimicifuga racemosa* L.—Black Cohosh. *Z Phytotherapie.* 1995;16:301–310.

Blumenthal M, ed. *The Complete German Commission E Monographs: Therapeutic Guide to Herbal Medicines.* Boston, Mass: Integrative Medicine Communications; 1998.

Daiber W. Climacteric Complaints: success without using hormones. *Ärztliche Praxis.* 1983;35:1946–1947.

Lieberman S. A review of the effectiveness of *Cimicifuga racemosa* (black cohosh) for the symptoms of monopause. *J Womens Health.* 1998;5:525–529.

Murray MT, Pizzorno J. *Encyclopedia of Natural Medicine.* Rocklin, Calif: Prima Publishing; 1998.

Newall CA, Anderson LA, Phillipson DJ. *Herbal Medicines: A Guide for Health-Care Professionals.* London, England: The Pharmaceutical Press; 1996.

Ringer DL, ed. *Physicians' Guide to Nutriceuticals.* Omaha, Neb: Nutritional Data Resources LP; 1998.

Schulz V, Hänsel R, Tyler VE. *Rational Phytotherapy.* Berlin, Germany: Springer-Verlag; 1998.

Stoll W. Phytopharmacon influences atrophic vaginal epithelium: Double blind-study—cimicifuga vs. estrogenic substances. *Therapeuticum.* 1987;1:23–31.

Taylor M. Alternatives to Hormone Replacement Therapy. *Comprehensive Therapy.* 1997;23:514–532.

Tyler VE. *Herbs of Choice: The Therapeutic Use of Phytomedicinals.* New York, NY: Pharmaceutical Products Press; 1994.

Warnecke G. Influencing menopausal symptoms with a phytotherapeutic agent: successful therapy with *Cimicifuga* mono-extract. *Med Welt.* 1985;36:871–874.

■ BURDOCK
Arctium lappa/Arctium minus/Arctium tomentosum (Botanical)
Asteraceae (Plant Family)
Bardanae radix (Pharmacopeial)

OVERVIEW
During the Middle Ages, burdock was valued for treating a host of ailments. English herbalists even preferred burdock root over sarsaparilla in remedies for boils, scurvy, and rheumatism. Burdock played an important role in Native American medical botany, and American herbalists have used the roots and seeds of this plant for two centuries.

Burdock root is traditionally classified as an alterative (blood purifier) and analgesic. It also acts as a diaphoretic (promoting profuse perspiration). While the leaf and root have similar pharmacological properties, most herbal remedies call for burdock root.

Burdock root is listed in the *Eclectic Materia Medica,* the *U.S. Pharmacopoeia,* and the official pharmacopoeia of several other countries. The root is used in remedies for arthritis, gout, and related inflammatory conditions. Diuretics are made from powdered burdock seeds, which yield a yellow bland fixed product called oil of lappa.

MACRO DESCRIPTION
Burdock is a biennial common weed native to Europe and northern Asia, but now widespread throughout the United States. A member of the thistle family, it is a stout, dull pale-green plant with many spreading branches. It reaches a height of three to four feet, and its purple flowers bloom between June and October. Burdock has alternate, wavy, heart-shaped leaves that are green on the top and whitish on the bottom. The deep roots are brownish-green, or nearly black on the outside.

This plant is rarely cultivated because it easily flourishes in the wild, and it grows optimally in light, well-drained soils. The leaves are collected during the first year of growth. The roots are harvested in the fall of the first year (or in the following spring before the flowers bloom), and then air-dried.

PART USED/PHARMACEUTICAL DESIGNATIONS
- Leaves
- Roots (rhizome)
- Whole herb

CONSTITUENTS/COMPOSITION
Sesquiterpene lactones; polyynes (mainly trideca-1,11-dien-3,5,7,9-tetrain); caffeic acid derivatives (including chlorogenic acid, isochlorogenic acid); carbohydrates (45% to 50% inulin [fructosan], mucilages); volatile oil of complex composition (phenylacetaldehyde, benzaldehyde, 2-alkyl-3-methoxy-pyrazines); phytosterols, tannins.

COMMERCIAL PREPARATIONS
Commercial preparations are made from the fresh or dried underground parts (usually from Arctium lappa but sometimes from the related species Arctium minus and/or Arctium tomentosum).

MEDICINAL USES/INDICATIONS
Burdock was historically used for pulmonary catarrh, arthritis and rheumatic conditions, scurvy, and venereal eruptions. It was externally applied for skin problems and applied to the forehead and soles to lessen symptoms of fever.

Burdock's traditional herbal actions are alterative, diuretic, laxative, digestive bitter, cholagogue, lymphatic cleanser, and diaphoretic. Herbalists use burdock root and leaves as a poultice for infected wounds and pimples, and it has traditionally been used as a part of blends for cancer therapy such as the Essiac formula. Herbalists warn that large doses can precipitate skin eruptions, headache, and aching joints due to excessive elimination.

Today, burdock is clinically used for a variety of skin problems, including psoriasis, eczema, contact dermatitis, skin eruptions (particularly on the head and neck), osteo and rheumatoid arthritis, and gout.

PHARMACOLOGY
Investigations conducted in the mid-1940s indicated that burdock leaf is active against gram-negative bacteria. While burdock root has only shown antibacterial activity against gram-negative strains, the leaf and flower exhibited anti-bacterial effects against both gram-negative and gram-positive strains. The roots and leaves have antifuruncalous effects and are used to treat furuncles, or boils.

Burdock reportedly has hypoglycemic properties, but the findings are contradictory. In one study, burdock extract produced a prolonged reduction in blood-sugar concentration accompanied by a rise in carbohydrate tolerance. However, in another investigation, burdock actually aggravated the diabetic condition in streptozotocin diabetic mice. In this study, burdock adversely affected parameters of glucose homeostasis, including basal glucose, basal insulin, insulin-induced hypoglycemia, and pancreatic insulin concentration.

In an in vivo experiment, both fresh and boiled burdock plant juice significantly lowered 7,12-dimethylbenz[a]anthracene (DMBA)-induced chromosome aberrations in rat bone marrow cells. DMBA usually produces chromosome aberrations of gaps and breaks, and only rarely causes more serious chromosome damage in the form of exchanges. Burdock suppressed the incidence of DMBA-induced aberrant metaphase cells (excluding cells with gaps). This suggests that burdock may block the onset of chemically induced carcinogenesis. In another investigation, burdock decreased the mutagenicity caused by *Salmonella* mutagens and toxins (both S9-metabolic-activating and non–S9-metabolic activating mutagens).

DOSAGE RANGES AND DURATION OF ADMINISTRATION
Recommended dosage:
- Dried root 2 to 6 g in decoction tid
- Tincture (1:5) 8 to 12 ml tid
- Fluid extract (1:1) 2 to 6 ml tid
- Tea: 2 to 6 g in 500 ml water

SIDE EFFECTS/TOXICOLOGY
Adverse side effects have been reported for an isolated case of a patient taking burdock. However, experts eventually concluded that the adverse reaction was not due to burdock, but instead to contamination from solanaceous alkaloids (probably in belladonna leaf).

WARNINGS/CONTRAINDICATIONS/PRECAUTIONS

According to the German Commission E, there are no known risks associated with the use of burdock. However, skin contact with burdock root has the potential for sensitization. There is a very slight risk of contact dermatitis when using burdock root plasters. Burdock should not be taken by pregnant and lactating women since this plant has in vivo uterine stimulant effects. As a general precaution, excessive amounts of burdock root should not be consumed because the toxicology of this plant is not well understood.

INTERACTIONS

Excessive intake of burdock may interfere with hypoglycemic (antidiabetic) medications.

REGULATORY AND COMPENDIAL STATUS

The U.S. FDA classifies burdock as a dietary supplement. The root and leaf are on the General Sale List, Schedule 1, Table A [R1a] in the UK. Burdock root is sold as a nonpresription drug in France and Germany.

REFERENCES

Blumenthal M, ed. *The Complete German Commission E Monographs.* Therapeutic Guide to Herbal Medicines. Boston, Mass: Integrative Medicine Communications; 1998:318.

Bradley P, ed. *British Herbal Compendium.* Dorset, England: British Herbal Medicine Association; 1992:1:46–49.

British Herbal Pharmacopoeia. 4th ed. Dorset, England: British Herbal Medicine Association; 1996:47–49.

De Smet PAGM, Keller K, Hänsel R, Chandler RF, eds. *Adverse Effects of Herbal Drugs.* Berlin, Germany: Springer-Verlag; 1997:231–237.

Dombradi CA, et al. Screening report on the antitumor activity of purified *Arctium Lappa* extracts. *Tumori.*1966;52:173–175.

Grases F, et al. Urolithiasis and phytotherapy. *Int Urol Nephrol.* 1994;26:507–511.

Grieve M. *A Modern Herbal.* New York, NY: Dover; 1971:1:143–145.

Gruenwald J, Brendler T, Jaenicke C. *PDR for Herbal Medicines.* Montvale, NJ: Medical Economics Company; 1998:656–657

Hutchens A. *Indian Herbalogy of North America.* Boston, Mass: Shambhala Publications; 1991:62–65.

Ito Y, et al. Suppression of 7,12-dimethylbenz(a)anthracene-induced chromosome aberrations in rat bone marrow cells by vegetable juices. *Mutat Res.* 1986;172:55–60.

Lapinina L, Sisoeva T. Investigation of some plants to determine their sugar lowering action. *Farmatevt Zh.* 1964;19:52–58.

Lin CC, et al. Anti-inflammatory and radical scavenge effects of *Arctium lappa.* *Am J Chin Med.* 1996;24:127–137.

Millspaugh C. *American Medicinal Plants.* New York, NY: Dover Publications; 1974:360–362.

Mowry D. *The Scientific Validation of Herbal Medicine.* New Canaan, Conn: Keats Publishing; 1986:3–6, 57–63.

Newall C, Anderson L, Phillipson J. *Herbal Medicines: A Guide for Health-care Professionals.* London, England: Pharmaceutical Press; 1996:52–53.

Swanston-Flatt SK, Day C, Flatt PR, Gould BJ, Bailey CJ. Glycaemic effects of traditional European plant treatments for diabetes. Studies in normal and streptozotocin diabetic mice. *Diabetes Res.* 1989;413:69–73.

Tyler V. *The Honest Herbal: A Sensible Guide to the Use of Herbs and Related Remedies.* 3rd ed. Binghampton, NY: Pharmaceutical Products Press; 1993:63–64.

■ CAT'S CLAW
Uncaria tomentosa (Botanical)
Rubiaceae (Plant Family)

OVERVIEW

Used in the rainforest for over 2,000 years by indigenous tribes, cat's claw has anti-inflammatory, cytotoxic, and antiviral properties. Traditional indications include sexually-transmitted diseases, arthritis, gastritis, contraception (a reported three-year hiatus in fertility), and cancer. Purported attributes drew attention from the Westernized world: in 1997, it was on the top-ten list of herb sales in natural food stores in the U.S.

In 1989 the methods for extracting the immune-stimulant oxindole alkaloid constituents in cat's claw root bark were patented. Primarily the work of Hildebert Wagner at the Institute for Pharmaceutical Biology, Munich, and Klaus Keplinger at Innsbruck University, studies revealed that cat's claw was antiviral in the feline crown virus, the lamb Maed visna virus, human herpesvirus, and effective against neurobronchitis and allergies. Injections of the alkaloids raised T-4 lymphocyte counts, and cat's claw preparations stimulated enhanced phagocytosis, and reduced both the progression of the AIDS virus and side effects of the therapies used to treat AIDS patients. It also reduced the side effects of radiation in cancer therapy.

Today, very few studies of cat's claw in humans exist. International research institutes and manufacturing companies currently conduct studies on the pharmacokinetics and mechanisms of action for cat's claw and its isolated constituents. Results of placebo controlled, phase II trials using cat's claw in the treatment of patients with HIV and rheumatoid arthritis have not yet been published.

MACRO DESCRIPTION

Cat's claw is a climbing shrub with woody, thick vines. Growing as high as 100 feet in the Amazon rainforest and tropical countries in South America and Central America, the vines have curved, claw-like thorns where leaves meet the stem. Inside the stem is a bitter-tasting, water-like liquid reportedly drunk as refreshment to relieve fatigue.

Two Uncaria species are called cat's claw, which are differentiated by their flowers: *U. tomentosa* has yellow-white flowers; *U. guianensis,* reddish-orange flowers. Phytochemically, *U. guinanesis* contains tetracyclic oxindoles not found in the therapeutically superior *U. tomentosa.*

The root bark is the source of medicine. Because harvesting the root destroys the plant, the inner bark of the vine may be used as well. It is unclear whether this is an equal substitute.

PART USED/PHARMACEUTICAL DESIGNATIONS
- Roots
- Bark
- Vine
- Inner bark

CONSTITUENTS/COMPOSITION
- Pentacyclic oxindole alkaloids (alloisopteropodine, alloteropdine, isomitraphylline, isorhynchophylline, mitraphylline, rhyncophylline)
- Tannins (epicatechin and procyandins)
- Quinovic acid glycosides
- Polyhydroxilated triterpenes

COMMERCIAL PREPARATIONS

Crude bark as tea or in tablets; aqueous-alcohol extracts standardized to oxindole alkaloids, in liquid form or dried encapsulations

MEDICINAL USE/INDICATIONS

Traditional: anti-inflammatory, antiviral; used for arthritis, dysentery, gastric ulcer, diabetes, cancer, menstrual disorders, convalescence, general debility, gonorrhea, cirrhoses

Conditions: acne, asthma, arthritis, bone pain, cancer, depression, fungus, fistulas, gastritis, gastric ulcer, hemorrhoids, herpes, inflammation of the urinary tract, immune system disorders, menstrual irregularities, neuralgias, rheumatism, shingles, wounds

Clinical Applications (pursuant to future research): disorders of the digestive tract; hypertension, and heart disease; HIV, AIDS, and cancers; drug or radiation side effects; allergy, herpes, shingles, arthritis, tumors, cysts, and to treat reduced physical and mental stamina

PHARMACOLOGY

Cat's claw has immune stimulant, anti-inflammatory, and antimutagenic actions.

Pentacyclic oxindole alkaloids stimulate phagocytosis and activate T-lymphocytes and macrophages. Quinovic acid glycosides act as an antiviral against rhinovirus type 1B and vesicular stomatitis virus. The oxindoles suppress growth in tumor cell lines; five are anti-leukemic. Root and bark extracts are anti-tumor.

In one study, mutagenic metabolites normally formed in the urine of smokers were absent following dosing with cat's claw.

Anti-inflammatory actions may be due to the quinovic acid glycosides, which demonstrate 46% to 69% inhibition of inflammation in vivo and in vitro. The sterols beta-sitosterol, stigmasterol, and campesterol are moderately anti-inflammatory.

Cat's claw may reduce side effects from chemotherapy, including hair loss, weight loss, nausea, secondary infections, and skin problems. Cat's claw may also have cardiovascular effects: Oxindole alkaloids rhynocophylline, hirsitume, and mitraphylline are hypotensive and vasodilative.

Rhynophylline inhibits platelet aggregation, prevents blood clots, relaxes endothelial blood vessels, dilates peripheral blood vessels, lowers heart rate, and lowers blood cholesterol.

DOSAGE RANGES AND DURATION OF ADMINISTRATION

Traditional use for treating conditions listed above:
- 3 to 25 g dried bark as tea or tablets
- 20 to 30 g finely chopped bark, boiled in a liter of water for 20 to 30 minutes. Take liquid tid.

Conventional use for treating mild stomach pains, sore throats, and colds; immune function; and minor injuries:
- Tea: 1 g root bark to 250 ml water, boil for 10 to 15 minutes, cool, and strain. Drink 1 cup, tid.

- Tincture: 1 to 2 ml bid to tid.
- Dry, encapsulated, standardized extract: 20 to 60 mg daily

SIDE EFFECTS/TOXICOLOGY

Nontoxic in traditional lore. Loose stools or diarrhea have been noted. The American Herbal Products Association (AHPA) safety rating: class 4 (indicating lack of data). Tannin content cautionary. More research could change this safety rating.

WARNINGS/CONTRAINDICATIONS/PRECAUTIONS

At this time, cat's claw should not be used in skin graft or organ transplant patients. Its use in patients with HIV, AIDS, and tuberculosis is controversial. Not for children under 3, or during pregnancy or breastfeeding.

INTERACTIONS

Pending further research, cat's claw should not be used with immunizations, cryoprecipitates, fresh blood plasma, or drugs that use animal protein or peptide hormones (animal sera, intravenous hyperimmunoglobulin therapy, intravenous thymic extracts, bovine/porcine insulin).

REGULATORY AND COMPENDIAL STATUS

U.S. FDA: Dietary supplement.

German Commission E: Not included in phytomedicinal monographs.

REFERENCES

Aquino R, De Simone F, Pizza C, Conti C, Stein ML. Plant metabolites. Structure and in vitro activity of quinovic acid glycosides from *Uncaria tomentosa* and Guettarda platypoda. *J Nat Prod.* 1989;52:679–685.

Aquino R, De Simone F, Vincieri FF, Pizza C, Gacs-Baitz C. New polyhydroxylated triterpenes from *Uncaria tomentosa. J Nat Prod.* 1990;53: 559–564.

Blumenthal M, ed. *The Complete German Commission E Monographs.* Boston, Mass: Integrative Medicine Communications; 1998.

Blumenthal M. Herbal update: Una de gato (cat's claw): Rainforest herb gets scientific and industry attention. *Whole Foods Magazine.* 1995: 62–68, 78.

Blumenthal M, Riggins C. *Popular Herbs in the U.S. Market: Therapeutic Monographs.* Austin, Tex: The American Botanical Council; 1997.

Davis BW. A "new" world class herb for applied kinesiology practice: *Uncaria tomentosa*—a.k.a. Una de Gato (UDG). Collected Papers of the International College of Applied Kinesiology. 1992.

de Matta SM, Monache FD, Ferrari F, Marini-Bettolo GB. Alkaloids and procyanidine of an Uncaria sp. from Peru. *Farmaco* [Sci]. 1976;31:527–535.

Keplinger K, et al. *Uncaria tomentosa* (Willd.) DC.—ethnomedicinal use and new pharmacological, toxicological and botanical results. *J Ethnopharmacol.* 1999;64:23–34.

Lemaire I, et al. Stimulation of interleukin-1 and -6 production in alveolar macrophages by the neotropical liana, *Uncaria tomentosa. J Ethnopharmacol.* 1999;64:109–115.

Lininger S, Wright J, Austin S, Brown D, Gaby A. *The Natural Pharmacy.* Rocklin, Calif: Prima Health; 1998:246.

McGuffin M, Hobbs C, Upton R, Goldberg A. *American Herbal Products Association's Botanical Safety Handbook.* Boca Raton, Fla: CRC Press; 1997.

Ozaki Y. Pharmacological studies of indole alkaloids obtained from domestic plants, Uncaria rhynchophylla Miq. And Amsonia elliptica Roem. et Schult. *Nippon Yakurigaku Zasshi.* 1989;94:17–26.

Sandoval-Chacon M, et al. Anti-inflammatory actions of cat's claw: the role of NF-kappaB. *Aliment Pharmacol Ther.* 1998;12:1,279–1,289.

Senatore A, Cataldo A, Iaccarino FP, Elberti MG. Phytochemical and biological study of *Uncaria tomentosa. Boll Soc Ital Biol Sper.* 1989;65:517–520.

Sheng Y, et al. Induction of apoptosis and inhibition of proliferation in human tumor cells treated with extracts of *Uncaria tomentosa. Anticancer Res.* 1998;18:3,363–3,368.

Steinberg PN. Cat's claw: medicinal properties of this Amazon vine. *Nutrition Science News.* 1995.

Wurm M, et al. Pentacyclic oxindole alkaloids from *Uncaria tomentosa* induce human endothelial cells to release a lymphocyte-proliferation-regulating factor. *Planta Med.* 1998;64:701–704.

Yepez AM, de Ugaz OL, Alvarez CM, De Feo V, Aquino R, De Simone F, Pizza C. Quinovic acid glycosides from *Uncaria guianensis. Phytochemistry.* 1991;30:1,635–1,637.

■ CAYENNE (PAPRIKA)

Capsicum frutescens/Capsicum spp. (Botanical)
Solanaceae (Plant Family)
Capsicum (Pharmacopeial)

OVERVIEW

Cayenne, also known as red pepper, was first introduced to the world by the Caribbean Indians, who gave it to Columbus. Since then its popularity has spread, and it has become an important spice particularly in cajun and creole cooking, and in the cuisines of southeast Asia, China, southern Italy, and Mexico. Capsaicin is the most important ingredient in cayenne and gives it its spiciness. Although spiciness is associated with heat, capsaicin stimulates a section of the hypothalmus which effectively lowers body temperature. Natives of subtropical and tropical climates consume it regularly because it helps them tolerate the heat. As well as being an important spice in many ethnic cuisines, cayenne has many important medicinal properties, including supporting and stimulating the cardiovascular system, acting as a long-lasting topical analgesic, improving digestion, and acting as an expectorant, antioxidant, and antibacterial. Cayenne is very beneficial for the cardiovascular system. A study done on natives of Thailand, who ingest cayenne every day in their meals, shows that they have much lower rates of cardiovascular disease than Americans. Cayenne lowers levels of blood cholesterol. It helps prevent blood clots as well. These properties greatly reduce the likelihood of developing atherosclerosis.

The capsaicin in cayenne has very powerful analgesic properties when applied topically. It works primarily by decreasing pain transmitters in the body, making it an excellent solution for the pain caused by postherpetic neuralgia, diabetic neuropathy, toothache and trigeminal neuralgia, post-mastectomy and other surgical trauma or stump pain, headaches, psoriasis, and osteoarthritis and rheumatoid arthritis. Capsaicin also reduces inflammation in joint tissues, which aggravates arthritic conditions. Use of capsaicin-laced taffy to relieve mouth pain from chemotherapy and radiation has been very effective.

Cayenne stimulates saliva and stomach secretions which promotes digestion. Its antibacterial power also fights infection in the gastrointestinal tract and can relieve infectious diarrhea. As an expectorant, it thins mucus and helps move it out of the respiratory tract, making it helpful for emphysema. Its strong antioxidants also protect lung tissue from cellular damage.

MACRO DESCRIPTION

Shrubby, tropical perennial. Can grow up to two feet. Branches and stems are hardwood and angular. Flowers bloom in pairs or clusters, greenish or yellowish-white. Leaves broad, elliptical, puffy, wrinkled. Fruit pendulous, podlike, shiny, red, orange, and yellow when ripe. Flowers in summer. Indigenous to Mexico and Central America, but now grows in subtropical and tropical zones of Europe, Asia, Africa, and North America.

PART USED/PHARMACEUTICAL DESIGNATIONS

- Seeds
- Fruit

CONSTITUENTS/COMPOSITION

Capsaicin (0.1% to 1.5%), carotenoids, vitamins A and C, flavonoids, volatile oil, steroidal saponins (capsidicins—in seeds only).

COMMERCIAL PREPARATIONS

Fruit eaten raw or cooked. Fruit dried and powdered. Powder can be added to foods, stirred into juice, tea, or milk, or taken in capsule form.

Capsaicin cream: Zostrix, Axsain, Capzasin-P (should contain at least 0.025% capsaicin).

MEDICINAL USES/INDICATIONS

Traditional: antioxidant, expectorant, anti-hypertensive, topical analgesic, stomachic, carminative, gastrointestinal stimulant, rubefacient, antibacterial, circulatory stimulant, diaphoretic, used to strengthen integrity of veins, capillaries and arteries. Historically used to treat ulcers.

Clinical applications: emphysema, high blood pressure, rheumatoid arthritis, osteoarthritis, carpal tunnel syndrome, fever, cluster headaches, migraine, shingles, indigestion, artherosclerosis, psoriasis, flatulent dyspepsia

Can also be used topically with caution for the following: post-herpetic neuralgia, trigeminal neuralgia, post-mastectomy pain, mouth pain from chemotherapy or radiation, diabetic neuropathy, psoriasis

PHARMACOLOGY

Capsaicin is the most important pharmacological ingredient in cayenne. Cayenne contains high levels of vitamin C and A, and its carotene molecules act as an antioxidant. Cayenne supports and stimulates the cardiovascular system in several ways. It helps prevent artherosclerosis by lowering blood cholesterol and triglyceride levels, which reduces blood pressure as well. It also increases fecal excretions of free cholesterol, preventing absorption of cholesterol. It has an anti-aggregation effect on platelets and increases fibrinolytic activity.

Cayenne contains six pain-relieving compounds and seven anti-inflammatory ones, the most important of which is capsaicin. It also contains salicylates which are similar to salicin, the herbal equivalent of aspirin. Capsaicin inhibits pain by causing an initial increase in substance P and then a depletion of it in the sensory nerves. Because of the initial stimulation of substance P, it takes several days for the pain release to become effective, but it is very helpful for chronic pain sufferers. The depletion of substance P is also thought to decrease inflammation in joint tissues affected by osteoarthritis and rheumatoid arthritis. Because cayenne is a rubefacient, it helps to increase blood flow to painful joints or cold extremities, and reduces the scaling and redness of psoriasis, although it may cause some initial burning and itching.

The capsaicin in cayenne stimulates the cooling center of the hypothalmus, which decreases body temperature. Its salicylate content and stimulation of sweat glands help reduce fever as well.

The gastric and duodenal mucosae have capsaicin-sensitive areas which respond to stimulation from capsaicin by increasing mucosal blood flow and vascular permeability, inhibiting gastric mobility and activating duodenal motility. This aids digestion and protects against acid- and drug-induced ulcers.

DOSAGE RANGES AND DURATION OF ADMINISTRATION

As an external analgesic, apply capsaicin cream (0.025% to 0.075% capsaicin) directly to affected area up to qid. Also used as tincture: 1:5, 1 ml tid.

SIDE EFFECTS/TOXICOLOGY

Cayenne pepper is generally regarded as safe in the U.S. Topical applications may cause temporary burning sensation or redness, but this should subside without complication. Keep cayenne away from eyes, as the capsaicinoids are a strong irritant to mucosal membranes. Chronic overuse of capsaicin can be toxic.

WARNINGS/CONTRAINDICATIONS/PRECAUTIONS

Wash hands well after use and avoid touching the eyes. Not very soluble in water, so use vinegar to remove it best. Cream may cause skin irritation in some people. Test on small area of skin before extended use. If causes irritation, discontinue use. May cause gastro-intestinal irritation, although does not influence duodenal ulcers. Do not use for children under age 2. Safe for use during pregnancy. It is not known if the spicy compounds are transferred through breast-feeding.

INTERACTIONS

May interfere with MAOIs and antihypertensive therapy. May increase hepatic metabolism of drugs.

REGULATORY AND COMPENDIAL STATUS

On U.S. FDA list of herbs generally regarded as safe. FDA approval of capsaicin creams, Zostrix and Axsain, for chronic pain.

REFERENCES

Boone CW, Kelloff GJ, Malone WE. Identification of candidate cancer chemopreventive agents and their evaluation in animal models and human clinical trials: a review. *Cancer Res.* 1990;50:2–9.

Chevallier A. *The Encyclopedia of Medicinal Plants.* London, England: DK Publishing Inc; 1996.

Duke J. *The Green Pharmacy.* Emmaus, Pa: Rodale Press; 1997.

Hot peppers and substance P. *Lancet.* 1983;I:1198. Editorial.

Gruenwald J, Brendler T, Jaenicke C et al, eds. *PDR for Herbal Medicines.* Montvale, NJ: Medical Economics Company; 1998.

Heinerman J. *Heinerman's Encyclopedia of Fruits, Vegetables and Herbs.* Englewood Cliffs, NJ: Prentice Hall; 1988.

Kowalchik C, Hylton W, eds. *Rodale's Illustrated Encyclopedia of Herbs.* Emmaus, Pa: Rodale Press; 1987.

Locock RA. Capsicum. *Can Pharm J.* 1985;517–519.

Munn, S.E., et al. The effect of topical capsaicin on substance P immunoreactivity: A clinical trial and immuno-hisochemical analysis [letter]. *Acta Derm Venereol (Stockh).* 1997;77:158–159.

Murray M. *The Healing Power of Herbs.* Rocklin, Calif: Prima Publishing; 1995.

Newall C, et al. *Herbal Medicines.* London, England: Pharmaceutical Press; 1996.

Tandan R, et al. Topical capsaicin in painful diabetic neuropathy. Controlled study with long-term follow-up. *Diabetes Care.* 1992;15:8–14.

Tyler V. *The Honest Herbal.* New York, NY: Pharmaceutical Products Press; 1993.

Visudhiphan S, et al. The relationship between high fibrinolytic activity and daily capsicum ingestion in Thais. *Am J Clin Nutr.* 1982;35:1452–1458.

Vogl T. Treatment of hunan hand. *N Engl J Med.* 1982;306:178.

Yeoh KG, et al. Chili protects against aspirin-induced gastroduodenal mucosal injury in humans. *Dig Dis Sci.* 1995;40:580–583.

■ CELERY SEED
Apium graveolens (Botanical)
Apiaceae (Plant Family)
Apii fructus (Pharmacopeial)

OVERVIEW
Celery seed is one of the lesser-known herbs in Western herbal medicine. However, it has been known for thousands of years in other parts of the world for its varied uses. During ancient times, Ayurvedic physicians (vaidyas) used celery seed to treat people with colds, flu, water retention, poor digestion, various types of arthritis, and certain ailments of the liver and spleen. Modern research has documented that there may indeed be a pharmacological basis for most of these uses. In addition, laboratory studies on animals indicate that celery seed may be useful for treating hypertension, and even in the prevention of cancer.

Celery seed has significant diuretic properties, which may be why it decreases hypertension. (It also contains constituents that are directly hypotensive, as well as significant amounts of calcium, which also lowers blood pressure.) In addition, the diuretic action combined with the presence of bactericidal compounds in celery seed support its usefulness in treating urinary tract infection.

Scientific evidence also shows that celery seed may aid in the prevention of cancer. A number of studies have examined the ability of whole celery seed extract or its individual constituents to prevent tumor formation in animals. The results of these studies have been positive. The phthalides, which determine the characteristic odor of celery, are especially potent as anti-tumor agents.

These compounds also stimulate the production of the enzyme glutathione-S-transferase. This enzyme helps break down many toxic substances in the body and may help support the traditional application of celery seed for treating disorders such as arthritis and cancer in these cases.

MACRO DESCRIPTION
The seed of a biennial slender plant which can grow to 60 cm in height, with three to five segmented leaves; small white flower petals; seeds are very small with a distinctive odor. Grows in northern warm or temperate zones.

PART USED/PHARMACEUTICAL DESIGNATIONS
The seeds of the celery plant have traditionally been used. (The plant and roots contain many of the same active constituents, however; essential oils made from the plant have occasionally been used in traditional medicine.)

CONSITUENTS/COMPOSITION
- Volatile oils (including apiol)
- Flavonoids
- 3-N-butyl-phthalide
- Alpha-linolenic-acid
- Beta-eudesmol
- Guaiacol
- Isoimperatorin
- Isoquercitrin
- P-cymene
- Umbelliferone

COMMERCIAL PREPARATIONS
- Fresh or dried seeds
- Tablets, various concentrations
- Celery seed oil capsules
- Alcohol or glycerine extract

MEDICINAL USES/INDICATIONS
- Hypertension (celery seed contains both diuretic and directly hypotensive constituents)
- Arthritis/rheumatism (anti-inflammatory and analgesic constituents)
- Liver disorders (hepatoprotective and detoxifying constituents)
- Nervous restlessness (nervine and sedative constituents)
- Muscle spasms (spasmolytic, anti-inflammatory, and analgesic constituents)
- Gout and calculi (said to increase elimination of uric acid)
- Urinary tract infections (bactericidal and diuretic constituents)
- Digestive tonic and carminative
- Emmenogogue (uterine stimulant)
- Galactogogue
- May be useful cancer preventative (constituents that stimulate detoxifying enzymes; others with anti-tumor-promoting properties)
- Used as aphrodisiac in traditional medicine
- Anti-inflammatory

PHARMACOLOGY
Arthritis and muscle spasm: Alpha-linoleic acid and umbelliferone have been shown to have anti-inflammatory activity. Umbelliferone is also an anti-prostaglandin, which may contribute to celery seed's effects on inflammation and arthritis. P-cymene is analgesic and antirheumatologic. Apiol, limonene, and umbelliferone are all antispasmodic. The high levels of calcium in celery seed may also aid in relaxing muscle spasm.

Urinary tract infections: Celery seed contains a number of consituents that have anti-bacterial properties. It also is a diuretic, which increases urine output to clear bacteria from the urinary tract. P-cymene, guaiacol, limonene, terpinen-4-ol, and umbelliferone are all bactericidal. Isoquercitrin and terpinen-4-ol have both bactericidal and diuretic properties. Apiol is also a diuretic.

Lowering of blood pressure: Alpha-linolenic acid has hypotensive properties; apiol and terpinen-4-ol act as diuretics; and isoquercitin has both hypotensive and diuretic activities. Celery seed also contains high levels of calcium, which may play a significant role in reducing blood pressure.

Liver disorders: In studies on rats, liver damage induced by hepatotoxins is inhibited by extracts of celery seed. Beta-eudesmol has hepatoprotective properties.

Uterine disorders: Apiol is a uterotonic and an emmenagogue (promotes menstruation). It also acts as an abortifacient, thereby contraindicating celery seed for use in pregnancy.

Anxiety and stress relief: Limonene has sedative properties. In addition, celery seeds contain high levels of calcium, which also tend to have a relaxing effect.

Anti-tumor and anti-oxidant properties: The phthalides, bitter liminoids, and sedanolide in celery seed stimulate the activity of the detoxifying enzyme glutathione S-transferase (GST). Compounds with this activity are potent anti-tumor agents. A number of other compounds found in celery seed also have anti-carcinogenic activity, including alpha-linoleic acid, isoimperatorin, isoquercitrin, limonene, and umbelliferone. In addition, alpha-linolenic acid has anti-metastatic lymphocytogenic, and immunostimulant properties.

DOSAGE RANGES AND DURATION OF ADMINISTRATION

- The dosages found in different preparations on the market vary. Recommended dosage is to take the equivalent of 1 to 3 g dried seed tid.
- Tablets: various concentrations available. Take 1 to 3 g tid
- Celery seed oil capsules: one to two capsules tid
- Celery seed extract: $1/4$ to $1/2$ tsp. tid, with 8 oz. juice or water
- Prepare a tea by pouring boiling water over 1 tsp. of freshly crushed seeds, 1 to 3 g dried seed tid. Let steep for 10 to 20 minutes before drinking.

SIDE EFFECTS/TOXICOLOGY

None reported

WARNINGS/CONTRAINDICATIONS/PRECAUTIONS

Do not use in pregnancy.

Do not use seed sold for horticultural use. They are usually treated with fungicide.

Do not use with active kidney inflammation. Phototoxic warnings as with St. John's wort are warranted here (i.e., not with UV therapy or with tanning booths).

INTERACTIONS

None reported

REGULATORY AND COMPENDIAL STATUS

N/A

REFERENCES

Appel LJ, Moore TJ et al. A clinical trial of the effects of dietary patterns on blood pressure. *N Engl J Med.* 1997;336:1117–1124. Abstract.

Atta AH, et al. Anti-nociceptive and anti-inflammatory effects of some Jordanian medicinal plant extracts. *J Ethnopharmacol.* 1998;60:117–124.

Balch J, Balch P. *Prescription for Nutritional Healing: A-to-Z Guide to Drug-Free Remedies Using Vitamins, Minerals, Herbs, & Food Supplements.* New York, NY: Avery Publishing Group; 1990.

Banerjee S, Sharma R, Kale RK, Rao AR. Influence of certain essential oils on carcinogen-metabolizing enzymes and acid-soluble sulfhydryls in mouse liver. *Nutr Cancer.* 1994;21:263–269. Abstract.

Duke JA. *Handbook of Phytochemical Constituents of GRAS Herbs and Other Economic Plants.* Boca Raton, Fla: CRC Press; 1992.

Ko FN, et al. Vasodilatory action mechanisms of apigenin isolated from *Apium graveolens* in rat thoracic aorta. Biochim Biophys Acta. November 14; 1991;1115:69–74.

Lewis, DA, et al. The anti-inflammatory activity of celery *Apium graveolens* L. *Int J Crude Drug Res.* 1985;23.

Mills SY. *Dictionary of Modern Herbalism: A Comprehensive Guide to Practical Herbal Therapy.* Rochester, Vt: Healing Arts Press; 1988.

Singh A, Handa SS. Hepatoprotective activity of Apium graveolens and Hygrophila auriculata against paracetamol and thioacetamide intoxication in rats. *J Ethnopharmacol.* 1995;49:119–126.

Steinmetz KA, Potter JD. Vegetables, fruit, and cancer. II. Mechanisms. *Cancer Causes Control.* 1991;2:427–442. Abstract.

Tsi D, et al. Effects of aqueous celery *(Apium graveolens)* extract on lipid parameters of rats fed a high fat diet. *Planta Med.* 1995;61:18–21.

Zheng GQ, et al. Chemoprevention of benzo[a]pyrene-induced forestomach cancer in mice by natural phthalides from celery seed oil. *Nutr Cancer.* 1993;19:77–86.

Zheng GQ, Kenney PM, Zhang J, Lam LK. Chemoprevention of benzo[a]pyrene-induced forestomach cancer in mice by natural phthalides from celery seed oil. *Nutr Cancer.* 1993;19:77–86.

■ CHAMOMILE, GERMAN
Matricaria recutita (Botanical)
Asteraceae (Plant Family)
Matricariae flos (Pharmacopeial)

OVERVIEW
German chamomile is used to relieve both external and internal inflammation. Externally, it reduces swelling caused by abrasions, exposure to chemicals or radiation, fungal invasion, or subdermal spasm or infection, and targets skin, mucous membranes, gums, and ano-genital areas. Inhaled, chamomile reduces spasm and inflammation of the respiratory tract. Used internally, it relieves colic and ulcers. It has been recommended for for carpal tunnel syndrome, insect bites, insomnia, gingivitis, and heartburn.

Beginning with the ancient Egyptians, Romans, and Greeks, who used chamomile flowers to relieve sun stroke, fevers, and colic, chamomile has held a prominent place in history. It is regarded by modern Europeans with a reverence similar to that given to ginseng by Asians. Germans describe chamomile as "alles zutraut," meaning that it is capable of anything. Most important, however, is that clinical studies support chamomile's broad range of use.

German chamomile is one of two chamomile species used medicinally. The hollow receptacle that lies beneath the flowers of *M. retutica* differentiates this species from Roman, or English, chamomile *(Chamaemelum nobile)*, which has a solid receptacle. Both chamomiles produce similar bioactive constituents and are used for similar ailments. They also share non-medicinal uses: chamomile extracts are added to hair dyes and shampoos to highlight hair or improve blonde tones, and chamomile oils add apple scents to soaps and perfumes.

MACRO DESCRIPTION
Leaves, alternate, with thread-like divisions, grow from a light green, smooth, striated stem. From spring through summer, 10 to 20 cream-colored or silver-white petals bloom around a swollen, yellow central disk, or receptacle. Diameter of flower heads is $1/2$ to $5/8$ of an inch. The plant can grow to 2 or 3 feet but is often found low to the ground in native Europe, Africa, and Asia, and in North and South America where it has been naturalized.

PART USED/PHARMACEUTICAL DESIGNATIONS
- Flower

CONSTITUENTS/COMPOSITION
0.25% to 1% volatile oils including alpha-bisabolol, chamazulene; 2.4% flavonoids including apigenin; 5% to 10% pectin-like mucilage; also contains coumarins (umbelliferone, methyl ether heniarin), polysaccharide, anthemic acid, tricontane. Chamazulene, present in chamomile volatile oil, is blue, and is formed from its precursor, matricin, upon steam distillation of the oil.

COMMERCIAL PREPARATIONS
Crude dried flowers are available to buy in bulk. Chamomile tea is readily available, also aqueous or alcohol extracts and topical ointments. Because of its popular use with children, chamomile is also one of the most available herbs in glycerite form.

MEDICINAL USES/INDICATIONS
- Traditional: anti-inflammatory, diuretic, vulnerary, antimicrobial, mildly sedative, carminative, aromatic, diaphoretic, and digestive tonic; actions, according to the German Commission E monograph,

include antipholigistic, musculotropic, antispasmodic, deodorant, antibacterial, bacteriostatic
- Conditions: peptic ulcers, colic, childhood sleeplessness, hemorrhoids, spasmodic cough, excess gas, abrasions of the skin; skin irritation due to chemicals, radiation, fungi, subdermal spasm, infection; for respiratory tract irritation, insomnia, gingivitis or other oral cavity inflammation and pain
- Clinical Applications: inflammatory conditions of the skin, gastrointestinal, ano-genital, and respiratory tracts, including colic, ulcers, excess gas, heartburn, irritation from chest colds, slow-healing wounds, abcesses, fistulae, oral cavity/gum inflammation, skin inflammation due to X ray or other radiation (as for cancer patients), psoriasis, eczema, vaginal inflammations, and children's skin conditions such as impetigo, hives, chicken pox, infant acne, heat rash, diaper rash

PHARMACOLOGY
Whole extract and individual constituents have been studied for topical and internal antispasmodic, anti-inflammatory, and carminative effects. Chamazulene, alpha-bisabolol, and apigenin have the highest anti-inflammatory actions against pro-inflammatory agents used on laboratory rats. Matricin, the precursor of chamazulene, demonstrates anti-inflammatory activity superior to chamazulene. Chamazulene (azulene) has been reported to inhibit histamine release, alpha-bisabolol and cis-spiroether, another component of the volatile oil, blocked carrageenan-induced rat paw edema and demonstrated muscle relaxant actions.

Alpha-bisabolol prevented the formation of indomethacin, stress, or alcohol-induced ulcers in laboratory animals.

In vitro tests show that chamomile oil is actively antibacterial and fungicidal at concentrations of at least 25 mg/ml, as is bisabolol at concentrations of at least 1 mg/ml. Whole extracts and isolated flavonoid and bisabolol constituents also inhibit spasm in guinea pig intestine: 10 mg apigenin reduced spasm comparably to 1 mg papaverine. Volatile oil increases bile secretion in cats and dogs.

Human studies demonstrate therapeutic efficiency for European propriety chamomile formulas used in weeping skin disorders, bedsores, contact dermatitis, eczema, and post-irradiation dermatitis. Chamomile was also antispasmodic and anti-inflammatory in both human duodenum and stomach; oral extracts promoted deep sleep in 10 out of 12 patients having cardiac catheterization; and topical ointments soothed and enhanced healing in patients using chamomile as adjunctive therapy for skin infections of the leg.

DOSAGE RANGES AND DURATION OF ADMINISTRATION
- To relieve spasms or inflammations of the gastrointestinal tract: tea, 2 to 3 g herb steeped in hot water, tid or qid between meals; 1:5 tincture (5 ml tid), glycerite 1 to 2 ml tid for children
- To use as a gargle, prepare tea as above, cool, and gargle
- To use for respiratory tract inflammation, pour a few drops of essential oil into steaming water and inhale; or prepare tea and inhale steam
- For bath, to sooth inflammations of the skin, use $1/4$ lb. dried flowers per bath made into a tea by slow cooking; or use essential oils in tub,

instructing patient to enter tub only after sufficient water is mixed with oils.

- Douches, for vaginal inflammation, use 3% to 10% infusion
- Poultices for external application to skin inflammation, use 3% to 10% infusion
- For psoriasis, eczema, or dry, flaky skin, use creams with 3% to 10% crude drug content

SIDE EFFECTS/TOXICOLOGY

The American Herbal Products Association (AHPA) gives chamomile a class 1 safety rating: safe with appropriate use. The AHPA also notes that highly concentrated tea is reportedly emetic (flower heads contain anthemic acid).

WARNINGS/CONTRAINDICATIONS/PRECAUTIONS

Persons allergic to members of the aster family (ragweed) may have an allergic reaction to chamomile; two cases of anaphylactic reactions have been reported, and in both cases there was a pre-determined allergy to ragweed.

According to the AHPA, in Germany chamomile labels are required to warn against using infusions near the eyes.

Avoid excessive use during pregnancy and lactation.

INTERACTIONS

No interactions with other herbs or drugs are currently known, but because chamomile contains coumarins, it may interfere with anticoagulant therapy.

REGULATORY AND COMPENDIAL STATUS

In the United States, German chamomile is a dietary supplement and GRAS in the food industry; in England, German chamomile is a licensed product; and the Commission E approves of topical and internal use for inflammatory conditions in Germany.

REFERENCES

Achterrath-Tuckermann U, et al. Pharmacological investigations with compounds of chamomile. V. Investigations on the spasmolytic effect of compounds of chamomile and Kamillosan on the isolated guinea pig ileum. *Planta Med.* 1980;39:38–50.

Blumenthal M, ed. *The Complete German Commission E Monographs.* Boston, Mass: Integrative Medicine Communications; 1998.

de la Motte S, Bose-O'Reilly S, Heinisch M, Harrison F. Doppelblind-vergleich zwischen einem apfelpektin/kamillenextrakt-präparat und plazebo bei kindern mit diarrhoe. *Arzneimittelforschung.* 1997;47:1247–1249.

Duke JA. *The Green Pharmacy.* Emmaus, Pa: Rodale Press; 1997.

Foster S. *Herbal Renaissance: Growing, Using and Understanding Herbs in the Modern World.* Salt Lake City, Utah: Gibbs-Smith; 1993.

Glowania HJ, Raulin C, Swoboda M. Effect of chamomile on wound healing - a clinical double-blind study. *Z Hautkr.* 1987; 62:1262, 1267–1271.

Kowalchik C, Hylton W, eds. *Rodale's Illustrated Encyclopedia of Herbs.* Emmaus, Pa: Rodale Press; 1998.

McGuffin M, Hobbs C, Upton R, Goldberg A. *American Herbal Products Associations's Botanical Safety Handbook.* Boca Raton, Fla: CRC Press; 1996.

Newall CA, Anderson LA, Phillipson JD. *Herbal Medicines: A Guide for Health Care Professionals.* London, England: The Pharmaceutical Press; 1996.

Salamon I. Chamomile: A medicinal plant. *Herb, Spice, and Medicinal Plant Digest.* 1992;10:1–4.

Schultz V, Hansel R, Tyler V. *Rational Phytotherapy: A Physician's Guide to Herbal Medicine.* Heidelberg: Springer; 1998.

Viola H, et al. Apigenin, a component of *Matricaria recutita* flowers, is a central benzodiazepine receptors-ligand with anxiolytic effects. *Planta Med.* 1995;61:213–216.

■ CHAMOMILE, ROMAN

Chamaemelum nobile (Botanical)
Asteraceae (Plant Family)
Chamomillae romanae flos (Pharmacopeial)

OVERVIEW

Roman, or English, chamomile reportedly reduces intestinal gas, calms muscle spasms, quells nausea and vomiting, induces a mild sedation, and has anti-inflammatory effects on skin and mucous membranes. Because of the similarity of its volatile oils, Roman chamomile acts similarly, if not identical to, German chamomile *(Matricaria recutita)*. It is used less often, however, because there exists less scientific documentation of its therapeutic effects. The origin of its many applications is largely empirical. Nevertheless, its high demand exceeds crop yields in native northern European countries, and chamomile is now exported from Argentina and Egypt.

At the dawn of the 20th century, chamomile was used as a folk medicine to restore tranquility and calm. Although more apt to be regarded in the United States as a pleasant-tasting tea with a nice aroma, chamomile is used medicinally today in Europe. There it is used not only as a mild sedative, but also as a tonic to speed recovery from numerous ailments. In particular, indications for use are indigestion caused by nervousness or mental stress accompanied by flatulence.

Roman chamomile differs from German chamomile in that the receptacle below the flower head is solid instead of hollow, and its leaf segments are thicker. The plant itself is lower to the ground. Double or semi-double flower heads are used in the commercial preparation of volatile oil. Both chamomiles share cosmetic, beverage, and food use; chamomile oils are added to hair dyes, ointments, shampoos, soaps, perfumes, liqueurs, and baked goods.

MACRO DESCRIPTION

Perennial herb with a creeping rhizome. Grows low to the ground but sometimes reaches up to one foot in height. Stems are hairy, and either drooping or erect. Grayish-green leaves are alternate, segmented. Flower heads emit an apple-like fragrance. Disk flowers yellow, ray flowers white, and the cone-shaped receptacle is solid. Roman chamomile is native to northwestern Europe and Northern Ireland but has been cultivated throughout Europe, the United States, and parts of South America.

PART USED/PHARMACEUTICAL DESIGNATIONS

- Flower

CONSTITUENTS/COMPOSITION

0.4% to 1.75% volatile oil containing angelic and tiglic acid esters; 1,8-cineole, farnesol, nerolidol, sesquiterpenes chamazulene, alpha-bisabolol; amyl/isobutlyl alcohols; flavonoids (apigenin, luteolin, quercetin, and their glycosides); coumarins, anthemic acid, phenolic/fatty acids; phytosterol. Chamazulene is formed from matricin upon steam distillation. Volatile oil is blue.

COMMERCIAL PREPARATIONS

Crude dried flowers are available to buy in bulk; also, tea, tincture; Roman chamomile may be an additive in topical ointments and cosmetics.

MEDICINAL USES/INDICATIONS

- Traditional: tonic, stomachic, diaphoretic, soporific, antispasmodic, and folk remedy for colic

- Conditions: ulcer, gastritis, slow-healing wounds, heartburn
- Clinical Applications: Roman chamomile is used alone or as a component of a number of European treatments for heartburn, anorexia, post-prandial bloating and fullness, nausea, newborn colic, spastic constipation, menstrual disorders, frontal sinus catarrh, hay fever, nasal and pharngeal mucositis, ear inflammation, wounds, burns, rashes, bedsores, hemorrhoids, Romeheld's syndrome, and diseases of the liver, and gallbladder. Due to lack of documentation, these uses are not approved by the German Commission E.

PHARMACOLOGY

In experiments with rats, Roman chamomile has been shown to reduce carrageenan-induced paw edema, a standard test for anti-inflammatory activity. Rat tests also demonstrate Roman chamomile-induced sedative and antidiuretic effects. Antitumor and cytotoxic activity have been demonstrated in vitro for various chamomile constituents. Farnesol is sedative and spasmolytic in vitro; and apigenin is associated with reductions in inflammation, spasm, and infection. However, Roman chamomile has not been tested as extensively as German chamomile, and it occurs as an unapproved botanical in the German Commission E monographs because of the lack of human data.

The volatile oil of Roman chamomile contains the same active constituents as German chamomile, and Commission E notwithstanding it has been assumed to have similar pharmacological actions.

Chamomiles are used in Europe in dermatology, pulmology, pediatrics, gynecology, gastroenterology, and otolaryngology. Their actions span a broad range of therapeutics, blocking convulsion, microbes, sepsis, inflammation, spasms, and viruses. Tests on humans demonstrate that German chamomile reduces inflammations in mucous membranes and on the skin that may be due to cuts, burns, yeasts, or other fungal growths. When it is inhaled, the volatile oil quells respiratory inflammations associated with colds. Investigations demonstrate that these actions are stimulated by volatile oil constituents chamazulene and alpha-bisabolol, and flavonoids and coumarins, also found in Roman chamomile.

DOSAGE RANGES AND DURATION OF ADMINISTRATION

To reduce intestinal colic, flatulence, digestive disturbance, lack of appetite, painful menstruation, gingivitis, or oral inflammation, choose from the following.

- Dried flowers, as tea, 1 to 4 g tid
- 70% alcohol extract, 1 to 4 ml tid

For hemorrhoids/skin inflammation, add a few teabags or chamomile tincture to bathwater. Ointments should contain 3% to 10% crude drug.

SIDE EFFECTS/TOXICOLOGY

Roman chamomile has a class 2b safety rating from The American Herbal Products Association (AHPA). Class 2b indicates that the AHPA advises against use during pregnancy, and lists it as a potential abortifacient due to its action on uterine smooth muscle and tendency to induce menstruation when taken at high doses. Normal dietary intake of Roman chamomile in tea is not associated with these actions. Roman chamomile in high doses may also stimulate emesis, due to anthemic acid in the flower heads.

One case of anaphylaxis reportedly resulted from Roman chamomile tea ingestion in patients with ragweed allergy.

WARNINGS/CONTRAINDICATIONS/PRECAUTIONS

Avoid use in patients with known allergies to the aster family (ragweed). In laboratory tests, cross reactions were noted with German chamomile, yarrow, lettuce, and chrysanthemum. Allergic rhinitis may develop in patients with atopic reactions to mugwort.

Do not use during pregnancy or lactation.

INTERACTIONS

No interactions with other herbs or drugs are currently known, but chamomile contains coumarins, which may interfere with anticoagulant therapy.

REGULATORY AND COMPENDIAL STATUS

Roman chamomile is on the General Sales List in England. The German Commission E does not approve of its medicinal use due to lack of demonstrated efficacy, but use of flower head as tea is permitted.

REFERENCES

Achterrath-Tuckermann U, et al. Pharmacologisch untersuchungen von kamillen-inhal-testoffen. *Planta Med.* 1980;39:38-50.

Berry M. The chamomiles. *Pharm J.* 1995;254:191–193.

Blumenthal M, ed. *The Complete German Commission E Monographs.* Boston, Mass: Integrative Medicine Communications; 1998.

Bradley PR. *British Herbal Compendium.* Dorset, England: British Herbal Medicine Association; 1992:1.

DeSmet PAGM, Keller K, Hansel R, Chandler RF. *Adverse Effects of Herbal Drugs.* New York, NY: Springer-Verlag; 1992:2.

Evans WC. *Trease and Evans' Pharmacognosy.* 13th ed. London, England: Bailliere Tindall; 1989.

Foster S. *Herbal Renaissance: Growing, Using and Understanding Herbs in the Modern World.* Salt Lake City, Utah: Gibbs-Smith; 1993.

Harborne J, Baxter H. *Phytochemical Dictionary: A Handbook of Bioactive Compounds from Plants.* Washington, DC: Taylor and Francis; 1993.

Harris B, Lewis R. Chamomile part 1. *Int J Alt Comp Med.* September 1994;12.

Hausen BM, et al. The sensitizing capacity of Compositae plants. *Planta Med.* 1984;50.

Leung A, Foster S. *Encyclopedia of Common Natural Ingredients Used in Food, Drugs, and Cosmetics.* 2nd ed. New York, NY: Wiley & Sons; 1996.

McGuffin M, Hobbs C, Upton R, Goldberg A. *American Herbal Products Association's Botanical Safety Handbook.* Boca Raton, Fla: CRC Press; 1996.

Newall CA, Anderson LA, Phillipson JD. *Herbal Medicines: A Guide for Health Care Professionals.* London, England: The Pharmaceutical Press; 1996:72–73.

Opdyke DLJ. Chamomile oil roman. *Food Cosmet Toxicol.* 1974;12:853.

Weiss RF. *Herbal Medicines.* Beaconsfield, England: Beaconsfield Publishers, Ltd; 1988.

■ COMFREY LEAF/COMFREY ROOT

Symphytum officinale (Botanical)
Boraginazeae (Plant Family)
Symphyti folium/Symphyti radix (Pharmacopeial)

OVERVIEW

Comfrey is a herbaceous perennial native to Europe and temperate Asia. It is now naturalized in the United States. Also known as knitbone, comfrey has traditionally been used to treat superficial wounds as well as the inflammation of sprains and broken bones.

Allantoin, a key constituent found in the roots and leaves, is a cell proliferant that promotes wound healing and tissue regeneration. Comfrey leaf contains rosmarinic acid, which decreases inflammation and microvascular pulmonary injury. The mucilages in comfrey are responsible for its efficacy as a local demulcent (a slippery medicine for inflamed surfaces).

Although many traditional herbalists consider comfrey a beneficial herb, several pharmacological studies show that it is potentially quite toxic. Comfrey preparations, especially those taken internally, have been associated with veno-occlusive disease and even death. Many comfrey species contain poisonous pyrrolizidine alkaloids, compounds known to be highly toxic to the liver. Echimidine is one of the most toxic pyrrolizidine alkaloids. Dangerously high levels of this alkaloid have been found in both prickley comfrey *(Symphytum asperum)* and Russian comfrey *(S. uplandicum)*. Although common comfrey *(S. officinale)* does not usually contain echimidine, other harmful pyrrolizidine alkaloids have been isolated from it. According to some research, small quantities of echimidine have been detected in about 25% of samples of common comfrey. Products made from the root should be used with extreme caution since the quantity of pyrrolizidine alkaloids in comfrey root is nearly ten times that in the leaves.

While *S. officinale* is the preferred source of comfrey herbal products, some comfrey preparations sold in the United States and Europe may unknowingly be made from Russian and prickley comfrey. Collectors who harvest raw plant material are not always able to identify different species of comfrey. Consequently, there are mislabeled comfrey products on the market that do not actually come from *S. officinale,* but instead come from other *Symphytum* species containing high echimidine levels. For this reason, special care must be taken in determining the source and botanical authenticity of commercial comfrey products.

■ MACRO DESCRIPTION

Fond of moist soils, comfrey has an erect and stiff-haired stem, and it grows to a height of 20 to 120 cm. Its flowers are dull purple, violet, or whitish, and densely arranged in clusters. The wrinkly and hairy leaves are oblong, and often differ in appearance depending upon their position on the stem: the lower leaves are broad at the base and tapered at the ends while the upper leaves are broad throughout and narrowed only at the ends. The slimy roots show a horn-like appearance when dried. The root has a black exterior and fleshy whitish interior filled with a glutinous juice.

PART USED/PHARMACEUTICAL DESIGNATIONS

• Leaves
• Roots (rhizome)
• Aerial parts

CONSTITUENTS/COMPOSITION

Pyrrolizidine-type alkaloids (0.3%), including symphytine, symlandine, echimidine, intermidine, lycopsamine, myoscorpine, acetyllycopsamine,

acetylintermidine, lasiocarpine, heliosupine, viridiflorine, echiumine; carbohydrates (gum, mucilage); pyrocatechol-type tannins (2.4%); triterpenes (phytosterols, steroidal saponins, isobauerenol); allantoin (0.75 to 2.55%), caffeic acid, carotene (0.63%), chlorogenic acid, choline, lithospermic acid, rosmarinic acid, silicic acid.

COMMERCIAL PREPARATIONS

Comfrey ointments (containing 5% to 20% of the drug), creams, mucilaginous decoctions, poultices, and liniments are made from the fresh or dried aerial parts, fresh or dried leaf, and/or root of comfrey species and are used for external application. Experts advise using only products made from the mature leaves of *S. officinale.* Root preparations are available but are not recommended for either internal or external use. PA-free comfrey preparations are also available.

MEDICINAL USES/INDICATIONS

Traditional herbal actions: demulcent; internal and external vulnerary (wound healer), relaxing expectorant, astringent, emollient, pectoral tonic.

Comfrey preparations are used externally (only on intact skin) for bruising, pulled muscles and ligaments, sprains, and blunt injuries. The root has anti-inflammatory, callus-promoting, and antimitotic action.

Clinical applications: Comfrey is a stimulant to fibroblast, osteoblast, and chrondroblast activity, and is thus used for fractures, sprains, and strains. The pyrrolizidine alkaloid-free form is used internally for ulceration or erosion of the gut wall and congestive bronchial conditions.

PHARMACOLOGY

In in vivo studies, unsaturated pyrrolizidine alkaloids isolated from comfrey have been shown to have hepatotoxic, carcinogenic, and mutagenic effects. In experiments in animals, comfrey extract given orally to rats had wound healing and analgesic properties and stimulated the actions of the drug-metabolizing enzyme, aminopyrine N-demethylase in the liver. In in vitro research, comfrey extract increased uterine tone.

Rosmarinic acid isolated from comfrey is responsible for in vitro anti-inflammatory effects. In other studies, pyrrolic esters found in comfrey exhibited weak antimuscarinic effects in clinical trials. Sarracine and platyphylline are nonhepatotoxic pyrrolizidine alkaloids used clinically to treat gastrointestinal hypermotility and peptic ulcers in human patients.

DOSAGE RANGES AND DURATION OF ADMINISTRATION

Herb and leaf ointments—root extracts and semi-solid products for external use: 5% to 20% dried drug or equivalent preparation. Daily dosage should not exceed 100 mcg of pyrrolizidine alklaoids with 1,2-unsaturated necine structure, including their N-oxides, for more than four to six weeks per year. Comfrey is also available as a 1:5 tincture of root and leaves (PA-free tincture, 1 to 2 ml tid). Capsules are not currently available due to concerns about PA content.

SIDE EFFECTS/TOXICOLOGY

Comfrey is basically safe if taken within recommended therapeutic dosages and if used only as external preparations on unbroken skin. However, internal consumption of comfrey over prolonged periods of time may cause hepatic veno-occlusive disease. Oral intake of comfrey is also associated with several cases of atropine poisoning. However, reported cases of atropine toxicity may have been due to deadly nightshade (belladonna leaf) contaminants in raw plant material used to manufacture comfrey products. Contamination can occur because comfrey and belladonna leaves resemble each other.

WARNINGS/CONTRAINDICATIONS/PRECAUTIONS

Topical comfrey preparations should never be used on broken skin. Pregnant and lactating women should not use comfrey products under any circumstances.

INTERACTIONS

No interactions have been reported between comfrey and other drugs.

REGULATORY AND COMPENDIAL STATUS

Comfrey products are sold in the United Kingdom, France, and Germany as nonprescription drugs. The U.S. FDA classifies common comfrey as a dietary supplement.

REFERENCES

Behninger C, et al. Studies on the effect of an alkaloid extract of *Symphytum officinale* on human lymphocyte cultures. *Planta Med.* 1989;55:518–522.

Blumenthal M, ed. *The Complete German Commission E Monograph; Therapeutic Guide to Herbal Medicines.* Boston. Mass: Integrative Medicine Communications; 1998:115–116.

Bradley P. ed. *British Herbal Compendium. Vol. I.* Dorset, England: British Herbal Medicine Association; 1992:66–68.

Dorland's Illustrated Medical Dictionary. 25th ed. Philadelphia, Pa: WB Saunders; 1974

Furmanowa M, et al. Mutagenic effects of aqueous extracts of *Symphytum officinale* L. and of its alkaloidal fractions. *J Appl Toxico.* 1983;Jun;3(3):127-30.

Goldman RS, et al. Wound healing and analgesic effect of crude extracts of *Symphytum officinale. Fitoterapi.* 1985;(6):323–329.

Gruenwald J, Brendler T, Jaenicke C, eds. *PDR for Herbal Medicines.* Montvale, NJ: Medical Economics Co; 1998:1163–1166.

Heinerman J. *Heinerman's Encyclopedia of Fruits, Vegetables and Herbs.* Englewood Cliffs, NJ: Prentice Hall; 1988:112–113.

Newall CA, Anderson LA, Phillipson JD. eds. *Herbal Medicines: A Guide for Health-care Professionals.* London: Pharmaceutical Press; 1996:87–89.

Olinescu A, et al. Action of some proteic and carbohydrate components of *Symphytum officinale* upon normal and neoplastic cells. *Roum Arch Microbiol Immunol.* 1993;52:73–80.

Ridker PM, et al. Hepatic venocclusive disease associated with the consumption of pyrrolizidine-containing dietary supplements. *Gastroenterology.* 1985;(88):1050–1054.

Schulz V, Hänsel R, Tyler VE. *Rational Phytotherapy: A Physician's Guide to Herbal Medicine.* 3rd ed. Berlin: Springer; 1998:262.

Shealy C. *The Illustrated Encyclopedia of Healing Remedies.* Dorset, UK: Element Books; 1998:132.

Tyler VE. *Herbs of Choice: The Therapeutic Use of Phytomedicinals.* Binghamton, NY: Pharmaceutical Products Press; 1994:158–169.

Tyler VE. *The Honest Herbal: A Sensible Guide to the Use of Herbs and Related Remedies.* 3rd Ed. Binghamton, NY: Pharmaceutical Products Press; 1993:97–100.

■ DEVIL'S CLAW ROOT

Harpagophytum procumbens (Botanical)
Pedaliaceae (Plant Family)
Harpagophyti radix (Pharmacopeial)

OVERVIEW

Harpagophytum procumbens and a closely related plant, Harpagophytum zeyheri, are native to southern Africa and Madagascar. They are the only two species in *Harpagophytum*, a genus in the sesame family. Both species have comparable anti-inflammatory and pain-reducing activity, and both are used as a source of *Harpagophytum radix*.

According to traditional folklore, the Khoisan of the Kalahari used the dried root in remedies to treat pain, pregnancy complications, and skin disorders. Devil's claw has appetite stimulating and mildly analgesic pharmacological actions. Today, this bitter-tasting plant is sold in Europe and Canada as a digestive aid and appetite stimulant.

Devil's claw is collected from the savannas and outskirts of the Kalahari Desert in South Africa and Namibia. The drug is made from dried, secondary tubers. The root tubers are always sliced or pulverized before they are dried because they are nearly impossible to cut once they have dried.

MACRO DESCRIPTION

Devil's claw is a leafy perennial with a branched root system and branched shoots. The fruit consists of large woody grapples that are pointed and barbed. The secondary tuber roots grow out of the main and lateral roots. The root tubers (also called peripheral tubers) can reach a size of 20 cm long and 3 cm thick. The crude drug is made from the dried, yellowish-gray to bright pink tubers.

PART USED/PHARMACEUTICAL DESIGNATIONS

- Roots (rhizome)
- Dried secondary tubers

CONSTITUENTS/COMPOSITION

Monoterpenes include mainly harpagoside (0.5% to 1.6%; extremely bitter iridoid glycoside), harpagide, procumbide; phenylethanol derivatives include acteoside (verbascoside), isoaceteoside; oligossacharides; harpagoquinones; other compounds (carbohydrates, amino acids, flavonoids).

COMMERCIAL PREPARATIONS

Dried powder capsules and fluid extract preparations are made from dried secondary tubers.

MEDICINAL USES/INDICATIONS

Traditional herbal actions: antirheumatic, analgesic, sedative, diuretic, antipyretic, anti-inflammatory; Newall painful arthroses, tendinitis, dyspepsia, liver and gallbladder problems, loss of appetite (anorexia); supportive treatment for degenerative musculoskelatal conditions (disorders of locomotive system)

Clinical applications: Rheumatic and joint disorders such as rheumatoid arthritis, osteo arthritis, and gout. Conditions involving inflammation of connective tissues such as fibromyalgia, fibrositis, tendinitis, adhesions due to scar tissue. Liver, kidney, and bladder disorders; allergies; arteriosclerosis; lumbago; gastrointestinal problems; menstrual symptoms; neuralgia; headache; heartburn; nicotine poisoning

PHARMACOLOGY

Several in vitro and in vivo investigations confirm that aqueous extracts of devil's claw and its primary active principle, harpagoside, have anti-inflammatory and anti-exudative effects. In one study, devil's claw exhibited anti-inflammatory effects comparable to those of the antiarthritic drug, phenylbutazone. Anti-inflammatory effects have been strongest in semi-chronic rather than in acute inflammatory animal models. In another investigation, however, devil's claw failed to show anti-inflammatory properties when compared to aspirin and indomethacin. Other studies have not unequivocally shown that devil's claw reduces inflammation in either animals or humans. Inconsistent findings on efficacy may be due to different modes of administering the drug. Gastric juices apparently inactivate some of the active constituents. Therapeutic effects may be difficult to demonstrate in animal models unless devil's root extracts are protected from gastric enzymes.

In an in vitro experiment, indomethacin and aspirin caused a 5% inhibition of prostaglandin synthetase activity, but devil's claw did not produce a significant reduction in enzyme activity. In vitro research also shows that harpagoside diminished the contractile response of smooth muscle in isolated muscle preparations. Harpagoside and other active principles presumably are able to alter the contractile response by disrupting calcium influx. In addition, devil's claw extracts have weak antifungal properties.

Devil's claw extracts are cardioactive and have protective activity against ventricular arrhythmias. However, the cardioactive effects are not entirely due to harpagoside. Instead, cardioprotecive properties are attributed to a synergy between hapagoside and other active constituents in the crude extract.

The biochemical action of devil's claw on arachidonic acid metabolism apparently differs from the mechanisms of action found in NSAIDs. The therapeutic effects are perhaps explained by in vivo conversion (via enzymatic hydrolysis) of either harpagoside or harpagide into harpagogenin.

In a double-blind, placebo-controlled clinical study, 89 patients with rheumatoid symptoms were given two g of powdered devil's claw daily for two months. The treatment group had significant improvements compared to the placebo group in sensitivity to pain and in flexibility measured by fingertip-floor distance.

DOSAGE RANGES AND DURATION OF ADMINISTRATION

- Dried tuber: Take 0.1 to 0.25 g tid, encapsulated or as decoction.
- Fluid extract (1:1 in 25% alcohol): Take 0.1 to 0.25 ml tid.
- Tincture (1:5 in 25% alcohol): Take 0.5 to 1.0 ml tid.

SIDE EFFECTS/TOXICOLOGY

Most experts consider devil's claw nontoxic and safe.

WARNINGS/CONTRAINDICATIONS/PRECAUTIONS

No side effects have been reported for devil's claw root when it is administered in recommended therapeutic doses. However, this herb should not be used in excess because information on toxicology is limited. Cardioactivity makes it potentially risky for individuals with certain medical conditions because devil's claw stimulates gastric secretions. Individuals with gastric and/or duodenal ulcers, and/or gallstones should not take devil's claw without the advice of a physician or other qualified health care provider. Cinnamylic acid and terpene in devil's claw may trigger allergic effects. Despite a common misconception that devil's claw is an abortifacient, pharmacological research suggests that this plant does not induce abortion. However, digestive stimulants such as devil's claw should not be used in pregnancy because of the reflexive action on uterine muscle.

INTERACTIONS

None known

REGULATORY AND COMPENDIAL STATUS

The U. S. FDA classifies devil's claw as a dietary supplement. The plant is accepted in France for specified indications. It is approved by the German Commision E. Devil's claw is not included on the GSL in Britain.

REFERENCES

Baghdikian B, Lanhers M, Fleurentin J, et al. An analytical study, anti-inflammatory and analgesic effects of *Harpagophytum procumbens* and *Harpagophytum zeyheri*. *Planta Med.* 1997;63:171–176.

Blumenthal M, ed. *The Complete German Commission E Monographs: Therapeutic Guide to Herbal Medicines.* Boston, Mass: Integrative Medicine Communications; 1998.

Bradley P, ed. *British Herbal Compendium.* Dorset, England: British Herbal Medicine Association; 1992;1:96–98.

British Herbal Pharmacopoeia 1996. 4th ed. Dorset, England: British Herbal Medicine Association; 1996.

Costa de Pasquale R, Busa G, Circosta C, et al. A drug used in traditional medicine:

Harpagophytum procumbens DC. III. Effects on hyperkinetic ventricular arrhythmias by reperfusion. *J Ethnopharmacology.* 1985;(13):193-9.

Grahame R, Robinson B. Devil's claw (*Harpagophytum procumbens*): pharmacological and clinical studies. *Ann Rheum Dis.* 1981;40:632.

Guyader M. 1984. Les plantes antirhumatismales. Etude historique et pharmacologique, et etude clinique du nebulisat *d'Harpagophytum procumbens* DC chez 50 patients arthrosiques sivis en service hospitalier. Paris: Universite Pierre et Marie Curie.

Lanhers MC, Fleurentin J, Mortier F, Vinche A, Younos C. Anti-inflammatory and analgesic effects of an aqueous extract of *Harpagophytum procumbens. Planta Med.* 1992;58:117–123.

Mabberley DJ. *The Plant-Book: A Portable Dictionary of the Higher Plants.* Cambridge, England: Cambridge University Press; 1987.

McLeod D, et al. Investigations of *Harpagophytum procumbens* (Devil's Claw) in the treatment of experimental inflammation and arthritis in the rat. *Br J Pharmacol.* 1979;66:140P

Moussard C, Alber D, Toubin M, Thevenon N, Henry JC. A drug used in traditional medicine, *Harpagophytum procumbens:* no evidence for NSAID-like effect on whole blood eicosanoid production in human. *Prostaglandins Leukot Essent Fatty Acids.* 1992;46:283–286.

Newall C, Anderson L, Phillipson J. *Herbal Medicines: A Guide for Health-care Professionals.* London, England: Pharmaceutical Press; 1996.

Occhiuto F, Circosta C, Ragusa S, Ficarra P, Costa De Pasquale R. A drug used in traditional medicine: *Harpagophytum procumbens* DC. IV. Effects on some isolated muscle preparations. *J Ethnopharmacol.* 1985;13:201–208.

Schulz V, Hänsel R, Tyler VE. *Rational Phytotherapy: A Physician's Guide to Herbal Medicine.* 3rd ed. Berlin, Germany: Springer-Verlag; 1998.

Tyler VE. *The Honest Herbal: A Sensible Guide to the Use of Herbs and Related Remedies.* 3rd ed. Binghampton, NY: Pharmaceutical Products Press; 1993.

Whitehouse L, et al. Devil's Claw (*Harpagophytum procumbens*): no evidence for anti-inflammatory activity in the treatment of arthritic disease. *Can Med Assoc J.* 1983;129:249–251.

■ ECHINACEA ANGUSTIFOLIA HERB-ROOT/ECHINACEA PALLIDA HERB-ROOT/ ECHINACEA PURPUREA HERB-ROOT

Echinacea angustifolia/Echinacea pallida/Echinacea purpurea (Botanical)

Asteraceae (Plant Family)

Echinacea angustofoliae herba-radix/Echinacea pallidae herba-radix/Echinacea purpureae herba-radix (Pharmacopeial)

OVERVIEW

Echinacea may reduce the symptoms and duration of colds, flu, chronic infections of the respiratory tract, or infections of the lower urinary tract. Topically, it may speed the healing of chronic or slow-healing wounds. Its nonspecific, immune-stimulant activity is currently under investigation, yet it is believed to particularly activate phagocytosis and stimulate fibroblasts.

The species is named for the sharp, spiny pales of its large conical seed head, which resemble the spines of an angry hedgehog (*echinos* is Greek for hedgehog). Of nine species, the three noted above are used medicinally.

An archeological dig in the region of the Lakota Sioux unearthed echinacea dating to the 1600s. Native Americans used echinacea for snakebites, oral lesions and pain, sepsis, coughs, sore throat, colic, and stomachaches. It was also historically used for scarlet fever, syphillis, malaria, blood poisoning, and diphtheria. Through the 1800s, it was the most widely used plant drug in the United States, dispensed by both eclectic physicians and more traditional doctors. It remained on the national list of official plant drugs in the United States until the 1940s, most likely taken off this list because the conditions it had been used for were then being treated with antibiotics.

MACRO DESCRIPTION

Native to North America, echinacea consists of erect stems and alternate or opposite leaves that vary from appearing oval shaped, to oval-shaped ending in points, with varying degrees of teeth along the edges. Flowers grow singly on stem ends. Blooms are large, bear both ray and disk flowers, and have a characteristic cone-shaped receptacle. Roots grow either vertically or horizontally.

E. angustifolia has purplish-red ray flower with darker disk flowers; *E. purpurea* bears deep rose-purple ray flowers, and pales in the seed head may be tipped with orange. *E. pallida*'s flowers are pale rose, usually drooping.

PART USED/PHARMACEUTICAL DESIGNATIONS

- Flower
- Seeds
- Leaves
- Roots
- Stems

CONSTITUENTS/COMPOSITION

Polysaccharides, flavonoids, caffeic acid derivatives (echinoside, cichoric acid, chlorogenic acid, and isochlorogenic acids), essential oils, polyacetylenes, alkylamides, alkaloids

COMMERCIAL PREPARATIONS

Many dozens of preparations are available as urological, wound, and flu remedies, but preparations standardized to 1:2 tincture, with 50% alcohol, 3 to 5 ml qid, made from fresh root or fresh root and cone are preferred. Extracts, tinctures, tablets, capsules, ointments and stabilized fresh extracts are available. In Europe, intraperitoneal and intravenous forms are sometimes used.

MEDICINAL USES/INDICATIONS

Traditional herbal actions: anti-microbial, immunostimulant, anti-infective, anti-inflammatory, alterative

Clinical applications: Furunculosis and boils, septicemia, nasopharyngeal inflammation, pyorrhea, tonsillitis, carbuncles, abscesses, viral, fungal, and bacterial illness, chronic respiratory infection, colds and flu. Used topically for wounds and dermal ulceration.

PHARMACOLOGY

Echinacea is an immune stimulant with anti-inflammatory, antiviral, and antibacterial effects. These effects are largely due to nonspecific immune system activation. Carbon clearance tests have measured significant echinacea-induced macrophage activation. Echinacea's polysaccharides are immunostimulatory; its polyacetylenes are anti-inflammatory.

Echinacea increases phagocytosis; activates T lymphocytes; stimulates tumor necrosis factor, properdin, and interferon; inhibits hyaluronidase; and stimulates the adrenal cortex.

One in vitro study showed that when mouse cells were injected with echinacea extracts and incubated, a 24-hour period of resistance to influenza, herpes, and vesicular viruses resulted, likely due to nonspecific T-cell activation.

In animal studies, Echinacea's polysaccharides induce tissue regeneration; polyacetylenes are anti-inflammatory when injected. Echinacea also exerts spasmolytic effects to acetylcholine-induced spasm.

A lipid-soluble alkene, Z-1, 8-pentadecadiene exerts significant anticancer effects in vivo against Walker tumors in rats and P388 leukemia in mice.

In studies in humans, a respected double-blind trial using 100 patients and an initial 2-day dose of 30 ml of echinacea followed by 15 ml for 4 more days demonstrated that echinacea could reduce the duration of a cold from 10 days to 7. In a double-blind, placebo-controlled study of 180 patients, 450 mg doses of *E. purpurea* herb extract was as effective as placebo in providing flu relief, but patients receiving 900 mg doses reported significant relief. Prophylaxis was demonstrated in a double-blind, placebo-controlled study: of 108 cold-prone patients, those receiving 4 ml of a proprietary echinacea formula bid significantly reduced cold recurrence. Fifteen drops of *E. purpurea* tid reduced rheumatoid inflammation up to 21.8% in an uncontrolled study; effects were almost half those exerted by cortisone and prednisone and did not cause additional adverse effects.

As part of a proprietary microbicide, *E. purpurea* demonstrated possible applications against both acyclovir-resistant and acyclovir-susceptible herpes simplex virus. In a recent double-blind, placebo-controlled crossover trial, *E. angustifolia* significantly enhanced natural-killer-cell activity against HIV transinfected cells. Echinacea's therapeutic potential in these diseases deserves further study.

DOSAGE RANGES AND DURATION OF ADMINISTRATION

For immune stimulation during viral or bacterial infection, choose equivalent form of the following and take three times daily.

- 1 to 2 g dried root, as tea
- 2 to 3 ml of 22% ethanol extract standardized to contain 2.4% beta-1,2-fructofuranosides
- 200 mg of powdered extract containing 6.5:1, or 3.5%, echinacoside
- Fluid extract (1:1): .5 ml to 1 ml tid
- Tincture (1:5): 1 to 3 ml tid
- Stabilized fresh extract: .75 ml tid

Commission E advises to discontine use of internal *E. purpurea* and *E. pallida* after eight weeks, and parenteral *E. purpurea* after three weeks.

SIDE EFFECTS/TOXICOLOGY

The American Herbal Products Association safety rating is class 1 (safe with appropriate use).

Echinacea is a member of the *Compositae* family and as such may rarely cause allergic reaction.

WARNINGS/CONTRAINDICATIONS/PRECAUTIONS

Isobutylamides, found only in *angustifolia* roots and *purpurea* seed heads, are responsible for the characteristic numbing and burning sensations when echinacea herb and root extracts are placed on the tongue. Sensation dissipates quickly.

Rare reports of dermatitis. Not recommended for use in systemic diseases (tuberculosis, leukoses, diabetes, collagenosis, multiple sclerosis, AIDS, HIV infection, other autoimmune diseases) or during immunosuppressant therapy. Safety during pregancy has not been studied.

INTERACTIONS

Do not use with immunosuppressant therapy.

REGULATORY AND COMPENDIAL STATUS

Dietary supplement in the United States. *E. pallida* root approved by Germany's Commission E for relief during flu-like infections; *E. purpurea* approved topically for chronic ulcers and slow healing wounds, internally for flu-like infections. On the General Sales List in England.

REFERENCES

Berman S. Dramatic increase in immune-mediated HIV killing activity induced by *Echinacea angustifolia. Int Conf AIDS* 12 (582). Abstract 32309.

Blumenthal M, ed. *The Complete German Commission E Monographs: Therapeutic Guide to Herbal Medicine.* Boston, Mass: Integrative Medicine Communications; 1998.

Bräunig B, Dorn M, Knick E. *Echinacea purpurea radix* for strengthening the immune response in flu-like infections. *Z Phytotherapie.* 1992;13:7–13.

Dorn M, Knick E, Lewith G. Placebo-controlled, double-blind study of *Echinacea pallidae radix* in upper respiratory tract infections. *Complementary Therapies in Medicine.* 1997;5:40–42.

Hobbs C. Echinacea: a literature review. *Herbalgram* 1994;30:33–47.

Hoheisel O, Sandberg M, Bertram S, Bulitta M, Schäfer M. Echinagard treatment shortens the course of the common cold: a double-blind, placebo-controlled clinical trial. *European Journal of Clinical Research.* 1997;9:261–269.

Hyman R, Pankhurst R. *Plants and Their Names: A Concise Dictionary.* New York, NY: Oxford University Press; 1995.

McGuffin M, Hobbs C, Upton R, Goldberg A, eds. *American Herbal Products Association's Botanical Safety Handbook.* Boca Raton, Fla: CRC Press; 1996.

Melchart D, Walther E, Linde K, Brandmaier R, Lersch C. Echinacea root extracts for the prevention of upper respiratory tract infections: a double-blind, placebo-controlled randomized trial. *Arch Fam Med.* 1998;7:541–545.

Melchart D, Linde IK, Worku F, Sarkady L, Holzmann M, Jurcic K, et al. Results of Five Randomized Studies on the Immunomodulatory Activity of Preparations of Echinacea. *J Alt Comp Med.* 1995;1(2):145–160.

Murray MT. *The Healing Power of Herbs: The Enlightened Person's Guide to the Wonders of Medicinal Plants.* Rocklin, Calif: Prima Publishing; 1995.

Newall CA, Anderson LA, Phillipson JD. *Herbal Medicines: A Guide for Health-Care Professionals.* London: The Pharmaceutical Press; 1996.

Schulz V, Hänsel R, Tyler VE. *Rational Phytotherapy: A Physicians' Guide to Herbal Medicine.* 3rd ed. Berlin: Springer; 1998.

Snow JM. Echinacea. *Protocol J Botanical Medicine.* 1997;2:18–24.

Thompson KD. Antiviral activity of Viracea against acyclovir susceptible and acyclovir resistant strains of herpes simplex virus. *Antiviral Res.* 1998;39:55–61.

Tyler VE. *Herbs of Choice: The Therapeutic Use of Phytomedicinals.* Binghamton, NY: Pharmaceutical Products Press; 1994.

Verhoef MJ, Hagen N, Pelletier G, Forsyth P. Alternative therapy use in neurologic disease: use in brain tumor patients. *Neurology* 1999;52:617–622.

■ EUCALYPTUS LEAF/EUCALYPTUS OIL
Eucalyptus globulus/Eucalyptus fructicetorum/polybractea/smithii (Botanical)
Myrtaceae (Plant Family)
Eucalypti folium/Eucalypti aetheroleum (Pharmacopeial)

OVERVIEW

Eucalyptus leaf is antibacterial, antiseptic, and astringent. It was most likely first used by the Aborigines of Australia, who applied it as a poultice for wounds, abscesses, and fungal infections of the skin. They also drank eucalpytus leaf tea to reduce fevers. In 19th century England, eucalyptus oil was used in hospitals to clean urinary catheters. Today, herbalists use fresh leaves as a topical antiseptic for wounds and recommend eucalyptus gargles for sore throats, as well as inhalation of the essential oil vapors for the treatment of croup, bronchitis, asthma, nasal congestion, and flu. The oil is antiviral and expectorant; eucalyptus oil-based chest rubs and vapor inhalations relieve respiratory ailments.

Eucalyptus is added to perfumes, soaps, foods, and beverages. It's also found in wax candles and topical sprays to repel insects. Recent research suggests that washing bedclothes with eucalyptus oil may decrease asthmatic patients' exposure to dust mites. Its effects on insect habitats gave it the nickname Australian fevertree: eucalyptus trees dried marshes in which it was planted, so that malaria-bearing mosquitos could not proliferate. It also kills cockroaches. Eucalyptus oil is highly toxic to humans and should be used with care.

MACRO DESCRIPTION

There are over 500 species of eucalyptus plants, ranging in height from five-foot shrubs to 480-foot trees. Of these, blue gum is the most common. Reaching up to 230 feet in height, it has smooth, blue-gray bark that peels in shreds, revealing a cream-colored trunk beneath.

Young leaves are opposite and broad; mature 4- to 12-inch leaves are alternate, swordlike, thick, dark green, and shiny. Clusters of flowers grow near axils, bear no petals but white flower stamens, and give way to seeded fruits. The roots, which collect water, quench thirst. When one end of a root is blown into, water drips out the other end and can be collected in a vessel. Eucalpytus is native to Australia and cultivated in Europe, the U.S., China, Africa, and South America. The leaves and branch tips are the source of crude extracts and steam-distilled oil.

PART USED/PHARMACEUTICAL DESIGNATIONS

- Leaves
- Branch tips

CONSTITUENTS/COMPOSITION

Fresh and dried leaves and branch tips yield yellow, sometimes colorless, volatile oil which consists primarily of cineole (70% to 85%; formerly called eucalyptol); also, monoterpenes (borneol, terpenines, a-terpineol, citronellal, geraniol, iso-fenchone, limonene, linalool, myrcene, a-phellandrene, a- and b-pinene, camphene, trans-pinocarveol, piperitone); sesquiterpenes (aromadendrene, cadinene, caryophyllene, a-copaene, a-,b-, and gamma-eudesmol, globulol); alkanes; flavonoids (eucalyptin). Leaf contains tannins, flavonoids (procyanidin b-2,3'-O-galloyl, prodelphinidin b-2,3'-O-galloyl, prodelphinidin, quercetin, hyperoside, rutin).

COMMERCIAL PREPARATIONS

Liquid essential oil (dilute with water, oil, or rubbing acohol before using), topical creams containing essential oil. To be used commercially, eucalyptus oil must have a high percentage of cineole (not less than 70%).

Concentrations of phellandrene and aldehydes must be low. Crude leaf and aqueous extracts from leaf material are also available.

Commercial cough drops, syrups, vaporizer fluid, liniments, toothpaste, and mouthwash may contain eucalyptus oil or 1.8-cineole; both are also used in dentistry. Used in perfume, no more than 1.0% oil is allowed in products; 0.002% is the allowable limit for 1.8-cineole content in foods.

MEDICINAL USES/INDICATIONS

Traditional actions: oil—antiseptic, expectorant, antiviral, febrifuge; leaves—decongestant, astringent, stimulant. Eucalyptus was historically used for pulmonary tuberculosis, bacterial dysentery, and aching joints, but it is no longer used clinically for these conditions.

Eucalyptus leaves are currently used internally for bronchial and throat inflammation, excess mucus, congestive chest conditions, to combat colds and influenza. Eucalyptus oil is used externally for chest congestion, aches and pains, ringworm, tinnea, and as a deoderant.

Clinical applications: The German Commission E approves internal use of leaf extracts and steam inhalation of essential oil for catarrh of the upper respiratory tract, and dilute essential oil topical applications to relieve rheumatic discomfort.

PHARMACOLOGY

Essential oil is antibacterial against *Escherichia coli, Staphylococcus spp., Pseudomonas, Enterobacter species, Hemophilus influenzae, Proteus mirabilis,* and *Klebsiella* species in agar plate tests. It is antifungal to *Aspergillus aeguptiacus* and *Trichoderma viride.* Gram-positive bacteria are apparently the most sensitive to eucalyptus preparations. Oral doses and external application are expectorant.

Crude leaf extract lowers high blood sugar levels in rabbits. The flavonoids quercetin and hyperoside demonstrate in vitro anti-influenza (Type A) activity.

In humans, a combination formula including eucalyptus oil has been used to successfully treat suppurative otitis. Topical application inhibits prostaglandin synthesis, and stimulates mild hyperemic, expectorant, and secretolytic effects. Leaf extracts stimulate the same effects.

DOSAGE RANGES AND DURATION OF ADMINISTRATION

- Eucalyptus leaf as infusion: 1 to 2 g per cup tid
- Eucalyptus leaf tincture (for catarrh): $^{1}/_{2}$ to 1 ml/day
- Oil for topical application (sore joints or chest rub for catarrh): 30 ml oil to 500 ml lukewarm water.
- Eucalyptol (catarrh): 0.05 to 0.2 ml (1 to 2 drops per cup boiling water) daily
- Eucalyptus oil (for topical application): add $^{1}/_{2}$ to 1 ml (15 to 30 drops) of oil to $^{1}/_{2}$ cup of carrier oil (sesame, olive, etc.). For inhalation, add 5 to 10 drops of oil to 2 cups boiling water; place towel over head and inhale steam.

SIDE EFFECTS/TOXICOLOGY

When used externally, eucalyptus oil is non-toxic, non-sensitizing, and does not promote phototoxicity. Internally, eucalpytus oil is toxic and must be diluted. Ingestion of 3.4 ml oil has resulted in death.

The American Herbal Products Association gives eucalyptus leaf a class 2d safety rating, specifying gastric and bile duct inflammatory disease as contraindications, and cautioning against use on the faces of children under age 2. Tannins (comprising 11% of leaf extract constituents) in the leaves may cause gastrointestinal distress or kidney and liver damage if leaf preparations are ingested in large amounts.

Symptoms of poisoning include epigastric burning, miosis, cyanosis, and convulsions. Charcoal lavage, diazepam, atropine, electrolyte replenishment, sodium bicarbonate, intubation, or oxygen respiration may be required as treatments. Non-fatal doses of leaf extracts or essential oil caused nausea, vomiting, diarrhea.

WARNINGS/CONTRAINDICATIONS/PRECAUTIONS

Eucalyptus oil should not be ingested; should be in diluted form when used topically. Do not use while pregnant or breastfeeding. Not for use in patients with inflammatory disease of gastrointestinal tract or bile ducts, or severe liver disease. Eucalyptus oil should not be applied to the face of infants or young children, and especially not near the nose or mouth; glottal spasm, bronchial spasm, or asphyxiation may result.

INTERACTIONS

Eucalyptus extract and oil may interfere with hypoglycemic therapy.

REGULATORY AND COMPENDIAL STATUS

Approved for food use in appropriate quantities in the U.S., and also as a dietary supplement. Licensed through the General Sales List in England. Approved for the treatment of respiratory catarrh and rheumatic complaints by the German Commission E.

REFERENCES

Belzner S. [Eucalyptus oil dressings in urinary retention] Eukalyptusol-kompresse bei harnverhalten. *Pflege Aktuell.* 1997;51:386–387.

Benouda A, Hassar M, Menjilali B. In vitro antibacterial properties of essential oils, tested against hospital pathogenic bacteria. *Fitoterapia.* 1988;59:115119.

Blumenthal M, ed. T*he Complete German Commission E Monographs.* Boston, Mass: Integrative Medicine Communications; 1998.

Bremness L. *Herbs.* New York, NY: DK Publishing; 1994.

Burrow A, Eccles R, Jones AS. The effects of camphor, eucalyptus and menthol vapour on nasal resistance to airflow and nasal sensation. *Acta Otolaryngol (Stockh).* 1983;96(1-2):157–161.

Castleman M. *The Healing Herbs.* Emmaus, Pa: Rodale Press; 1991.

El-keltawi NEM, Megalla SE, Ross SA. Antimicrobial activity of some Egyptian aromatic plants. *Herba Pol.* 1980;26:245250.

Evans WC. *Trease and Evans' Pharmacognosy.* 13th ed. London, England: Bailliere Tindall; 1989.

Gruenwald J, Brendler T et al, eds. *PDR for Herbal Medicines.* Montvale, NJ: Medical Economics Company Inc; 1998.

Kumar A, et al. Antibacterial properties of some *Eucalyptus* oils. *Fitoterapia.* 1988;59:141-144.

Leung A, Foster S. *Encyclopedia of Common Natural Ingredients Used in Food, Drugs, and Cosmetics.* 2nd ed. New York, NY: Wiley & Sons; 1996.

McGuffin M, Hobbs C, Upton R, Goldberg A. *American Herbal Products Association's Botanical Safety Handbook.* Boca Raton, Fla: CRC Press; 1996.

Newall CA, Anderson LA, Phillipson JD. *Herbal Medicines: A Guide for Health Care Professionals.* London, England: The Pharmaceutical Press; 1996:72–73.

Nichimura H, Calvin M. Essential oil of Eucalyptus globulus in California. *J Agr Food Chem.* 1979;27:432–435.

Osawa K, et al. Macrocarpals H, I, and J from the Leaves of *Eucalyptus globulus. J Nat Prod.* 1996;59:823–827.

Tovey ER, McDonald LG. Clinical aspects of allergic disease: A simple washing procedure with eucalyptus oil for controlling house dust mites and their allergens in clothing and bedding. *J Allergy Clin Immunol.* 1997;100:464–467.

Whitman BW, Ghazizadeh H. Eucalyptus oil: therapeutic and toxic aspects of pharmacology in humans and animals [letter; comment]. *J Paediatr Child Health.* 1994;30(2):190–191.

■ EVENING PRIMROSE

Oenothera biennis (Botanical)
Onagraceae (Plant Family)

OVERVIEW

Currently, evening primrose seed oil (EPO) is used to treat atopic dermatitis and cyclical/non-cyclical mastalgia. It is also considered to be potentially useful for the treatment of premenstrual syndrome and many other inflammatory conditions. The plant that the seed oil comes from, evening primrose, has served as both food and medicine at previous times in history. Native Americans ate the boiled, nutty-flavored root, and used leaf poultices from the plant for bruises and hemorrhoids. European settlers took the root back to England and Germany, where it was introduced as food and became known as German rampion. The plant was also a Shaker medicine, sold commercially.

Recent investigation of dietary fatty acids and their roles in health stimulated interest in evening primrose. EPO contains the essential fatty acids linoleic acid (LA) and gamma-linolenic acid (GLA). GLA, an omega-6 series fatty acid, normally forms in the body during the desaturation of LA. Both GLA and its break-down product, dihomogamma-linolenic acid (DGLA), are involved with the formation of prostaglandins E1 (PGE1) and E2 (PGE2). PGE1 are vasodilatory, immune-modulating, and anti-inflammatory prostaglandins. They also inhibit platelet aggregation and phospholipase A2, block cholesterol synthesis, and lower blood pressure. PGE2 prostaglandins, on the other hand, tend toward the opposite of these actions.

EPO ingestion, and subsequent GLA and DGLA formation, may result in reductions to PGE2 stimulation by arachadonic acid. Tests demonstrate that DGLA-stimulated PGE1 reduces PGE2. EPO delivers GLA, bypasses conversion, and favors PGE1 formation over PGE2. The many potential uses of EPO include atopic eczema, diabetes, cardiovascular disease, high cholesterol, chronic fatigue syndrome, and cancer. Patients with some of these illnesses have demonstrated a slower LA-GLA conversion rate, as well as, in some cases, deficient levels of LA due to poor diet.

MACRO DESCRIPTION

Biennial plant native to North America, evening primrose grows a rosette of leaves in the first year, and creamy yellow or bright yellow flowers in the second. Flowers bloom after sunset, June through September, or on overcast days. Stems are branched, with alternate, lanceolate leaves; flowers contain a predominant X-shaped stamen and seeds. This monograph focuses on the seed from which the oil is extracted.

PART USED/PHARMACEUTICAL DESIGNATIONS

- Flower
- Leaves
- Roots
- Seed oil

CONSTITUENTS/COMPOSITION

Seed oil contains up to 25% fatty oil, which is extracted with hexane (except in the case of products labeled "hexane free") to produce a 60% to 80% linoleic acid/8% to 14% gamma-linolenic acid product.

COMMERCIAL PREPARATIONS

Standardized preparations (8% gamma-linolenic acid), in capsules or as oil.

MEDICINAL USES/INDICATIONS

Traditional actions of the leaf, flower, and root bark include vulnerary, stomachic, demulcent, and anti-inflammatory. Oil is used topically for infantile eczema. Conditions for which it is used clinically today include bruises, wounds, obesity, hemorrhoids, infantile eruptions.

In clinical applications, there are two categories of potential indications.

- Conditions associated with essential fatty acid deficiency or imbalance: acne, arthritis, rheumatoid arthritis, asthma, chronic fatigue syndrome, platelet aggregation and high blood pressure relative to congestive heart failure, diabetic neuropathy, developmental disorders, diabetes, dry scaly skin, eczema, fibrocystic breast disease, inflammation, intermittent claudication, hypercholesterolemia, mastalgia, metabolic disorders, migraine, multiple sclerosis, premenstrual syndrome, psoriases, psychological disorders, Raynaud's syndrome, Sjogren's syndrome
- Conditions associated with difficulty or inability to convert cis-linoleic acid to prostaglandin E1: aging-related disorders, alcoholism, cancer, poor nutrition, radiation damage

PHARMACOLOGY

Anti-inflammatory and relaxed smooth muscle response may result from alterations in prostaglandin biosynthesis. Effects of EPO vary and indicate a need for future research.

Placebo-controlled studies show positive effects for EPO in: rheumatoid arthritis patients (resulting in a lesser need for NSAIDs in 60% of RA patients despite the lack of changes in biochemical indicators); Sjogren's syndrome (mild increase in tear flow); irritable bowel syndrome (symptom improvement); chronic fatigue syndrome (symptom improvement); kidney transplant graft survival rate; endometriosis (90% symptom reduction in EPO group, versus 10% symptom reduction in placebo group); schitzophrenic symptoms (EPO/zinc/B$_6$/C/niacin combination, also improved tardive dyskenesia, memory loss); alcohol withdrawal; Alzheimer's disease.

Two large double-blind, placebo-controlled trials showed no effect of EPO on atopic dermatitis. Smaller studies, with severe cases, showed positive results.

Most studies support EPO in the treatment of non-cyclic breast pain and inflammation. A daily dosage of 3 g EPO had an equal effect to bromocriptine. Neither EPO nor bromocriptine were as effective as danazol, but the EPO recipients had significantly fewer side effects (4%) than did the pharmaceutical recipients (danazol: 30%; bromocriptine: 35%).

Both positive results and no results have been demonstrated in studies on the effects of EPO on premenstrual syndrome, and studies on EPO in multiple sclerosis also yield conflicting results; patients in early or less severe stages of the disease showed the greatest benefit.

Effects of EPO and GLA on human cancers are currently under study.

DOSAGE RANGES AND DURATION OF ADMINISTRATION

Products are standardized to contain 8% gamma-linolenic acid. A three-month treatment period may be necessary in order to achieve a clinical response. The recommended doses are as follows.

- Atopic dermatitis: 6 to 8 g (adult); 2 to 4 g (child)
- Cyclical and non-cyclical mastalgia: 3 to 4 g daily
- Premenstrual syndrome: 3 g daily

SIDE EFFECTS/TOXICOLOGY

American Herbal Products Association (AHPA) safety rating: class 1 (safe with appropriate use). Reported side effects are rare and mild, and include nausea, stomach pain, headache. Soft stool and abdominal pain indicate excess dosage.

WARNINGS/CONTRAINDICATIONS/PRECAUTIONS

EPO may trigger latent temporal lobe epilepsy. Schitzophrenics receiving phenothiazines are at greatest risk; occurrence not yet observed in non-phenothiazine therapy.

Breast milk contains LA and GLA; EPO safety while breastfeeding is inferred. During pregnancy, use with caution as for any herbal preparation or dietary supplement.

INTERACTIONS

Increases risk of temporal lobe epilepsy when used in combination with epileptogenic drugs for schizophrenia.

REGULATORY AND COMPENDIAL STATUS

In the Unites States, EPO is a dietary supplement. In England, a proprietary evening primrose oil is licensed for use in atopic eczema and mastalgia. Germany has approved evening primrose as a food, but the oil is not included in the Commission E monographs.

REFERENCES

Belch JJR, Ansell D, Madhok R, O'Dowd A, Sturrock RD. Effects of altering dietary essential fatty acids on requirements for NSAIDs in patients with rheumatoid arthritis. *Ann Rheum Dis.* 1988;47:96–104.

Blumenthal M, Riggins C. *Popular Herbs in the U.S. Market: Therapeutic Monographs.* Austin, Tex: The American Botanical Council; 1997.

Brehler R, Hildebrand A, Luger TA. Clinical reviews: recent developments in the treatment of atopic eczema. *J Am Acad Dermatol.* 1997; 36: 989–990.

Foster S. *Herbal Renaissance: Growing, Using and Understanding Herbs in the Modern World.* Salt Lake City, Utah: Gibbs-Smith; 1993.

Fugh-Berman A. Complementary and Alternative Therapies in Primary Care: Clinical trials of herbs. *Primary Care: Clinics in Office Practice.* 1997; 24: 889–903.

Graham-Brown R. Psychodermatology: Managing adults with atopic dermatitis. *Dermatologic Clinics.* 1996;14: 536.

Greenfield, S.M. et al. A randomized controlled study of evening primrose oil and fish oil in ulcerative colitis. *Aliment Pharmacol Ther.* 1993;7:159–166.

Horrobin DF. Interactions between n-3 and n-6 essential fatty acids (EFAs) in the regulation of cardiovascular disorders and inflammation. *Prostaglandins Leukot Essent Fatty Acids.* 1991;44:127–131.

Horrobin DF. The relationship between schizophrenia and essential fatty acid and eicosanoid metabolism. *Prostaglandins Leukot Essent Fatty Acids.* 1992;46:71–77.

Jamal GA, Carmichael H. The effect of γ-linolenic acid on human diabetic peripheral neuropathy: A double-blind placebo-controlled trial. *Diabetic Med.* 7:319-323.

Khoo, S.K., C. Munro, D. Battistutta. 1990. Evening primrose oil and treatment of premenstrual syndrome. *Med J Aust.* 153.

Leung A, Foster S. *Encyclopedia of Common Natural Ingredients Used in Food, Drugs, and Cosmetics.* 2nd ed. New York, NY: Wiley & Sons; 1996.

McGuffin M, Hobbs C, Upton R, Goldberg A. *American Herbal Products Associations' Botanical Safety Handbook.* Boca Raton, Fla: CRC Press; 1996.

Murray M. *The Encyclopedia of Nutritional Supplements.* Rocklin, Calif: Prima Publishing; 1996.

Newall CA, Anderson LA, Phillipson JD. *Herbal Medicines: A Guide for Health Care Professionals.* London, England: The Pharmaceutical Press; 1996.

Scarff DH, Lloyd DH. Double-blind, placebo-controlled crossover study of evening primrose oil in the treatment of canine atopy. *Veterinary.* 1992.

Schultz V, Hansel R, Tyler V. Rational Phytotherapy: *A Physician's Guide to Herbal Medicine.* Heidelberg: Springer-Verlag; 1998.

Stewart JCM, et al. Treatment of severe and moderately severe atopic dermatitis with evening primrose oil (Epogam): a multi-center study. *J Nut Med.* 1991;2:9–16.

■ FEVERFEW

Tanacetum parthenium/Chrysanthemum parthenium (Botanical)
Compositae (Plant Family)
Tanaceti parthenii herba (Pharmacopeial)

OVERVIEW

A wealth of scientific evidence shows that feverfew is an effective treatment and prophylactic for migraine headaches. Used for centuries in European folk medicine, feverfew was traditionally utilized for headache, arthritis, and fever. The word feverfew is a corruption of the Latin febrifuge, which literally means fever-reducing.

In a survey conducted in Britain in the 1980s, 70% of migraine sufferers who ate two to three fresh feverfew leaves daily experienced considerable relief from their headaches. A clinical study later revealed that feverfew significantly reduced the symptoms of migraine when compared with placebo. Feverfew also lessened accompanying symptoms of nausea and vomiting. In 1997, this medicinal herb ranked #19 on a list of the top herbs sold at health food stores in the United States.

Feverfew's anti-migraine activity comes from parthenolide, a sesquiterpene lactone. Parthenolide is a spasmolytic that makes smooth muscle in the walls of cerebral blood vessels less reactive to vasoconstrictors. Parthenolide helps prevent migraines and lessen the severity of existing migraines by acting as an antagonist to vasoconstrictors such as serotonin, prostaglandins, and norepinephrine.

Parthenolide and standardized extracts of feverfew containing parthenolide block the release of serotonin from blood vessels and prevent platelets from over-aggregating. Parthenolide also inhibits the actions of compounds released from cells that cause inflammation.

MACRO DESCRIPTION

Native to southeastern Europe, feverfew is now widespread throughout Europe, North America and Australia. It is a short, herbaceous, composite perennial. It is a member of the daisy family, and it blooms between July and October. This aromatic plant gives off a strong and bitter odor. Its yellow-green leaves are alternate and bipinnatifid. The small, daisy-like yellow flowers are arranged in a dense corymb.

PART USED/PHARMACEUTICAL DESIGNATIONS

- Leaves (dried leaves)
- Dried aerial parts

CONSTITUENTS/COMPOSITION

Flavonoids, polyenes, volatile oil (camphor, borneol, terpenes, various esters); sesquiterpene lactones (85% is parthenolide) (0.1% to 0.9% of plant); sesquiterpenes, monoterpenes, spiroketal enol ether polyenes.

COMMERCIAL PREPARATIONS

Parthenolide content varies tremendously and depends on geographical origin. Nearly 50% of feverfew products from Canada lacked parthenolide. And no parthenolide could be detected in samples from Mexico and Eastern Serbia. It is for this reason that feverfew preparations should be standardized for at least 0.2% parthenolide.

MEDICINAL USES/INDICATIONS

Traditional actions: relaxant, anti-inflammatory, vasodilator, digestive bitter, emmenagogue. Historically, feverfew was used for intestinal parasites, anemia, insect bites, irregular menses, stomachaches, and as an abortifacient, although it is rarely used this way now.

Clinical applications of feverfew include preventing and treating migraine, initial inflammatory stages of arthritis, rheumatic diseases, allergies, congestive dysmenorrhea, vertigo, and tinnitus.

Conditions: migraine, arthritis, rheumatic diseases, allergies

PHARMACOLOGY

In vitro and in vivo studies show that feverfew has anti-inflammatory activity and prophylactic action against migraines. The underlying cause of migraine headaches presumably involves two primary mechanisms: (1) over-aggregation of platelets; and (2) release of serotonin and inflammatory compounds from platelets. In vivo and in vitro studies show unequivocally that parthenolide disrupts both mechanisms.

Parthenolide apparently neutralizes sulfhydryl groups on enzymes crucial for platelet aggregation. And it probably achieves its prophylactic effects by suppressing the release of serotonin from platelets. In in vivo studies, extracts of feverfew blocked the synthesis of prostaglandin, thromboxane, and leukotriene.

In vitro findings indicate that feverfew may be beneficial for arthritis. The anti-arthritic effects may be due to the ability of feverfew to destroy peripheral blood mononuclear cells in the synovium.

The first human clinical study of feverfew involved a small sample of only 17 patients, but the results were dramatic. All patients enrolled in this study had taken feverfew for several years. Nine patients were given a placebo and eight were given 50 mg of feverfew daily. During the six-month study period, the patients remaining on feverfew experienced continued relief. Migraines increased almost threefold in the patients taking placebo. However, the increase in symptoms in the placebo group may have actually been part of a feverfew-withdrawal syndrome.

In a double-blind, placebo-controlled, crossover study of 72 migraine sufferers, the treatment group received 70 to 114 mg of feverfew. They had a 24% reduction in the number of migraines when compared with the placebo group. The treatment group had fewer symptoms, although the length of each individual migraine episode did not change.

In another investigation, feverfew showed no clear-cut clinical benefits for rheumatoid arthritis. However, a low dosage of powdered leaf product was used and the parthenolide content was not determined in this trial. Because of the limitations of this study, the efficacy of feverfew for arthritis is inconclusive.

DOSAGE RANGES AND DURATION OF ADMINISTRATION

Recommended dosage:
- Treatment and prevention of migraine: standardized feverfew extract (minimum 0.25 mcg parthenolide) bid
- Acute migraine attack: 1 to 2 g parthenolide daily
- For other conditions: 1 to 2 ml bid of 1:1 fluid extract; 2 to 4 ml bid of 1:5 tincture

SIDE EFFECTS/TOXICOLOGY

There are no long-term studies on feverfew toxicology. Minor side effects of nervousness and mild gastrointestinal irritation have been reported with use of standardized feverfew tablets. Adverse side effects of abdominal pain, indigestion, flatulence, diarrhea, nausea, and vomiting have also been observed. Mouth ulcerations, loss of taste, and swelling of the lips, tongue, and mouth occur in about 10% of individuals who chew the leaves.

In vivo studies revealed little evidence of negative reactions to feverfew in daily doses 100 times the dose given to humans. A histological examination of human lymphocytes showed that feverfew does not cause chromosomal abnormalities.

WARNINGS/CONTRAINDICATIONS/PRECAUTIONS

Feverfew is indicated for migraine sufferers who do not respond to conventional treatment. Because this herb can alter the menstrual cycle, menstruating women should use it with caution. Pregnant and lactating women and children under 2 years of age should not take feverfew.

INTERACTIONS

In vivo and in vitro findings suggest that feverfew may interact with antithrombotic drugs such as aspirin and warfarin. Individuals taking these medications should use feverfew only under the supervision of a qualified health care provider.

REGULATORY AND COMPENDIAL STATUS

The U.S. FDA classifies feverfew as a dietary supplement. Feverfew is used as a nonprescription drug for migraine headache in Britain and Germany.

REFERENCES

Blumenthal M, ed. *The Complete German Commission E Monographs. Therapeutic Guide to Herbal Medicines.* Boston, Mass: Integrative Medicine Communications; 1998:12.

Bradley P, ed. *British Herbal Compendium.* Dorset, England: British Herbal Medicine Association; 1992:1:96–98

Brown D. *Herbal Prescriptions for Better Health.* Rocklin, Calif: Prima Publishing; 1996:91–95

De Weerdt CJ, Bootsma HPR, Hendriks H. Herbal Medicines in migraine prevention. Randomized double-blind placebo controlled crossover trial of a feverfew preparation. *Phytomedicine.* 1996;3:225–230.

Grieve M. *A Modern Herbal.* New York, NY: Dover; 1971:1:309–310.

Gruenwald J, Brendler T, Jaenicke C et al, eds. *PDR for Herbal Medicines.* Montvale, NJ: Medical Economics Company; 1998:1171–1173.

Heptinstall S, Groenewegen W, Spangenberg P, Lösche W. Inhibition of platelet behavior by feverfew: a mechanism of action involving sulfhydryl groups. *Folia Haematol Int Mag Klin Morphol Blutforsch.* 1988;43:447–449.

Johnson ES, Kadam NP, Hylands DM, Hylands PJ. Efficacy of feverfew as prophylactic treatment of migraine. *Br Med J.* 1985;291:569–573.

Johnson ES. Patients who chew chrysanthemum leaves. *MIMS Magazine* May 15, 1983:32–35.

Murphy JJ, Heptinstall S, Mitchell JR. Randomised double-blind placebo-controlled trial of feverfew in migraine prevention. *Lancet.* 1988;2:189–192.

Murray MT. *The Healing Power of Herbs: The Enlightened Person's Guide to the Wonders of Medicinal Plants.* 2nd ed. Rocklin, Calif: Prima Publishing; 1995.

Newall CA, Anderson LA, Phillipson JD. *Herbal Medicines: A Guide for Health-care Professionals.* London, England: Pharmaceutical Press; 1996:119–120.

Palevitch D, Earon G, Carasso R. Feverfew *(Tanacetum parthenium)* as a prophylactic treatment for migraine: a double-blind controlled study. *Phytotherapy Res.* 1997;11:508–511.

Pattrick M, Heptinstall S, Doherty M. Feverfew in rheumatoid arthritis: a double-blind, placebo controlled study. *Ann Rheum Dis.* 1989;48:547–549.

Tyler VE. *Herbs of Choice: The Therapeutic Use of Phytomedicinals.* Binghamton, NY: Pharmaceutical Products Press; 1994:126–134.

Tyler VE. *The Honest Herbal: A Sensible Guide to the Use of Herbs and Related Remedies.* 3rd ed. Binghampton, NY: Pharmaceutical Products Press; 1993.

■ FLAXSEED

Linum usitatissimum (Botanical)
Linaceae (Plant Family)
Lini semen (Pharmacopeial)

OVERVIEW

Used by the ancient Egyptians, flax was originally grown in the Mediterranean and Western Europe for industrial, nutritional, and medicinal uses. It is now found as both a cultivated and semi-wild plant throughout temperate and tropical regions.

Flax is a rich source of dietary fiber that can lower cholesterol levels. The oil in flaxseed (linseed) is medicinally important for cardiovascular conditions and cancer prevention. Linseed oil contains both omega-3 fatty acids and omega-6 fatty acids as well as plant nutrients such as phytoestrogens. Linoleic and alpha-linolenic acid are essential fatty acids that the body requires for normal cellular function.

Alpha-linolenic acid (ALA) is an omega-3 oil while linoleic acid is an omega-6 oil. Flaxseed oil is nature's richest storehouse of omega-3 fatty acids. The content of omega-3 oils in flaxseed is more than double the quantity in fish oils. Experts think that the high amount of unsaturated fatty acids in flaxseed oil significantly reduces the risk for arteriosclerosis.

MACRO DESCRIPTION

Flax is an annual plant that grows up to five feet in height. It flourishes in deep moist soils rich in sand, silt, and clay. Ideally, flax should be quickly grown and harvested. Its gray-green leaves and delicate cordial blue (or sometimes white) flowers make it easily recognizable. The plant flowers only in the morning. The spherical, pea-size fruit contain flat, shiny, brown seeds filled with linseed oil. Mucilage is obtained from the husks of the seeds. Both the oil and mucilage of linseed are used for a variety of health conditions. The fruits are threshed to loosen the seeds, and the seeds do not actually ripen until after the plant has been harvested.

PART USED/PHARMACEUTICAL DESIGNATIONS

- Flowers (fresh flowering plant)
- Seeds (flaxseed oil)

CONSTITUENTS/COMPOSITION

Mucilages (3% to 10%); cyanogenic glycosides 0.05% to 0.1% (linustatin and neolinustin); fatty oil (30% to 45%), includes linolenic acid (40% to 70%), linoleic acid (10% to 25%), oleic acid (13% to 30%); mono- and triglycerides, free sterols, sterol esters, hydrocarbons: proteins (25%), ballast (25%), lignans, phenylpropane derivatives.

COMMERCIAL PREPARATIONS

Flaxseed is available as whole, bruised, or milled seeds. Linseed oil can be purchased in liquid form (to use in preparing food) or as soft gels for dietary supplementation. For optimal benefits, flaxseed oil should be added to foods (such as salad dressings) but not cooked or heated.

MEDICINAL USES/INDICATIONS

Traditional actions: whole seed, crushed seed, seed oil: bulking laxative, anti-inflammatory, demulcent, antitussive, emollient, vulnerary and expectorant. Was also historically used from gonorrhea, dysentery and diarrhea, although herbalists no longer use it for these conditions.

Internal conditions: whole or cracked seed preparations for chronic constipation, colon problems due to laxative abuse, irritable colon, diverticulitis, mucilage for gastritis and enteritis. Decoction used for cough and bronchial irritation, bladder or urinary tract inflammation.

External conditions: poultice for burns and scalds, local skin irritation, drawing poultices for local infections, pimples, boils, etc.

Clinical applications: elevated cholesterol and triglycerides; preventative for cardiovascular disease and cancer

PHARMACOLOGY

Epidemiological studies suggest that omega-3 oils significantly reduce the risk of heart disease. Omega-3 fatty acids lower LDL cholesterol and triglyceride levels. They also block platelet over-aggregation, reduce blood pressure in persons with hypertension, and lower fibrinogen levels. Consequently, omega-3 oils are clinically beneficial for hypercholesterolemia, angina, hypertension, psoriasis, eczema, cancer, and autoimmune disorders such as rheumatoid arthritis and multiple sclerosis.

ALA, the main fatty acid in linseed, improves arterial function by increasing the strength, flexibility, and permeability of cell membranes. ALA offers greater protection against heart attacks than oleic acid (found in canola and olive oil). But in one study, ALA was not responsible for the anti-arteriosclerosis effect in Type II flaxseed. ALA comprises only 2% to 3% of the total oil in Type II flaxseed.

Linolenic acid is a biologic precursor of prostaglandins. Prostaglandins are hormone-like substances that influence serum cholesterol levels, red blood cell aggregation, and smooth muscle function. Omega-3 oils help prevent cancer, stroke, and heart attacks by mediating the actions of prostaglandins. In other research, linseed oil had antibacterial action. Both linolenic acid and hydrolyzed linseed oil blocked the growth of methicillin-resistant strains of *Staphylococcus aureus*.

Flaxseed is a rich source of lignans. Lignans are platelet-activating factor-receptor antagonists that have recently sparked medical interest because of their role in improving cardiovascular health. The lignans in linseed oil have both estrogenic and anti-estrogenic effects. Phytoestrogens in linseed are thought to favorably reduce certain symptoms of menopause while other lignans act as weak estrogen antagonists.

There is new evidence that anti-estrogenic activity as well as other mechanisms inhibit carcinogenesis at various stages of tumor development. ALA and other compounds in linseed oil are known to have anti-cancer activity, particularly during the initiation and promotional stages of carcinogenesis. Lignans also suppress colon tumor growth, and it appears that flaxseed has both short-term and long-term protective effects against colon cancer.

In one investigation, the lignans enterolactone and enterodiol reduced the number of tumors observed in test animals genetically prone to developing mammary tumors. In another study, mice with experimentally-induced melanoma had flaxseed added to their diets. Flaxseed reduced metastasis and suppressed the development of metastatic secondary tumors in the animals. These findings strongly support the use of flaxseed as a complementary nutritional therapy for preventing metastasis in cancer patients. However, it should be noted that the correlations between dietary flaxseed supplements and cancer inhibition at various stages of carcinogenesis have been inconsistent.

DOSAGE RANGES AND DURATION OF ADMINISTRATION

Recommended dosage:

- Flaxseed: 1 tbsp. whole or bruised (but not ground) seed with 150 ml liquid bid to tid times a day for gastritis and enteritis; 2 to 3 tbsp. bulk seeds taken with 10 times the amount of water as a bulk laxative
- Poultice: 100 g soaked in boiling water for 10 to 15 minutes, strained, placed in cheesecloth and applied
- Decoction: 15 g of whole seed simmered in 1 cup water for 10 to 15 minutes
- Flaxseed oil: 1 tbsp. daily

SIDE EFFECTS/TOXICOLOGY

There are no side effects if flaxseed and linseed oil are taken within recommended therapeutic doses. However, large quantities of flaxseed consumed without sufficient fluid can cause ileus (constriction of the small intestine).

WARNINGS/CONTRAINDICATIONS/PRECAUTIONS

Contraindications include esophageal stricture, ileus, GI stricture, and acute intestinal inflammation. No contraindications for pregnant or lactating women.

INTERACTIONS

Flaxseed can delay the absorption of other drugs if taken simultaneously with them.

REGULATORY AND COMPENDIAL STATUS

The U.S. FDA classifies flaxseed as a dietary supplement.

REFERENCES

Allman MA, Pena MM, Pang D. Supplementation with flaxseed oil versus sunflowerseed oil in healthy young men consuming a low fat diet: effects on platelet composition and function. *Eur J Clin Nutr.* 1995;49:169–178.

Bierenbuam ML, Reichstein R, Watkins TR. Reducing atherogenic risk in hyperlipemic humans with flax seed supplementation: a preliminary report. *J Am Coll Nutr.* 1993;12:501–504.

Blumenthal M, ed. *The Complete German Commission E Monographs. Therapeutic Guide to Herbal Medicines.* Boston, Mass: Integrative Medicine Communications; 1998:47,132.

British Herbal Pharmacopoeia. 4th ed. Dorset, England: British Herbal Medicine Association; 1996.

Clark WF, et al. Flaxseed: a potential treatment of lupus nephritis. *Kidney International.* 1995;48:475–480.

Cunnane SC, et al. High alpha-linolenic acid flaxseed *(Linum usitatissimum):* some nutritional properties in humans. Br J Nutr. 1993;69:443–453.

Cunnane SC. Nutritional attributes of traditional flaxseed in healthy-young adults. *Am J Clin Nutr.* 1995;61:62–68.

De Smet P. *Adverse Effects of Herbal Drugs.* New York, NY: Springer-Verlag; 1997.

Grieve M. *A Modern Herbal.* New York, NY: Dover; 1971:1:309–310.

Gruenwald J. Brendler T, Christof J. *PDR for Herbal Medicines.* Montvale, NJ: Medical Economics Company; 1998:940–941.

Prasad K, Mantha S, Muir A, Westcott N. Reduction of hypercholesterolemic arteriosclerosis by CDC-flaxseed with very low alpha-linolenic acid. *Arteriosclerosis.* 1998;434:367–375.

Serraino M, Thompson L. The effect of flaxseed supplementation on the initiation and promotional stages of mammary tumorigenesis. *Nutr Cancer.* 1992;25:153–159.

Sung M, Lautens M, Thompson L. Mammalian lignans inhibit the growth of estrogen-independent human colon tumor cells. *Anticancer Research.* 1998;1346:1405–1408.

Thompson L, Richard S, Orcheson L, Seidl M. Flaxseed and its lignan and oil components reduce mammary tumor growth at a late stage of carcinogenesis. *Carcinogenesis.* 1996;434:1373–1376.

Yan L, Yee J, Li D, McGuire M, Thompson L. Dietary flaxseed supplementation and experimental metastasis of melanoma cells in mice. *Cancer Lett.* 1998;61:181–186.

■ GARLIC

Allium sativum (Botanical)
Alliaceae (Plant Family)
Allii sativi bulbus (Pharmacopeial)

OVERVIEW

Known for their pungent odor, garlic bulbs have been revered as both a food and medicine in many cultures for millennia. Construction workers who built the Egyptian pyramids were supposedly given huge rations of garlic to sustain their resistance against fevers. Legend has it that gravediggers in early eighteenth-century France drank a concoction of macerated garlic in wine to protect themselves against a plague. And during the two world wars, military physicians gave garlic to their patients as a preventive against gangrene.

The primary active compound in garlic is alliin, an odorless substance derived from the sulfur-containing amino acid, cysteine. However, alliin is found only within the intact cells of garlic. When garlic bulbs are crushed, the cell walls are broken, and an enzyme, allinase, converts alliin into a degradation product called allicin (diallyldisulfide-S-oxide). Allicin is an unstable compound that gives garlic its characteristic odor. Allicin is more active than alliin, and it readily forms other odorous sulfur-containing active constituents.

MACRO DESCRIPTION

Native to central Asia, garlic now grows worldwide as a cultivated plant. This perennial reaches a height of 25 to 70 cm (10 to 28 in). Its stem is either erect or crook-like, and its leaves are flat and broad. Topping the stalks are five to seven pale flowers with reddish or greenish white petals arranged in a loose globular cluster. The subterranean compound bulb has 4 to 20 cloves, or secondary bulbs, each one weighing about 1 g. Each clove is covered by a silky white or green skin.

PART USED/PHARMACEUTICAL DESIGNATIONS

• Bulbs

CONSTITUENTS/COMPOSITION

On average, 0.35% sulfur (1% of the dry weight). Alliin rapidly decomposes to form allicin which comprises 0.25% to 1.15% of garlic cloves. Alliin content is 0.7% to 1.7% in dried bulbous garlic. Other sulfur-containing constituents comprise about 25% to 35% of compounds in garlic after the cells have been damaged.

COMMERCIAL PREPARATIONS

Commercial preparations are manufactured from whole fresh bulbous garlic, dried bulbous garlic, or oil of garlic. The quantity of active principles in commercial products varies depending on the method of preparation and percentage of active compounds in fresh garlic cloves. This percentage reportedly varies by a factor of 10. Aged garlic products (garlic fermentation products) are odor-free. However, aged garlic products have limited therapeutic benefits because the active principles in them are usually converted into inert substances. Consumers should use standardized garlic products containing a specified concentration of allicin.

MEDICINAL USES/INDICATIONS

Historical uses: all infections both internally and as a poultice. Used as a warming herb and as preventive for colds and flu, menstrual pain, mouthwash, and as a douche. Anthelmintic (expels worms).

Traditional actions: antihypertensive, anticholesterolaemic, anti lipidaemic, reduces platelet aggregation, vasodilator, expectorant, antihistiminic, antimicrobial

Clinical Applications: treatment and prevention of atherosclerosis, elevated blood lipids, and thrombosis. Also used to stabilize blood sugar level, and for gastrointestinal infections by positively affecting intestinal flora.

PHARMACOLOGY

Numerous in vitro and in vivo investigations show that garlic has broad spectrum antimicrobial activity against bacteria, viruses, fungi, and intestinal parasites (helminths). Garlic also has immune-enhancing, antioxidant, and vasodilating activity. In both in vitro and in vivo studies, garlic produces anti-inflammatory, blood-sugar lowering (antidiabetic), and anti-cancer effects.

Research on garlic shows unequivocally that it can help prevent atherosclerosis through its effects on elevated lipids and blood pressure. Studies on both animals and humans indicate that garlic favorably shifted the high-density lipoprotein: low-density lipoprotein ratio toward lowered LDL and higher HDL values. It also lowered plasma viscosity and improved both blood fluidity and capillary blood flow. Garlic increased fibrinolytic activity, prolonged bleeding and clotting time, and inhibited platelet aggregations. Garlic consumption reduced blood pressure in hypertensive patients.

Double-blind clinical studies reveal that garlic lowered cholesterol and triglyceride levels in hyperlipidemic patients, and reduced blood pressure. In a 16-week, placebo-controlled trial involving 261 patients, the treatment group had a significant reduction in total cholesterol when compared with the placebo group. This trend has been confirmed by two meta-analyses of investigations on the influence of garlic on blood lipids. Garlic powder administered to patients for a minimum of four weeks resulted in an average decline of either 9% or 12% in total blood cholesterol. The average reduction in triglycerides was 13%.

Findings on the therapeutic effects of commercial garlic preparations were contradictory, presumably due to variable levels of active constituents in the commercial products used in the clinical trials. Garlic preparations can be dried (heated or freeze-dried), distilled, extracted with garlic oils, aged, or deodorized by unspecified processes. Allicin and ajoene (a self-condensation product of allicin) are absent in dried garlic preparations. Furthermore, allinase is unstable in the presence of gastric acids in the stomach. In order to be efficacious, dried garlic products must take the form of enteric-coated capsules or tablets.

Garlic has antioxidant properties, and antitoxic activity against carbon tetrachloride, isoproterenol, and heavy metal poisoning. It inhibits tumor proliferation in sarcoma, bladder tumors, isolated colon carcinoma cells, and liver cell carcinomas. In population studies in Asia, the incidence of stomach cancer deaths was lower in people who ate large quantities of garlic. The active principles in garlic may exert anti-cancer effects by stimulating the immune system to inhibit carcinogenesis.

Allicin probably accounts for antibiotic and antiplatelet activity. Allicin also lowers cholesterol levels by blocking lipid synthesis and by increasing the excretion of neutral and acidic sterols. Ajoene prevents blood clots by inhibiting platelet aggregation in vitro and in vivo in a dose-dependent and reversible manner. By inhibiting platelet aggregation, ajoene has a protective effect against atherosclerosis, coronary thrombosis, and stroke.

DOSAGE RANGES AND DURATION OF ADMINISTRATION

Recommended dosage (lower doses for prevention, higher doses for infection):

- 1,000 to 3,000 mg daily usually taken in encapsulated form (500 mg capsules)
- Oil: 0.03 to 0.12 ml tid

SIDE EFFECTS/TOXICOLOGY

Excessive dietary intake can cause stomach upset, and topical use of garlic can result in both burn-like skin lesions and allergic contact dermatitis.

WARNINGS/CONTRAINDICATIONS/PRECAUTIONS

Individuals prone to slow blood clotting should not take therapeutic doses of garlic. Excessive intake of either dietary or nondietary sources of garlic can increase the risk of hemorrhagic complications during surgery and postoperative bleeding. Pregnant and lactating women should also avoid consuming garlic in large quantities since it has abortifacient and uteroactive properties. Garlic can alter the menstrual cycle.

INTERACTIONS

Individuals taking anticoagulant drugs such as aspirin should not ingest excessive quantities of garlic.

REGULATORY AND COMPENDIAL STATUS

The U.S. FDA classifies garlic as a dietary supplement. Bulbous garlic products are sold as nonprescription drugs in France and Germany.

REFERENCES

Berthold, H.K. et al.. Effect of a garlic oil preparation on serum lipoproteins and cholesterol metabolism. *JAMA*. 1998;279.

Bradley PR, ed. *British Herbal Compendium*. Dorset, England: British Herbal Medicine Association; 1992:1:105–108.

DeSmet PAGM, Keller K, Hänsel R, Chandler RF, eds. *Adverse Effects of Herbal Drugs*. Berlin, Germany: Springer-Verlag; 1997:235–236.

Gruenwald J, Brendler T, Jaenicke C et al, eds. *PDR for Herbal Medicines*. Montvale, NJ: Medical Economics Company 1998:940–941.

Kiesewetter, H; Jung F, Mrowietz C, et al. Effects of garlic on blood fluidity and fibrinolytic activity: a randomised, placebo-controlled, double-blind study. *Br J Clin Pract*. 1990;44:24–29.

Mader FH. Treatment of hyperlipidaemia with garlic-powder tablets. Evidence from the German Association of General Practitioners' multicentric placebo-controlled double-blind study. *Arzneimittelforschung*. October 1990;40:1111–1116.

Murray MT. *The Healing Power of Herbs: The Enlightened Person's Guide to the Wonders of Medicinal Plants*. Second Ed. Rocklin, Calif: Prima Publishing; 1995:121–131.

Newall C, Anderson L, Phillipson J. *Herbal Medicines: A Guide for Health-care Professionals*. London, England: Pharmaceutical Press; 1996:129–133.

Orekhov A, Tertov V, Sobenin I, Pivovorava E. Direct antiatherosclerosis-related effects of garlic. *Ann Med*. 1995;37:63–65.

Schulz V, Hansel R, Tyler V. *Rational Phytotherapy: A Physician's Guide to Herbal Medicine*. 3rd ed. Berlin, Germany: Springer-Verlag; 1998:107–123.

Silagy C, Neil A. Garlic as a lipid lowering agent-a meta-analysis. *J R Coll Physicians Lond*. 1994;28:39–45.

Steiner M, Khan AH, Holbert D, Lin RI. A double-blind crossover study in moderately hypercholesterolemic men that compared the effect of aged garlic extract and placebo administration on blood lipids. *Am J Clin Nutr*. 1996;64:866–870.

Tyler V. *Herbs of Choice: The Therapeutic Use of Phytomedicinals*. Binghamton, NY: Pharmaceutical Products Press; 1994:104–115.

Tyler V. *The Honest Herbal: A Sensible Guide to the Use of Herbs and Related Remedies*. 3rd ed. Binghampton, NY: Pharmaceutical Products Press; 1993:139–143.

Warshafsky S, Kramer RS, Sivak SL. Effect of garlic on total serum cholesterol. *Ann Intern Med*. 1993;119:599–605.

■ GINGER ROOT

Zingiber officinale (Botanical)
Zingiberaceae (Plant Family)
Zingiberis rhizoma (Pharmacopeial)

OVERVIEW

Ginger root relieves nausea and emesis and may prevent or reduce the symptoms of motion sickness and seasickness. While nausea is currently the main indication for use, inhibition of cyclooxygenase and lipoxygenase inflammatory pathways and related prostaglandin synthetase and platelet aggregation support the use of ginger in colds, sore throats, flus, headaches, and some types of arthritis and muscular pain.

As a culinary spice, ginger was known for centuries to reduce flatulence, bloating, and indigestion, and to stimulate the appetite. It was highly sought after by Europeans, who traded with China and India during the sixteenth and seventeenth centuries and used it fresh, powdered, or crystallized in cooking. In 1884, England is said to have imported more than 5 million pounds of ginger.

Native to Asia where its use as a culinary spice spans at least 4,400 years, ginger grows in fertile, moist, tropical soil. It was transported as far west as Jamaica, where it became an export crop as early as 1547. Explorers and settlers brought it to southern Florida and further west to Mexico.

Ginger can be grown at home by planting rhizomes in soils of mixed loam, sand, peat moss, and compost in bright sun with plenty of water. Within a year, gnarled, branched rhizome spread throughout the soil, bearing numerous tubers.

MACRO DESCRIPTION

White, yellow, or greenish-yellow flowers, which may have a purplish tint at the edges, form at cone-shaped, three-inch spikes, off erect 6- to 12-inch stalks (cultivated ginger rarely flowers). Above ground leaves are dark green, narrow, lanceolate or linear-lanceolate, with a noticeable rib. The rhizome is light beige, aromatic, and has a sharp, spicy flavor.

PART USED/PHARMACEUTICAL DESIGNATIONS

• Roots (rhizome)

CONSTITUENTS/COMPOSITION

Volatile oil containing sesquiterpenes (zingiberene, bisabolene); oleoresin with pungent principles (gingerols, shogaols)

COMMERCIAL PREPARATIONS

Fresh or dried rhizome prepared as aqueous, aqueous-alcohol, glycerite, or dried powder liquid extracts including tinctures and syrups; oil; rhizome tea; dried, powdered tablets, capsules; crystallized ginger

MEDICINAL USES/INDICATIONS

Traditional herbal actions: carminative, diaphoretic, antispasmodic, antiemetic, cholagogue, circulatory stimulant, peripheral vasodilator, expectorant, antiseptic, topical rubifacient

Conditions: intestinal colic, flatulence, indigestion, headache, sore throat, arthritis, common cold, flu, delayed menstruation, pelvic congestion, menstrual cramps

Clinical Applications: motion sickness, nausea, vomiting, indigestion, flatulence, common cold, flu, dysmenorrhea; also used topically for arthritis, sore joints, and muscle sprains.

PHARMACOLOGY

Ginger root increases gastric motility, stimulates bile secretion, and is carminative and antiemetic. It promotes bile flow and reduces inflammation through prostaglandin inhibition.

In studies in animals, ginger or its oleoresin or volatile oil components are hypoglycemic, hypo- and hypertensive, anthelmintic (*Anisakis* larvae) in vitro, and positively inotropic. Ginger inhibits cholesterol absorption after time, increases bile flow, and inhibits hydrochloric acid/ethanol-induced gastric lesions. It also inhibits prostaglandin biosynthesis and platelet aggregation in vitro.

In humans, ginger relieves motion sickness comparably to dimenhydrinate (Dramamine), most likely through actions within the gastrointestinal tract and not on the central nervous system, at doses of up to 2 g every four hours or as needed. Its superiority to dimenhydrinate remains equivocal. Currently, at least one formulation awaits FDA approval for over-the-counter status for treating nausea and motion sickness.

High doses of ginger (10 to 20 g of fresh ginger per day, or 500 mg of dried ginger four times a day) were found to significantly reduce migraine intensity and rheumatoid arthritis pain, respectively. Rheumatoid arthritis patients receiving either 5 to 50 g of fresh ginger or 0.1 to 1.0 g of powdered root experienced significant reductions in joint pain and an increase in mobility. These effects may be due to cyclooxygenase and lipoxygenase pathway inhibition.

DOSAGE RANGES AND DURATION OF ADMINISTRATION

Daily dose:
• 2 to 4 g daily of fresh root (0.25 to 1.0 g of powdered root)
To relieve nausea, flatulence, or indigestion:
• 2 to 4 g daily of fresh root (0.25 to 1.0 g of powdered root) or 1.5 to 3.0 ml tincture daily, relative to the strength and processing of the tincture
To prevent emesis:
• 1g ginger (½ tsp.) every 4 hours as needed
• 2 ginger capsules (1 g) tid
• ¼ oz. piece of fresh ginger, chewed
To relieve cold symptoms, fever associated with flu, sore throat, menstrual cramps, headache:
• Steep 2 tbsp. of freshly shredded ginger in boiled water, bid to tid.
• Place a drop of ginger oil or a few slices of fresh rhizome in steaming water and inhale.
To relieve arthritis:
• Fresh ginger juice, extract, or tea, 2 to 4 g daily
• Use oil or fresh root in a warm poultice or compress and apply to painful areas. Place a drop of ginger oil in massage oil and rub into painful joints and muscles.

SIDE EFFECTS/TOXICOLOGY

American Herbal Products Association safety rating: fresh root, class 1 (safe with appropriate use); dried root, class 2b (not to be used during pregnancy). May cause mild heartburn.

WARNINGS/CONTRAINDICATIONS/PRECAUTIONS

Because ginger increases bile flow, gallstones contraindicate use.

The use of ginger to control morning sickness during pregnancy is controversial. Ginger obtained through food is not considered risky during pregnancy. Doses of 1 g dried ginger root to relieve morning sickness has not resulted in any reports of miscarriage or toxicity to either the fetus or the mother. The AHPA does not advise dried root during pregnancy.

Two Japanese studies showed in vitro mutagenicity for one of the pungent principles of ginger. Subsequent studies showed that risk to humans is diminished significantly by antimutagenic properties of other ginger constituents. Some Chinese sources claim that 20 to 28 g of ginger will cause miscarriage, presumably due to its effects on uterine smooth muscle tissue. Pregnant women are advised not to ingest more than normal dietary levels of ginger, such as those found in ginger ale, cookies, breads, and main dishes.

INTERACTIONS

In doses exceeding dietary intake, ginger may interfere with cardiac, anticoagulant, or antidiabetic medications due to in vitro actions on platelets and heart muscle and in vivo effects on blood sugar levels.

REGULATORY AND COMPENDIAL STATUS

Ginger is a GRAS (generally recognized as safe) food additive in the United States and the FDA categorizes it as a dietary supplement. Recently published United States Pharmacopeia (USP) Information Monographs do not recommend therapeutic use of ginger, citing insufficient scientific evidence; OTC approval by the FDA has not yet been granted. In England, ginger is licensed through the General Sales List, and in Germany it is approved as a nonprescription drug for dyspepsia and motion sickness by the Commission E.

REFERENCES

Awang DVC. Ginger. *Can Pharma J.* 1992:309–311.

Blumenthal M, ed. *The Complete German Commission E Monographs: Therapeutic Guide to Herbal Medicine.* Boston, Mass: Integrative Medicine Communications; 1998.

Blumenthal M, Riggins CW. *American Botanical Council's Popular Herbs in the U.S. Market: Therapeutic Monographs.* Austin, Texas: ABC; 1997:33–240.

Bremness L. Herbs. *The Visual Guide to More than 700 Herb Species from around the World.* London: Dorling Kindersley Limited; 1994.

Duke JA. *The Green Pharmacy.* Emmaus, Pa: Rodale Press; 1997.

USP publishes information monographs on ginger and valerian. *HerbalGram.* 1998;43:30, 57, 71.

Grontved A, et al. Ginger root against seasickness: a controlled trial on the open sea. *Acta Otolaryngol.* 1988;105:45-49.

Kowalchik C, Hylton W, ed. *Rodale's Illustrated Encyclopedia of Herbs.* Emmaus, Pa: Rodale Press; 1998.

McGuffin M, Hobbs C, Upton R, Goldberg A, eds. *American Herbal Products Association's Botanical Safety Handbook.* Boca Raton, Fla: CRC Press; 1997.

Nagabhushan M, Amonkar AJ, Bhide SV. Mutagenicity of gingerol and shogaol and antimutagenicity of zingerone in salmonella/microsome assay. *Cancer Lett.* 1987;36:221-233.

Nakamura H, Yamamoto T. Mutagen and anti-mutagen in ginger, *Zingiber officinale. Mutat Res.* 1982;103:119-126.

Newall CA, Anderson LA, Phillipson JD. *Herbal Medicines: A Guide for Health-care Professionals.* London: The Pharmaceutical Press; 1996:157–159.

Schulick P. The many roles of ginger. *Natural Foods Merchandiser's Nutrition Science News.* 1995:6–7.

Schulz V, Hänsel R, Tyler VE. *Rational Phytotherapy: A Physicians' Guide to Herbal Medicine.* 3rd ed. Berlin, Germany: Springer; 1998.

Yeung H. *Handbook of Chinese Herbs and Formulas.* Los Angeles, Calif: Los Angeles Institute of Chinese Medicine; 1985:1.

■ GINKGO BILOBA
Ginkgo biloba (Botanical)
Ginkgoaceae (Plant Family)
Ginkgo folium (Pharmacopeial)

OVERVIEW
Ginkgo biloba is one of the oldest living tree species, existing even before the Ice Age. Although Chinese herbal medicine has used both the ginkgo leaf and seed for centuries, modern research has focused on the standardized *Ginkgo biloba* extract (GBE), which is produced from the leaves. This extract is highly concentrated and much more effective than any other use of the leaves. More than 400 published studies have been done on GBE, making it one of the best researched of all herbal medicines. In Germany and France it is the most frequently prescribed herbal medicine and is in the top five of all medical prescriptions written in those countries. GBE is a powerful aid to circulatory problems, particularly cerebral insufficiency and peripheral arterial insufficiency seen most often in the elderly. It has strong antioxidant properties as well, protecting both the central nervous system and the cardiovascular system from damage and the effects of aging.

GBE improves circulation by strengthening the vascular system and inhibiting platelet aggregation, preventing atherosclerosis, which leads to cerebral insufficiency, coronary artery disease, peripheral arterial insufficiency, and strokes. Cerebral insufficiency can cause much of the mental deterioration or dementia associated with aging, including memory loss, vertigo, tinnitus, disorientation, and depression. GBE has been shown to increase blood flow to the brain, resulting in a marked improvement for many patients. It is also used effectively to prevent the onset of mental deterioration for those approaching old age. In a few small studies, GBE seemed to slow and even stop the progress of Alzheimer's disease, particularly in the early stages.

Peripheral arterial insufficiency is caused by arterial narrowing or obstruction and its most common symptom is intermittent claudication, particularly in the calves. GBE has been shown to improve blood flow in the limbs and increase walking tolerance at levels much higher than standard medical treatments. Other peripheral vascular disorders that respond to GBE include diabetic peripheral vascular disease, Raynaud's phenomenon, acrocyanosis, and postphlebitis syndrome. Because of its ability to improve circulation, GBE is being studied as an aid for impotence caused by impaired blood flow. Recent studies have shown good results, which are probably due to GBE's ability to increase blood flow without changing systemic blood pressure. There is evidence that GBE may also reduce certain PMS symptoms, including fluid retention, vascular congestion, and breast tenderness.

MACRO DESCRIPTION
Ginkgo biloba is a deciduous tree that can live up to 1,000 years and grow to a height of 120 feet. It has short branches with shoots that have fan-shaped, bilobed leaves. The fruit has a strong, unpleasant odor and is inedible, with an edible inner seed. Once common in North America and Europe, the Ice Age destroyed all but remnants that survived in China. Now grown in Asia, Europe, and North America.

PART USED/PHARMACEUTICAL DESIGNATIONS
- Seeds
- Leaves

CONSTITUENTS/COMPOSITION
Ginkgo flavone glycosides (quercetin, kaempferol, isorhamnetine, proanthocyandins), several terpene molecules unique to ginkgo (ginkgolides and bilobalide), organic acids

COMMERCIAL PREPARATIONS
Ginkgo biloba extract standardized to contain 24% ginkgo flavone glycosides (50:1 extract) and 6% terpene lactones. (There are several different brands of GBE available in the United States, but almost all of the scientific and clinical studies have been performed on the original German formula.) Encapsulated herb and tincture are also available.

MEDICINAL USES/INDICATIONS
Traditional herbal actions: circulatory stimulant, antidepressant, antithrombotic

Clinical applications: intermittent claudication, allergies, dementia, vertigo, vascular fragility, short-term memory loss, headache, depression, stroke, poor circulation, atherosclerosis, cerebral vascular insufficiency, Alzheimer's disease, tinnitus, cochlear deafness, macular degeneration, diabetic retinopathy, peripheral arterial insufficiency, impotence, PMS, Raynaud's phenomenon

PHARMACOLOGY
GBE strengthens tissue by stabilizing cell membranes, acting as an antioxidant, and inhibiting free radical damage. It also aids cell use of oxygen and glucose. These properties are particularly important for brain cell tissue, which is most vulnerable to free radical damage and oxygen deprivation. Brain cells are also protected by GBE's ability to improve blood circulation to the brain, particularly the hippocampus and striatum, areas most affected by micro-embolization. GBE has also been shown to increase the rate of transmission of information to the nerve cell level, enhancing memory ability. These combined effects allow GBE to reverse mental deterioration caused by vascular insufficiency. The mental deterioration caused by Alzheimer's seems to be significantly delayed by GBE's ability to enhance brain function, along with normalizing the acetylcholine receptors in the hippocamus and increasing cholinergic transmission.

GBE strengthens the vascular system by focusing on two areas: vascular endothelium and the system that regulates blood vessel tone. As a vasodilator, it stimulates the release of endothelium-derived relaxing factor and prostacyclin. GBE also restricts an enzyme that causes blood vessels to relax and stimulates greater tone throughout the vessels.

GBE greatly influences platelet function by inhibiting platelet aggregation, platelet adhesion, and degranulation. Along with its powers as an antioxidant, this influence seems to come from GBE's ability to inhibit a substance known as platelet-activating factor (PAF). PAF stimulates platelet aggregation, and causes inflammation and allergic reactions by increasing vascular permeability, activation of neutrophil, smooth-muscle contractions including bronchoconstriction, and reducing coronary blood flow. Higher PAF levels are also associated with aging. Many of GBE's clinical results may come from its ability to inhibit PAF and its effects. The unique terpene lactones in GBE, particularly the ginkgolides, are thought to be the main source of this ability to inhibit PAF.

The terpene lactones in GBE (ginkgolides and bilobalide) also protect nerve cells from damage during periods of ischemia or hypoxia. This hypoxic tolerance is seen particularly in cerebral tissue, making GBE an effective treatment for people who have suffered strokes or transient ischemic attacks.

DOSAGE RANGES AND DURATION OF ADMINISTRATION

- Take 120 mg daily in two divided doses of 50:1 extract standardized to 24% flavone glycodises. Patients with more serious dementia or Alzheimer's disease may need to work up to 240 mg daily in two to three divided doses. Results often take four to six weeks, but should continue to accumulate. Some dramatic changes may not appear for six months.
- Capsules of dried herb with 10 mg standardized extract (1 to 3 capsules tid)
- Tincture (1:5): 2 to 4 ml tid
- Fluid extract (1:1): 1 to 3 ml tid

SIDE EFFECTS/TOXICOLOGY

GBE is very safe and side effects are rare. In a few cases, gastrointestinal upset, headaches, and dizziness were reported. GBE has been shown not to alter heart rate and blood pressure or to change cholesterol and triglyercides levels. Because it decreases platelet aggregation, there is some concern that ginkgo may increase risk of intracranial hemorrhage. Use with caution in conjunction with other blood-thinning agents (i.e. Coumadin).

WARNINGS/CONTRAINDICATIONS/PRECAUTIONS

The fruit of *Ginkgo biloba* should not be handled or ingested. Ingesting the seed can cause severe adverse effects. The German Commission E reports the only contraindication for GBE is a hypersensitivity to Ginkgo biloba preparations. There are no known contraindications for pregnancy, but pregnant or lactating women should exercise caution since there is a lack of studies showing GBE's effects during pregnancy.

INTERACTIONS

None known

REGULATORY AND COMPENDIAL STATUS

The German Commission E approves specific GBE extracts for use in treating dementia, peripheral arterial insufficiency, vertigo, and tinnitus.

REFERENCES

Bauer U. Six-month double-blind randomized clinical trial of *Ginkgo biloba* extract versus placebo in two parallel groups of patients suffering from peripheral arterial insufficiency. *Arzneimittelforschung.* 1984;34:716–720.

Blumenthal M, ed. *The Complete German Commission E Monographs: Therapeutic Guide to Herbal Medicines.* Boston, Mass: Integrative Medicine Communications; 1998.

Brown D. *Herbal Prescriptions for Better Health.* Rocklin, Calif: Prima Publishing; 1996.

Carper J. *Miracle Cures.* New York, NY: HarperCollins, 1997.

DeSmet PAGM, Keller K, Hänsel R, Chandler RF, eds. *Adverse Effects of Herbal Drugs.* Berlin, Germany: Springer-Verlag; 1997.

Kinghorn, A., Ed. *Human Medicinal Agents from Plants.* Washington, DC: American Chemical Society, 1993.

Le Bars PL, Katz MM, Berman N, Itil TM, Freedman AM, Schatzberg AF. A placebo-controlled, double-blind, randomized trial of an extract of *Ginkgo biloba* for dementia. *JAMA.* 1997;278:1327–1332.

Murray M. *The Healing Power of Herbs: The Enlightened Person's Guide to the Wonders of Medicinal Plants.* 2nd ed. Rocklin, Calif: Prima Publishing; 1995.

Newall C, et al. *Herbal Medicines: A Guide for Health-care Professionals.* London, England: Pharmaceutical Press; 1996.

Peters H, Kieser M, Holscher U. Demonstration of the efficacy of *Ginkgo biloba* special extract Egb 761 on intermittent claudication a placebo-controlled, double-blind trial. *Vasa.* 1998;27:105–110.

Schulz V, Hänsel R, Tyler VE. *Rational Phytotherapy: A Physicians' Guide to Herbal Medicine.* Berlin, Germany: Springer-Verlag; 1998.

■ AMERICAN GINSENG
Panax quinquefolium (Botanical)
Araliaceae (Plant Family)
Ginseng radix (Pharmacopeial)

OVERVIEW

American ginseng stimulates convalescence, rehabilitation, stamina and strength through actions that are similar to those of its more famous Asian cousin, *Panax ginseng*. In Asian countries, ginseng is regarded as the king of herbs and is added to many everyday items, including beverages. The Chinese associated ginseng with longevity, virility, strength, and wisdom as early as 1 A.D., according to written accounts. As long as the roots are five or six years old, at which time they contain suitable amounts of active plant chemicals, American ginseng is considered similar enough to Asian ginseng chemically to be used interchangeably.

Ginseng can be difficult to cultivate. It is susceptible to blights, needs loamy, high-humus soil, and prefers 70% shade. This difficulty made it a good export crop early on in American history, because it was plentiful here. In 1718, American ginseng brought five dollars a pound in Canton, China. In 1773, 55 tons of American ginseng were sold to the Chinese. By 1824, 380 tons were exported. Even Daniel Boone traded ginseng.

Ginseng is classified as an adaptogen and antioxidant. Adaptogens increase physiological resistance to stressors. Antioxidants function similarly, reducing the negative consequences of free radicals. Modern research shows that ginseng improves resistance to bacterial, viral, emotional, cognitive, muscular, metabolic, and cardiovascular stressors, and suggests a plethora of ginseng or ginseng constituent actions. While the elderly take it to diminish debility from age-related illness, others take it to enhance physical and cognitive performance. Ongoing studies are looking into ginseng for the treatment of cancer, diabetes, cardiovascular disease, non-AIDS related immune system depression, infertility, aging, and depression.

According to alternative medicine practitioners, American and Asian ginsengs are indicated in stress, fatigue, convalescence and diabetes, and Siberian ginseng in stress, fatigue, atherosclerosis, and impaired kidney function. Confusion regarding which ginseng to use for stress, fatigue, and convalescence (American, Asian, or Siberian) stems from the suggestion that active components in one type are superior to those in another type, e.g., ginsenosides versus eleutherosides. Such superiority has not been demonstrated. Early Russian studies indicated that Siberian ginseng's positive effects exceed those of Asian ginseng's. These results are supported by empirical reports, but are challenged by investigators who question the validity of the studies and the quality of the Siberian ginseng preparation. At this time, all three ginsengs are regarded as adaptogens, all three share contraindication and side effect profiles, and despite qualitative differences, each is used for similar indications. Cost, standardization, and the reputation of the manufacturer may be the deciding points in determining which product to use.

MACRO DESCRIPTION

After two years' growth the leaves are five-lobed and palmate; after a few more years, leaflets develop on prongs. Stem grows from a tap root and can reach up to 16 inches in height. Small, greenish-white flowers grow in clusters and produce red berries with two seeds.

Light beige, variably thick, gnarled root can appear similar in shape to the human body, and has offshoots with long stringy hairs that can look like arms and legs. The root is harvested at 4 to 6 years' age; age is determined by the numbers of wrinkles on the neck of the root. The crude drug is prepared from the lateral root and root hairs.

PART USED/PHARMACEUTICAL DESIGNATIONS

- Roots

CONSTITUENTS/COMPOSITION

Dried root contains ginsenosides (Rb1 as marker); polysaccharide glycans (quinquefolan A, B, and C)

COMMERCIAL PREPARATIONS

White ginseng (dried, peeled) is prepared as liquid extracts, powders, or capsules.

MEDICINAL USES/INDICATIONS

Traditional:
- Adaptogen
- Bitter tonic
- Restorative
- Alterative

Clinical applications:
- Diabetes
- Ulcer
- Edema
- Cancer
- Hypercholesterolemia
- Infertility
- Fatigue
- Frequent colds or viral illness
- Rehabilitation after acute illness
- To increase stamina and well being

PHARMACOLOGY

American ginseng reduces stress and fatigue and improves physical and mental function. In studies in humans, American ginseng improves cholesterol ratios, increases blood alcohol clearance, reduces liver toxicity, improves psychomotor performance, helps control asthma, lowers blood sugar levels, and regulates blood pressure and adrenocorticotropic hormone. Studies in humans also indicate that American ginseng may be used as adjunctive therapy in the treatment of diabetic neuropathy, reactive depression, psychologically-induced impotence, and psychological disorders in children. Many of these studies involve other species of ginseng, in particular, *Panax ginseng* (Asian ginseng). However, while further study is needed for clarification, the two species do exert similar actions.

Non-insulin-dependant diabetes is perhaps the condition most often used to study the effects of constituents specific to American ginseng. The polysaccharide glycans, quinquefolans A, B, and C are hypoglycemic in mice. Ginsenoside Rb1 reduces concentrations of islet insulin to practically nothing.

DOSAGE RANGES AND DURATION OF ADMINISTRATION

White ginseng standardized to 0.03% ginsenosides, designated as Rb1.The recommended dose is: 1 to 2 g fresh root, 0.6 to 2 g dried root, or 200 to 600 mg liquid extract daily. Healthy persons using

American ginseng for enhanced physical or mental performance or to improve resistance to stressors should take these doses in cycles of 15 to 20 days followed by two-week breaks.

For rehabilitation after an illness, the elderly should take 0.5 g bid 2 for three months; or, take 0.5 g bid for one month, followed by a two-month break, and repeat cycle if desired.

SIDE EFFECTS/TOXICOLOGY

American ginseng is not considered to have side effects when used at the recommended daily dose.

The American Herbal Products Association (AHPA) rates American ginseng as class 2d: 2d indicates that specific restrictions apply; hypertension is the specific restriction.

WARNINGS/CONTRAINDICATIONS/PRECAUTIONS

Similar contraindications to those for Asian ginseng may be applicable to American ginseng: patients with acute illness, cardiovascular disease, diabetes, or blood pressure disorders should use caution when taking ginseng. Pregnant women should not take ginseng because its safety during pregnancy has not been determined.

American ginseng is currently on the United Plant Savers (UpS) at-risk list, meaning that the species is endangered due to overharvesting or lack of habitat. Wisconsin currently produces the most ginseng, which is still sent primarily to China. In 1905 the state passed a law that made it illegal to dig ginseng roots until after they've been allowed to set seed (August 1). Poaching roots and spreading fungus from cultivated to wild crops are as much of a threat to the species as is overharvesting.

INTERACTIONS

American ginseng may increase the effects of caffeine or other stimulants as well as phenelzine (Nardil), antipsychotics, or blood pressure, anti-diabetic, or steroidal medications.

REGULATORY AND COMPENDIAL STATUS

The U.S. FDA classifies ginseng as a dietary supplement. In Germany, Asian ginseng root is approved with nonprescription status, and in the United Kingdom it is licensed on the General Sales List.

REFERENCES

Bahrke M, Morgan P. Evaluation of the ergogenic properties of ginseng. *Sports Medicine.* 1994;18:229–248.

Blumenthal M, ed. *The Complete German Commission E Monographs.* Boston, Mass: Integrative Medicine Communications; 1998.

Blumenthal M, Riggins C. *Popular Herbs in the U.S. Market: Therapeutic Monographs.* Austin, Tex: The American Botanical Council; 1997.

Chen X, et al. The effects of Panax quinquefolium saponin (PQS) and its monomer ginsenoside on heart. *Chung Kuo Chung Yao Tsa Chih.* 1994;19:617–20, 640.

Foster S. *Herbal Renaissance: Growing, Using and Understanding Herbs in the Modern World.* Salt Lake City, Utah: Gibbs-Smith; 1993.

Huang KC. *The Pharmacology of Chinese Herbs.* Boca Raton, Fla: CRC Press; 1993.

Kowalchik C, Hylton W, eds. *Rodale's Illustrated Encyclopedia of Herbs.* Emmaus, Pa: Rodale Press; 1998.

Kwan CY. Vascular effects of selected antihypertensive drugs derived from traditional medicinal herbs. *Clin Exp Pharmacol Physiol.* 1995;(suppl 1):S297–S299. Review.

Li J, et al. Panax quinquefolium saponins protects low density lipoproteins from oxidation. *Life Sci.* 1999;64:53–62.

McGuffin M, Hobbs C, Upton R, Goldberg A. *American Herbal Products Association's Botanical Safety Handbook.* Boca Raton, Fla: CRC Press; 1996.

Murphy LL, et al. Effect of American ginseng (Panax quinquefolium) on male copulatory behavior in the rat. *Physiol Behav.* 1998;64:445–450.

Murray M. *The Healing Power of Herbs: the Enlightened Person's Guide to the Wonders of Medicinal Plants.* Rocklin, Calif: Prima Publishing; 1995.

Newall CA, Anderson LA, Phillipson JD. *Herbal Medicines: A Guide for Health Care Professionals.* London, England: The Pharmaceutical Press; 1996.

Oshima Y. Isolation and hypoglycemic activity of quinquefolans A, B, and C, glycans of *Panax quinquefolium* roots. J Nat Prod. 1987;50:188–190.

Schultz V, Hansel R, Tyler V. *Rational Phytotherapy: A Physician's Guide to Herbal Medicine.* New York, NY: Springer; 1998.

Thornton L. The ethics of wildcrafting. *The Herb Quarterly.* 1998:41–46.

Waki I. Effects of a hypoglycemic component of Ginseng radix on insulin biosynthesis in normal and diabetic animals. *J Pharmacobiodyn.* 1982;5:547–554.

Yuan CS, et al. Modulation of American ginseng on brainstem GABAergic effects in rats. *J Ethnopharmacol.* 1998;62:215–222.

■ ASIAN GINSENG
Panax ginseng (Botanical)
Araliaceae (Plant Family)
Ginseng radix (Pharmacopeial)

OVERVIEW

Ginseng is recommended to help the body recover from disease, and to improve mental and physical performance. Benefits attributed to it from over 2,000 years of use have been discussed in numerous studies. In Asian countries, ginseng is regarded as the king of herbs and is added to many every day items, including beverages. The Chinese have associated ginseng with longevity, virility, strength, and wisdom since at least 1 A.D., according to written accounts.

The scientific name given to ginseng by Swedish botanist Carl Linnaeus in 1753 uses the Greek words *pan* (all) and *ax* (akos; cure) to mean the root that cures all ills. More recently, ginseng is classified as an adaptogen and antioxidant. Adaptogens are substances that increase physiological resistance to stressors. Antioxidants function similarly, decreasing circulating free radicals and reducing their negative effects on the body. Modern research shows that ginseng increases the body's ability to fight against bacterial, viral, emotional, cognitive, muscular, metabolic, and cardiovascular stressors.

Elderly persons take ginseng to induce a feeling of well-being, increase stamina, and combat the negative physical and mental effects of recent or chronic age-related degenerative conditions. Younger persons take it to increase athletic strength and sexual virility and to improve intellectual performance. Ongoing studies are looking into the effects of ginseng as adjunctive therapy for cancer, diabetes, cardiovascular disease, non–AIDS related immune system disorders, male and female infertility, aging, menopause, and depression.

American and Asian ginsengs are indicated in stress, fatigue, convalescence and diabetes, and Siberian ginseng in stress, fatigue, atherosclerosis, and impaired kidney function. Confusion regarding which ginseng to use for stress, fatigue, and convalescence (American, Asian, or Siberian) stems from the suggestion that active components in one type are superior to those in another type, e.g., ginsenosides versus eleutherosides. Such superiority has not been demonstrated. Early Russian studies indicated that Siberian ginseng's positive effects exceed those of Asian ginseng's. These results are supported by empirical reports, but are challenged by investigators who question the validity of the studies and the quality of the Siberian ginseng preparation. At this time, all three ginsengs are regarded as adaptogens, all three share contraindication and side effect profiles, and despite qualitative differences, each is used for similar indications.
Cost, standardization, and the reputation of the manufacturer may be the deciding points in determining which product to use.

MACRO DESCRIPTION

The ginseng root is harvested at 4 to 6 years' age. Mature herbaceous plants bear five-lobed palmate leaves, which circle a stem that grows from a tap root and can reach up to 16 inches in height. At the fourth year, the plant produces a small, greenish-white umbel-shaped flower cluster at the junction of the leaves and stem. These produce red berries.

Light beige, variably thick, gnarled root can appear similar in shape to the human body and has offshoots with long stringy hairs that can look like arms and legs. Age is determined by the numbers of wrinkles around the neck of the root. The crude drug is prepared from the lateral root and root hairs.

PART USED/PHARMACEUTICAL DESIGNATIONS

• Roots

CONSTITUENTS/COMPOSITION

Dried root contains at least 1.5% ginsenosides (Rg1 as marker); glycans (panaxans) up to 0.05% volatile oil; polysaccharide fraction DPG-3-2; peptides; and maltol.

COMMERCIAL PREPARATIONS

White ginseng (dried, peeled) or red ginseng (unpeeled root steamed before drying) is prepared as aqueous, aqueous-alcohol or alcohol liquid extracts, and as powders or capsules.

MEDICINAL USES/INDICATIONS

Traditional: adaptogen, tonic, restorative, alterative, anodyne, appetite-stimulant, aphrodisiac, antidepressant, cardiotonic, carminative, expectorant, hormone restorative, nervine, sedative, sialogogue, stimulant, stomachic.

Clinical applications: Rehabilitation; to increase stamina and well-being, particularly in the elderly. German Commission E monograph describes ginseng as a "tonic to counteract weakness and fatigue, as a restorative for declining stamina and impaired concentration, and as an aid to convalescence." Also used to treat diabetes, ulcer, edema, cancer, hypercholesterolemia, infertility, fatigue, frequent colds or viral illness, menopause, and red blood cell depletion.

PHARMACOLOGY

In 37 clinical studies published between 1968 and 1990, ginseng improved physical and cognitive performance, mood, or metabolism.
Still other studies suggest a plethora of ginseng actions.
- ginseng improves cholesterol ratios
- elevates blood alcohol clearance
- reduces liver toxicity
- improves psychomotor performance
- helps control asthma and chronic respiratory disease (200 mg per day improved respiratory strength, oxygenation capacity, and walking distance in chronic respiratory disease patients)
- lowers blood sugar levels
- regulates blood pressure and adrenocorticotropic hormone
- enhances athletic stamina.

Studies in humans also indicate that ginseng may be used as adjunctive therapy in the treatment of diabetic neuropathy, reactive depression, psychologically-induced impotence, and psychological disorders in children.

Asian ginseng stimulates the central nervous system, neurotransmitters, oxygen metabolism, and glycogen stores. Antidiabetic effects may be due to hypoglycemic actions of panaxans and ginseng polysaccharide fraction DPG-3-2. Virility may be related to increases in both male and female hormones in gonads. The beneficial effects of ginseng in treating cardiovascular disease may be due to decreases in serum levels of cholesterol, triglyceride, and fatty acids, and increases in high-density lipoprotein.

Studies in mice have shown that ginseng elevates antibody levels, improves cell-mediated immunity and natural-killer-cell activity, lymphocytes, phagocytosis, in vitro; stimulates interferon production in the spleen. Polysaccharides in leaves and roots enhance macrophage binding. Also in mice, ginseng extracts inhibit DMBA-, urethane-, and aflatoxin B1-induced tumors; injections of ginseng administered along with radiation prevent radiation-induced bone marrow death and increase liver cell recovery. Ginseng also stimulates red blood cell formation in bone marrow.

DOSAGE RANGES AND DURATION OF ADMINISTRATION

White or red ginseng standardized to 1.5% ginsenosides, designated as Rg1. The recommended dose is 1 to 2 g fresh root, or 0.6 to 2 g dried root, or 200 to 600 mg liquid extract daily. Healthy persons using ginseng for enhanced physical or mental performance or to improve resistance to stressors should take these doses in cycles of 15 to 20 days followed by two-week breaks.

For rehabilitation after an illnes, the elderly should take 0.5 g bid for three months; or take 0.5 g bid for one month, followed by a two-month break, and repeat cycle if desired.

SIDE EFFECTS/TOXICOLOGY

The German Commission E cites no adverse effects with recommended daily dose. Agitation, addiction, changes in blood pressure, or "Ginseng Abuse Syndrome" are no longer associated with the normal use of ginseng. Adulterants, such as caffeine, are thought to cause these effects; NSAID adulterants may cause ginseng-associated Stevens–Johnson syndrome.

The American Herbal Products Association (AHPA) rates ginseng as a class 2d herb. 2d indicates that specific restrictions apply; in the case of ginseng, hypertension is the specific restriction.

WARNINGS/CONTRAINDICATIONS/PRECAUTIONS

Patients with acute illness, cardiovascular disease, diabetes, or blood pressure disorders should use caution when taking ginseng. Pregnant women should not take ginseng because its safety during pregnancy has not been determined.

INTERACTIONS

Red ginseng may increase the effects of caffeine or other stimulants. Any ginseng product may increase the effects of phenelzine (Nardil) or other antipsychotics, or blood pressure, antidiabetic or steroidal medications.

REGULATORY AND COMPENDIAL STATUS

The U.S. FDA classifies ginseng as a dietary supplement. In Germany the ginseng root is approved with nonprescription status, and in the United Kingdom it is licensed on the General Sales List.

REFERENCES

Bahrke M, Morgan P. Evaluation of the ergogenic properties of ginseng. *Sports Medicine.* 1994;18:229–248.

Blumenthal M, ed. *The Complete German Commission E Monographs.* Boston, Mass: Integrative Medicine Communications; 1998.

Blumenthal M, Riggins C. *Popular Herbs in the U.S. Market: Therapeutic Monographs.* Austin, Tex: The American Botanical Council; 1997.

Choi HK, Seong DH, Rha KH. Clinical Efficacy of Korean red ginseng for erectile dysfunction. *Int J Impotence Res.* 1995;7:181–186.

D'Angelo L, et al. A double-blind, placebo-controlled clinical study on the effect of a standardized ginseng extract on psychomotor performance in healthy volunteer. *J Ethnopharmacol.* 1986;16:15–22.

Dega H, Laporte JL, Frances C, Herson S, Chosidow O. Ginseng as a cause for Stevens-Johnson Syndrome? *Lancet.* 1996;347:1344.

De Smet PAGM, Keller K, Hansel R, Chandler RF, eds. *Adverse Effects of Herbal Drugs.* New York, NY: Springer-Verlag; 1992:1.

Dorling E. Do ginsenosides influence the performance? Results of a double-blind study. *Notabene medici.* 1980;10:241–246.

Foster S. *Asian Ginseng.* Austin, Tex: The American Botanical Council; 1996.

Gross D, Krieger D, Efrat R, Dayan M. Ginseng extract G115 for the treatment of chronic respiratory diseases. *Schweizerische Zeitschrift fur Ganzheits Medizin.* 1995;1(95):29–33.

Huang KC. *The Pharmacology of Chinese Herbs.* Boca Raton, Fla: CRC Press; 1993.

Kowalchik C, Hylton W, eds. *Rodale's Illustrated Encyclopedia of Herbs.* Emmaus, Pa: Rodale Press; 1998.

McGuffin M, Hobbs C, Upton R, Goldberg A. *American Herbal Products Association's Botanical Safety Handbook.* Boca Raton, Fla: CRC Press; 1996.

Murray M. *The Healing Power of Herbs: the Enlightened Person's Guide to the Wonders of Medicinal Plants.* Rocklin, Calif: Prima Publishing; 1995.

Newall CA, Anderson LA, Phillipson JD. *Herbal Medicines: A Guide for Health Care Professionals.* London, England: The Pharmaceutical Press; 1996.

Quiroga HA, Imbriano AE. The effect of *Panax ginseng* extract on cerebrovascular deficits. *Orientacion Medica.* 1979;1208:86–87.

Quiroga HA. Comparative double-blind study of the effect of Ginsana Gii5 and Hydergin on cerebrovascular deficits. *Orientacion Medica.* 1982;1281:201–202.

Choi HK, Seong DH, Rha KH. Clinical efficacy of Korean red ginseng for erectile dysfunction. *Int J Impotence Res.* 1995;7:181-186.

Schultz V, Hansel R, Tyler V. *Rational Phytotherapy: A Physician's Guide to Herbal Medicine.* New York, NY: Springer; 1998.

Sun XB, Matsumoto T, Yamada H. Purification of immune complexes clearance enhancing polysaccharide from the leaves of *Panax ginseng*, and its biological activities. *Phytomedicine.* 1994;1:225–231.

Tang W, Eisenbrand G. *Chinese Drugs of Plant Origin: Chemistry, Pharmacology, and Use in Traditional and Modern Medicine.* New York, NY: Springer; 1992.

You JS, Hau DM, Chen KT, Huang HF. Combined effects of ginseng and radiotherapy on experimental liver cancer. *Phytotherapy Research.* 1995;9:331–335.

■ SIBERIAN GINSENG

Eleutherococcus senticosus/Acanthopanax senticosus (Botanical)
Araliaceae (Plant Family)
Eleutherococci radix (Pharmacopeial)

OVERVIEW

Explored in the 1950s as an alternative to Asian ginseng, which was expensive and difficult to grow, Siberian ginseng is used today to increase physical and mental stamina, speed convalescence, and provide resistance to the detrimental effects of stress. Mirroring the functions of Asian and American ginseng, these uses also reflect thousands of years' use by the people of Russia and China.

All three types of ginseng occur in the same plant family, Araliaceae. While their constituents differ, studies conducted in Russia since the late 1950s conclude that like its distant cousins, Siberian ginseng has similar adaptogenic functions. Adaptogens increase physiologic resistance to stressors. They also normalize processes within the body that may have been altered in response to those stressors, and are nontoxic and nonspecific in action. By 1985, studies of Siberian ginseng conducted in the Soviet Union, with the involvement of over 4,300 healthy and diseased subjects, confirmed these effects. In 1962, consequent to approval of 33% alcohol Siberian ginseng extract for human use by the Pharmacological Committee of USSR Ministry of Health, 3 million Soviets were estimated to be taking it regularly. Among these were Soviet astronauts and Olympic team members. Ongoing studies are looking into the effects of ginseng in terms of its adjunctive therapeutic use for diabetes, infertility, atherosclerosis and rheumatic heart disease, cancer, and conditions due to depressed immune function, such as chronic fatigue syndrome.

American and Asian ginsengs are indicated in stress, fatigue, convalescence and diabetes, and Siberian ginseng in stress, fatigue, atherosclerosis, and impaired kidney function. Confusion regarding which ginseng to use for stress, fatigue, and convalescence (American, Asian, or Siberian) stems from the suggestion that active components in one type are superior to those in another type, e.g., ginsenosides versus eleutherosides. Such superiority has not been demonstrated. Early Russian studies indicated that Siberian ginseng's positive effects exceed those of Asian ginseng's. These results are supported by empirical reports, but are challenged by investigators who question the validity of the studies and the quality of the Siberian ginseng preparation. At this time, all three ginsengs are regarded as adaptogens, all three share contraindication and side effect profiles, and despite qualitative differences, each is used for similar indications. Cost, standardization, and the reputation of the manufacturer may be the deciding points in determining which product to use.

MACRO DESCRIPTION

Siberian ginseng is cultivated from a shrub that grows one to three meters in height. Palmate leaves with five serrated, thorny-veined leaflets are attached to long petioles that are covered with bristles. Petioles are attached to stems, which are noted for their backward-pointing prickles. Stem bark is gray-brown.

Flowers grow in umbels from a peduncle; male flowers are violet, female flowers, yellow. These produce round black berries.

The Siberian ginseng root is 1.5 to 4 cm long, brown to brownish gray, with lengthwise wrinkles. It is twisted, variably branched with a few rootlets. It smells aromatic and tastes bitter and astringent.

PART USED/PHARMACEUTICAL DESIGNATIONS

• Roots

CONSTITUENTS/COMPOSITION

Root contains 0.6% to 0.9% eleutheroside components common to many plant species. Many are glycosides. Eleutheroside A is a sterol (daucosterol); B is a phenylopropanoid (syringin); B_1 (isofraxidin) and B_3 are coumarins; C is a monosaccharide (methyl-alpha-D-galactoside); B_4, D, and E (acanthoside D) are lignans; and I, K, L, and M are triterpene saponins. Root also contains aglycones, polysaccharide glycans (eleuthocans A-G) and various sugars, phenylpropanoids, oleanolic acid, dihydroxybenzoic acid (DBA), and volatile oil.

COMMERCIAL PREPARATIONS

• Crude drug (bark, whole root and rhizome)
• Aqueous-alcohol liquid extracts
• Solid extracts
• Powders
• Capsules
• Tablets

MEDICINAL USES/INDICATIONS

Traditional:
• Stimulant
• Tonic
• Diuretic
• To treat insomnia
• To enhance virility
• To increase the body's resistance to stress

Clinical applications:
• Stress
• Fatigue
• Atherosclerosis
• Impaired kidney function
• Lower back/kidney pain
• Anorexia
• Rheumatoid arthritis
• Chronic fatigue syndrome
• Blood pressure disorders
• Symptoms of coronary arteriosclerosis
• Symptoms of radiotherapy- and chemotherapy-induced leukopenia
• ADHD
• Debility
• Diminished capacity for work or concentration
• To help during convalescence

PHARMACOLOGY

Siberian ginseng has normalizing, stress-resistant, and immune stimulant effects. In studies involving over 4,300 subjects, Siberian ginseng was administered orally to determine its effects on disease, or to assess its ability to help the body tolerate stress. Subjects who had atherosclerosis, pyelonephritis, diabetes mellitus, hypertension, hypotension, craniocerebral trauma, neurosis, rheumatic heart disease, chronic bronchitis, and pulmonary tuberculosis noted overall improvements in their condition. Healthy subjects in these studies were exposed to extremes in temperature, sound, working conditions, exercise, and deep-sea diving decompression. They noted enhanced physical labor and stamina, mental concentration and acuity. They were better able to tolerate to extreme conditions, had improved capillary function, and improved resistance to hypoxemia. New blood formation was enhanced in blood donors. In both healthy and non-healthy subjects, a 33% alcohol extract was used, for up to 39 days followed by a two-to-three week break if the study was to be continued.

Immune stimulant effects, noted through increases in lymphocyte count (particularly T-lymphocytes) were reported in a double-blind, placebo-controlled study of healthy subjects.

In studies in animals, Siberian ginseng polysaccharides were immunostimulating. Intraperitoneal injection resulted in eleutheran-stimulated hypoglycemia in alloxan-induced hyperglycemic mice. DBACK reduced collagen- and ADP- induced platelet aggregation comparably to aspirin.

Infusions of Siberian ginseng increased stress resistance in rats and improved work performance in mice. Intraperitoneal injections increased gonadotrophic action in both male and female mice. Mineralcorticoid, glucocorticoid, and steroid receptor binding was observed. Siberian ginseng had sedative and CNS stimulant effects, and caused both increases and reduction in barbiturate sleeping time. It was antileukemic and reduced toxicity caused by antitumor and antileukimic agents (rybromycin, thio-TEPA, Dopan, 6-mercaptopurine, cyclophosan, ethymidine, benzo-TEPA, sarcolysin; chlorofos s.c., malonic acid).

DOSAGE RANGES AND DURATION OF ADMINISTRATION

- Dried root (tea, or in capsules): 2 to 3 g daily or equivalent preparations
- Tincture: 5 ml tid
- 33% aqueous-alcohol extract, 2 to 4 ml, one to three times daily
- Solid extract (dried, powdered), with at least 1% eleutheroside F: 100 to 200 mg tid

Note: Take before 3 P.M. to avoid insomnia; A three-month course, followed by a two-to-three week Siberian ginseng–free interval, or occasional use for one month, followed by two-month Siberian ginseng–free intervals, should be observed.

SIDE EFFECTS/TOXICOLOGY

American Herbal Products Association safely rating: class 1 (safe with appropriate use); German Commission E lists no side effects. High doses (4.5 to 5 ml tid) may cause insomnia, irritability, melancholy, anxiety; in studies conducted in the Soviet Union, some patients with rheumatic heart disease noted pericardial pain, high blood pressure, headaches, and palpitations.

WARNINGS/CONTRAINDICATIONS/PRECAUTIONS

Hypertension (>180/90 mm Hg) contraindicates use. Although studies in animals suggest Siberian ginseng is nonteratogenic, its safety during pregnancy has not been determined.

INTERACTIONS

Siberian ginseng may potentiate the effects of caffeine and other stimulants and should not be taken with antipsychotic drugs, steroids, or hormones.

REGULATORY AND COMPENDIAL STATUS

U.S. FDA: dietary supplement; German Commission E: approved for non-prescription use; not licensed through the General Sales List in the United Kingdom.

REFERENCES

Asano K, et al. Effect of *Eleutherococcus senticosus* extract on human physical working capacity. *Planta Medica.* 1986;3:175–177.

Awang D. Siberian ginseng toxicity may be case of mistaken identity. *Can Med Assoc J.* 1996;155:1237.

Blumenthal M, Riggins C. *Popular Herbs in the U.S. Market: Therapeutic Monographs.* Austin, Tex: The American Botanical Council; 1997.

Blumenthal M, ed. *The Complete German Commission E Monographs.* Boston, Mass: Integrative Medicine Communications; 1998.

Farnsworth N, Wagner H, Kikino H. *Economic and Medicinal Plant Research.* London, England: Academic Press Inc; 1985:1.

Foster S. *Siberian Ginseng (Eleutherococcus senticosus).* Austin, Tex: American Botanical Council; 1990.

Hacker B, Medon P. Cytotoxic effects of *E. sentococcus aqueous* extract against L1210 leukemia cells. *J Pharm Sci.* 1984;73:270–272.

Hebel S, ed. Eleutherococcus. *The Lawrence Review of Natural Products.* Facts and Comparisons; 1996:1–3.

Kaloeva ZD. Effect of glycosides from *Eleutherococcus senticosus* on the parameters of hemodynamics in patients with hypotension. *Farmakol Toksikol.* 1986;49:73.

Leung A, Foster S. *Encyclopedia of Common Natural Ingredients Used in Food, Drugs, and Cosmetics.* 2nd ed. New York, NY: John Wiley & Sons, Inc; 1996.

McGuffin M, Hobbs C, Upton R, Goldberg A. *American Herbal Products Association's Botanical Safety Handbook.* Boca Raton, Fla: CRC Press; 1996.

Murray M. *The Healing Power of Herbs: the Enlightened Person's Guide to the Wonders of Medicinal Plants.* Rocklin, Calif: Prima Publishing; 1995.

Newall CA, Anderson LA, Phillipson JD. *Herbal Medicines: A Guide for Health Care Professionals.* London, England: The Pharmaceutical Press; 1996.

Novozhilov GN, Sil'chenko KI. The mechanism of adaptogenic action of *Eleutherococcus senticosus* extract on the human body under thermal stress. *Fiziol Cheloveka.* 1985;11:303–306.

Schultz V, Hansel R, Tyler V. *Rational Phytotherapy: A Physician's Guide to Herbal Medicine.* New York, NY: Springer; 1998.

Wu Jia Seng: Acanthopanax senticosus [in Chinese]. Heilungkiang Institute of Traditional Chinese Medicine. [No date].

Xiao, P-G. et al. Immunological aspects of Chinese medicinal plants as antiaging drugs. *J Ethnopharmacol.* 1993;38:167–175.

■ GOLDENSEAL
Hydrastis canadensis (Botanical)
Ranunculaceae (Plant Family)
Hydrastis rhizoma (Pharmacopeial)

OVERVIEW

Goldenseal was originally a Native American medicinal herb, introduced to early settlers by Cherokee and Iroquois tribes. They used it as a yellow dye, as well as a wash for skin diseases and sore eyes, and various forms of catarrh. It has acquired a considerable reputation as a general bitter tonic, anti-infective, and remedy for various gastric and genitourinary disorders. In recent years it has been over-harvested and is now considered a threatened species. Fortunately, commercial cultivation has alleviated the shortage, but it is still quite expensive.

Goldenseal is an herb that is particularly applicable to disorders and infections of the mucous membranes. It is thought to strengthen the immune system, potentiate the effects of insulin, and cleanse the system. Extensive laboratory research has shown that the alkaloid constituents of goldenseal possess anti-inflammatory and antibiotic properties. One of the main ingredients in goldenseal, berberine, has been shown to have activity against a broad range of microbes, from trichomonas to giardia to candida to tapeworms.

Goldenseal is considered by naturopathic physicians to be astringent and healing to the gut wall and other mucous membranes, making it useful for disorders of the intestine and stomach. It also is considered to act as a digestive stimulant and cholagogue, a laxative, and as a stimulating adjunct to other remedies for the lungs, kidneys, and reproductive tract. Goldenseal may be especially useful for congestion and chronic inflammation of the respiratory and urogenital tracts; catarrhal affliction of the nose; chronic gastritis and enteritis; catarrh of the bladder; hepatic congestion; eye inflammation; inflammation of the vagina, uterus, and urethra; chronic constipation; hemorrhoids; and anal fissures.

Externally, goldenseal is valuable for chronic inflammation of mucous membranes, cracks and fissures of the nipples, indolent ulcers, and as a lotion to stop profuse sweating. It is also useful as an eyewash.

MACRO DESCRIPTION

Goldenseal is a small perennial plant, with a single hairy stem producing two five-lobed, serrated leaves and a small single apetalous flower with greenish sepals. These give way to a raspberry-like fruit. The rhizome is a bright yellow-brown in color, twisted, and wrinkled with many fine rootlets attached. This breaks easily to reveal a dark yellow interior. The taste is bitter. Goldenseal can be found growing wild in rich, shady woodlands throughout northern North America. It is now also commercially cultivated.

PART USED/PHARMACEUTICAL DESIGNATIONS

- Root/rhizomes

CONSTITUENTS/COMPOSITION

Alkaloids: berberine, canadine, corypalmine, hydrastine, reticuline
Also contains: tannins, vitamins, minerals

COMMERCIAL PREPARATIONS

Goldenseal is available in the following forms.
- Dried root/rhizomes
- Tablets, various concentrations
- Powdered root in capsules, various concentrations
- Alcoholic tinctures
- Low-alcohol extracts

MEDICINAL USES/INDICATIONS

Traditional herbal actions: cholagogue, astringent, digestive bitter, vulnerary (heats ulcerated surfaces internally and externally), laxative, anti-pathogenic
Clinical applications:
- For gastric and enteric inflammations (e.g., gastritis, enteritis, diarrhea, peptic ulcers)
- Useful for colds, flu, and glandular swelling
- Acts as a cholagogue, improves digestion and reduces food sensitivities
- May be helpful in diabetes
- Used as a nasal infusion to reduce excess mucous
- As external application for lacerations, abrasions, abscesses, boils, and other skin eruptions
- As a rinse for throat, gum, and mouth inflammation or sores, use extract or tincture as mouthwash, or prepare a rinse as follows: In 1 cup of warm water, mix 1/4 tsp. salt and 1/2 tsp., or the contents of 1 capsule of goldenseal powder. (It will not dissolve completely.)
- For vaginal problems, use tea or extract, or the rinse described above as a douche. (Strain out suspended particles before using.)
- For middle-ear inflammation and congestion, mix with olive oil and use several drops in each ear.
- For mild conjunctivitis or eye irritation, use sterile water to make the rinse above and use as eyewash. (Discard if the solution becomes cloudy, indicating bacterial growth.)

■ PHARMACOLOGY

- Antibiotic, anti-infective: Berberine has been shown to have antibacterial, antifungal, and antiprotozoal properties. It has been shown to inhibit the growth of *Giardia lamblia, Trichomonas vaginalis,* and *Entamoeba histolytica* in culture, as well as numerous other bacteria and microorganisms, including *Candida, C. vibrio,* and trypanosomes. It may also be an immune stimulant. Hydrastine has been found to kill tapeworms, and also has bactericidal properties. Reticuline has bactericidal properties as well.
- Anti-diabetic/hypoglycemic: Berberine is known to be effective in lowering blood glucose.
- Anti-diarrheal: Berberine has been shown to have antidiarrheal properties. In addition to its antimicrobial properties, laboratory studies have shown that it can halt the excessive intestinal secretion of electrolytes caused by endotoxins from bacteria such as *E. coli.*
- Anti-inflammatory/analgesic: Berberine has been found to have anti-inflammatory properties. One study found that this may arise in part from the inhibition of DNA-synthesis in activated lymphocytes. Berberine and reticuline both have analgesic and antispasmodic properties. Berberine and corypalmine are both antioxidant, which may also help reduce inflammation.
- Carminative and cholagogue: Berberine has both carminative and cholagogic actions.

DOSAGE RANGES AND DURATION OF ADMINISTRATION

- Tincture (1:5): 60% alcohol .5 to 1.5 ml tid
- Tablets or powder/capsules: 0.5 to 2 g tid

- Tea, 1/4 tsp. to 1/2 tsp. powdered root per cup, steeped 10 minutes. Up to 2 cups/day.
- Extract: 0.03 to 0.12 g tid

SIDE EFFECTS/TOXICOLOGY

In very large doses, goldenseal may cause convulsions and over-stimulation of the nervous system. Long-term use of high dosages have caused elevated white blood cell counts. Signs of toxicity take the form of irritation of the mouth and throat, diarrhea, and vomiting. Ulceration can occur internally and externally with severe overdosing.

WARNINGS/CONTRAINDICATIONS/PRECAUTIONS

- Not recommended for use in pregnancy—contains berberine which has abortifacient properties.
- Not recommended for use in presence of hypertension.
- Long-term use may weaken the beneficial bacterial flora of the digestive tract. Acidophilus capsules or yogurt should therefore be taken to restore proper balance of probiotic flora.
- Extended consumption of large amounts of this herb have been shown to lower B vitamin absorption and utilization.

INTERACTIONS

There is debate as to whether goldenseal acts as a brain tonic when combined with gotu kola.

REGULATORY AND COMPENDIAL STATUS

Goldenseal has been officially recognized by most Western pharmacopeias.

However, a federal interagency committee has recommended that the National Toxicology Program review and possibly test goldenseal for its potential to cause developmental problems or cancer of the reproductive system or both.

REFERENCES

Balch J, Balch P. *Prescription for Nutritional Healing: A-to-Z Guide to Drug-Free Remedies Using Vitamins, Minerals, Herbs, & Food Supplements.* New York, NY: Avery Publishing Group; 1990.

Duke JA. *Handbook of Phytochemical Constituents of GRAS Herbs and Other Economic Plants.* Boca Raton, Fla: CRC Press; 1992.

Foster S. Goldenseal. *American Botanical Council: Botanical Series No. 309.*

Genest K, Hughes DW. Natural products in Canadian pharmaceuticals, *Hydrastis canadensis. Can J Pharm Sci.* 1969;4.

Kaneda Y, Tanaka T, Saw T. Effects of berberine, a plant alkaloid, on the growth of anaerobic protozoa in axenic culture. *Tokai J Exp Clin Med.* 1990;15:417–423.

Mills SY. *Dictionary of Modern Herbalism: A Comprehensive Guide to Practical Herbal Therapy.* Rochester, Vt: Healing Arts Press; 1988.

Nishino H, et al. Berberine sulfate inhibits tumor-promoting activity of teleocidin in two-stage carcinogenesis on mouse skin. *Oncology.* 1986;43:131–134.

Shideman FE. A review of the pharmacology and therapeutics of Hydrastis and its alkaloids, hydrastine, berberine and canadine. *Comm on Nat Formulary Bull.* 1950;18:3–19.

Sun D, Courtney HS, Beachey EH. Berberine sulfate blocks adherence of Streptococcus pyogenes to epithelial cells, fibronectin, and hexadecane. *Antimicrob Agents Chemother.* 1988;32:1370–1374.

Swanston-Flatt SK, et al. Evaluation of traditional plant treatments for diabetes: studies in streptozotocin diabetic mice. *Acta Diabetol Lat.* 1989;26:51–55.

Zhu B, Ahrens FA. Effect of berberine on intestinal secretion mediated by Escherichia coli heat-stable enterotoxin in jejunum of pigs. *Am J Vet Res.* 1982; 43:1594–1598.

■ GRAPE SEED
Vitis vinifera (Botanical)
Vitaceae (Plant Family)

OVERVIEW

Grapes reach far back into history. Fossilized leaves and seeds from the Miocen and Teriary periods have been unearthed in Europe, Iceland, and North America; in Switzerland from the period of the Bronze Age; and in Egyptian tombs and hieroglyphics. Grapes are noted in the Bible. Homer drank wine made from grapes, circa 700 B.C.

All parts of the plant have been used for medicinal use. Sap was used in Europe for eye and skin ailments. Leaves had astringent and hemostatic actions. Grapes that were not yet ripe were used for sore or infected throats. Raisins had therapeutic applications, too—for instance, in the treatment of consumption, constipation, and thirst. Ripe grapes, however, had a plethora of applications, including cancer, cholera, smallpox, nausea, ophthalmia, and skin, kidney, and liver diseases. Similar and additional applications were prevalent in the Middle East, India, and China. Grapes have also been listed in many pharmacopoeias.

Today, however, grapes are rarely, if ever, used for any of these purposes. Apart from being source materials in the manufacture of food and beverage uses, grapes are harvested because they are a source of oligomeric proanthocyanidins (OPCs), therapeutically active antioxidants. Compared to most botanical products used for their own individual therapeutic properties, grape seed is used for the OPCs it contains. These polyphenolic constituents are also found in green tea and maritime pine bark. Extracts made from each of these plants contain similar OPC values and may be used interchangeably for specific indications, including chronic venous insufficiency and some opthalmologic conditions. Effects have not been evaluated by Germany's Commission E, and in the United States, the use of pine bark (pycnogenol) for OPCs is much more prevalent than grape seed OPCs.

MACRO DESCRIPTION

Grapes are the fruit of *Vitis vinifera,* native to Asia but naturalized to most other continents in temperate regions. The perennial consists of a woody, climbing vine. The stem produces a peeling bark, and the large, circular to circular-ovate leaves are dentate or jagged at the margins, pale green on the top, and grayer underneath. Fruits are oval, and may be green, red, or purple. OPCs occur on the outside of the grape seeds as well as on the inner grape skin.

PART USED/PHARMACEUTICAL DESIGNATIONS

- Seeds
- Fruit skin

CONSTITUENTS/COMPOSITION

OPCs, also called procyandins, consist of a variable number of flavan units, and are dimeric, trimeric, tetrameric, and oligomeric, depending on the length of the bonds that link them. A patented process, developed by French biochemist Jaques Mesquelier in 1970, assures that each of these chains is present in a grape seed product.

COMMERCIAL PREPARATIONS

Extracts are standardized to 95% OPC content.

MEDICINAL USES/INDICATIONS

Grape plants were originally used for purposes described in the overview. Because OPCs were not isolated from grape seed until 1970, there was no traditional folk use of OPCs.

Clinical applications: Results from controlled trials support the use of grape seed OPCs for impaired visual function due to macular degeneration and chronic venous insufficiency. In addition, lymphedema, acrocyanosis, varicose veins, telangiectases, capillary fragility and permeability secondary to diabetes, cancer, premenstrual syndrome, and dental caries are some of the many indications for which grape seed OPCs might prove useful.

PHARMACOLOGY

Pharmacologic activities of OPCs are numerous. In vitro, OPCs' antioxidant activity is 50 times greater than vitamin E's and 20 times greater than vitamin C's, in both lipid and aqueous phases. OPCs significantly and dose-dependently prevent vitamin E loss, and lower blood cholesterol levels through possible reversal of cholesterol transport, and by increasing both intestinal cholesterol absorption and bile acid excretion. OPCs also inhibit angiotensin I converting enzyme, ascorbic acid oxidase, histidine decarboxylase, and prevents histamine release and arterial damage. OPCs are thought to prevent atherosclerosis by inhibiting platelet aggregation and vascular constriction. They stabilize capillary walls and prevent xylene-induced capillary permeability. OPCs also demonstrate anti-mutagenic activity, and inhibit carageenan-induced rat paw edema.

In a double-blind, placebo controlled trial, grape seed extract was an effective prophylactic against post-operative facial swelling. In an open trial, venolymphatic symptoms of premenstrual syndrome in 165 study subjects were relieved with grape seed OTC therapy. Capillary resistance in 28 diabetic and hypertensive patients rose significantly in an open trial that provided patients with 150 mg OPCs daily. It is also effective in relieving upper extremity lymphedema secondary to radical mastectomy.

DOSAGE RANGES AND DURATION OF ADMINISTRATION

- As a preventive for atherosclerosis, ophthalmologic disorders, or other conditions: 50 mg standardized extract/day.
- For therapeutic purposes: 150 to 300 mg/day.

SIDE EFFECTS/TOXICOLOGY

None known

WARNINGS/CONTRAINDICATIONS/PRECAUTIONS

None known

INTERACTIONS

None known

REGULATORY AND COMPENDIAL STATUS

In the United States, grape seed OPC is a dietary supplement. It was not reviewed by Germany's Commission E.

REFERENCES

Amsellem M, et al. Endotelon in the treatment of venolymphatic problems in premenstrual syndrome: multi-center study on 165 patients. *Tempo Medical*. 1987;282.

Ariga TK, Hamano M. Radical scavenging action and its mode in procyanidins B-1 and B-3 from azuki beans to peroxyl radicals. *Agricultural Biological Chemistry*. 1990;54:2499–2504.

Baruch J. Effect of grape seed extract in postoperative edema [in French]. *Ann Chir Plast Esthet*. 1984;4.

Blumenthal M, Riggins C. *Popular Herbs in the U.S. Market: Therapeutic Monographs*. Austin, Tex: American Botanical Council; 1997.

Bombardelli E, Morazzoni P. *Vitis vinifera L. Fitoterapia*. 1995; 66:291–317.

Chang WC, Hsu FL. Inhibition of platelet aggregation and arachidonate metabolism in platelets by procyanidins. *Prostagland Leukotri Essential Fatty Acids*. 1989;38:181–188.

Corbe C, Boissin JP, Siou A. Light vision and chorioretinal circulation: study of the effect of procyanidolic oligomers (Endotelon) [in French]. *J Fr Ophthalmol*. 1988;11:453–460.

Delacrois P. Double-blind study of grape seed extract in chronic venous insufficiency. *La Revue De Med*. 1981;28–31.

Fromantin M. Les oligomeres procyanidoliques dans le traitement de la fragilite capillaire et de la retinopathie chez les diabetiques: a propos de 26 cas. *Med Int*. 1982;16.

Kashiwada Y, et al. Antitumor agents, 129: tannins and related compounds as selective cytotoxic agents. *J Nat Prod*. 1992;55:1033–1043.

Lagrua G, et al. A study of the effects of procyanidol oligomers on capillary resistance in hypertension and in certain nephropathis. *Sem Hop*. 1981;57:1399–1401.

Maffei FR, Carini M, Aldini G, Bombardelli E, Morazzoni P, Morelli R. Free radical scavenging action and anti-enzyme activities of procyanidins from *Vitis vinifera*: a mechanism for their capillary protective action. *Arzneimittelfarichung*. May 1994; 44:592–601.

Maffei FR, Carini M, Aldini G, Bombardelli E, Morazzoni P. Sparing effect of procyanidins from *Vitis vinifera* on vitamin E: in vitro studies. *Planta Med*. 1998;64:343–347.

Masquelier J. Comparative action of various vitamin P related factors on the oxidation of ascorbic acid by cupric ions. *Bulletin de la Societe de Chimie Biologique*. 1951;33:304–305.

Masquelier J. Natural products as medicinal agents. *Planta Med*. 1980;242S–256S.

Meunier, M.T., et al. Inhibition of angiotensin I converting enzyme by flavonolic compounds: *in vitro* and *in vivo* studies. *Planta Med*. 1987;53: 12–15.

Murray M. *The Healing Power of Herbs: the Enlightened Person's Guide to the Wonders of Medicinal Plants*. Rocklin, Calif: Prima Publishing; 1995.

Schultz V, Hänsel R, Tyler V. *Rational Phytotherapy: A Physician's Guide to Herbal Medicine*. New York, NY: Springer-Verlag; 1998.

Schwitters B, Masquelier J. *OPC in Practice: The Hidden Story of Proanthocyanidins, Nature's Most Powerful and Patented Antioxidant*. Rome, Italy: Alfa Omega Publishers; 1995.

Tebib, K, et al. Dietary grape seed tannins affect lipoproteins, lipoprotein lipases, and tissue lipids in rats fed hypercholesterolemic diets. *J Nutr*. 1994; 124: 2451–2457.

Tebib K, et al. Polymeric grape seed tannins prevent plasma cholesterol changes in high-cholesterol-fed rats. *Food Chem*. 1994;49:403–406.

Walker, Morton. The nutritional therapeutics of Masquelier's oligomeric proanthocyanidins (OPCs). *Townsend Letter for Doctors and Patients*. 1996;175/76: 84–92.

Zafirov D, Bredy-Dobreva G, Litchev V, Papasova M. Antiexudative and capillaritonic effects of procyanidines isolated from grape seeds *(V. vinifera)*. *Acta Physiol Pharmacol Bulg*. 1990;16:50–54.

■ GREEN TEA
Camellia sinensis (Botanical)

OVERVIEW

Native to eastern Asia, tea was originally grown in China at least 5,000 years ago. Today, tea is widely cultivated in Asia and parts of the Middle East and Africa. Green tea is unfermented, while black tea is fermented. Oolong tea is semifermented. In green tea the fresh leaves are slightly steamed and then quickly dried. This process inactivates enzymes that oxidize polyphenols to derivative compounds.

Polyphenols have antioxidant and anticancer activities, but their conversion products do not. Green tea polyphenols (GTP) surpass vitamins C and E in their antioxidant protective properties. In black teas, the leaves are dried slowly, allowing them to ferment. The polyphenol conversion products in black tea have no significant therapeutic benefits.

Green tea is used in traditional Chinese medicine to promote digestion, counter flatulence, stimulate mental function, improve eyesight, and regulate body temperature. It is also thought to strengthen the arteries, reduce excess fats, clear phlegm, and neutralize poisons. The tannins in green tea have antidiarrhea activity. The longer tea leaves are brewed, the greater the tannin content.

MACRO DESCRIPTION

The tea plant is a large shrub with evergreen leaves that can reach a height of 30 feet. However, it is usually pruned to two to three feet. The flowers have five or six white petals and multiple yellow stamens. The branches are smooth and covered by shiny, dark green, hairy leaves. The age of the leaf can be determined by its position on the harvested stem. The leaf buds, young leaves, and stem are the preferred plant parts for making teas.

PART USED/PHARMACEUTICAL DESIGNATIONS

- Leaves
- Leaf buds

CONSTITUENTS/COMPOSITION

Purine alkaloids (caffeine [2.9 to 4.2%], theophylline [0.02 to 0.04%], theobromine [0.15 to 0.2%]; polyphenols (including (+)-catechin, d-catechin, + catechin, (-)-epicatechin (EC), (-)epicatechin gallate (ECG), (-) epigallocatechin (EGC), (-) epigallocatechin-gallate (EGCG), and other catechin derivatives; phenolic acids; terpenoids; indole; anorganic ions.

COMMERCIAL PREPARATIONS

Commercial preparations consist of dried leaf tea as well as extracts made from the leaves and leaf buds. The leaves are harvested, immediately heated, and then rolled and crushed to prevent enzymatic changes from altering the color and natural constituents. Green tea has 300 to 400 mg polyphenols and 50 to 100 mg caffeine per cup. Decaffeinated products contain concentrated polyphenols (60% to 89% total polyphenols). Both the epigallocatechin and total polyphenol content should be considered when purchasing commercial products.

MEDICINAL USES/INDICATIONS

Traditional herbal actions: astringent, bronchodilator, antiviral, antiarteriosclerotic, anticholesteremic

Current clinical applications: cancer prevention, coughs, colds, asthma, diarrhea, bacterial dysentery, and adjunct to radiation treatment (reduces tissue damage).

PHARMACOLOGY

Green tea taken as a beverage has antioxidant, anticancer, antimutagenic, antibacterial, antifungal, and antiviral properties. Population studies show that green tea use correlated with lowered serum cholesterol totals and triglyceride levels, lowered LDL levels, and increased HDL levels. Green tea probably prevents atheroslerosis by blocking the oxidation of LDL. Purine alkaloids isolated from green tea have a relaxing effect on bronchial smooth muscle. Purine alkaloids also enhance cornary blood flow and simulate cardiac muscle. They may even account for the diuretic effects of green tea. One of the catechins in green tea, EGCG, had an antiplatelet aggregation effect comparable to aspirin.

Other population studies suggest that green tea taken daily as a beverage prevents cancer. Black tea consumption, on the other hand, correlated with increased risk of cancers of the rectum, gallbladder, and endometrium. GTP suppressed the activation and formation of cancer-causing substances. The cancer-prevention effects of green tea are strongest against cancers of the gastrointestinal tract, lung, and breast.

In in vitro experiments, GTP blocked the growth of mammary cancer cell lines. Green tea apparently disrupts interactions among tumor promoters, hormones, growth factors, and their receptors. In animal models, green tea extracts administered to mice in doses comparable to the amount consumed by humans blocked the formation of ultraviolet B (UVB)-induced sunburn lesions and skin tumors. And in both animal and human investigations, green tea beverages ingested with meals inhibited the formation of carcinogenic nitrosamines.

In vivo research revealed that green tea polyphenols (GTP) enhanced the catalytic activity of key enzymes involved in the synthesis of glutathione and quinone in the liver, small intestine, and lungs. EGCG showed potent antitumorigenesis in skin. In human investigations, GTP had significant antimutagenic properties against carcinogens formed through the process the cooking meats and fish. Polyphenols also scavenged free radicals such as hydrogen peroxide and superoxide anions. In other research, epicatechin derivatives decreased lipid peroxidation in epidermal microsomes. And GTP significantly decreased dental carries by inhibiting Streptococcus mutans, the bacterium that causes dental cavities.

DOSAGE RANGES AND DURATION OF ADMINISTRATION

Green tea is not usually prescribed as a medication even though it has therapeutic benefits.
Recommended dosage:
- Tea beverage: 3 cups/day (3 g soluble components, or 240 to 320 g polyphenols)
- Standardized green tea extract (80% total polyphenols and 55% epigallocatechin): 300 to 400 mg/day.
- Capsules and liquid preparations are also available.

SIDE EFFECTS/TOXICOLOGY

Quantities of greater than 5 cups of tea consumed as a beverage (equivalent to more than 300 mg caffeine taken daily) are considered overdoses. Intake above this level can produce side effects of restlessness, tremor, and heightened reflex excitability. Long-term daily dosage beyond 1.5 g of caffeine can induce irritability, insomnia, palpitation, vertigo, vomiting, diarrhea, loss of appetite, and headache. Vomiting and abdominal spasm are indications of potential caffeine overdose.

WARNINGS/CONTRAINDICATIONS/PRECAUTIONS

Individuals who have sensitive stomachs should limit their intake of green tea. The chlorogenic acid and tannins in tea can cause hyperacidity, gastric irritation, reduced appetite, and diarrhea. Tea should also be used with caution by people who have cardiovascular complications, kidney disorders, overactive thyroids, and a tendency toward spasm. Because caffeine overdoses can lead to anxiety attacks, persons prone to panic or other similar psychiatric disorders should exercise caution in drinking tea.

Pregnant women should avoid caffeine. At the very least, they should limit their intake to a maximum of 200 mg/day, or 3 cups taken at evenly spaced intervals during the day. Nursing mothers who drink tea put their infants at risk for sleep disorders.

INTERACTIONS

Individuals taking alkaline drugs should not use tea products. Tea beverages can delay the resorption of alkaline medications because tannins bind with alkaline compounds.

REGULATORY AND COMPENDIAL STATUS

The U.S. FDA classifies green tea as a dietary supplement. Green tea is not usually sold as an herbal medicine. It is approved as a nonprescription traditional diuretic in Belgium.

REFERENCES

Ali M, et al. A potent thromboxane inhibitor in green tea. *Prostaglandins Leukot Essent Fatty Acids*. 1990;40:281–283.

Blumenthal M, ed. *The Complete German Commission E Monographs*. Therapeutic Guide to Herbal Medicines. Boston, Mass: Integrative Medicine Communications; 1998:47, 132.

Bradley P, ed. *British Herbal Compendium*. Dorset, England: British Herbal Medicine Association; 1992:1:96–98.

Heinerman J. *Heinerman's Encyclopedia of Fruits, Vegetables and Herbs*. Englewood Cliffs, NJ: Prentice Hall; 1988:112–113.

Imai K, Nakachi K. Cross sectional study of effects of drinking green tea on cardiovascular and liver diseases. *BMJ*. 1995;310:693–696.

Murray M. *The Healing Power of Herbs: The Enlightened Person's Guide to the Wonders of Medicinal Plants*. Second Ed. Rocklin, Calif: Prima Publishing; 1995.

Poppel Piet A, van den Brandt. Consumption of black tea and cancer risk: a prospective cohort study. *J Natl Cancer Inst*. 1996;88:93–100.

Shim JH, Kang MG, Kim YH, Roberts C, Lee IP. Chemopreventive effect of green tea (*Camellia sinensis*) among cigarette smoke. *Cancer-Epidemio-Biomarkers-Prev*. 1995;Jun; 4(4): 387-91.

Sirving K. Drinking black tea may cut risk of stroke. *AMA Arch Intern Med*. March 25, 1998.

Snow J. Camellia sinensis (L.) Kuntze (Theaceae). *The Protocol Journal of Botanical Medicine*. 1995;1:47–51.

Tamozawa H, et al. Natural antioxidants I. Antioxidant components of tea leaf (Thea sinensis L.). *Chem Pharm Bull*. 1984;32:2011–2014.

Tyler V. *Herbs of Choice: The Therapeutic Use of Phytomedicinals*. Binghamton, NY: Haworth; 1994.

Wang Z, et al. Antimutagenic activity of green tea polyphenols. *Mutation Research*. 1989;223:273–285.

Windridge C. *The Fountain of Health. An A-Z of Traditional Chinese Medicine*. London, England: Mainstream Publishing; 1994:259.

■ HAWTHORN BERRY/HAWTHORN FLOWER/HAWTHORN LEAF/HAWTHORN LEAF WITH FLOWER

Crataegus monogyna/Crataegus laevigata (Botanical)

Rosaceae (Plant Family)

Crataegi fructus/crataegi flos/crataegi folium/crataegi folium cum flore (Pharmacopeial)

OVERVIEW

Hawthorn improves cardiac function in patients with New York Heart Association stage II heart failure. Clinical trials support a minimum dose of 300 mg hawthorn extract to reduce debility from cardiac insufficiency. Various tolerance markers (standard bicycle ergometry, spiroergometry, radionucleotide ventriculography, and subjective complaints) support this conclusion. Further study is required to determine the effects of hawthorn on other cardiovascular conditions (hypertension, arteriosclerosis, angina pectoris, and paroxysmal tachycardia) considered by herbalists to be indications for hawthorn therapy.

MACRO DESCRIPTION

Hawthorn is a thorny, deciduous shrub up to five feet tall, found in deciduous forests of North America, Europe, North Africa, and western Asia. Flower clusters, which bloom in May, have five petals, five sepals, and numerous stamens. Leaves are variable, toothed or lobed, and alternate. Oval or round fruit (haws), which are red when ripe, contain five nutlets. Crude drug is prepared from leaves, white flowers, and berries.

PART USED/PHARMACEUTICAL DESIGNATIONS

- Flowers
- Leaves
- Fruit

CONSTITUENTS/COMPOSITION

Flavonoids (e.g., hyperoside, vitexin rhamnoside, rutin, vitexin, kaempferol, apigenin); oligomeric procyanidins (e.g., epicatechin, catechin)

Leaves and flowers in crude drug contain about 1% flavonoids (hyperoside as marker), 1% to 3% oligomeric procyanidins (epicatechin as marker); berries in crude drug contain about 0.1% hyperoside.

COMMERCIAL PREPARATIONS

Aqueous, aqueous-alcohol, solid, glycerite, dried (powdered), and compounded extracts are available as liquid, tablet, or capsule, standardized to flavonoid/oligomeric procyanidin content

MEDICINAL USES/INDICATIONS

Traditional: cardiotonic, hypotensive, coronary vasodilator, mild diuretic, astringent

Conditions: coronary artery disease, congestive heart failure, essential hypertension, angina pectoris, postmyocardial infarction rehabilitation, cardiac weakness following infectious disease, antiarrythmias, possibly varicose veins, thrombosis

Clinical applications: for diminishing or deteriorating cardiac capacity due to stage II heart failure, according to New York Heart Association standards

PHARMACOLOGY

Animal studies originated with a 1966 genetic experiment that focused on gypsy moths. The colony, about to die due to inbreeding and a diet of alder leaves, recovered completely when fed hawthorn leaves, and also became stronger and larger. Subsequent in vivo and in vitro animal experiments showed that hawthorn extracts increase coronary blood flow, cause vasodilation (and hypotension), reduce peripheral resistance, benefit peripheral blood flow (and circulation), and have positive inotropic effects (increasing rat myocyte efficiency more than isoprenaline). Hawthorn extracts also block beta-adrenoceptors, are antiarrhythmic, and, in rat hearts subject to ischemia and reperfusion, increase recovery rate, reduce lactate release, reduce ventricular fibrillation, and prolong survival.

In humans, hawthorn, a positive inotropic agent, increases the refractory period that cardiac glycosides shorten, reducing the probability of arrhythmia while stabilizing heart rhythm. Also a peripheral vasodilator, hawthorn reduces blood pressure and increases coronary flow. It has positive dromotropic effects and negative bathmotropic effects, and increases coronary and myocardial circulatory perfusion. Actions may be due to cAMP (cyclic adenosine monophosphate)—or TXA_2 (thromboxane$_2$)—inhibition or to other undetermined actions.

DOSAGE RANGES AND DURATION OF ADMINISTRATION

To decrease NYHA stage II cardiac insufficiency:

- 160 to 900 mg standardized (4 to 20 mg flavonoids/30 to 160 mg oligomeric procyanidins) fluid crude extract daily for at least six weeks
- 120 to 240 mg extract, standardized to 1.8% vitexin rhamnoside/ 10% procyanidins three times daily for at least six weeks.

SIDE EFFECTS/TOXICOLOGY

American Herbal Products Association (AHPA) safety rating: class 1 (safe with appropriate use)

Infrequent side effects: Two of 367 subjects in placebo-controlled trials reported nausea, headache, migraine, palpitations, and soft stools.

Toxicity: After IP dosing of 3 g per kg body weight (rats and mice), toxicity was indicated by sedation, difficulty breathing, and tremors, but not death. Oral doses—30, 90, or 300 mg per kg body weight administered to rats and dogs for 26 weeks and 300 to 600 mg per body weight administered for one month—were nonfatal and nontoxic.

WARNINGS/CONTRAINDICATIONS/PRECAUTIONS

Advise patients not to self-medicate. If symptoms do not improve after six weeks of treatment, reevaluate the condition. Encourage frequent follow-ups. Take appropriate precautions regarding potential heart failure, imminent surgery, and prescription change.

Patients should not use hawthorn during pregnancy.

INTERACTIONS

Hawthorn may increase the effects of digitalis. Hawthorn is sometimes combined with other supplements and herbs for stronger effect.

REGULATORY AND COMPENDIAL STATUS

In the United States, the FDA classifies hawthorn as a dietary supplement; in Canada, it has new-drug status and is not approved for self-treatment of cardiovascular disease. Hawthorn is not licensed through the General Sales

List (GSL) in England, and while the Commission E in Germany approves the use of hawthorn leaf and flower for the treatment of NYHA stage II heart failure, it does not approve the use of hawthorn berry.

REFERENCES

Bahorun T, Gressier B, Trotin F, et al. Oxygen species scavenging activity of phenolic extracts from hawthorn fresh plant organs and pharmaceutical preparations. *Arzneimittelforschung.* 1996;46:1086–1089.

Blumenthal M, ed. *The Complete German Commission E Monographs: Therapeutic Guide to Herbal Medicines.* Boston, Mass: Integrative Medicine Communications; 1998.

Blumenthal M, Riggins C. *American Botanical Council's Popular Herbs in the U.S. Market. Therapeutic Monographs.* Austin Tex: ABC; 1997.

Chaterjee SS. In vitro and in vivo studies on the cardioprotective action of oligomeric procyanidins in a crataegus extract of leaves and blooms. *Arzneimittelforschung.* 1997;47:821–825.

The Criteria Committee of the New York Heart Association I. *Diseases of the Heart and Blood Vessels: Nomenclature and Criteria for Diagnosis.* 6th ed. Boston, Mass: Little, Brown; 1964.

Hoffmann D. Hawthorn: The Heart Helper. *Alternative & Complementary Therapies.* 1995;4:191–192.

Kowalchik C, Hylton W, eds. *Rodale's Illustrated Encyclopedia of Herbs.* Emmaus, Pa: Rodale Press; 1998.

Leuchtgens H. Crataegus special extract WS 1442 in NYHA II heart failure. A placebo controlled randomized double-blind study [in German]. *Fortschr Med.* 1993;111:352–354.

Loew D, Albrecht M, Podzuweit H. Efficacy and tolerability of a Hawthorn preparation in patients with heart failure stage I and II according to NYHA—a surveillance study. Presented at the Second International Congress on Phytomedicine; 1996; Munich, Germany.

McGuffin M, Hobbs C, Upton R, Goldberg A. *American Herbal Products Association's Botanical Safety Handbook.* Boca Raton, Fla: CRC Press; 1997.

Nasa Y, Hashizume AN, Hoque E, Abiko Y. Protective effect of crataegus extract on the cardiac mechanical dysfunction in isolated perfused working rat heart.

Arzneimittelforschung. 1993;42II(9):945–949.

Newall CA, Anderson LA, Phillipson JD. *Herbal Medicines: A Guide for Health Care Professionals.* London, England: The Pharmaceutical Press; 1996.

Nikolov N, Wagner H, Chopin J, Della Monica G, Chari VM, Seligmann O. Recent investigations of crataegus flavonoids. Proceedings of the International Bioflavonoid Symposium; 1981; Munich, Germany.

Popping S, Rose H, Ionescu I, Fischer Y, Kammermeier H. Effect of a hawthorn extract on contraction and energy turnover of isolated rat cardiomyocytes. *Arzneimittelforschung.* 1995;45:1157–1161.

Schmidt U, Kuhn U, Ploch M, Hubner WD. Efficacy of the hawthorn (crataegus) preparation LI 132 in 78 patients with chronic congestive heart failure defined as NYHA functional class II. *Phytomedicine.* 1994;1:17–34.

Schultz V, Hansel R, Tyler V. *Rational Phytotherapy: A Physician's Guide to Herbal Medicine.* Heidelberg: Springer; 1998.

Schussler M, Holzl J, Fricke U. Myocardial effects of flavonoids from crataegus species. *Arzneimittelforschung.* 1995;45:842–845.

Tauchert M, Ploch M, Hubner WD. Effectiveness of hawthorn extract LI 132 compared with the ACE inhibitor Captopril: Multicenter double-blind study with 132 NYHA stage II. *Muench Med Wochenschr.* 1994;136 (suppl):S27–S33.

Vibes J, Lasserre B, and Gleye J. Effects of a methanolic extract from *Crataegus oxycantha* blossoms on TXA2 and PGI2 synthesizing activities of cardiac tissue. *Med Sci Res.* 1993;21:534–436.

Vibes J, Lasserre B, Gleye J, Declume C. Inhibition of thromboxane A2 biosynthesis I vitro by the main components of *Crataegus oxyacantha* (hawthorn) flower heads. *Prostaglandins, Leukotrienes and Essential Fatty Acids.* 1994;50:174–175.

Weikl A, Assmus KD, Neukum-Schmidt A, et al. Crataegus special extract WS 1442. Assessment of objective effectiveness in patients with heart failure. *Fortschr Med.* 1996;114:291–296.

Weiss R F. *Herbal Medicine.* Beaconsfield, England: Beaconsfield Publishers, Ltd; 1988:162–169.

Werbach M. *Botanical Influences on Illness.* Tarzana, Calif: Third Line Press; 1994.

Zapfe G, Assmus KD, Noh HS. Placebo-controlled multicenter study with Crataegus special extract WS 1442: clinical results in the treatment of NYHA II cardiac insufficiency. Presented at the Fifth Congress on Phytotherapy; June 11, 1993; Bonn, Germany.

■ KAVA KAVA
Piper methysticum (Botanical)
Piperaceae (Plant Family)
Piperis methystici rhizoma (Pharmacopeial)

OVERVIEW

Kava root preparations reduce stress-related anxiety and the effects of anxiety disorders. Studies show that these antianxiety effects are significant, superior to placebo, and similar to effects of benzodiazepines used in the treatment of anxiety without causing similar adverse side effects. Kava also reduces anxiety associated with or precipated by menopause, and it is a topical oral anaesthetic. Kava promotes sleep in larger doses and a state of calm in smaller doses. The effects of kava are relaxing, not stupefying; it disposes users to sociability, not hostility.

The kava plant comes from Oceania, the geographical area of Polynesia, Micronesia, and Melanesia in the Pacific Ocean. Kava consumption among native peoples was first discovered during Captain James Cook's *Endeavour* voyage (1768 to 1771). The Swedish botanists who accompanied Captain Cook recorded kava as an indigenous intoxicant. Tribes used kava as a ceremonial as well as social drink, with different purposes and rituals surrounding its use, including which members were allowed to drink it. Despite the efforts of the 19th century Christian missionaries to quash kava use, today kava is available at kava bars on some islands and provides a good living for exporters, who cultivate kava commercially. It is often presented as a gift of honor and goodwill to dignitaries and foreigners at welcoming ceremonies. President and Mrs. Lyndon B. Johnson, Hillary Rodham Clinton, and Pope John Paul II have participated in kava ceremonies.

Kava was available in some parts of Germany by the late 19th century, but it was rare. Despite its long-standing use in Hawaii, Kava has caught on only recently in the mainland U.S. as a popular herbal medicine. In the past three years, kava has been the subject of intense marketing and may soon exceed South Pacific supply. Its safety and regulation are also current points of controversy. While side effects effects are mild (the most frequently reported are GI discomfort, headache, dizziness, or skin rash, and these occur in a small percentage of study participants), excess amounts of kava impair driving ability. Yellowing of the skin, hair, and nails, and drying and cracking of the skin, is seen in some chronic users, as is disturbance to vision or oculomotor equilibrium. And because so many recovered substance abusers are taking kava daily, its addictive potential is still under question, despite the lack of demonstrable evidence from a 1994 addiction potential study.

MACRO DESCRIPTION

Kava is an erect, branching shrub with prominent, succulent leaves. It grows up to six meters in damp tropical climates. The heart-shaped green leaves are smooth and pointed; erect yellow-green inflorescence develops at axils. The rhizome is harvested when it is five to eight cm thick, after three to five years' growth, when the plant is two to two and a half meters tall. Numerous long, bundled, tuberous hairs grow from the rhizome.

PART USED/PHARMACEUTICAL DESIGNATIONS

- Roots[rhizome]

CONSTITUENTS/COMPOSITION

Dried herb contains 3.5% kavapyrones, including 1% to 2% kawain, 0.6% to 1% dihydrokawain, 1.2% to 2% methysticin, and 0.5% to 0.8% dihydromethysticin.

COMMERCIAL PREPARATIONS

In some cultures, the method of preparation involved chewing the root and spitting the juice into a bowl; saliva served as a macerate. Today, manufacturers use alcohol-water or acetate macerations or percolations to extract kava's active constituents from ground rhizome. Kava is available as aqueous-alcohol extracts and encapsulations, standardized to 70% kavalactone content, and as tinctures, tablets, and dried root.

MEDICINAL USES/INDICATIONS

Traditional Actions: Antispasmodic, nervine, relaxant, anti-anxiety, anaestetic, diuretic. Historically used for gonorrhea, chronic cystitis or other urinary tract symptoms, menstrual disorder and migraines, but it is not used for this now. Currently used as a relaxant of skeletal muscles for pain and stiffness, anxiety, insomnia, menopausal anxiety, uncontrolled epilepsy, pain, and jet lag.
Conditions: anxiety, insomnia
Clinical Applications: stress-related anxiety, anxiety disorder, phobias, restlessness, insomnia

PHARMACOLOGY

By 1998, six human double-blind, controlled trials on kava's therapeutic effects had been conducted. These trials demonstrate consistent, significant antianxiety effects of kava, although the methodologies of some are questionable. One recent study (1997) found a standardized, 70% kavalactone kava extract superior to placebo in treating non-psychotic patients. Of 101 outpatients who met DSM-III-R criteria and participated in the study, 52 received kava, and symptoms in the majority of this group improved throughout the 25-week study, some noting improvements by week eight. Results from the Hamilton Anxiety Scale, somatic and psychic anxiety, Clinical Global Impression, Self-Report Symptoms Inventory, and Adjective Mood Scale not show only kava's superiority to placebo in the treatment of non-psychotic anxiety, but also support kava's use in lieu of tricyclic antidepressants and benzodiazepine drugs.

Individual effects of kava constituents have also been investigated. The kavapyrones (kawain, dihydrokawain, methysticin, dihydromethysticin) are anticonvulsant, central muscle relaxants (similar to mephenesin) and locally anesthetic. They are also superior to strychnine antagonists in preventing strychnine poisoning in animal tests. In rabbits, these constituents diminish excability to the limbic system similar to benzodiazepines, and are also neuroprotective in mice and rats. In addition, nine studies have analyzed the effects of isolated dihydrokawin (DL-kawain) in anxiety disorder, with results similar to those of whole extract preparations.

DOSAGE RANGES AND DURATION OF ADMINISTRATION

To relieve anxiety and insomnia, and reduce stress, standard dose is 2.0 to 4.0 g as decoction up to three times daily, or standardized formulas (containing 70% kavalactones) for a daily intake of 60 to 600 mg kavalactones. Treatment length varies: it may take four weeks to reach peak therapeutic effect. In Germany and Australia, patients are advised not to continue dosing longer than three months.

SIDE EFFECTS/TOXICOLOGY

Typical side effects are mild, and include allergy (skin rash), headache, gastrointestinal distress, and dizziness. The American Herbal Products

Association recommends that kava not be used during pregnancy or while breast-feeding (class 2b and 2d); also, do not drive when using excessive dosages (class 2d).

Extreme doses of 13 liters per day—300 to 400 g dried rhizome per week—resulted in yellowing of the skin, ataxia, rash, hair loss, and changes in vision, appetite, and respiration. This dose exceeds recommended doses by 100 times.

WARNINGS/CONTRAINDICATIONS/PRECAUTIONS

Do not use during pregnancy or while breast-feeding. Do not exceed recommended dose or length of treatment.

INTERACTIONS

May potentiate effects of barbiturates or alcohol.

REGULATORY AND COMPENDIAL STATUS

Kava is a dietary supplement in the U.S. and approved for use by the German Commission E in the treatment of anxiety and restlessness. Not approved in Canada for non-medicinal inclusion in oral preparations.

REFERENCES

Blumenthal M, ed. *The Complete German Commission E Monographs: Therapeutic Guide to Herbal Medicines.* Boston, Mass: Integrative Medicine Communications; 1998.

Foster S. *101 Medicinal Herbs.* Loveland, Colo: Interweave Press; 1998.

Kinzler E, Kromer J, Lehmann E. Effect of a special kava extract in patients with anxiety-, tension, and excitation states of non-psychotic genesis. Double blind study with placebos over four weeks [in German]. *Arzneimforsch.* 1991;41:584–588.

Lehmann E, et al. Efficacy of special kava extract *(Piper methysticum)* in patients with states of anxiety, tension and excitedness of non-mental origin—A double blind placebo controlled study of four weeks treatment. *Phytomedicine.* 1996;3:113–119.

Lindenberg Von D, Pitule-Schodel H. D, L-Kavain in comparison with oxazepam in anxiety states. Double-blind clinical trial. *Forschr Med.* 1990;108:50–54.

McGuffin M, Hobbs C, Upton R, Goldberg A. *American Herbal Products Associations's Botanical Safety Handbook.* Boca Raton, Fla: CRC Press; 1996.

Munte TE, Heinze HJ, Matzke M, et al. Effects of oxazepam and an extract of kava roots *(Piper methysticum)* on event-related potentials in a word recognition task. *Neuropsychobiology.* 1993;27:46–53.

Schulz V, Hänsel R, Tyler V. *Rational Phytotherapy: A Physician's Guide to Herbal Medicine.* New York, NY: Springer-Verlag; 1998.

Singh YD, Blumenthal M. Kava: An overview. *HerbalGram.* 39:34–55.

Volz HP, Kieser M. Kava-kava extract WS 1490 versus placebo in anxiety disorders—a randomized placebo-controlled 25-week outpatient trial. *Pharmacopsychiatry.* 1997;30:1–5.

Warnecke G. Psychosomatic dysfunction in the female climacteric. Clinical effectiveness and tolerance of kava extract WS 1490 [in German]. *Fortschr Med.* 1991;109:119–122.

■ LEMON BALM
Melissa officinalis (Botanical)
Lamiaceae (Plant Family)
Melissae folium (Pharmacopeial)

OVERVIEW

Lemon balm—mildly sedating, antiviral, and carminative—is used commonly as tea, tincture, and ointment throughout Western Europe, where it was named Europe's plant of the year in 1988. In the United States, herbalists recommend lemon balm for a broad range of indications, including insomnia, dyspepsia, infant colic, anxiety, depression, and chronic fatigue syndrome.

Lemon balm is also used to reduce the pain and swelling of arthritis; to alleviate headaches; to desensitize individuals prone to allergy, eczema, and asthma; to relax uterine smooth muscle tissue during premenstrual syndrome; and to regulate hot flashes during menopause. While many of these uses have not been corroborated with controlled trials, studies with laboratory animals and tissue cultures have supported the empirical results of traditional uses of lemon balm.

In the 1970's, lemon balm volatile oil was demonstrated to exact nonspecific sedative actions. Its effects on the gastrointestinal tract are apparently due to smooth muscle relaxation. Studies also demonstrate modulation of thyroid stimulating in relation to lemon balm administration. And current research supports its use for cold sores or lesions due to herpes virus types 1 and 2.

Lemon balm has been used for thousands of years. The Greek physician Dioscorides used it for dog and scorpion bites. In the Middle Ages, Eau de Melissa was commonly used as a sedative. The 17th century English herbalist, Nicholas Culpepper, claimed that lemon balm could lift spirits, prevent fainting, stimulate clear thinking, and precipitate menstruation. American eclectic physicians used lemon balm during the 19th century as a mild stimulant. European colonists used it to sweat out fevers. Lemon balm's scientific name, Melissa, is derived from the Greek word for bee: bees are attracted to its odor. It is added to cosmetics, furniture polish, insect repellant, and food.

MACRO DESCRIPTION

Erect perennial, growing up to two feet in height, with branching, hairy, square stems. Oval/heart shaped leaves, wrinkled, opposite, broad, toothed, grow one to three inches long, and smell like lemon. White-yellow flower clusters bloom at leaf axils July through September and sometimes become light blue. Native to Southern Europe and North Africa. Cultivated around the world.

PART USED/PHARMACEUTICAL DESIGNATIONS

• Leaves

CONSTITUENTS/COMPOSITION

Leaves contain a minimum of 0.05% volatile oil, with citronellal, citral a and b, geraniol, neral, caryophyllene, linalool, and limonene primary terpenoid constituents; also, phenol carboxylic acids and estimated 4% rasmarinic acid; and bitter principles, flavonoids, and tannins.

COMMERCIAL PREPARATIONS

Dried leaf, tea, capsules, extracts, creams, and oil, and combined with other sedative or carminative botanical preparations.

MEDICINAL USES/INDICATIONS

Traditional: carminative, diaphoretic, febrifuge; essential oil is sedative, spasmolytic, antibacterial; poultices used for sores, tumors, headaches, stomach and menstrual complaints, insect bites

Conditions: catarrh, influenza, painful or delayed menstruation, nervous unrest or insomnia, gastrointestinal discomfort (internal administration); wounds or lesions (topical application)

Clinical applications: Lemon balm leaf preparations are approved in Germany as treatment for nervous sleep disorders, appetite loss, and for symptoms of functional gastrointestinal disorders (flatulence, abdominal bloating). There is promise of potential usefulness in treatment of cold sore/Herpes simplex symptoms

PHARMACOLOGY

Components in lemon balm essential oil cause mild, nonspecific sedation when given at dosage ranges of 3 to 100 mg/kg (laboratory animals). Citronellal, a terpene in the volatile oil, may be the primary sedating constituent. In a study to determine the effects of 178 herbal extracts on herpes, influenza, and polio viruses, lemon balm's phenol constituents showed significant antiviral effects. The oil also has antibacterial activity, and tannins are currently considered the antiviral agents that speed healing from cold sores and herpes.

A multicenter, double-blind study showed that a concentrated ointment (700 mg crude drug per g ointment), applied bid to qid for 5 to 10 days, began to relieve symptoms by the second day of treatment. By the fifth day, 50% more participants applying lemon balm versus placebo noted full symptom relief, and recovery involved less scabbing than with placebo. Both patients and their doctors preferred the lemon balm treatment. Lemon balm ointment at this level of concentration is not currently available in the United States. Tea can be used when cooled and applied topically.

Freeze-dried liquid extracts are both antithyrotropic and antigonadotropic in laboratory tests. Lemon balm extract interferes with thyroid stimulating hormone binding with Graves' immunoglobulin (Graves'-specific IgG), and consequent thyroid activation, a finding that supports lemon balm's use in the treatment of Grave's disease.

Eugenol, geraniol, and nerol, constituents in many plant volatile oils in addition to lemon balm's, have been evaluated individually. Eugenol, which is used in dentistry as an antiseptic and anesthetic, has convulsant, antioxidant, hypothermic, spasmolytic, central nervous system depressant, and platelet aggregation suppressant actions. Spasmolytic actions pertained to general smooth muscle activity in both human and animal experimental models; platelet aggregation provoked by arachidonate, adrenaline, and collagen was blocked in vitro. Geraniol's antiseptic actions are seven times more potent than phenol. Antibacterial actions of both geraniol and nerol are under investigation.

DOSAGE RANGES AND DURATION OF ADMINISTRATION

• For difficulty in sleeping, or to reduce symptoms of gastrointestinal distress: 1.5 to 4.5 g dried herb as tea several times daily or as directed by physician, or tincture, 2 to 5 ml tid, or equivalent in fluid extract or encapsulated form.

- For cold/herpes sores: Steep 2 to 4 tsp. dried leaf in 1 cup boiling water for 10 to 15 minutes, cool, apply topically throughout the day.

SIDE EFFECTS/TOXICOLOGY

The American Herbal Products Association safety rating for lemon balm is class 1, safe with appropriate use. The German Commission E cites no associated toxicity or side effects.

WARNINGS/CONTRAINDICATIONS/PRECAUTIONS

Emmenagogue; do not use during pregnancy.

INTERACTIONS

May interfere with thyroid treatments, other Graves' disease therapy.

REGULATORY AND COMPENDIAL STATUS

Dietary supplement in U.S.; leaf preparations are approved for use as tea in the treatment of functional digestive distress and insomnia by the German Commission E.

REFERENCES

Auf'mkolk M, Ingbar JC, Kubota K, et al. Extracts and auto-oxidized constituents of certain plants inhibit the receptor-binding and the biological activity of Graves' immunoglobulins. *Endocrinology.* 1985;116:1687–1693.

Auf'mkolk M; H; Hesch RD; Ingbar SH Ingbar JC; Amir SM; Winterhoff H; Sourgens. Inhibition by certain plant extracts of the binding and adenylate cyclase stimulatory effect of bovine thyrotropin in human thyroid membranes. *Endocrinology.* 1984;115:527–534.

Blumenthal M, ed. *The Complete German Commission E Monographs.* Boston, Mass: Integrative Medicine Communications; 1998.

Bremness L. *Herbs.* New York, NY: DK Publishing, 1994.

Castleman M. *The Healing Herbs.* Emmaus, Pa: Rodale Press; 1991.

Duke JA. *The Green Pharmacy.* Emmaus, Pa: Rodale Press; 1997.

Foster S. *Herbal Renaissance: Growing, Using and Understanding Herbs in the Modern World.* Salt Lake City, Utah: Gibbs-Smith; 1993.

Kowalchik C and Hylton W, eds. *Rodale's Illustrated Encyclopedia of Herbs.* Emmaus, Pa: Rodale Press; 1998.

Leung A, Foster S. *Encyclopedia of Common Natural Ingredients Used in Food, Drugs, and Cosmetics.* 2nd ed. New York, NY: Wiley & Sons; 1996.

May G, Willuhn G. Antiviral effect of aqueous plant extracts in tissue culture [In German]. *Arzneimittelforschung.* 1978;28:1–7.

McCaleb R. Melissa relief for herpes sufferers. *HerbalGram.* 1995;34.

McGuffin M, Hobbs C, Upton R, Goldberg A. *American Herbal Products Associations's Botanical Safety Handbook.* Boca Raton, Fla: CRC Press; 1996.

Perry EK, et al. Medicinal plants and Alzheimer's disease: Integrating ethnobotanical and contemporary scientific evidence. *J Altern Complement Med.* 1998;4:419–428.

Schultz V, Hansel R, Tyler V. *Rational Phytotherapy: A Physician's Guide to Herbal Medicine.* New York, NY: Springer-Verlag; 1998.

Soulimani R, et al. Neurotropic action of the hydroalcoholic extract of *Melissa officinalis* in the mouse. *Planta Med.* 1991;57:105–109.

Tagashira M, Ohtake Y. New Antioxidative 1,3-Benzodioxole from *Melissa officinalis.* *Planta Med.* 1988;64:555–558.

Taylor L. *Herbal Secrets of the Rainforest.* Rocklin, Calif: Prima Publishing; 1998.

Tyler VE. Phytomedicines in Western Europe: their potential impact on herbal medicine in the United States. Presented at: Human Medicinal Agents from Plants, The American Chemical Society, 1992. *HerbalGram* 30, 67.

Vogt HJ, Tausch I, Wöbling RH, Kaiser PM. Melissenextrakt bei Herpes simplex. *Der Allgemeinarzt.* 1991;13:832–841.

Wöbling RH, Leonhardt K. Local therapy of herpes simplex with dried extract from *Melissa officinalis. Phytomedicine.* 1994;1:25–31.

■ LICORICE

Glycyrrhiza glabra (Botanical)
Fabaceae (Plant Family)
Liquiritiae radix (Pharmacopeial)

OVERVIEW

Glycyrrhiza glabra, or Spanish licorice, grows wild in some areas of Europe and Asia. It is one of several important medicinal plant species belonging to the *Glycyrrhiza genus.* Numerous pharmacological studies conducted over the past 50 years show that licorice has both therapeutic uses and adverse side effects.

Glycyrrhizin, one of the active components in licorice root, consists of glycyrrhizic acid in a mixture of potassium and calcium salts. Glycyrrhizin is 50 times sweeter than sugar and gives licorice its characteristic sweet taste. The active ingredient in licorice root is glycyrrhetic acid, a triterpene glycoside with saponin-like properties formed from the hydrolysis of glycyrrhizin. Both glycyrrhizin and glycyrrhetic acid are efficacious in treating peptic ulcers. However, both compounds can also cause mineralocorticoid side effects, including lethargy, headache, sodium and water retention, excess potassium excretion, and high blood pressure.

MACRO DESCRIPTION

Spanish licorice is a perennial that grows three to seven feet in height. It has a root system comprised of taproots, branch rootstock, and runners, or underground woody stems that grow horizontally. The long, cylindrical roots are straight pieces of wrinkled, fibrous wood 14 to 20 m in length and 5 to 20 mm in diameter. The rootstock has a yellowish-brown exterior and yellow interior.

PART USED/PHARMACEUTICAL DESIGNATIONS

- Roots (rhizome): rhizome, root, and stolon

CONSTITUENTS/COMPOSITION

Terpenoids (glycyrrhizic acid [yields glycyrrhetinic acid and glucuronic acid upon hydrolysis], glycyrrhetol, glabrolide, licoric acid, liquiritic acid, beta-amyrin); coumarins (glycyrin, heniarin, liqcoumarin, umbelliferone, GU-7); flavonoids (flavonols, isoflavones); volatile oil; amino acids, amines, sterols, gums, lignin.

COMMERCIAL PREPARATIONS

Licorice products are made from both peeled and unpeeled dried roots, and the underground roots, stolons, and rhizomes of several varieties of *Glycyrrhiza glabra.* Commercial preparations consist of powdered root, finely cut roots, dry extracts, and liquid extracts. Deglycyrrhizinated licorice (DGL) is usually manufactured as an extract. DGL is free of adverse side effects and is used to treat gastric and duodenal ulcers.

MEDICINAL USES/INDICATIONS

Traditional herbal actions: expectorant (cough remedy), demulcent (soothing topical medication), antispasmodic, anti-inflammatory, laxative, adaptogen, antihepatatoxin, antiviral, antitumor, antipyretic, relaxing expectorant. It is also used to normalize immune function.

Clinical applications: allergies, autoimmune conditions, especially those that affect connective tissue (for example, lupus scleroderma), bronchitis, peptic ulcer, chronic gastritis, rheumatism, arthritis, primary adrenocortical insufficiency, chronic esophageal and gastric inflammation, asthma, used as antimicrobial and antiviral.

PHARMACOLOGY

In in vivo research, glycyrrhizin had antitoxic activity against diphtheria, tetanus, and tetrodotoxin. The isoflavonoid constituents account for the in vitro antimicrobial effects of licorice alcohol extracts against *Staphylococcus aureus, Streptococcus mutans, Mycobacterium smegmatis,* and *Candida albicans.* In other in vivo investigations, glycyrrhetic acid blocked free radical formation that can lead to chemically-induced liver toxicity.

In in vitro experiments, glycyrrhizin and its derivative showed antimicrobial activity against numerous bacteria, fungi, and viruses (including HIV, hepatitis A, and several herpes viruses). Glycyrrhetinic acid significantly reduced tumor promoter activity both in vitro and in vivo, and it inhibited the growth of various cancer cell lines.

Glycyrrhizin and glycyrrhetic acid have moderate binding affinity for glucocorticoid and mineralocorticoid receptors, and weak affinity for estrogen, sex-hormone-binding globulin, and corticosteroid-binding globulin. Licorice inhibits estrogen metabolism when estrogen levels are high, and it enhances estrogen metabolism when estrogen levels are low. The estrogenic activity of licorice probably comes from isoflavones.

The steroid-like activity of glycyrrhizin and glycyrrhetic acid is responsible for the anti-inflammatory properties of licorice root. Licorice extends the half-life of cortisol by suppressing the metabolism of cortisol in the liver. In studies in humans, oral intake of glycyrrhizin increased the plasma levels of prednisolone administered intravenously. And glycyrrhetinic acid enhanced the pharmacological activity of hydrocortisone on the lungs. Topical glycyrrhetinic acid enhances the action of hydrocortisone on inflammatory conditions of the skin.

In other human research, glycyrrhizin products taken intravenously resolved at least some liver function damage in about 40% of hepatitis patients. Both oral and topical licorice preparations have been shown to be effective in treating canker sores, eczema and psoriasis, herpes simplex, premenstrual syndrome, and Addison's Disease. Other studies reveal that the efficacy of DGL in treating gastric ulcers can be comparable to that of Tagamet and Zantac.

Licorice achieves its anti-ulcer effect by accelerating the secretion rate of mucus by the gastric mucosa. Glycyrrhetic acid in particular has a therapeutic effect on peptic ulcers. It helps maintain high levels of prostaglandin in the stomach by blocking the activity of two crucial enzymes involved in the metabolism of prostaglandins E and F_2-alpha. This is a key mechanism since elevated prostaglandin levels in the stomach protect the gastric mucosa.

The pharmacological activity of DGL is due to flavonoids, and unlike glycyrrhizin and licorice extracts, DGL is virtually free of the adverse mineralocorticoid side effects.

DOSAGE RANGES AND DURATION OF ADMINISTRATION

Recommended dosage:
- Dried root: 1 to 5 g as infusion or decoction tid
- Licorice tincture 1:5: 2 to 5 ml tid
- DGL extract: 0.4 to 1.6 g tid for peptic ulcer

• DGL extract 4:1: in chewable tablet form 300 to 400 mg 20 minutes before meals for peptic ulcer

SIDE EFFECTS/TOXICOLOGY

Oral intake of more than 20 g/day of licorice can cause adverse effects. Excessive consumption of glycyrrhizin causes pseudoaldosteronism, a condition characterized by over-sensitization to the hormone aldosterone from the adrenal cortex. Pseudoaldosteronism produces the mineralocorticoid symptoms of headache, lethargy, hypertension, sodium and water retention, elevated potassium secretion, and sometimes even cardiac arrest. Symptoms usually manifest within one week if the daily ingestion is over 100 g. The adverse effects of licorice resemble symptoms associated with injections of deoxycorticosterone (ACTH) given in large doses.

Death occurs only rarely from ingesting licorice, but side effects such as lethargy and muscular weakness may occur with excess consumption. Muscle pain occurs about one third of the time, and numbness in the extremities is seen about one fourth of the time with moderate intake. Other side effects include weight gain and, on rare occasions, myoglobinuria.

WARNINGS/CONTRAINDICATIONS/PRECAUTIONS

Persons who consume large quantities of licorice, chew tobacco, or use other licorice-flavored products are at risk for licorice toxicity. Adverse reactions to ingesting licorice products have been reported for individuals who have hypertension, kidney or heart disorders, hypokalemia, cirrhosis of the liver or cholestatic liver diseases, and hypertonia. Licorice is also contraindicated for pregnant women. High doses of licorice products should not be used for longer than four to six weeks.

INTERACTIONS

Interactions with thiazide diuretics can cause potassium loss, which can lead to increased sensitivity to digitalis glycosides.

REGULATORY AND COMPENDIAL STATUS

The U.S. FDA classifies licorice root as a dietary supplement. The German Commission E approves the herb for use in catarrhs of the upper respiratory tract and for gastric/duodenal ulcers.

REFERENCES

Acharya SK; Dasarathy S, Tandon A, Joshi YK, Tandon BN. A preliminary open trial on interferon stimulator (SNMC) derived from *Glycyrrhiza glabra* in the treatment of subacute hepatic failure. Indian *J Med Res.* 1993;98:69–74.

Arase Y, et al. The long term efficacy of glycyrrhizin in chronic hepatitis C. *Cancer.* 1997;79:1494–1500.

Blumenthal M, ed. *The Complete German Commission E Monographs: Therapeutic Guide to Herbal Medicines.* Boston, Mass: Integrative Medicine Communications; 1998:161–162.

Bradley P, ed. *British Herbal Compendium.* Dorset, England: British Herbal Medicine Association; 1992:1:145–148.

Chen M, et al. Effect of glycyrrhizin on the pharmokinetics of prednisolone following low dosage of prednisolone hemisuccinate. *J Clin Endocrinol Metab.* 1990;70:1637–1643.

De Smet PAGM, Keller K, Hänsel R, Chandler RF, eds. *Adverse Effects of Herbal Drugs.* Berlin, Germany: Springer-Verlag; 1997:67–87.

Gruenwald J, Brendler T, Christof J, Jaenicke C, eds. *PDR for Herbal Medicines.* Montvale, NJ: Medical Economics Co.; 1998:875–879.

Hattori T, et al. Preliminary evidence for inhibitory effect of glycyrrhizin on HIV replication in patients with aids. *Antiviral Research.* 1989;II:255–262.

Heinerman J. *Heinerman's Encyclopedia of Fruits, Vegetables and Herbs.* Englewood Cliffs, NJ: Prentice Hall; 1988.

Kinghorn A, Balandrin M, eds. *Human Medicinal Agents from Plants.* Washington DC: American Chemical Society; 1993: chap 3.

Mori, K. et al. Effects of glycyrrhizin (SNMC: stronger neo-minophagen C) in hemophilia patients with HIV-I infection. Tohoku *J. Exp. Med.* 1990;162:183–193.

Murray MT. *The Healing Power of Herbs: The Enlightened Person's Guide to the Wonders of Medicinal Plants.* 2nd ed. Rocklin, Calif: Prima Publishing; 1995:228–239.

Newall CA, Anderson LA, Phillipson JD, eds. *Herbal Medicines: A Guide for Health-care Professionals.* London: Pharmaceutical Press; 1996:183–186.

Ohuchi K, et al. Glycyrrhizin inhibits prostaglandin E2 formation by activated peritoneal macrophages from rats. *Prostagland Med.* 1981; 7:457–463.

Snow JM. Glycyrrhiza glabra L. (Leguminaceae). *Protocol J Botan Med.* 1996;1:9–14.

Turpie A, Runcie J, Thomson T. Clinical trial of deglycyrrhizinate liquorice in gastric ulcer. *Gut.* 1969;10:299–303.

Tyler VE. *Herbs of Choice: The Therapeutic Use of Phytomedicinals.* Binghamton, NY: Pharmaceutical Products Press; 1994:197–199.

■ MILK THISTLE FRUIT/MILK THISTLE HERB
Silybum marianum (Botanical)
Asteraceae (Plant Family)
Cardui mariae fructus/Cardui mariae herba (Pharmacopeial)

OVERVIEW

Milk thistle seed protects the liver and restores the liver's ability to detoxify harmful substances. Used for centuries in the ancient world, milk thistle was touted by Greek and Medieval physicians as a remedy for snakebites, jaundice, and other liver diseases. Its uses in Western folk medicine were versatile, and nursing mothers took milk thistle leaf to increase their milk flow. Extensive research conducted over the past 30 years shows that milk thistle seed extract is an effective treatment for cirrhosis of the liver, hepatitis, and inflammatory liver conditions.

Silymarin is a group of flavonoid-like compounds extracted from the small hard fruits (kenguil seeds) of milk thistle. The liver-protecting and liver-repairing functions of silymarin are due to two main actions: antioxidant and protein-restoring activities. The antioxidant activity of silymarin is ten times more powerful than vitamin E. Antioxidants scavenge free radicals that damage cells and cause lipid peroxidation. In lipid peroxidation, unstable free radicals attack the cell membrane. Silymarin prevents toxic and foreign substances from penetrating liver cells by stabilizing the outer membrane of liver cells. The active constituents displace toxins by binding to proteins and receptors on the cell membrane. Silymarin also stimulates protein synthesis in ribosomes so that new liver cells can grow and damaged liver cells can be replaced. Because silymarin acts mainly on the liver and kidneys, it is an effective antidote against poisonous substances that accumulate in the liver.

MACRO DESCRIPTION

Native to the Mediterranean, milk thistle is now widespread in many areas, including eastern Europe, Asia, the eastern United States, and California. It grows wild in dry sunny areas with well-drained soils, but is usually cultivated in northern regions. This biennial or annual stout thistle has broad, wavy, lanceolate leaves; large, prickly, leaves marbled with white; and red-purple flowers. The stem branches at the top, reaching heights of 4 to 10 feet. The small, hard-skinned fruits are brown, spotted, and shiny. This plant is easy to grow, and it matures rapidly, usually in less than a year.

PART USED/PHARMACEUTICAL DESIGNATIONS
- Flowers
- Stems
- Seeds
- Leaves
- Fruits (kenguel seed or compressed achenes)

CONSTITUENTS/COMPOSITION

Fruit contains 1.5% to 3% silymarin (flavonolignans, consisting of 50% silybarin [silybin] and lesser amounts of isosilybin, dehydrosilybin, silydianin, silychristin); tyramine, histamine, essential oils, lipids (20% to 30%), sugars, alkaloids, saponins, mucilages, vitamins C, E, and K, flavonoids.

COMMERCIAL PREPARATIONS

Milk thistle is prepared for oral use as capsules of concentrated extract of standardized dried herb (70% to 80%, or about 140 mg silymarin); tincture (liquid extract). There are several teas containing the standardized extract. Silymarin must be concentrated because it is poorly absorbed from the gastrointestinal tract.

MEDICINAL USES/INDICATIONS

- Traditional herbal actions: promotes milk production; jaundice; chologue and choleretic (promotes bile production for obstructive liver and gallbladder disorders); hepato-restorative, galactagogue, and demulcent.
- Clinical applications: for chronic liver and gallbladder disorders such as cirrhosis, damage from harmful chemicals and alcohol abuse, cholangitis, pericholangitis, gallstones, and chronic hepatitis B, C, D, E, and as a supportive in acute hepatitis A; for topical use in skin conditions such as psoriasis, eczema, aging skin, erythema, burns, wounds, and sores.

PHARMACOLOGY

Milk thistle extract (silymarin) has a liver-protecting effect against toxic chemicals (carbon tetrachloride, galactosamine, praseodymium, thioacetamide, acetaminophen). It is the most important antidote in modern medicine to poisoning from deathcap mushroom (*Amanita phalloides*). Milk thistle extract is so effective that it counteracts *Amanita* toxins even if it is taken 10 minutes after mushrooms are consumed.

Silymarin has antioxidant effects in both in vitro and in vivo studies. Glutathione is an antioxidant that helps the liver detoxify harmful chemicals, drugs, and hormones. Silymarin keeps glutathione levels from dropping too low, and in healthy humans it raises glutathione levels in the liver by as much as 35%.

In several experiments, silymarin protected against ulcers and gastrointestinal problems, relieved allergies by blocking histamine release, and decreased the activity of tumor-promoting agents. Silymarin also increased the movement of human polymorphonuclear leukocytes (PML's) blocked by harmful substances. And a silymarin-phospholipid complex had anti-inflammatory activity.

In humans, milk thistle seed extract improved fatty liver caused by chemical and alcohol damage. And in several double-blind, placebo-controlled studies, milk thistle extract improved liver dysfunction in patients with hepatitis B, chronic alcoholic liver disease, alcohol-induced liver disease, chronic exposure to organophosphates, toxic liver disorders, and chronic hepatitis. Silymarin also lowered the death rate of alcoholic patients compared to controls over a two to four year period, and it reduced the symptoms of hepatitis (abdominal upset, decreased appetite, fatigue). Silymarin increased serum bilirubin levels and liver enzymes when compared to controls, and it had a favorable effect on Type II hyperlipidemia, low platelet count, and psoriasis. Benefits of milk thistle extract have been reported for subclinical cholecstasis of pregnancy, cholangitis, and pericholangitis.

DOSAGE RANGES AND DURATION OF ADMINISTRATION

- Recommended dosage: 1 to 4 g dried fruit (seeds), (200 to 400 mg silymarin)
- Protective dosage for healthy people: silymarin 120 mg bid; Tincture (1:5): L 2 to 6 ml tid
- Restorative dosage for people with liver disorders: silymarin 120 mg tid. Silymarin-phosphatidylcholine complex (in 1:1 ratio) is absorbed better and has more clinical benefits than silymarin alone. (Phosphatidylcholine is a key element in cell membranes.)

Decoction: 1 to 4 g of fruit in 500 ml water tid

• Recommended dosage for complex: 100 to 200 mg bid

SIDE EFFECTS/TOXICOLOGY

No toxicity has been reported for long-term use in test animals (20 g/kg in mice; 1 g/kg in dogs), and long term use does not seem to pose any danger. Milk thistle occasionally has a mild laxative effect due to increased bile flow and secretion. Dietary fiber (guar gum, psyllium oat bran, pectin) can be taken to stop loose stools and mucosal irritation.

WARNINGS/CONTRAINDICATIONS/PRECAUTIONS

Alcohol-based extracts are not recommended for severe liver problems.

INTERACTIONS

None noted

REGULATORY AND COMPENDIAL STATUS

The U.S. FDA classifies milk thistle as a dietary supplement. In Germany, milk thistle is used as a nonprescription drug for inflammatory liver disease and cirrhosis.

REFERENCES

Alarcón de la Lastra A, Martín M, Motilva V, et al. Gastroprotection induced by silymarin, the hepatoprotective principle of Silybum marianum in ischemia-reperfusion mucosal injury: role of neutrophils. *Planta Med.* 1995;61:116–119.

Dorland Newman WA, ed. Dorland's Illustrated Medical Dictionary. 25th ed. Philadelphia, Pa: WB Saunders. 1974.

Feher J, Deak G, Muzes G, Lang I, Neiderland V, Nekan K, et al. Hepatoprotective activity of silymarin therapy in patients with chronic alcoholic liver disease. *Orv Hetil.* 1990;130:51.

Ferenci P, Dragosics B, Dittrich H, Frank H., Benda L, Lochs H, et al. Randomized controlled trial of silymarin treatment in patients with cirrhosis of the liver. *J Hepatol.* 1989;9:105-13.

Flora K, Hahn M, Rosen H, Benner K. Milk thistle (Silybum marianum) for the therapy of liver disease. *Am J Gastroenterol.* 1998;93:139–43.

Hobbs C. *Milk Thistle: The Liver Herb.* 2nd ed. Capitola, Calif: Botanica Press; 1992.

Hocking G. A Dictionary of Natural Products. Medford, NJ: Plexus; 1997.

Kinghorn A, Balandrin M, eds. *Human Medicinal Agents from Plants.* Washington, DC: American Chemical Society; 1993.

Magliulo E, Gagliardi B, Fiori GP. Results of a double blind study on the effect of silymarin in the treatment of acute viral hepatitis, carried out at two medical centres. *Med Klinik.* 1978;73:1060–1065.

Morazzoni P, Bombardelli E. *Silybum marianum (Carduus marianus). Fitoterapia.* 1995;LXVI.

Murray M. *The Healing Power of Herbs: The Enlightened Person's Guide to the Wonders of Medicinal Plants.* 2nd ed. Rocklin, Calif: Prima Publishing; 1995.

Murray M, Pizzorno J. *Encyclopedia of Natural Medicine.* 2nd ed. Rocklin, Calif: Prima Publishing; 1998.

Palasciano G, Portincasa P, Palmieri V, Ciani D, Vendemiale G, Altomare E. The effect of silymarin on plasma levels of malon-dialdehyde in patients receiving long-term treatment with psychotropic drugs. *Curr Therapeut Res.* 1994;55(5):537-545.

Schulz V, Hansel R, Tyler V. *Rational Phytotherapy: A Physician's Guide to Herbal Medicine.* 3rd ed. Berlin, Germany: Springer-Verlag; 1998.

Tyler V. *The Honest Herbal: A Sensible Guide to the Use of Herbs and Related Remedies.* 3rd ed. New York, NY: Pharmaceutical Products Press; 1993:chap 3.

■ PAU D'ARCO
Tabebuia avellanedae(Botanical)
Bignoniaceae(Plant Family)

OVERVIEW

Pau d'arco is the name of a tea derived from the bark of several *Tabebuia* species. There are over 100 species of evergreen trees and shrubs in the *Tabebuia* genus, all of them native to tropical regions of Central and South America. Pau d'arco often comes from *Tabebuia avellanedae,* a tree found in the Amazonian rain forest. However, according to some, the correct scientific name for pau d'arco is *Tabebuia impetiginosa.* Other sources claim that *Tabebuia chrysata* is also marketed in the United States as pau d'arco.

Traditional herbalists in the Brazilian Amazonian rain forest make an infusion from either *Tabebuia avellanedae* or *Tabebuia altissima* to treat ulcers, diabetes, rheumatism, cancer, and ringworm. The popularity of this tree for treating cancer, malignant tumors, and Candida fungal infections has soared over the past decade. Increasing demand for pau d'arco has only intensified stripping the bark from the trees, making *Tabebuia* one of the most exploited plant groups in the Amazon. *Tabebuia* species are now seriously threatened by extinction.

Extracts of *Tabebuia avellanedae* have anti-inflammatory, antimicrobial, and anticancer effects. The inner part of the bark supposedly contains lapachol, an active principle that has been shown to be an effective anticancer agent. However, the scientific evidence for the anticancer effects of pau d'arco is weak. While the bark of *Tabebuia* species does contain lapachol derivatives, only trace amounts of the anticancer compound, lapachol, are actually present. To further complicate matters, most of the research on the chemistry of *Tabebuia* has been done on the heartwood rather than the bark. But it is the bark that is medicinally important. Critics point out that the relatively high cost and lack of evidence to support therapeutic claims, combined with the fact that pau d'arco is potentially an endangered species, make it a less-than-desirable herbal supplement.

MACRO DESCRIPTION

Most species in the *Tabebuia genus* are broad-leaf evergreen trees. *Tabebuia avellanedae* grows to a height of 125 feet and is distinguished by rose-to-violet colored flowers. It has exceptionally hard wood that is disease-resistant and does not easily decay.

PART USED/PHARMACEUTICAL DESIGNATIONS

- Inner bark

CONSTITUENTS/COMPOSITION

Tabebuia avellanedae heartwood: naphthoquinones (lapachol, 2 to 7%; menaquinone-1, deoxylapachol, beta-lapachone, alpha-lapachone, dehydro-alpha-lapachone); anthraquinones (2-methylanthraquinone, 2-hydroxymethylanthraquinone, 2-acetoxymethylanthraquinone, anthraquinone-2-aldehyde, 1-hydroxyanthraquinone, 1-methoxyanthraquinone, 2-hydroxy-3-methylquinone, tabebuin).

COMMERCIAL PREPARATIONS

Pau d'arco products are not usually standardized for lapachol or naphthoquinone content. Some pau d'arco herbal teas are not authentic, but are derived from the bark of *Tecoma curialis.* Since *Tabebuia* and *Tecoma* species are in the same botanical family (Bignoneaceae), they often contain some of the same active principles. Consequently, remedies made from *Tecoma* and *Tabebuia* tree bark sometimes have similar therapeutic activities.

MEDICINAL USES/INDICATIONS

Traditional use: tonic, blood builder, rheumatism, cystitis, prostatitis, bronchitis, gastritis, ulcers, liver disorders, asthma, gonorrhea, ringworm, hernias; breast, liver, and prostate cancers

Traditional herbal actions: immune tonic, antimicrobial, antifungal, antineoplastic, antiviral

Clinical applications: cancer, *Candida albicans* infections (used internally and topically for internal and topical vaginal candidiasis), oral thrush candidiasis, infections of the genito-urinary tract (cystitis, prostatitis), herpes, stomatitis, lupus, Hodgkins disease

PHARMACOLOGY

In the mid 1950s, Brazilian researchers reported that lapachol isolated from *Tabebuia avellanedae* had antimicrobial effects against gram-positive and acid-fast bacteria. Lapachol also showed strong antimicrobial effects against Brucella, and it had fungistatic (fungus-inhibiting) properties. However, these effects decreased as the extract was progressively purified to yield a higher content of lapachol but lower quantity of other constituents. Ongoing studies have since confirmed that *Tabebuia avellanedae* extracts contain not only lapachol, but other active constituents as well. These additional compounds include active quinones such as alpha-lapachone, beta-lapachone, and xyloidone.

Lapachol and other quinones in *Tabebuia avellanedae* showed antiviral activity against herpes simplex types I and II, influenza virus, poliovirus, and vesicular stomatitis virus. Beta-lapachone produced an antiviral effect by blocking crucial viral enzymes, including DNA and RNA polymerases, as well as retrovirus reverse transcriptase.

Lapachol also had antiparasitic activity against the larvae that cause schistosomiasis, a water-borne disease. When taken orally, lapachol is secreted into the skin where it provides a barrier to the larvae of schistosomes. Beta-lapachone destroys the parasite responsible for trypanosomiasis (Chagas' disease).

In other studies, pau d'arco extracts were effective in reducing inflammation associated with cervicitis and cervicovaginitis. Although extracts reportedly had low toxicity in several investigations, lapachol is known to be toxic when administered as an isolated active principle. Lapachol destroys vitamin K activity. Interestingly, pau d'arco contains a vitamin K–like compound that probably compensates for the anti–vitamin K action of lapachol. This may explain why remedies made from the whole plant do not interfere with vitamin K activity.

In in vivo studies, lapachol exhibited anticancer effects against Walker 256 carinosarcoma, Yoshida sarcoma, and Murphy-Sturm lymphosarcoma. Despite these promising results, lapachol is not a practical cancer therapy. When given at therapeutically effective doses, lapachol produces the adverse side effects of nausea, vomiting, anemia, and a tendency to bleed. Monkeys given daily doses of 0.0625 to 0.25 g/kg of lapachol developed severe anemia, especially during the initial two weeks of treatment.

Lapachol seemed to be a promising new drug when Phase I clinical trials on its safety were first launched at the National Cancer Institue (NCI) in 1968, but researchers soon discovered that therapeutic doses produced mildly toxic side effects. There have been no clinical investigations on the efficacy of lapachol for treating cancer and other diseases because this compound is too toxic for human consumption. However, the anthraquinones in pau d'arco exhibited vitamin K–like activity. It is possible that anti–vitamin K adverse side effects may not have occurred in the NCI study had the whole plant been used instead of lapachol, the isolated compound.

DOSAGE RANGES AND DURATION OF ADMINISTRATION

- One cup decocted bark 2 to 8 times/day (1 tsp. pau d'arco boiled in 1 cup water 5 to 15 min)
- Tincture 1:5: 1 ml tid or qid
- Capsules: 1,000 mg tid

SIDE EFFECTS/TOXICOLOGY

- Large doses can cause nausea.
- Whole bark decoctions do not appear to be toxic for human consumption even though lapachol, one of the active constituents, causes adverse side effects.

WARNINGS/CONTRAINDICATIONS/PRECAUTIONS

Individuals prone to blood-clotting conditions should consult with their health care practitioner before using pau d'arco.

INTERACTIONS

No interactions have been reported.

REGULATORY AND COMPENDIAL STATUS

The U.S. FDA classifies pau d'arco as a dietary supplement.

REFERENCES

Anesini C, et al. Screening of plants used in Argentine folk medicine for antimicrobial activity. *J Ethnopharmacol.* 1993;39:119–128.

Block J, Sterpick A, Miller W; Wiernik P. Early clinical studies with lapachol (NSC-11905). *Cancer Chemother Rep.* 1974;4(part 2):27–28.

Gershon H, Shanks L. Fungitoxicity of 1,4-naphthoquinones to *Candida albicans* and *Trichophyton mentagrophytes. Can J of Microbio.* 1975;21:1317–1321.

Duke J, Vasquez R. *Amazonian Ethnobotanical Dictionary.* Boca Raton, Fla: CRC Press; 1994:164.

Kinghorn AD, Balandrin MA, eds. *Human Medicinal Agents from Plants.* Washington, DC: American Chemical Society; 1993:16–17.

Murray MT. *The Healing Power of Herbs: The Enlightened Person's Guide to the Wonders of Medicinal Plants.* 2nd ed. Rocklin, Calif: Prima Publishing; 1995:220–227.

Nakona K, et al. Iridoids From *Tabebuia Avellanedae. Phytochemisty.* 1993;32:371–373.

Perez H, et al. Chemical Investigations and in Vitro Antimalarial Activity of *Tabebuia ochracea* ssp. Neochrysanta. *International Journal of Pharmacognosy.* 1997;35:227–231.

Schultes RE, Raffauf RF. *The Healing Forest: Medicinal and Toxic Plants of the Northwest Amazonia.* Portland, Ore: Dioscorides Press; 1990:107–109.

Shealy CN. *The Illustrated Encyclopedia of Healing Remedies.* Dorset UK: Element Books; 1998:132.

Tyler VE. *Herbs of Choice: The Therapeutic Use of Phytomedicinals.* Binghamton, NY: Pharmaceutical Products Press; 199:180.

Tyler VE. *The Honest Herbal: A Sensible Guide to the Use of Herbs and Related Remedies.* 3rd ed. Binghamton, NY: Pharmaceutical Products Press; 1993:239–240.

Ueda S, et al. Production of anti-tumour-promoting furanonaphthoquinones in *Tabebuia avellanedae* cell cultures. *Phytochemistry.* 1994;36:323–325.

■ PEPPERMINT LEAF/PEPPERMINT OIL

Mentha x piperita (Botanical)
Lamiaceae (Plant Family)
Menthae piperitae folium/Menthae piperitae aetheroleum (Pharmacopeial)

OVERVIEW

Peppermint is widely used for its antispasmodic, antiseptic, carminative, anaesthetic, and choleretic properties. It aids digestion and is held to be helpful for many stomach problems, irritable bowel syndrome, nausea, morning sickness, dysmenorrhea, diarrhea, constipation, and flatulence. In larger doses, it may have an emmenagogic effect. Studies show that peppermint oil acts as a choleretic, stimulating the flow of bile, which improves digestion. Peppermint oil also has antiviral properties, inhibiting many viruses that cause digestive problems.

Menthol, a major constituent of peppermint oil, is well known for its external analgesic counterirritant effects. It cools as well as numbs the skin, producing effective relief from the itching caused by hives and poison ivy. A combination of peppermint oil's analgesic and antispasmodic properties also make it an effective remedy for headaches. Studies suggest that correct use of the oil can be as effective as taking 1 g of acetaminophen.

Peppermint and menthol appear most frequently in cold medicines, where they are effective as decongestants. The strong antiviral properties of peppermint are most concentrated in the tea form, and drinking it will restrict the growth of many cold and flu viruses. It is also very effective for a dry cough, because it calms the throat muscles, and as an expectorant, because menthol thins the mucus.

MACRO DESCRIPTION

Square stems grow up to two feet tall. Flowers are tiny, purple, in whorls and terminal spikes, with four stamens. Leaves are opposite, simple, toothed, and very fragrant. It blooms from July through August. Peppermint is native to Europe and Asia; some types are indigenous to South Africa, South America, and Australia. It is naturalized in North America and cultivated primarily in Oregon, Washington, and Wisconsin.

PART USED/PHARMACEUTICAL DESIGNATIONS

- Flower
- Leaves
- Oil

CONSTITUENTS/COMPOSITION

The herb consists of the leaves and flowering tops of *Mentha x piperita* (family Lamiaceae) and is made up of volatile oil (0.5% to 4%) composed of 50% to 78% menthol and 5% to 20% menthol esterfied with various organic acids, such as acetic and bovaleric. Also flavonoids (luteolin, menthoside), phenolic acids, and triterpenes.

COMMERCIAL PREPARATIONS

Packaged peppermint tea is widely available or may be made from dried fresh peppermint leaves.

Tinctures: Peppermint spirit is an alcoholic solution containing 10% peppermint oil and 1% peppermint leaf extract. To make a tincture, add one part peppermint oil to nine parts pure grain alcohol. Enteric-coated capsules (0.2 ml of peppermint oil per capsule)

Creams or ointments (should contain 1% to 16% menthol): Mentholatum or Vicks VapoRub

MEDICINAL USES/INDICATIONS

Traditional: antispasmodic, carminative, choleretic, antibacterial, decongestant, external analgesic, antiemetic, aromatic, emmenagogue, antiparasitic, stimulant

Conditions: irritable bowel syndrome, nausea, morning sickness, diarrhea, dysmenorrhea, constipation, flatulence, gallstones, headache, hives, nasal congestion, dry cough

Clinical applications: spastic complaints of gastrointestinal tract and bile ducts, irritable colon, catarrhs of respiratory tract, inflammation of oral mucosa, myalgic and neuralgic conditions

PHARMACOLOGY

Peppermint's primary active component is menthol, the focus of most scientific experiments, which have determined it to be effective internally as an antispasmodic, carminative, choleretic, decongestant, and antibacterial, and externally as an analgesic.

Peppermint's carminative properties work by relaxing the esophageal sphincter, allowing gas pressure to escape the stomach. Because of this, peppermint should not be used in case of gastro-esophageal reflux disease because it may exacerbate the condition. Peppermint oil antagonizes the spasmogenic action of barium chloride, pilocarpine, and physostigmine. It also acts competitively with nifedipine and blocks $Ca\ 2^+$—exciting stimuli, thereby inhibiting muscle contractions. A recent study reported that 89.5% of patients with irritable bowel syndrome showed significant improvement in abdominal symptoms after being treated with enteric-coated peppermint oil capsules. The enteric coating allows the peppermint oil to reach the intestines without being absorbed into the stomach. In the intestines, the oil is believed to inhibit the hypercontractility of intestinal smooth muscle and restore proper muscle tone.

In vitro studies show that peppermint oil can inhibit and destroy influenza A viruses, herpes simplex, mumps virus, *Streptococcus pyogenes, Staphylococcus aureus, Pseudomonas aeruginosa,* and *Candida albicans.* The menthol and related terpenes found in peppermint oil have been shown by several studies to dissolve gallstones by lowering bile cholesterol levels while raising bile acid and lecithin levels in the gallbladder.

Peppermint works as an external analgesic by blocking muscle contractions caused by serotonin and substance P, but it also stimulates cold receptors on the skin, which may influence the spinal cord's pain transmissions. The oil also relaxes the pericranial muscles and increases blood flow to the capillaries, making it an effective treatment for headaches.

DOSAGE RANGES AND DURATION OF ADMINISTRATION

- For digestion and upset stomach, peppermint tea (infusion), 1 to 2 tsp. of dried leaves per 8 oz. of water, 3 to 4 cups daily between meals; peppermint glycente for children, 1 to 2 ml daily
- For gallstones and irritable bowel syndrome, 1 to 2 enteric-coated capsules tid between meals
- As an external analgesic, menthol in a cream or ointment form no more than tid to qid
- For upset stomach or vomiting, 3 to 6 g of leaf, or 5 to 15 drops of tincture

• For tension headaches, tincture of peppermint oil. Apply light coating to entire forehead with fingertips or small sponge. If there is occipital pain, apply to back of neck as well. Allow to evaporate.

SIDE EFFECTS/TOXICOLOGY

When taken as a tea, peppermint is usually considered safe, although hypersensitivity reactions have been reported. Rare negative reactions to enteric-coated peppermint oil capsules may include skin rash, heartburn, bradycardia (slowed heartbeat), and muscle tremors. Menthol or peppermint oil applied topically could cause contact dermatitis or rash. Peppermint oil should be diluted and taken in small amounts, as excessive ingestion could cause interstitial nephritis and acute renal failure. An estimated fatal dose of menthol is 2 to 9 g if taken internally. There are no known mutagenic or carcinogenic effects.

WARNINGS/CONTRAINDICATIONS/PRECAUTIONS

No contraindications to peppermint as an herb. Peppermint oil is contraindicated by biliary tract obstruction, cholecystitis, and severe liver damage. Infants and small children should not use peppermint tea or oil. Pregnant or nursing mothers should use peppermint tea only in small doses and those with a history of miscarriage should avoid it. Do not mistake oil for tincture preparations.

INTERACTIONS

None known.

REGULATORY AND COMPENDIAL STATUS

On the U.S. FDA's list of herbs, peppermint is generally regarded as safe as a dietary supplement. The German Commission E approves it for internal use as an antispasmodic, carminative, choleretic, and decongestant, and for external use as an analgesic.

REFERENCES

Blumenthal M, ed. *The Complete German Commission E Monographs*. Boston, Mass: Integrative Medicine Communications; 1998.

Castleman M. *The Healing Herbs*. New York, NY: Bantam Books; 1991.

Dew MJ, Evans BK, Rhodes J. Peppermint oil for the irritable bowel syndrome: a multi-centre trial. *Br J Clin Pract*. 1984;(11–12):394, 398.

Duke J. *The Green Pharmacy*. Emmaus, Pa: Rodale Press; 1997.

Feng XZ. Effect of Peppermint oil hot compresses in preventing abdominal distension in postoperative gynecological patients [In Chinese]. *Chung Hua Hu Li Tsa Chih*. 1997; 32:577–578.

Hills J. The mechanism of action of peppermint oil on gastrointestinal smooth muscle. *Gastroenterology*. 1991;101:55–65.

Koch TR. Peppermint oil and irritable bowel syndrome [In Process Citation]. *Am J Gastroenterol*. 1998;93:2304–2305.

Kowalchik C, Hylton W, eds. *Rodale's Illustrated Encyclopedia of Herbs*. Emmaus, Pa: Rodale Press; 1987.

Lawson MJ, Knight, RE, Tran K, Walker G, Robers-Thompson, IC. Failure of enteric-coated peppermint oil in the irritable bowel syndrome: a randomized double-blind crossover study. *J Gastroent Hepatol*. 1988;3:235-238.

Mowrey D. *The Scientific Validation of Herbal Medicine*. New Canaan, Conn: Keats Publishing, Inc; 1986.

Murray MT. *The Healing Power of Herbs*. Rocklin, Calif: Prima Publishing; 1995.

Pittler MH, Ernst E. Peppermint oil for irritable bowel syndrome: a critical review and metaanalysis. *Am J Gastroenterol*. 1998;93:1131–1135.

Rees W. Treating irritable bowel syndrome with peppermint oil. *Br Med J*. 1979;II:835–836.

Schulz V, Hänsel R, Tyler V. *Rational Phytotherapy*. Berlin, Germany: Springer; 1998.

Tyler V. *Herbs of Choice: The Therapeutic Use of Phytomedicinals*. New York, NY: Pharmaceutical Products Press; 1994.

■ SAW PALMETTO BERRY
Serenoa repens/Sabal serrulata (Botanical)
Aracaceae (Plant Family)
Sabal fructus (Pharmacopeial)

OVERVIEW

Saw palmetto is a leading treatment for benign prostatic hyperplasia (BPH) in Germany and Austria, and is among the top five dietary supplements sold in the United States. It relieves bladder and urinary disturbances associated with stage I and II BPH. Stage I symptoms include frequent urination, nocturea, delayed urination, low urinary force, and post-void dribbling; stage II symptoms herald bladder function debility and include urgency and incomplete emptying of the bladder. Sexual dysfunction has also been reported. The majority of men over 60 are considered to have urinary symptoms attributable to BPH. The condition may progress to prostate cancer, bladder infections, and damaged kidneys if left untreated.

First used in the treatment of BPH late in the nineteenth century, saw palmetto has been the subject of at least 20 laboratory studies and 18 clinical studies. These experiments demonstrated saw palmetto's antiestrogenic and antiandrogenic effects and confirmed that the berry extract reduces 5-alpha-reductase. These are considered significant interventions in the treatment of BPH.

Most recently, researchers assessed the results of 18 controlled trials and concluded that saw palmetto can be as effective as finasteride in improving BPH-affected urine flow and urgency. Compared to placebo, saw palmetto relieved nocturia by 25%, urinary tract symptoms by 28%, increased peak urine flow by 28%, and decreased residual volume by 43%. Finasteride does shrink the prostate, however, and saw palmetto does not.

Saw palmetto berries provided food and medicine for Native Americans for centuries. Aside from their nutritional value, the berries were considered expectorant, sedative, and diuretic by traditional folk healers. It was used to reduce inflammation in genitourinary catarrh and to treat breast disorders in women. Some herbalists claim that saw palmetto can increase breast size, and that it is an aphrodisiac. These claims are unsubstantiated, however.

From 1906 to 1916, saw palmetto berries were listed in the U.S. Pharmacopoeia and were described as effective remedies for chronic and subacute cystitis, chronic bronchitis, laryngitis, catarrh that accompanies asthma, and enlarged prostate glands. It was also in the National Formulary from 1926 to 1950.

MACRO DESCRIPTION

The saw palmetto shrub is a fan palm that grows from 6 to 10 feet in warm climates, from South Carolina to Mississippi and throughout Florida. Lush palmate leaves have lance-shaped leaflets and are supported by spiny stems. Flowers are white and develop yellow olive-like berries, which become bluish-black when ripe and have an oily sheen attributable to their fatty acid content.

PART USED/PHARMACEUTICAL DESIGNATIONS

- Berries

CONSTITUENTS/COMPOSITION

Saturated and unsaturated, mostly free fatty acids (capric, caprylic, caproic, lauric, palmitic, and oleic acids); free and conjugated sterols; fruits also contain high-molecular weight polysaccharides and flavonoids. Fat-soluble extracts are standardized to contain 85% to 95% fatty acids and sterols.

COMMERCIAL PREPARATIONS

Crude dried berries, tea, powdered encapsulations, tablets, tinctures, and liposterolic extracts standardized to contain 85% to 95% fatty acids and sterols.

MEDICINAL USES/INDICATIONS

Saw palmetto was historically used as an expectorant and to treat general debility, respiratory catarrh, and muscle wasting due to age or menopause.

Traditional herbal actions: Tonic for both female and male reproductive systems and urinary tracts, nourishing tonic, anti-inflammatory, urinary antiseptic, relaxant, diuretic.

Clinical applications: Used for the relief of symptoms of stage I and II BPH. Future research may lead to the treatment of female androgen excess disorders, such as hirsutism and polycystic ovary disease. Increases milk flow in nursing mothers, used to treat infections of the genito-urinary system, such as cystitis, urethritis, and salpingitis.

PHARMACOLOGY

Liposterolic extracts act at the cytosolic, androgenic receptor of prostate tissue in vitro to inhibit 5-alpha-reductase, block adrenergic receptors, and inhibit DHT-producing enzymes. Inhibition of dihydrotestosterone (DHT) and 5-alpha-reductase may have a positive effect in the treatment of BPH. Finasteride inhibits 5-alpha-reductase, which in turn blocks testosterone from transforming into DHT, and DHT may be responsible for the hyperproliferation of prostate cells involved in the etiology of BPH.

Despite evidence of estrogenic activity, liposterolic extracts also significantly stimulate antiestrogenic effects; it blocked nuclear estrogen receptors in prostatic tissue samples of patients with BPH. After a 90-day treatment period, researchers analyzed the function of androgen, estrogen, and progesterone receptor tissues in 35 study participants. The group given saw palmetto extract had lower cellular and nuclear estrogen and progesterone receptor values than the placebo group. Cellular androgen levels remained the same, but nuclear androgen levels declined. Estrogen may promote BPH due to inhibition of hydroxylation and elimination of DHT. Some investigators feel that estrogen's role in BPH is more significant than that of DHT.

DOSAGE RANGES AND DURATION OF ADMINISTRATION

To reduce symptoms associated with stages I and II BPH: 160 mg liposterolic extract, standardized to contain 85% to 95% fatty acids and sterols, or equivalent, bid.
- Tincture (1:4): 2 to 4 ml tid
- Fluid extract of dried berry pulp (1:1): 1 to 2 ml tid
- Capsules: 1,000 mg tid
- Tea: 2 tsp. dried berry with 24 oz. water, simmer slowly until liquid is reduced by half, take 4 oz. tid. The tea tastes vile but is effective.

SIDE EFFECTS/TOXICOLOGY

Adverse effects are very rare and include mild stomach upset. The American Herbal Products Association gives saw palmetto a class 1 safety rating, indicating that it is safe with appropriate use.

WARNINGS/CONTRAINDICATIONS/PRECAUTIONS

Before self-medicating with saw palmetto, patients should get a firm diagnosis of BPH. Although saw palmetto relieves symptoms, it does not shrink the prostate; therefore, the condition should be closely monitored by a health care provider.

Saw palmetto has hormonal effects and should not be used during pregnancy or lactation until specific studies prove otherwise.

INTERACTIONS

Saw palmetto may interfere with hormonal therapies such as contraceptive pills and patches and hormone-replacement therapy.

REGULATORY AND COMPENDIAL STATUS

Dietary supplement in the U.S., saw palmetto is approved for use in the treatment of stage I and II BPH by Germany's Commission E, and is on the General Sales List (GSL) in England.

REFERENCES

Blumenthal M, ed. *The Complete German Commission E Monographs:Therapeutic Guide to Herbal Medicine.* Boston, Mass: Integrative Medicine Communications; 1998.

Braeckman J. The extract of *Serenoa repens* in the treatment of benign prostatic hyperplasia: A multicenter open study. *Curr Therapeut Res* 1994;55:776–785.

Carilla E, Briley M, Fauran F, et al. Binding of Permixon, a new treatment for prostatic benign hyperplasia, to the cytosolic androgen receptor in the rat prostate. *J Steroid Biochem* 1984;20:521-523.

Carraro JC, et al. Comparison of phytotherapy (Permixon) with finasteride in the treatment of benign prostate hyperplasia: a randomized international study of 1,098 patients. *The Prostate.* 1996;29(4):231-240.

Di Silverio F, D'Eramo G, Lubrano C, et al. Evidence that *Serenoa repens* extract displays an antiestrogenic activity in prostatic tissue of benign prostatic hypertrophy patients. *Eur Uro.*1992;21:309-314.

el-Sheikh M, Dakkak MR, Saddique A. The effect of permixon on androgen receptors. *Acta Obstet Gynecol Scand.* 1988;67:397–399.

Hutchens AR. *Indian Herbalogy of North America.* Boston, Mass: Shambhala Publications; 1973:243–244.

Leung A, Foster S. *Encyclopedia of Common Natural Ingredients Used in Food, Drugs, and Cosmetics.* 2nd ed. New York, NY: John Wiley & Sons; 1996:467–468.

McGuffin M, Hobbs C, Upton R, Goldberg A. *American Herbal Products Association's Botanical Safety Handbook.* Boca Raton, Fla: CRC Press; 1996.

Murray MT. *The Healing Power of Herbs: Tthe Enlightened Person's Guide to the Wonders of Medicinal Plants.* Rocklin, Calif: Prima Publishing; 1995.

Newall CA, Anderson LA, Phillipson JD. *Herbal Medicines: A Guide for Health-Care Professionals.* London, England: The Pharmaceutical Press; 1996,

Schulz V, Hänsel R, Tyler VE. *Rational Phytotherapy: A Physicians' Guide to Herbal Medicine.* Berlin, Germany: Springer-Verlag; 1998.

Sökeland J, Albrecht J. A combination of *Sabal* and *Urtica* extracts vs. finasteride in BHP (stage I to II acc. to Alken): A comparison of therapeutic efficacy in a one-year double-blind study. *Urologe A.* 1997;36:327–333.

Mandressi A, et al. Treatment of uncomplicated benign prostatic hypertrophy BPH by an extract of *Serenoa Repens* clinical results. *J Endocrinol Invest.* 1987;10(suppl 2):49.

Wilt TJ, Ishani A, Stark G, et al. Saw palmetto extracts for treatment of benign prostatic hyperplasia: a systematic review. *JAMA.* 1998;280:1604–1609.

Wood HC, Osol A. *United States Dispensatory.* 23rd ed. Philadelphia, Pa: J.B. Lippincott; 1943;971–972.

Champault G, Patel JC, Bonnard AM. A double-blind trial of an extract of the plant *Serenoa repens* in benign prostatic hyperplasia. *Br J Clin Pharmacol.* 1984;18:461-462.

■ STINGING NETTLE HERB/STINGING NETTLE LEAF/STINGING NETTLE ROOT

Urtica dioica/Urtica urens (Botanical)
Urticaceae (Plant Family)
Urticae herba/Urticae folium/Urticae radix (Pharmacopeial)

OVERVIEW

Stinging nettle usually refers to *Urtica dioica*, but it can also include a closely related species, *Urtica urens*, known as garden nettle, and hybrids of these two species. *Urtica dioica* is an annual native to the temperate regions of Eurasia, now found throughout the world.

Healers from many cultures use nettle branches as part of a whipping technique called flagellation or urtification. Whipping paralyzed limbs and other afflicted or painful body parts supposedly activates the muscles and stimulates the organs. Hot leaf poultices and pounded leaves made from nettle were traditionally used as topical treatments for rheumatic pain. The herb was also historically used to treat uterine hemorrhage (particularly after childbirth) and as a snuff for nosebleeds. Today, nettle root is an effective therapy for treating the symptoms of benign prostatic hyperplasia (BPH).

MACRO DESCRIPTION

Stinging nettle *(Urica dioica)*, or common nettle, is an herbaceous shrub that reaches a height of nearly 3 feet. It prefers nitrogen-rich soil and blooms between June and September. The heart-shaped, finely toothed, tapered leaves are alternate and elliptical. The small green flowers are incomplete, and multiple types of flowers are often found on a single plant. The entire plant, especially the leaves and stem, is sparsely covered with stinging hairs that are painful when touched.

The stings are glandular hairs, or sharp, polished spines. Each hair contains an acrid fluid filled with histamine and formic acid. These chemical substances are released whenever the plant is forcefully applied to the skin, and they immediately irritate and inflame the skin. Histamine is probably responsible for the initial stinging sensation. However, nettle stings can have a therapeutic effect by acting as counter-irritants. Ironically, nettle juice can also be used as an antidote to painful nettle stings.

PART USED/PHARMACEUTICAL DESIGNATIONS

- Seeds
- Leaves
- Roots (rhizome) and underground parts (fresh and dried)

CONSTITUENTS/COMPOSITION

Flavonoids (in flowers) include glycosides of quercetins (isoquercitin, rutin), kaempferol, isohamnetin; amines (in stinging hairs) consist of small quantities of histamine, choline, acetylcholine, serotonin); chlorophylls; vitamins; triterpenes; sterols; carboxylic acids; minerals (high potassium and calcium salt content, silicic acid).

COMMERCIAL PREPARATIONS

Commercial preparations are made from fresh or dried aerial parts of *Urtica dioica, Urtica urens,* hybrids gathered during the flowering season, or from dried root/rhizome. Tinctures and tea products are available, as are capsules made from dried or freeze-dried herb.

MEDICINAL USES/INDICATIONS

Traditional herbal actions: nutritive, alterative, circulatory stimulant, galactagogue, hypo-glycemic, topical rubefacient (fresh leaves, only with caution), anti-histaminic and antidote to stings (fresh juice)

Clinical applications: supportive treatments (internal and external) for rheumatic ailments; irrigation therapy for inflammatory diseases of lower urinary tract; prevention and treatment of kidney gravel. Diuretic effect if taken with sufficient fluid. Treatment of seasonal allergies, non-insulin-dependent diabetes. Root is used to treat micturition (urinary) disorders in BPH stages 1 and 2, while the leaf is used for urinary tract infections, kidney and bladder stones, and rheumatism. It is also used as a topical compress or cream for arthritic joints, gout, sprains and strains, neuralgia, sciatica, tendonitis, burns, hemorrhoids, and insect bites. Fresh expressed juice is used for anemia and cardiac insufficiency with edema.

PHARMACOLOGY

Open, observational, and placebo-controlled double-blind studies confirm that nettle root extract is efficacious for several conditions, including BPH. In vivo studies have shown that nettle herb has diuretic activity, presumably due to the presence of flavonoids and high potassium content. An aqueous root extract exhibited mild anti-inflammatory effects in a carrageenan-induced animal edema model.

In other animal studies, nettle had CNS-depressant, analgesic, hypoglycemic, and hyperglycemic effects. Urticin has been identified as the hypoglycemic principle responsible for lowering blood sugar levels in rabbits. Nettle herb extracts showed uterine activity in both pregnant and nonpregnant mice. The uteroactive effect was attributed to betaine and serotonin.

Stinging nettle root has a favorable effect on BPH by increasing urinary volume and maximum urinary flow while reducing residual urine. Although nettle root extract lessens the symptoms of enlarged prostate, it does not actually decrease the enlargement.

Prostate enlargement has been linked to elevated testosterone levels, specifically to increased activity of enzymes involved in testosterone production. An active principle in nettle is thought to either lower the amount of free testosterone or inhibit a crucial enzyme, such as aromase, required for testosterone production.

Nettle root extract interferes with testosterone synthesis by competitively displacing sex-hormone-binding globulin (SHBG). However, the effective concentration needed for competitive displacement may be much greater than the concentration available in therapeutic doses.

The active constituent responsible for the anti-BPH effect has not been unequivocally determined, but it may consist of an agglutinin (a protein mixture called UDA) and several polysaccharides isolated from nettle root. Lectin induces interferon production by human lymphocytes and triggers nonspecific agglutination of erythrocytes. In an in vitro study, a component of UDA from nettle inhibited virus-induced cell damage caused by HIV-1, HIV-2, CMV, RSV, and influenza A.

In human clinical trials, nettle herb juice produced marked diuresis in patients with myocardial and chronic venous insufficiency, and showed hemostatic activity. And in a double-blind investigation, nettle herb was mildly efficacious in the treatment of allergic rhinitis.

DOSAGE RANGES AND DURATION OF ADMINISTRATION

- Seeds Dried herb: 2 to 4 g tid as infusion
- Seeds Fluid extract (1:1): 2 to 4 ml tid
- Seeds Tincture (1:5): 4 to 8 ml tid
- Seeds Fresh leaf infusion: 8 to 12 g fresh plant and ample liquid (at least 2 liters/day or equivalent)
- Seeds Root tincture/spiritus (1:10), for external use: 4 to 6 g/day or equivalent preparations (may be difficult to acquire in the U.S. except in blends)
- Seeds Topical compress, for external use: 4 to 6 g of herb in infusion

SIDE EFFECTS/TOXICOLOGY

No major side effects. Skin exposure to Urtica dioica can cause a stinging sensation (contact urticaria). Nettle root tea taken orally can cause mild gastrointestinal complaints, gastric irritation, burning sensation of the skin, edema, and oliguria (decreased urine output in relation to fluid intake). Allergic reactions (edema, skin afflictions) to leaf preparations have been reported in rare cases.

WARNINGS/CONTRAINDICATIONS/PRECAUTIONS

Irrigation therapy should not be used if edema is present. The massive amounts of fluids required for irrigation therapy can cause fluid retention due to reduced cardiac or renal activity. Nettle has abortifacient activity, and it can alter the menstrual cycle. Pregnant women should not use nettle, and lactating women should avoid excessive use of this herb.

INTERACTIONS

Excessive use of nettle may interfere with the actions of hypoglycemic, hyperglycemic, antidiabetic, and CNS depressive drugs.

REGULATORY AND COMPENDIAL STATUS

The U. S. FDA classifies stinging nettle as a dietary supplement. It is listed on the General Sale List (GSL) in Britain. In Germany, nettle root is used as a therapy for urinary complaints during early stages of BPH. Stinging nettle is approved by the German Commission E.

REFERENCES

Balzarini J, Neyts J, Schols D, Hosoya M, Van Damme E, Peumans W, De Clercq E. The mannose-specific plant lectins from Cymbidium hybrid and Epipactis helleborine and the (N-acetylglucosamine) n-specific plant lectin from *Urtica dioica* are potent and selective inhibitors of human immunodeficiency virus and cytomegalovirus replication in vitro. *Antiviral Research.* 1992;18:191–207.

Belaiche P, Lievoux O. Clinical Studies on the Palliative Treatment of Prostatic Adenoma with Extract of Urtica Root. *Phytotherapy Research.* 1991;5:267-269.

Blumenthal M, ed. *The Complete German Commission E Monographs. Therapeutic Guide to Herbal Medicines.* Boston, Mass: Integrative Medicine Communications; 1998:47, 132.

Bradley P, ed. *British Herbal Compendium.* Dorset, England: British Herbal Medicine Association; 1992;1:166–167.

Chrubasik S, Enderlein W, Bauer R, Grabner W. Evidence for antirheumatic effectiveness of Herba *Urticae dioica* in acute arthritis: A pilot study. *Phytomedicine.* 1997;4:105–108.

Grieve M. A Modern Herbal. New York, NY: Dover; 1971;2:574-579

Gruenwald J, Brendler T, Christof J. *PDR for Herbal Medicines.* Montvale, NJ: Medical Economics Company; 1998:1197–1199.

Hutchens A. *Indian Herbalogy of North America.* Boston, Mass: Shambhala; 1991:204–206.

Krzeski T, Kazon M, Borkowski A, Witeska A, Kuczera J. Combined extracts of *Urtica dioica* and *Pygeum africanum* in the treatment of benign prostatic hyperplasia: double-blind comparison of two doses. *Clin Ther.* 1993;15:1011–1020.

Millspaugh C. *American Medicinal Plants.* New York, NY: Dover; 1974:611–614.

Newall C, Anderson L, Phillipson J. *Herbal Medicines: A Guide for Health-Care Professionals.* London, England: Pharmaceutical Press; 1996:201–202.

Oliver F, Amon E, Breathnach A, Francis D, Sarathchandra P, Black A, Greaves M. Contact urticaria due to the common stinging nettle *(Urtica dioica*—histological, ultrastructural and pharmacological studies. *Clin Exp Dermatology.* 1991;267:1–7.

Schneider H, Honold E, Masuhr T. Treatment of benign prostatic hyperplasia. Results of a treatment study with the phytogenic combination of Sabal extract WS 1473 and Urtica extract WS 1031 in urologic specialty practices. *Fortschr Med.* 1995;267:37–40.

Schulz V, Hänsel R, Tyler VE. *Rational Phytotherapy: A Physician's Guide to Herbal Medicine. 3rd* ed. Berlin, Germany: Springer-Verlag; 1998:228–238.

S̆okeland J, Albrecht J. Lignans from the roots of *Urtica dioica* and their metabolites bind to human sex hormone binding globulin (SHBG). *Planta Med.* 1997;36:529–532.

Tyler VE. *Herbs of Choice: The Therapeutic Use of Phytomedicinals.* Binghamton, NY: Haworth; 1994:84–85.

Wylie G, et al. A comparative study of Tenidap, a cytokine-modulating anti-rheumatic drug, and diclofenac in rheumatoid arthritis: a 24 week analysis of a 1-year clinical trial. *Br J Rheumatol.* 1995;34:554–563.

■ ST. JOHN'S WORT

Hypericum perforatum (Botanical)
Hypericaceae (Plant Family)
Hyperici herba (Pharmacopeial)

OVERVIEW

Medicinal use of St. John's wort dates back to ancient Greece. The renowned physicians Dioscorides and Hippocrates used it to treat various illnesses, and it was long believed to rid the body of evil spirits. Belief in the herb's powers continued through the Middle Ages, but by the end of the 19th century, interest in it—and most other medicinal plants—had waned. Recent research on St. John's wort has focused attention on the herb, and it has become extremely popular with health product consumers in the United States. In Europe, where St. John's wort has a longer history of use, it is used to treat wounds, gastritis, kidney and lung problems, insomnia, and depression.

Most clinical studies of St. John's wort have focused on its use in treating mild to moderate depression. In a 1996 meta-analysis, researchers examined 23 randomized trials of St. John's wort in 1,757 patients with mild to moderate depression. Acknowledging the limitations of using pooled data from studies that used different dosages and preparations, experimental designs and patient populations, the researchers still concluded that St. John's wort is better than placebo in treating some types of depression. However, they could not draw firm conclusions about whether St. John's wort is as effective as standard antidepressants. The analysis did find that St. John's wort causes fewer side effects than standard antidepressants.

The National Institute of Mental Health (NIMH) does not currently recommend the use of St. John's wort for treatment of depression and has called for more rigorous research on the herb. Along with two other branches of the National Institutes of Health—the Office of Alternative Medicine and the Office of Dietary Supplements—NIMH has funded a three-year controlled clinical study of the herb in clinically depressed patients.

In at least one controlled trial, patients with seasonal affective disorder (SAD) responded well to treatment with St. John's wort, and the herb seems to be even more effective when used in combination with light therapy.

The antiretroviral activity of St. John's wort has raised hopes for using it to treat acquired immunodeficiency syndrome (AIDS). Results of small pilot studies have been promising, with patients showing stable or increased helper T cell counts, improved helper-to-suppressor T cell ratios, and low incidence of opportunistic infection, but larger and longer-term studies are still needed.

Topical preparations of St. John's wort have shown antibacterial and wound-healing activity and have been used to treat burns, muscle pain, and hemorrhoids. Topical preparations also have been used to reduce pain, inflammation, and to promote nerve-tissue regeneration. Interestingly, debate continues over the most active ingredient in St. John's wart, although its therapeutic effects are widely accepted and acknowledged.

MACRO DESCRIPTION

St. John's wort is a shrubby perennial with flat-topped clusters of bright yellow flowers. The plant is native to Britain and Europe but now grows wild in many other parts of the world, including the United States. It grows best in sunny sites with dry, gravelly, or chalky soil.

PART USED/PHARMACEUTICAL DESIGNATIONS

- Leaves
- Flowering tops

CONSTITUENTS/COMPOSITION

The best-studied active components are hypericin and pseudohypericin, found in both the leaves and flowers. There has been recent research to suggest that these best-studied components may not be the most active in the plant, with significant debate ensuing within the industry. Other components include flavonoids, xanthones, phenolic carboxylic acids, essential oils, carotenoids, alkanes, phloroglucinol derivatives, phytosterols, and medium-chain fatty acid alcohols.

COMMERCIAL PREPARATIONS

St. John's wort is available in various forms, including dried herb (chopped or powdered), capsule, liquid extract, tincture, infused oil, and tea infusion.

The recommended preparation of St. John's wort currently accepted by the industry is an extract standardized to contain 0.3% hypericin.

MEDICINAL USES/INDICATIONS

- Reduces symptoms of anxiety, depression, apathy, anorexia, and feelings of worthlessness
- Relieves insomnia and hypersomnia
- In topical form, promotes healing of wounds and burns; antimicrobial; reduces swelling
- Shows promise as adjuvant therapy for viral infections such as herpes simplex, influenza, mononucleosis, AIDS, M.S., Fibromyalgia, and neuro-muscular inflammations

PHARMACOLOGY

- Antidepressant activity. Initial research suggested that hypericin acts as a monoamine oxidase (MAO) inhibitor, but more recent work shows that xanthones and flavonoids may be responsible for this activity. The most recent studies indicate that hypertorin, a phoraglucinal, is partly responsible for the anti-depressant activity.
- Antibacterial activity. Extracts show broad-spectrum antimicrobial activity against such organisms as Escherichia coli, Staphylococcus aureus, Streptococcus mutans, Pseudomonas aeruginosa, and Proteus vulgaris in-vitro.
- Antiviral activity. Active components hypericin and pseudohypericin show antiviral activity against herpes simplex virus types 1 and 2, Epstein-Barr virus, influenza types A and B, and vesicular stomatitis virus in vitro. These components have also been shown to be active against a number of retroviruses, including the human immunodeficiency virus (HIV).

DOSAGE RANGES AND DURATION OF ADMINISTRATION

As an antidepressant, RDA is 300 to 500 mg of a 0.3% standardized extract, tid with meals, for a minimum of four to six weeks.

SIDE EFFECTS/TOXICOLOGY

St. John's wort causes severe photosensitivity in grazing animals that eat large amounts of the plant. Such reactions are rare in humans and have been seen only in people taking very large doses for HIV infection.

However, as a precaution, people with fair skin and people who take St. John's wort in large doses or over long periods should use a sunscreen with a skin protection factor (SPF) of at least 15 and should not use sunlamps or tanning beds or booths while taking the herb.

Other side effects are usually mild. They may include:
- Abdominal pain, bloating, constipation
- Nausea, vomiting
- Dizziness
- Dry mouth
- Itching, hives, skin rash
- Sleep problems
- Elevated blood pressure
- Unusual tiredness

WARNINGS/CONTRAINDICATIONS/PRECAUTIONS
- Take with food to reduce chances of gastric upset.
- Do not take during pregnancy or while breast-feeding.

INTERACTIONS
- May interact with L-dopa, 5-hydroxytryptophan
- Should be taken cautiously with MAO inhibitors such as furazolidone (Furoxone), isocarboxazid (Marplan), moclobemide (Manerex), phenelzine (Nardil), procarbazine (Matulane), selegiline (Eldepryl) or tranylcypromine (Parnate)
- Can be effective complement to selective serotonin reuptake inhibitors (SSRIs) such as fluoxetine (Prozac), paroxetine (Paxil) or sertraline (Zoloft). Debate exists whether they may be taken in combination if under careful observation.

REGULATORY AND COMPENDIAL STATUS
St. John's wort is labeled as a dietary supplement by the U.S. Food and Drug Administration.

REFERENCES
Bombardelli E, Morazzoni P. *Hypericum perforatum. Fitoterapia.* 1995;LXVI:43–68.

Degar S, et al. Inactivation of the human immunodeficiency virus by hypericin: Evidence for phytochemical alterations of p24 and a block in uncoating. *AIDS Res Hum Retroviruses.* 1992;8:1929–1936.

De Smet P, Peter AGM, Nolen WA. St. John's wort as an antidepressant. *Br Med J.* 1996;313:241–247.

Furner V, Bek M, Gold JA. A phase I/II unblinded dose ranging study of hypericin in HIV-positive subjects. *Int Conf AIDS.* 1991;7:199.

Cott JM. In vitro receptor binding and enzyme inhibition by *Hypericum perforatum* extract. *Pharmacopsychiatry.* 1997;30(suppl 2):108–112.

Gulick R, et al. Human hypericism: A photosensitivity reaction to hypericin (St. John's wort). *Int Conf AIDS.* 1992; 8:B90.

Lavie G, et al. Studies of the human mechanism of action of the antiviral agents hypericin and pseudohypericin. *Proc Natl Acad Sci USA.* 1989;86:5963–5967.

Linde K, Ramirez G, Mulrow CD, et al. St. John's wort for depression: an overview and meta-analysis of randomised clinical trials. *BMJ.* 1996;313:253–257.

Martinez B, Kasper S, Ruhrmann S, Moller HJ. Hypericum in the treatment of seasonal affective disorders. *J Geriatr Psychiatry Neurol.* 1994;7(Suppl 1):S29–33.

Meruelo D, Lavie G, Lavie D. Therapeutic agents with dramatic antiretroviral activity and little toxicity at effective doses: Aromatic polycyclic diones hypericin and pseudohypericin. *Proc Natl Acad Sci USA.* 1988;85:5230–5234.

Muller WE, Rolli M, Schafer C, Hafner, U. Effects of *hypericum* extract (LI 160) in biochemical models of antidepressant activity. *Pharmacopsychiatry.* 1997;30(suppl):102–107.

Murray MT. *The Healing Power of Herbs: The Enlightened Person's Guide to the Wonders of Medicinal Plants.* Rocklin, Calif: Prima Publishing; 1995.

Rasmussen P. St. John's wort: a review of its use in depression. *Australian Journal of Medical Herbalism.* 1998;10:8–13.

Tyler VE. *The Honest Herbal: A Sensible Guide to the Use of Herbs and Related Remedies.* Binghamton, NY: Pharmaceutical Products Press; 1993.

■ VALERIAN ROOT
Valeriana officinalis (Botanical)
Valerianaceae (Plant Family)
Valerianae radix (Pharmacopeial)

OVERVIEW
Valerian root relieves anxiety and nervousness-related chronic and periodic insomnia. Herbalists have understood the mildly sedating, sleep-enhancing properties of valerian for centuries, and also recommend its use for mild stomach pains, headaches, and menstrual pain. Currently, the FDA is considering the approval of valerian root as an OTC sleep aid.

MACRO DESCRIPTION
This three-to-five-foot herbaceous perennial has erect grooved, hollow stems that are hairy at the base and branch out toward the top. Dark green leaves grow in four to eight pairs from each stem; simple, pinnately lobed, and opposite, with hairy leaf veins on underside. Small fragrant flowers are white, lavender, or pink with three stamens and bloom in June in four-inch-wide panicles. Ornamental and medicinal, this perennial grows wild in damp, elevated locations.

Rhizomes, roots, and occasional stolons are sources of the crude drug. Superior preparations are light brown with a faint scent; darker, more pungent scents are considered inferior. The rhizome is one to two inches tall, ovoid, cylindrical, and light grayish-brown; with a "dirty sock" smell when dried. Darker offshoots of multiple joints with coarse longitudinal wrinkles grow from the rhizome. Stolons are gnarled and also light grayish-brown. Fresh root tastes sweet, spicy, and bitter. Soils rich in minerals grow healthier roots and provide stronger tinctures. These roots have sweeter taste and reduced "dirty sock" smell.

PART USED/PHARMACEUTICAL DESIGNATIONS
• Roots

CONSTITUENTS/COMPOSITION
The rhizome contains 0.8% to 1% iridoid valepotriates, 80% to 90% of which occur as valtrates (didrovaltrate, isovaltrate) and other iridoids. Many of these preparations no longer contain all of these constituents.

Rhizome hypodermis contains 0.3% to 0.8% volatile oil, which consists of monoterpenes and sesquiterpenes, which occur mostly as esters, including 0.1% to .03% valerenic (sometimes called valeric) as well as acetoxy-valerenic acids in medicinal valerian, as well as bornyl isovalerate, bornyl acetate, and bornyl formate. Valerian also contains alkaloids—including actinidine, valerine, and valerianine—and polyphenolic acids (caffeic and chlorogenic acids), tannins, gum, and resin.

COMMERCIAL PREPARATIONS
Aqueous, aqueous-alcohol, and glycerite extracts, which are standardized to contain 0.8% valerenic acid content, are available in liquid, tablet, or capsule form. Non-standardized dried-root material is available cut and sifted (for tea) or in capsules. *Valeriana officinalis* is the species most frequently used in the United States, often compounded with other sedative herbs (passionflower, hops, lemon balm, kava) to enhance relaxation and provide mild sedation.

MEDICINAL USES/INDICATIONS
Traditional: sedative, mild hypnotic, carminative, antispasmodic, bactericide, anodyne (pain relief), nervine

Conditions: insomnia, nervousness, stress-related anxiety, migraine, stomach or intestinal cramps, hysteria, exhaustion, and abdominal, pelvic, or menstrual cramps

Clinical applications: insomnia, anxiety, stress, fever, convulsions, neuralgia, spastic muscles, night leg cramps

PHARMACOLOGY
The whole root drug is mildly sedating and reduces smooth muscle spasms. Actions may be due to increased concentrations of GABA (gamma-aminobutyric acid) in the synaptic cleft; increased GABA concentrations may decrease CNS activity, result in sedation, and reduce anxiety. Components in valerian extracts apparently decrease GABA catabolism, inhibit GABA uptake and release (secondary to a reversal of the NA(+) and Ca(2+)-independent GABA carrier release of [3H]GABA), and trigger peripheral nervous system spasmolytic effects.

Individual components of volatile oil and iridoids depress the central nervous system, reduce smooth muscle spasms in laboratory animals, with positive inotropic/negative chronotropic effects on coronary smooth muscle, and reduce arrhythmia and convulsion.

In human studies, valerian enhances sleep, reduces nighttime sleep disturbances, and improves overall sleep quality (in geriatric sleep-disturbed patients, nonelderly chronic insomniacs, and periodic insomniacs) and mood.

Although clinical trials are not yet conclusive, early results suggest that valerian can be as effective as benzodiazepines for sleep disorders, without benzodiazepine "hangover" or addiction risk.

DOSAGE RANGES AND DURATION OF ADMINISTRATION
To reduce nervousness, anxiety, or headache or menstrual pain, any of the following forms and dosages may be used. Dosages repeated three times a day will also reduce sleeplessness. To relieve insomnia, patients must take a dosage at least 30 to 45 minutes before bedtime. For chronic insomnia, allow two weeks of continued use to achieve optimum therapeutic effect, then continue use for another two to four weeks.
• 2 to 3 g dried root in tea, up to several times daily
• 1/4 to 1/2 tsp. (1 to 3 ml) tincture, up to several times daily
• 1/4 tsp. (1 to 2 ml) fluid extract (1:1)
• 150 to 300 mg valerian extract, dried or liquid, standardized to contain 0.8% valerenic acid, 1% to 1.5% valtrates

SIDE EFFECTS/TOXICOLOGY
Valerian is a safe, mild, herbal medicine. The German Commission E lists no side effects. The American Herbal Products Association (AHPA) rates valerian class 1 (safe when used appropriately). Mild gastrointestinal upset infrequently reported. Reports that chronic use (longer than two to four months) causes insomnia are controversial. Some individuals develop a "paradoxical reaction" of nervousness and excitability with valerian (rare).

WARNINGS/CONTRAINDICATIONS/PRECAUTIONS
Valerian has not posed risks to fetuses or breast-fed newborns, but all pregnant and lactating women should consult with a professional when considering taking any herb.

Valepotriates, valtrate, didrovaltrate, dihydrovaltrate, and isovaltrate have cytotoxic and mutagenic properties in vitro on specific cultured tumor cells and strains of bacteria. In humans, the degradation of these substances into baldrinals and possible polymers are believed to form nonmutagenic metabolites. Although the specific risks to human stomach, liver, and intestines have not been proven, species with high valepotriate content (e.g., Mexican and Indian valerian) are not recommended, and valerenic acid preparations, such as *V. officinalis*, are advised.

INTERACTIONS

Valerian may interfere with anxiolytics, hypnotics, analgesics, and antiepileptics, and may enhance effects of kava, passionflower, lemon balm, hops, poppy, and skullcap.

REGULATORY AND COMPENDIAL STATUS

Valerian is considered a dietary supplement and GRAS (generally recognized as safe) as a food additive in the United States. It is awaiting FDA approval as an over-the-counter sleep aid. Valerian is approved in Germany by the German Commission E to treat nervous restlessness and sleeping disorders and in Canada as a sedative and spasmolytic.

REFERENCES

Balderer G, Borbely AA. Effect of valerian on human sleep. *Psychopharmacol.* 1985;87:406–409.

Blumenthal M, ed. *The Complete German Commission E Monographs.* Boston, Mass: Integrative Medicine Communications; 1998.

Blumenthal M, Riggins C. *Popular Herbs in the U.S. Market: Therapeutic Monographs.* Austin, Tex: The American Botanical Council; 1997.

Brown D. *Herbal Prescriptions for Better Health.* Rocklin, Calif: Prima Publishing; 1996.

DeSmet PAGM,ed. *Adverse Effects of Herbal Drugs.* New York, NY: Springer-Verlag; 1997:3.

Diefenbach K, et al. Valerian effects on microstructure of sleep in insomniacs. (2nd Congress of the European Assoc. for Clinical Pharmacology and Therapeutics, Berlin, Germany, Sept. 17-20.) *Eur J Clin Pharmacol.* 1997;52 (suppl):A169.

Hobbs C. *The Herbal Prescriber.* Santa Cruz, Calif. Botanica Press; 1995.

Kowalchik C, Hylton W, eds. *Rodale's Illustrated Encyclopedia of Herbs.* Emmaus, Pa: Rodale Press; 1998:495–496.

Leathwood PD. Aqueous extract of valerian root (*Valeriana officinalis* L.) improves sleep quality in man. *Pharmacol Biochem Behav.* 1982;17:65–71.

Leung A, Foster S. *Encyclopedia of Common Natural Ingredients Used in Food, Drugs, and Cosmetics.* 2nd ed. New York, NY: John Wiley and Sons; 1996.

Lindahl O, Lindwall L. Double-blind study of a valerian preparation. *Pharmacol Biochem Behav.* 1989;32:1065–1066.

Lindahl O, Lindwall L. Double–blind study of valopotriates by hairy root cultures of *Valeriana officinalis* var. sambucifolia. *Planta Med.* 1992;58:A614.

McGuffin M, Hobbs C, Upton R, Goldberg A. *American Herbal Products Association's Botanical Safety Handbook.* Boca Raton, Fla: CRC Press; 1997:120.

Murray, MT. *The Healing Power of Herbs: The Enlightened Person's Guide to the Wonders of Medicinal Plants.* Rocklin, Calif: Prima Publishing; 1995.

Newall CA, Phillipson JD. Interactions of Herbs with Other Medicines. Kings Centre for Pharmacognosy, the School of Pharmacy, University of London. *The European Phytojournal.* 1998; 1. Available at: www.ex.ac.uk/phytonet/phytojournal.

Petkov V. Plants with hypotensive, antiatheromatous and coronarodilating actions. *Am J Chin Med.* 1979;7:197–236.

Samuelsson G. *Drugs of Natural Origin: A Textbook of Pharmacognosy.* Stockholm, Sweden: The Swedish Pharmaceutical Press; 1992.

Santos MS. Synaptosomal GABA release as influenced by valerian root extract—involvement of the GABA carrier. *Arch Int Pharmacodyn Ther.* 1994; 327:220–231.

Schultz V, Hansel R, Tyler V. *Rational Phytotherapy: A Physician's Guide to Herbal Medicine.* New York, NY: Springer-Verlag; 1998.

Seifert T. Therapeutic effects of valerian in nervous disorders: a field study. *Therapeutikon.* 1988;2(94).

Schultz H, Stolz C, Muller J. The effect of valerian extract on sleep polygraph in poor sleepers: a pilot study. *Pharmacopsychiatry.* 1994;27:147–151.

Wagner et al. Comparative studies on the sedative action of valeriana extracts, valepotriates, and their degradation products. *Planta Med.* 1980;39:358–365.

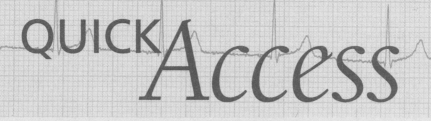

QUICK Access

SUPPLEMENTS

5-Hydroxytryptophan (5-HTP)
Alpha-Linolenic Acid (ALA)
Alpha-Lipoic Acid
Brewer's Yeast
Bromelain
Calcium
Cartilage
Chromium
Copper
Creatine
Dehydroepiandrosterone (DHEA)
Ethylenediaminetetraacetic Acid (EDTA)
Flaxseed Oil
Gamma-Linolenic Acid (GLA)
Glutamine
Iron
Lipase
Lysine
Magnesium
Manganese
Melatonin
Phenylalanine
Phosphorus
Potassium
Psyllium
Selenium
Spirulina
Sulfur
Tyrosine
Vanadium
Vitamin A (Retinol)
Vitamin B1 (Thiamine)
Vitamin B2 (Riboflavin)
Vitamin B3 (Niacin)
Vitamin B5 (Pantothenic Acid)
Vitamin B6 (Pyridoxine)
Vitamin B9 (Folic Acid)
Vitamin B12 (Cobalamin)
Vitamin C (Ascorbic Acid)
Vitamin D
Vitamin E
Vitamin H (Biotin)
Vitamin K
Zinc

■ 5-HYDROXYTRYPTOPHAN (5-HTP)

OVERVIEW

5-hydroxytryptophan (5-HTP) is an amino acid that occurs in the body. It is the immediate precursor of the brain neurotransmitter serotonin. 5-HTP is well-absorbed with approximately 70% of an oral dose reaching the bloodstream. Some orally administered 5-HTP is rapidly decarboxylated to serotonin in the "peripheral vasculature" (before reaching the brain), and some crosses the blood-brain barrier and increases synthesis of serotonin. In the process of serotonin biosynthesis, tryptophan is hydroxylated to 5-HTP and then decarboxylated to serotonin (5-HT). The tryptophan hydroxylase enzyme catalyzes tryptophan's conversion to 5-HTP, and the 5-hydroxytryptophan decarboxylase enzyme catalyzes 5-HTP's conversion to 5-HT. The conversion of tryptophan to 5-HTP is the rate-limiting step in the production of serotonin from tryptophan.

The 5-HTP decarboxylase enzyme is widely distributed in the body with highest activity in the gut wall and liver. Peripheral serotonin does not cross the blood-brain barrier. 5-HTP Decarboxylase inhibitors are sometimes given in conjunction with 5-HTP to inhibit peripheral conversion and help insure that adequate levels of serotonin are produced in the brain. However, studies indicate that 5-HTP works as well, if not better, when used without decarboxylase inhibitors.

DIETARY SOURCES

Griffonia simplicifolia seed

CONSTITUENTS/COMPOSITION

Dietary supplements of 5-HTP should be manufactured to 99% or higher purity levels.

COMMERCIAL PREPARATIONS

5-HTP is extracted from the seeds of the African *Griffonia simplicifolia* plant using an alcoholic extraction process that produces an oily solid. The oily extract is then purified into a dry solid. Standard preparations available as 25, 50, and 100 mg capsules or tablets.

THERAPEUTIC USES

Bipolar (manic) depression: 5-HTP (200 mg tid) with lithium has proven helpful in the treatment of bipolar disorder.

Depression: 5-HTP has been shown to be effective in treating mild to moderate depression in 5-HT deficient individuals. Its effects are similar to those observed with the anti-depressant drugs Imipramine and Fluvoxamine. Treatment with 5-HTP (ranging from 150 to 300 mg per day for one to six weeks) improved depressed mood, anxiety, insomnia, and physical symptoms.

Fibromyalgia: Numerous clinical studies suggest that low serotonin levels cause symptoms of fibromyalgia. Treatment with 5-HTP enhances serotonin synthesis which increases pain tolerance and sleep quality. 5-HTP treatment (300 mg tid for 30 to 90 days) has been shown to improve symptoms of depression, anxiety, insomnia, and somatic pain (number of painful areas and morning stiffness) in patients with fibromylagia.

Insomnia: 5-HTP has been shown to reduce the time required to fall asleep and improve sleep quality in numerous double-blind, clinical trials.

Migraine Headache: 5-HTP (200 to 600 mg/day for two to six months), has been shown to reduce the frequency and severity of migraine headaches in several clinical trials. Significantly fewer side effects were observed with 5-HTP compared to other migraine headache drugs.

Obesity: 5-HTP treatment causes decreased carbohydrate intake and may result in weight loss in obese patients. It is hypothesized that 5-HTP may promote weight loss by promoting satiety. In one study, overweight persons were given 300 mg 5-HTP three times daily, for six weeks with no dietary restriction. For the second six weeks of the trial, they were placed on a 1,200 calorie-per-day diet in addition to the 5-HTP treatment. At the end of the 12 weeks, the 5-HTP group had lost an average of 11.63 pounds, while the placebo group had lost only 1.87 pounds. Early satiety was reported by 100% of the participants during the first six-week period, and by 90% of the participants on 5-HTP during the second six-week period. In another study, 5-HTP (750 mg per day for two weeks) administered to 25 overweight NIDDM patients caused a significant reduction in daily energy intake (from fat and carbohydrate) and body weight.

Headaches in children: Children with sleep disorder-related headaches have been shown to respond favorably to 5-HTP treatment.

DOSAGE RANGES AND DURATION OF ADMINISTRATION

The therapeutic dose, and length of treatment, will depend on the condition being treated. In clinical trials, dosages ranged from 150 to 900 mg per day and lasted for two weeks to six months.

SIDE EFFECTS/TOXICOLOGY

Relatively few adverse effects are associated with its use in the treatment of depression. 5-HTP causes mild gastrointestinal disturbances in some people. These side effects include mild nausea, heartburn, flatulence, feelings of fullness, and rumbling sensations. Side effects are reduced after extended treatment (four to six weeks).

WARNINGS/CONTRAINDICATIONS/PRECAUTIONS

Individuals taking anti-depressant drugs, such as MAOIs or selective serotonin reuptake inhibitor (SSRIs), or other prescription drugs, should consult with their physician before taking 5-HTP. Excessive 5-HTP stimulation may cause "serotonin syndrome" (excess accumulation of serotonin in the synapses), characterized by altered mental states, autonomic dysfunction, and neuromuscular abnormalities.

INTERACTIONS

May potentiate the effects of St. John's wort.

Vitamin B$_6$, niacin, and magnesium serve as cofactors in the conversion of 5-HTP to serotonin.

REFERENCES

Angst J, et al. The treatment of depression with L-5-hydroxytryptophan versus imipramine. Results of two open and one double-blind study. *Arch Psychiatr Nervenkr.* 1977;224:175–186.

Birdsall TC. 5-Hydroxytryptophan: a clinically-effective serotonin precursor. *Altern Med Rev.* 1998;3:271–280.

Byerley WF, et al. 5-Hydroxytryptophan: a review of its antidepressant efficacy and adverse effects. *J Clin Psychopharmacol.* 1987;7:127–137.

Cangiano C, et al. Effects of oral 5-hydroxy-tryptophan on energy intake and macronutrient selection in non-insulin dependent diabetic patients. *Int J Obes Relat Metab Disord.* 1998; 22:648–654.

Cangiano C, Ceci F, Cascino A, et al. Eating behavior and adherence to dietary prescriptions in obese adult subjects treated with 5-hydroxytryptophan. *J Clin Nutr.* 1992;56:863–867.

Caruso I, Sarzi Puttini P, Cazzola M, et al. Double-blind study of 5-hydroxytryptophan versus placebo in the treatment of primary fibromyalgia syndrome. *J Int Med Res.* 1990;18:201–209.

Ceci F, Cangiano C, Cairella M, Cascino A, et al. The effects of oral 5-hydroxytryptophan administration on feeding behavior in obese adult female subjects. *J Neural Transm.* 1989;76:109–117.

DeBenedittis G, Massei R. Serotonin precursors in chronic primary headache. A double-blind cross-over study with L-5-hydroxytryptophan vs. placebo. *J Neurosurg Sci*. 1985; 29:239–248.

DeGiorgis, G, et al. Headache in association with sleep disorders in children: a psychodiagnostic evaluation and controlled clinical study—L-5-HTP versus placebo. *Drugs Exp Clin Res*. 1987;13:425–433.

Ganong WF. *Review of Medical Physiology*. 13th ed. San Mateo, Calif: Appleton & Lange; 1987.

Juhl JH. Primary fibromyalgia syndrome and 5-hydroxy-L-tryptophan: a 90-day open study. *Altern Med Rev*. 1998;3:367–375.

Magnussen I, Nielson-Kudsk F. Bioavailability and related pharmacokinetics in man of orally administered L-5-Hydroxytryptophan in steady state. *Acta Pharmacol et Toxicol*. 1980;46:257–262.

Martin TG. Serotonin syndrome. *Ann Emerg Med*. 1996;28:520–526.

Murray MT, Pizzorno JE. *Encyclopedia of Natural Medicine*. 2nd ed. Rocklin, Calif: Prima Publishing; 1998.

Nicolodi M, Sicuteri F. Fibromyalgia and migraine, two faces of the same mechanism. Serotonin as the common clue for pathogenesis and thearpy. *Adv Exp Med Biol*. 1996;398:373–379.

Puttini PS, Caruso I. Primary fibromyalgia and 5-hydroxy-L-tryptophan: a 90-day open study. *J Int Med Res*. 1992;20:182–189.

Reibring L, Agren H, Hartvig P, et al. Uptake and utilization of [beta-11c] 5-hydroxytryptophan (5-HTP) in human brain studied by positron emission tomography. *Pyschiatry Research*. 1992;45:215–225.

Shils ME, Olson JA, Shike M, eds. *Modern Nutrition in Health and Disease*. 8th ed. Media, Pa: Williams & Wilkins; 1994:1.

Takahashi S, et al. Measurement of 5-hydroxindole compounds during L-5-HTP treatment in depressed patients. *Folia Psychiatr Neurol Jpn*. 1976;30:461–473.

Van Hiele IJ. L-5-hydroxytryptophan in depression: the first substitution therapy in psychiatry? *Neuropsychobiology*. 1980; 6:230–240.

Van Praag HM. Management of depression with serotonin precursors. *Biol Psychiatry*. 1981;16:291–310.

Zmilacher K, et al. L-5-hydroxytryptophan alone and in combination with a peripheral decarboxylase inhibitor in the treatment of depression. *Neuropsychobiology*. 1988;20:28–33.

■ ALPHA-LINOLENIC ACID (ALA)

OVERVIEW

The fatty acid alpha-linolenic acid (ALA) is an essential nutrient. It is the 18-carbon polyunsaturated fatty acid (PUFA) in the omega-3 series found in unhydrogenated oils derived from plants. ALA is found primarily in margarines as well as as rapeseed (canola), flaxseed, and soybean oils.

ALA is a "parent" fatty acid. Our bodies convert it into the longer-chain omega-3 fatty acids (such as docosahexaenoic acid [DHA] and eicosapentaenoic acid [EPA]), which are found primarily in fish oils. Scientists studying DHA and EPA have shown that omega-3 oils have several beneficial effects. Because these fatty acids are produced by ALA, this research can be applied to ALA as well.

The beneficial effects of omega-3 series oils include: lowering cholesterol and triglyceride levels, reducing the risk of heart disease, lowering blood pressure, improving rheumatoid arthritis, and protecting myelin formation and function. Omega-3 oils may also be helpful in treating multiple sclerosis and diabetes, and in preventing cancer.

ALA may help prevent coronary heart disease, and inhibit atherosclerosis. In one small study, 15 obese persons took 20 g of ALA from margarine products based on flax oil daily. As a result, the subjects showed improvement in arterial compliance, and thus had a decreased risk of cardiovascular disease, despite a rise in LDL oxidizability. At the same time, insulin sensitivity and HDL cholesterol diminished. Another study found that ALA supplements from vegetable oil and EPA and DHA supplements from a fish source have largely parallel effects on hemostatic factors. Other research has indicated that ALA acts equivalently to n-6 fatty acids with respect to lipid and lipoprotein effects. However, very large amounts of ALA, which is plant-based, were needed to reduce tricylglycerol concentrations, which is the hallmark effect of the fish-based omega-3 fatty acids. The study concluded that plant-derived ALA is not equivalent to fish-based acids in its effect on lipoprotein metabolism. Scientists agree that the relationship among the fatty acids and the ratio of ALA to linoleic acid in the diet is an important area for further study.

Scientists are also investigating other uses for ALA. The anti-inflammatory and immunoregulatory effects of ALA, and its successor fatty acids, have been demonstrated. Successful treatment of migraines and alleviation of depression with ALA have been reported. Topical application of ALA inhibits melanin production and accelerates turnover of the stratum corneum, thus aiding in the removal of melanin pigment from the epidermis.

DIETARY SOURCES

- Flax seeds
- Flaxseed oil
- Linseed oil
- Canola (rapeseed) oil
- Soybean oil
- Margarine, if based on canola or soybean oil
- Pumpkin
- Walnuts

CONSTITUENTS/COMPOSITION

Alpha-linolenic acid is a long-chain polyunsaturated fatty acid with 18 carbon atoms. It is the parent fatty acid in the omega-3 series. It is converted to eicosapentaenoic acid (EPA), then to decosahexaenoic acid (DHA), then to the prostaglandin E_3 series (PGE_3). Some fish products (e.g., mackerel and salmon) can introduce EPA and DHA directly into the body.

The essential fatty acids, including ALA, are known as vitamin F. The Food and Drug Administration prohibits the use of the term "vitamin F" in advertising, because foods like french fries could be advertised as being "vitamin enriched" because they were fried in oil containing these fatty acids.

COMMERCIAL PREPARATIONS

ALA is commercially prepared in two ways.

- Cooking oils (canola oil, soybean oil, margarines made from these oils). Hydrogenated products are not preferred.
- Medicinal oil (flaxseed oil, gelatin capsules of flaxseed oil)

Several manufacturing methods can destroy the nutritional value of the products. Some preferred manaufacturers use proprietary names for their packaging processes. Bio-Electron Process (Barlean's Organic Oils), Spectra-Vac (Spectrum Naturals), or Omegaflo (Omega Nutrition) are some examples. Generally, a high quality oil will be certified as organic by a reputable third party, is packaged in light-resistant containers, may be refrigerated, and will be dated.

THERAPEUTIC USES

The primary uses of ALA and other omega-3 oils include the following.

- Cardiovascular disease: reducing cholesterol levels and blood pressure
- Allergic and inflammatory conditions: e.g., for treatment of psoriasis and eczema
- Autoimmune diseases: e.g., for treatment of multiple sclerosis, lupus, and cancer

DOSAGE RANGES AND DURATION OF ADMINISTRATION

There is no recommended dietary allowance of ALA.

A healthy person eating a normal diet should consume fewer saturated fats and more polyunsaturated essential fatty acids.

SIDE EFFECTS/TOXICOLOGY

N/A

WARNINGS/CONTRAINDICATIONS/PRECAUTIONS

Total fat intake should be considered.

The ratio of ALA to other essential fatty acids may be important in treating some conditions.

INTERACTIONS

ALA interacts with other fatty acids.

REFERENCES

Ando H, Ryu A, Hashimot A, Oka M, Ichihashi M. Linoleic acid and alpha-linolenic acid lightens ultraviolet-induced hyperpigmentation of the skin. *Arch Dermatol Res.* 1998;290:375–381.

Billeaud C, Bougle D, Sarda P, et al.. Effects of preterm infant formula supplementation with alpha-linolenic acid with a linoleate/alpha-linoleate ration of 6. *Eur J Clin Nutr.* August 1997;51:520–527.

DeDeckere EA, Korver O, Verschuren PM, Katan MB. Health aspects of fish and n-3 polyunsaturated fatty acids from plant and marine origin. *Eur J Clin Nutr.* 1998;52:749–753.

Edwards R, Peet M, Shay J, Horrobin D. Omega-3 polyunsaturated fatty acid levels in the diet and in red blood cell membranes of depressed patients. *J Affect Disord.* 1998;48:149–155.

Ensminger AH, Ensminger ME, Konlande JE, Robson JRK. *Foods & Nutrition Encyclopedia.* 2nd ed. Baton Rouge, Fla: CRC Press, Inc; 1994:1:684–708.

Ferretti A, Flanagan VP. Antithromboxane activity of dietary alpha-linolenic acid. *Prostaglandins Leukot Essent Fatty Acids.* 1996;54:451–455.

Freese R, Mutanen M. Alpha-linolenic acid and marine long-chain n-3 fatty acids differ only slightly in their effects on hemostatic factors in healthy subjects. *Am J Clin Nutr.* 1997;66:591–598.

Garrison Jr RH, Somer E. *The Nutrition Desk Reference.* 3rd ed. New Canaan, Conn: Keats Publishing, Inc; 1995:23–64.

Haas EM. *Staying Healthy with Nutrition.* Berkley, Calif: Celestial Arts Publishing; 1992:65–79.

Harris WS. N-3 fatty acids and serum lipoproteins: human studies. *Am J Clin Nutr.* 1997;65:1645S (10).

de Lorgeril M, Renaud S, Mamelle N, et al. Mediterranean alpha-linolenic acid-rich diet in secondary prevention of coronary heart disease. *Lancet.* 1994;343:1454–1459.

Mantzioris E., James MJ, Gibson RA, Cleland LG. Dietary subsitutions with an alpha-linolenic acid-rich vegetable oil increases eicosapentaenoic acid concentrations in tissues. *Am J Clin Nutr.* 1994;59:1304–1309.

Murray MT. *Encyclopedia of Nutritional Supplements.* Rocklin, Calif: Prima Publishing; 1996:239–278.

Nestel PJ, Pomeroy SE, Sasahara T, et al. Arterial compliance in obese subjects is improved with dietary plant n-3 fatty acid from flaxseed oil despite increased LDL oxidizability. *Arterioscler Thromb Vasc Biol.* 1997;17:1163–1170.

Newstrom H. *Nutrients Catalog.* Jefferson, NC: McFarland & Co, Inc; 1993:103–105.

Simon JA, Fong J, Bernert JT Jr, Browner WS. Serum fatty acids and the risk of stroke. *Stroke.* 1995;26:778–782.

Shils ME, Olson JA, Shike M, Ross AC. *Modern Nutrition in Health and Disease.* 9th ed. Baltimore, Md: Williams & Wilkins; 1999:90–92, 1377–1378.

Voskuil DW, Feskens EJM, Katan MB, Kromhout D. Intake and sources of alpha-linolenic acid in Dutch elderly men. *Eur J Clin Nutr.* 1996;50:784–787.

Wapnir RA. Copper absorption and bioavailability. *Am J Clin Nutr.* 1998;67:1054s.

Wagner W, Nootbaar-Wagner U. Prophylactic treatment of migraine with gamma-linolenic and alpha-linolenic acids. *Cephalalgia.* April 1997;17:127–130.

Werbach MR. *Nutritional Influences on Illness.* 2nd ed. Tarzana, Calif: Third Line Press; 1993:13–22; 655–671.

Yehuda S, Rabinovitz S, Carasso RL, Mostofsky DI. Fatty acids and brain peptides. *Peptides.* 1998;19:407–419.

■ ALPHA-LIPOIC ACID

OVERVIEW

In recent years, increasing attention has been paid to the group of vitamins, minerals, and enzymes known as antioxidants. Some of the better known antioxidants are vitamins A, C and E, beta-carotene, selenium, and melatonin. Antioxidants play an important role in preventing aging-related degenerative conditions through their actions in fighting free radicals. Free radicals are wastes generated by the regular metabolic processes in the cells. Free radicals are normally present in the body and actually serve useful purposes, such as aiding in the production of hormones and activating enzymes. However, when there is an excess of free radicals in the body, they become destructive.

In addition to being by-products of normal metabolic processes, free radicals also can result from exposure to radiation, toxic chemicals (such as those contained in cigarette smoke, automobile exhaust, and other environmental pollutants), and from overexposure to the sun's rays. Free radicals are atoms or molecules that contain unpaired electrons. They tend to bind to other molecules, causing chemical reactions that can be destructive to the body. They can damage cells, interfere with the immune system, and contribute to degenerative diseases such as cancer and cardiovascular disease. In fact, free radical damage may be the basis for the aging process. Antioxidants bind with these reactive molecules to counteract their harmful effect.

The antioxidant alpha-lipoic acid (also called thioctic acid) is made by the body and directly supports detoxifying abilities of the liver. It enhances the antioxidant functions of vitamins C and E and glutathione. Alpha-lipoic acid (ALA) has growth-stimulating properties, prevents cell damage, regulates blood sugar, and chelates toxic metals out of the blood. In animal studies, it has been shown to enhance cognitive function as well. It is also involved in the production of muscular energy and directs calories toward energy production. Because it is both water- and fat-soluble, ALA is able to function in almost any part of the body, including the brain.

DIETARY SOURCES

Dietary sources of alpha-lipoic acid include the following:
- Spinach
- Broccoli
- Beef
- Yeast
- Kidney
- Heart

CONSTITUENTS/COMPOSITION

Alpha-lipoic acid, along with glutathione, is one of the thiol antioxidants. It is a carboxy acid with two sulfur atoms in its molecule, and occurs as an amide in plant and animal tissues.

COMMERCIAL PREPARATIONS

Alpha-lipoic acid is available commercially in capsule form.

THERAPEUTIC USES

Because alpha-lipoic acid relieves stress on the liver and directly supports its detoxifying functions, it has been used in the treatment of chronic hepa-titis and Amanita (a particularly toxic mushroom) poisoning. It is able to bind to toxic metals and is used for heavy metal detoxification. Alpha-lipoic acid can help eliminate toxic effects of anasthesia, analgesics, or other drugs used in the course of surgery, and to ease subsequent pain. A recommended dose is two 100-mg capsules tid one week before surgery and two weeks postoperatively.

The thiols are central to antioxidant defense in the brain. Alpha-lipoic acid has a low molecular weight; it is readily absorbed from nutritional sources and crosses the blood-brain barrier. Current research indicates that alpha-lipoic acid and its metabolite dihydrolipoate have protective effects on brain and neural tissue. Preliminary human studies support conclusions of animal and in vitro studies showing a role for ALA in the treatment of stroke and other brain disorders involving free radical damage. In an animal study, treatment with ALA was associated with a four-fold increase in stroke survival.

Alpha-lipoic acid has shown great promise in the treatment of nerve dysfunction in diabetics. Diabetes mellitus is associated with free radicals; studies with diabetics have revealed oxidative stress loads. In more than one study, treatment with alpha-lipoic acid has significantly reduced the pain, burning, paresthesia, and numbness associated with diabetic neuropathy. Alpha-lipoic acid has also been shown to increase glucose transport in diabetics, and to lead to improved heart rate variability.

DOSAGE RANGES AND DURATION OF ADMINISTRATION

Currently, no recommended dosages have been established for ALA. ALA manufacturers suggest one or two 50-mg capsules daily as a dietary supplement.

SIDE EFFECTS/TOXICOLOGY

Studies investigating the effects of alpha-lipoic acid on nerve damage related to diabetes found no side effects at the dosage levels they were testing.

WARNINGS/CONTRAINDICATIONS/PRECAUTIONS

Diabetics should take ALA with caution as it can cause hypoglycemia.

INTERACTIONS

Alpha-lipoic acid enhances the functions of antioxidant vitamins C and E, and of glutathione (another thiol produced by the body). While there have been claims of alpha-lipoic acid's ability to regenerate vitamin E, this has not been supported by animal studies.

REFERENCES

Hocking GM. *A Dictionary of Natural Products*. Medford, NJ: Plexus Publishing; 1997:39;449,797.

Mindell E, Hopkins V. *Prescription Alternatives*. New Canaan, Conn: Keats Publishing; 1998:55–56.

Packer J, Tritschler HJ, Wessel K. Neuroprotection by the metabolic antioxidant alpha-linoic acis. *Free Radic Biol Med*. 1997;22:359–378.

Walker LP, Brown E. *The Alternative Pharmacy*. Paramus, NJ: Prentice Hall; 1998:36, 78, 216, 326, 362, 375.

Ziegler D, Gries FA. Alpha-lipoic acid in the treatment of diabetic peripheral and cardiac autonomic neuropathy. *Diabetes*. 1997;46 (suppl 2):S62–66.

■ BREWER'S YEAST

OVERVIEW

Brewer's yeast, which is often called nutritional yeast, was originally a by-product of the brewing of beer. While still used for brewing, it is also now produced for its nutritional value. Nutritional yeast is not exactly the same as brewer's yeast. Brewer's yeast was originally used as a nutritional supplement, then other yeasts were made available for this purpose. Brewer's yeast differs from live baker's yeast in that its live yeast cells have been destroyed, leaving the nutrients behind. Live yeast cells can actually deplete the body of B vitamins and other nutrients.

Nutritional yeast contains high levels of many important nutrients, including all of the B vitamins (except for B$_{12}$), 16 out of 20 amino acids, and 14 different minerals. The amino acids in yeast are protein components which help the body repair tissue and fight disease. Brewer's yeast has a high protein content, with one tbsp. providing 4.6 g, making it a rich source of protein for vegetarians. It is also high in phosphorus.

Because yeast is such a rich source of the B vitamin family, it enhances the roles these vitamins play in the body. The B-complex vitamins support and optimize carbohydrate, fat, and protein metabolism. They also support the nervous system and maintain tonicity in gastrointestinal muscles. Different B vitamins play different roles, particularly in their support of the nervous system. They relieve stress, depression, irritability, and fatigue, and also help protect against aging. When under the pressures of stress or infection, the body needs higher supplies of these important vitamins. The body does not store excess B vitamins, so they must be continually replenished. B vitamins can also help deter morning sickness.

Biotin, one of the B vitamins that brewer's yeast supplies, has been shown to strengthen brittle nails and improve the health of hair. It also improves the metabolism of scalp oils, which make it an important treatment for seborrheic dermatitis, a condition seen most often in infants ("cradle cap") and the elderly. Biotin is also used to treat diabetes, since it enhances insulin sensitivity, increases glucokinase activity, and is helpful for treating diabetic neuropathy.

Brewer's yeast is also an important source of chromium. There is no official RDA for chromium, but the U.S. FDA recommends 120 mcg daily. However, 90% of Americans are deficient in this important mineral. Chromium has the ability to significantly lower low density lipoprotein (LDL) levels in the blood and raise high density lipoprotein (HDL) levels. Studies have shown that cardiac patients can have 40% lower blood levels of chromium than those without coronary artery disease. Some research has suggested that brewer's yeast also contains other hypocholesterolemic factors beyond its rich chromium content.

Chromium is also an important supplement for those with Type II (adult onset) diabetes. It can significantly lower blood glucose levels by aiding transmission of insulin into the cells. Researchers have been able to lower some glucose levels in diabetics to almost normal levels with daily chromium doses of 1,000 mcg. Chromium supplementation should be considered as an adjunct to started medications.

Even if blood glucose levels are normal, skin glucose tolerance appears to be impaired in cases of acne. Several studies have tested the use of chromium for acne treatment, with good results. Chromium's ability to increase the effectiveness of insulin's activity in the body has also led to its use as a weight loss aid. Chromium can be difficult for the body to absorb, but brewer's yeast is one of most absorbable ways to take it.

CONSTITUENTS/COMPOSITION

Chromium, thiamine, nicotinic acid, riboflavine, pyridoxine, pantothenic acid, biotin, folic acid, cyanocobalamin, aminobenzoic acid, and inositol.

COMMERCIAL PREPARATIONS

Brewer's yeast comes in powder, flake, tablet, and liquid form.

THERAPEUTIC USES

- As a source of chromium: to reduce blood sugar levels in Type II diabetics, to lower blood cholesterol levels, to aid in weight loss, and to aid in the treatment of acne
- As a source of B vitamins: to relieve stress, depression, irritability, and fatigue
- As a source of biotin: to strengthen hair and nails and treat seborrheic dermatitis and diabetes

DOSAGE RANGES AND DURATION OF ADMINISTRATION

Can be taken in juice or water. Four tbsp. per day are recommended. If the body's diet is low in B vitamins, this amount may cause gas. It is best to begin with 1 tsp. in a glass of juice and work slowly up to 4 tbsp. Nutritional yeast may be taken as a source of chromium to assist weight loss and treat impaired glucose tolerance, or of biotin to promote strong nails and healthy hair and treat cradle cap, diabetes, and diabetic neuropathy.

SIDE EFFECTS/TOXICOLOGY

Brewer's yeast has no known side effects.

WARNINGS/CONTRAINDICATIONS/PRECAUTIONS

Be cautious with yeast products if you have an overgrowth of intestinal yeast (*Candida albicans or rhodotorula* yeast). People with osteoporosis should avoid yeast because of its high levels of phosphorus. If taking a yeast supplement, also take extra calcium.

INTERACTIONS

None reported

REFERENCES

Balch J, Balch P. *Prescription for Nutritional Healing.* Garden Park City, NY: Avery Publishing Group; 1997.

Bentley JP, Hunt TK, Weiss JB, et al. Peptides from live yeast cell derivative stimulate wound healing. *Arch Surg.* 1990;125:641–646.

Chromium necessary to regulate blood sugar. *Conscious Choice: The Journal of Ecology and Natural Living.* June 1998;11:33.

Hegoczki J, Suhajda A, Janzso B, Vereczkey G. Preparation of chromium enriched yeasts. *Acta Alimentaria.* 1997;26:345–358.

Li Y-C. Effects of brewer's yeast on glucose tolerance and serum lipids in Chinese adults. *Biol Trace Elem Res.* 1994;41:341–347.

McCarty MF. Insulin resistance in Mexican Americans: a precursor to obestity and diabetes? *Med Hypotheses.* 1993;41:308–315.

Murray M. Biotin: An overlooked essential B vitamin. *The America Journal of Natural Medicine.* May 1996;3:5–6.

Murray M. The chromium connection. *Health Counselor.* March 1997;9:48–59.

Rabinowitz MB, Gonick HC, Levin SR, Davidson MB. Effects of chromium and yeast supplements on carbohydrate and lipid metabolism in diabetic men. *Diabetes Care.* 1983;6:319–327.

■ BROMELAIN

OVERVIEW

Bromelain is a proteolytic digestive enzyme that is extracted from the stem and the fruit of the pineapple plant *(Ananas comosus)*. It is best known as a digestive aid and for its anti-inflammatory effects in soft tissue injury and edema. However, bromelain has been used successfully to treat a number of disorders including cardiovascular disease, joint disease, upper respiratory tract infection, and Peyronie's disease. Bromelain has also been used successfully to debride wounds and to potentiate the actions of antibiotics and chemotherapeutic agents.

DIETARY SOURCES

Bromelain is one of the simple digestive enzymes that is extracted from tropical fruits, in this case pineapples.

CONSTITUENTS/COMPOSITION

Bromelain A and B, the proteolytic enzymes of pineapples, constitute bromelain. Bromelain also consists of peroxidase, acid phosphatase, protease inhibitors, and calcium.

COMMERCIAL PREPARATIONS

Bromelain is available in tablet (500 mg) or capsule form for oral use.

THERAPEUTIC USES

- Traumatic injuries and surgery. Bromelain's anti-inflammatory effects reduce the pain, bruising, and swelling from trauma (e.g., sports injuries) or surgery and speed the healing process. (The pain reduction is probably due to decreased tissue inflammation rather than to a direct analgesic effect.)
- Digestive aid. Bromelain has been used as a digestive enzyme, especially in patients with pancreatic insufficiency. It has been known to relieve gastrointestinal upset in humans and to heal ulcers in experiments in animals.
- Cardiovascular disease. Bromelain can relieve the symptoms of angina pectoris, inhibit platelet aggregation and clot formation, and break down arterial plaques by promoting fibrolysis; thus, it can be used to treat angina, thrombosis, thromophlebitis, varicose veins, and atherosclerosis.
- Joint inflammation. Because bromelain's anti-inflammatory effects reduce joint inflammation, it can be used for rheumatoid arthritis, osteoarthritis, sciatica, bursitis, tendinitis, and scleroderma.
- Potentiation of antibiotics and chemotherapeutic agents. By increasing absorption and tissue penetration, bromelain may potentiate the actions of chemotherapeutic agents and antibiotics. It has been shown to result in tumor regression when used in combination with selected chemotherapeutic agents.
- AIDS. Bromelain is a natural protease inhibitor (a protein-digesting enzyme) that may prove useful in the treatment of AIDS patients to control the replication of HIV. It is less expensive and is associated with fewer side effects than the protease inhibitors that are currently used for this function. More study is needed on bromelain's clinical usefulness in treating persons with HIV and AIDS.
- Upper respiratory tract infections. Bromelain has demonstrated effectiveness in suppressing mucolytic cough and decreasing bronchial secretions, resulting in increased lung function in patients with upper respiratory tract infections. It has also proved effective in patients with sinusitis.
- Peyronie's disease. The deposition of fibrin, which is responsible for the thickening of the fibrous connective tissue in the penis, can be prevented with bromelain.
- Wound debridement. Bromelain as a topical agent can accelerate the healing of burns.
- Anti-metastatic. Several studies suggest use as an anti-metastatic agent with chemotherapy.

DOSAGE RANGES AND DURATION OF ADMINISTRATION

For use as a digestive aid, 500 mg with meals are recommended. For other uses, the following dosages are recommended.

- Traumatic injuries—500 mg qid on an empty stomach
- Cardiovascular disease—500 to 750 mg tid on an empty stomach
- Joint inflammation—500 to 2,000 mg/day in two doses
- Antitumor activity—1,000 mg/day

The standard duration of administration is 8 to 10 days, but longer periods are tolerated.

■ SIDE EFFECTS/TOXICOLOGY

Bromelain may cause nausea, vomiting, diarrhea, metrorrhagia, and hypermenorrhea, but no serious side effects have been reported in humans. Experiments in animals have not shown bromelain to cause cancer or birth defects.

WARNINGS/CONTRAINDICATIONS/PRECAUTIONS

- Allergic reactions, including skin reactions and asthma, may occur if the patient is allergic to pineapples.
- Caution must be used in patients with coagulation disorders and liver or kidney disease.
- Caution must be used in patients with hypertension.
- No data are available for use during pregnancy.

INTERACTIONS

- Increased bleeding may result if given simultaneously with anticoagulants.
- Bromelain can potentiate the blood levels of tetracyclines.
- Tachycardia may result when given to patients with hypertension.

REFERENCES

Bromelain. *Alternative Medicine Review.* August 1998;3:302–305.

Desser L, Rehberger A, Kokron E, Paukovits W. Cytokine synthesis in human peripheral blood mononuclear cells after oral administration of polyenzyme preparations. *Oncology.* 1993;50:403–407.

Haas EM. *Staying Healthy with Nutrition: The Complete Guide to Diet and Nutritional Medicine.* Berkeley, Calif: Celestial Arts; 1992:257–258.

Harborne J, Baxter H, eds. *Phytochemical Dictionary: A Handbook of Bioactive Compounds from Plants.* London, England: Taylor & Francis; 1993:376.

Masson M. Bromelain in blunt injuries of the locomotor system. A study of observed applications in general practice. *Fortschr Med.* 1995;113:303–306.

Murray MT. *Encyclopedia of Nutritional Supplements: The Essential Guide for Improving Your Health Naturally.* Rocklin, Calif: Prima Publishing; 1996:429.

Murray MT, Pizzorno JE. *Encyclopedia of Natural Medicine.* 2nd ed. Rocklin, Calif: Prima Publishing; 1998:208,297–298,568,807,829–830.

Reynolds JEF, ed. *Martindale: The Extra Pharmacopoeia.* 31st ed. London, England: Royal Pharmaceutical Society; 1996:1681.

Taussig SJ, Batkin S. Bromelain, the enzyme complex of pineapple (Ananas comosus) and its clinical application. An update. *J Ethnopharmacol.* 1998;22:191–203.

Uhlig G, Seifert J. The effect of proteolytic enzymes (traumanase) on posttraumatic edema. *Fortschr Med.* 1981;99:554–556.

Walker JA, Cerny FJ, Cotter JR, Burton HW. Attenuation of contraction-induced skeletal muscle injury by bromelain. *Med Sci Sports Exerc.* 1992;24:20–25.

Werbach MR. *Nutritional Influences on Illness: A Sourcebook of Clinical Research.* New Canaan, Conn: Keats Publishing; 1987:64–65,268–269,386.

■ CALCIUM

OVERVIEW

Calcium is critical to the development and maintenance of bones and teeth. It also plays an important role in controlling the heartbeat, maintaining proper blood pressure, clotting blood, transmitting nerve impulses, contracting and relaxing muscles, maintaining the integrity of mucosal membranes and cell walls, and activating enzymes such as lipase, adenosine triphosphatase (ATPase), succinate dehydrogenase, and choline acetylase.

Calcium comprises approximately 2% of an adult's body weight, more than any other mineral; the amount of calcium in an infant's body is approximately 0.8%. The rate of absorption is greatest in childhood (50% to 70% of the calcium ingested), decreasing in adults to 10% to 40%. As the intake of calcium increases, the percent absorbed decreases. Vitamin D (especially D_3, or cholecalciferol) is the most important vitamin for assisting in the absorption of calcium. The antioxidant vitamins A, C, and E are also important. Lactose aids absorption, improving the value of milk as a source of calcium. Magnesium and phosphorus are significant in assisting in proper absorption. Recommended ratios of calcium to each of these minerals range from 1:2 to 2:1, but are currently under review. Iron, zinc, and manganese play a less important role. Stress and lack of exercise can cause negative calcium balances.

Parathyroid hormone (PTH), vitamin D, and the thyroid hormone calcitonin act to maintain normal blood calcium levels of 9 to 11 mg/100 ml. PTH stimulates the release of calcium from bone and decreases excretion from the kidney, and it acts with vitamin D to increase the rate of absorption, if blood levels are reduced. Calcitonin lowers blood calcium levels that are too high by inhibiting calcium release from bone.

Average dietary calcium intakes in Americans are lower than recommended levels; the problem is particularly acute with women. Calcium deficiency has been linked to stunted growth, bone deformities, rickets, osteoporosis, osteomalacia, muscle spasms, leg cramps, high blood pressure, and colon cancer. Recent studies question the role of calcium in decreasing the incidence of colon cancer. Although kidney stones can result from toxic levels of calcium in certain susceptible individuals, high calcium intake can actually decrease the risk of kidney stones, and large calcium supplements are accepted therapy for kidneys stones associated with intestinal hyperoxalosis.

DIETARY SOURCES

- Rich sources: cheeses (especially Parmesan, Romano, Gruyère, Swiss, provolone, Monterey Jack, Edam, Cheddar, Muenster, Gouda, Tilsit, Colby, Caraway, Brick, Roquefort, Port du Salut, Cheshire, Havarti, Fontina, Mozzarella, Feta), wheat-soy flour, blackstrap molasses, rennin
- Good sources: almonds, Brazil nuts, caviar, dried figs, dark greens (turnip, dandelion, collard, mustard), hazelnuts, ice cream, kale, bok choy, broccoli, cabbage, milk, oysters, sardines, soybean flour, yogurt (Milk and dairy products account for about 75% of dietary calcium in Americans; butter, cream cheese, and other high-fat dairy products contain little or no calcium.)
- Many herbs, spices, and seaweeds supply calcium (e.g., basil, chervil, cinnamon, dill weed, fennel, fenugreek, ginseng, kava kava, kelp, marjoram, oregano, parsley, poppy seed, sage, savory).

CONSTITUENTS/COMPOSITION

The mineral calcium is the fifth most prevalent element in the biosphere. The calcium ion (Ca^{2+}) can form bonds with up to 12 oxygen atoms and is nearly unique in its ability to interact with the peptide chain.

COMMERCIAL PREPARATIONS

Calcium citrate: soluable (optimizing absorption); most bioavailable; safe levels of lead; easily digested. It is recommended for elderly patients and persons taking acid-lowering medications, and it may be more effective in hypertension control than calcium carbonate. The citrate effects may inhibit kidney stone formation.

Calcium carbonate: Lead levels are safe if it is a refined product. Some antacids (Rolaids/Tums) contain 500 mg of calcium carbonate.

Calcium gluconate and calcium lactate: soluble; safe levels of lead

Calcium chloride: not recommended (irritates the gastrointestinal tract)

Homeopathic calcium medications and their uses:
- *Calcarea carbonica:* backache, pain
- *Calcarea fluorica:* tissue elasticity
- *Calcarea phosphorica:* fatigue, discontentment, discomfort, pain
- *Calcarea sulfurica:* sores, wounds, abscesses, boils, cysts

THERAPEUTIC USES

- Osteoporosis: to preserve adequate mineral mass, prevent loss of structural bone components, maximize repair of damaged bones, prevent loss of bone mass
- Hypertension: to reduce blood pressure (most effective in elderly, African Americans, and salt-sensitive hypertension patients, but not in salt-resistant hypertensive patients)
- Premenstrual syndrome (PMS): to relieve menstrual cramps, irritability or apprehension, muscle cramps
- Pregnancy: to reduce pregnancy-induced hypertension and prevent preeclampsia
- Menopause: to reduce headaches, irritability, insomnia, depression
- Dental: to improve loose teeth, gingivitis, periodontal disease
- Cardiovascular: to reduce heart irregularity, lower cholesterol

DOSAGE RANGES AND DURATION OF ADMINISTRATION

Recommendations for adequate calcium intakes promulgated by the National Academy of Science Food and Nutrition Board in 1997:
Infants:
- birth to 6 months: 210 mg/day
- 6 months to 1 year: 270 mg/day

Children:
- 1 to 5 years: 500 mg/day
- 6 to 8 years: 800 mg/day

Adolescents:
- 9 to 18 years: 1,300 mg/day

Adults:
- 19 to 50 years: 1,000 mg/day
- Over 50 years: 1,200 mg/day

Lactating or pregnant women:
- 14 to 18 years: 1,300 mg/day
- 19 years and older: 1,000 mg/day

Ideally, supplements should be taken in small doses throughout the day, and six to eight 8-oz. glasses of water should be consumed to avoid constipation.

SIDE EFFECTS/TOXICOLOGY

Nutritional toxicity is an increase in blood calcium levels (hypercalcemia) because intake is too high, or an increase of urine calcium excretion resulting in calcification of the kidneys or development of renal stones. Results of hypercalcemia include decreased gastrointestinal and muscle tone, kidney failure, emotional deterioration, large urine volumes, constipation, nausea, confusion, coma, and ultimately death. Doses of 5,000+ mg/day are toxic. Osteopetrosis may result from continuous high calcium intake.

WARNINGS/CONTRAINDICATIONS/PRECAUTIONS

- Unrefined calcium carbonate, especially if derived from limestone or oyster shells, Dolomite, and bone meal calcium supplements may contain toxic levels of lead.
- Doses above 2,000 mg/day may increase the risk of kidney stones and soft-tissue calcification.
- Calcium chloride is contraindicated in hypocalcemia caused by renal insufficiency.

INTERACTIONS

Increased calcium loss through urine is caused by:
- Sodium
- Phosphorus
- Aluminum-containing antacids
- Sugar
- Saturated fat
- Caffeine
- Alcohol
- High protein intake from supplements or special diets

Calcium absorption inhibitors include:
- Alcohol
- Aspirin
- Barbituates
- Neomycin
- Strong sedatives
- Oxalic acid (chocolate, rhubarb, spinach, chard, sweet potatoes, dried beans)
- Phytic acid (grains)
- Uronic acid (hemicellulose fibers in fruits and vegetables)

Excess calcium can interfere with absorption of iron, zinc, magnesium, iodine, manganese, and copper.

REFERENCES

Cappuccio FP, Elliott P, Allender PS, et al. Epidemiologic association between dietary calcium intake and blood pressure: a meta-analysis of published data. *Am J Epidemiol.* 1995;142:935–945.

Devine A, Dick IM, Heal SJ, et al. A 4-year follow-up study of the effects of calcium supplementation on bone density in elderly postmenopausal women. *Osteoporosis Int.* 1997;7:23–28.

Ensminger AH, Ensminger ME, Konlande JE, Robson JRK. *Foods and Nutrition Encyclopedia.* 2nd ed. Baton Rouge, Fla: CRC Press Inc; 1994;2:1338–1341.

Garrison Jr RH, Somer E. *The Nutrition Desk Reference.* 3rd ed. New Canaan, Conn: Keats Publishing Inc; 1995:158–165.

Hardman JG, Gilman AG, Limbird LE, eds. *Goodman and Gilman's Pharmacological Basis of Therapeutics.* 9th ed. New York, NY: McGraw-Hill; 1996:839–874.

Heinerman J. *Heinerman's Encyclopedia of Nature's Vitamins and Minerals.* Paramus, NJ: Prentice Hall Inc; 1998:296–302.

Murray MT. *Encyclopedia of Nutritional Supplements.* Rocklin, Calif: Prima Publishing; 1996:159–175.

Nicar MJ, Pak CY. Calcium bioavailability from calcium carbonate and calcium citrate. *J Clin Endocrinol Metab.* 1985;61(2):391–393.

Rodrâiguez JA, Novik V. Calcium intake and bone density in menopause. Data of a sample of Chilean women followed-up for 5 years with calcium supplementation. *Rev Med Chil.* 1998;126:145–150.

Shils ME, Olson JA, Shike M, Ross AC. *Modern Nutrition in Health and Disease.* 9th ed. Baltimore, Md: Williams & Wilkins; 1999:169–192, A127–A128.

Thys-Jacobs S, Starkey P, Bernstein D, Tian J. Calcium carbonate and the premenstrual syndrome: effects on premenstrual and menstrual symptoms. Premenstrual Syndrome Study Group. *Am J Obstet Gynecol.* 1998;179:444–452.

Werbach MR. *Nutritional Influences on Illness.* 2nd ed. Tarzana, Calif: Third Line Press; 1993:655–680.

■ CARTILAGE

OVERVIEW

Cartilage is elastic, translucent connective tissue found in animals and man. Most cartilage is converted to bone as an animal matures, but some remains in such sites as the nose, ears, knees, and other joints. Cartilage extracts and supplements are made from cows (bovine cartilage), whose bodies contain both cartilage and bone, and sharks (shark cartilage), whose bodies contain cartilage and no bone.

Cartilage supplements are said to shrink tumors; to cure, or at least slow the development of, cancers; to reverse bone diseases such as osteoporosis; and to treat other conditions, such as macular degeneration and psoriasis, in which overgrowth of blood vessels causes disease symptoms.

The notion of using cartilage medicinally began in 1954, when bovine tracheal cartilage was found to promote wound healing. Since then, clinical trials have shown this substance to be effective against a broad range of conditions ranging arthritis to cancers. In studies at the Comprehensive Medical Clinic in Southern California, patients reported pain relief in as little as three weeks, though patients should be cautioned against expecting rapid relief. Early reports claimed that sharks do not get cancer, which proved to be untrue, although it is true that the incidence of cancer in sharks is low.

Shark cartilage that has been dried and pulverized into fine powder for use as a supplement contains many active components. Among the most important is an angiogenesis inhibitor (a protein that, at least in laboratory research, suppresses the development of new blood vessels). In cancer, this angiogenesis inhibitor deprives tumors of nutrients by blocking their ability to develop new blood vessels. In macular degeneration, it prevents blindness by blocking the uncontrolled growth of blood vessels in the eye. These effects have been demonstrated in the laboratory but have not yet been proven in human trials. Phase III clinical trials began in December 1998 on a liquid antiangiogenesis drug called Neovastat, which is made from shark cartilage. The 550 patients with small-cell lung cancer who participated were given chemotherapy; half were also given Neovastat, the other half a placebo. The joint studies are being conducted by the U. S. National Cancer Institute and a biotechnology company.

Bovine cartilage that has been cleaned, dried, and powdered to be used as a supplement helps to accelerate wound healing and reduce inflammation. Bovine tracheal cartilage was initially called catrix (from the Latin *cicatrix*, which refers to a healed wound). Today it is recognized as one of the few substances that speed wound healing. Both shark and bovine cartilage are beneficial for psoriasis, rheumatoid arthritis, and ulcerative colitis.

DIETARY SOURCES

Commercially prepared supplements of bovine or shark cartilage.

CONSTITUENTS/COMPOSITION

Shark cartilage contains angiogenesis inhibitor proteins; approximately 16% calcium and 8% phosphorus, which are absorbed as nutrients; and immune system-stimulating mucopolysaccharides, carbohydrates that form chemical bonds with water.

Bovine cartilage is believed to inhibit tumor growth, and the polysaccharides it contains are believed to combat cancer by stimulating the immune system.

COMMERCIAL PREPARATIONS

Neither shark nor bovine cartilage is U.S. FDA-approved for safety or effectiveness. (Shark cartilage was under study by the National Cancer Institute when it was discovered that every one of the cartilage supplements provided for the study had been contaminated. The trials were stopped.)

Both shark and bovine cartilage may be obtained at health stores or by mail-order as nutritional supplements. They maybe purchased in powder or capsule form under a variety of brand names, typically in capsules of 750 mg.

THERAPEUTIC USES

Shark and/or bovine cartilage is used to:

- Treat or prevent cancer by stopping the growth of blood vessels upon which tumors depend for nutrients
- Arrest the growth of new blood vessels in macular degeneration
- Treat arthritis
- Treat psoriasis
- Treat regional enteritis
- Relieve or reduce pain, inflammation, and joint damage associated with osteoarthritis and rheumatoid arthritis

■ DOSAGE RANGES AND DURATION OF ADMINISTRATION

When using shark or bovine cartilage as a dietary supplement, 3 to 4 capsules per day.

When using shark or bovine cartilage to treat cancer, the normal supplement dose may increase by 3 fold.

SIDE EFFECTS/TOXICOLOGY

Some shark cartilage products have a strong fish odor and flavor that may be unpleasant. Taken in large doses, shark cartilage has a very unpleasant taste and often causes nausea.

WARNINGS/CONTRAINDICATIONS/PRECAUTIONS

With their providers' approval, most people can take shark cartilage safely as an adjunct to conventional treatments for arthritis and cancer; however, cartilage supplements should not be used in place of conventional treatments. Shark cartilage should not be used by:

- Children
- Pregnant women
- Patients who recently underwent surgery
- Patients who recently survived a heart attack

INTERACTIONS

Bovine cartilage is not known to interfere with other medications. Shark cartilage is believed to be safe when taken with other medications.

People who ingest large quantities of shark cartilage may also need extra magnesium and potassium supplements to maintain the body's correct mineral balance.

REFERENCES

Balch J, Balch P. *Prescription for Nutritional Healing.* 2nd ed. Garden City Park, NY: Avery Publishing Group; 1997.

Burton Goldberg Group. *Alternative Medicine: The Definitive Guide.* Puyallup, Wash: Future Medicine Publishing, Inc; 1994.

Cassileth BR. *The Alternative Medicine Handbook.* New York, NY: W. W. Norton & Company; 1998.

Dupont E, Savard PE, Jourdain C, et al. Antiangiogenic properties of a novel shark cartilage extract: potential role in the treatment of psoriasis. *J Cutan Med Surg.* 1998;2:146–152.

Horsman MR, Alsner J, Overgaard J. The effect of shark cartilage extracts on the growth and metastatic spread of the SCCVII carcinoma. *Acta Oncol.* 1998;37:441–445.

Kriegal H, John Prudden and Bovine Tracheal Cartilage Research. *Alternative & Complementary Therapies*. April/May 1995.

Miller DR, Anderson GT, Stark JJ, Granick JL, Richardson D. Phase I/II trial of the safety and efficacy of shark cartilage in the treatment of advanced cancer. *J Clin Oncol*. 1998;16:3649–3655.

Moss R. *Cancer Therapy*. Brooklyn, NY: Equinox Press Inc; 1992.

Murray M. *Encyclopedia of Nutritional Supplements*. Rocklin, Calif: Prima Publishing; 1996.

Prudden JF. The treatment of human cancer with agents prepared from bovine cartilage. *Biol Response Mod*. 1985;4:551–584.

Romano CF, Lipton A, Harvey HA, Simmonds MA, Romano PJ, Imboden SL. A phase II study of Catrix-S in solid tumors. *J Biol Response Mod*. 1985;4:585–589.

Sheu JR, Fu CC, Tsai Ml, Chung WJ. Effect of U-995, a potent shark cartilage-derived angiogenesis inhibitor, on anti-angiogenesis and anti-tumor activities. *Anticancer Res*. 1998;18:4435–4441.

■ CHROMIUM

OVERVIEW

Chromium is an essential trace element for humans. Chromium in tissue is highest during infancy and decreases steadily with age. The average adult body contains about 600 mcg of chromium. Absorption occurs primarily in the jejunum and is affected by interactions with other metals, such as zinc, iron, and vanadium, and chelating agents, such as oxalate and phytate. After absorption, transferrin binds trivalent chromium and transports it to body tissues. Absorbed chromium is excreted primarily in the urine, with small amounts lost in hair, perspiration, and bile. Unabsorbed chromium (>99%) is lost in the feces.

Chromium must be converted to a biologically active form for physiological function. Glucose tolerance factor (GTF), a biologically active form isolated from brewer's yeast, contains chromium (III), nicotinic acid, and the amino acids glycine, glutamic acid, and cysteine. GTF potentiates insulin's actions and therefore influences carbohydrate, lipid, and protein metabolism. It works with insulin to facilitate glucose uptake, regulate blood sugar levels, and stimulate protein synthesis. The exact nature of the chromium-insulin interaction is unknown. Chromium may potentiate insulin action through direct action on insulin or its receptor, or it may regulate the synthesis of a molecule that potentiates insulin action. In clinical studies, GTF chromium has been shown to potentiate the effects of insulin and decrease serum cholesterol and triglycerides.

It is estimated that as many as 90% of all American diets are low in chromium. Individuals often consume less than the suggested minimum intake for chromium. The trend toward consuming highly processed foods may be a major contributing factor to this problem; appreciable losses of chromium occur in the refining of foods. Children with protein-calorie malnutrition, diabetics, and older individuals may be especially susceptible to chromium deficiency. Stressors such as elevated simple sugars, strenuous physical exercise or work, infection, and physical trauma may increase the loss of chromium, thereby increasing the need for chromium. Symptoms of chromium deficiency include glucose intolerance, elevated circulating insulin, glycosuria, fasting hyperglycemia, impaired growth, decreased longevity, elevated serum cholesterol and triglycerides, increased incidence of aortic plaques, peripheral neuropathy, brain disorders, decreased fertility and sperm count, negative nitrogen balance, and decreased respiratory quotient.

DIETARY SOURCES

- Brewer's yeast (best dietary source when grown on chromium-rich medium)
- Lean meats (especially processed meats)
- Cheeses
- Pork kidney
- Whole-grain breads and cereals
- Molasses
- Spices
- Some bran cereals

Vegetables, fruits, and most refined and processed foods (except for some processed meats, which contain high amounts of chromium) contain low amounts of chromium. Hard tap water can supply 1% to 70% of one's daily intake. Cooking in stainless steel cookware increases the chromium content of food.

CONSTITUENTS/COMPOSITION

Chromium is a white, hard, brittle metal that occurs in any oxidation state from -2 to +6. Trivalent chromium is the most stable and biologically active oxidation state and forms compounds with other organic compounds.

COMMERCIAL PREPARATIONS

Chromium is available commercially in several forms, including chromium polynicotinate, chromium picolinate, chromium-enriched yeast, and chromium chloride. Chromium is available in multivitamins and alone in tablet and capsule forms. Daily preparation doses are typically between 15 and 200 mcg chromium in multivitamins.

THERAPEUTIC USES

Diabetes. Chromium supplementation may improve glucose tolerance in healthy individuals and Type II diabetics with low chromium levels, and older individuals with abnormal glucose tolerance. Not all healthy individuals show a response to chromium supplementation. Individuals with low chromium levels appear to benefit the most from supplementation.

Poor dietary intake of chromium results in impaired glucose tolerance and symptoms similar to those of Type II diabetes mellitus. Individuals with marginally elevated blood glucose concentrations may benefit from chromium supplementation. One study assessed the effects of chromium supplementation (200 mcg chromium chloride per day) on 20 normal subjects with marginally impaired glucose tolerance. By the end of the three-month trial, 18 of the 20 subjects exhibited significant improvement in glucose tolerance.

Supplementation with chromium has also been shown to improve glucose tolerance in some diabetic patients. There is some indication that Type II diabetics may have an increased requirement for chromium. In one study, diabetic patients with severe complications, such as retinopathy and nephropathy, showed lower blood concentrations of chromium.

Older individuals are more susceptible to low tissue chromium levels, abnormal glucose tolerance, and increased incidence of diabetes and cardiovascular disease. Several studies have examined the correlation between low chromium levels and impaired glucose tolerance. In one clinical study, chromium supplementation improved glucose tolerance in 50% of older subjects (> age 70) tested. Older individuals with mild abnormalities in glucose metabolism appear to benefit more from supplementation than those with extreme diabetic-like abnormalities in glucose intolerance.

Chromium is also used to treat the following conditions.

- Hypoglycemia. Chromium deficiency may be an underlying contributing factor of hypoglycemia in some individuals. Supplementation with 200 mcg of chromium improves the symptoms of hypoglycemia in some individuals.
- Cardiovascular disease. A low amount of chromium in the diet is associated with increased blood cholesterol and increased risk of developing cardiovascular disease. Supplementation with chromium has been shown to increase HDL cholesterol and lower triglyceride and total cholesterol levels in diabetics and in individuals with impaired glucose tolerance.
- Glaucoma. Chromium affects insulin receptors in the eye. There is a strong association between chromium deficiency and increased risk of glaucoma.

- Obesity. Preliminary evidence suggests that chromium supplementation may help reduce body fat and increase lean body mass in some individuals. Chromium's ability to increase insulin sensitivity may explain these effects.
- Osteoporosis. Chromium picolinate has been shown to decrease urinary excretion of calcium and hydroxy-proline in women, and may help preserve bone density in postmenopausal women.

DOSAGE RANGES AND DURATION OF ADMINISTRATION

There are no RDAs established for chromium. The estimated safe and adequate daily dietary intakes of chromium are as follows:

- Infants birth to 6 months: 10 to 40 mcg
- Infants 6 to 12 months: 20 to 60 mcg
- Children 1 to 3 years: 20 to 80 mcg
- Children 4 to 6 years: 30 to 120 mcg
- Children 7 to 10 years: 50 to 200 mcg
- 11+ years: 50 to 200 mcg

Dosage for disease prevention and treatment is typically 200 mcg chromium one to three times a day.

SIDE EFFECTS/TOXICOLOGY

Excess intake or tissue accumulation of chromium can inhibit the effectiveness of insulin.

WARNINGS/CONTRAINDICATIONS/PRECAUTIONS

Hexavalent chromium is more toxic than trivalent. Industrial exposure to high amounts of chromium, usually airborne, can result in toxicity symptoms, including allergic dermatitis, skin ulcers, and bronchogenic carcinoma. Trivalent chromium, the form found in foods, is poorly absorbed; thus, extremely high amounts are necessary to attain toxic levels. Gastric irritation can occur at extremely high doses.

INTERACTIONS

Chromium combines with niacin to form glucose tolerance factor (GTF). Calcium carbonate and antacids reduce the absorption of chromium.

REFERENCES

Anderson RA, Cheng N, Bryden NA, et al. Elevated intakes of supplemental chromium improve glucose and insulin variables in individuals with type 2 diabetes. *Diabetes.* 1997;46:1,786–1,791.

Anderson RA, Polansky MM, Bryden NA, Bhathena SJ, Canary JJ. Effects of supplemental chromium on patients with symptoms of reactive hypoglycemia. *Metabolism.* 1987;36:351–355.

Bahadori B, Wallner S, Schneider H, Wascher TC, Toplak H. Effect of chromium yeast and chromium picolinate on body composition of obese, non-diabetic patients during and after a formula diet. *Acta Med Austriaca.* 1997;24:185–187.

Friedman E, ed. *Biochemistry of the Essential Ultratrace Elements.* New York, NY: Plenum Press; 1984.

Fujimoto S. Studies on the relationships between blood trace metal concentrations and the clinical status of patients with cerebrovascular disease, gastric cancer, and diabetes mellitus. *Hokkaido Igaku Zasshi.* 1987;62:913–932.

Krause MV, Mahan LK. *Food, Nutrition, and Diet Therapy.* 7th ed. Philadelphia, Pa: WB Saunders Co; 1984.

McCarty MF. Anabolic effects of insulin on bone suggests a role for chromium picolinate in preservation of bone density. *Med Hypotheses.* 1995;45:241–246.

Murray MT, Pizzorno JE. *Encyclopedia of Natural Medicine.* 2nd ed. Rocklin, Calif: Prima Publishing; 1998.

Shils ME, Olsen JA, Shike M, eds. *Modern Nutrition in Health and Disease.* 8th ed. Media, Pa: Williams and Wilkins Co; 1994:1.

Somer E. *The Essential Guide to Vitamins & Minerals.* New York, NY: HarperCollins Publishers; 1992

Urberg M, Zemel MB. Evidence for synergism between chromium and nicotinic acid in the control of glucose tolerance in elderly humans. *Metabolism.* 1987;36:896–899.

Wilson BE, Gondy A. Effects of chromium supplementation on fasting insulin levels and lipid parameters in healthy, non-obese young subjects. *Diabetes Res Clin Pract.* 1995;28:179–184.

■ COPPER

OVERVIEW

Copper is an essential nutrient required for hemoglobin formation and many other functions. Copper is involved in producing and releasing energy through enzymes in the cytochrome system of cell respiration. It is essential for the development and maintenance of skeletal structures; specifically, copper helps to form collagen, especially in the bone and connective tissues. In the nervous system, copper conducts electrical impulses and helps maintain the myelin sheath around nerve fibers through the synthesis of phospholipids. In addition, copper has been linked to anti-inflammatory effects through oxygen-free radical metabolism and control of histamine levels. Copper is involved in iron metabolism and may play a role in thermal regulation, glucose metabolism, and blood clotting. Recent evidence suggests it also plays a role in proper functioning of the immune system.

The average daily intake by individuals consuming a typical Western diet has now been established as 1.0 to 1.5 mg. This is lower than the 1.5 to 3.0 mg per day recommended to be safe and adequate. Pregnant women have higher needs, and greater supplementation may be indicated.

Copper deficiency in human beings is considered rare. Anemia resulting from copper deficiency has been found in individuals who have undergone intestinal bypass surgery, in patients receiving parenteral nutrition, in malnourished infants, and in persons ingesting excessive amounts of zinc. Copper deficiency in human beings has been linked to anemia, red blood cell rupture, demyelination and degeneration of the nervous system, pigmentation abnormalities in both skin and hair, abnormalities of the immune system, poor collagen integrity, faulty bone development, reduced activity of the antioxidant selenoglutathione peroxidase, elevated LDL cholesterol and reduced HDL cholesterol, and leukopenia (particularly granulocytopenia). Copper is important for converting T_3 to T_4, so low copper levels may reduce thyroid function. Animal studies indicate that copper deficiency results in central nervous system disturbances similar to Parkinson's disease, including symptoms of ataxia, tremors, and uncontrolled movements.

Wilson's disease, a genetic disorder, affects copper metabolism and leads to low serum and hair copper levels with high liver and brain copper levels. Serious problems, such as irreversible liver, kidney and brain damage, and even death, may result. It is treated with chelating agents; penicillamine is most often used as it binds copper in the gut and carries it out. Copper levels may be reduced through a low-copper diet, combined with more zinc and manganese in the diet and as supplements.

In Menkes disease, a rare problem of copper malabsorption in infants, that can often be fatal, decreased intestinal absorption causes copper to accumulate in the intestinal lining.

Indian childhood cirrhosis, a hereditary disease with accumulating copper in the liver, used to be fatal, but can now be treated with chelators. The incidence of ICC in India has decreased in recent years, but similar diseases have appeared elsewhere.

DIETARY SOURCES

Copper is found in many varied food sources. The best sources include:

- Seafood (especially raw oysters; also squid, whelk, lobster, mussels, crab)
- Organ meats (beef liver, kidneys, heart)
- Nuts (e.g., cashews, filberts, macadamia nuts, pecans, almonds, pistachio nuts)
- Legumes (especially lentils, navy beans, peanuts)
- Chocolate (unsweetened or semisweet baker's chocolate, cocoa]
- Cereals (e.g., bran flakes, shredded wheat, raisin bran)
- Fruits and vegetables (e.g., dried fruits, mushrooms, tomatoes, potatoes, bananas, grapes, avocado)
- Blackstrap molasses
- Black pepper

An additional source is water that flows through copper piping.

CONSTITUENTS/COMPOSITION

Copper is the third most abundant essential trace mineral. (Iron and zinc are first and second.) In biologic systems, copper is primarily found as $Cu2^+$, although it can appear as Cu^+ or even Cu^{3+}.

COMMERCIAL PREPARATIONS

Copper is available combined with sulfate, picolinate, gluconate, and amino acids. Data is not available to evaluate one form against another.

Superoxide dismutase (SOD), with copper, has been used to treat arthritis. Stability in the stomach and small intestine is an issue, however, and oral use may be contraindicated. Enteric-coated tablets of active SOD may improve suitability for oral treatment of arthritis and other inflammatory disorders. In a Danish study, arthritis patients who were treated with injections of SOD obtained relief from many of their symptoms, such as joint swelling, pain, and morning stiffness.

THERAPEUTIC USES

Therapeutic uses for copper include:

- Arthritis: Copper bracelets have been shown to reduce pain and inflammation associated with arthritis, although the exact mechanism is unknown. Recent research suggests that copper salicylate used to treat arthritis reduces symptoms more effectively than either copper or aspirin alone. SOD injections have reportedly provided relief in several European studies.
- Leukopenia and anemia
- Chemical hypersensitivity
- Cardiovascular disease: to prevent aortic aneurysms, treat high cholesterol
- Where copper levels are low, used to treat vitiligo, fatigue, allergies, and stomach ulcers

DOSAGE RANGES AND DURATION OF ADMINISTRATION

- Daily dietary copper intake recommended by the National Research Council of the United States: 1.5 to 3.0 mg per day for adults. For children 2 to 11 years, 1.5 to 2.5 mg. Not recommended for children under 2.
- A zinc-to-copper ratio in the range of 8:1 to 15:1 is consistently recommended.
- For leukopenia and anemia, daily doses up to 0.1 mg/kg of cupric sulfate orally, or 1 to 2 mg per day added to nutrient solution of nutrients for parenteral administration.

SIDE EFFECTS/TOXICOLOGY

Copper toxicity is rare. Circumstances in which acute copper poisoning has occurred include accidental consumption by children, ingestion of several grams in suicide attempts, application of copper salts to burned skin, drinking water from contaminated water supplies, and consumption of acidic food or beverages stored in copper containers.

Toxicity results in nausea, vomiting, epigastric pain, headache, dizziness, weakness, diarrhea, and a characteristic metallic taste. In severe (but rare) cases, tachycardia, hypertension, jaundice, uremia, coma, or death can result.

WARNINGS/CONTRAINDICATIONS/PRECAUTIONS

Chronic copper toxicosis has been observed in dialysis patients following months of hemodialysis when copper tubing was used and in vineyard workers using copper compounds as pesticides.

Copper is an emetic. As little as 10 mg usually produces nausea, and 60 mg usually produces vomiting. The lethal dose for copper may be as little as 3.5 g. Copper supplements should be kept away from children.

INTERACTIONS

Excess copper can interfere with absorption of zinc.

Copper deficiency may be aggravated by:
- Alcohol
- Egg
- Fructose

Excretion losses may be increased by:
- Molybdenum

Copper absorption may be adversely affected by:
- Calcium
- Iron
- Manganese
- Tin
- Zinc
- Phytates

- Vitamin B$_6$
- Vitamin C (high levels of supplementation)
- Cysteine
- Antacids in very high amounts

REFERENCES

Asseth J, Haugen M, et al. Rheumatoid arthritis and metal compounds—perspectives on the role of oxygen radical detoxification. *Analyst.* 1998;123:3–6.

Ensminger AH, Ensminger ME, Konlande JE, Robson JRK. *Foods and Nutrition Encyclopedia.* 2nd ed. Baton Rouge, Fla: CRC Press Inc; 1994;1:476–479.

Garrison Jr RH, Somer E. *The Nutrition Desk Reference.* 3rd ed. New Canaan, Conn: Keats Publishing Inc; 1995:188–192.

Haas EM. *Staying Healthy With Nutrition.* Berkley, Calif: Celestial Arts Publishing; 1992:190–194.

Hardman JG, Gilman AG, Limbird LE, eds. *Goodman and Gilman's Pharmacological Basis of Therapeutics.* 9th ed. New York, NY: McGraw-Hill; 1996:1325–1326.

Heinerman J. *Heinerman's Encyclopedia of Nature's Vitamins and Minerals.* Paramus, NJ: Prentice Hall Inc; 1998:250–255.

Mazzetti I, Grigolo B, Borzai RM, Meliconi R, Facchini A. Serum copper/zinc superoxide dismutase levels in patients with rheumatoid arthritis. *J Clin Lab Res.* 1996;26(4):245–249.

Murray MT. *Encyclopedia of Nutritional Supplements.* Rocklin, Calif: Prima Publishing, 1996:199–203.

Newstrom H. *Nutrients Catalog.* Jefferson, NC: McFarland & Co. Inc; 1993:141–151.

Olivares M, Uauy R. Copper as an essential nutrient. *Am J Clin Nutr.* 1996;63:791S–796S.

Pennington JA, Schoen SA. Total diet study: estimated dietary intakes of nutritional elements. *Int J Vitam Nutr Res.* 1996;66:350–362.

Shils ME, Olson JA, Shike M, Ross AC. *Modern Nutrition in Health and Disease.* 9th ed. Baltimore, Md: Williams & Wilkins; 1999:241–252.

Uauy R, Olivares M, Gonzalez M. Essentiality of copper in humans. *Am J Clin Nutr.* 1998;67(5 suppl):952S–959S.

Wapnir RA. Copper absorption and bioavailability. *Am J Clin Nutri.* May 1998;67;5:1054s.

Werbach MR. *Nutritional Influences on Illness.* 2nd ed. Tarzana, Calif: Third Line Press; 1993:655–680.

■ CREATINE

OVERVIEW

Creatine is an amino acid (a protein building block) which is absorbed into the bloodstream in the small intestine and excreted as the by-product creatinine in the urine. Creatine in the form of creatine phosphate (phosphocreatine) is an important form of high-energy phosphate found in skeletal muscle cells. During high-intensity exercise lasting for a short time (15 to 30 seconds), phosphocreatine is broken down into phosphate and creatine. The energy released is used to regenerate ATP, the primary source of energy. As phosphocreatine becomes depleted, output power drops because ATP cannot be regenerated fast enough. Therefore, more energy is available for use. In short-duration, high-intensity anaerobic sports such as weight lifting or sprinting, it is logical that more creatine phosphate in the muscles would allow greater ATP regeneration to produce more energy and increase performance.

Research has shown that taking creatine monohydrate supplements enhances performance for athletes who participate in high-intensity, short-duration sports. Several studies have been recently conducted to study a variety of sports and various dosages of creatine. The results are generally concurrent. After an initial "loading" phase of about a week, a "maintenance" phase keeps most athletes' muscle concentrations of creatine high enough to see noticeable changes in endurance and strength, and also an increase in lean muscle mass. However, some individuals are genetically predisposed to have high stores of creatine already in their muscles, or have a high efficiency or inefficiency in producing ATP. These people will not see a dramatic ergogenic (energy-producing) effect from creatine monohydrate supplementation.

DIETARY SOURCES

About half of an individual's daily need of creatine is synthesized in the liver, kidneys, and pancreas from the amino acids glycine, arginine, and methionine. The other half is provided from the diet.

Meat or fish are the best natural sources of creatine. There is about 1 g of creatine in a half pound of raw meat. However, for purposes of "loading" the skeletal muscles to gain ergogenic benefits, it is not feasible to get extra creatine from the diet alone. Supplementation is necessary.

CONSTITUENTS/COMPOSITION

There are three different forms of creatine. Creatine is primarily stored in the skeletal muscles as free creatine and phosphocreatine. Creatine monohydrate is the form primarily used for supplementation to increase the skeletal muscles' stores of both free creatine and the phosphorylized form used to fuel energy release during the conversion of ATP.

COMMERCIAL PREPARATIONS

Creatine monohydrate is available in a variety of forms. The most common form is a powder which is ingested by mixing with juice or water. Generally, about 1 tsp. provides a 5 g dose of creatine monohydrate. Liquid creatine monohydrate, a more recently marketed preparation, is now competing with the powdered form. Claimed benefits of the liquid form are faster absorption and convenience over the powdered variety. Creatine monohydrate is also available in tablets, capsules, energy "bars," chews, drink mixes, and other preparations. Since combining creatine monohydrate with glucose is reported to be more effective than taking creatine alone, there are many preparations with differing combinations of creatine and glucose or other carbohydrates.

THERAPEUTIC USES

- Primarily used by athletes as a supplement to "load" muscle stores of creatine to improve strength, endurance, and lean muscle mass for high-intensity, short-duration exercise
- May reduce blood lipids
- May improve glucose metabolism
- Reduces muscle wasting in post-surgical patients
- May benefit heart patients by increasing myocardial metabolism and reducing fibrillation as well as allowing increased exercise capacity
- May provide anti-inflammatory and analgesic activity

DOSAGE RANGES AND DURATION OF ADMINISTRATION

The typical loading regimen for the average weight athlete consists of taking creatine monohydrate supplements in the dose of 5 g, qid (20 g/day) for seven days, depending on body weight. After that, the maintenance phase consists of 2 to 5 g/day to sustain the stores of creatine in the muscles.

SIDE EFFECTS/TOXICOLOGY

The only well-documented side effect has been weight gain. This is due to water being stored in the muscle cells (volumization), general water weight gain, and also an increase in lean muscle tissue.

Unsubstantiated side effects which have been reported include greater incidence of muscle cramping, strains and pulls; gastrointestinal distress; kidney impairment; and liver damage. However, studies have been done which negate these claims.

WARNINGS/CONTRAINDICATIONS/PRECAUTIONS

Not useful to increase performance in endurance (aerobically oriented) exercise.

INTERACTIONS

Caffeine has been proven to negate any of the ergogenic effects of creatine supplementation. Coffee, tea, and soft drinks should be avoided. Creatine monohydrate in combination with glucose seems to be more effective in increasing muscle energy and endurance than just supplementing with creatine monohydrate alone.

REFERENCES

Bosco C, et al. Effect of oral creatine supplementation on jumping and running performance. *Int J Sports Med.* 1997;18:369–372.

Earnets, C.P.; Almada, A.L.; Mitchell, T.L. High-performance capillary electrophoresis: pure creatine monohydrate reduces blood lipids in men and women. *Clin Sci.* 1996;91:113–118.

Grindstaff PD, et al. Effects of creatine supplementation on repetitive sprint performance and body composition in competitive swimmers. *Int J Sport Nutr.* 1997;7:330–346.

Juhn, MS, Tarnopolsky M. 1998. Potential side effects of oral creatine supplementation: a critical review. *Clin J Sport Med.* 1998;8:298–304.

Juhn, MS, Tarnopolsky M. Oral creatine supplementation and athletic performance: a critical review. *Clin J Sport Med.* 1994;8:286–297.

Kreider RB, Ferreira M, et al. Effects of creatine supplementation on body composition, strength and sprint performance. *Med Sci Sports Exerc.* 1998;30(1):73–82.

Kreider RB, Rasmussen C, Ransom J, Almada AL. Effects of creatine supplementation during training on the incidence of muscle cramping, injuries and GI distress. Presented at the National Strength and Conditioning Association Convention; June 24–28, 1998; Nashville, Tenn. Accessed at www.eas.com/research/creatine/0698.html on February 21, 1999.

Kreider RB, Ferreira M, Wilson M, et al. Effects of creatine supplementation on body composition, strength, and sprint performance. *Med Sci Sports Exerc.* 1998;30:73–82

Lawrence SR, et al. The effect of oral creatine supplementation on maximal exercise performance in competitive rowers. *Sports Medicine, Training and Rehabilitation.* 1997;7:243–253.

McNaughton LR, Dalton B, Tarr J. The effects of creatine supplementation on high–intensity exercise performance in elite performers. *Eur J Appl Physiol.* 1998;78:236–240.

Odland LM, et al. Effect of oral creatine supplementation on muscle [PCr] and short-term maximum power output. *Med Sci Sports Exerc.* 1997;29:216–219.

Poortmans JR, et al. Effect of short-term creatine supplementation on renal responses in men. *Eur J Appl Physiol.* 1997;76:566–567.

Prevost MC, Nelson AG, Morris GS. Creatine supplementation enhances intermittent work performance. *Res Q Exerc Sport.* 1997;68:233–240.

Schneider DA, et al. Creatine supplementation and the total work performed during 15-s and 1-min bouts of maximal cycling. *Aust J Sci Med Sport.* 1997;29:65–68.

Smith, J.C., et al. Effect of oral creatine ingestion on paarameters of the work rate-time relationship and time to exhaustion in high-intensity cycling. *Eur J Appl Physiol.* 1998;77:360–365.

Thompson CH, et al. Effect of creatine on aerobic and anaerobic metabolism in skeletal muscles in swimmers. *Br J Sports Med.* 1996;30:222–225.

Vandenberghe K, et al. Caffeine counteracts the ergogenic action of muscle creatine loading. *J Appl Physiol.* 1996;80:452–457.

Vandebuerie F, Vanden Eynde B, Vandenberghe K, Hespel P, et al. Effects of creatine loading on endurance capacity and sprint power in cyclists. *Int J Sports Med.* 1998;19:490–495.

Vandenberghe K, et al. Long-term creatine intake is beneficial to muscle performance during resistance training. *J Appl Physiol.* 1997;83:2055–2063.

Volek JS, et al. Creatine supplementation enhances muscular performance during high-intensity resistance exercise. *J Am Diet Assoc.* 1997;97:765–770.

Werbach MR. *Nutritional Influences on Illness: A Sourcebook of Clinical Research.* New Canaan, Conn: Keats Publishing, Inc; 1988.

■ DEHYDROEPIANDROSTERONE (DHEA)

OVERVIEW

Dehydroepiandrosterone (DHEA) is the most abundant androgen (15 to 30 mg/day) secreted by the adrenal glands and to some extent by the ovaries and testes. It is a precursor for other steroid hormones, such as testosterone and estrogen. Peak levels of DHEA occur at age 25. By age 80, DHEA levels have decreased to 10% to 20% of the peak level. DHEA has been called an antiaging hormone because deficiencies of DHEA in old age may make individuals more susceptible to cancer of the breast, prostate, bladder; atherosclerosis; hypertension; autoimmune diseases (e.g., diabetes, lupus erythematosus, rheumatoid arthritis); osteoporosis; high cholesterol; obesity; memory disturbances; chronic fatigue; and manifestations of aging (older persons with these conditions have been found to have low levels). When given to older patients, DHEA increased feelings of physical and psychological well-being; increased immune cell production; and enhanced mood, energy, and sleep. Older individuals with higher DHEA levels are often in better heath than individuals with lower levels. The two most important factors concerning DHEA are its decline in old age and its deficiency in several major disease states.

DIETARY SOURCES

Most of the DHEA on the market is made in laboratories from sterols (especially diosgenin) extracted from wild yams found in Mexico. Some extracts from wild yams are marketed as "natural DHEA." These extracts of diosgenin are supposedly converted into DHEA by the body. However, because it takes several chemical reactions to covert diosgenin into DHEA, it is unlikely that the body can make this conversion. Thus, only pharmaceutical grade DHEA should be used.

CONSTITUENTS/COMPOSITION

DHEA is a weak androgen synthesized in large quantities by the adrenal cortex. However, it can be converted into more potent androgens (testosterone and estrogen) throughout the body as needed. Only a small percentage of the body's DHEA (5%) is in the active form; the rest (95%) is attached to sulfur molecules (DHEA-S)—that is, it is sulfated by the liver—and serves as a reserve to be converted to the active form when needed. When blood levels of DHEA are measured, DHEAS is usually the measurement taken.

COMMERCIAL PREPARATIONS

DHEA is available in capsules, chewing gum, or drops that are placed under the tongue. DHEA is either natural or synthetic. However, it is debatable whether the body can process diosgenin into steroid hormones. Thus, it is recommended that only "pharmaceutical grade" DHEA be taken.

THERAPEUTIC USES

- Heart disease. Men with heart disease have low levels of DHEAS. In one study, healthy men with low levels of DHEAS were three times more likely to eventually die of heart disease than those with high levels of DHEAS.
- Obesity. Experimental animals given DHEA did not become obese, but a control group given no supplements did become obese when given the same amount of food. In human studies, DHEA has not demonstrated a beneficial effect on body composition, even at high doses.
- Aging. Significant positive changes (e.g., less muscle wasting, less memory loss, improved mood and energy) have been seen in elderly men given DHEA.
- Osteoporosis. DHEA given to postmenopausal women increases bone mass. However, supplementation is not recommended until more extensive human trials have been conducted.
- Cancer. Experimental animals bred for breast cancer did not develop cancer when given DHEA supplements. Also, women with breast cancer have low levels of DHEA.
- Autoimmune disease. Low levels of DHEA have been found in patients with autoimmune disorders (e.g., lupus erythematosus, rheumatoid arthritis, multiple sclerosis, ulcerative colitis, AIDS). DHEA supplements improved stamina and overall sense of well-being in patients with autoimmune disorders. Patients with lupus treated with DHEA have shown symptomatic improvement, especially of kidney function, often permitting a reduction of their corticosteroids.
- Depression. DHEA has been used experimentally, to treat depressed patients. Improvements in both depression and memory were observed.
- AIDS. DHEA treatment in AIDS patients may have promise since low DHEA levels have been correlated with decreased immune function. However, controlled trials have not been conducted to investigate this supposition.
- Performance enhancement. Because DHEA is thought to build muscle mass, reduce fat, and reduce recovery time following injury, it is popular with athletes. However, human studies are needed to verify these claims. DHEA is also used to enhance sexual performance.

DOSAGE RANGES AND DURATION OF ADMINISTRATION

DHEA is available without a prescription. Dosages for men and women differ; men seem to tolerate higher doses. Men can safely take up to 50 mg/day; women should not take more than 25 mg/day. Positive effects have been noted at dosages as low as 5 mg/day. Because the long-term effects of DHEA supplementation have not been studied and data from clinical trials is virtually nonexistent, the safety and efficacy of DHEA has not been determined.

SIDE EFFECTS/TOXICOLOGY

High doses of DHEA are associated with negative side effects for both men and women. However, the administration of high doses may be appropriate when treating serious illness (e.g., autoimmune diseases). High doses may inhibit the body's natural ability to synthesize DHEA and may be heptaotoxic. In addition, women should be alert for any signs of masculinization because the end products of DHEA in women are androgens (male hormones). Possible signs include loss of hair on the head, hair growth on the face, weight gain around the waist, and acne. Men should also be alert for signs of excess testosterone (e.g., sexual aggressiveness, testicular atrophy, aggressive tendencies, male pattern baldness, and high blood pressure). Blood levels of DHEA should be checked every six months.

WARNINGS/CONTRAINDICATIONS/PRECAUTIONS

Because DHEA is a precursor of estrogen and testosterone, patients with hormone-sensitive cancers (e.g., breast, prostate, ovarian, testicular) should avoid taking DHEA.

DHEA is not recommended for people under the age of 40, unless DHEA levels are known to be low (< 130 mg/dL in women and < 180 mg/dL in men).

The International Olympic Committee and the National Football League recently banned the use of DHEA by athletes because its effects are very similar to anabolic steroids.

INTERACTIONS

One study indicated that vitamin E may protect against the oxidative damage associated with DHEA treatment.

Alcohol can potentiate the effects of DHEA.

REFERENCES

Balch JF, Balch PA. *Prescription for Nutritional Healing.* 2nd ed. Garden City Park, NY: Avery Publishing; 1997:544–555.

Mindell E, Hopkins V. *Prescriptions Alternatives.* New Canaan, Conn: Keats Publishing; 1998:473–476.

Reynolds JE. *Martindale: The Extra Pharmacopoeia.* 31st ed. London, England: Royal Pharmaceutical Society; 1996:1504.

Shealy CN. *The Illustrated Encyclopedia of Healing Remedies.* Shaftesbury, England: Element Books; 1998:273.

Thompson G. Doctors warn of dangers of muscle-building drugs. *The New York Times.* March 2, 1999.

■ ETHYLENEDIAMINETETRAACETIC ACID (EDTA)
OVERVIEW

EDTA is a synthetic amino acid compound administered intravenously. This procedure, called chelation therapy, is a non-surgical treatment for coronary artery disease and a wide variety of vascular disorders. By binding to toxic and excess metals in the bloodstream, EDTA allows for their elimination from the body through urine. Their removal, in turn, reduces the activity of damaging free radicals. It is these free radicals that create dangerous, artery-clogging plaque. The end result of chelation therapy is an improved blood supply to the legs, heart, and other organs.

More than 40 million Americans face coronary artery disease, and many of them (more than 400,000 annually) undergo coronary artery bypass surgery. Many health care professionals recognize EDTA as a preventive measure as well as an effective alternative treatment for some of these patients. EDTA administration occurs on an outpatient basis in a health care provider's office. Since hospitalization is unnecessary, chelation therapy is more comfortable, less invasive, and much less expensive than traditional bypass surgery. Administering health care providers should make themselves aware of the protocol set by the American College of Advancement of Medicine (ACAM) and the American Board of Chelation Therapy (ABCT).

Researchers developed EDTA chelation therapy as a treatment for metal toxicity, such as lead poisoning. It has also been used in response to digitalis toxicity. Again, the process is one of binding to, and thus removing, injurious metals from the body. Administration of EDTA also positively affects cerebrovascular insufficiency, arthritis, multiple sclerosis, Parkinson's disease, and Alzheimer's disease, and it may lower cancer mortality.

Making healthful dietary changes (e.g., eating fewer saturated fats and increasing the consumption of plant foods and fiber) contributes to the success of chelation therapy. Researchers also recommend the addition of nonprescription nutritional supplements, such as an anti-oxidant formula and a multi-vitamin.

EDTA is not, at this time, approved by the FDA as an alternative to bypass surgery. It is a controversial option among healthcare professionals due to risk concerns. An overdose (administered too quickly or too often) of EDTA chelation therapy could, in theory, lead to kidney failure or even death. However, no such toxicity has occurred in the hundreds of thousands of cases of properly performed therapy in the past 25 years. Currently, government-authorized investigational trials are underway which are likely to confirm the safety of EDTA and lead to FDA approval.

Healthcare professionals also express concerns about the lack of demonstrated clinical proof of efficacy. Analysis of recent studies, however, revealed a high correlation between treatment and patient improvement. Anecdotal evidence also leans heavily in favor of EDTA.

EDTA chelation therapy is FDA-approved and available as treatment for heavy metal and digitalis toxicity.

DIETARY SOURCES

EDTA is a synthetic amino acid and has no natural sources.

CONSTITUENTS/COMPOSITION

The chelating agent ethylenediaminetetraacetic acid (EDTA) is a synthetic amino acid usually combined with vitamins and minerals (such as vitamin C and magnesium), and delivered intravenously.

COMMERCIAL PREPARATIONS

The patent on EDTA is long expired. This generic, synthetic amino acid may be manufactured and sold by any drug company under the names ethylenediaminetetraacetic acid, edetic acid, tetracemic acic, and edathamil.

THERAPEUTIC USES

Heart disease: By binding to heavy metals, toxins, and metabolic wastes, EDTA counters free-radical damage, clears clogged arteries, and improves blood flow to the heart. Chelation therapy, then, is offered as a preventive for atherosclerosis, an alternative to heart bypass treatment, and/or a post-surgical procedure for patients with (or at risk for) cardiovascular disease.

Metal toxicity: Chelation therapy is one of the only recognized (and FDA-approved) antidotes to lead, mercury, or arsenic poisoning. Research confirms that children with lead poisoning experience healthy growth spurts after undergoing EDTA chelation therapy. EDTA is also indicated as a chelating solution to digitalis toxicity.

EDTA's metal cleansing mechanisms may have a positive effect on Alzheimer's disease, which may be worsened by aluminum in the brain. Additionally, the improved blood flow brought about by a course of intravenous EDTA can significantly improve conditions as varied as multiple sclerosis, gangrene, and macular degeneration. Chelation therapy also impedes the activity of damaging free radicals that lead to or exacerbate cancer, lupus, and arthritis.

DOSAGE RANGES AND DURATION OF ADMINISTRATION

EDTA is usually administered intravenously, with magnesium and vitamin C, over a period of three to four hours. Doses of 2.5 g in 500 ml $^1/_2$N saline have achieved favorable results. Only one dose of EDTA should be dispensed in a single 24-hour period; two to three weekly treatments are typical. Most patients require 20 to 30 infusions in response to coronary artery disease.

One gram intravenous EDTA delivered over one hour is the recommended adult dosage as an antidote for heavy metal toxicity.

Administering physicians should consult with ACAM or ABCT regarding more specific dosage protocol.

SIDE EFFECTS/TOXICOLOGY

EDTA infusions must be given slowly and at least 24 hours apart in order to avoid potentially dangerous side effects, such as kidney failure, other organ damage, seizure, or death.

WARNINGS/CONTRAINDICATIONS/PRECAUTIONS

The American College of Advancement of Medicine (ACAM) provides training and chelation therapy protocol.

Additionally, the administering physician should monitor or measure blood pressure and circulation; cholesterol and other blood compounds; blood sugar and nutritional levels; kidney and other organ function; pre- and post-vascular function; and tissue minerals before, during, and after EDTA delivery.

INTERACTIONS

EDTA chelation therapy is most effective when combined with a diet low in saturated fats and high in fiber, and fortified by an anti-oxidant formula and a multivitamin.

Efficacy of intravenous delivery is apparently boosted by inclusion of IV vitamins and minerals, such as vitamin C and magnesium.

REFERENCES

Burns CB, Currie B. The efficacy of chelation therapy and factors influencing mortality in lead intoxicated petrol sniffers. *Aust N Z J Med.* 1995;25:197–203.

Chappell LT, Stahl JP. The correlation between EDTA chelation therapy and improvement in cardiovascular function: a meta-analysis. *J Adv Med.* 1993;6:139–160.

Carey C, Lee H, and Woeltje K, eds. *Washington Manual of Medical Therapeutics.* 29th ed. Philadelphia, Penn: Lippincott-Raven; 1998.

Cranton E, Brecher A. *Bypassing Bypass.* Norfolk, Va: Donning Co; 1989.

Cranton E. *A Textbook on EDTA Chelation.* New York, NY: Humay Sciences Press; 1989.

Guldager B, Brixen KT, Jorgensen SJ, Nielsen HK, Mosekilde L, Jelnes R. Effects of intravenous EDTA treatment on serum parathyroid hormone (1-84) and biochemical markers of bone turnover. *Dan Med Bull.* 1993;40:627–630.

Hancke C, Flytlie K. Benefits of EDTA chelation therapy on arteriosclerosis. *J Adv Med.* 1993;6:161–172.

Lin JL, Ho HH, Yu CC. Chelation therapy for patients with elevated body lead burden and progressive renal insufficiency. A randomized, controlled trial. *Ann Intern Med.* 1999;130:7–13.

Murray, M. *Encyclopedia of Nutritional Supplements: The Essential Guide for Improving Your Health Naturally.* Rocklin, CA: Prima Publishing; 1996:435–436.

Olszewer E, Sabag FC, Carter JP. A pilot double-blind study of sodium-magnesium EDTA in peripheral vascular disease. *J Natl Med Assoc.* 1990;82:173–177.

Olszewer E, Carter JP. EDTA chelation therapy in chronic degenerative disease. *Med Hypotheses.* 1988;27:41–49.

Reynolds JEF, ed. *Martindale: The Extra Pharmacopoeia.* 31st ed. London, England: Royal Pharmaceutical Society; 1996.

Sloth-Nielson J, Guldager B, Mouritzen C, et al. Arteriographic findings in EDTA chelation therapy on peripheral arteriosclerosis. *Am J Surg.* 1991;162:122–125.

■ FLAXSEED OIL

OVERVIEW

Flaxseed oil is a rich source of alpha-linolenic acid (ALA), an omega-3 fatty acid. Omega-3 fatty acids (n-3) constitute one of two major families of polyunsaturated fatty acids, the other family being omega-6 (n-6). ALA is the parent substance of the n-3 fatty acid family. Linoleic acid is the parent substance for the n-6 fatty acid family. These two families have very different biochemical roles in the body. ALA is an essential fatty acid and is necessary for the normal function of all tissues. Through a series of steps, it is metabolized to eicosapentaenoic acid (EPA), docosahexaenoic acid (DHA), and prostaglandins in the body. Prostaglandins are hormone-like compounds that help regulate blood pressure, blood clotting, heart rate, vascular dilation, lipolysis, and immune response.

American diets are typically high in n-6 fatty acids and low in n-3 fatty acids. The average diet supplies only 0.15 g of n-3 fatty acids per day. A high ratio of n-6:n-3 fatty acid may encourage production of proinflammatory metabolites (arachidonic acid, prostaglandin E1, and prostaglandin E2) and negatively affect the body's response to disease. Changing the intake of dietary fatty acids may modify the body's response to disease, injury, and infection. Clinical trials indicate that supplementation with n-3 fatty acids from plants such as flaxseed can encourage production of the anti-inflammatory metabolites and inhibit the production of proinflammatory metabolites.

ALA is used as a source of energy by the body and partly as a precursor of the metabolites. Most studies indicate that a certain amount of ALA is converted to EPA in the body but conversion to DHA is limited. Results of one study showed that with a diet high in saturated fat conversion to EPA and DHA is approximately 6% and 3.8%, respectively. With a diet rich in n-6 polyunsaturated fatty acids, conversion is reduced by 40% to 50%. Flaxseed oil raises tissue EPA levels comparably to fish oil when dietary linoleic acid is restricted. In one study, the degree of conversion was proportional to a weekly portion (50 to 100 g) of fatty fish depending on the fat content of the fish. In some instances, ALA may be an effective alternative to fish oil supplements. However, a high ratio of ALA:linoleic acid may be necessary to produce the effects demonstrated after feeding fish oils.

Deficiencies in essential fatty acid can reduce both primary and secondary immune responses and modify the inflammatory response in animals. Symptoms associated with a deficiency in n-3 fatty acids include neurological changes (parasthesias, weakness, pain in the legs, inability to walk) and impaired vision.

DIETARY SOURCES

Ground flaxseed or flaxseed meal

CONSTITUENTS/COMPOSITION

Flaxseed contains 55% to 65% essential fatty acids, beta-carotene, and mixed carotenoids. Some processors add vitamin E to increase the oil's stability and shelf life.

COMMERCIAL PREPARATIONS

- Flaxseed oil is easily destroyed by heat, light, and oxygen.
- For optimal stability, seeds should be fresh pressed at low temperatures in the absence of light, extreme heat, or oxygen.
- Flaxseed oil is available in liquid and softgel capsule form, and should be refrigerated to prevent rancidity.
- Liquids require bottling in nonreactive, opaque or dark containers to prevent transmission of light. Capsules require similar packaging.

- Flaxseed oil can be used on salads and cooked vegetables or added to foods after they have been cooked. Flaxseed oil should not be heated since this destroys its anti-inflammatory qualities.

THERAPEUTIC USES

- **Inflammation.** Arachidonic acid and its proinflammatory metabolites are released from membrane phospholipids during an inflammatory reaction. EPA and DHA decrease the production of proinflammatory prostaglandins and thromboxanes from arachidonic acid. EPA competes with liberated arachidonic acid and induces the production of less inflammatory and chemotactic derivatives. A 1:1 or 1.3:1 ratio of ALA:linoleic acid may be optimal for reducing arachidonic acid production. This gives flax oil a use in inflammatory conditions such as arthritis, asthma, allergies, and dysmenorrhea
- **Skin disorders.** A small amount of research indicates that n-3 fatty acids may be of value in alleviating certain skin diseases such as psoriasis.
- **Immune system.** Studies in humans and animals have demonstrated that flaxseed oil is as effective as EPA at inhibiting the autoimmune reaction. This may prove useful in such conditions as rheumatoid arthritis and ulcerative colitis.
- **Hypertension.** Fish oil or flaxseed oil appear to be very effective in lowering blood pressure. One tablespoon of flaxseed oil per day can lower both the systolic and diastolic readings by up to 9 mm Hg.
- **Cardiovascular disease.** n-3 fatty acids have been shown to improve lipid profiles in hundreds of studies. The majority of studies used fish oils, not flaxseed oil. The few studies conducted with flaxseed oil indicate that it is not equivalent to fish oil. Large quantities of flaxseed oil are required to induce similar effects seen with fish oils. Flaxseed may offer some cardiovascular protection by improving arterial circulation and arterial function in high-risk subjects.
- **Diabetes.** Flaxseed oil may be a safer alternative to fish oil supplements in diabetics with altered lipid metabolism. High doses of fish oils have been shown to increase blood lipids and worsen blood sugar control in some individuals. However, some Type II diabetics may have low delta-6-desaturase activity, which prevents them from efficiently converting ALA to EPA in the body; flaxseed oil may not be an effective therapy in these individuals.
- **Nephritis.** Flaxseed oil reduced glomerular filtration injury and declining renal function in a rat-5/6 renal ablation model. Blood pressure, plasma lipids, and urinary prostaglandins were also favorably affected by the flaxseed oil treatment.
- **Drug resistance.** ALA, gamma-linolenic acid, EPA, and DHA have been shown to reverse tumor cell drug resistance in vitro.

DOSAGE RANGES AND DURATION OF ADMINISTRATION

One to three teaspoons liquid flaxseed oil per day, or 3,000 mg (capsules) bid, as a starting dose is most recommended.

Dosage for disease prevention and treatment will vary depending on fatty acid content of the diet, individual body physiology (ALA conversion to EPA), and the type of disorder.

SIDE EFFECTS/TOXICOLOGY

There are no side effects or toxicity associated with increased intake of flaxseed oil.

WARNINGS/CONTRAINDICATIONS/PRECAUTIONS

Flaxseed oil can add additional calories and fat to the diet if there is not a compensatory reduction in other fats.

INTERACTIONS

May increase vitamin E requirements. Reduced platelet aggregation due to lowered prostaglandin species may increase bleeding time. Begin with a lower dose for those on blood-thinning medication or with a bleeding disorder.

REFERENCES

Allman-Farinelli MA, Hall D, Kingham K, Pang D, Petocz P, Favaloro EJ. Comparison of the effects of two low fat diets with different alpha-linolenic acid ratios on coagulation and fibrinolysis. *Atherosclerosis.* 1999;142:159–168.

Bierenbuam ML, Reichstein R, Watkins TR. Reducing atherogenic risk in hyperlipemic humans with flaxseed supplementation: a preliminary report. *J Am Coll Nutr.* 1993;12:501–504.

Clark WF, Parbtani A, Hugg MW, et al. Flaxseed: a potential treatment of lupus nephritis. *Kidney Int.* 1995;48:475–480.

Cunnane SC, Ganguli S, Menard C, et al. High alpha-linolenic acid flaxseed (Linum usitatissimum): some nutritional properties in humans. *Br J Nutr.* 1993;69:443–453.

Cunnane SC, Hamadeh MJ, Liede AC, Thompson LU, Wolever TM, Jenkins DJ. Nutritional attributes of traditional flaxseed in healthy-young adults. *Am J Clin Nutr.* 1995;61:62–68.

Das UN, Madhavi N, Sravan KG, Padma M, Sangeetha P. Can tumor cell drug resistance be reversed by essential fatty acids and their metabolites? *Prostaglandins Leukot Essent Fatty Acids.* 1998;58:39–54.

Dox IG, Melloni BJ, Eisner GM. *The HarperCollins Illustrated Medical Dictionary.* New York, NY: HarperCollins Publishers; 1993.

Gerster H. Can adults adequately convert alpha-linolenic acid (18:3n-3) to eicosapentaenoic acid (20:5n-3) and docosahexaenoic acid (22:6n-3)? *Int J Vitam Nutr Res.* 1998;68:159–173.

Harris WS. N-3 fatty acids and serum lipoproteins: human studies. *Am J Clin Nutr.* May 1997;65(5 suppl):1645S–1654S.

Heller A, Koch T, Schmeck J, Van Ackern K. Lipid mediators in inflammatory disorders. *Drugs.* 1998;55:487–496.

Ingram AJ, Parbtani A, Clark WF, Spanner E, Huff MW, Philbrick DJ, Holub BJ. Effects of flax oil diets in a rat-5/6 renal ablation model. *Am J Kidney Dis.* 1995;25:320–329.

Kaminskas A, Levaciov, Lupinovic V, Kuchinskene Z. The effect of linseed oil on the fatty acid composition of blood plasma low- and very low-density lipoproteins and cholesterol in diabetics [in Russian]. *Vopr Pitan.* 1992;5–6:13–14.

Leece EA, Allman MA. The relationships between dietary alpha-linolenic: linoleic acid and rat platelet eicosapentaenoic and arachidonic acids. *Br J Nutr.* 1996;76:447–452.

Mantzioris E, James MJ, Gibson RA, Cleland LG. Differences exist in the relationships between dietary linoleic and alph-linolenic acids and their respective long-chain metabolites. *Am J Clin Nutr.* 1995;61:320–324.

Mayser P, Mrowietz U, Arenberger P, et al. Omega-3 fatty acid-based lipid infusion in patients with chronic plaque psoriasis: results of a double-blind, randomized, placebo-controlled, multicenter trial. *J Am Acad Dermatol.* 1998;38:539–547

Murray MT, Pizzorno JE. *Encyclopedia of Natural Medicine.* 2nd ed. Rocklin, Calif: Prima Publishing; 1998.

Nestel PJ, et al. Arterial compliance in obese subjects is improved with dietary plant n-3 fatty acid from flaxseed oil despite increased LDL oxidizabilty. *Arterioscler Thromb Vasc Biol.* 1997;17:1163–1170.

Norman AW, Litwack G. *Hormones.* Orlando, Fla: Academic Press, Inc; 1987.

Orten JM, Neuhaus OW, eds. *Human Biochemistry.* 10th ed. St. Louis, Mo: The C.V. Mosby Company; 1982.

Prasad K. Dietary flaxseed in prevention of hypercholesterolemic atherosclerosis. *Atherosclerosis.* 1997;132:69–76.

Shils ME, Olson JA, Shike M, eds. *Modern Nutrition in Health and Disease.* 8th ed. Media, Pa: Williams and Wilkins Co; 1994:1.

Schmidt MA. *Smart Fats: How Dietary Fats and Oils Affect Mental, Physical and Emotional Intelligence.* Berkeley, Calif: Frog, Ltd; 1997.

Valsta LM, Salminen I, Aro A, Mutanen M. Alpha-linolenic acid in rapeseed oil partly compensates for the effect of fish restriction on plasma long chain n-3 fatty acids. *Eur J Clin Nutr.* 1996;50:229–235.

∎ GAMMA-LINOLENIC ACID (GLA)

OVERVIEW

Gamma-linolenic acid (GLA) is a polyunsaturated fatty acid (PUFA) in the omega-6 series. It is derived from linoleic acid, and it is the precursor of arachidonic acid and the prostaglandin E_1 series.

Direct supplementation of GLA is ordinarily in the form of evening primrose oil, black currant seed oil, and borage oil. These sources also provide linoleic acid. For example, evening primrose oil is 72% linoleic acid.

People who have diabetes are less able to convert linoleic acid to GLA than healthy individuals. Other conditions that appear to reduce the capacity to convert linoleic acid to GLA include aging, alcoholism, atopic dermatitis, premenstrual syndrome, rheumatoid arthritis, cancer, and cardiovascular disease.

GLA is of benefit to diabetics by improving nerve conduction and preventing diabetic neuropathy. One animal study suggests that the combination of GLA and ascorbate is particularly advantageous.

Upon ingestion, GLA is elongated rapidly to dihomo-gamma-linolenic acid (DGLA). DGLA is efficacious in vasodilation, lowering of blood pressure, and the prevention of atherosclerosis.

GLA has an anti-inflammatory effect in humans. The mechanism is not completely understood, but oral administration of GLA can help suppress T-cell proliferation; GLA and DGLA suppress T-cell activation. In at least one study, rheumatoid arthritis patients taking GLA for a year improved over time, suggesting that GLA can function as a slow-acting, disease-modifying antirheumatic drug. The hope is to establish a therapeutic GLA dose that will reduce the need for other medication in persons with rheumatoid arthritis. This would help reduce the gastrointestinal problems associated with the use of non-steroidal anti-inflammatory drugs (NSAIDs). Research results are, however, somewhat controversial. There is some evidence that the effect of long-term supplementation actually may be contrary to the desired results of reducing inflammation. Nevertheless, GLA supplementation is particularly popular with persons with rheumatoid arthritis.

Corroborated studies suggest that GLA is unique among the omega-6 PUFA series in suppressing tumor growth and metastasis. It inhibits both motility and invasiveness of human colon cancer, breast cancer, and melanoma cells. Whether DGLA and prostaglandin E are involved in the process remains to be determined.

Recent animal research has suggested that GLA, in combination with eicosapentaenoic acid (EPA), can be beneficial in senile osteoporosis because it enhances absorption and retention of calcium. In addition, a pilot study done on elderly women suggested that GLA and eicosapentaenoic acid (EPA) reduce bone turnover rates and have beneficial effects on bone density and calcium absorbtion.

A recent Japanese study showed that evening primrose oil may be beneficial for hemodialysis patients with uremic skin symptoms. Patients given evening primrose oil showed significant improvement in skin dryness, pruritis, and erythema; and an increase in plasma concentration of a wide variety of essential fatty acids, more than patients who were given linoleic acid.

The ratio of omega-6 oils to omega-3 oils should be 4:1. However, the American diet provides more than 10 times the needed amount of omega-6 oils in the form of linoleic acid. This is because they comprise the primary oil ingredient added to most processed foods and are found in commonly used cooking oils. The total intake of linoleic acid is approximately 100 times the GLA intake. Because GLA is not found in abundance in common foods, supplementation may be necessary to mimic clinical dosages.

DIETARY SOURCES

In addition to the plant seed oils of evening primrose, black currant, borage, and fungal oils, GLA is found in human milk and, in small amounts, in a wide variety of common foods, particularly organ meats.

CONSTITUENTS/COMPOSITION

Gamma-linolenic acid is a long-chain polyunsaturated fatty acid with 18 carbon atoms. It is derived from linoleic acid; it is elongated to dihomo-gamma-linolenic acid (DGLA), then desaturated to arachidonic acid, and then is converted to the prostaglandin E_1 series (PGE_1).

GLA is available directly from evening primrose oil (7% to 10% GLA), black current seed oil (15% to 20% GLA), borage oil (18% to 26% GLA), and fungal oil (23% to 26% GLA). GLA bioavailability may be related to the precise triacylglycerol composition. Although the GLA concentration in borage oil appears to be twice as high as in evening primrose oil, research has shown that the GLA effects, such as formation of prostaglandin E_1, are comparable for both on a gram-for-gram basis.

The essential fatty acids are known as vitamin F. The Food and Drug Administration prohibits the term "vitamin F" for advertising purposes, because of problems with foods such as french fries being advertised as "vitamin enriched" because they were fried in oil.

COMMERCIAL PREPARATIONS

- Evening primrose oil
- Black currant seed oil
- Borage oil
- Borage oil capsules

THERAPEUTIC USES

- Rheumatoid arthritis: GLA may reduce inflammation by suppressing T-cell proliferation and activation.
- Diabetes: GLA supplementation assists nerve function and helps prevent nerve disease in diabetics.
- Cancer: GLA may suppress tumor growth and metastasis, particularly in colon cancer, breast cancer, and melanoma.
- Heart disease: GLA may prevent heart disease by inhibiting plaque formation, increasing vasodilation, and lowering blood pressure.
- Eyes: GLA is beneficial in Sjogren's syndrome and may be useful in other dry eye conditions.
- Supplementation may alleviate the symptoms of aging, alcoholism, atopic dermatitis, osteoporosis, and premenstrual syndrome.
- Menstrual problems (amenorrhea, dysmenorrhea): Essential fatty acids such as those found in flaxseed, evening primrose, and borage oils reduce inflammation and support hormone production. Dosage is 1,000 to 1,500 mg daily or bid.

DOSAGE RANGES AND DURATION OF ADMINISTRATION

There is no recommended dietary allowance (RDA) for GLA.

A recommended dosage for rheumatoid arthritis is 1.4 g/day. As the cost of oils can be prohibitive, and lower doses are usually effective, an acceptable clinical dosage of evening primrose, black currant, or borage oil would be 1,500 mg daily or bid.

Studies have shown that up to 2.8 g of GLA/day is well tolerated.

SIDE EFFECTS/TOXICOLOGY

Dietary sources of GLA appear to be completely nontoxic. A healthy person eating a normal diet should consume fewer saturated fats and more polyunsaturated essential fatty acids.

WARNINGS/CONTRAINDICATIONS/PRECAUTIONS

N/A

INTERACTIONS

No significant interactions are noted.

REFERENCES

Bolton-Smith C, Woodward M, Tavendale R. Evidence for age-related differences in the fatty acid composition of human adipose tissue, independent of diet. *Eur J Clin Nutr.* 1997;51:619–624.

Brzeski M, Madhok R, Capell HA. Evening primrose oil in patients with rheumatoid arthritis and side-effects of non-steroidal anti-inflammatory drugs. *Br J Rheumatol.* 1991;30:370–372.

Brown NA, Bron AJ, Harding JJ, Dewar HM. Nutrition supplements and the eye. *Eye.* 1998;12(pt 1):127–133.

Ensminger AH, Ensminger ME, Konlande JE, Robson JRK. *Foods & Nutrition Encyclopedia.* 2nd ed. Baton Rouge, Fla: CRC Press, Inc; 1994:1:684–708.

Fan YY, Chapkin RS. Importance of dietary gamma-linolenic acid in human health and nutrition. *J Nutr.* 1998;128:1411–1414.

Garrison RH Jr, Somer E. *The Nutrition Desk Reference.* 3rd ed. New Canaan, Conn: Keats Publishing, Inc; 1995:23–64.

Haas EM. *Staying Healthy with Nutrition.* Berkley, Calif: Celestial Arts Publishing; 1992:65–79.

Jamal GA, Carmichael H. The effects of gamma-linolenic acid on human diabetic peripheral neuropathy: a double-blind placebo-controlled trial. *Diabet Med.* 1990;7:319–323.

Jiang WG, Hiscox S, Bryce RP, Horrobin DF, Mansel RE. The effects of n-6 polyunsaturated fatty acids on the expression of nm-23 in human cancer cells. *Br J Cancer.* 1998;77:731–738.

Jiang WG, Hiscox S, Bryce RP, Horrobin DF, Mansel RE. Gamma linolenic acid regulates expression of maspin and the motility of cancer cells. *Biochem Biophys Res Commun.* 1997;237:639–644.

Kruger MC, Coetzer H, deWinter R, Gericke G, Papendorp DH. Calcium, gamma-linolenic acid and eicosapentaenoic acid supplementation in senile osteoporosis. *Aging (Milano).* 1998;10:385–394.

Leventhal LJ, Boyce EG, Zurier Rb. Treatment of rheumatoid arthritis with blackcurrant seed oil. *Br J Rheumatol.* 1994;33:847–852.

Murray MT. *Encyclopedia of Nutritional Supplements.* Rocklin, Calif: Prima Publishing; 1996:239–278.

Newstrom H. Nutrients Catalog. Jefferson, NC: McFarland & Co., Inc; 1993:103–105.

Puolakka J, Makarainen L, Viinikka L, Ylikorkala O. Biochemical and clinical effects of treating the premenstrual syndrome with prostaglandin synthesis precursors. *J Reprod Med.* 1985;30:149–153.

Shils ME, Olson JA, Shike M, Ross AC. *Modern Nutrition in Health and Disease.* 9th ed. Baltimore, Md: Williams & Wilkins; 1999:90–92; 1377–1378.

Wagner W, Nootbaar-Wagner U. Prophylactic treatment of migraine with gamma-linolenic and alpha-linolenic acids. *Cephalalgia.* 1997;17:127–130.

Werbach MR. *Nutritional Influences on Illness.* 2nd ed. Tarzana, Calif: Third Line Press; 1993:13–22; 655–671.

Zurier RB, Rossetti RG, Jacobson EW, et al. Gamma-Linolenic acid treatment of rheumatoid arthritis. A randomized, placebo-controlled trial. *Arthritis Rheum.* 1996;39:1808–1817.

■ GLUTAMINE
OVERVIEW

Glutamine is an amino acid, one of the building blocks of protein that are linked together by peptide bonds in specific chemical arrangements to form proteins. It is found in both plant and animal proteins and is available in a variety of supplemental forms. Glutamine helps the body maintain the correct acid-alkaline balance and is a necessary part of the synthesis of RNA and DNA. Glutamine also helps promote a healthy digestive tract.

Unlike other amino acids that have a single nitrogen atom, glutamine contains two nitrogen atoms that enable it to transfer nitrogen and remove ammonia from body tissues. Glutamine readily passes the blood-brain barrier and, within the brain, is converted to glutamic acid, which the brain needs to function properly. It also increases gamma-aminobutyric acid (GABA) in the brain, which is also needed for proper mental activity.

Glutamine is the most plentiful free amino acids in muscles. Its ability to help build and maintain muscle makes glutamine especially attractive to dieters and muscle-builders, but that same ability also helps prevent muscle-wasting associated with prolonged inactivity, disease, and stress. With sufficient glutamine in the bloodstream, muscle loss that would otherwise be caused by injury, surgery, trauma, prolonged illness, or stress can be prevented. The body uses glutamine and glucose to make glucosamine, an amino sugar that plays a key role in the formation of nails, tendons, skin, eyes, bones, ligaments, heart valves, and mucous secretions throughout the body.

Conditions that have been treated with L-glutamine supplements include fibrosis, autoimmune diseases, arthritis, intestinal ailments, peptic ulcers, diseases of the connective tissues, tissue damage caused by radiation treatment, developmental disabilities, epilepsy, schizophrenia, fatigue, and impotence.

Because L-glutamine possibly reduces sugar and alcohol cravings, it could be considered for treating recovering alcoholics. Suggested dose: 1,000 mg tid with 50 mg of vitamin B_6, on an empty stomach.

DIETARY SOURCES

Glutamine is found in animal proteins and vegetable proteins. Natural sources of glutamine include soy proteins, milk, meats, raw spinach, raw parsley, and cabbage.

Nutrition experts recommend choosing supplements whose label describes the contents as USP pharmaceutical grade L-crystalline amino acids.

The purest form of amino acid supplements is called free-form and is available in powder or encapsulated powder. Free-form amino acids are readily absorbed and nonallergenic, and are stable at room temperature but destroyed by high temperatures ($350°$ to $660°$ F) typical of cooking.

CONSTITUENTS/COMPOSITION

Glutamine is available as an isolated amino acid or in combination amino acid and protein supplements.

L-forms of amino acid supplements such as L-glutamine are believed to be more compatible with human biochemistry than D-forms because the chemical structure spirals to the left.

COMMERCIAL PREPARATIONS

Glutamine is available in a variety of foods and food supplements, protein mixtures, amino acid formulas, and individual supplements in liquid, powder, tablets, and capsules. Supplemental forms of glutamine are sold in vitamin and mineral sections of most pharmacies and health food stores.

THERAPEUTIC USES

- Glutamine is not one of the nine essential amino acids (which must be ingested because the body cannot manufacture them). However, extreme stress and prolonged illness may cause glutamine to become an essential amino acid, and hence a valuable dietary component.
- Glutamine aids recovery after surgery, wounds or injury, hemorrhage, prolonged illness including AIDS and cancer, and chemotherapy.
- In one recent study, glutamine reduced mouth pain by 4.5 days compared to placebo users in 24 methotrexate chemotherapy patients suffering from mouth sores and difficulty swallowing.
- Glutamine speeds healing of peptic ulcers.
- Because glutamine is one of the primary fuels used by intestinal lining cells, supplementation with glutamine helps restore gastric mucosa and improves mucosa metabolism. Glutamine also helps repair the gastrointestinal lining after damage caused by radiation or leaky gut syndrome, and benefits chronic GI diseases such as colitis, AIDS, cancer, and Crohn's disease. Large doses (more than 1,000 mg tid) helped protect chemotherapy patients' stomach linings, according to a 1996 study.
- Glutamine helps suppress food cravings.

DOSAGE RANGES AND DURATION OF ADMINISTRATION

- Glutamine supplements, like all amino acid supplements, should be taken on an empty stomach, preferably in the morning or between meals.
- For peptic ulcers, 500 mg daily, taken on an empty stomach, is recommended.
- To curb food cravings, 1,000 mg daily is recommended.
- To treat irritable bowel syndrome (IBS), eliminate foods that trigger symptoms and take glutamine (500 mg tid) and peppermint oil (1 capsule three to six times daily).
- For stasis ulcers (open sores on the leg that are caused by poor blood flow), take each day: glutamine (500 mg) with a basic nutritional supplement program and vitamin C (2,000 mg in divided doses with meals and at bedtime), vitamin A (10,000 IU), zinc (22.5 to 50 mg), and vitamin E (400 IU orally and additional vitamin E oil squeezed from capsules onto the wound to aid healing and prevent recurrence).
- To aid wound healing, take glutamine (500 mg) with a basic vitamin-mineral formula and vitamin C (2,000 mg divided at meals and bedtime), vitamin A (10,000 IU), zinc (22.5 to 50 mg), vitamin E (400 IU), and vitamin B_3 (100 mg) daily.

SIDE EFFECTS/TOXICOLOGY

Glutamine can worsen damage caused by any disease that allows ammonia to accumulate to excess in the blood. It is not recommended in patients who have Reye's syndrome, kidney disease, cirrhosis of the liver, or other illnesses that cause overload of ammonia in the body.

Proteins (taken as a source of amino acid glutamine) should not be overused. In healthy persons, protein is safely metabolized and broken down by the liver into glucose and ammonia, which is a toxin. If one consumes an excessive amount of protein or if digestion is poor or liver function is impaired, ammonia can accumulate in the body and cause damage. Strenuous exercise can also promote excess ammonia in the body. Too much ammonia can cause encephalopathy or hepatic coma, or it can pose serious health threats. As ammonia is broken down by the body into urea, the urea can cause kidney inflammation and back pain.

WARNINGS/CONTRAINDICATIONS/PRECAUTIONS

- Glutamine supplements must be kept completely dry because moisture causes glutamine powder to break down into ammonia and pyroglutamic acid.
- Glutamine in foods is readily destroyed by cooking.
- Despite the similarity of their names, the following substances are different and are not interchangeable: glutamine; glutamic acid, also called glutamate; glutathione; gluten; and monosodium glutamate.

INTERACTIONS

Glutamine is absorbed more readily when taken with vitamin B_6 and vitamin C.

REFERENCES

Balch J, Balch P. *Prescription for Nutritional Healing.* 2nd ed. Garden City Park, NY: Avery Publishing Group; 1997.

Castell LM, Newsholme EA. The effects of oral glutamine supplementation on athletes after prolonged, exhaustive exercise. *Nutrition.* 1997;13:738–742.

Den Hond E. Hiele M, Peeters M, Ghoos Y, Rutgeerts P. Effect of long-term oral glutamine supplements on small intestinal permeability in patients with Crohn's disease. *J Parenter Enteral Nutr.* 1999;23:7–11.

Giller R, Matthews K. *Natural Prescriptions.* New York, NY: Carol Southern Books/Crown Publishers; 1994.

Gottlieb B. *New Choices in Natural Healing.* Emmaus, Pa.: Rodale Press, Inc.; 1995.

Haas R. *Eat Smart, Think Smart.* New York, NY: HarperCollins; 1994.

Kirschmann G, Kirschmann J. *Nutrition Almanac.* 4th ed. New York, NY: McGraw Hill; 1996.

LaValle J. Natural agents for a healthy GI tract. *Drug Store News.* January 12, 1998;20.

Li J, Langkamp-Henken B, Suzuki K, Stahlgren LH. Glutamine prevents paranteral nutrition-induced increases intestinal permeability. *J Parenter Enteral Nutr.* 1994;18:303–307.

Napoli M. Chemo effect alleviated. *Health Facts.* October 1998;23:6.

Noyer CM, Simon D, Borczuk A, Brandt LJ, Lee MJ, Nehra V. A double-blind placebo-controlled pilot study of glutamine therapy for abnormal intestinal permeability in patients with AIDS. *Am J Gastroenterol.* 1998;93:972–975.

Shabert JK, Wilmore DW. Glutamine deficiency as a cause of human immunodeficiency virus wasting. *Med Hypotheses.* March 1996; 46:252–256.

Yoshida S, Matsui M, Shirouzu Y, Fujita H, Yamana H, Shirouzu K. Effects of glutamine supplements and radiochemotherapy on systemic immune and gut barrier function in patients with advanced esophageal cancer. *Ann Surg.* 1998;227:485–491.

■ IRON

OVERVIEW

Iron is an essential mineral that has many physiologic functions. It can be found in two forms in the body: heme and nonheme. Heme iron is part of the hemoglobin and myoglobin molecules. Hemoglobin is the oxygen-carrying pigment of erythrocytes. Myoglobin transports and stores oxygen within muscle and releases it to meet increased metabolic demands during muscle contraction. Several enzymes contain iron both in the heme and nonheme forms. These enzymes are involved in a variety of processes in the body including cellular respiration, detoxification, and protection against free radical damage.

Iron is absorbed from the diet by the mucosal cells of the small intestine. The amount of iron absorbed depends on the body's store of iron: an individual with iron deficiency can absorb 50% of dietary iron while an individual with sufficient iron stores may absorb only 5% to 15%. Heme iron, which comes from hemoglobin and myoglobin in meat products, and nonheme iron, which comes from plant and dairy products, are absorbed by two different mechanisms. While heme iron usually accounts for only 15% of iron in the diet, it is absorbed two to three times more readily than nonheme iron. Nonheme iron accounts for approximately 85% of iron in the diet but its absorption from the small intestine is dependent on "solubility enhancers and inhibitors" that are consumed during the same meal. Ascorbic acid and factors present in meat enhance absorption by keeping it soluble and stimulating the secretion of gastric juices, respectively. Dietary inhibitors of nonheme iron absorption include calcium phosphate, tannins, phytic acids (present in unprocessed whole-grain products), and polyphenols (present in tea and some vegetables).

Transferrin, the iron-specific plasma transport protein, transports iron to tissues. The transferrin receptor regulates the entry of iron into tissues: when tissues are in an iron-rich environment, the cell surface transferrin receptor is downregulated; when tissues are in an iron-poor environment, the transferrin receptor is upregulated.

The storage forms of iron are called ferritin and hemosiderin. They are present in the liver, bone marrow, spleen, and muscle. Ferritin and hemosiderin are mobilized for hemoglobin production and other cellular iron needs.

Iron deficiency manifests itself as hypochromic microcytic anemia and is most common in infants and children (6 months to 4 years), adolescents especially girls, and pregnant women. It is characterized by reduced work capacity in adults and a reduced ability to learn in children. The inability to maintain body temperature in a cold environment and decreased resistance to infection may also result from iron deficiency. Cardiovascular and respiratory changes that can lead to cardiac failure is the end result of progressive, untreated anemia.

Hemochromatosis—the excess storage of iron in the body—can lead to organ damage. It is most prevalent in individuals who have a genetic defect that causes the body to absorb more iron than normal, and may be the most common autosomal recessive disease in humans. Other causes of iron overload are excessive oral intake and repeated transfusions. Individuals with hemochromatosis are at a higher risk for hepatic carcinoma.

At least two of the following tests should be performed to diagnose iron deficiency (the most common cause of anemia) or overload.
- Plasma ferritin—measures iron stores
- Transferrin saturation—measures iron supplies to the tissues
- Erythrocyte protoporphyrin—measures the ratio of zinc protoporphyrin to heme. (Zinc is incorporated into protoporphyrin when iron stores are too low.)
- Hemoglobin or hematocrit measurement—8 to 11 g/dL of hemoglobin is considered anemic

DIETARY SOURCES

The best source of iron in the diet is heme iron, which comes from the hemoglobin and myoglobin of animal protein. Heme iron is more readily absorbed and less affected by other dietary constituents than nonheme iron. Some good sources of heme iron are:
- Liver
- Lean red meat
- Poultry
- Fish
- Oysters
- Shellfish
- Kidney
- Heart

Nonheme iron absorption is affected by a number of factors. The best enhancer of nonheme iron absorption is vitamin C. Nonheme protein absorption is also enhanced by factors in meat. Inhibitors of nonheme protein absorption include calcium phosphate, bran, phytic acid, polyphenols, and tannins. The following are good nonheme sources of iron.
- Dried beans
- Fruits
- Vegetables

Foods with added iron include the following.
- Egg yolks
- Dried fruits
- Dark molasses
- Whole-grain and enriched bread
- Wines
- Cereals

CONSTITUENTS/COMPOSITION

Iron occurs in foodstuffs as heme and nonheme iron. Heme iron, contained in food products from animals, is in the form of hemoglobin or myoglobin. Nonheme iron is iron salts and is contained in plant and dairy products. Nonheme iron makes up the majority of dietary iron, but heme iron is better absorbed.

COMMERCIAL PREPARATIONS

Ferrous sulfate is used to fortify infant formula and canned foods, while foods stored in air-permeable packages are fortified with elemental iron powders (North America) or ferric pyrophosphate and ferric orthophosphate (Europe). Ferrous sulfate (FEOSOL and others) is the most widely used oral supplement, but other ferrous salts such as fumarate, succinate, and gluconate are absorbed equally as well. Iron dextran injection (INFED) is the parenteral preparation currently used in the United States.

THERAPEUTIC USES

To replete iron stores in iron-deficient anemia. Underlying causes of iron-deficient anemia include the following:
- Chronic blood loss (hemorrhoids, parasites, bleeding peptic ulcer, malignancy)
- Inadequate iron intake or inefficient absorption (iron-poor diet, chronic gastrointestinal disturbances)
- Increased iron requirement due to expanded blood volume (infancy, adolescence, pregnancy)

DOSAGE RANGES AND DURATION OF ADMINISTRATION

Recommended Daily Allowances of iron are as follows.

- Neonates to 6 months: 6 mg
- Infants 6 mos. to 1 year: 10 mg
- Children 1 to 10 year: 10 mg
- Men 11 to 18 year: 12 mg
- Men 19+ years: 10 mg
- Women 11 to 50 years: 15 mg
- Women 51+ years: 10 mg
- Pregnant women: 30 mg
- Lactating women: 15 mg

SIDE EFFECTS/TOXICOLOGY

Oral iron therapy:

- Gastrointestinal disturbances (nausea, diarrhea, constipation, heartburn, upper gastric discomfort)
- Hemochromatosis from long-term excessive intake
- Iron toxicity- causes severe organ damage and death. The most pronounced effects are hemorrhagic necrosis of the gastrointestinal tract, which manifests as vomiting and bloody diarrhea. (Lethal dose: 200 to 250 mg/kg; therapeutic dose: 2 to 5 mg/kg/day)

Parenteral iron therapy:

- Headache, malaise, fever, generalized lymphadenopathy, arthralgias, urticaria, exacerbation of rheumatoid arthritis, phlebitis, and in rare instances anaphylactic reactions.

WARNINGS/CONTRAINDICATIONS/PRECAUTIONS

- Iron supplements should be kept in childproof bottles and out of the reach of children. Children between the ages of 12 and 24 months are at the highest risk of iron poisoning due to accidental ingestion.
- Parenteral iron therapy should be used only when there are specific indications due to rare anaphylactic reactions, which can be fatal despite treatment.

INTERACTIONS

- Vitamin C enhances absorption of iron from the diet.
- The antacid magnesium trisilicate, H_2 blockers, and protonpump inhibitors reduce absorption of oral iron.
- Disodium etidronate, levodopa, penicillamine, ciprofloxacin, norfloxacin, ofloxacin, and tetracycline absorption is reduced by iron.

REFERENCES

Belton N. Iron deficiency in infants and young children. *Professional Care of Mother and Child.* 1995;5:69–71.

Cook JD, Skikne BS. Intestinal regulation of body iron. *Blood Rev.* 1987;1:267–272.

Ekhard ZE, Filer LJ, eds. *Present Knowledge in Nutrition.* 7th ed. Washington, DC: ILSI Press; 1996:191–201.

Fleming DJ, Jacques PF, Dallal GE, et al. Dietary determinants of iron stores in a free-living elderly population: the Framingham Heart Study. *Am J Clin Nutr.* 1998;67:722–733.

Hardman JG, Limbird LE, eds. *Goodman and Gillman's The Pharmacological Basis of Therapeutics.* 9th ed. New York: McGraw-Hill; 1996:1326–1333.

Mahan LK, Arlin MT, eds. *Krause's Food, Nutrition, and Diet Therapy.* 8th ed. Philadelphia, Pa: WB Saunders Co.; 1992:96–97.

National Research Council. *Recommended Dietary Allowances.* 10th ed. Washington, DC: National Academy Press; 1989:158–165.

Mason P. *Nutrition and Dietary Advice in the Pharmacy.* Oxford, UK: Blackwell Scientific; 1994:234–235.

Recommendations to Prevent and Control Iron Deficiency in the United States. Atlanta, Ga: Centers for Disease Control and Prevention. Morbidity and Mortality Weekly Report; April 3, 1998;47(RR-3):1–29.

The Food and Nutrition Information Center. National Agricultural Library (NAL), United States Department of Agriculture's (USDA) Agricultural Research Service (ARS). Accessed at *www.nal.usda.gov/fnic/Dietary/rda.html* on January 8, 1999.

Tzonou A, Lagiou P, Trichopoulou A, et al. Dietary iron and coronary heart disease: a study from Greece. *Am J Epidemiol.* 1998;147:161–166.

■ LIPASE
OVERVIEW

Lipases are one of three categories of enzymes manufactured by the pancreas. The pancreas also secretes the hormones insulin and glucagon, which are needed to metabolize sugar, into the bloodstream. The other two enzymes include amylases, which break starch molecules into more simple sugars, and proteases, which break protein molecules into single amino acids. The most common dietary fats, triglycerides, comprise 95% of all ingested fats and are comprised of a glycerol molecule combined with three fatty acid molecules. The lipases aid the digestion of fats by hydrolyzing the glycerol linkage within the chain to create more assimilable free fatty acids and monoglycerides. These components are then transported in the body by lipoproteins. Pancreatic lipase and bile salts are required for intestinal digestion and absorption.

DIETARY SOURCES

This enzyme is manufactured by the pancreas. It does not come from diet, but may be supplemented by animal enzymes.

CONSTITUENTS/COMPOSITION

Gastric and pharyngeal (salivary) lipases are different from pancreatic lipase. They have lower molecular weights, a lower pH optimum (4 to 6 vs. 6 to 8), and a greater stability at pH 3. Gastric lipase is produced in the stomach and cleaves triglycerides at Sn-3 position within the stomach and duodenum. Pharyngeal lipase is produced in the oral cavity, also cleaving triglycerides at Sn-3 position within the mouth, esophagus, and stomach. Pancreatic lipase is produced in the pancreas, splitting Sn-1 and Sn-3 positions within the duodenum.

These lipases are important in the hydrolysis of triglycerides in milk during infancy, when the secretion of pancreatic lipase is not fully developed. In adults, as much as 10% to 15% of ingested fat may be partially hydrolyzed in the stomach.

Hepatic lipase has also been shown to impact aspects of blood lipid metabolism. It facilitates the clearance of potentially artherogenic lipoproteins by the liver and impacts the levels of the protective high-density lipoproteins.

COMMERCIAL PREPARATIONS

Lipase tablets are available in units of 6,000 Lus, and 1 to 2 capsules are recommended daily, to be taken before meals.

THERAPEUTIC USES

Tablets or capsules of pancreatic enzyme extracts with meals can be used to treat impaired digestion, malabsorption, and subsequent nutrient deficiencies. Some consider pancreatic enzymes of value in treating autoimmune disorders, inflammatory diseases, and food allergies. They have been most studied in treating early diagnosed celiac disease by enhancing the benefit of a gluten-free diet.

A reduction in lipase activity is unlikely to induce malabsorption in an adult, because pancreatic lipase is usually secreted in abundant amounts. Deficiency of pancreatic lipase of clinical significance only when its secretion is below 10% to 15% of normal levels.

DOSAGE RANGES AND DURATION OF ADMINISTRATION

Recommended treatment with lipase to aid fat digestion is 1 to 2 capsules of 6,000 LUs tid before meals. Lipase can also be found combined with protease and amylase.

SIDE EFFECTS/TOXICOLOGY

None reported

WARNINGS/CONTRAINDICATIONS/PRECAUTIONS

Lipase and other pancreatic enzyme supplements are not associated with side effects.

INTERACTIONS

None reported

REFERENCES

Berkow R, ed. *The Merck Manual of Medical Information.* Home Ed. Whitehouse Station, NJ: Merck Research Laboratories; 1997.

Mahan KL, Marian A. *Krause's Food Nutrition and Diet Therapy.* 8th ed. Philadelphia, Pa: WB Saunders Co; 1993.

Murray MT. *Encyclopedia of Nutritional Supplements.* Rocklin, Calif: Prima Publishing; 1986.

Shils ME, Olson JA, Shike M, eds. *Modern Nutrition in Health and Disease.* 8th ed. Philadelphia, Pa.: Lea and Febiger; 1994

■ LYSINE

OVERVIEW

Lysine is an essential amino acid that is not synthesized in adequate amounts by the body, so it must be obtained from dietary sources. Lysine furnishes the structural components for the synthesis of carnitine, which promotes fatty acid synthesis within the cell. It is particularly important for proper growth. Lysine also regulates calcium absorption and plays an important role in the formation of collagen.

A vegetarian diet may not provide sufficient lysine. Among protein sources, plants often contain insufficient sources of lysine. Lysine is the limiting amino acid of many cereals. In many areas of the world where diets are grain-based, this becomes important as a lysine deficiency can create a negative nitrogen balance and lead to kidney stones. Lysine deficiency may be characterized by fatigue, nausea, dizziness, appetite loss, emotional agitation, decreased antibody formation, decreased immunity, slow growth, anemia, reproductive disorders, pneumonia, acidosis, and bloodshot eyes.

Lysine has been used to treat herpes infections caused by both herpes simplex viruses and herpes zoster. Supplementation can improve recovery speed and suppress recurrences of infections. Some studies have found lysine of potential benefit in treating cardiovascular disease, osteoporosis, asthma, migraines, nasal polyps, and postepisiotomy pain.

DIETARY SOURCES

Generally, lysine is found in the following foods:
- Meat, particularly red meats
- Cheeses
- Poultry
- Sardines
- Nuts
- Eggs
- Soybeans

The most concentrated sources are torula yeast, dried and salted cod, soybean protein isolate, soybean protein concentrate, Parmesan cheese, pork loin (excluding fat), dried and frozen tofu, freeze-dried parsley, defatted and low-fat soybean flour, fenugreek seed, and dried spirulina seaweed.

CONSTITUENTS/COMPOSITION

Lysine is an essential amino acid. Chemically, lysine is unique among the amino acids in that it possesses two amino (NH_2) groups. The extra amino group can react with other substances, such as glucose or lactose, creating an amino-sugar complex that cannot be split by digestive enzymes, thus reducing the availability of lysine.

Lysine is also known as LYS, amino acid K, and 2-diamino-hexanoic acid. Its chemical composition is $C_6H_{13}NO_2$.

COMMERCIAL PREPARATIONS

- L-lysine acetylsalicylate (LAS)
- Lysine clonixinate (LC)
- L-lysine monohydrochlorine (LMH)

THERAPEUTIC USES

- Asthma: LAS, when administered by inhalation, has been shown to protect against histamine-induced bronchoconstriction.
- Herpes: Supplementation may improve recovery speed and suppress recurrences of infections.
- Migraine: Treatment with a combination of LAS and metoclopramide may be effective.
- Nasal polyps: Recent research suggests that LAS may prevent relapses of nasal polyps.
- Postepisiotomy pain: 125 mg/day of LC was found to reduce postepisiotomy pain in primiparous patients with moderate to severe postepisiotomy pain.

DOSAGE RANGES AND DURATION OF ADMINISTRATION

The following are the recommended dietary allowances, according to the National Research Council.
- Birth to 4 months: 103 mg/kg/day
- 5 months to 2 years: 69 mg/kg/day
- 3 to 12 years: 44 mg/kg/day
- Adults and teenagers: 12 mg/kg/day

Based on obligatory amino acid losses (including data from amino acid tracer studies), it has been suggested that adults need 30 mg/kg/day.

Nutritional doses are 1 to 3 g per day.

SIDE EFFECTS/TOXICOLOGY

Lysine appears to be nontoxic.

WARNINGS/CONTRAINDICATIONS/PRECAUTIONS

L-lysine may increase cholesterol and triglyceride levels.

INTERACTIONS

Vitamin C aids lysine in collagen formation.

REFERENCES

Bruzzese N, Sica G, Iacopino F, et al. Growth inhibition of fibroblasts from nasal polyps and normal skin by lysine acetylsalicylate. *Allergy.* 1998;53:431–434.

De los Santos AR, Marti MI, Espinosa D, Di Girolamo G, Vinacur JC, Casadei A. Lysine clonixinate vs. paracetamol/codeine in postepisiotomy pain. *Acta Physiol Pharmacol. Ther Latinoam.* 1998;48:52–58.

Ensminger AH, Ensminger ME, Konlande JE, Robson JRK. *Foods & Nutrition Encyclopedia.* 2nd ed. Baton Rouge, Fla: CRC Press, Inc; 1994:1,2:60–64, 1,748.

Flodin NW. The metabolic roles, pharmacology, and toxicology of lysine. *J Am Coll Nutr.* 1997;16:7–21.

Garrison Jr RH, Somer E. *The Nutrition Desk Reference.* 3rd ed. New Canaan, Conn: Keats Publishing, Inc; 1995:39–52.

Haas EM. *Staying Healthy With Nutrition.* Berkeley, Calif: Celestial Arts Publishing; 1992.

Hugues FC, Lacoste JP, Danchot J, Joire JE. Repeated doses of combined oral lysine acetylsalicylate and metoclopramide in the acute treatment of migraine. *Headache.* 1997;37:452–454.

Newstrom H. *Nutrients Catalog.* Jefferson, NC: McFarland & Co; 1993:303–312.

Shils ME, Olson JA, Shike M, Ross AC. *Modern Nutrition in Health and Disease.* 9th ed. Baltimore, Md: Williams & Wilkins; 1999:41, 1,010.

Werbach MR. *Nutritional Influences on Illness.* 2nd ed. Tarzana, Calif: Third Line Press; 1993:159–160, 384, 434, 494–495, 506, 580, 613–614, 636.

■ MAGNESIUM
OVERVIEW

Magnesium is essential to many metabolic reactions, including lipid metabolism, amino acid activation, the glycolytic cycle, and the citric acid cycle. Its primary function is as an enzyme cofactor, thus producing energy, synthesizing lipids and proteins, regulating calcium flow and parathyroid hormone (PTH) secretion, forming urea, and relaxing muscles. Vitamin B_6 works with magnesium in many enzyme systems and assists in the body's accumulation of magnesium.

Dietary intake is generally thought to be insufficient, although clinical depletion is rare in Americans. One problem in determining actual dietary intake is that a number of foods have not been thoroughly analyzed, and laboratory analysis of magnesium contents often do not agree with food composition tables. However, inadequate dietary intake is not usually the sole cause of deficiency. Proper balance also depends on efficient intestinal and renal absorption and excretion. Risk factors for depletion include gastrointestinal disorders, such as inflammatory bowel disease, pancreatitis, fatty acid malabsorption, ileal dysfunction, and gastrointestinal infections (viral, bacterial, or protozoan) that result in malabsorption or vomiting and diarrhea; renal dysfunction with excessive urine loss; nephrotoxic and diuretic drugs; and endocrine disorders, such as hyperthyroidism, diabetes mellitus, and hyperparathyroidism with hypercalcemia.

Magnesium deficiency most severely affects cardiovascular, neuromuscular, and renal tissues, and has been linked to agitation, anemia (hemolytic), anorexia, anxiety, ataxia, cardiac arrhythmias, confusion, Crohn's disease, depression, disorientation, fasciculations, hallucinations, heart disease, heart attacks resulting from coronary artery spasm, heart failure from defibrillation, hyperactivity, hypertension, insomnia, irritability, kidney stones, muscle pains, muscular weakness, nausea and vomiting, nervousness, nystagmus, neuromuscular irritability, organic brain syndrome, paresthesias, pronounced startle response, restlessness, seizures, sonophobia, tachycardia, increased triglyceride levels, and vertigo.

Increased levels of magnesium sulfate from treatment of preeclampsia or other problems of pregnancy have been associated with significantly reduced risks of cerebral palsy and possibly mental retardation in very low-birth-weight infants; however, a preliminary report of a recent study is contradictory. Use of magnesium to prevent premature labor at less than 34 weeks gestation in women who are not pre-eclamptic is disputed. In a recent study, use of $MgSO_4$ (magnesium sulfate) as a randomized treatment for such women was associated with higher infant mortality, and the study was stopped.

DIETARY SOURCES

- Rich sources: tofu, legumes, whole grains, green leafy vegetables, wheat bran, Brazil nuts, soybean flour, almonds, cashews, blackstrap molasses, pumpkin and squash seeds, pine nuts, black walnuts
- Good sources: peanuts, whole wheat flour, oat flour, beet greens, spinach, pistachio nuts, shredded wheat, bran cereals, oatmeal, bananas, baked potatoes (with skin)
- Many herbs, spices, and seaweeds supply magnesium (e.g., agar seaweed, coriander, dill weed, celery seed, sage, dried mustard, basil, cocoa powder, fennel seed, savory, cumin seed, tarragon, marjoram, poppy seed)

CONSTITUENTS/COMPOSITION

The magnesium ion (Mg^{2+}) forms complexes with many types of organic molecules. It binds with phosphates, and weakly with carboxylates and hydroxyls. Magnesium stabilizes many ribonucleotides and deoxyribonucleotides, inducing important physicochemical changes.

COMMERCIAL PREPARATIONS

Supplementary magnesium is available in several varieties of salts.
- Magnesium citrate, magnesium gluconate, and magnesium lactate are more soluble and bioavailable than magnesium oxide.
- Magnesium chloride is more soluble than magnesium oxide, gluconate, citrate, hydroxide, and sulfate, and does not require stomach acid for solubility, but its use is limited due to its hygroscopic properties.
- Magnesium hydroxide (milk of magnesia)
- Magnesium sulfate (Epsom salts)

THERAPEUTIC USES

- Cardiovascular: to prevent atherosclerosis and myocardial infarction, reduce high blood pressure, treat angina, prevent strokes, improve cholesterol and triglyceride levels
- Cardiac arrhythmia: to inhibit triggered beats arising from early afterdepolarizations, treat congenital long QT syndrome (torsade de pointes)
- Lung function: to halt acute asthma attacks and acute exacerbations of chronic obstructive pulmonary disease, reduce recurrence of apnea in infants
- Diabetes: to improve insulin action and glucose metabolism, decrease insulin need, ease diabetic blood pressure
- Hearing: to prevent noise-induced hearing loss
- Glaucoma: to improve peripheral circulation and visual field
- Fatigue: to improve sleep, restore normal energy level
- Mental health: to reduce nervousness, anxiety, and depression
- Migraines: to treat food-allergy-induced migraine headaches using ionized magnesium
- Pregnancy: to lower blood pressure, prevent preeclampsia and eclampsia
- Renal: to prevent kidney stones
- Menstruation and premenstrual syndrome (PMS): to relieve menstrual cramps, irritability, fatigue, depression, and water retention

DOSAGE RANGES AND DURATION OF ADMINISTRATION

Recommendations for adequate magnesium intake promulgated by the Food and Nutrition Board of the Institute of Medicine in 1997:
Infants:
- Birth to 6 months: 30 mg/day
- 6 months to 1 year: 75 mg/day
Children:
- 1 to 3 years: 80 mg/day
- 4 to 8 years: 130 mg/day
- 9 to 13 years: 240 mg/day
Adolescents:
- 14 to 18 years (men): 410 mg/day
- 14 to 18 years (women): 360 mg/day
Adults:
- 19 to 30 years (men): 400 mg/day
- 19 to 30 years (women): 310 mg/day
- 31+ years (men): 420 mg/day
- 31+ years (women): 320 mg/day
Pregnant women:
- Up to 18 years: 400 mg/day
- 19 to 30 years: 350 mg/day
- 31 to 50 years: 360 mg/day

Lactating women:
- Up to 18 years: 360 mg/day
- 19 to 30 years: 310 mg/day
- 31 to 50 years: 320 mg/day

These represent significant increases for adolescents and adults from the Recommended Dietary Allowance promulgated by the National Academy of Sciences in 1989. Supplementation should be in small doses three to six times throughout the day with a full glass of water to reduce chance of diarrhea.

SIDE EFFECTS/TOXICOLOGY

Nutritional toxicity is rare. Symptomatic magnesium excess may occur in patients with gastrointestinal disorders and renal insufficiency when magnesium-based laxatives or antacids are taken. With increasing hypermagnesemia, the effects are lowered blood pressure, nausea, vomiting, brachycardia and urinary retention (serum levels as low as 3 mEq/L), mental status changes, electrocardiogram changes (longer P-R and Q-T intervals), central nervous system depression, severe respiratory depression, coma, and cardiac arrest (at or near 15 mEq/L).

WARNINGS/CONTRAINDICATIONS/PRECAUTIONS

Individuals with severe heart disease (such as high-grade atrioventricular block) should take magnesium only on the advice of their physician. Individuals with kidney disease should not take more than 3,000 mg per day. Overuse of magnesium hydroxide (milk of magnesia) as a laxative or antacid, or magnesium sulfate (Epsom salts) as a laxative and tonic, may cause deficiencies of other minerals or lead to toxicity.

INERACTIONS

Increased magnesium loss can be caused by:
- Sodium
- Sugar
- Caffeine
- Alcohol
- Fiber
- Folic acid
- Riboflavin in high dosages
- Insulin
- Diuretics
- Digitalis

Magnesium absorption or transport inhibitors include:
- Calcium
- Iron
- Manganese
- Phosphorus
- Zinc
- Fat

REFERENCES

Britton J, Pavord I, Richards K, Wisniewski A, Knox A, Lewis S. Dietary magnesium, lung function, wheezing, and airway hyperactivity in a random adult population sample. *Lancet.* 1994; 344:357–362.

Ensminger AH, Ensminger ME, Konlande JE, Robson JRK. *Foods and Nutrition Encyclopedia.* 2nd ed. Baton Rouge, Fla: CRC Press Inc; 1994;2:1338–1341.

Garrison Jr RH, Somer E. *The Nutrition Desk Reference.* 3rd ed. New Canaan, Conn: Keats Publishing Inc; 1995:158–165.

Hardman JG, Gilman AG, Limbird LE, eds. *Goodman and Gilman's Pharmacological Basis of Therapeutics.* 9th ed. New York, NY: McGraw-Hill; 1996:839–874.

Heinerman J. *Heinerman's Encyclopedia of Nature's Vitamins and Minerals.* Paramus, NJ: Prentice Hall Inc; 1998:296–302.

Murray MT. *Encyclopedia of Nutritional Supplements.* Rocklin, Calif: Prima Publishing; 1996:159–175.

Posaci C, Erten O, Uren A, Acar B. Plasma copper, zinc and magnesium levels in patients with premenstrual tensions syndrome. *Obstetricia et Gynecologica Scandinavica.* 1994; 73:452–455.

Romano TJ. Magnesium deficiency in systemic lupus erythematosus. *J Nutr Environ Med.* 1997;7:107–111.

Romano TJ, Stiller JW. Magnesium deficiency in fibromyalgia syndrome. *J Nutr Med.* 1994;4:165–167.

Sacks FM, Willett WC, Smith A, Brown LB, Rosner B, Moore TJ. Effect on blood pressure of potassium, calcium, and magnesium in women with low habitual intake. *Hypertension.* 1998;31:131–138.

Shils ME, Olson JA, Shike M, Ross AC. *Modern Nutrition in Health and Disease.* 9th ed. Baltimore, Md: Williams & Wilkins; 1999:169–192, A127–A128.

Werbach MR. *Nutritional Influences on Illness.* 2nd ed. Tarzana, Calif: Third Line Press; 1993:655–680.

■ MANGANESE
OVERVIEW

Manganese is a trace element. It occurs widely in plant and animal tissues and is an essential element for many animal species. Manganese absorption occurs throughout the small intestine. The exact mechanism of absorption is unknown, although it is thought to occur by a two-step mechanism that involves an initial uptake from the lumen followed by active transport across the mucosal cells. A specific manganese-carrying plasma protein called transmanganin has been identified. Almost all absorbed manganese is excreted with the feces; only trace amounts are found in the urine. Absorption efficiency is estimated to be roughly 5% and may decline as dietary intake increases. The retention of manganese is estimated to be 10%, 14 days after feeding. The human body contains a mere 20 milligrams of manganese, mostly in cell mitochondria. Organs rich in mitochondria, such as liver, kidney, and pancreas have relatively high manganese concentrations. Bone has the highest concentration of manganese.

Manganese serves two primary biochemical functions in the body, (1) it activates specific enzymes, and (2) it is a constituent of several metalloenzymes. The enzymes manganese activates include hydrolases, decarboxylases, kinases, and transferases. Certain other ions (cobalt, magnesium) can replace its function in this capacity. The manganese metalloenzymes include arginase, pyruvate carboxylase, glutamine synthetase, and manganese superoxide dismutase.

Manganese participates in numerous biochemical functions in the body including steroid and sulfomucopolysacchride biosynthesis, carbohydrate and lipid metabolism, and bone, blood clot, and protein formation. It is also essential for normal brain function, possibly through its role in biogenic amine metabolism. Many of the precise biochemical roles of manganese have not been determined.

Manganese deficiency has been induced in several animal species, but not in humans. Deficiency symptoms in animals include skeletal abnormalities, impaired growth, disturbed or depressed reproductive function, ataxia of the newborn, and defects in lipid and carbohydrate metabolism. Although frank deficiency symptoms have not been observed in humans, biochemical evidence has established its essentiality in humans. Impaired fertility, growth retardation, birth defects, bone malformations, seizures, and general weakness may result from manganese deficiencies.

DIETARY SOURCES

- Nuts (especially pecans, almonds)
- Wheat germ and whole grains
- Unrefined cereals
- Leafy vegetables
- Liver
- Kidney
- Legumes
- Dried fruits

Refined grains, meats, and dairy products contain only small amounts of manganese. Highly refined diets contain significantly less manganese (0.36 to 1.78 mg) than diets high in unrefined foods (8.3 mg).

CONSTITUENTS/COMPOSITION

Mn^{2+} is the characteristic oxidative state of manganese in solution, in metal enzyme complexes, and in metalloenzymes. Mn^{3+} is the oxidative state in the enzyme manganese superoxide dismutase (MnSOD), and the form that binds to transferrin and interacts with Fe^{3+}.

COMMERCIAL PREPARATIONS

Manganese is available commercially in a wide variety of forms including manganese salts (sulfate and chloride) and manganese chelates (gluconate, picolinate, aspartate, fumarate, malate, succinate, citrate, and amino acid chelate). Preparation doses are typically between 2 and 20 mg.

THERAPEUTIC USES

- Diabetes: Type I and II diabetics have significantly less manganese than healthy individuals. Diabetics with liver disorders and those not on insulin therapy may excrete more manganese. Manganese appears to have a hypoglycemic effect and may decrease blood glucose levels in insulin-resistant diabetics.
- Rheumatoid Arthritis: RA, as well as other inflammation brought on by strains and sprains may respond well to manganese treatment. Levels of MnSOD may be significantly decreased in individuals with rheumatoid arthritis. Manganese supplementation increases MnSOD activity.
- Epilepsy: An important study in the early 1960s demonstrated that manganese-deficient rats were more susceptible to seizures, and had EEG tracings consistent with seizure activity. People who have schizophrenia may also respond well to magnesium supplementation.
- Osteoporosis: Manganese, and other trace elements, increase spinal bone mineral density in postmenopausal women.
- Immunocompetence and cancer: Adequate manganese is necessary for normal antibody production. Excessive or inadequate manganese intakes may affect neutrophil and macrophage function.
- Cadmium toxicity: Manganese reduces toxic effects of cadmium in rats.
- Other conditions: Manganese is also used to treat atherosclerosis, hypercholesterolemia, tinnitus, and hearing loss.
- Total parenteral nutrition (TPN): Bone changes may occur in patients given TPN solutions containing inadequate quantities of manganese. In contrast, cholestatic and nervous system disorders have been associated with high blood concentrations of manganese from long-term TPN treatment. Children's TPN solutions should contain low-dose manganese (0.018 mumol/kg per 24 hours).

DOSAGE RANGES AND DURATION OF ADMINISTRATION

The exact amount of manganese required by the human body is not known. The Food and Nutrition Board (FNB) of the National Research Council (NRC) has established estimated safe and adequate daily intakes for manganese as follows:

- Infants 0 to 0.5 years: 0.3 to 0.6 mg
- Infants 0.5 to 1 year: 0.6 to 1.0 mg
- Children and adolescents 1 to 3 years: 1.0 to 1.5 mg
- Children and adolescents 4 to 6 years: 1.5 to 2.0 mg
- Children and adolescents 7 to 10 years: 2.0 to 3.0 mg
- Children and adolescents 11+ years: 2.0 to 5.0 mg
- Adults: 2.0 to 5.0 mg.

These estimates are based on the assumption that most dietary intakes fall in this range and do not result in deficiency or toxicity signs. The estimates may be modified as additional information becomes available. More manganese (10 mg/day) should be consumed if the diet contains high amounts of substances that inhibit manganese absorption. In therapeutic use for epilepsy, inflammation, or diarrhea, the dose may be increased three-to-sixfold.

SIDE EFFECTS/TOXICOLOGY

Manganese is one of the least toxic of the trace elements, though excessive intake may produce toxic effects. There are only a few reports of oral manganese poisoning in man. Manganese toxicity is more common in humans chronically exposed to manganese dust found in steel mills and mines and certain chemical industries. Toxicity principally affects the brain, causing severe psychiatric abnormalities, but may also increase blood pressure in the doses used to treat schizophrenia.

WARNINGS/CONTRAINDICATIONS/PRECAUTIONS

The FNB of the NRC recommends that the upper limits for the trace elements should not be habitually exceeded because the toxicity levels may be only several times usual intakes.

INTERACTIONS

Calcium, copper, iron, magnesium, and zinc compete for absorption in the small intestines. Excess intake of one can reduce absorption of the others. Excess manganese may produce iron-deficiency anemia.

REFERENCES

Davis CD, Greger JL. Longitudinal changes of manganese-dependent superoxide dismutase and other indexes of manganese and iron status in women. *Am J Clin Nutr.* 1992;55:747–752.

el-Yazigi A, Hannan N, Raines DA. Urinary excretion of chromium, copper, and manganese in diabetes mellitus and associated disorders. *Diabetes Res.* 1991;18:129–134.

Fell JM, Reynolds AP, Meadows N, et al. Manganese toxicity in children receiving long-term parenteral nutrition. *Lancet.* 1996;347:1218–1221.

Friedman E, ed. *Biochemistry of the Essential Ultratrace Elements.* New York, NY: Plenum Press; 1984.

Goering PL, Haassen CD. Mechanism of manganese-induced tolerance to cadmium lethality and hepatotoxicity. *Biochem. Pharmacol.* 1985;34:1371-1379.

Itokawa Y. Trace elements in long-term total parenteral nutrition [in Japanese]. *Nippon Rinsho.* 1996;54:172–178.

Johnson MA, Smith MM, Edmonds JT. Copper, iron, zinc, and manganese in dietary supplements, infant formulas, and ready-to-eat breakfast cereals. *Am J Clin Nutr.* 1998;67(suppl):1035S–1040S.

Krause, MV., & Mahan, L.K. *Food, Nutrition, and Diet Therapy.* 7th ed. Philadelphia, Pa: WB Saunders Co., 1984.

Orten JM., Neuhaus OW, eds. *Human Biochemistry.* 10th ed. St. Louis, MO: The C.V. Mosby Co; 1982.

Pasquier C, Mach PS, Raichvarg D, Sarfati G, Amor B, Delbarre F. Manganese-containing superoxide-dismutase deficiency in polymorphonuclear leukocytes of adults with rheumatoid arthritis. *Inflammation.* 1984;8:27–32.

Saltman PD, Strause LG. The role of trace minerals in osteoporosis. *J Am Coll Nutr.* 1993;12:384–389.

Shils ME, Olsen JA, Shike M, eds. *Modern Nutrition in Health and Disease.* 8th ed. Media, Pa: Williams and Wilkins Co; 1994:1.

Shvets NV, Kramarenko LD, Vydyborets SV, Gaidukova SN. Disordered trace element content of the erythrocytes in diabetes mellitus [in Russian]. *Lik Sprava.* 1994;1:52–55.

Somer E. *The Essential Guide to Vitamins & Minerals.* New York, NY: HarperCollins Publishers; 1992.

Whitney EN, Hamilton EN. *Understanding Nutrition.* 3rd ed. St. Paul, Minn: West Publishing Co; 1984.

■ MELATONIN

OVERVIEW

Melatonin is an important hormone that is secreted by the pineal gland in the brain. Since its identification in 1958, studies have shown that melatonin plays a crucial role in ordering the complex hormone secretion patterns that regulate the body's circadian rhythm. Melatonin also helps control sleeping and waking periods, because its release is stimulated by darkness and suppressed by light. It also controls the timing and release of female reproductive hormones, affecting menstrual cycles, menarche, and menopause.

Overall levels of melatonin in the body also contribute to the process of aging. The standard rhythmic pattern of melatonin levels are absent until about 3 months of age. After that, the nocturnal levels of melatonin are at their highest for the first few years and then begin to decline as puberty begins. After puberty, nocturnal melatonin levels are relatively stable throughout adulthood and then fall as people age. In old age, the nocturnal rise in melatonin may be barely detectable. Because melatonin opposes the degeneration caused by high levels of corticosteroids (i.e. protein catabolism, suppressed immune function, and altered blood glucose metabolism), higher melatonin levels may help promote health and extend life-span.

Studies show that jet lag is most likely caused by a disrupted circadian rhythm that can be effectively adjusted by using melatonin. Insomnia that is seen in the elderly and in some children with sleeping disorders is usually caused by low melatonin levels. That, too, can be treated with the proper supplementation. Childhood diseases that may cause melatonin-related sleep disorders include autism, epilepsy, Down syndrome, and cerebral palsy. Melatonin supplementation can also benefit blind people whose sleeping rhythms are disturbed. Melatonin is not effective as a sleeping aid for persons with normal melatonin levels.

Several studies have shown how melatonin levels shift during monthly menstrual cycles. Nocturnal melatonin is highest during the premenstrual period and lowest during the midmenstrual period. It is thought that rising melatonin levels may bring on menstruation and lowering ones may bring on a surge of luteinizing hormone and ovulation. Administering melatonin prior to the midcycle surge of luteinizing hormone appears to block ovulation, leading to speculation about the use of melatonin as a natural contraceptive.

Melatonin also has antioxidant, antiestrogenic, and oncostatic properties, which may produce some of its anticancer effects. As an antioxidant, melatonin appears to be able to neutralize hydroxyl, the most damaging of all oxygen-based free radicals. Studies show that melatonin can help prevent and treat some hormonally related cancers, such as breast cancer and prostate cancer. The most promising results are seen when melatonin is used in conjunction with interferon or interleukin-2, anticancer agents that are much less effective without melatonin. Melatonin not only enhances the use of interleukin-2, an important immune cytokine, but it also reduces the numerous side effects often associated with it.

Many studies have shown that some patients suffering from depression have lower-than-normal melatonin levels. Seasonal affective disorder (SAD) is often effectively treated with phototherapy, and research has shown that SAD patients often have delayed melatonin rhythms in the winter. While some forms of depression may have direct links to melatonin levels, other types of depression have not responded well to melatonin treatment. Exaggerated depressive symptoms have been reported in some cases of depressed patients receiving daytime melatonin supplements. Melatonin has increased psychotic behavior in some schizophrenic patients.

DIETARY SOURCES

N/A

CONSTITUENTS/COMPOSITION

Melatonin is a hormone manufactured by serotonin and secreted by the pineal gland. It is an indole, like the simple amino acid, tryptophan.

COMMERCIAL PREPARATIONS

Melatonin can be taken in tablet, capsule, and sublingual tablet form.

THERAPEUTIC USES

- Used to restore sleeping patterns and fatigue caused by jet lag
- As a sleeping aid for those who suffer from insomnia as a result of low melatonin levels (i.e. elderly and some children with sleep disorders)
- Inhibits initiation and growth of some hormonally related cancers and non-small cell lung cancer, particularly in conjunction with interferon or interleukin 2 treatment
- May be beneficial for treatment of depression related to low melatonin levels (i.e. SAD)
- Preliminary studies show it may be useful in multiple sclerosis, SIDS, coronary heart disease, epilepsy and post-menopausal osteoporosis.

DOSAGE RANGES AND DURATION OF ADMINISTRATION

Official dosage ranges have not yet been set for melatonin supplementation. Sensitivity to melatonin may vary from individual to individual. For those especially sensitive to it, lower doses may work more effectively than the standard amount. Higher doses could cause anxiety or irritability.

For treatment of insomnia, a dose of 3 mg taken an hour before bedtime is usually effective, although dosages as low as 0.1 to 0.3 mg may improve sleep for some people. If 3 mg a night is not effective after three days, try 6 mg one hour before bedtime. An individually effective dose should produce restful sleep and no daytime irritability or fatigue. For treatment of jet lag, take 5 mg of melatonin one hour before bedtime upon arrival at new location; repeat for the first five days. Dosages for anticancer treatment may be much higher (i.e. 10 to 50 mg per day). Long-term melatonin supplementation should not be carried out without a health care provider's supervision.

SIDE EFFECTS/TOXICOLOGY

There are no known serious side effects to regulated melatonin supplementation. Some people may experience vivid dreams or nightmares. Overuse or incorrect use of melatonin could disrupt circadian rhythms. Long term effects have not been well studied. In rats, melatonin decreases T_4 and T_3 uptake levels.

WARNINGS/CONTRAINDICATIONS/PRECAUTIONS

Melatonin can cause drowsiness if taken during the day. If morning drowsiness is experienced after taking melatonin at night, reduce dosage levels. In some cases of depression, daytime doses of melatonin can increase depression. May be contraindicated for those with autoimmune disorders and immune system cancers (i.e. lymphoma, leukemia). Because melatonin suppresses corticosteroid activity, those who are taking corticosteroids for anti-inflammatory or immune suppressive purposes (i.e. transplant patients) should exercise caution with melatonin supplementation.

Melatonin could interfere with fertility. It is also contraindicated during pregnancy and lactation. Lack of sleep and insufficient exposure to darkness may suppress natural production of melatonin.

INTERACTIONS

- Vitamin B_{12} influences melatonin secretion in the body. Low levels of melatonin will often reflect low vitamin B_{12} levels as well. Taking vitamin B_{12} (1.5 mg of methylcobalamin per day) can improve sleeping disorders.
- Protein, vitamin B_6, niacinamide, and acetyl carnitine all support melatonin production.
- Nonsteroidal anti-inflammatory drugs (NSAIDs) reduce melatonin secretion in the body.
- Beta blockers inhibit the nocturnal rise of melatonin levels
- Tricyclics, monoamine oxidase inhibitors, and some antidepressants increase the levels of brain melatonin.
- Benzodiazepines, like Xanax and Valium, interfere with melatonin production.
- Alcohol and caffeine can interfere with melatonin production.
- Diuretics and calcium channel blockers can interfere with melatonin production.

REFERENCES

Atkins R. *Dr. Atkin's Vita-Nutrient Solution.* New York, NY: Simon and Schuster. 1998.

Balch J and Balch P. *Prescription for Nutritional Healing.* Garden City Park, NY: Avery Publishing Group; 1997.

Lissoni, P, Vigore L, Rescaldani R, et al. Neuroimmunotherapy with low-dose subcutaneous interleukin-2 plus melatonin in AIDS patients with CD4 cell number below 200/mm3: a biological phase-II study. *J Biol Regul Homeost Agents.* 1995;9:155–158.

MacIntosh A. Melatonin: clinical monograph. *Q Rev Nat Med.* 1996; 47–60.

Mindell E and Hopkins V. *Prescription Alternatives.* New Canaan, Conn: Keats Publishing, Inc.; 1998.

Murphy P, Myers B, Badia P. NSAIDs suppress human melatonin levels. *Am J Nat Med.* 1997; iv: 25.

Murray, M. *Encyclopedia of Nutritional Supplements.* Rocklin, Calif: Prima Publishing; 1996.

Petrie K, Conaglen JV, Thompson L, Chamberlain K. Effect of melatonin on jet lag after long haul flights. *BMJ.* 1989;298:705–707.

Rosenfeld, I. *Dr. Rosenfeld's Guide to Alternative Medicine.* New York, NY: Random House; 1996.

Tzischinsky O, Lavie P. Melatonin possesses time-dependent hypnotic effects. *Sleep.* 1994;17:638–645.

Zhdanova IV, Wurtman RJ, Morabito C, Piotrovska VR, Lynch HJ. Effects of low oral doses of melatonin, given 2-4 hours before habitual bedtime, on sleep in normal young humans. *Sleep.* 1996;19:423–431.

Zhdanova IV, Wurtman RJ, Lynch HJ, et al. Sleep-inducing effects of low doses of melatonin ingested in the evening. *Clin Pharmacol Ther.* 1995; 57:552–558.

■ PHENYLALANINE

OVERVIEW

Phenylalanine is an essential amino acid that is not synthesized in adequate amounts by the body, so it must be obtained from dietary sources. In healthy individuals, phenylalanine is converted by the body into tyrosine. Tyrosine is the parent compound for the manufacturing of the hormones norepinephrine and epinephrine by the adrenal medulla and of the hormones thyroxine and triiodothyronine by the thyroid gland. In adults, approximately 90% of the recommended dietary allowance (RDA) of phenylalanine is hydroxylated to form tyrosine. The remaining 10% is used for tissue protein synthesis. In children, 60% of the RDA is used for tissue protein synthesis, and the remaining 40% is hydroxylated to form tyrosine.

The inability to convert excess phenylalanine to tyrosine is the underlying cause of phenylketonuria (PKU), the most common metabolic genetic defect. PKU is actually a group of inherited disorders involving phenylalanine metabolism. Patients with PKU have one or more of a number of enzyme defects associated with a corresponding recessive gene. The disease appears in infants 3 to 6 months old. As it must be treated before 3 months of age, PKU screening is done during the first 48 hours of life. The incidence of PKU is approximately 1 in 10,000 Caucasian infants and 1 in 132,000 black infants. Mental retardation, usually severe, is the primary manifestation of untreated PKU. Other manifestations may include seizures, muscular hypertonicity, exaggerated tendon reflexes, tremors, and hyperactivity. A skin condition similar to eczema occurs in 15% to 20% of untreated patients.

Treatment for PKU-positive patients is a phenylalanine-restricted, tyrosine-supplemented diet to maintain adequate blood phenylalanine levels for optimum brain development and growth. There is some disagreement about whether these diets can be discontinued without adverse effect and, if so, at what age. Some studies have shown significant differences in mental functioning, in both performance and intelligence, between those who have discontinued the diet and those who have maintained the diet. In adults who have discontinued the diet, severe agoraphobia has been reported, which is reversible with a return to the phenylalanine-restricted diet.

Pregnant women with PKU that is untreated at the time of conception and during gestation give birth to infants with poor intrauterine growth, microcephaly, and congenital abnormalities that are often severe.

Symptoms of phenylalanine deficiency may include confusion, emotional agitation, depression, decreased alertness, decreased memory, behavioral changes, decreased sexual interest, bloodshot eyes, and cataracts. If not corrected by supplemental dietary phenylalanine and tyrosine, the deficiency may lead to restricted weight gain and stunted growth, osteopenia, anemia, alopecia, and even death.

Aspartame (Nutrasweet), the synthetic sweetener, is formed by combining phenylalanine and aspartic acid. The FDA maintains that it is safe; however, there continues to be controversy over its use, and relatively little is known about its effect during pregnancy in the general population.

DIETARY SOURCES

Generally, phenylalanine is found in cheeses; nuts and seeds; milk chocolate; meat (excluding fat), particularly organ meats; poultry (excluding skin); fish, including shellfish; milk; and eggs. The most concentrated sources are torula yeast, soybean protein isolate, soybean protein concentrate, peanut flour, dried spirulina seaweed, defatted and low-fat soybean flour, dried and salted cod, defatted soy meal, dried and frozen tofu,

Parmesan cheese, almond meal, dry roasted soybean nuts, dried watermelon seeds, and fenugreek seeds.

CONSTITUENTS/COMPOSITION

Phenylalanine is an essential amino acid. It is also known as PHA, PHE, amino acid F, and 2-amino-3-phenyl propanoic acid. Its chemical composition is $C_9H_{11}NO_2$.

COMMERCIAL PREPARATIONS

- D-phenylalanine capsules
- L-phenylalanine capsules
- D,L-phenylalanine capsules (50/50 blend of D-phenylalanine and L-phenylalanine)
- Topical creams

THERAPEUTIC USES

- Cancer: Restriction of phenylalanine and tyrosine may help decrease tumor growth and metastasis, particularly in malignant melanoma.
- Depression: L-phenylalanine has been used in treating bipolar disorders with both manic and depressive states combined with vitamins B_6; and D.
- Inflammation: Supplementation in the form of D-phenylalanine may be beneficial.
- Multiple sclerosis: Supplementation has been shown to improve bladder control, increase mobility, and ameliorate depression.
- Pain: Supplementation has been effective for chronic pain, particularly for osteoarthritis; use in doses of 250 mg 15 to 30 minutes before meals tid for a period of at least two days and up to three weeks.
- Parkinson's disease: Supplementation in the form of D-phenylalanine may reduce rigidity, walking disabilities, and speech difficulties.
- Rheumatoid arthritis: Supplementation in the form of D,L-phenylalanine was shown to be beneficial in one study.
- Vitiligo: Beneficial effects have been shown given treatment with oral L-phenylalanine, topical cream containing 10% phenylalanine, and ultraviolet-A radiation.

DOSAGE RANGES AND DURATION OF ADMINISTRATION

The following are the recommended dietary allowances for phenylalanine plus tyrosine, according to the National Research Council.

- Birth to 4 months: 125 mg/kg/day
- 5 months to 2 years: 69 mg/kg/day
- 3 to 12 years: 22 mg/kg/day
- Adults and teenagers: 14 mg/kg/day

Based on obligatory amino acid losses (including data from amino acid tracer studies), it has been suggested that adults need 39 mg/kg/day.

Nutritional doses are 0.75 to 2 g per day; therapeutic doses are 2 to 3 g per day; experimental doses are 4 to 5 g per day.

SIDE EFFECTS/TOXICOLOGY

See "Warnings/Contraindications/Precautions"

WARNINGS/CONTRAINDICATIONS/PRECAUTIONS

- Anxiety, headaches, and hypertension are possible side effects of supplementation.
- Individuals with PKU and women who are lactating or pregnant should avoid supplementation.
- L-dopa competes with phenylalanine and should not be taken at the same time of day.

• Little is known about the use of aspartame (Nutrasweet) during pregnancy.

INTERACTIONS

• Vitamins B$_6$ and C help the body absorb phenylalanine.
• Increased amounts of other amino acids will inhibit phenylalanine.

REFERENCES

Bugard P, Bremer HJ, Buhrdel P, et al. Rationale for the German recommendations for phenylalanine level control in phenylketonuria 1997. *Eur J Pediatr.* 1999;158:46–54.

Ensminger AH, Ensminger ME, Konlande JE, Robson JRK. *Foods & Nutrition Encyclopedia.* 2nd ed. Baton Rouge, Fla: CRC Press, Inc; 1994:1,2:60–64, 1,748.

Garrison Jr RH, Somer E. *The Nutrition Desk Reference.* 3rd ed. New Canaan, Conn: Keats Publishing, Inc; 1995:39–52.

Haas EM. Staying Healthy With Nutrition. Berkeley, Calif: Celestial Arts Publishing; 1992.

Herbert V, Subak-Sharpe GJ, eds. *Total Nutrition (Mount Sinai School of Medicine).* New York, NY: St. Martin's Press; 1995:318–320.

Newstrom H. *Nutrients Catalog.* Jefferson, NC: McFarland & Co; 1993:303–312.

Pietz J. Neurological aspects of adult phenylketonuria. *Curr Opin Neurol.* 1998;11:679–688.

Pietz J, Dunckelmann R, Rupp A, et al. Neurological outcome in adult patients with early-treated phenylketonuria. *Eur J Pediatr.* 1998;157:824–830.

Shils ME, Olson JA, Shike M, Ross AC. *Modern Nutrition in Health and Disease.* 9th ed. Baltimore, Md: Williams & Wilkins; 1999:41, 1,010.

Start K. Treating phenylketonuria by a phenylalanine-free diet. *Prof Care Mother Child.* 1998;8:109–110.

Werbach MR. *Nutritional Influences on Illness.* 2nd ed. Tarzana, Calif: Third Line Press; 1993:159–160, 384, 434, 494–495, 506, 580, 613–614, 636.

■ PHOSPHORUS

OVERVIEW

Next to calcium, phosphorus is the most abundant mineral in the body, making up about 1% of total body weight. Most of it is found in bones and teeth. Phosphorus is present in the body as phosphates and, in addition to its role in bone formation, it is vital to energy production and exchange. Phosphorus helps in muscle contraction and nerve conduction. It aids kidney function and helps maintain the body's pH balance. Phospholipids are fat molecules that play a role in the maintenance of cell membranes. As a component of adenosine triphosphate (ATP), phosphorus is involved in the body's primary metabolic cycles and in protein synthesis for growth, maintenance, and repair of all body tissues and cells, as well as in the production of the nucleic acids in DNA and RNA. It is also necessary for the absorption of many vitamins and minerals, including vitamin D, calcium, iodine, magnesium, and zinc.

The parathyroid hormone (PTH) regulates the metabolism of phosphorus and calcium in the body. About two-thirds of phosphorus is absorbed from the intestine, the rate depending to some extent on levels of calcium and vitamin D, as well as the activity of PTH. While 85% of phosphorus is deposited in bones and teeth, the remainder is found in cells and other body tissues. The blood contains about 3.5 mg of phosphorus per 100 ml of plasma; total blood phosphorus is between 30 and 40 mg. Together, calcium and phosphorus assure the formation and maintenance of strong bones. The ideal dietary ratio of Ca/P is 1:1. A low Ca/P ratio can lead to bone resorption as the body draws upon existing calcium stores in the bone to pair with excess phosphorus. Not only is phosphorus absorbed more efficiently than calcium, but people are likely to get more phosphorus from their diets. The typical American diet has Ca/P ratios ranging from 1:2 to 1:4. The growing consumption of soft drinks, which are buffered with phosphates (as much as 500 mg in one serving), and high consumption of red meat and poultry, which contain 10 to 20 times as much phosphorus as calcium, are largely responsible for this imbalance. Decreased Ca/P ratios due to excess dietary phosphorus impair calcium absorption, which contributes to bone loss, osteoporosis, and periodontal disease. Low Ca/P ratios have also been associated with an increased incidence of hypertension and elevated risk for colon-rectal cancer.

Phosphorus deficiency, or hypophosphatemia, is rare except in people affected by certain diseases, in those receiving parenteral nutrition, or in those who have received phosphate-binding agents that contain aluminum for extended periods. It has been associated with anorexia, anxiety, apprehension, bone pain, bone fragility, stiffness in the joints, fatigue, irregular breathing, irritability, numbness, paresthesias, weakness, and weight change. In children, decreased growth, poor bone and tooth development, and symptoms of rickets may be signs of phosphorus deficiency. A greater concern for physicians is hyperphosphatemia, or an excess of phosphorus. This is most often the result of dietary imbalance. This has a negative result in terms of bone density and is of particular concern to women. Acute or chronic renal failure may also lead to hyperphosphatemia; in these cases restricting phosphorus intake to 800 to 1,000 mg is indicated.

DIETARY SOURCES

Dietary sources of phosphorus include the following.

- Red meat and poultry
- Dried milk and milk products
- Wheat germ
- Yeast
- Grains
- Hard cheeses
- Canned fish
- Nuts
- Potatoes
- Eggs
- Soft drinks

CONSTITUENTS/COMPOSITION

Elemental phosphorus, a white or yellow waxy substance that burns on contact with air (thus the term phosphorescent), is used in some homeopathic remedies. However, because it is highly toxic, it is no longer used in medicine. Instead, inorganic phosphates are used to treat phosphate deficiency. The following forms are used.

- Dibasic potassium phosphate
- Monobasic potassium phosphate
- Dibasic sodium phosphate
- Monobasic sodium phosphate
- Tribasic sodium phosphate

COMMERCIAL PREPARATIONS

Phosphorus is available over-the-counter in capsules. Because it is readily available in a variety of foods, phosphorus supplementation is usually confined to athletes who take it to reduce muscle pain and fatigue.

THERAPEUTIC USES

Phosphorus, by itself, is used in the treatment of only a few medical conditions. Along with calcium, however, it can help in healing bone fractures and in the treatment of osteomalacia, osteoporosis, and rickets. Regulating the ratio of calcium/phosphorus intake through dietary sources can reduce stress and alleviate problems like arthritis, which are related to calcium metabolism.

Hypophosphatemia can cause an impaired response to insulin for which supplementation with dibasic calcium phosphate (2 g tid with meals) has shown good results. Phosphate supplementation is also used in the treatment of diabetic ketoacidosis (DKA), and in constipation due to hypercalcemia. Mono- and dibasic sodium phosphates may be used as mild laxatives administered by mouth or rectally. Elemental phosphorus is used in homeopathic treatments for coughs and some types of acute gastroenteritus.

DOSAGE RANGES AND DURATION OF ADMINISTRATION

The U.S. RDA for phosphorus is 800 to 1,200 mg daily. The RDA for those up to age 24 and during pregnancy and lactation is 1,200 mg daily.

SIDE EFFECTS/TOXICOLOGY

Phosphates can be toxic at levels over 1 g/day, leading to diarrhea, calcification of organs and soft tissue, and preventing the absorption of iron, calcium, magnesium, and zinc. High levels of phosphorus can promote the loss of calcium through nutritional hyperparathyroidism.

WARNINGS/CONTRAINDICATIONS/PRECAUTIONS

The overconsumption of foods high in phosphorus can drain calcium resources and lead to reduced bone mass. American dietary habits, particularly the high consumption of meat and soft drinks, makes low Ca/P ratios quite common. This imbalance may be the source of the high incidence of osteoporosis in the U.S. and other affluent nations where similar dietary habits prevail. Some researchers have identified this as the likely mechanism contributing to low bone mass in American women. Further retrospective studies are needed to investigate this hypothesis. Low ratios of dietary Ca/P also reduce the efficacy of treatments for osteoporosis. A 1986 experimental study of 158 females, aged 20 to 75, found that treatment of osteoporosis may in fact be fruitless when dietary Ca/P ratios exceed

1:1.25. Patients need to be aware of the dietary sources of both calcium and phosphorus so that they can take a more active role in balancing these two elements in their diet.

INTERACTIONS

Overuse of aluminum-containing antacids can result in phosphorus deficiency. Iron and magnesium interfere with phosphorus absorption, and caffeine increases phosphorus excretion by the kidneys. Low vitamin D intake can also contribute to phosphorus deficiency.

REFERENCES

Anderson JJB. Calcium, phosphorus, and human bone development. *J Nutr.* 1996;126:1153S–1158S.

Berner YN, Shike M. Consequences of phosphate imbalance. *Annu Rev Nutr.* 1988;8:121–148.

Carey CF, Lee HH, Woeltje KF, eds. *The Washington Manual of Medical Therapeutics.* 29th ed. New York, NY: Lippincott-Raven; 1998:230–237,444–448.

da Cunha DF, dos Santos VM, Monterio JP, de Carvalho da Cunha SF. Miner *Electrolyte Metab.* 1998;24:337–340.

Kuntziger H, Altman JJ. Hyperphosphoremia and hypophosphoremia [in French]. *Rev Prat.* 1989;39:949–953.

Metz JA, Anderson JJB, Gallagher Jr PN. Intakes of calcium, phosphorus, and protein, and physical activity level are related to radial bone mass in young adult women. *Am J Clin Nutr.* 1993;58: 537–542.

Mindell E, Hopkins V. *Prescription Alternatives.* Canaan, Conn: Keats Publishing Inc; 1998:495–496.

Reynolds JEF, ed. *Martindale: The Extra Pharmacopoeia.* 31st ed. London, Great Britain: Royal Pharmaceutical Society; 1996:1181–1182, 1741.

Shires R, Kessler GM. The absorption of tricalcium phosphate and its acute metabolic effects. *Calcif Tissue Int.* 1990;47:142–144.

Villa ML, Packer E, Cheema M, et al. Effects of aluminum hydroxide on the parathyroid-vitamin D axis of postmenopausal women. *J Clin Endocrinol Metab.* 1991;73:1256–1261.

Walker LP, Brown EH. *The Alternative Pharmacy.* NJ: Prentice-Hall; 1998:97.

Werbach MR. *Nutritional Influences on Illness: A Sourcebook of Clinical Research.* Canaan, Conn: Keats Publishing Inc; 1987.

■ POTASSIUM

OVERVIEW

Potassium is the principal cation (positively charged element of an electrolyte) of intracellular fluid with a concentration of 140 mmol/L. The extracellular fluid potassium concentration is 3.5 to 5.5 mmol/L, making it thirty-fold less concentrated than the intracellular fluid. Together with sodium, the principal cation of the extracellular fluid, potassium maintains the potential difference across cell membranes. The importance of potassium's contribution to this function is best demonstrated by the consequences of hyperkalemia (increase in extracellular potassium concentration) and hypokalemia (decrease in extracellular potassium concentration) on the heart. Both conditions result in abnormal depolarization and repolarization of cardiac cells, leading to potentially fatal cardiac arrhythmias and conduction disturbances.

Other physiologic functions in which potassium plays a role include energy metabolism, membrane transport, normal water balance, acid-base balance, and osmotic equilibrium. The relationship of potassium and sodium is essential to good health, with a ratio of dietary potassium to sodium recommended at 5:1.

Recent studies have provided strong evidence that potassium may have an anti-hypertensive function. A meta analysis of 33 randomized controlled clinical trials with about 2,600 participants demonstrated that potassium supplementation was associated with a significant reduction in mean systolic and diastolic blood pressure. The mechanisms behind the blood pressure-lowering effects of potassium include effects on natriuresis, the renin-angiotensin-aldosterone system, direct vasodilatatory functions, baroreflex sensitivity, and catecholaminergic functions as well as an improvement of glucose tolerance.

Other studies suggest that there may be a role for potassium together with glucose and insulin in the reduction of acute myocardial infarction (AMI) mortality. Glucose-insulin-potassium (GIK) treatment was shown to decrease AMI mortality by itself or in combination with thrombolytic therapy, revascularization procedures, or both. A possible mechanism of GIK action is decrease of circulating levels of free fatty acids (FFA) and myocardial uptake of FFA.

Studies have revealed that the elderly are at high risk for hyperkalemia. The aging process alters normal renal function, leading to an inhibition of normal potassium excretion. In this setting of impaired renal function, several drugs which are commonly prescribed to the elderly can further alter the kidney's ability to excrete potassium, leading to hyperkalemia and a potentially life-threatening situation.

DIETARY SOURCES

The richest dietary sources of potassium are fresh unprocessed food including meats and fish, vegetables (especially potatoes), fruits (especially avocados), and citrus juices. Ample potassium can be obtained by a varied diet with adequate intake of milk, meats, cereals, vegetables, and fruits.

CONSTITUENTS/COMPOSITION

Potassium is a metallic element of the alkali group with an atomic weight of 39 and atomic symbol of K. It is the chief intracellular cation; 98% of total body potassium is found in the intracellular fluid.

COMMERCIAL PREPARATIONS

Potassium supplements are usually available in the form of potassium salts or potassium bound to mineral chelates. These include the following.

- Potassium acetate
- Potassium bicarbonate and potassium citrate effervescent
- Potassium chloride
- Potassium gluconate

Potassium is also sometimes included in multivitamin preparations.

THERAPEUTIC USES

- To treat the symptoms of hypokalemia
- To control and prevent hypertension
- To reduce the mortality associated with AMI (used in combination with glucose and insulin)
- To counteract glucose intolerance
- To protect against stroke
- To treat cardiac arrhythmias
- To treat muscle weakness
- To assist in the treatment of diabetes mellitus

DOSAGE RANGES AND DURATION OF ADMINISTRATION

The average potassium intake estimated by the National Research Council is as follows.

- In infants: 780 mg/day
- In children: 1,600 mg /day
- In adults: 3,500 mg/day

There is no recommended increased intake of potassium during pregnancy and lactation.

SIDE EFFECTS/TOXICOLOGY

Side effects from prescribed use include the following.

- Gastrointestinal (stomach pain, nausea, vomiting, diarrhea, flatulence)
- Cardiovascular (bradycardia)
- Metabolic, endocrine (hyperkalemia)
- Respiratory (weakness, difficult breathing)
- Local tissue necrosis with extravasation

Toxic effects due to overdose include the following.

- Muscle weakness
- Lethargy
- Gastric hypomotility
- Paralysis
- Cardiac arrhythmia
- Conduction disturbances
- Death

WARNINGS/CONTRAINDICATIONS/PRECAUTIONS

Use with caution in patients with renal insufficiency. Should not be used in patients with severe renal impairment. Because renal function declines with age, the elderly are at high risk of renal insufficiency. Care should be taken when prescribing potassium supplements to the elderly.

INTERACTIONS

- Potassium-depleting drugs include thiazides, furosemide, ethacrynic acid, and bumetanide
- Carbonic anhydrase inhibitors such as acetazolamide
- Potassium-sparing diuretics such as spironolactone, triamterene, amiloride
- NSAIDS
- ACE inhibitors
- Beta-blocking agents
- Heparin
- Digoxin
- Trimethoprim

REFERENCES

Ascherio A, Rimm EB, Hernan MA, et al. Intake of potassium, magnesium, calcium, and fiber and risk of stroke among U.S. men. *Circulation*. 1998;98:1198–1204.

Brancati FL, Appel LJ, Seidler AJ, Whelton PK. Effect of potassium supplementation on blood pressure in African Americans on a low-potassium diet. *Arch Intern Med*. 1996;156:61–72.

Luft F, Ekhard ZE, Filer LJ, eds. *Present Knowledge in Nutrition*. 7th ed. Washington, DC: ILSI Press; 1996:272–276.

Mahan LK, Arlin MT, eds. *Krause's Food, Nutrition, and Diet Therapy*. 8th ed. Philadelphia, Pa: WB Saunders Co.; 1992:147, 390.

National Research Council: Recommended Dietary Allowances. 10th ed. Washington, DC: National Academy Press; 1989:255–257.

Ganong WF. *Review of Medical Physiology*. 18th ed. Stamford, Conn: Appleton & Lange; 1997: 677.

Apstein C. Glucose-Insulin-Potassium for accute myocardial infraction: remarkable results from a new prospective, randomized trial. *Circulation*. 1998;98:2223–2226.

Perazella M, Mahnensmith R. Hyperkalemia in the elderly. *J Gen Intern Med*. 1997;12:646–656.

Sacks FM, Willett WC, Smith A, et al. Effect on blood pressure of potassium, calcium, and magnesium in women with low habitual intake. *Hypertension*. 1998;31(1):131–138

Singh RB, Singh NK, Niaz MA, Sharma JP. Effect of treatment with magnesium and potassium on mortality and reinfarction rate of patients with suspected acute myocardial infarction. *Int J Clin Pharmacol Thera*. 1996;34:219–225.

Suter PM. Potassium and Hypertension. *Nutrition Reviews*. 1998;56:151–133.

Young DB, Lin H, McCabe RD. Potassium's cardiovascular protective mechanisms. *Am J Physiology*. 1995;268(part 2):R825–R837.

■ PSYLLIUM

OVERVIEW

Psyllium, also called psyllium seed, is a soluble fiber that comes from a perennial weed, a relative of the common plantain herb of the family Plantaginaceae, of which there are about 250 species worldwide. (It is not the same as the edible plantain Musa paradisiacae.) Psyllium seeds are coated in mucilage, 1.5 to 3.5 mm, oval or boat-shaped, and dark ruddy brown in color, and produce no odor and almost no taste.

Psyllium seeds or husks can be purchased in bulk from health stores or pharmacies. Psyllium can also be found as an ingredient in commercially prepared laxative products such as Metamucil (which contains psyllium hydrophilic muciloid), which undergo more processing than all-natural products.

Used as a dietary fiber, psyllium is a bowel tonic and gentle bulk laxative that attracts water and creates larger, softer stools. Doctors and herbalists recommend psyllium as a stool softener and bulking agent to relieve constipation, diarrhea, hemorrhoids, irritable bowel syndrome, hemorrhoids, and Crohn's disease. Considered a good intestinal cleanser and stool softener, psyllium is one of the most popular fibers available. Unlike bran fiber, psyllium does not cause excessive gas and bloating.

Soluble fibers such as psyllium can help prevent the intestine from absorbing cholesterol, and several studies have found that adding psyllium to the diet can produce a significant reduction in serum cholesterol in the absence of other dietary modifications and can increase cholesterol reduction when coupled with cholesterol-lowering medication.

High-fiber foods, including psyllium, aid in reducing the risk of hypertension, heart disease, and even some cancers. Studies examining the effects of psyllium husks on colon cancer have found that the fiber strongly reduces the ability of a carcinogen to cause colon cancer. Animal studies found that rats fed psyllium husks produced the highest fecal bacteria counts and the bulkiest and most moist stools. Animal studies also showed that the greater the fiber intake, the lower the rate of fatal colon disease. Other studies have shown that high-fiber diets appear to be protective against breast and other cancers as well.

Several studies have shown that adding fiber to the diet can significantly increase weight loss even in the absence of calorie restriction. Clinical studies have shown that fiber supplements enhance blood sugar control and reduce calorie absorption by as much as 30 to 180 calories a day, which would result in a 3- to 18-pound weight loss over the course of a year. Both soluble and insoluble fibers aid weight loss. Water-soluble fibers such as psyllium, taken with water before meals, create a feeling of fullness by expanding to a gelatinous mass in the stomach, causing the dieter to consume smaller quantities of food. Fiber supplements also aid blood sugar and insulin control. Because fiber supplements absorb water rapidly, people who use fiber as a weight-reducing aid must take care to be well hydrated by drinking at least six to eight full glasses of water each day.

DIETARY SOURCES

Psyllium seed or husk (from plantain herb)

CONSTITUENTS/COMPOSITION

Psyllium is available as psyllium seed or husk, or as a combination of the two. Its constituents include acids, alkaloids, amino acids, fixed oil, protein, iridoids, tannins, flavonoids, and a variety of sugar and polysaccharide components and other plant carbohydrates in the seed mucilage.

COMMERCIAL PREPARATIONS

Psyllium is an ingredient in some commercially prepared laxatives, including Metamucil.

It is also found in some combination herbal remedy products, such as Aerobic Bulk Cleanse (ABC), which contains blond psyllium seed husks and licorice and hibiscus herbs. ABC is used to heal and cleanse the colon and to treat diarrhea and constipation.

THERAPEUTIC USES

- Relieves constipation as a stool softener and gentle, bulk laxative
- Relieves diarrhea
- Cleanses and helps heal the colon
- Acts as a fiber supplement
- Lowers cholesterol
- Treats irritable bowel syndrome
- Treats hemorrhoids
- Aids weight reduction
- Acts as a cancer inhibitor

DOSAGE RANGES AND DURATION OF ADMINISTRATION

There is no RDA for psyllium, but herbal and health professionals recommend using $1/2$ to 2 tsp. of psyllium one or two times a day.

Add $1/2$ to 2 tsp. of psyllium seed to 1 cup (8 ozs.) of warm water, mix well, then drink immediately (before it becomes too thick to consume; psyllium thickens rapidly when exposed to water). It may be beneficial to begin with a low dose, such as 1 tsp. in an 8-oz. glass of water, then increase to 2 tsp. if needed.

For irritable bowel syndrome, take psyllium fiber daily, starting with 1 tsp. in water once a day, then gradually increase psyllium intake: every three or four days, increase the amount by 1 tsp. in another glass of water up to a maximum of four glasses every day.

Psyllium may be taken first thing in the morning or at bedtime.

SIDE EFFECTS/TOXICOLOGY

If taken at the same time or within one hour of taking medications, psyllium can interfere with their absorption and effectiveness.

It is possible to develop sensitivity to psyllium in breakfast cereal, according to a 1990 *Journal of the American Medical Association* report, which described a nurse who had in the past dispensed laxatives that contained psyllium and later suffered anaphylaxis upon exposure to a breakfast cereal that contained psyllium.

WARNINGS/CONTRAINDICATIONS/PRECAUTIONS

Use in children only under the direction of a qualified health care provider.

Psyllium must always be taken with at least a full 8 ozs. (1 cup) of water.

Do not take guar, another soluble fiber supplement whose mechanism is similar, at the same time as psyllium; use one or the other, but not both.

Diabetics should use caution when taking herbs such as psyllium (also marshmallow root and flax) that have a high mucilage content because they may affect blood sugar.

INTERACTIONS

Psyllium should be taken at least one hour after taking prescription or over-the-counter drugs. If drugs and psyllium are taken too close together, psyllium can interfere with the drug's absorption and effectiveness.

Conflicting studies have linked fiber supplements, and specifically the phytates in grain fiber products, to impaired absorption of minerals, which can potentially result in mineral deficiencies, although, it should be noted, wheat bran was most strongly linked to this effect, and the effect itself has not been clearly proven. Fiber as a dietary component was not linked to mineral absorption problems and did not appear to interfere with minerals in other foods.

REFERENCES

Alabaster O, Tang ZC, Frost A, Sivapurkar N. Potential synergism between wheat brain and psyllium: enhanced inhibition of colon cancer. *Cancer Lett.* 1993;75:53–58.

Ashraf W, Park F, Lof J, Quigley EM. Effects of psyllium therapy on stool characteristics, colon transit and anorectal function in chronic idiopathic constipation. *Aliment Pharmacol Ther.* 1995;9:639–647.

Balch J, Balch P. *Prescription for Nutritional Healing.* 2nd ed. Garden City Park, NY: Avery Publishing Group; 1997.

Fernandez-Banares F, Hinojosa J, Sanchez-Lombrana JL, et al. Randomized clinical trials of Platago ovata seeds (dietary fiber) as compared with mesalaminein maintaining remission in ulcerative colitis. *Am J Gastroenterol.* 1999;94:427–433.

Giller R, Matthews K. *Natural Prescriptions.* New York, NY: Carol Southern Books; 1994.

Kirschmann G, Kirschman J. *Nutrition Almanac.* 4th ed. New York, NY: McGraw-Hill; 1996.

McRorie JW, Daggy BP, Morel JG, Diersing PS, Miner PB, Robinson M. Psyllium is superior to docusate sodium for treatment of chronic constipation. *Aliment Pharmacol Ther.* 1998;12:491–497.

Moss R. *Cancer Therapy.* Brooklyn, NY: Equinox Press, Inc.; 1992.

Murray M. *Encyclopedia of Nutritional Supplements.* Rocklin, Calif: Prima Publishing; 1996.

The Review of Natural Products. St. Louis, Mo: Facts and Comparisons; 1998.

Rodrigues-Moran M, Guerrero-Romero F, Lazcano-Burciaga G. Lipid- and glucose-lowering efficacy of Plantago Psyllium in type II diabetes. *J Diabetes Complications.* 1998;12:273–278.

■ SELENIUM

OVERVIEW

Selenium is a trace mineral and an important part of the enzyme glutathione peroxidase. It is an effective antioxidant, especially when combined with vitamin E. Working as part of this enzyme, selenium or, more specifically, the organic complex selenocysteine, helps protect intracellular structures by preventing the formation of damaging free radicals. Like other antioxidant supplements, selenium slows chemical aging and helps maintain elasticity of bodily tissues, organs, and the cardiovascular system.

Extreme selenium deficiency can lead to a rare heart disorder known as Keshan disease, which results in congestive heart failure and is most evident in parts of China where soil-selenium levels are low. More commonly, though, selenium deficiency is indicated in high rates of cancer, heart disease, and immunodepression. Selenium is frequently lacking in Western diets, again due to mineral-poor farmland. Typical consumption in the U.S. is estimated at 100 mcg/day. Many of selenium's antioxidant and anti-carcinogenic functions require much greater augmentation (>200 mcg/day).

Numerous animal and human studies conclude that fortifying the diet with added selenium, vitamin E, and other vital antioxidants boosts the immune system by stimulating white blood cell development and thymus function. In this way, selenium significantly challenges cancerous tumor incidence and development, and contributes to myriad other immune system benefits. Conversely, research finds low levels of selenium and glutathione peroxidase in cancer patients.

Selenium also plays a crucial role in preventing or managing coronary heart disease, stroke, and cardiovascular disease both before and after heart attacks, especially for patients who smoke, due to its antioxidant mechanisms and its role in lowering LDL cholesterol levels. Selenium also appears to inhibit platelet aggregation, increasing its significance in cardiovascular health.

Other studies have determined that selenium improves liver and metabolic function, even in extreme cases of alcoholic cirrhosis of the liver, and enhances pancreatic function. Additionally, sufficient selenium intake has been indicated in prostrate health and sperm motility, plays a prominent role in skin health and elasticity, and protects against cataract formation. Selenium acts as an antagonist to heavy metals.

DIETARY SOURCES

Brewer's yeast and wheat germ, liver, butter, fish and shellfish, garlic, grains, sunflower seeds, and Brazil nuts are all food sources for naturally occurring selenium. Herbal sources include alfalfa, burdock root, catnip, fennel seed, ginseng, raspberry leaf, and yarrow.

The amount of selenium in foodstuffs corresponds directly to selenium levels in soil. Deficiencies are noted in parts of China and the U.S. where soil-selenium ratios are low.

Food-source selenium is destroyed during processing. Therefore, a varied diet of whole foods is recommended. (Whole foods are those eaten in their original form, rather than canned, frozen, or otherwise commercially processed or prepared.)

CONSTITUENTS/COMPOSITION

Selenium occurs most commonly in nature as inorganic sodium selenite. Other, more absorbable and active forms include selenomethione or selenocysteine and selenium-rich yeast.

COMMERCIAL PREPARATIONS

Selenium is available as part of many vitamin-mineral supplements, all nutritional antioxidant formulas, and, increasingly, as an independent supplement. Suggested intake is between 50 and 200 mcg per day for adults. Men apparently require more than women, because stores are lost with ejaculation. Selenium should be taken with vitamin E, as the two act synergistically, and without vitamin C, which decreases absorbability and is likely to increase risk of selenium toxicity.

THERAPEUTIC USES

Clinical trials suggest that supplemental selenium well beyond daily dietary intake (>100 mcg) is necessary to support at least some of the following functions. Selenium deficiency is most evident in a positive response to supplemental selenium therapy. Blood and urinary levels are inadequate indicators of selenium intake and tissue levels.

- Cancer. Acts as an anti-cancer antioxidant, protecting against or reducing the incidence of breast, colon, liver, skin, and respiratory tumors and cancers.
- Heart disease. Prevents and manages coronary heart disease, cardiovascular disease, and stroke by helping to lower LDL cholesterol and reduce platelet aggregation. Reduces post-heart attack mortality. Successful in treatment of Keshan disease.
- Immunodepression. Boosts immune function and white blood cell development. Suggested in the treatment of depressed immune disorders such as lupus. Contributes to body's ability to fight bactericidal action of phagocytes. Counters heavy metal toxicity such as lead, mercury, and cadmium poisoning. Stimulates antibody formation in response to vaccinations.
- Liver disease. Effective against alcohol-induced cirrhosis of the liver and alcoholic cardiomyopathy. Promotes proper liver and metabolic function.
- Skin disorders. Indicated for treatment of acne, eczema, psoriasis, vasculitis, and other skin disorders. Responds to vitamin E deficiencies in combination with vitamin E supplementation. Prevents premature aging.
- Muscular and inflammatory illness. Effective in treating all major symptoms of myotonic dystrophy. Suggested in the treatment of inflammatory conditions such as rheumatoid arthritis.
- Eyesight. Required for the antioxidant protection of the lens; helps prevent cataract formation.
- Reproductive Health. May assist in male fertility, prostate function, and sperm motility.
- Promotes healthy fetal development and may help in prevention of SIDS.

DOSAGE RANGES AND DURATION OF ADMINISTRATION

A minimum RDA for selenium is as follows.
- Neonates to 6 months: 10 mcg.
- Infants 6 months to 1 year: 15 mcg
- Children 1 to 6 years: 20 mcg
- Children 7 to 10 years: 30 mcg
- Males 11 to 14 years: 40 mcg
- Males 15 to 18 years: 50 mcg
- Males over 19 years: 70 mcg
- Females 11 to 14 years: 45 mcg
- Females 15 to 18 years: 50 mcg
- Females over 19 years: 55 mcg

- Pregnant females: 65 mcg
- Lactating females: 75 mcg
- Usual dosage for children: 30 to 150 mcg or 1.5 mcg per pound of body weight. For adults: 50 to 200 mcg/day.

SIDE EFFECTS/TOXICOLOGY

Long-term ingestion of excessive levels of selenium (>1,000 mcg/day) may produce fatigue, depression, arthritis, hair or fingernail loss, garlicky breath or body odor, gastrointestinal disorders, or irritability. Such high intakes and chronic toxicity are rare.

WARNINGS/CONTRAINDICATIONS/PRECAUTIONS

Studies found high hair selenium levels in children with learning disabilities and behavioral problems. Extremely high doses may cause cumulatively toxic effects over time.

INTERACTIONS

Vitamin E and other antioxidant nutrients increase selenium's effectiveness in promoting glutathione peroxidase activity. Use and absorption of selenium are hampered by high doses of vitamin C, heavy metals and, possibly, high intakes of zinc and other trace minerals. Vitamin C may also increase risk of selenium toxicity. Chemotherapy drugs may increase selenium requirements.

REFERENCES

Balch JF, Balch PA. *Prescription for Nutritional Healing.* 2nd ed. Garden City Park, NY: Avery Publishing Group; 1997:28.

Clark LC, Combs GF Jr, Turnbull BW, et al. Effects of selenium supplementation for cancer prevention in patients with carcinoma of the skin. *JAMA.* 1996;276:1957–1963.

Combs GF, Clark LC. Can dietary selenium modify cancer risk? *Nutr Rev.* 1985;43:325–331.

Dworkin BM. Selenium deficiency in HIV infection and the acquired immunodeficiency syndrome (AIDS). *Chem Biol Interact.* 1994;91:181–186.

Garland M, Morris JS, Stampfer MJ, et al. Prospective study of toenail selenium levels and cancer among women. *J Natl Cancer Inst.* 1995;8:497–505.

Haas EM. *Staying Healthy with Nutrition: The Complete Guide to Diet and Nutritional Medicine.* Berkeley, Calif: Celestial Arts; 1992:211–216.

Murray MT. *Encyclopedia of Nutritional Supplements: The Essential Guide for Improving Your Health Naturally.* Rocklin, Calif: Prima Publishing; 1996:10–13, 222–228.

National Research Council, Diet and Health. *Implications for Reducing Chronic Disease Risk.* Washington, DC: National Academy Press; 1989:376–379.

Prasad K, ed. *Vitamins, Nutrition and Cancer.* New York, NY: Karger; 1984.

Walker LP, Hodgson Brown E. *The Alternative Pharmacy.* Paramus, NJ: Prentice Hall Press; 1998:313.

Wasowicz W. Selenium concentration and glutathione peroxidase activity in blood of children with cancer. *J Trace Elem Electrolytes Health Dis.* 1994;8:53–57.

Werbach MR. *Nutritional Influences on Illness: A Sourcebook of Clinical Research.* New Canaan, Conn: Keats Publishing; 1988.

Yang GQ, Xia YM. Studies on human dietary requirements and safe range of dietary intakes of selenium in China and their application in the prevention of related endemic diseases. *Biomed Environ Sci.* 1995;8:187–201.

Yoshizawa K, Willett WC, Morris SJ, et al. Studies of prediagnostic selenium level in toenails and the risk of advanced prostrate cancer. *J Natl Cancer Inst.* 1998;90:1219–1224.

■ SPIRULINA

OVERVIEW

Spirulina is a type of blue-green algae of which there are several species. It grows best in a warm climate and in warm alkaline water. Spirulina was historically used by the Mexican (Aztec, Mayan), African, and Asian peoples, who consumed it as a staple for thousands of years.

Spirulina is a rich source of nutrients, especially protein. Its antiviral and anticancer properties are a result of its being rich in phycocyanin, a blue polypeptide that gives spirulina its blue-green color. Phycocyanin has the ability to stimulate the production and activity of both white and red blood cells and to increase the production of antibodies and cytokines, which help fight foreign invasions. Because of these properties, spirulina has been used extensively in Russia to treat the victims, especially children, of the nuclear disaster at Chernobyl. In these children whose bone marrow had been damaged from radiation exposure, spirulina promoted the evacuation of radionucleotides and stimulated T-cell production, which boosted the immune system of these patients.

DIETARY SOURCES

Spirulina is a microalgae that flourishes in warm climates and warm alkaline water. It is available dried and freeze-dried.

CONSTITUENTS/COMPOSITION

Spirulina is a complete protein—62% of it is made up of essential and nonessential amino acids. It is also thought to provide the entire B complex of vitamins, though its vitamin B_{12} content has been called into question. It is also rich in phycocyanin, chlorophyll, beta-carotene and other carotenoids, vitamin E, minerals (e.g., zinc, manganese, copper, iron), trace minerals (e.g., selenium), and essential fatty acids (e.g., gamma-linolenic acid). Because the cell walls of spirulina are made of complex proteins and sugars (unlike other species of blue-green algae whose walls are made up of cellulose), it is very easily digested. The exact nutrient profile depends on the species.

COMMERCIAL PREPARATIONS

Most spirulina consumed in the United States is cultivated scientifically. There are many different spirulina species, only some of which are identified on commercial preparations. *Spirulina maxima* (cultivated in Mexico) and *Spirulina platensis* (cultivated in California) are the most popular.

THERAPEUTIC USES

Currently, spirulina has the following uses:

- AIDS and other viruses (e.g., herpes simplex, human cytomegalovirus, influenza virus, mumps, measles). Spirulina has the ability to inhibit viral replication as well as strengthen the immune system by stimulating T-cell, macrophage, bone marrow stem cell, and natural-killer-cell production and activity. Data from one study indicate that calcium spirulina (Ca-Sp), a component of spirulina, is a powerful antiviral agent against HIV-1 and HSV-1.
- Cancer. Spirulina causes regression and inhibition of some cancers in experimental animals by stimulating enzyme activity (e.g. endonuclease), which is responsible for repairing damaged DNA. A study performed in India showed that *Spirulina fusiformis* supplementation reversed oral leukoplakia in tobacco chewers.

- Anemia. Spirulina promotes hematopoiesis (formation and development of blood cells).
- Skin disorders. Because spirulina is rich in gamma-linolenic acid, it helps to maintain healthy skin and treat several skin disorders (such as eczema and psoriasis).
- Vitamin A deficiency. Studies in India determined that *Spirulina fusiformis* is an effective source of dietary vitamin A.
- Colitis. One study showed that a component of spirulina, C-phycocyanin, reduced inflammation caused by acetic acid-induced colitis in rats. It also showed some reduction in colonic damage.

Clinical applications of spirulina include malabsorption syndrom with gas and bloating, general immune support, and as an easily absorbed protein supplement for people with a lack of appetite. It is also used in the treatment of Candida and hypoglycemia. It is often used by weight lifters as a protein source.

DOSAGE RANGES AND DURATION OF ADMINISTRATION

Patients should consult their health care providers for the correct dosage of spirulina. However, a standard dose of spirulina is 4 to 6 500 mg tablets per day.

SIDE EFFECTS/TOXICOLOGY

No adverse effects were found after high-dose experiments in animals.

WARNINGS/CONTRAINDICATIONS/PRECAUTIONS

No fetotoxicity nor teratogenicity was found when high-doses of spirulina were administered to pregnant animals.

INTERACTIONS

None reported

REFERENCES

Annapurna VV, Deosthale YG, Bamji MS. Spirulina as a source of vitamin A. *Plant Foods Hum Nutr.* 1991;41:125–134.

Chamorro G, Salazar M, Favila L, Bourges H. Pharmacology and toxicology of Spirulina alga. *Rev Invest Clin.* 1996;48:389–399. *Abstract.*

Chamorro G, Salazar M. Teratogenic study of spirulina in mice. *Arch Latinoam Nutr.* 1990;40:86–94.

Spirulina: good source of beta-carotene, but no miracle food. *Environ Nutr.* 1995;18:7.

Gonzalez R, Rodriguez S, Romay C, et al. Anti-inflammatory activity of phycocyanin extract in acetic acid-induced colitis in rats. *Pharmacol Res.* 1999;39:1055–1059.

Hayashi K, Hayashi T, Kojima I. A natural sulfated polysaccharide, calcium spirulan, isolated from *Spirulina platensis*: in vitro and ex vivo evaluation of anti-herpes simplex virus and anti-human immunodeficiency virus activities. *AIDS Res Hum Retroviruses.* 1996;12:1463–1471.

Mathew B, Sankaranarayanan R, Nair PP, et al. Evaluation of chemoprevention of oral cancer with *Spirulina fusiformis. Nutr Cancer.* 1995;24:197–202.

Qureshi MA, Garlich JD, Kidd MT. Dietary *Spirulina platensis* enhances humoral and cell-mediated immune functions in chickens. *Immunopharmacol Immunotoxicol.* 1996;18:465–476.

Romay C, Armesto J, Remirez D, Gonzalez R, Ledon N, Garcia I. Antioxidant and anti-inflammatory properties of C-phycocyanin from blue-green algae. *Inflamm Res.* 1998;47:36–41.

Salazar M, Martinez E, Madrigal E, Ruiz LE, Chamorro GA. Subchronic toxicity study in mice fed *Spirulina maxima. J Ethnopharmacol.* 1998;62:235–241.

Shealy NC. *The Illustrated Encyclopedia of Healing Remedies.* Boston, Mass: Element Books; 1998:277.

Walker LP, Brown EH. *The Alternative Pharmacy.* Paramus, NJ: Prentice Hall Press; 1998:51–53.

■ SULFUR

OVERVIEW

The mineral sulfur has been used medicinally for more than 2,000 years. In *The Odyssey,* Homer describes burning sulfur to purify the air. This same practice was used during times of plague in Europe to disinfect contaminated areas. It is a constituent of the amino acids cystine, cysteine, and methionine, present in all cells of the body. It is considered non-toxic as any excess not used by the body is excreted in the urine and feces. Recognized as a "macromineral," it is found in significant amounts (>5g) in the body. About 0.25% of our body weight is sulfur. It is most prevalent in the keratin of skin, hair, and nails. It also is found as a component of the anti-coagulant heparin, and as chondriotin sulfate found in healthy bones and cartilage. Known as "nature's beauty mineral" it is fundamental for the synthesis of collagen which keeps the skin elastic and young-looking. Today, it is primarily used as a treatment for skin ailments such as eczema and other itchy skin conditions. It also aids oxidation reactions and protects the body against toxins which are increasingly present in our environment.

Arthritis sufferers flock to therapeutic sulfur hot springs to benefit from their pain-reducing effect, whether it be solely through the sulfur content, or through some action of other minerals. A 1992 Russian study determined that sulfur baths significantly lowered the pain sensitivity of patients with rheumatic diseases. An early study determined that taking sulfur baths raises the body's blood level of sulfur, in effect acting as a supplement, while other research indicates that sulfur is a desensitizing agent for the pain and discomfort experienced by cancer patients undergoing radiation therapy. Recent research suggests the reported beneficial effects of garlic (such as lowering cholesterol, blood pressure, and blood sugar) are at least partly due to the sulfur it contains.

DIETARY SOURCES

Because sulfur is a constituent of the amino acids cystine, cysteine, and methionine, it is found in protein-rich foods such as meat, organ meats, poultry, fish, eggs, cooked dried beans and peas, and milk and milk products. Other good sources include garlic, onions, brussel sprouts, asparagus, kale, and wheat germ.

CONSTITUENTS/COMPOSITION

Sulfur in its elemental form is a mineral found in rock beside hot springs and volcanic craters. It is found sparsely in elemental form, but is widely seen combined with other metals. The sulfur used in homeopathic treatment is a yellow-green powder extracted from the mineral. The characteristic "rotten egg" smell is caused from sulfur dioxide gas.

COMMERCIAL PREPARATIONS

Supplementation of sulfur is usually not necessary because most people get the required amount from dietary protein, but certain commercial preparations are available. To ease skin rashes, ointments, creams, lotions and dusting powders containing sulfur as the active ingredient are available. Organic sulfur in the form of MSM (metylsulfonylmethane) is available as a dietary supplement in tablets and capsules.

THERAPEUTIC USES

- Used to ease the red, itchy rash of eczema, candidiasis, dry scalp, diaper rash, hemorrhoids, and similar conditions
- Aids in digestive disorders, especially regurgitation of food, indigestion made worse by milk, and chronic diarrhea and vomiting in the morning
- To help gynecological complaints such as PMS and menopause symptoms
- To ease the symptoms of rheumatism, osteoarthritis, rheumatoid arthritis
- Can help acne; used as a topical antiseptic similar to benzoyl peroxide, but not as potent or irritating to the skin
- May aid mental stress such as depression, irritability, forgetfulness, disturbed sleep
- Good for eye health
- Can help treat offensive body odors
- Reported to reduce reaction to radiation therapy used in cancer treatment

DOSAGE RANGES AND DURATION OF ADMINISTRATION

There is no specific RDA established for sulfur. It is thought that approximately 850 mg/day is needed, considering the daily turnover of sulfur in the body.

For arthritis patients, 500 to 1,000 mg/day is the pharmacologic dosage range.

SIDE EFFECTS/TOXICOLOGY

No toxicity symptoms have been reported for elemental sulfur specifically since all excesses are excreted. However, some people are highly allergic to relatives of sulfur such as sulfites and sulfa drugs. Sulfites, sulfur-containing food preservatives, can trigger asthma and other allergic reactions in susceptible individuals. The major side effect of sulfa drugs is hypoglycemia, although other reactions include skin rashes, headache, fever, fatigue, and gastric distress. Sulfur-sensitive patients should avoid these drugs.

WARNINGS/CONTRAINDICATIONS/PRECAUTIONS

- Regarding sulfa drugs: Do not use during long-term corticosteroid use or pregnancy.
- Persons who are allergic to various sulfur containing compounds such as sulfites, sulfates and sulfa drugs, should probably avoid sulfur supplements as a precaution.
- Use sulfa drugs with caution in those who are elderly, alcoholic, or have impaired kidney or liver function.

INTERACTIONS

- Sulfur is a component of vitamin B_1, biotin, and the active form of pantothenic acid (also called co-enzyme A), which are required for metabolism and nerve health.
- Too much selenium can compete with sulfur. It can substitute itself for sulfur in the proteins of some enzymes, altering their functions.
- Arsenic poisoning is a result of arsenic's ability to bind with the sulfur portion of some amino acids, thus inactivating them.

REFERENCES

Balch J, Balch P. *Prescription for Nutritional Healing.* 2nd ed. Garden City, NY: Avery Publishing Group; 1997.

Eades MD. *The Doctor's Complete Guide to Vitamins and Minerals.* New York, NY: Dell Publishing; 1994.

Haas EM. *Staying Healthy with Nutrition.* Berkeley, Calif: Celestial Arts; 1992.

Lockie A. Geddes N. *The Complete Guide to Homeopathy.* New York, NY: DK Publishing; 1995.

Lester MR. Sulfite sensitivity: significance in human health. *J Am Coll Nutr.* 1995;14(3):229-32.

Mahan LK, Arlin MT. *Krause's Food, Nutrition and Diet Therapy.* 8th ed. Philadelphia, Pa: WB Saunders Company (Harcourt, Brace, Jovanovich, Inc.); 1992.

Martensson J. The effect of fasting on leucocyte and plasma glutathione and sulfur amino acid concentrations. *Metabolism.* 1986;35:118–121.

Midell E, Hopkins V. *Prescription Alternatives.* New Canaan, Conn: Keats Publishing; 1998.

The Mineral Connection website. MSM, Biologicial Sulfur supplements. Accessed at *www.mineralconnection.com/msm.htm* on March 5, 1999.

Murray MT; Pizzorno JE. *Encyclopedia of Natural Medicine.* Rev. 2nd edition. Rocklin, Calif: Prima Publishing; 1998.

Nutrition Search, Inc.. *Nutrition Almanac.* Rev. ed. New York, NY: McGraw-Hill; 1979.

Pratsel HG, Eigner UM, Weinert D, Limbach B. The analgesic efficacy of sulfur mud baths in treating rheumatic diseases of the soft tissues [In Russian]. *Vopr Kurortol Fizioter Lech Fiz Kult.* 1992;1992:37–41.

Roediger WE, Moore J, Babidge W. Colonic sulfide in pathogenesis and treatment of ulcerative colitis. *Dig Dis Sci.* 1997;42:1571–1579.

Rossi A, Kaitila I, Wilcox WR, et al. Proteoglycan sulfation in cartilage and cell cultures from patients with sulfate transporter chondrodysplasias: relationship to clinical severity and indications on the role of intracellular sulfate production. *Matrix Biol.* 1998;17:361–369.

Shealy CN. *The Illustrated Encyclopedia of Healing Remedies.* Boston, Mass: Element Books, Inc; 1998.

Smith SM, McDonald A, Webb D. *Complete Book of Vitamins and Minerals.* Lincolnwood, Ill: Publications International, Ltd; 1998.

Smirnova OV, Saliev VP, Klemparskaia NN, Dobronravova NN. Purified sulfur as an agent to relieve the side effects in the radiation therapy of cervical cancer [In Russian]. *Med Radiol Mosk.* 1991;36:16–19.

Somer E. *The Essential Guide to Vitamins and Minerals.* New York, NY: Harper Collins Publishers Inc; 1995.

Sukenik S, Giryes H, Halevy, et al. Treatment of psoriatic arthritis at the Dead Sea. *J Rheumatol.* 1994;21:1305–1309.

Weiner M. *The Complete Book of Homeopathy.* New York, NY: MJF Books; 1989.

Werbach MR. *Nutritional Influences on Illness: A Sourcebook of Clinical Research.* New Canaan, Conn: Keats Publishing, Inc; 1988.

■ TYROSINE

OVERVIEW

Tyrosine is a nonessential amino acid. It is synthesized in the body from phyenylalanine and is a precursor of adrenaline (epinephrine), norepinephrine, dopamine, thyroid hormones, and some types of estrogen. In order for tyrosine to metabolize into these substance, folic acid, niacin, vitamin C, and copper are needed. Low levels of tyrosine can lead to deficiencies in norepinephrine and dopamine—neurotransmitters that regulate mood. Depression can result. Animal studies have demonstrated that stressed animals have reduced levels of norepinephrine; however, administration of tyrosine prevented a norepinephrine deficiency. Tyrosine deficiency is also associated with low blood pressure, low body temperature, and restless leg syndrome.

Tyrosine aids in the the production of melanin (pigment responsible for hair and skin color) and in the functions of the adrenal, thryroid, and pituitary glands. A deficiency of tyrosine has been associated with hypothyroidism.

Because tyrosine binds unstable molecules that can potentially cause damage to the cells and tissues, it is considered a mild antioxidant. Thus, it may be useful in heavy smokers and in individuals exposed to chemicals and radiation.

DIETARY SOURCES

Although tyrosine is found in soy products, chicken, fish, almonds, avocados, bananas, dairy products, lima beans, pumpkin seeds, and sesame seeds, it is difficult to get therapeutic amounts of it from food. It is also produced from phenylalanine in the body.

CONSTITUENTS/COMPOSITION

N/A

COMMERCIAL PREPARATIONS

Many tyrosine supplements are available.

THERAPEUTIC USES

- Depression. Tyrosine appears to be a safe and effective treatment for depression; however, symptoms of depression recur when tyrosine is discontinued. Most data regarding tyrosine's efficacy in treating depression are anecdotal.
- Stress. Tyrosine seems to relieve the physical symptoms of stress if administered before the stressful situation, though limited human studies have been performed.
- Premenstrual syndrome (PMS). Though most data are anecdotal, tyrosine appears to help reduce the irritability, depression, and fatigue associated with PMS.
- Low sex drive. Tyrosine appears to stimulate the libido.
- Parkinson's disease. Parkinson's disease is treated with L-dopa, which is made from tyrosine; thus, the effects of tyrosine supplementation is being studied in Parkinson's disease patients.
- Weight loss. Tyrosine is an appetite suppressant and helps to reduce body fat.

- Chronic fatigue and narcolepsy. Tyrosine appears to have a mild stimulatory effect on the central nervous system.
- Drug detoxification. Tyrosine appears to be a successful adjunct for the treatment of cocaine abuse and withdrawal. It is often used in conjunction with tryptophan and imipramine (an antidepressant). In one study, 75% to 80% of patients treated with tyrosine stopped cocaine use completely or decreased usage by 50%. Successful withdrawal from caffeine and nicotine has also been anecdotally reported.
- Phenylketonuria (PKU). Tyrosine supplementation is advocated in patients with PKU; however, it is necessary to control plasma tyrosine levels (normal: 45 micromole/L) before tyrosine supplementation is considered.

DOSAGE RANGES AND DURATION OF ADMINISTRATION

- For depression, premenstrual syndrome, and chronic fatigue, a 500 to 1,000 mg dose before each of three meals is recommended.
- For stress, 1500 mg/day is recommended.
- For low sex drive, Parkinson's disease, drug detoxification, and weight loss, 1 to 2 g/day in divided doses is recommended.
- It appears that up to 12 g/day of tyrosine can be ingested safely. However, high-dose therapy should be monitored by a health care provider.

SIDE EFFECTS/TOXICOLOGY

- Migraine headache
- High blood pressure
- Mild gastric upset
- Promotes cancer cell division

WARNINGS/CONTRAINDICATIONS/PRECAUTIONS

Tyrosine should not be given to patients who are taking monoamine oxidase (MAO) inhibitors for depression or to patients with high blood pressure because it can cause dangerously high blood pressure elevations. Tyrosine may also promote the growth of malignant melanoma by promoting the division of cancer cells.

Amino acids should not be taken regularly; ingestion may inhibit the body's natural production of these chemicals.

INTERACTIONS

Some researchers feel that tyrosine is more effective if it is taken with up to 25 mg of vitamin B_6. It should be taken 30 minutes before meals three times a day on an empty stomach (with juice or water). Tyrosine should not be taken with other amino acids or proteins such as milk.

REFERENCES

Balch JF, Balch PA. *Prescriptions for Nutritional Healing.* 2nd ed. Garden City Park, NY: Avery Publishing; 1997:42.

Haas EM. *Staying Healthy with Nutrition.* Berkeley, Calif: Celestial Arts; 1992:51.

Mindell E, Hopkins V. Prescription Alternatives. New Canaan, Conn: Keats Publishing; 1998:398.

Shealy CN. *The Illustrated Encyclopedia of Healing Remedies.* Shaftesbury, England: Element; 1998:269

Werbach MR. *Nutritional Influences on Illness.* New Canaan, Conn: Keats Publishing, 1987:162.

■ VANADIUM

OVERVIEW

Vanadium is an essential trace mineral. Although scientists know very little about how vanadium functions in humans, they believe that at the very least it is necessary for bone and tooth formation. One hundred years ago, vanadium was administered as a cure for various diseases, but it was toxic at the high doses that were prescribed. Based on animal studies, scientists believe that a lack of vanadium may result in high cholesterol and triglyceride levels, poor blood sugar control (e.g., diabetes or hypoglycemia), and cardiovascular and kidney disease.

Some experts believe that most American diets provide from 20 to 60 mcg of vanadium per day; others believe that the amount is many times that. At any given time, the body contains 25 to 100 mg of vanadium. It is present in varying amounts in the soil and in many foods. It can also be inhaled from the air as a result of burning petroleum or petroleum products. Deficiency states in humans have not been described, and no RDA has been established. Vanadium is poorly absorbed by the body once ingested, with as much as 95% eliminated.

Recently, a derivative of vanadium, peroxovanadium, has been used in experimental animals. It was 50 times more potent than vanadate in normalizing blood sugar without the toxicity shown by vanadium. Tests in humans have not been completed.

DIETARY SOURCES

While vanadium is found in many foods, the best sources are sunflower, safflower, corn, and olive oils, as well as buckwheat, parsley, oats, rice, green beans, carrots, cabbage, pepper, and dill. It is also found in shellfish. Vanadium supplementation for a healthy person is rarely necessary. Eating any of the above foods should supply a sufficient quantity.

CONSTITUENTS/COMPOSITION

Vanadium exists in several forms including vanadyl or vanadate. Vanadyl sulfate is most commonly found in nutritional supplements. There are at least three other forms of vanadium less biologically significant.

COMMERCIAL PREPARATIONS

Over-the-counter doses of vanadium are 30 to 60 mg/day in pill form.

THERAPEUTIC USES

- Diabetes (15 to 100 mg/day). Vanadium improves insulin sensitivity and glucose tolerance in type I and type II diabetes mellitus in experimental animals; however, supporting data on humans are not available.
- Bones and teeth. Vanadium improves the mineralization of bones and teeth in experimental animals.
- Body building (0.5 mg/kg/day). Studies have been unable to determine definitively any performance-enhancing effects of vanadium.
- High cholesterol. Vanadium seems to have the ability to reduce cholesterol in experimental animals.
- Heart disease. Rates of heart disease are low in areas of the world (e.g., South America) where the soil contains high levels of vanadium.

DOSAGE RANGES AND DURATION OF ADMINISTRATION

Taking 50 to 100 mcg/day of vanadium is enough to meet or exceed nutritional requirements, without risking toxicity. Some manufacturers promote high dosages (15 to 100 mg) of vanadyl sulfate per day, but clinical data do not warrant such dosages at this time. Because deficiency states have not been described and nontoxic therapeutic dosages have not been determined, caution should be taken when using vanadium as a nutritional supplement. Bodybuilders and persons with diabetes are tempted to take high doses because of its purported ability to improve or mimic insulin action.

SIDE EFFECTS/TOXICOLOGY

Animal studies have not been successful in proving the efficacy and safety of vanadium. Death rates for laboratory animals are high when doses required to reduce blood sugar are administered. In lower doses, high blood pressure elevation and tremor have also been reported. High levels of vanadium may also contribute to some bone and kidney diseases. Additional problems reported include:

- Gastrointestinal upset with low doses
- Manic depression with high doses
- Inhibition of protein synthesis
- Pulmonary irritation from inhaled vanadium dust (e.g., petroleum workers)
- Oxidative damage to beta cells

WARNINGS/CONTRAINDICATIONS/PRECAUTIONS

Although vanadium is inhaled wherever petroleum is burned, it is not usually a cause for concern. However, extremely high doses (e.g., in workers who clean petroleum storage tanks) appear to irritate the lungs and may turn the tongue green, but neither symptom appears to cause any long-term or serious problem. High levels of vanadium may cause manic depression.

INTERACTIONS

- The effects of vanadium are reduced by some psychiatric medications (e.g., phenothiazines, monoamine oxidase inhibitors).
- Vanadium inhibits sodium-potassium pump activity; however, lithium, which is used in the treatment of manic depression, can reverse or reduce this inhibition.
- Ascorbic acid, ethylenediaminetetraacetic acid (EDTA), and methylene blue decrease vanadium levels in the body and thus are effective in treating manic depression in which vanadium levels are high.
- Tobacco decreases vanadium uptake.
- Vanadium and chromium should not be taken together.

REFERENCES

Balch JF, Balch PA. *Prescription for Nutritional Healing.* Garden City Park, NY: Avery Publishing; 1997:29.

Bender DA, Bender AE. *Nutrition: A Reference Handbook.* New York, NY: Oxford University Press; 1997:424.

Murray MT. *Encyclopedia of Nutritional Supplements.* Rocklin, Calif: Prima Publishing; 1996:232–234.

Murray MT, Pizzorno JE. *Encyclopedia of Natural Medicine.* 2nd ed. Rocklin, Calif: Prima Publishing; 1998:283–284.

Shealy CN. *The Illustrated Encyclopedia of Healing Remedies.* Boston, Mass: Element Books; 1998:268.

Role of vanadium as a mimic of insulin. *Nutri Res Newslett.* 1998;17:11.

Werbach MR. *Nutritional Influences on Illness.* New Canaan, Conn: Keats Publishing; 1987:87–88, 159.

Yale J-F, Lachance D, Bevan AP. Hypoglycemic effects of peroxovanadium compounds in Sprague-Dawley and diabetic BB rats. *Diabetes.* 1995;44:1274–1276.

■ VITAMIN A (RETINOL)

OVERVIEW

Vitamin A is a fat-soluble vitamin necessary for maintaining vision, epithelial (mucous) membranes, bone growth, and immunity. Most commonly known for its importance in preventing "night-blindness," vitamin A is an important part of the visual pigment molecules present in all retinal cells (both rods and cones) and plays a vital role in both day and night vision. Vitamin A has long been known as the "anti-infective" vitamin and plays an important role in the proper functioning of the immune system. Vitamin A maintains the integrity of all mucous membranes, which is the body's first line of defense against infection. When the body is deficient in vitamin A, mucus-producing cells are replaced by keratin-producing cells. The secretion of mucus diminishes and the mucous membranes become tough and relatively inflexible, leaving the body defenseless against invading organisms. Vitamin A stimulates white blood cell function and increases antibody response.

Vitamin A is required during the growth of cell membranes and also for repair of cell membranes during wound healing. Other functions of vitamin A include glycogen synthesis, protein metabolism, hormone synthesis, and as a coenzyme in the skin, bone, retina, liver, and adrenal glands.

DIETARY SOURCES

Vitamin A is only found in foods of animal origin. Beef, calf, and chicken liver are the richest sources. Vitamin A is also found naturally in whole milk and butter. Lowfat and skim milk is fortified to replace the vitamin A that is lost when the fat is removed from the milk. Dairy products supply about half of the vitamin A consumed by most individuals. The other half is supplied by fruits and vegetables that are rich in beta-carotene, the vitamin A precursor that is readily converted to vitamin A in the body. Beta-carotene is abundant in orange and dark green leafy vegetables and fruits. Refer to the section on beta-carotene for a full listing of good food sources.

CONSTITUENTS/COMPOSITION

There are three different forms of vitamin A: retinol, retinal, and retinoic acid. Retinal and retinoic acid appear to be the active forms of retinol. Retinal is primarily involved with vision and reproduction, while retinoic acid is important for growth and cell differentiation.

COMMERCIAL PREPARATIONS

Natural vitamin A is available as retinol or retinyl palmitate. All forms are easily absorbed. Supplemental vitamin A is available in tablets or capsules of 10,000 IU, 25,000 IU or 50,000 IU.

THERAPEUTIC USES

- Treatment of skin disorders, primarily acne and psoriasis
- Immune system enhancement, especially against viral infections
- Reduces infant mortality from measles
- Treatment of severe burns and other wounds
- Night blindness; hyperkeratosis

DOSAGE RANGES AND DURATION OF ADMINISTRATION

As of 1980, vitamin A is measured as *retinol equivalents* or RE. One RE corresponds to the biological activity of 1 mcg of retinol. However, supplemental vitamin A is still most commonly expressed in *international units* or IU. One RE is equal to 3.33 IU of retinol.

The current RDA's expressed in RE are 1,000 mcg RE for men, and 800 mcg RE for women. However, for convenience in determining supplement dosages, the following RDA information is expressed in both RE and IU.

• Infants up to 1 year:	1,875 IU	400 mcg RE
• 1 to 3 years:	2,000 IU	400 mcg RE
• 4 to 6 years:	2,500 IU	500 mcg RE
• 7 to 10 years:	3,500 IU	700 mcg RE
• Males over 10 years:	5,000 IU	1,000 mcg RE
• Females over 10 years:	4,000 IU	800 mcg RE
• Pregnant women:	5,000 IU	1,000 mcg RE
• Lactating women:	6,500 IU	1,200 mcg RE

To reverse vitamin A deficiency or to prevent deficiency during acute viral infection, a single oral dose of 50,000 IU for one or two days is safe even for infants. Adults and children over 8 years can tolerate up to 50,000 IU daily for up to two weeks. In general, daily doses of up to five times the RDA (25,000 IU for adults and 12,000 IU for children) have been found to be safe. However, a health care provider must continue to monitor any high dose therapy. This applies especially to treatments for skin disorders. For other health issues, beta-carotene is the preferred supplement, as it may be administered in significantly higher doses without the same risk of toxicity. Pregnant women must avoid any type of vitamin A supplements (beyond what is found in prenatal vitamins), due to the higher risk of birth defects.

SIDE EFFECTS/TOXICOLOGY

Vitamin A toxicity (hypervitaminosis A) has been widely studied. Tolerance varies among individuals and may be related to liver function status as well as other variables such as body weight. Doses of 1 million IUs taken daily for five years have been tolerated by some people, while others show symptoms of toxicity with doses as low as 25,000 IU per day. Children are most susceptible to vitamin A toxicity, especially if they take multiple vitamins along with fortified foods. Vitamin A toxicity in the fetus can occur if pregnant women take more than 6,000 IU per day.

Overdoses or chronic excesses affect the same body systems that are affected by vitamin A deficiency, and some of the symptoms of toxicity and deficiency are the same. The most common symptom of toxicity is increased intracranial pressure exhibited as chronic headache. Other symptoms of vitamin A toxicity and deficiency are as follows. Abdominal pain, muscle and joint pain, fatigue, dry, cracking skin and lips, dry eyes, conjunctivitis, alopecia, anorexia, nausea, diarrhea, leukocytosis, and bone fractures.

WARNINGS/CONTRAINDICATIONS/PRECAUTIONS

Supplementation with vitamin A over 6,000 IU/day is associated with birth defects, and pregnant women should avoid any vitamin A treatments or supplements beyond what is contained in prenatal vitamins.

Patients must be closely monitored by their provider for any symptoms of toxicity during high dose therapy for skin conditions using isotretinoin (Accutane).

Most multivitamins contain the RDA of 5,000 IU of vitamin A. Dairy products and fortified foods contribute an additional 2,500 IU/day or more. Patients should be careful of using additional fish liver oil supplements or products formulated for "eye health," "immune system enhancement," "skin formulas," "acne formulas," or "bone or joint repair." Any of these formulas are likely to contain additional vitamin A. Always check the labels for vitamin A content, and be careful that daily intake does not exceed the recommended safety levels.

Vitamin A is contraindicated for use in individuals with chronic kidney or liver disease.

Overuse of alcohol makes vitamin A toxicity more likely to occur.

INTERACTIONS

In general, adequate intake of fat, protein, vitamin E, and zinc are needed for the body to properly absorb and use vitamin A. Vitamin E enhances the body's use of vitamin A. Supplementation with high doses of vitamin E decreases vitamin A stores in the body.

Adequate zinc and protein are required to produce retinol-binding protein, which picks up vitamin A in the liver and carries it into the blood stream. A minimum intake of 7 oz/day of protein is necessary for proper vitamin A usage.

Some medications, such as estrogens and oral contraceptives, may increase plasma retinol levels.

REFERENCES

Eades MD. *The Doctor's Complete Guide to Vitamins and Minerals.* New York, NY: Dell Publishing; 1994:48.

Fawzi WW. Vitamin A supplementation and child mortality. *JAMA.* 1993;269:898–903.

Fawzi WW, Mbise RL, Hertzmark E, et al. A randomized trial of vitamin A supplements in relation to mortality among human immunodeficiency virus-infected and uninfected children in Tanzania. *Pediatr Infect Dis J.* 1999;18:127–133.

Fortes C, Forastiere F, Agabiti N, et al. The effect of zinc and vitamin A supplementation on immune response in an older population. *J Am Geriatr Soc.* 1998;46:19–26.

Futoryan T, Gilchrest BA. Retinoids and the skin. *Nutr Rev.* 1994;52:299–310.

Kindmark A, Rollman O, Mallmin H, et al. Oral isotretinoin therapy in severe acne induces transient suppression of biochemical markers of bone turnover and calcium homeostasis. *Acta Derma Venereol.* 1998;78:266–269.

Melhus H, Michaelsson K, Kindmark A, et al. Excessive dietary intake of vitamin A is associated with reduced bone mineral density and increased risk for hip fracture. *Ann Intern Med.* 1998;129:770–778.

Murray M. *Encyclopedia of Nutritional Supplements.* Rocklin, Calif: Prima Publishing; 1996.

Nursing '93 Drug Handbook. Springhouse, Pa: Springhouse Corporation; 1993.

Semba RD. Vitamin A, immunity and infection. *Clin Infect Dis.* 1994;19:489–499.

Whitney E, Cataldo C, Rolfes S. *Understanding Normal and Clinical Nutrition.* St. Paul, Minn: West Publishing Company; 1987.

■ VITAMIN B₁ (THIAMINE)

OVERVIEW

Vitamin B_1 (thiamine) is a water-soluble vitamin. Intake of vitamin B_1 is required on a regular basis due to the body's inability to store it in large amounts. Vitamin B_1 is absorbed from the lumen of the intestine by an active transport process. In the mucosal cells of the duodenum, vitamin B_1 is phosphorylated resulting in thiamine monophosphate (TMP), thiamine pyrophosphate (TPP), and thiamine triphosphate (TTP). The most physiologically active and abundant form of the vitamin in the body is TPP. In carbohydrate metabolism, TPP functions as a coenzyme in the decarboxylation of alpha-ketoacids such as pyruvate and in transketolation. Decarboxylation of alpha-ketoacids produces energy, which can be used by cells, and transketolation reactions yield pentoses, which can be used for nucleic acid synthesis, and NADPH, which is used in fatty acid synthesis. In neuronal cells, a noncoenzymatic role for vitamin B_1, in which it modulates brain chloride channels, has also been described.

The disease of vitamin B_1 deficiency is called beri beri. Beri beri is characterized by neurological symptoms ('dry' beri beri) and cardiovascular symptoms ('wet' beri beri). Beri beri became widespread in East Asia in the nineteenth century when polished rice, which lacked the vitamin B_1-rich husks, became a diet staple. Major causes of vitamin B_1 deficiency in today's society are alcoholism and inadequate intake of vitamin B_1; the latter cause occurring mostly in less industrialized countries. Treating beri beri patients with vitamin B_1 reduces the symptoms of the disease.

Recent studies suggest a role for vitamin B_1 in the management of congestive heart failure. Patients given the loop diuretic furosemide may be at greater risk for vitamin B_1 deficiency through urinary loss, which can lead to wet beri beri and can contribute to cardiac insufficiency. In these patients, supplementation with thiamine results in improved cardiac conditions.

Vitamin B_1 may also play a negative role in cancer chemotherapy. Researchers have found that the overadministration of vitamin B_1 to chemotherapy patients may aid the tumor cells by providing ribose via transketolation as a substrate for nucleic acid synthesis and ultimately tumor growth.

NATURAL SOURCES

- Pork
- Wheat germ
- Grain cereals
- Brewer's yeast
- White enriched rice
- Soy milk
- Sunflower seeds
- Beans
- Pasta
- Peanuts (unroasted)

Brewer's yeast is the richest source of vitamin B_1. Although milk, fruits, and vegetables are not rich in vitamin B_1, they contribute significantly to the recommended daily allowance of vitamin B_1 when consumed in sufficient amounts.

CONSTITUENTS/COMPOSITION

The vitamin B_1 molecule consists of pyrimidine and thiazole rings connected by a methylene bridge. In its pure form, thiamine hydrochloride is a crystalline yellowish-white powder with a salty, nut-like taste. It is fairly stable in dry form and is only heat stable in acid form. Its stability in prepared food is dependent on cooking time and temperature, pH, amount of water used and discarded, and whether the water used was chlorinated.

Sulfites, which are used in the production and processing of food, destroy the biological activity of vitamin B_1 by splitting the molecule into its pyrimidine and thiazole moieties.

COMMERCIAL PREPARATION

Vitamin B_1 is available commercially in salt form as thiamine hydrochloride and thiamine mononitrate. Standard preparations are available as 50-mg, 100-mg, and 300-mg doses in vitamin B_1 tablets or capsules; 50-mg, 125-mg, and 150-mg doses in B-complex capsules or tablets, and in 1.5-mg doses in multivitamins (both adult and children's chewable).

THERAPEUTIC USES

Therapeutic uses are limited to conditions that are caused by vitamin B_1 deficiency and prophylactic treatment of vitamin B_1 deficiency.

- Dry beri beri. Symptoms of dry beri beri include peripheral neuritis with sensory disturbances in the extremities, convulsions, exaggeration of tendon reflexes, and the "burning feet syndrome." This is usually observed in chronic alcoholics. Chronic alcoholics with these symptoms should receive up to 40 mg of oral vitamin B_1 daily.

- Wernicke's encephalopathy. This is a vitamin B_1 deficiency that affects the central nervous system. Classic symptoms are confusion, ophthalmoplegia, nystagmus, and ataxia. A typical treatment consists of 100 mg of intravenous vitamin B_1 daily for three days. If left untreated, Wernicke's encephalopathy can lead to Korsakoff's psychosis, which is characterized by confabulation and in most cases is not treatable once established.

- Cardiovascular disease. This is also called wet beri beri and is characterized by heart hypertrophy, dilatation, tachycardia, respiratory distress, and edema of the legs. Treatment with vitamin B_1 will lead to striking recovery if vitamin B_1 deficiency is the true cause of the disease. A typical therapy regimen is 10 to 30 mg of parenteral vitamin B_1 tid until symptoms reverse.

- Infantile beri beri. Infantile beri beri is seen mostly in breast-fed infants of vitamin B_1-deficient mothers, which mainly occurs in less industrialized countries. Symptoms include loss of appetite, vomiting, constipation, greenish stools, and progressive edema. Loss of laryngeal nerve function, which leads to aphonia, is a diagnostic feature. In acute disease decreased urine output and cardiac failure occurs. Infants with a mild form of the disease can be treated with 10 mg of oral vitamin B_1 daily. Twenty-five mg of intravenous vitamin B_1 should be administered to infants with acute cardiac failure, although the prognosis is poor. This treatment should be conducted only under physician supervision.

- Gastrointestinal disorders. In some patients vitamin B_1 deficiency affects the gastrointestinal tract. When this occurs, vitamin B_1 replacement can relieve symptoms such as ulcerative colitis, diarrhea, and gastrointestinal hypotonia.

- Neuritis of pregnancy. This is caused by hyperemesis gravidarum or low vitamin B_1 intake. If vitamin B_1 deficiency is the cause of the neuritis, clinical improvement will be seen following vitamin B_1 therapy. A typical therapy regimen is 5 to 10 mg of vitamin B_1 daily, given parenterally if vomiting is severe.

- Congenital defects. Maple syrup disease, congenital lactate acidosis, subacute necrotizing encephalopathy, and vitamin B_1-responsive megaloblastic anemia are inherited diseases with congenital defects in vitamin B_1 metabolism. Vitamin B_1 therapy has been reported to improve these conditions.

- Prophylaxis. Patients receiving parenteral nutrition and those whose vitamin B_1 status is suspect (comatose patients, alcoholics) should be given vitamin B_1 supplementation before receiving dextrose-containing solutions.

DOSAGE RANGES AND DURATION OF ADMINISTRATION

- Neonates to 6 months: 0.3 mg/day
- Infants 6 months to 1 year: 0.4 mg/day
- Children 1 to 3 years: 0.7 mg/day
- Children 4 to 6 years: 0.9 mg/day
- Children 7 to 10 years: 1.0 mg/day
- Boys over 11 years, men 18 to 50 years: 1.5 mg/day
- Men over 50 years: 1.2 mg/day
- Girls over 11 years, women 18 to 50 years: 1.1 mg/day
- Women more than 51 years: 1.0 mg/day
- Pregnant women: 1.5 mg/day; lactating women: 1.6 mg/day.

SIDE EFFECTS/TOXICOLOGY

Vitamin B_1 is relatively nontoxic. Some gastric disturbance may be seen at very high oral doses. Exceeding the RDA for vitamin B_1 by more than 100-fold has in rare instances led to an allergic reaction.

WARNINGS/CONTRAINDICATIONS/PRECAUTIONS

Vitamin B_1 may play a role in failed chemotherapy in cancer patients who receive doses that are 200-fold over the RDA.

INTERACTIONS

Furosemide may lead to vitamin B_1 deficiency in patients with congestive heart failure. Chronic alcoholism inhibits absorption of vitamin B_1 from the intestinal lumen.

REFERENCES

Hardman JG, Limbird LE, eds. *Goodman and Gilman's The Pharmacological Basis of Therapeutics.* 9th ed. New York, NY: McGraw-Hill; 1996:1555–1558.

Mahan LK, Arlin MT, eds. *Krause's Food, Nutrition and Diet Therapy.* 8th ed. Philadelphia, Pa: WB Saunders;1992:85–87.

Ekhard ZE, Filer LJ, eds. *Present Knowledge in Nutrition.* 7th ed. Washington, DC: ILIS Press; 1996:160–166.

Mason P. *Nutrition and Dietary Advice in the Pharmacy.* Oxford, UK: Blackwell Scientific; 1994:269–271.

Boros LG, Brandes JL, Lee W-N P, et al. Thiamine supplementation to cancer patients: a double-edged sword. *Anticancer Res.* 1998;18:595–602.

Leslie D, Gheorghiade M. Is there a role for thiamine supplementation in the management of heart failure? *Am Heart J.* 1996;131:1248–1250.

Lindberg MC, Oyler RA. Wernick's encephalopathy. *Am Fam Physician.* 1990;41:1205–1209.

National Academy of Science. Recommended Daily Allowances. Accessed at www.nal.usda.gov/fnic/dietary/rda.html on January 4, 1999.

■ VITAMIN B₂ (RIBOFLAVIN)

OVERVIEW

Riboflavin is a water-soluble, heat-stable vitamin. It is a component of two flavin coenzymes, flavin-adenine dinucleotide (FAD) and flavin mononucleotide (FMN). These coenzymes are intermediaries in electron transport in many oxidative-reduction reactions throughout the body. Riboflavin is essential to tissue respiration and to the generation of energy metabolism from carbohydrates, proteins, and fats. Riboflavin is necessary for normal development and repair of the immune system and of body tissues such as skin, hair, nails, and connective tissue. Recent studies suggest that riboflavin may be an effective low-cost preventive treatment for migraine headaches. A proposed mechanism for this effect suggests that migraines result from a reduction of energy production in the mitrocondria, and riboflavin increases mitocondrial energy efficiency. In a 1998 study from Belgium, patients who suffered from migraines were given 400 mg of riboflavin a day for three months. Other patients also received a daily dose of aspirin. Fifty-nine percent of patients in the riboflavin groups showed at least a 50% improvement compared to 15% in the placebo group.

Animal studies suggest that elevated riboflavin levels protect against oxidative damage. Studies have shown reduced myocardial damage after an ischemic event, prevention of nerve damage after stroke, and minimization of oxidative damage resulting from the introduction of toxins.

Riboflavin supplements may help in the treatment of sickle cell anemia. They may also help in the treatment of anemia by enhancing the efficacy of iron.

Riboflavin, in combination with B₆, helps relieve the symptoms of carpal tunnel syndrome.

Some studies suggest that riboflavin abnormalities are associated with cataract development. A New York State Lens Opacities Case-Control Study evaluated the risk factors for various types of cataracts. Among the 1,380 participants (ages 40 to 79 years), they found that the risk for cataracts increased if the levels of certain nutrients, including riboflavin, were low. Glutathione, an enzyme that helps protect the eye, requires riboflavin to work effectively. Other studies have suggested no relationship between riboflavin and cataracts; some studies suggest that high-dose riboflavin can induce cataracts. Thirty-three percent of the geriatric population has riboflavin deficiency. High-level supplementation in this population, however, may be contraindicated.

A recent study evaluated the links between rheumatoid arthritis and riboflavin status in individuals with and without the disease. Biochemical riboflavin deficiency was more frequent in those with active disease. Riboflavin deficiency may reduce the activity and effect of glutathione, an enzyme that works to prevent inflammation involved in rheumatoid arthritis.

Frank deficiency of riboflavin is rare. However, subclinical deficiency is common in certain populations, including those with lactose intolerance, malabsorptive disorders, diarrhea, and irritable bowel syndrome. The elderly, whose diets are low in red meats and dairy products, may also be at risk for mild riboflavin deficiency. Systemic infection, with or without gastrointestinal tract involvement, may increase the body's need for riboflavin. Symptoms of riboflavin deficiency include cracking of lips and corner of the mouth, swollen, inflamed tongue, visual disturbances such as sensitivity to light and cataract formation, anemia, and dermatitis.

DIETARY SOURCES

- Brewer's yeast
- Almonds
- Organ meats
- Whole grains
- Wheat germ
- Wild rice
- Mushrooms
- Soybeans
- Milk
- Spinach

Flours and cereals are enriched with riboflavin. Riboflavin is destroyed by light and alkalis, but not by heat, although it will leach into cooking water. To retain riboflavin content, foods should be stored in dark containers.

CONSTITUENTS/COMPOSITION

Riboflavin supplements are available in two forms: simple riboflavin or riboflavin-5-phosphate (the activated form).

COMMERCIAL PREPARATIONS

Riboflavin is available in multivitamin preparations, in B-complex vitamins, and as riboflavin and activated riboflavin, in 25-, 50-, and 100-mg tablets.

THERAPEUTIC USES

- Indicated for sickle cell anemia
- Preventive measure for migraine headaches
- May relieve rheumatoid arthritis
- May be useful in treating cataracts secondary to deficiency
- Part of therapy to relieve carpal tunnel syndrome
- Reduces the effects of stress
- Skin problems such as acne (especially acne rosacea), dermatitis, eczema, and ulcers may improve with supplementation
- May improve muscle cramps
- Indicated when initiating any B vitamin supplementation
- Enhances immune function
- Preventive against free radical damage

DOSAGE RANGES AND DURATION OF ADMINISTRATION

RDA for riboflavin is listed below.
- Children 1 to 3 years: 0.5 mg/day
- Children 4 to 8 years: 0.6 mg/day
- Children 9 to 13 years: 0.9 mg/day
- Men 14 years and older: 1.3 mg/day
- Women 14 to 19 years: 1.0 mg/day
- Women during pregnancy: 1.4 mg/day
- Women during lactation: 1.6 mg/day

SIDE EFFECTS/TOXICOLOGY

The body does not absorb high doses (>20 mg) of riboflavin well, making toxicity rare. Reactions to excess doses may include itching, numbness, burning or prickling sensations, and sensitivity to light.

WARNINGS/CONTRAINDICATIONS/PRECAUTIONS

Urine will become discolored with high doses of riboflavin. This can affect urinalysis results.

INTERACTIONS

- Riboflavin is essential to the activation of B₆ (pyridoxine) and interacts with B₁ (thiamine).

- Riboflavin is vital to the conversion of tryptophan to B$_3$ (niacin).
- Riboflavin metabolism can be affected by sulfa drugs, anti-malaria drugs, estrogen, cathartic agents, and alcohol.
- The effectiveness of the anticancer drug methotrexate may be reduced by high doses of riboflavin.
- Riboflavin excretion many be increased by taking some antibiotics and phenothiazine drugs.
- Riboflavin is activated in the liver. Major tranquilizers and some antidepressants may inhibit this activation.
- Riboflavin status may be adversely affected by long-term use of barbituates.
- Riboflavin may be destroyed during treatment of neonatal jaundice.

REFERENCES

Schoenen J, Jacquy J, Lenaerts M. Effectiveness of high-dose riboflavin in migraneprophilaxis. A randomized controlled trial. *Neurology.* February 1998;50:466–470.

Realey N. *Vitmains Etc.* Melbourne, Australia: Bookman Press; 1998.

Murray MT. *Encyclopedia of Nutritional Supplements.* Rocklin, Calif: Prima Health; 1996.

1999 Drug Facts and Comparisons. New York, NY: J.B. Lippincott Company; 1998.

Christenson, H. Riboflavin can protect tissues from oxidative injury. *Nutr Rev.* May 1993;51:149–150.

Matarese L, Gottschlich M. *Contemporary Nutrition Support Practice. A Clinical Guide.* Philadelphia, Pa: WB Saunders Company; 1998.

Duyff R. *The American Dietary Association Complete Food and Nutrition Guide.* Minneapolis, Minn: Cronimed Publishing; 1996.

Food and Nutrition Board, Institute of Medicine. Dietary Reference Intakes for Thiamin, Riboflavin, Niacin, Vitamin B6, Folate, Vitamin B12, Pantothenic Acid, Biotin, and Choline. Washington, DC: National Academy Press; 1998.

■ VITAMIN B₃ (NIACIN)

OVERVIEW

Vitamin B₃ (niacin) is a water-soluble vitamin, absorbed in the small intestine and excreted in the urine. Because it is not stored, it is needed in frequent, small doses. Because it is easily excreted, it is also less likely to reach toxic levels; however, therapeutic dosing in the treatment of high blood cholesterol levels can cause dangerous side effects, especially liver problems, and must be monitored closely.

The human body uses niacin in more than 50 chemical reactions. Working together with various enzymes (co-enzyme activity), niacin is instrumental in the release of energy from carbohydrates which fuels all body systems. It is necessary for proper central nervous system (brain) function. It is also involved in fat and cholesterol metabolism and the manufacture of many body compounds including sex and adrenal hormones. Other functions of vitamin B₃ include the regulation of blood sugar, antioxidant mechanisms, and detoxification reactions.

DIETARY SOURCES

Fifty percent of the niacin used by the body comes from the conversion of the amino acid tryptophan. Therefore, the richest sources of niacin are protein-rich foods such as extra-lean meats, chicken, fish, eggs, cooked dried beans and peas, brewer's yeast, liver and other organ meats, nonfat/lowfat milk and cheese, soybeans, and nuts. Other sources are enriched bread and cereals, and whole grains (except corn). The most abundant vegetable sources are mushrooms and greens. It is better to steam, bake, or stir-fry vegetables, as niacin may be lost in cooking water.

CONSTITUENTS/COMPOSITION

There are two main forms of vitamin B₃: niacin (nicotinic acid, nicotinate) and niacinamide (nicotinamide). The amide form (niacinamide) has no vasodilator action nor any effect on serum lipids in the treatment of high cholesterol. Therefore, niacin is the form prescribed for lowering cholesterol levels, while niacinamide is preferred for arthritis and Type 1 diabetes. Preformed niacin is available from vegetable sources such as brewer's yeast, wheat germ, and nuts; however, most of the niacin our bodies use is that which is converted from the amino acid tryptophan provided by protein sources.

COMMERCIAL PREPARATIONS

Niacin is available in the following forms.
- Tablets: 25 mg, 50 mg, 100 mg, 250 mg, 500 mg
- Elixer: 50 mg/5 ml
- Injection: 30 ml vials, 100 mg/ml

Timed-release capsules and tablets are widely available and were devised to help reduce "niacin flush" (a flushing of the face caused by capillary dilation). However, several studies have shown a significant increase in liver damage associated with the use of this type of preparation. Most literature suggests that sustained-release niacin should not be used because of its potential damage to the liver. Two recent eastern European studies indicate that wax-coated sustained-release niacin does not have undesirable side effects. But until further studies can be done, it would be prudent to avoid timed-release preparations of niacin.

Niacinamide is available in the following forms:
- Tablets: 50 mg, 100 mg, 500 mg
- Tablets (timed-release): 1,000 mg
- Injection: 100 mg/ml

Niacin is also available as inositol hexaniacinate, a preparation developed in Europe. Inositol hexaniacinate is a natural sustained-release delivery method that is not thought to lead to liver disorders.

THERAPEUTIC USES

Niacin:
- Effective in reduction of LDL and triglyceride levels
- Increases HDL levels
- Reduces the risk of developing cardiovascular disease
- Has a synergystic effect when combined with other cholesterol-reducing medications

Niacinamide:
- May help osteoarthritis and rheumatoid arthritis
- May be effective in treatment and control of early-onset insulin-dependent (Type I) diabetes
- In combination with vitamins A and E, niacin (nicotinic acid) helps prevent and treat heart disease
- Varying success in treatment of schizophrenia, anxiety, depression, and other mental illnesses
- Used in the treatment of alcoholism
- May be beneficial in the treatment of hypoglycemia
- Has been used as a treatment for insomnia due to its sedative effects

DOSAGE RANGES AND DURATION OF ADMINISTRATION

Because niacin can be obtained from tryptophan, it is measured in "niacin equivalents" and is based on estimates from overall calorie consumption. The niacin RDA is 6.6 mg equivalents/1,000 kcals, or a minimum of 13 mg daily, which should be consumed to maintain tissue store in healthy adults. The 1989 RDAs for niacin are:
- Infants up to 6 months: 5 mg
- Infants 6 months to 1 year: 6 mg
- Children 1 to 3 years: 9 mg
- Children 4 to 6 years: 12 mg
- Children 7 to 10 years: 13 mg
- Males 11 to 14 years: 17 mg
- Males 15 to 18 years: 20 mg
- Males 19 to 50: 19 mg
- Males 50+: 15 mg
- Females 11 to 18 years: 15 mg
- Females 19 to 50: 15 mg
- Females 50+: 13 mg
- Females pregnant: 17 mg
- Females lactating: 20 mg

Requirements may be higher for those who have cancer, those who are being treated with isoniazid (for tuberculosis), women taking oral contraceptives, and people with protein deficiencies.

Therapeutic dosing in the treatment of high blood cholesterol levels is within the range of 1,500 to 2,000 mg of pure crystalline niacin daily in divided dosage. This level should be reached gradually over a period of four to six weeks. It should be taken with meals to minimize GI irritation.

Therapeutic doses of 150 mg/day have been reported to aid in migraine relief.

SIDE EFFECTS/TOXICOLOGY

The most common side effect of niacin at doses of 75 mg or more is "niacin flush," a sometimes painful tingling sensation and flushing of the face and upper torso caused by dilation of capillaries. Onset of niacin flush is seen 15 to 30 minutes after ingestion. While generally not harmful, it can be uncomfortable or frightening for some people. Niacin flush can be reduced or sometimes eliminated by the ingestion of 80 to 325 mg of aspirin 30 minutes prior to taking the niacin.

The most serious problem associated with high-dose niacin therapy is the risk of liver toxicity. Doses over 2,000 mg increase the risk of abnormal liver function and necessitate frequent monitoring. Side effects can be reduced by developing tolerance to niacin supplementation over several weeks. Starting at low doses and increasing every four to seven days up to a therapeutic dose (500 to 2 g/day) may help reduce the amount of flushing and also reduce the risk of liver toxicity. Niacin flush is caused by a release of histamines; therefore, asthma sufferers should avoid high doses.

Other side effects of high doses of niacin include heartburn, nausea, vomiting, diarrhea, ulcers, liver malfunction, low blood pressure, and fainting. High doses of niacin (nicotinic acid) can also increase the blood levels of uric acid and glucose, leading to possible misdiagnosis of diabetes or gout.

Niacinamide does not cause niacin flush even at high doses, but also does not provide the beneficial cholesterol-lowering effects of niacin. Niacinamide can also have a sedative effect. Inositol hexaniacinate is an effective delivery method not thought to cause liver problems.

WARNINGS/CONTRAINDICATIONS/PRECAUTIONS

Niacin supplementation at therapeutic doses can cause liver damage and peptic ulcers; therefore, persons with a history of these ailments should not take large doses. Asthma sufferers should not take more than 75 mg of niacin due to histamine release, but can safely take niacinamide for dietary supplementation or other purposes. Diabetics, gallbladder patients, and gout patients should be supervised closely by a health care practitioner if taking therapeutic doses of niacinamide. Due to side effects, therapeutic dosing needs to be monitored closely by a health care practitioner to avoid toxic effects. Liver function and blood glucose should be closely monitored in all patients early in therapy.

INTERACTIONS

- Vitamin B_3 (niacin) is intrinsically involved with other B vitamins to maintain proper cell function and energy release.
- Vitamin B_2 is required for conversion of tryptophan to niacin.
- Niacin can be combined with other lipid-reducing drugs to promote efficacy in treatment of high cholesterol.
- Niacin may reduce the toxic effects of adriamycin in cancer treatment.
- Niacinamide may enhance effectiveness of anti-epileptic medications such as phenobarbitol or primidone.
- Tryptophan competes with another amino acid, leucine; therefore, chronic excess intake of leucine can cause secondary tryptophan and niacin deficiency.
- When taken with antihypertensive drugs (sympathetic blocking type), it may have an additive vasodilating effect and cause postural hypotension. Use together cautiously.
- Excessive alcohol intake can diminish stores or interfere with absorption of niacinamide.

REFERENCES

Aronov DM, Keenan JM, Akhmedzhanov NM, Perova NV, Oganove RY, Kiseteva NY. Clinical trial of wax-matrix sustained-release niacin in a Russian population with hypercholesterolemia. *Arch Fam Med.* 1996;5:567–575.

Berge KG, Canner PL. Coronary drug project: experience with niacin. Coronary Drug Project Research Group. Eur J Clin Pharmacol. 1991;40(suppl 1):S49–S51.

Boden G, Chen X, Igbal N. Acute lowering of plasma fatty acids lowers basal insulin secretion in diabetic and nondiabetic subjects. *Diabetes.* 1998;47:1609–1612.

Capuzzi DM, Guyton JR, Morgan JM, et al. Efficacy and safety of an extended-release niacin (Niaspan): a long-term study. *Am J Cardiol.* Dec 17, 1998;82:74U–81U.

Chojnowska-Jezierska J, Adamska-Dyniewska H. Prolonged treatment with slow-release nicotinic acid in patients with type II hyperlipidemia. *Pol Arch Med Wewn.* 1997;98:391–399.

Eades MD. *The Doctor's Complete Guide to Vitamins and Minerals.* New York, NY: Dell Publishing; 1994.

Gardner SF, Schneider EF, Granberry MC, Carter IR. Combination therapy with low-dose lovastatin and niacin is as effective as higher-dose lovastatin. *Pharmacotherapy.* 1996;16:419–423.

Guyton JR. Effect of niacin on atherosclerotic cardiovascular disease. *Am J Cardiol.* Dec 17, 1998;82:18U–23U.

Guyton JR, Capuzzi DM. Treatment of hyperlipidemia with combined niacin-statin regimens. *Am J Cardiol.* Dec 17, 1998;82:82U–84U.

Hendler SS. *The Doctor's Vitamin and Mineral Encyclopedia.* New York, NY: Simon and Schuster; 1990.

Hocking GM. *A Dictionary of Natural Products.* Medford, NJ: Plexus Publishing, Inc; 1997.

Harborne JB, Baxter H, eds. *Phytochemical Dictionary: A Handbook of Bioactive Compounds from Plants.* Rev. ed. London, England: Taylor & Francis; 1995.

Lieberman S, Bruning N. *The Real Vitamin and Mineral Book.* Garden City Park, NY: Avery Publishing Group, Inc; 1990.

Lomnicky Y, Friedman M, Luria MH, Raz I, Hoffman A. The effect of the mode of administration on the hypolipidaemic activity of niacin: continuous gastrointestinal administration of low-dose niacin improves lipid-lowering efficacy in experimentally-induced hyperlipidaemic rats. *J Pharm Pharmacol.* 1998;50:1233–1239.

Mostaza JM, Schulz I, Vega GL, Grundy SM. Comparison of pravastatin with crystalline nicotinic acid monotherapy in treatment of combined hyperlipidemia. *Am J Cardiol.* 1997;79:1298–1301.

Murray MT. *Encyclopedia of Nutritional Supplements.* Rocklin, Calif: Prima Publishing; 1996.

Nursing 93 Drug Handbook. Springhouse, Pa: Springhouse Corporation; 1993.

Nutrition Search, Inc. *Nutrition Almanac.* Rev. ed. New York, NY: McGraw-Hill, 1979.

O'Keefe Jr JH, Harris WS, Nelson J, Windsor SL. Effects of pravastatin with niacin or magnesium on lipid levels and postprandial lipemia. *Am J Cardiol.* 1995;76:480–484.

Smith SM, McDonald A, Webb D. *Complete Book of Vitamins and Minerals.* Lincolnwood, Ill: Publications International, Ltd; 1998.

Somer E. *The Essential Guide to Vitamins and Minerals.* New York, NY: Harper Collins Publishers Inc; 1995.

Vacek J, Dittmeier G, Chiarelli T, White J, Bell HH. Comparison of lovastatin (20 mg) and nicotinic acid (1.2 mg) with either drug alone for type II hyperlipoproteinemia. *Am J Cardiol.* 1995;76:182–184.

Werbach MR. *Nutritional Influences on Illness: A Sourcebook of Clinical Research.* New Canaan, Conn: Keats Publishing, Inc; 1988.

Whitney E, Cataldo C, Rolfes S. *Understanding Normal and Clinical Nutrition.* 2nd ed. St. Paul, Minn: West Publishing Co; 1987.

Zeman F. *Clinical Nutrition and Dietetics.* 2nd ed. New York, NY: Macmillan Publishing Company; 1991.

■ VITAMIN B₅ (PANTOTHENIC ACID)

OVERVIEW

Known as the "antistress" vitamin, vitamin B₅ (or pantothenic acid) plays an important role in adrenal function and cellular metabolism. This water-soluble B vitamin is converted into a substance called coenzyme A. Coenzyme A is essential to the metabolism of fats, carbohydrates, and proteins for energy. It is required in the synthesis of fatty acids, cholesterol, steroids, bile, phospholipids, red blood cells, hormones, and neurotransmitters. Vitamin B₅ as coenzyme A is needed for proper adrenal cortex function. It supports the adrenal glands in the making of cortisone and other adrenal hormones that counteract the stress response and enhance metabolism. Also extremely important, coenzyme A is needed to convert choline, a nutrient, into acetylcholine, an important neurotransmitter involved with neuromuscular reactions. Vitamin B₅ is necessary for proper functioning of the immune system. Research has demonstrated that a deficiency of this nutrient impairs immune system function and is therefore necessary for proper immune response. Another important discovery about vitamin B₅ is that it seems to help decrease the painful symptoms of rheumatoid arthritis.

The most well known research on the role of vitamin B₅ in combatting stress occurred more than 30 years ago. This study showed that rats given large doses of vitamin B₅ survived twice as long when forced to remain in cold water than did rats who did not receive the vitamin. Other animal and human studies trying to support the claim that vitamin B₅ increases endurance and stamina have been too few to positively confirm this theory. There is no argument over the fact that vitamin B₅ is needed for proper adrenal function, but whether or not supplementation can enhance adrenal function is not yet proven.

The most promising recent study in this area showed that athletes who received vitamin B₅ supplements performed better than those who received placebos. Those who received vitamin B₅ used 8% less oxygen and had 17% less lactic acid buildup. These differences are significant, but need to be confirmed by further studies.

In 1980, the General Practitioner Research Group conducted a double-blind study showing that calcium pantothenate supplementation significantly reduced the severity of rheumatoid arthritis symptoms. This supports the use of vitamin B₅ supplementation along with herbs and other natural therapies in the treatment of this disease.

DIETARY SOURCES

Pantothenic acid derives its name from the Greek word *pantos,* meaning "everywhere," referring to its wide availability in foods. Deficiency is very uncommon, but possible for those who have diets dominated by highly processed foods. Large amounts of vitamin B₅ are lost in the milling and refining of grains and in canning, freezing, cooking, or otherwise processing of vegetables and other foods. Vitamin B₅ is not replaced in the "enrichment" of refined flour, bread, rice, and noodles, and these are poor sources of the vitamin. The best dietary sources are brewer's yeast, liver, eggs, fish, chicken, cheese, milk, mushrooms, whole-grain breads and cereals, dried beans and peas, nuts (peanuts, pecans, hazelnuts), potatoes, avocados, cauliflower, oranges, and bananas.

CONSTITUENTS/COMPOSITION

Vitamin B₅ is most commonly available as calcium pantothenate. Recently, a metabolite of pantothenic acid, called pantethine, has become available. Research has shown this substance to have significant cholesterol-and lipid-lowering activity, and research continues in the areas of cardiovascular disease prevention, and immune system stimulation.

COMMERCIAL PREPARATIONS

Vitamin B₅ is available in supplement form as calcium pantothenate, which is 92% pantothenic acid and 8% calcium. It is available in 100, 250, and 500 mg capsules. It is also usually included in vitamin B complex formulas.

THERAPEUTIC USES

Vitamin B₅ has become increasingly popular as a nutritional supplement due to claims that it boosts energy, increases stamina and athletic performance, rejuvenates skin and hair, and decreases the symptoms of allergies, asthma, and psoriasis (due to its support of corticosteroid synthesis).

Some of these claims arise from studies that have shown that vitamin B₅ deficiency in rats caused increased graying of fur, decreased growth, and destruction of adrenal glands.

Human studies have shown that a deficiency of vitamin B₅ results in fatigue, depression, digestive problems, problems with blood sugar metabolism (most commonly hypoglycemia), loss of nerve function, and depressed cellular and antibody immune response. These problems may manifest symptoms such as vomiting, abdominal cramps, tingling or burning hands or feet, skin problems, muscle cramps, recurring infections, and worsening of allergy or asthma symptoms.

Some health care providers recommend the use of vitamin B₅ to treat allergies (to support the manufacture of adrenocorticosteroids, thereby reducing allergy symptoms). There are no clinical trials that judge the validity of this application.

There is documented clinical evidence to support the following uses of vitamin B₅.
Pantothenic acid:
- To reduce pain and swelling of rheumatoid arthritis
- To improve wound healing

Pantethine:
- To significantly lower blood cholesterol levels
- Particularly beneficial for diabetics—to lower blood lipids without negatively affecting blood sugar control and to improve platelet function
- To speed up the detoxification of alcohol

DOSAGE RANGES AND DURATION OF ADMINISTRATION

There is no RDA for vitamin B₅, but the 1989 Safe and Adequate Intakes are as follows:
- Birth to 6 months: 2 mg
- 6 months to 1 year: 3 mg
- 1 to 6 years: 3 to 4 mg
- 7 to 10 years: 4 to 5 mg
- 11 years and older: 4 to 7 mg

Americans consume an average of 4 to 10 mg/day. Individual needs vary according to food intake and the amount of stress (physical, environmental, or emotional/mental) one is undergoing.

Therapeutic dosages range from 250 to 500 mg of pantothenic acid daily for general adrenal support to 2,000 mg daily for rheumatoid arthritis. The recommended dose of pantethine for lowering cholesterol and triglycerides is 300 mg three times daily (900 mg/day).

SIDE EFFECTS/TOXICOLOGY

There is no documented toxicity with even large doses of vitamin B₅.

WARNINGS/CONTRAINDICATIONS/PRECAUTIONS

There are no significant safety issues documented for vitamin B5. However, research has not been adequate enough to assess the safety of large doses over the long term. It is recommended that vitamin B5 be supplemented along with the rest of the B vitamin family to prevent metabolic imbalance.

INTERACTIONS

There are no documented adverse interactions with any herbs or drugs.

REFERENCES

Arsenio L, et al. Effectiveness of long-term treatment with pantethine in patients with dyslipidemia. *Clin Ther.* 1986;8:537–545.

Bertolini S, Donati C, Elicio N, et al. Lipoprotein changes induced by pantethine in hyper-lipoproteinemic patients: adults and children. *Int J Clin Pharmacol Ther Toxicol.* 1986;24:630–637.

Binaghi P, Cellina G, Lo Cicero G, et al. Evaluation of the cholesterol-lowering effectiveness of pantethine in women in perimenopausal age [in Italian]. *Minerva Med.* 1990;81:475–479.

Coronel F, Tornero F, Torrente J, et al. Treatment of hyperlipemia in diabetic patients on dialysis with a physiological substance. *Am J Nephrol.* 1991;11:32–36.

Gaddi A, et al. Controlled evaluation of pantethine, a natural hypolipidemic compound in patients with different forms of hyperlipoproteinemia. *Atherosclerosis.* 1984;50:73–83.

Gensini GF, et al. Changes in fatty acid composition of the single platelet phospholipids induced by pantethine treatment. *Int J Clin Pharmacol Res.* 1985;5:309–318.

Haas E. *Staying Healthy with Nutrition: The Complete Guide to Diet and Nutritional Medicine.* Berkeley, Calif: Celestial Arts Publishing; 1992.

Hendler SS. *The Doctors' Vitamin and Mineral Encyclopedia.* New York, NY: Fireside Press; 1991.

Lieberman S, Bruning N. *The Real Vitamin and Mineral Book.* 2nd ed. New York, NY: Avery Publishing Group; 1997.

Murray M. *Encyclopedia of Nutritional Supplements.* Rocklin, Calif: Prima Publishing; 1996.

Prisco D, Rogasi PG, Matucci M, et al. Effect of oral treatment with pantethine on platelet and plasma phospholipids in IIa hyperlipoproteinemia. *Angiology.* 1987;38:241–247.

Somer E. *The Essential Guide to Vitamins and Minerals.* New York, NY: HarperCollins Publishers, Inc; 1995.

Vaxman F, Olender S, Lambert A, et al. Effect of pantothenic acid and ascorbic acid supplementation on human skin wound healing process. A double-blind, prospective and randomized trial. *Eur Surg Res.* 1995;27:158–166.

■ VITAMIN B₆ (PYRIDOXINE)

OVERVIEW

Vitamin B₆ is a water-soluble vitamin that occurs naturally in three forms: pyridoxine (PN), pyridoxal (PL), and pyridoxamine (PM). The basic structure of vitamin B₆ is a pyridine ring with a substituted four position. Substitution with a hydroxymethyl group leads to PN; substitution with a formyl group leads to PL; and substitution with an aminomethyl group leads to PM. All three forms can also be phosphorylated at position 5, which results in PLP, PMP, and PNP. PLP and PMP are the active coenzyme forms of the vitamin.

Absorption of vitamin B₆ takes place in the jejunum by a passive, nonsaturable process. In the blood, vitamin B₆ is transported in the plasma and red blood cells. Ninety percent of circulating vitamin B₆ is in the form of PL and PLP. The liver absorbs most of the circulating vitamin B₆ and converts it to PLP, which (after hydrolysis of the phosphate group) is then available to other tissues. The phosphorylation and hydrolysis of PL in the liver is just one example of how the metabolism of vitamin B₆ from absorption through storage is highly regulated by phosphorylation. The liver is also the conversion site for 40% to 60% of the daily vitamin intake to 4-pyridixic acid (4-PA), which is excreted in the urine. The major storage depot of vitamin B₆ in the body is muscle tissue, which contains 80% to 90% of the total body pool, most of it in the form of PLP bound to glycogen phosphorylase.

The active coenzyme forms of vitamin B₆, PLP and PMP, take part in enzymatic reactions that affect several cellular and systemic processes throughout the body. The primary reactions involve aminotransferases, decarboxylations, side chain cleavages, and dehydratases.

Vitamin B₆ is involved with the following cellular and systemic processes.

- Gluconeogenesis—through transamination reactions and as the essential coenzyme of glycogen phosphorylase
- Niacin formation—during the enzymatic conversion of tryptophan to niacin
- Lipid metabolism—phospholipid biosynthesis is PLP-dependent
- Nucleic acid synthesis and immune system processes—serine transhydroxymethylase, a PLP-dependent enzyme is involved in 1-carbon metabolism and therefore DNA synthesis. Normal DNA synthesis is an important process in proper immune function.
- Hormone modulation—PLP modulates the expression of cytosolic aspartate aminotransferase by preventing the glucocorticoid receptor from binding to the glucocorticoid response element of the aspartate aminotransferase gene.
- Nervous system processes—PLP is involved in several enzymatic reactions that result in the production of neurotransmitters such as gamma-aminobutyric acid, dopamine, norepinephrine, serotonin, and histamine.

Decreased plasma PLP concentrations have been reported in many disease states. These include renal disease, alcoholism, coronary heart disease, breast cancer, Hodgkin's disease, and diabetes. The finding of decreased plasma PLP in many of these studies must be taken in the context that the other vitamers of B₆ were not measured, leaving open the possibility that vitamin B₆ levels are not truly lowered in these conditions.

DIETARY SOURCES

The best sources of vitamin B₆ are chicken, fish, kidney, liver, pork, and eggs. The following are also good sources.

- Yeast
- Wheat germ
- Whole grain cereals
- Legumes
- Potatoes
- Bananas
- Oatmeal

PL and PLP are the predominate forms of vitamin B₆ found in animal food products. PM and PN and their phosphorylated forms are the predominant forms found in plant food products. A glucoside form of the vitamin in which a glucose is linked to the five position is also found in vegetables, but this form of the vitamin is not efficiently absorbed by the human body.

CONSTITUENTS/COMPOSITION

Pyridoxine is a white, crystalline, odorless compound that is readily soluble in water and alcohol. Food processing and storage can result in considerable loss of active vitamin B₆. The range of vitamin B₆ losses during freezing are from 36% to 55%.

COMMERCIAL PREPARATIONS

Pyridoxine hydrochloride is the most commonly found commercial preparation of vitamin B₆. It is formulated into tablets in multivitamin form (including chewable children's multivitamins), B-complex form, or by itself in doses ranging from 1 to 150 mg.

THERAPEUTIC USES

- Prophylactic use in multivitamin form to prevent the symptoms of vitamin B₆ deficiency such as stomatitis, glossitis, cheilosis, irritability, depression, and confusion
- Counteracts sideroblastic anemia that occurs with the use of the anti-tuberculin drugs isoniazid and pyrazinamide, and the peripheral neuritis that occurs with isoniazid use
- Treatment of isoniazid overdose
- Counteracts antivitamin B₆ activity of penicillamine, cycloserine, and hydralazine
- To control pyridoxine-dependent seizures that occur in neonates, infants, and toddlers. These seizures result from an inborn error of metabolism that causes abnormal binding of PLP to glutamic acid decarboxylase and results in a reduction of gamma-aminobutyric acid (GABA) synthesis
- To control the nausea and vomiting of pregnancy. Doses of 30 to 75 mg per day benefit some women, and doses of up to 40 mg per day have not been proven to be teratogenic. Careful consideration should be taken when prescribing more than the RDA of vitamin B₆ because of the risk of neurologic problems with excessive doses
- Some premenstrual syndromes can be improved by vitamin B₆ at a dose of 150 mg per day. Vitamin B₆ therapy at these doses must be used with caution because of the risk of neurologic symptoms.
- Together with folic acid and vitamin B₁₂, vitamin B₆ reduces high plasma levels of homocysteine, which is an independent risk factor for cardiovascular disease.

DOSAGE RANGES AND DURATION OF ADMINISTRATION

As one's protein intake increases, so too does the requirement for vitamin B₆. The RDA for vitamin B₆ has been established as that needed for two times the RDA of protein intake.

RDA for:

• Neonates to 6 mos.	0.3 mg
• Infants 6 mos. to 1 year	0.6 mg
• Children: 1 to 3 years	1.0 mg
• 4 to 6 years	1.1 mg
• 7 to 10 years	1.4 mg
• Boys: age 11 to 14 years	1.7 mg

- Men: age 15 years +   2.0 mg
- Girls: age 11 to 14 years   1.4 mg
- Women age 15 to 18 years   1.5 mg
- Women age 19 years +   1.6 mg
- Pregnant women   2.2. mg
- Lactating women   2.1 mg

SIDE EFFECTS/TOXICOLOGY

Prolonged ingestion of high doses of vitamin B_6 (as little as 200 mg of pyridoxine per day) can result in severe sensory neuropathy and ataxia. Discontinuing the use of vitamin B_6 supplements can result in a complete recovery within 6 months.

WARNINGS/CONTRAINDICATIONS/PRECAUTIONS

- Because of the risk of neurotoxicity from chronic use of large daily doses of vitamin B_6, caution must be used when prescribing vitamin B_6 therapy for premenstrual syndrome, and the nausea and vomiting of pregnancy.
- Vitamin B_6 enhances the peripheral decarboxylation of levodopa thereby reducing its effectiveness in treating Parkinson's disease.

INTERACTIONS

- Isoniazid, cycloserine, penicillamine, pyrazinamide, and hydralazine interfere with vitamin B_6 metabolism or action.

REFERENCES

Berger AR, Schaumburg HH, Schroeder C, Apfel S, Reynolds R. Dose response, coasting and differential fiber vulnerability in human toxic neuropathy: a prospective study of pyridoxine neurotoxicity. *Neurology.* 1992;42:1367–1370.

Brush MG, Bennett T, Hansen K. Pyridoxine in the treatment of premenstrual syndrome: a retrospective survey in 630 patients. *Br J Clin Pract.* 1998;42:448–452.

Diegoli MS, da Fonseca AM, Diegoli CA, Pinoltti JA. A double-blind trial of four medications to treat severe premenstrual syndrome. *Int J Gynaecol Obstet.* 1998;62:63–67.

Ekhard ZE, Filer LJ, eds. *Present Knowledge in Nutrition.* 7th ed. Washington, DC: ILSI Press; 1996:191–201.

Folsom AR, Nieto FJ, McGovern PG, et al. Prospective study of coronary heart disease incidence in relation to fasting total homocysteine, related genetic polymorphisms, and B vitamins: the atherosclerosis risk in communities. *Circulation.* 1998;98:204–210.

Hardman JG, Limbird LE, eds. *Goodman and Gillman's Pharmacological Basis of Therapeutics.* 9th ed. New York: McGraw-Hill; 1996:1326–1333.

Keniston RC, Nathan PA, Leklem JE, Lockwood RS. Vitamin B6, vitamin C, and carpal tunnel syndrome. A cross-sectional study of 441 adults. *J Occup Environ Med.* 1997;39:949–959.

Mahan LK, Arlin MT, eds. *Krause's Food, Nutrition, and Diet Therapy.* 8th ed. Philadelphia, Pa: WB Saunders Co; 1992:96–97.

National Research Council: Recommended Dietary Allowances. 10th ed. Washington, DC: National Academy Press; 1989: 158–165.

Ballal RS, Jacobsen DW, Robinson K. Homocysteine: update on a new risk factor. *Cleve Clin J Med.* 1997;64:543–549.

Gospe SM. Current perspectives on pyridoxine-dependent siezures. *J Pediatr.* 1998;132:919-923.

Murphy PA. Alternative therapies for nausea and vomiting of pregnancy. *Obstet Gynecol.* 1998; 91:149-155.

O'Connell BJ. The pediatrician and the sexually active adolescent: treatment of common menstrual disorders. *Pediatr Clin North Am.* 1997;44:1391–1404.

Recommended Dietary Allowance. American Academy of Sciences. Accessed at www.nal.usda.gov/fnic/Dietary/rda.html on January 8, 1999.

■ VITAMIN B$_9$ (FOLIC ACID)
OVERVIEW

Folic acid functions with vitamin B$_{12}$ in many genetic, metabolic, and nervous system processes. Folic acid helps protect against heart disease, birth defects, osteoporosis, and certain cancers. It is vital to DNA and RNA synthesis, and therefore is critical to cell division, maintenance of the genetic code, regulation of cell division, and transfer of inherited characteristics. As many as 15% of people may have a genetic mutation causing higher homocysteine levels. This results in an increased risk for heart disease, and, in women, increased risk of having children with neural tube defects. Folic acid is essential to protein metabolism, notably for its role in reducing homocysteine levels by converting it to methionine.

A 1998 study published in *British Medical Journal* found that in 1,114 people in 12 trials, folic acid supplementation reduced homocysteine levels by 25%. The Framingham Heart Study (1998) revealed similar findings. In 1998, researchers at the Harvard School of Public Health published data from the Nurses Health Study showing that intake of folic acid and vitamin B$_6$ well above the current RDA reduced the risk of congestive heart disease (CHD) by about 30%. The study tracked 80,082 women over a 14-year period.

Deficiency of folic acid has been linked to several birth defects, including the neural tube defect spina bifida. Up to half of neural tube defects are believed to be preventable if women of childbearing age supplement their diet with folic acid. Adequate intake of folic acid should begin several weeks before, and continue through at least the first four weeks of pregnancy. Women who have previously had a child with neural tube defect can reduce the risk of recurrence by about 70% through supplementation with up to 4 mg folic acid per day. Studies suggest that the levels of folic acid necessary to prevent neural tube defects are more easily derived from fortified foods and supplements than from natural food sources alone.

Increased homocystiene concentrations in the blood may also play a role in osteoporosis by interfering with collagen cross-linking, leading to a defective bone matrix. Folic acid helps produce neurotransmitters such as serotonin and dopamine. These regulate brain functions including mood, sleep, and appetite. Correcting folic acid deficiency has reversed mental or psychological symptoms in some, particularly in the elderly. Folic acid exerts a mild antidepressant effect. Supplementation optimizes the effect of the drug Prozac.

At particular risk for folate deficiency are the elderly, alcoholics, psychiatric patients, people taking certain medications, and women taking contraceptive pills. Folic acid is required for the formation of healthy red and white blood cells. Folic acid deficiency causes macrocytic anemia in which the red blood cells are fewer in number, larger in size, and contain less oxygen-carrying hemoglobin than normal cells. Folic acid deficiency may play a role in cancer development, particularly cancers of the cervix, lung, and colon, possibly through its action in DNA synthesis. In a study published in 1996, researchers examined the relationship between folate status and colorectal cancer in male smokers involved in the alpha-tocopherol beta-carotene (ATBC) study. Those with diets higher in folic acid had significantly reduced risk of colon cancer. Low blood levels of folic acid may increase the risk of cervical dysplasia. Low folic acid intake may also contribute to rheumatoid arthritis, constipation, cataracts, headaches, and infertility.

DIETARY SOURCES
- Liver
- Lentils
- Rice germ
- Brewer's yeast
- Soy flour
- Black-eyed peas
- Navy beans
- Kidney beans
- Peanuts
- Spinach
- Turnip greens
- Lima beans
- Whole wheat
- Asparagus

Food processing (e.g., boiling, heating) can destroy folic acid. Food stored at room temperature for long periods can also lose its folic acid content.

As of January 1998, commercial grain products have been fortified with 140 mcg of folic acid per 100 g of grain product. This will result in an average increase in folic acid intake of 100 mcg per day.

CONSTITUENTS/COMPOSITION
Folic acid occurs in food in its unactivated form (folate).

B$_9$ supplements are available as both folic acid and folinic acid (5-methyl-tetra-hydrofolate). While folic acid is the more stable compound, folinic acid is the most efficient at raising body stores.

COMMERCIAL PREPARATIONS
Folic acid is widely available in multivitamin and B-complex preparations. Standard over-the-counter preparations include 400 mcg and 800 mcg tablets. Prescription folic acid is available in 1 mg tablets in packages of 30, 100, 1,000, and UD 100, as injections of 5mg/ml in 10 vials. Folinic acid is available as 5 mg, 15 mg and 25 mg tablets in 30s, 100s, and UD 50s. Injections (3 mg/ml) are available.

THERAPEUTIC USES
- Supplementation indicated for women of childbearing age to prevent neural tube birth defects
- Protects against heart disease and stroke
- Protects against osteoporosis
- Indicated for prevention and treatment of cervical dysplasia
- Helps prevent cervical, lung, and colon cancer
- May relieve depression
- Indicated for mental or psychiatric symptoms in elderly
- May improve acne
- Supplementation indicated for individuals with AIDS
- Indicated, with B$_{12}$, for macrocytic anemia
- Aids in the formation of healthy red blood cells, preventing macrocytic anemia
- Indicated for candidiasis
- Helps prevent and treat rheumatoid arthritis
- May aid constipation
- Adjunctive therapy of cataracts
- May relieve headaches
- Part of therapy for treatment of infertility
- May decrease risk of stroke
- Used in treatment of sickle cell anemia

DOSAGE RANGES AND DURATION OF ADMINISTRATION
The RDA for folic acid follows.
- Infants under 6 months: 25 mcg
- 6 to 12 months: 35 mcg

- Children 1 to 3 yrs: 50 mcg
- Children 4 to 6 years: 75 mcg
- Children 7 to 10 yrs: 100 mcg
- Male and female 11 to 14: 150 mcg
- Males 15+: 400 mcg
- Females 15+: 400 mcg
- Pregnant females: 400 mcg
- Lactating females: 280 mcg
- Tolerable upper intake: 1,000 mcg/day

SIDE EFFECTS/TOXICOLOGY

Folic acid toxicity is rare. High doses (>15 mg) can cause gastrointestinal disturbances, sleep problems, and allergic skin reactions.

WARNINGS/CONTRAINDICATIONS/PRECAUTIONS

Folic acid supplementation can mask vitamin B_{12} deficiency. Vitamin B_{12} deficiency can lead to irreversible neurological damage. Therefore, folic acid supplementation should always include vitamin B_{12}.

High dosage folic acid supplementation should be used with extreme caution in those with epilepsy. It may increase seizure activity.

INTERACTIONS

Folic acid needs niacin, vitamin B_{12}, choline, and vitamin C to be converted to the biologically active form. Vitamin C helps reduce the amount of folic acid lost to excretion. Zinc absorption may be reduced with folic acid intake.

Estrogens, alcohol, some chemotherapy drugs, sulfasalazine, barbiturates, and anticonvulsant drugs interfere with folate absorption.

Aspirin, ibuprofen, acetaminophen and other NSAIDS can increase the body's need for folic acid if taken for long periods.

REFERENCES

Bendich A, Deckelbaum R, eds. *Prevention Nutrition: The Comprehensive Guide for Health Professionals.* Totowa, NJ: Humana Press; 1997.

Bronstrup A, Hages M, Prniz-Langenohl R, Pietrzik K. Effects of folic acid and combinations of folic acid and vitamin B12 on plasma homocysteine concentrations in healthy, young women. *Am J Clin Nutr.* 1998;68:1104–1110.

Cancers, Nutrition and Food. Washington, DC: World Cancer Research Fund/American Institute for Cancer Research; 1997.

Ebly EM, Schaefer JP, Campbell NR, Hogan DB. Folate status, vascular disease and cognition in elderly Canadians. *Age Ageing.* 1998;27:485–491.

1999 Drug Facts and Comparisons. Facts and Comparisons; 1998.

Giles WH, Kittner SJ, Croft JB, Anda RF, Casper ML, Ford ES. Serum folate and risk for coronary heart disease: Results from a cohort of US adults. *Ann Epidemiol.* 1998;8:490–496.

Lewis DP, Van Dyke DC, Stumbo PJ, Berg MJ. Drug and environmental factors associated with adverse pregnancy outcomes. Part II: Improvement with folic acid. *Ann Pharmacother.* 1998;32:947–961.

Malinow MR, Duell PB, Hess DL, et al. Reduction of plasma homocyst(e)ine levels by breakfast cereal fortified with folic acid in patients with coronary heart disease. *N Engl J Med.* 1998;338:1009–1015.

Morgan SL, Baggott JE, Lee JY, Alarcon GS. Folic acid supplementation prevents deficient blood folate levels and hyperhomocysteinemia during long-term, low-dose methotrexate therapy for rheumatoid arthritis: implications for cardiovascular disease prevention. *J Rheumatol.* 1998;25:441–446.

Murray MT. *Encyclopedia of Nutritional Supplements.* Rocklin, Calif: Prima Health; 1996.

Ortiz Z, Shea B, Suarez-Almazor ME, et al. The efficacy of folic acid and folinic acid in reducing methotrexate gastrointestinal toxicity in rheumatoid arthritis. A metaanalysis of randomized controlled trials. *J Rheumatol.* 1998;25:36–43.

Reavley N. *Vitamins, etc.* Melbourne, Australia: Bookman Press; 1998.

Rimm EB, Willett WC, Hu FB, et al. Folate and vitamin B6 from diet and supplements in relation to risk of coronary heart disease among women. *JAMA.* 1998;279:359–364.

Ringer D, ed. *Physician's Guide to Nutriceuticals.* St. Joseph, Mich: Nutritional Data Resources; 1998.

Watkins ML. Efficacy of folic acid prophylaxis for the prevention of neural tube defects. *Ment Retard Dev Disab Res Rev.* 1998;4:282–290.

Wolf PA. Prevention of stroke. *Lancet.* 1998;352 (suppl III):15–18.

VITAMIN B$_{12}$ (COBALAMIN)

OVERVIEW

Vitamin B$_{12}$ (cobalamin) is a water-soluble vitamin, first defined in 1926 as the extrinsic factor in liver that could cure the then-fatal pernicious anemia. Vitamin B$_{12}$ is obtained from animal protein products in the diet. In the stomach it binds to a glycoprotein called intrinsic factor (IF), which is secreted from the parietal cells of the gastric mucosa. The IF-B$_{12}$ complex binds to specific receptors on ileal mucosal cells and is transported to the circulation. In the circulation, vitamin B$_{12}$ binds to the plasma globulin transcobalamin II for transport to cells, where it carries out its metabolic function, or to the liver, where it is stored until it is needed by other tissues. Because the liver can store 1 to 10 mg of vitamin B$_{12}$, and vitamin B$_{12}$ can be reabsorbed from the bile in the enterohepatic circulation, strict vegetarians who eat little or no animal products may only gradually (after 20 to 30 years) develop any vitamin B$_{12}$ deficiency.

Vitamin B$_{12}$ is an essential coenzyme for the normal function of all cells. It affects cell growth and replication. The active coenzyme forms of vitamin B$_{12}$ are 5-deoxyadenosylcobalamin and methylcobalamin. 5-deoxyadenosyl-cobalamin is required for the conversion of L-methylmalonyl CoA to succinyl CoA, which is an important reaction in the degradation of certain amino acids and carbohydrate and lipid metabolism. Methylcobalamin aids in the synthesis of methionine by transferring a methyl group from methyl-folate (folic acid) to homocysteine to form methionine.

This reaction has two important consequences. First, methionine is converted to S-adenosyl-methionine, which is an intermediate in methylation reactions and protein synthesis. Second, by transferring the methyl group from methylfolate, vitamin B12 regenerates tetrahydrofolate, which is needed for DNA synthesis. Since methylfolate is the predominant form of folate in the serum, a deficiency of vitamin B$_{12}$ leads to folate being "trapped" as methylfolate, which results in defective DNA synthesis and ultimately megaloblastic (pernicious) anemia.

This process provides a common basis for the development of megaloblastic anemia from either a vitamin B$_{12}$ or folic acid deficiency. The increase in homocysteine levels and decrease in S-adenosyl-methionine levels that are also a consequence of vitamin B$_{12}$ deficiency may play a role in the neurologic symptoms seen in pernicious anemia.

Most deficiencies of vitamin B$_{12}$ seen today are not due to a dietary deficiency but to inadequate absorption. Gastric atrophy or gastric surgery can inhibit the secretion of IF and lead to vitamin B$_{12}$ deficiency. Gastric atrophy is a common cause of vitamin B$_{12}$ deficiency in the elderly as it is a progressive, genetically determined, age-dependent disease that occurs as a person ages. Less common etiologies of vitamin B$_{12}$ deficiency are pancreatic disorders, which affect the secretion of pancreatic enzymes that are needed to release vitamin B$_{12}$ from salivary proteins (so that it can bind to IF), and a congenital absence of transcobalamin II.

DIETARY SOURCES

The best sources of vitamin B$_{12}$ include the following.
- Liver
- Kidney
- Milk
- Eggs
- Fish
- Cheese

CONSTITUENTS/COMPOSITION

Vitamin B$_{12}$ is a red crystalline water-soluble substance that contains a corrin nucleus linked to a central cobalt atom. In the coenzymatically active forms of vitamin B$_{12}$, a methyl group or a 5-deoxyadenosyl group is bound to the cobalt atom.

COMMERCIAL PREPARATIONS

Vitamin B$_{12}$ is commercially available as cyanocobalamin. This is the most stable form of the vitamin. It is formulated into tablets, softgels, and lozenges in multivitamin form (including chewable children's multivitamins and drops), B-complex form, or by itself.

THERAPEUTIC USES

The therapeutic uses of vitamin B$_{12}$ are limited to conditions that are caused by B$_{12}$ deficiency and prophylactic treatment of B$_{12}$ deficiency. The method of treating the deficiency depends on its underlying etiology. Symptoms of vitamin B$_{12}$ deficiency caused by insufficient intake of vitamin B$_{12}$ can be alleviated by oral vitamin B$_{12}$ therapy, whereas a deficiency due to malabsorption of the vitamin must be treated parenterally.

Pernicious anemia is the most notable disease of vitamin B$_{12}$ deficiency. Pernicious anemia is caused by malabsorption of vitamin B$_{12}$, most commonly due to a lack of availability of intrinsic factor. It is characterized by pallor, glossitis, achlorhydria, gastric mucosal atrophy, weakness, and neurologic symptoms. Neurologic symptoms include paresthesias of the hands and feet, unsteadiness, decreased deep-tendon reflexes, and, in later stages of disease, confusion, loss of memory, and moodiness. Patients can become delusional and psychotic.

The hematopoietic symptoms such as megaloblastic anemia usually precede neurologic disorders. Uncomplicated pernicious anemia, which is characterized by mild or moderate anemia without leukopenia, thrombocytopenia or neurologic symptoms, can be treated with 1 to 10 mcg of vitamin B$_{12}$ a day. It is not pertinent that treatment be given immediately; treatment can wait until other causes of anemia are ruled out.

Emergency treatment including vitamin B$_{12}$ and folic acid supplementation as well as blood transfusions is needed for patients who exhibit neurologic symptoms, thrombocytopenia, leukopenia, infection, or bleeding. Elderly patients with severe anemia may also have tissue hypoxia, cerebrovascular insufficiency, and congestive heart failure. A typical initial treatment consists of 100 mcg of cyanocobalamin and 1 to 5 mg of folic acid given intramuscularly. Daily intramuscular injections of 100 mcg of cyanocobalamin and 1 to 2 mg of oral folic acid should be continued for one to two weeks. Subjective responses to therapy include the patient's increased sense of well-being within the first 24 hours of therapy. Disappearance of megaloblastic morphology of the bone marrow is the first objective hematologic response. Improvement of neurologic symptoms depend on the duration and severity of the abnormality. Full return to normal function can occur if the abnormality was present only for a few months; however, patients with abnormalities present for many months or years may never have a full recovery.

Once started, vitamin B$_{12}$ therapy for pernicious anemia must be continued throughout life. Treatment consists of a monthly intramuscular injection of cyanocobalamin. Patients should be monitored every three to six months to ensure the effectiveness of the therapy.

Vitamin B$_{12}$ therapy has been used with some success in the treatment of children with methylmalonic aciduria.

Together with folic acid and vitamin B6, vitamin B12 has been shown to reduce high plasma levels of homocysteine, which is an independent risk factor for cardiovascular disease.

DOSAGE RANGES AND DURATION OF ADMINISTRATION

The RDA for vitamin B12 is as follows.

- Neonates to 6 months.: 0.3 mcg
- Infants 6 months to 1 year: 0.5 mcg
- Children 1 to 3 years: 0.7 mcg
- Children 4 to 6 years: 1.0 mcg
- Children 7 to 10 years: 1.4 mcg
- Men age 11 years and over: 2.0 mcg
- Women age 11 years and over: 2.0 mcg
- Pregnant women: 2.2 mcg
- Lactating women: 2.6 mcg

SIDE EFFECTS/TOXICOLOGY

Daily oral ingestion of up to 100 mcg of vitamin B12 has no known toxic effects.

WARNINGS/CONTRAINDICATIONS/PRECAUTIONS

Parenteral cyanocobalamin given for vitamin B12 deficiency caused by malabsorption should be given intramuscularly or by the deep subcutaneous route but never intravenously.

INTERACTIONS

Doses of vitamin C 500 mg or greater have been shown to destroy intrinsic factor and convert vitamin B12 to inactive or anti-vitamin B12 active analogues. Persons ingesting these amounts of vitamin C should be monitored for vitamin B12 deficiency.

The antihyperglycemia drug metformin impairs intestinal absorption of vitamin B12 and is associated with a low frequency of megaloblastic anemia.

REFERENCES

Ballal RS, Jacobsen DW, Robinson K. Homocysteine: update on a new risk factor. *Cleve Clin J Med.* 1997;64:543–549.

Committee on Dietary Allowances. *Recommended Dietary Allowances.* National Academy of Sciences. Accessed at *www.nal.usda.gov/fnic/Dietary/rda.html* on January 8, 1999.

Ekhard ZE, Filer LJ, eds. *Present Knowledge in Nutrition.* 7th ed. Washington, DC: ILSI Press; 1996:191–201.

Hardman JG, Limbird LE, eds. *Goodman and Gillman's The Pharmacological Basis of Therapeutics.* 9th ed. New York, NY: McGraw-Hill; 1996:1326–1333.

Mahan LK, Arlin MT, eds. *Krause's Food, Nutrition, and Diet Therapy.* 8th ed. Philadelphia, Pa: WB Saunders Co; 1992:96–97.

Dorland Newman WA, ed. *Dorland's Illustrated Medical Dictionary.* 28th ed. Philadelphia, Pa: WB Saunders Co; 1994:73.

Ingram CF, Fleming AF, Patel M, Galpin JS. The value of intrinsic factor antibody test in diagnosing pernicious anaemia. *Cent Afr J Med.* 1998;44:178–181.

Lobo A, Naso A, Arheart K, et al. Reduction of homocysteine levels in coronary artery disease by low-dose folic acid combined with levels of vitamins B6 and B12. *Am J Cardiol.* 1999;83:821–825.

Lee AJ. Metformin in noninsulin-dependent diabetes mellitus. *Pharmacotherapy.* 1996;16:327–351.

National Research Council. *Recommended Dietary Allowances.* 10th ed. Washington, DC: National Academy Press; 1989:158–165.

Nilsson-Ehle H. Age-related changes in cobalamin (vitamin B12) handling. Implications for therapy. *Drugs Aging.* 1998;12:277–292.

Remacha AF, Cadafalch J. Cobalamin deficiency in patients infected with the human immunodeficiency virus. *Semin Hematol.* 1999;36:75–87.

van Asselt DZ, van den Broek WJ, Lamers CB, et al. Free and protein-bound cobalamin absorption in healthy middle-aged and older subjects. *J Am Geriatr Soc.* 1996;44:949–953.

■ VITAMIN C (ASCORBIC ACID)

OVERVIEW

Vitamin C functions primarily to form collagen, the primary protein used to make connective tissue and form scar tissue, and is needed to form bone, and cartilage. Vitamin C is also an antioxidant which protects all cells from oxidative damage. It also protects other vitamins such as vitamin E and A from oxidation as well. Research has shown that vitamin C protects the body against heart disease and many types of cancer. It is essential to proper wound healing, and has shown benefit for use in treating exercise-induced asthma. Most importantly, it is now known that vitamin C is critical to proper immune system function. Infection and inflammation rapidly deplete vitamin C from the body. Constant replacement is needed in order to maximize immune function and overcome infection.

Probably the biggest controversy surrounding vitamin C in the past few decades is whether or not it prevents colds. Research has shown that vitamin C does reduce the formation of histamine, which may help reduce cold symptoms. Clinical studies have shown that although vitamin C can reduce the length and severity of cold symptoms, it has not yet been proven to prevent colds. However, maintaining a strong and healthy immune system which increases resistance to all types of infection and disease is a good reason for consuming adequate amounts of vitamin C. The latest research on vitamin C shows that it is protective against sunburn and reduces the development of nitrate tolerance during nitroglycerin therapy in congestive heart failure patients.

DIETARY SOURCES

Vitamin C is present in many fruits and vegetables. The following foods are excellent sources of vitamin C: orange juice, green peppers, watermelon, papaya, grapefruit juice, grapefruit, cantaloupe, strawberries, mango, broccoli, tomato juice, Brussels sprouts, cauliflower, and cabbage.
Vitamin C is also found in raw and cooked leafy greens, (turnip greens, spinach), canned or fresh tomatoes, potatoes, winter squash, raspberries, and pineapple. Vitamin C is sensitive to light, air, and heat. Eating vegetables raw, or minimally cooked, increases their vitamin C content.

CONSTITUENTS/COMPOSITION

Vitamin C is ascorbic acid. It becomes dehydroascorbic acid when it is oxidized by the body. Ascorbic acid is the form that is used for supplements and as a food additive to protect against oxidative spoilage.

COMMERCIAL PREPARATIONS

You can purchase either natural or synthetic ascorbic acid in a wide variety of supplement forms. Tablets, capsules, and chewable tablets are probably the most popular, but vitamin C also comes in powdered crystalline, effervescent tablet and liquid form. You can purchase dosages from 25 mg to 1,000 mg per tablet; the most common are 100 mg, 250 mg, 500 mg, and 1,000 mg. "Buffered" C is available for those who find regular ascorbic acid is too harsh for their stomachs. "Ester-C" is a form of vitamin C composed of esters, which is promoted to be better absorbed by the body. Laboratory testing has challenged this claim, showing that absorption did not differ significantly from regular vitamin C.

THERAPEUTIC USES

- Boosts immune functions
- Protects against cancer
- Necessary for wound healing
- Helps prevent cataract development
- Increases HDL (good) cholesterol
- Decreases risk of cardiovascular disease
- Reduces blood pressure

- Decreases histamine levels (useful in treating allergies)
- Reduces capillary fragility
- Counteracts asthma (reduces airway spasms)
- Helps overcome male infertility
- Used in treatment of cervical dysplasia
- Helps protect diabetics against long-term complications by lowering sorbitol levels and reducing glycosylation of proteins
- Protects against sunburn and its effects
- Increases integrity of connective tissue, assisting treatment of bleeding gums, bruising, and arthritis
- Is anti-inflammatory
- Protects fat-soluble anti-oxidants (e.g. vitamin E) from oxidation

DOSAGE RANGES AND DURATION OF ADMINISTRATION

The range of safe Vitamin C intake appears to be very broad, and research has proved that even very high daily doses over 10 g (10,000 mg) for extended periods of time are usually well tolerated. Although the minimum daily requirement is 60 mg/day, physical stresses such as exertion, illness, infection, surgery, wound healing, exposure to toxic chemicals and metals, high or low temperatures, smoking, and chronic use of medication all increase the need for vitamin C. The amount needed varies with the severity of the stress, but may be as high as 1,000 mg/day or even higher. While consuming 60 mg/day of vitamin C may be sufficient to prevent deficiency symptoms, at least 100 to 250 mg is needed to saturate the tissues. And, since vitamin C is water-soluble and not stored in the body, the tissue supply requires constant replacement. Eating foods rich in vitamin C and/or dividing a supplement dose to be taken bid or tid is optimal. General recommendations for vitamin C intake is 250 to 500 mg/day for the average healthy adult. Some nutritionists recommend 500 to 1,000 mg tid (with each meal) for recovery after illness surgery, or severe injury.

SIDE EFFECTS/TOXICOLOGY

Vitamin C is considered non-toxic; excesses are excreted by the body. High doses of vitamin C can cause diarrhea, and nutritionists state that this side effect is useful in assessing an individual's tolerance and optimal daily allowance for proper tissue saturation. Diarrhea, gas, or other intestinal disturbances are harmless and reversible with lower dosing. Although the literature is full of speculated warnings, no harmful effects even from long-term "megadosing" have been observed.

WARNINGS/CONTRAINDICATIONS/PRECAUTIONS

Individuals with a history of kidney problems of any kind may not be candidates for vitamin C supplements due to increased urinary oxalate formation in oxalate kidney stone formers. Infants born to mothers taking 6 g or more of vitamin C may develop rebound scurvy after birth, due to the sudden drop in intake.

INTERACTIONS

- Works synergistically with other antioxidant nutrients, most notably vitamin E, selenium and beta-carotene
- Increases iron absorption
- Decreases copper absorption
- Interferes with blood test for vitamin B_{12} and bilirubin
- No documented adverse interactions with any drugs or herbs
- High doses interfere with stool occult blood tests

It should be noted that vitamin C is used by the liver to detoxify drugs and other chemicals. Individuals on any type of drug therapy should consult with a professional before taking high doses of vitamin C.

REFERENCES

Cohen H, Neuman I, Nahum H. Blocking effect of Vitamin C in exercise-induced asthma. *Arch Pediatr Adolesc Med.* 1997;151:367–370.

Eades MD. *The Doctor's Complete Guide to Vitamins and Minerals.* New York, NY: Dell Publishing; 1994.

Eberlein-Konig B, Placzek M, Przybilla B. Protective effect against sunburn of combined systemic ascorbic acid (vit.C) and D-alpha-tocopherol (vit.E). *J Am Acad Dermatol.* 1998;38:45–48.

Galley HF, Thornton J, et al. Combination oral antioxidant supplementation reduces blood pressure. *Clin Sci.* 1997;92:361–365.

Hendler SS. *The Doctors' Vitamin and Mineral Encyclopedia.* New York, NY: Fireside Press, 1991.

Lieberman S, Bruning N. *The Real Vitamin & Mineral Book.* 2nd ed. New York, NY: Avery Publishing Group; 1997.

Mahan K, Arlin M, eds. *Krause's Food, Nutrition and Diet Therapy.* 8th ed. Philadelphia, Pa: WB Saunders Company; 1992.

Mosca L, et al. Antioxidant nutrient supplementation reduces the susceptibility of low density lipoprotein to oxidation in patients with coronary artery disease. *J Am Coll Cardiol.* 1997;30:392–399.

Murray MT. *Encyclopedia of Nutritional Supplements.* Rocklin, Calif: Prima Publishing; 1996.

Watanabe H, Kakihana M, Ohtusuka S, Sugishita Y. Randomized, double blind, placebo-controlled study of ascorbate on the preventive effect of nitrate tolerance in patients with congestive heart failure. *Circulation.* 1998;97:886–891.

Whitney E, Cataldo C, Rolfes S. *Understanding Normal and Clinical Nutrition.* St. Paul, Minn: West Publishing Company; 1987.

■ VITAMIN D

OVERVIEW

Vitamin D is fat-soluble and the only vitamin whose active form (calcitrol) is a hormone. Its most important role is to maintain serum calcium and phosphorus levels within an acceptable range, which is critical for many body functions, including the normal development of bones and teeth, normal cell growth, and regulation of the immune and nervous systems. Low levels of vitamin D lead to osteomalacia, a mineralization deficit of the bones, associated with osteoporosis, osteoarthritis, rheumatoid arthritis, multiple sclerosis, diabetes, heart disease, and an overactive parathyroid.

The elderly, particularly those in northern climates and those who are house-bound, are at significant risk for vitamin D deficiency. A 1998 study in the *New England Journal of Medicine* found vitamin D deficiency in 57% of a random group of 290 hospitalized patients over age 65. Studies support vitamin D supplementation for the prevention and treatment of osteoporosis in postmenopausal women. In a 1997 study by Tufts University, supplementation with calcium (500 mg) and vitamin D (700 IU/day) was provided to 176 men and 213 women over age 65. The results were a significant increase in bone mass and a 50% reduction in fracture rate after three years.

Vitamin D is involved in cell growth and maturation and has shown anti-cancer properties. In vitro studies have suggested that vitamin D inhibits growth of breast and prostate cancer cells. The Physicians Health Study, published in 1996, found links between dietary vitamin D and a slightly decreased risk of prostate cancer. A 1996 epidemiological study in Sweden and the 1996 Harvard Nurses Study found that dietary vitamin D decreased the risk of colorectal cancer.

Vitamin D is involved in regulating the immune system and is being considered as a therapy for autoimmune disorders and to suppress rejection of transplanted organs. Vitamin D analogs have successfully been used to treat the skin disorder psoriasis.

DIETARY SOURCES

- Cod liver oil
- Salmon
- Tuna
- Fortified milk
- Oysters
- Mushrooms
- Fortified cereals
- Egg yolk

Few foods are natural sources. The primary source for humans has traditionally been sunlight. A fair-skinned person can receive adequate vitamin D through the skin with 20 to 30 cumulative minutes of daily sun exposure. A dark-skinned person may require three hours for a similar dose. Clouds, smog, clothing, sunscreen, and window glass all filter the ultraviolet light necessary for vitamin D_3 to be synthesized by provitamin D in the skin. Latitude, time of day, and season of the year also impact synthesis.

CONSTITUENTS/COMPOSITION

There are three forms of vitamin D.

- D_1: calciferol, found in some foods
- D_2: ergocalciferol, the form most widely found in food and most commonly added to food and nutritional supplements
- D_3: cholecalciferol, originates in the skin

All these forms of vitamin D are converted into calcitriol, the active form of the vitamin, in the liver and kidney

COMMERCIAL PREPARATIONS

- Supplemental vitamin D is available in natural and synthetic forms.
- Fish liver oil is the common natural source and provides vitamin D_2.
- Over-the counter preparations of vitamin D_2 are available in 50 IU, 100 IU, 400 IU, 500 IU, 600 IU, and 1,000 IU dosage as soft gel capsules, tablets, and liquid.
- Prescription preparations of vitamins D_2 and D_3 are available in tablets from 400 IU to 50,000 IU.
- Synthetic dihydrotachysterol is a reduction product of a close isomer to vitamin D_2, available by prescription.

THERAPEUTIC USES

- Protects against rickets, osteomalacia, osteoporosis, and osteopenia
- Protects against bone fractures in the elderly
- Recommended in the treatment of osteoporosis in postmenopausal women
- Recommended during fall and winter months for the elderly in northern climates and for those who do not receive daily exposure to direct sunlight
- Indicated for those with fat malabsorption disorders, including celiac disease, tropical sprue, cystic fibrosis, pancreatic disease, and short bowel syndrome
- Indicated for those on anticonvulsant drug therapy or glucocorticoid therapy
- Recommended for those on strict vegan diets
- Helps prevent some cancers by inhibiting the growth of human leukemia, colon cancer, skin cancer, and breast cancer cells
- Involved in the regulation of the immune system; may be indicated to treat autoimmune disorders and to suppress rejection of transplanted organs
- Plays a role in the secretion of insulin, thus aiding regulation of blood sugar
- Suppresses action of parathyroid hormone and may play a role in the treatment of an overactive parathyroid
- May reduce cartilage damage in osteoarthritis
- May decrease disease activity for rheumatoid arthritis
- May protect against multiple sclerosis
- May prevent diabetes mellitus
- May decrease the risk of arteriosclerosis
- May help prevent inflammatory bowel disease, tuberculosis, stroke, and high blood pressure

DOSAGE RANGES AND DURATION OF ADMINISTRATION

Adequate Daily Intake (AI)* is as follows.

- Infants and children: 5 mcg (200 IU)
- Adults up to age 50: 5 mcg (200 IU)
- Adults ages 51 to 70: 10 mcg (400 IU)
- Adults over age 70: 15 mcg (600 IU)

RDA:

- Infants up to 6 months: 7.5 mcg (300 IU)
- Children: 10 mcg (400 IU)
- Adults up to age 25: 10 mcg (400 IU)
- Adults age 25 and older: 5 mcg (200 IU)

SIDE EFFECTS/TOXICOLOGY

High daily more than doses (1,000 IU) of vitamin D can be toxic. The range between therapeutic and toxic doses is narrow. The major effect of toxicity is hypercalcemia, with symptoms of excessive thirst, metallic taste,

*AI reflects a level at which normal values and functional indicators of nutrition are maintained.

bone pain, fatigue, sore eyes, itching skin, vomiting, diarrhea, urinary urgency, impaired muscle function, and cardiovascular and renal failure. Prolonged exposure to sunlight does not result in vitamin D toxicity.

WARNINGS/CONTRAINDICATIONS/PRECAUTIONS

Vitamin D should not be given to those with high blood calcium levels or high blood phosphorus levels. Vitamin D should be given with caution to those suffering from cardiac or kidney diseases.

INTERACTIONS

- Vitamin D is necessary for calcium and phosphorus metabolism.
- Pantothenic acid is necessary for the synthesis of vitamin D.
- Cholestyramine interferes with the absorption of vitamin D.
- Mineral oil interferes with the absorption of vitamin D.
- Alcohol interferes with the conversion of vitamin D to its biologically active form.
- Certain anticonvulsant therapies, such as phenytoin, may decrease the activity of vitamin D by increasing its metabolism.
- Mineral imbalances may result from use of vitamin D in those taking magnesium-containing antacids, digitalis glycosides, verapamil, and thiazide diuretics.

REFERENCES

American Academy of Sciences. *Dietary Reference Intakes: Calcium Phosphorus, Magnesium, Vitamin D, and Fluoride.* National Academy Press; 1997.

Bendich A, Deckelbaum R, eds. *Preventive Nutrition: The Comprehensive Guide for Health Professionals.* Totowa, NJ: Humana Press; 1997.

Brenner RV, Shabahang M, Schumaker LM, et al. The antiproliferation effect of vitamin D analogs on MCF-7 human breast cancer cells. *Cancer Lett.* 1995;92:77–82.

Dawson-Hughes B, Harris SS, Dallal GE. Plasma calcidiol, season, and serum parathyroid hormone concentrations in healthy elderly men and women. *Am J Clin Nutr.* 1997;65:67–71.

Dawson-Hughes B, Harris SS, Krall EA, etal. Effect of calcium and vitamin D supplementation on bone density in men and women 65 years of age and older. *N Engl J Med.* 1997;337:670–676.

Deroisy R, Collette J, Chevallier T, et al. 1998. Effects of two 1-year calcium and vitamin D₃ treatments on bone remodeling markers and femoral bone density in elderly women. *Curr Thera Res.* 59(12):850–862.

Drug Facts and Comparisons 1999. St. Louis, Mo: A. Wolters Kluwer Company; 1998.

Heikkinen AM, Tuppurainen MT, Niskanen L, et al. Long-term vitamin D₃ supplementation may have adverse effects on serum lipids during menopause hormone replacement therapy. *J Endocrinology.* 1997;137:495–502.

Kizaki M, Ikeda Y, Simon KJ, et al. Effect of 1,25-dihydroxyvitamin D₃ and its analogs on human immunodeficiency virus infection in monocytes-macrophages. *Leukemia.* 1993;7:1525–153.

Kitch BT, Vamvakas EC, Dick IM, et al. Hypovitaminosis D in medical implants. *N Engl J Med.* 1998;338:777–783.

Langman M, Boyle P, et al. Chemoprevention of colorectal cancer. *Gut.* 1998;43:578–585.

Mahan K, Arlin M. *Krause's Food, Nutrition and Diet Therapy.* 8th ed. Philadelphia, Pa: WB Saunders Company; 1992.

Martinez ME, Giovannucci EL Colditz GA, et al. Calcium, vitamin D, and the occurrence of colorectal cancer among women. *JNCI.* 1996;88:1375–1382.

Reavley N. *Vitamins, Etc.* Melbourne, Australia: Bookman Press; 1998.

Thomas MK., Lloyd-Jones DM, Thadhani RI, et al. Hypovitaminosis D in medical inpatients. *N Engl J Med.* 1998;338:777–783.

■ VITAMIN E
OVERVIEW

Vitamin E is an important antioxidant which protects cells from free radical damage, thereby prolonging cell life and slowing the aging process. Research has shown this nutrient plays a vital role in the prevention and treatment of cardiovascular disease, cancer, immune system disorders, and aging-related degenerative diseases.

Three major clinical studies (The Nurses Health Study, The Physicians' Health Study, and a study done by the University of Texas Southwestern Medical Center) have provided evidence supporting the benefits of vitamin E supplementation in the prevention of heart disease. Vitamin E blocks the oxidation of LDL cholesterol, thereby reducing arterial damage and plaque formation. A study at the University of South Carolina School of Medicine showed that 100 IU of vitamin E daily actually may have reversed arterial blockage. A World Health Organization Study showed that supplemental vitamin E was more likely to prevent fatal heart attacks than by lowering blood cholesterol, presumably because it prevents oxidation of cholesterol into its most toxic form.

Vitamin E has long been recognized as an anti-clotting agent, thereby reducing risk of heart attack and stroke. Studies have shown vitamin E's important role in cancer prevention and in the benefits of use during cancer treatment. Animal and human studies have concluded that the nutrient blocks the initiation of carcinogenesis and reduces the incidence of skin, oral, stomach, colon, and breast cancer. Other studies have suggested that vitamin E may also reduce the risk of lung, esophageal, and cervical cancer. Researchers have found that during cancer treatment, vitamin E supplementation protects normal cells from the damaging effects of chemotherapy without protecting the cancer cells, which reduces side effects without reducing efficacy. New research suggests that vitamin E interferes with oxygen-controlled signals which promote cancer cell growth.

The most recent studies have shown vitamin E supplementation may reduce the incidence of prostate cancer, reverse diabetic neuropathy in Type II diabetics, may increase/improve insulin's effect in Type II diabetes, and significantly improve immune status in aging adults. Preliminary research suggests the nutrient may slow or prevent the progress of degenerative brain diseases.

DIETARY SOURCES

Food sources of vitamin E include wheat germ oil, margarine, soybean oil, almonds, safflower oil, hazelnuts, corn oil, peanuts, cottonseed oil, walnuts, canola oil, mayonnaise, sunflower seeds, spinach, kale, sweet potatoes, yams.

Vitamin E is destroyed when vegetable oils are processed and bleached; only cold-pressed vegetable oils are a good source. Wheat germ oil is the richest source of natural vitamin E.

CONSTITUENTS/COMPOSITION

Vitamin E occurs in several forms with varying biologic activity. Alpha-tocopherol is the most common, most potent, and best absorbed form. Other forms include beta-, delta-, and gamma-tocopherol, and alphatocotrienol.

COMMERCIAL PREPARATIONS

Supplemental Vitamin E is available in both natural and synthetic forms.
- Natural Vitamin E (d-alpha-tocopherol) has been the preferred form, and it is available with mixed tocopherols added.
- The synthetic form is dl-alpha-tocopherol.
- Standard preparations are available in 50 IU, 100 IU, 200 IU, 400 IU, 500 IU, 600 IU, and 1,000 IU softgels, tablets, and capsules.
- Vitamin E succinate ("dry-E") is water soluble and best tolerated by those with fat malabsorption syndromes.

THERAPEUTIC USES

Vitamin E may have the following therapeutic effects.
- Slows the aging process of all cells/tissues
- Protection against environmental pollutants and toxins
- Protects integrity of red blood cells and aids in prevention of hemolytic anemia
- Supplementation indicated for all fat malabsorption disorders, including celiac disease, tropical sprue, cystic fibrosis, and pancreatic disease
- Indicated for use in the treatment of most skin disorders, i.e. acne, eczema, psoriasis
- Prevention against atherosclerosis or its progression by helping reduce/reverse plaque formation
- Prevents oxidation of LDL cholesterol
- Improves arterial response when atherosclerosis is present
- Reduces tissue damage associated with ischemia during heart surgery; indicated for use before and after any surgery
- Promotes proper wound healing
- Anticlotting agent useful in prevention of pulmonary embolism, thrombosis, and stroke; indicated for use for angina, atherosclerosis, intermittant claudication, and for women using hormonal contraceptives
- Aids in prevention of cataracts and macular degeneration
- Indicated for use in all reproductive disorders
- Reduces symptoms associated with premenstrual syndrome
- Effective against fibrocystic breast disease
- Protects against initiation of carcinogenesis
- Indicated for use in cancer prevention and treatment
- May slow progression of mental deterioration associated with Alzheimer's, degenerative, or arteriosclerotic brain disease
- Significantly improves age-related immune response dysfunction
- Indicated for use in Type II diabetes
- Significantly decreases symptoms of lupus erythematosis with dose of 1,200 IU/day

DOSAGE RANGES AND DURATION OF ADMINISTRATION

Recommended Dietary Allowances (RDAs) are as follows.
- Neonates to 6 months: 4 IU
- Infants 6 months to 1 year: 6 IU
- Children 1 to 3 years: 9 IU
- Children 4 to 10 years: 10 IU
- Children over 10 years and adults: 12 IU for females, 15 IU for males.

Note: 1mg vitamin E equals 1.5 IU.
Based on clinical trials, the recommended dose for disease prevention and treatment for adults is 400 to 800 IU/day.

SIDE EFFECTS/TOXICOLOGY

Vitamin E is relatively nontoxic. Adverse effects which may occur with very high doses (more than 1,200 IU/day) include nausea, flatulence, diarrhea, heart palpitations.

WARNINGS/CONTRAINDICATIONS/PRECAUTIONS
- Increased blood pressure. Individuals with hypertension may show an increase in blood pressure if starting dose is too high. Recommendation is for initial dose of 100 IU/day, increasing as tolerated up to 400 IU/day with monitoring as dosage is increased.
- Prolonged bleeding time.
- High doses of vitamin E may interfere with vitamin K activity.

- Caution with Warfarin use.
- Extreme doses (more than 800 IU) over time may have detrimental effects, although toxicity per se has not been documented.

INTERACTIONS

- May exacerbate vitamin K deficiency; assessment of vitamin K status is recommended if deficiency is suspected
- Concommitant use with anticoagulant drugs increases risk of abnormal bleeding
- Iron supplementation destroys vitamin E and increases its requirement
- Cholestyramine and colestipol may decrease absorption of vitamin E
- Vitamin E enhances and increases the body's use of vitamin A; excessive intakes of vitamin E reduces/depletes vitamin A stores
- Selenium enhances vitamin E's antioxidant activity
- Chronic alcoholism depletes vitamin E stores in the liver

REFERENCES

Balch J, Balch, P. *Prescription for Nutritional Healing: A-to-Z Guide to Supplements.* New York, NY: Avery Publishing Group; 1998.

Chan AC. Vitamin E and atheroschlerosis. *J Nutr.* 1998;128:(10):1593–1596.

Feltman J. *Prevention's Food & Nutrition.* Emmaus, Pa: Rodale Press; 1993.

Klatz R. Vitamin E. *Total Health.* Sept/Oct 97: 28.

Leske MC, Chylack Jr LT, He Q, et al. Antioxidant vitamins and nuclear opacities: the longitudinal study of cataract. *Ophthalmology.* 1998;105:831–836.

Lieberman S, Bruning N. *The Real Vitamin & Mineral Book.* 2nd ed. New York, NY: Avery Publishing Group; 1997.

Liebman B. Vitamin E and Fat. *Nutrition Action Healthletter.* Jul/Aug 96:10

Mahan K, Arlin M, eds. *Krause's Food, Nutrition and Diet Therapy.* 8th ed. Philadelphia, Pa: WB Saunders Company; 1992.

Meydani SN, Meydani M, Blumberg JB, et al. Assessment of the safety of supplementation with different amounts of vitamin E in healthy older adults. *Am J Clin Nutr.* 1998;68:311–318.

Meydani SN, Meydani M, Blumberg JB, et al. Vitamin E supplementation and in vivo immune response in healthy elderly subjects. A randomized controlled trial. *JAMA.* 1997;277:1380–1386.

Nursing 93 Drug Handbook. Springhouse, Pa: Springhouse Corporation; 1993.

Pronsky Z. *Food-Medication Interactions.* 9th ed. Pottstown, Pa: 1995.

Whitney E, Cataldo C, Rolfes S. *Understanding Normal and Clinical Nutrition.* St. Paul, Minn: West Publishing Co; 1987.

■ VITAMIN H (BIOTIN)

OVERVIEW

Biotin is a water-soluble vitamin whose primary function is as a coenzyme in carbohydrate, amino acid, and lipid metabolism. Biotin is essential for cell growth and replication through its role in the manufacturing of DNA and RNA. Biotin has been shown to improve blood glucose control in diabetes by enhancing insulin sensitivity and increasing the activity of glucokinase, the enzyme responsible for the first step in the utilization of glucose by the liver. Studies have observed improvements with doses from 9 mcg to 16 mcg. High doses of biotin may also be useful in the treatment of diabetic neuropathy. Healthy hair and nails require biotin. Supplementation (up to 2,500 mcg/day) has been effective in treating frail, splitting, or thin toenails or fingernails and in improving hair health (through its action on the metabolism of scalp oils). Biotin has also been used to combat premature graying of hair, though it's likely to be useful only for those with a biotin deficiency.

Biotin is synthesized in the intestinal microflora. For this reason, deficiency states are rare. A vegetarian diet enhances the synthesis and absorption of biotin. Those at risk for biotin deficiency include infants with inherited deficiency disorders, babies fed biotin-deficient formula, people who eat large amounts of raw egg whites, which inactivate biotin, and people who are fed intravenously. Symptoms include hair loss, a dry, scaly dermatitis, anorexia, nausea, and depression. Biotin deficiency can exacerbate seborrheic dermatitis (cradle cap) in infants. Several case histories reveal the successful treatment of cradle cap in infants with biotin through direct supplementation to either the infant or the mother if she is breast-feeding. In adults with seborrheic dermatitis, biotin supplementation in conjunction with vitamin B-complex supplementation is necessary. Biotin deficiency also impacts the immune system.

DIETARY SOURCES

- Liver
- Nuts
- Kidney
- Egg yolks
- Brewer's yeast
- Chocolate
- Whole grains and whole grain breads
- Beans
- Fish

Food-processing techniques can destroy biotin, therefore less-processed products will have a greater percentage of their biotin intact.

CONSTITUENTS/COMPOSITION

Biotin is available as isolated biotin or as biocytin, a complex in brewer's yeast, composed of 65.6% biotin.

COMMERCIAL PREPARATIONS

Biotin is available in multivitamin and vitamin B complexes, and in individual supplements.

Standard preparations are available in 10 mcg, 50 mcg, 100 mcg, and 500 mcg tablets.

THERAPEUTIC USES

Biotin can be used to treat:

- Infants with a potentially fatal genetic abnormality, which leads to an inability to utilize biotin
- Some skin disorders, such as seborrheic dermatitis (cradle cap)
- Blood glucose control in diabetics
- Diabetic neuropathy
- Frail, splitting, or thin nails
- Hair loss due to deficiency
- Gray hair (in some instances)
- Metabolic abnormalities in Duchenne muscular dystrophy
- Fat metabolism in weight-loss programs (normalizes)
- Intestinal candidiasis

DOSAGE RANGES AND DURATION OF ADMINISTRATION

Due to biotin's synthesis in the gut, an RDA has not been set. The adequate intake for biotin has been estimated at 30 to 100 mcg per day. Average daily biotin intake in the American diet has been estimated to be 28 to 42 mcg.

SIDE EFFECTS/TOXICOLOGY

There have been no reported toxic effects, even at high doses.

WARNINGS/CONTRAINDICATIONS/PRECAUTIONS

No contraindications have been identified.

INTERACTIONS

- Biotin works closely with folic acid, pantothenic acid, vitamin B12, and coenzyme Q10—all must be present for activity.
- Biotin lessens the symptoms of pantothenic acid and zinc deficiencies.
- Raw egg white contains a protein called avidin that prevents biotin absorption.
- Sulfa drugs, estrogen, and alcohol may raise biotin requirements.
- Prolonged use of anticonvulsant drugs may lead to biotin deficiency.
- Long-term use of antibiotics can affect the balance of the digestive system and reduce or stop the manufacturing of biotin by bacteria.

REFERENCES

Bendich A, Deckelbaum R. *Preventive Nutrition: The Comprehensive Guide for Health Professionals.* Totowa, NJ: Humana Press; 1997.

Houchman LG, et al. Brittle nails: response to biotin supplementation. *Cutis.* 1993;51:303–307.

Jung U, Helbich-Endermann M, Bitsch R, et al. Are patients with chronic renal failure (CRF) deficient in biotin and is regular biotin supplementation required? *Z Ernahrungswiss.* 1998;37:363–367.

Koutsikos D, Agroyannis B, Tzanatos-Exarchou H. Biotin for diabetic peripheral neuropathy. *Biomed Pharmacother.* 1990;44:511–514.

Koutsikos D, Fourtounas C, Kapetanaki A, et al. Oral glucose tolerance test after high-dose i.v. biotin administration in normoglucemic hemodialysis patients. *Ren Fail.* 1996;18:131–137.

Messina M. *The Dietitian's Guide to Vegetarian Diets: Issues and Applications.* Gaithersburg, Md: Aspen Publishers, Inc; 1996.

Murray M. *Encyclopedia of Nutritional Supplements.* Rocklin, Calif: Prima Publishing; 1997.

Reavley N. *Vitamins etc.* Melbourne, Australia: Bookman Press; 1998.

Ringer DL. *Physicians Guide to Nutraceuticals.* Omaha, Neb: Nutritional Data Resources; 1998.

Schulpis KH, Nyalala JO, Papakonstantinou ED, et al. Biotin recycling impairment in phenylketonuric children with seborrheic dermatitis. *Int J Dermatol.* 1998;37:918–921.

Zempleni J, Mock DM. Advanced analysis of biotin metabolites in body fluids allows a more accurate measurement of biotin bioavailability and metabolism in humans. *J Nutr.* 1999;129:494–497.

■ VITAMIN K

OVERVIEW

Vitamin K is fat-soluable and has an important role in making prothrombin and other proteins that help with blood clotting. Injections of vitamin K may be given before or after surgery to prevent hemorrhaging. Patients at risk of excessive bleeding because of liver disease, jaundice, malabsorption, or prolonged use of aspirin or antibiotics may also receive injections. Vitamin K has been used to treat heavy menstrual bleeding. It has also been used with vitamin C to treat morning sickness.

This vitamin is not readily transferred from mother to child. Without the intestinal bacteria necessary to synthesize vitamin K, newborns are at increased risk for hemorrhage. In these cases, newborns are often given vitamin K injections. Additionally, premature babies are at high risk for brain hemorrhage. Vitamin K supplements are often given to women at high risk of delivering prematurely. Women taking anti-epileptic drugs during pregnancy are often given supplements of vitamin K as their babies are at particular risk for deficiency. In the early 1990s, researchers reported a possible increase in risk for childhood cancers in children who were given vitamin K injections at birth. Results of recent studies, however, have been inconclusive. Some research suggests that oral supplements in three doses of 1 to 2 mg, may be an acceptable alternative to injections.

Vitamin K inhibits the formation of calcium oxalate stones by synthesizing urinary proteins essential to kidney function. Vegetarians, whose diets are often high in vitamin K, have a low incidence of kidney stones.

Vitamin K is necessary for the conversion of osteocalcin, a protein that regulates the function of calcium in bone turnover and mineralization, to its active form. Vitamin K supplements may improve bone mineralization in postmenopausal women by increasing blood levels of osteocalcin and also by lowering the amount calcium excreted in the urine. Research suggests that vitamin K intakes much higher than the current recommendations improve biochemical markers of bone formation as well as bone density. Large supplemental doses of vitamin K have been useful in the treatment of osteoporosis. Low levels of vitamin K have been found in those with osteoporosis. In a Japanese study published in 1997, researchers found that, in a group of post-menopausal and peri-menopausal women with menopausal symptoms receiving hormone replacement therapy, those with reduced bone mineral density had lower levels of vitamin K_1 and K_2 than those with normal bone mineral density. Low levels of vitamin K have also been found in men with osteoporosis. A 1998 study suggested that vitamin K supplementation improves bone health in female elite athletes with amenorrhea. A 1998 study from the University of Pittsburgh suggests a synthetic form of vitamin K may stop liver cancer cell growth.

DIETARY SOURCES

- Chlorophyll
- Green tea
- Turnip greens
- Broccoli
- Spinach
- Cabbage
- Asparagus
- Dark green lettuce

Freezing foods may destroy vitamin K. However, heating does not affect it.

CONSTITUENTS/COMPOSITION

Vitamin K occurs in three forms. Vitamin K_1 (phylloquinone) is made by plants and is considered the preferred form; vitamin K_2 (menaquinone) is made by animals, birds, and by bacteria in the intestinal tract; and vitamin K_3 (menaphthone or menadione), is synthetic.

COMMERCIAL PREPARATIONS

- Supplemental vitamin K is available in both natural and synthetic forms.
- Supplements of fat-soluble chlorophyll are an excellent source of K_1.
- The water-soluble chlorophyll form of vitamin K is commonly sold in stores. Because this form cannot be absorbed in the gastrointestinal tract, its use is limited to the treatment of skin wounds.
- K_1 and K_3 are available in multivitamin complexes, and as 5-mg tablets.
- K_1 injections are found in 2 mg/ml in 0.5-ml amps, and in 10 mg/ml in 1-ml ampules, and 2.5-ml and 5-ml vials.

THERAPEUTIC USES

- Helps prevent hemorrhage in surgical patients.
- Reduces risk of excessive bleeding in those with liver disease, jaundice, malabsorption and kidney disease.
- Reduces excessive bleeding in those on long-term aspirin or antibiotic therapy.
- Treats heavy menstrual bleeding.
- Used with vitamin C to treat morning sickness.
- Is a preventive measure for hemorrhage in newborns.
- May prevent calcium oxalate stones in the kidney.
- Supplements may improve bone mineralization.
- Large supplemental doses have been used to treat osteoporosis.
- A vitamin K analog, K compound 5, may stop liver cancer growth.
- Some forms (water-soluble chlorophyll) helps to control body, fecal, and urinary odor.
- Water-soluble forms are used in the treatment of skin wounds.

DOSAGE RANGES AND DURATION OF ADMINISTRATION

Recommended Dietary Allowances (RDAs) are as follows.
- Neonates to 6 months: 5 mcg
- Infants 6 to 12 months:10 mcg
- Children 1 to 3 years: 15 mcg
- Children 4 to 6 years: 20 mcg
- Children 7 to 10 years: 30 mcg
- Men: 80 mcg
- Women: 65 mcg
- Pregnancy: 65 mcg
- Lactation: 65 mcg

Three doses are recommended to prevent neonatal hemorrhage: 1 to 2 mg, the first given at the first feeding, the second at two to four weeks, and the third at eight weeks.

SIDE EFFECTS/TOXICOLOGY

Natural vitamin K is rarely toxic. However, large amounts of menadione, a synthetic form of vitamin K, may cause liver damage and hemolytic anemia. Intravenous injection of vitamin K can cause flushing, sweats, chest pain, and constricted breathing. Hemolysis, jaundice, and hyperbilirubinemia have been observed in newborns after the administration of vitamin K. Pain, swelling, and eczema may result from intramuscular injections.

WARNINGS/CONTRAINDICATIONS/PRECAUTIONS

- Vitamin K can interfere with the action of anticoagulants such as warfarin or coumadin.
- X rays and radiation can raise vitamin K requirements.
- Vitamin K is excreted in breast milk, and crosses the placenta.

Use with caution in women who are pregnant or breast-feeding in conditions where there is concern for excess vitamin K.

INTERACTIONS

- Aspirin, cholestyramine, phenytoin, and mineral oil laxatives can increase the amount of vitamin K needed in the body.
- Vitamin K is injected to stop the bleeding caused by some snake venoms. These venoms destroy vitamin K, and prevent blood from clotting.
- Extended use of antibiotics may result in vitamin K deficiency. These drugs kill not only harmful bacteria, but also beneficial, vitamin K-activating bacteria.
- Taking large amounts of vitamin E and vitamin A may interfere with vitamin K function.

REFERENCES

Bendich A, Decklebaum R. *Preventive Nutrition: The Comprehensive Guide for Health Professionals.* Totowa, NJ: Humana Press; 1997.

Drug Facts and Comparisons 1999. St. Louis, Mo: Facts and Comparisons; 1998: 270–272.

Craciun AM, Wolf J, Knapen MH, Brouns F, Vermeer C. Improved bone metabolism in female elite athletes after vitamin K supplementation. *Int J Sports Med.* 1998;19:479–484.

Feskanich D, Weber P, Willett WC, Rockett H, Booth SL, Colditz GA. Vitamin K intake and hip fractures in women: a prospective study. *Am J Clin Nutr.* 1999;69:74–79.

Jatoi A, Lennon C, O'Brien M, Booth SL, Sadowski J, Mason JB. Protein-calorie malnutrition does not predict subtle vitamin K depletion in hospitalized patients. *Euro J Clin Nutri.* 1998; 52:934–937.

Jie KG, Bots ML, Vermeer C, Witteman JC, Grobbee DE. Vitamin K status and bone mass in women with and without aortic atherosclerosis: a population-based study. *Calcif Tissue Int.* 1996;59:352–356.

Kohlmeier M, Saupe J, Shearer MJ, Schaefer K, Asmus G. Bone health of adult hemodialysis patients is related to vitamin K status. *Kidney Int.* 1997;51:1218–1221.

Krummel D, Kris-Etherton P. *Nutrition in Women's Health.* Gaithersburg, Md: Aspen Publishers; 1996:434–435.

Lubetsky A, Dekel-Stern E, Chetrit A, Lubin F, Halkin H. Vitamin K intake and sensitivity to warfarin in patients consuming regular diets. *Thromb Haemost.* 1999;8:396–399.

Murray M. *Encyclopedia of Nutritional Supplements.* Rocklin, Calif: Prima Publishing; 1996:54–58.

Novel form of vitamin K may stop liver cancer cell growth. *Oncology.* 1998;12:1541.

Reavley N. *Vitamins, Etc.* Melbourne, Australia: Bookman Press; 1998

Shils ME, Olson JA, Shike M, Ross CA, eds. *Modern Nutrition in Health and Disease.* 9th ed. New York, NY: Lippincott, Williams & Wilkins; 1998.

Tamatani M, Morimoto S, Nakajima M, et al. Decreased circulating levels of vitamin K and 25-hydroxyvitamin D in osteopenic elderly men. *Metabolism.* 1998;47:195–199.

Which vitamin K preparation for the newborn? *Drug Ther Bull.* March 1998;36:17–19.

■ ZINC

OVERVIEW

Zinc is an essential trace mineral, which, next to iron, is the second most abundant trace mineral in the body. It is a component in over 200 enzymes. Zinc is stored primarily in muscle but high concentrations are also found in red and white blood cells, and the retina. It is also found in bones, skin, kidney, liver, and pancreas. In men, the prostate gland contains more zinc than any other organ.

Zinc is a part of some important antioxidant compounds, including superoxide dismutase (SOD) and zinc monomethionine. It protects the liver from chemical damage, helping with detoxification of the body. It is required for a healthy immune system. Taking zinc supplements has been shown to reduce infection and speed wound healing. Studies have shown it helps treat and prevent acne. It is essential for proper growth and development, especially early in life. It is necessary to maintain proper vision, taste, and smell.

Zinc deficiency may be a more common problem than previously thought, especially as people age. In clinical studies on the effects of zinc supplementation in the elderly, zinc improved immune system function, reduced the incidence of illness, and decreased the incidence of anorexia.

Recent research has been conducted to determine the true value of zinc lozenges in preventing or reducing cold symptoms.

DIETARY SOURCES

Zinc absorption from foods varies from 20% to 40% of ingested zinc. Zinc from animal foods is the best-absorbed form. When bound with the phytates or oxalates in vegetable sources, zinc is less available, and vegetable fiber itself impedes the absorption of zinc. Dairy products and eggs contain fair amounts of zinc, but again, it may be poorly absorbed from these sources.

The following foods contain high amounts of zinc in the most absorbable form.
- Oysters (richest source)
- Red meats
- Shrimp, crab, and other shellfish

Other good sources, but which may be less absorbable, include legumes (especially lima beans, black-eyed peas, pinto beans, soybeans, peanuts) whole grains, miso, tofu, brewer's yeast, cooked greens, mushrooms, green beans, and pumpkin seeds.

CONSTITUENTS/COMPOSITION

Zinc is a metallic element present in soil.

COMMERCIAL PREPARATIONS

The most commonly used zinc supplement has been zinc sulfate. This is the least expensive form, but it may cause gastric irritation and is less absorbable than other forms. It is usually prescribed as 220 mg zinc sulfate, which provides approximately 55 mg of elemental zinc. More absorbable forms such as the following are available.
- Zinc picolinate
- Zinc citrate
- Zinc acetate
- Zinc glycerate
- Zinc monomethionine

These forms come in capsules supplying 30 or 50 mg of elemental zinc. The amount in milligrams per capsule of these other zinc compounds can vary, according to the percentage of elemental zinc contained. Zinc lozenges are also available which supply varying amounts of zinc and used for treating colds.

THERAPEUTIC USES

Benefits of zinc include the following.
- Treats depressed immunity
- Improves wound healing
- Treats and may prevent acne
- May prevent macular degeneration
- Treats anorexia nervosa (anorexia is a symptom of zinc deficiency, and the teenage population is at higher risk for zinc deficiency due to dietary habits)
- Improves male fertility and sexual function, especially among smokers
- Treats rheumatoid arthritis
- Treats Wilson's disease (a disorder of excess copper storage)
- Decreases taste alteration during cancer treatments
- Improves sense of taste and smell

Some conditions may impair zinc absorption, or increase the need for zinc. Individuals with the following conditions may benefit from zinc supplementation.
- Acrodermatitis eteropathica (the inherited disease of zinc malabsorption)
- Pregnancy, lactation
- Alcoholism
- Diabetes
- Kidney disease, dialysis
- Celiac disease
- Inflammatory bowel disease, ulcerative colitis
- Chronic diarrhea
- Pancreatic insufficiency
- Oral contraceptive use
- Prostate problems (BPH, prostatitis, cancer)

DOSAGE RANGE AND DURATION OF ADMINISTRATION

The RDA for zinc is as follows.
- Infants to 1 year: 5 mg
- 1 to 10 years: 10 mg
- Males over 10 years: 15 mg
- Females over 10 years: 12 mg
- Pregnant females: 15 mg
- Lactating females: (0 to 6 months) 19 mg, (6 to 12 months) 16 mg

Therapeutic ranges (elemental zinc):
- Men: 30 to 60 mg daily
- Women: 30 to 45 mg daily

Doses over this amount should be limited to only a few months under the supervision of a health care professional.

SIDE EFFECTS/TOXICOLOGY

Zinc is the least toxic trace mineral. Symptoms of toxicity are GI irritation and vomiting, usually occurring after a dose of 2,000 mg or more has been ingested. Studies have confirmed that up to 10 times the RDA (150 mg) taken even over time was not toxic. Doses this high are unnecessary and interfere with the assimilation of other trace minerals such as copper and iron.

Too much zinc (over 150 mg/day over time) lowers HDL cholesterol and raises LDL cholesterol, an undesirable affect. Megadoses of zinc are reported to depress immune function. Studies on this have been inconclusive, and further research is needed.

Zinc sulfate can cause gastric irritation, but another form can be used instead if this occurs. Other reported side effects of zinc toxicity are dizziness, headache, drowsiness, increased sweating, muscular incoordination, alcohol intolerance, hallucinations, and anemia.

WARNINGS/CONTRAINDICATIONS/PRECAUTIONS

Because of the multiple interactions zinc has with other nutrients, it is advisable to take a balanced multiple vitamin/mineral preparation that contains zinc as well as copper, iron, and folate, to help prevent deficiencies of these nutrients.

INTERACTIONS

- Excess zinc can interfere with copper absorption and cause a copper deficiency which indirectly affects iron status and can lead to anemia.
- Excess copper intake interferes with zinc absorption.
- Iron supplements can impair zinc absorption. Optimally, zinc supplements should be taken at a separate time from iron-containing supplements.
- Calcium may interfere with zinc absorption at high doses.
- Zinc interferes with folate absorption.
- Dietary fiber (present in vegetables and, to a lesser degree, fruit) interferes with the absorption of zinc.

REFERENCES

Eby GA. Zinc ion availability—the determinant of efficacy in zinc lozenge treatment of common colds. *J Antimicrob Chemother.* 1997;40:483–493.

Feltman J. *Prevention's Food & Nutrition.* Emmaus, Pa: Rodale Press; 1993.

Fortes C, Forastiere F, Agabiti N, et al. The effect of zinc and vitamin A supplementation on immune response in an older population. *J Am Geriatr Soc.* 1998;46:19–26.

Garland ML, Hagmeyer KO. The role of zinc lozenges in treatment of the common cold. *Ann Pharmacother.* 1998;32:63–69.

Golik A, Zaidenstein R, Dishi V, et al. Effects of captopril and enalapril on zinc metabolism in hypertensive patients. *J Am Coll Nutr.* 1998;17:75–78.

Haas E. *Staying Healthy with Nutrition, The Complete Guide to Diet and Nutritional Medicine.* Berkeley, Calif: Celestial Arts Publishing; 1992.

Hendler SS. *The Doctors' Vitamin and Mineral Encyclopedia.* New York, NY: Fireside Press; 1991.

Lieberman S, Bruning N. *The Real Vitamin & Mineral Book.* 2nd ed. New York, NY: Avery Publishing Group; 1997.

Murray M. *Encyclopedia of Nutritional Supplements.* Rocklin, Calif: Prima Publishing; 1996.

Pronsky Z. *Food-Medication Interactions.* 9th ed. Pottstown, Pa: Food-Medicine Interactions; 1995.

Sazawal S, Black RE, Jalla S, et al. Zinc supplementation reduces the incidence of acute lower respiratory infections in infants and preschool children: a double-blind, controlled trial. *Pediatrics.* 1998;102(part 1):1–5.

Shealy CN. *The Illustrated Encyclopedia of Healing Remedies.* Boston, Mass: Element Books Inc.; 1998.

Somer E. *The Essential Guide to Vitamins and Minerals.* New York, NY: HarperCollins Publishers, Inc.; 1995.

Whitney E, Cataldo C, Rolfes S. *Understanding Normal and Clinical Nutrition.* St. Paul, Minn: West Publishing Co.; 1987.

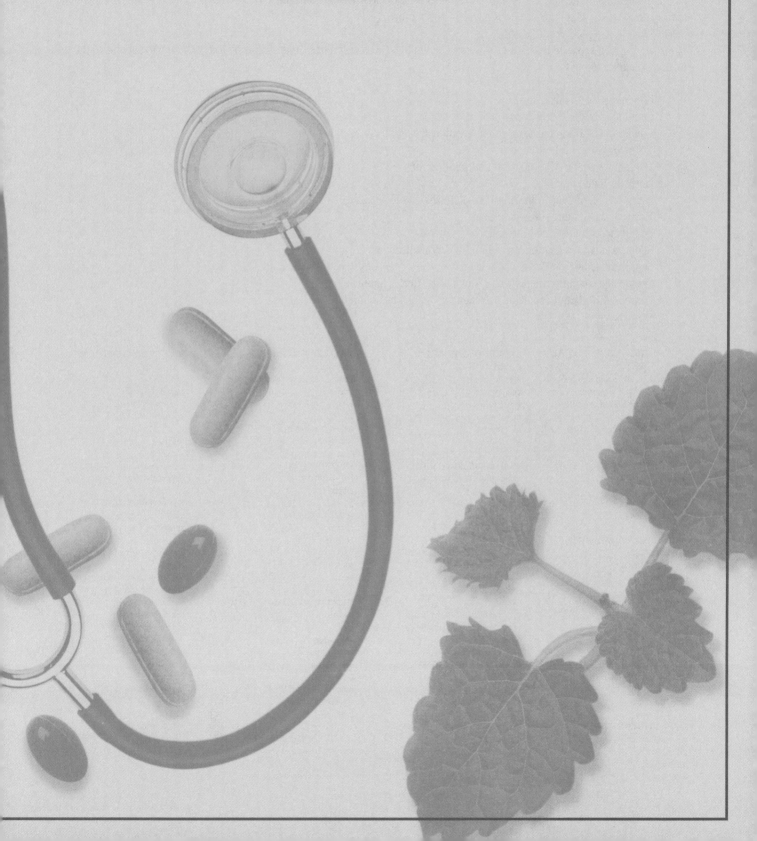

QUICK Access

CROSS-REFERENCE GUIDE

This comprehensive Cross-Reference Guide allows for a quick search of category lists drawn from the *Quick Access* monographs. At a glance, you can review the herbs or supplements used in treating a particular condition, the contraindications of using a particular herb or supplement, and much more. Once you have found what you are looking for in the Cross-Reference Guide, refer to the appropriate monograph for detail.

As an example, you may care to quickly review all of the herbs and supplements that may be used to treat benign prostatic hyperplasia. Using one of the many search lists included, you will find a list that includes vitamins, amino acids, herbs, and micro-nutrients. Reference back to the monograph on BPH to review more detail, or reference back to the monograph on the individual herb or supplement mentioned. The majority of those most often used or prescribed herbs and supplements are currently in *Quick Access* monograph system, with future editions supplying even more.

There are thirteen separate lists that can be searched in this Cross-Reference Guide, allowing easy and targeted access to the information you are looking for.

- Conditions by Medical Category
- Conditions by Signs and Symptoms
- Conditions by Herb and Supplement Treatment Options
- Herbs by Uses and Indications
- Herbs by Warnings, Precautions, Contraindications
- Herbs by Side Effects
- Herbs by Interactions with Other Drugs, Herbs, Supplements
- Herbs by Taxonomic Cross-Reference
- Supplements by Uses and Indications
- Supplements by Warnings, Precautions, Contraindications
- Supplements by Side Effects
- Supplements by Interactions with Other Drugs, Herbs, Supplements
- Combined Herb and Supplement Treatment Options by Condition

■ CONDITIONS BY MEDICAL CATEGORY

This list takes the condition monograph topics and organizes them into respective medical systems or categories.

BRAIN AND NERVOUS SYSTEM CONDITIONS
dementia
headache, migraine
headache, sinus
headache, tension
Parkinson's disease
seizure disorders

DIGESTION AND ABSORPTION CONDITIONS
cirrhosis of the liver
constipation
diarrhea
dysphagia
gallbladder disease
gastritis
gastroesophageal reflux disease
hepatitis, viral
intestinal parasites
irritable bowel syndrome
peptic ulcer
ulcerative colitis

ENDOCRINE CONDITIONS
diabetes mellitus
hyperthyroidism
hypothyroidism
thyroiditis

EYE/EAR/NOSE/THROAT CONDITIONS
allergic rhinitis
conjunctivitis
laryngitis
otitis media
pharyngitis
sinusitis

GENITOURINARY CONDITIONS
benign prostatic hyperplasia
prostatitis
urethritis
urinary incontinence
urolithiasis

GYNECOLOGIC CONDITIONS
amenorrhea
dysmenorrhea
endometriosis
menopause
preeclampsia
urinary tract infection in women
vaginitis

HEART and CIRCULATORY CONDITIONS
angina
atherosclerosis
congestive heart failure
hypertension
endocarditis
myocardial infarction
pericarditis

INFECTIOUS DISEASES
candidiasis
herpes zoster (varicella-zoster)
virus
herpes simplex virus
HIV and AIDS
Reiter's syndrome
Roseola

INTEGUMENTARY CONDITIONS
alopecia
burns
cutaneous drug reactions
dermatitis
eczema
insect bites
psoriasis
warts

MUSCULOSKELETAL CONDITIONS
bursitis
gout
low back pain
osteoarthritis
osteomyelitis
osteoporosis
rheumatoid arthritis
sprains and strains
tendinitis

PSYCHIATRIC CONDITIONS
anorexia nervosa
anxiety
depression-unipolar mood
disorders

PULMONARY CONDITIONS
asthma
bronchitis
chronic obstructive
pulmonary disease
common cold
cough
influenza
pertussis
primary pulmonary hypertension
pulmonary edema

OTHER CONDITIONS
anemia
attention-deficit/hyperactivity
disorder
chronic fatigue syndrome
edema
fever of unknown origin
fibromyalgia syndrome
food allergy
hemorrhoids
hypercholesterolemia
hyperkalemia
hypoglycemia
infantile colic
insomnia
motion sickness
obesity
Raynaud's phenomenon
sexual dysfunction
sleep apnea

■ **CONDITIONS BY SIGNS AND SYMPTOMS**

This list extracts the individual signs and symptoms included in each condition monograph and combines them to create a collection of all medical conditions that may be considered when a particular sign or symptom presents.

ABDOMINAL CRAMPING
allergic rhinitis
diarrhea
food allergy
insect bites
ulcerative colitis

ABDOMINAL CRAMPING, LOW
dysmenorrhea
irritable bowel syndrome
urinary tract infection in women

ABDOMINAL DISCOMFORT
hepatitis, viral

ABDOMINAL PAIN
anemia
cirrhosis of the liver
gastritis
HIV and AIDS
hypercholesterolemia
seizures

ABDOMINAL PAIN, LOW
benign prostatic hyperplasia

ABDOMINAL PAIN, RADIATING ANTERIORLY
urolithiasis

ABDOMINAL PAIN, UPPER RIGHT
preeclampsia

ABDOMINAL SWELLING
constrictive pericarditis

ABDOMINAL TENDERNESS
endometriosis

ABSCESS
candidiasis

ABSCESS, TISSUE AROUND PAINFUL BONE
osteomyelitis

ABSENTMINDEDNESS
seizures

ACHE RADIATING TO LOWER BACK, GROIN, LEGS
dysmenorrhea

ACHILLES TENDINITIS
Reiter's syndrome

ACNE
amenorrhea

ACNEIFORMS
cutaneous drug reactions

AGITATION
hyperthyroidism, thyroid storm

AGNOSIA
dementia

ALERTNESS, CHANGE IN
sleep apnea

ALLERGIES
chronic fatigue syndrome

ALLODYNIA
fibromyalgia syndrome

AMENORRHEA
menopause

ANAL FISSURES
hemorrhoids

ANAL INFECTIONS
herpes simplex virus, genital

ANAPHYLAXIS
insect bites

ANEMIA
ulcerative colitis

ANEMIA, NORMOCHROMIC
rheumatoid arthritis

ANEMIA, NORMOCYTIC
rheumatoid arthritis

ANGINA
anemia
pulmonary edema

ANGIOEDEMA
food allergy
insect bites

ANGIOMAS, SPIDER
cirrhosis of the liver

ANOREXIA
amenorrhea
cirrhosis of the liver
congestive heart failure
gallbladder disease
gastritis
hepatitis, viral
pericarditis
pertussis
Reiter's syndrome
ulcerative colitis

ANTERIOR FONTANELLE, BULGING
roseola

ANXIETY
congestive heart failure
dementia
hypoglycemia
myocardial infarction
pericarditis
pulmonary edema
sexual dysfunction

ANXIETY, ANTICIPATORY
insomnia

AORTITIS
Reiter's syndrome

APHASIA
dementia
endocarditis

APHONIA
laryngitis

APNEA
pertussis
seizures

APNEA SYNDROME, INFANTS
gastroesophageal reflux disease

APPETITE, INCREASED
hyperthyroidism

APPETITE LOSS
allergic rhinitis
severe herpes simplex virus
neonatal herpes simplex virus
oral-facial herpes zoster
   (varicella-zoster)
influenza

APRAXIA
dementia

ARCHED BACK AND CLENCHED FISTS
infantile colic

ARRHYTHMIA
myocardial infarction
Reiter's syndrome

ARTERIES, HARDENED FEEL OF
atherosclerosis

ARTHRALGIAS
chronic fatigue syndrome
hepatitis, viral
ulcerative colitis

ARTHRITIC DISORDERS
Reiter's syndrome

ARTHRITIS (THREE JOINTS OR MORE)
rheumatoid arthritis

ARTHUS REACTION
insect bites

ASCITES, PORTAL HYPERTENSION
cirrhosis of the liver

ASPIRATION
dysphagia, oropharyngeal

ASPIRATION, RECURRENT
gastroesophageal reflux disease

ASTHMA
insect bites

ASYMMETRICAL SIGNS
Reiter's syndrome

AURA
migraine headache
seizures

AUTOMATISMS
seizures

AVERSION TO CIGARETTES
hepatitis, viral

BACK PAIN
anemia
endocarditis
low back pain
osteoporosis
prostatitis

BACK PAIN, PERSISTENT
osteomyelitis

BALANCE, POOR
Parkinson's disease

BALDNESS, FEMALE DIFFUSE
alopecia

BALDNESS, MALE PATTERN
alopecia

BALD PATCHES
alopecia

BELCHING
gastroesophageal reflux disease
infantile colic

BILIARY COLIC
gallbladder disease

BIZARRE BEHAVIOR
hypoglycemia

BLADDER FUNCTION PAIN
endometriosis

BLADDER OUTLET OBSTRUCTION
benign prostatic hyperplasia
prostatitis

BLEPHAROSPASM
Parkinson's disease

BLINDNESS
herpes simplex virus, eye

BLINKING, INFREQUENT
hyperthyroidism

BLISTERS
burns
dermatitis
psoriasis

BLOATING
constipation
edema
intestinal parasites
irritable bowel syndrome

BLOOD PRESSURE, HIGH
preeclampsia
seizures

BLOOD PRESSURE, RAPID DROP
food allergy

BLOOD PRESSURE ABNORMALITIES
amenorrhea

BLURRED VISION
diabetes
herpes simplex virus
HIV and AIDS
hypoglycemia

BODY-MASS INDEX (BMI) OVER 25 OR 30
obesity

BONE PAIN AND SENSATION OF HEAT
osteomyelitis

BONY CREPITUS
osteoarthritis

BONY HYPERTROPHY
osteoarthritis

BOWEL EMPTYING, INCOMPLETE
constipation
irritable bowel syndrome

BOWEL FUNCTION PAIN
endometriosis

BOWEL HABIT CHANGES
irritable bowel syndrome

BOWEL MOVEMENT, RELIEF OF PAIN AFTER
irritable bowel syndrome

BOWEL MOVEMENT, UPON WAKING OR AFTER EATING
irritable bowel syndrome

BOWEL MOVEMENTS, DIFFICULTY
constipation

BOWEL MOVEMENTS, MUCUS DISCHARGE
ulcerative colitis

BRADYKINESIA
Parkinson's disease

BREAST ENLARGEMENT
amenorrhea

BREATH, SHORTNESS OF
asthma
bronchitis
food allergy
endocarditis

BREATHING DIFFICULTY
edema
HIV and AIDS
hyperkalemia
laryngitis
Parkinson's disease
pharyngitis

BREATHING SPLINTED
pericarditis

BRONCHIAL INFECTION, RECURRENT
chronic obstructive
  pulmonary disease

BRONCHITIS-LIKE SYMPTOMS
pertussis

BRONCHOSPASM
gastroesophageal reflux disease

BRUIT, OVER THYROID GLAND
hyperthyroidism

BRUIT OVER NARROWED VESSEL
atherosclerosis

CARDIOVASCULAR FAILURE
insect bites

CARPAL TUNNEL SYNDROME
hypothyroidism

CERVICAL ADENOPATHY
herpes simplex virus, oral-facial

CERVICAL LESIONS
herpes simplex virus, genital

CERVICITIS
urethritis in women

CHEST, BURNING SENSATION
bronchitis

CHEST, HYPERINFLATED
asthma

CHEST, PRESSURE SENSATION
dysphagia, esophageal

CHEST PAIN
angina
atherosclerosis
gastroesophageal reflux disease
HIV and AIDS
myocardial infarction
pericarditis

CHEST PAIN, PLEURITIC
primary pulmonary hypertension

CHEST TIGHTNESS
asthma
pulmonary edema

CHILLS
chronic fatigue syndrome
cough
diarrhea
gout
endocarditis
influenza
pharyngitis
prostatitis
urinary tract infection in women
urolithiasis

CHOKING
dysphagia
oropharyngeal
pertussis

CIRCINATE BALANITIS
Reiter's syndrome

CIRCULATORY COLLAPSE
herpes simplex virus, neonatal

CIRRHOSIS
amenorrhea

CIRRHOSIS OF LIVER
alcoholism

COLD, DAMP WEATHER PAIN
sinus headache

COLD AND CYANOSED FEET AND HANDS
migraine headache

COLD HANDS AND FEET
menopause

COLD INTOLERANCE
hypothyroidism

COMA
diabetes
hypoglycemia
seizures

CONCENTRATION, IMPAIRED
anxiety
chronic fatigue syndrome
depression-unipolar mood
  disorders

CONFUSION
hyperthyroidism
hypothyroidism

CONGESTIVE HEART FAILURE
cough

CONJUNCTIVITIS
herpes simplex virus, eye
Reiter's syndrome

CONSCIOUSNESS, ALTERING
pericardial effusion

CONSCIOUSNESS, LOSS OF
seizures

CONSCIOUSNESS, LOSS OF, INFANTS
pertussis

CONSTANT MOTION TO LESSEN PAIN
urolithiasis

CONSTANT STARE
hyperthyroidism

CONSTIPATION
dysmenorrhea
hemorrhoids
hypothyroidism
irritable bowel syndrome
Parkinson's disease
seizures

CORNEAL LESIONS
herpes simplex virus, eye

CORNEAL ULCERATION
Reiter's syndrome

CORONARY HEART DISEASE
menopause

COSTOCHONDRITIS
Reiter's syndrome

COUGH
asthma
chronic obstructive pulmonary
  disease
common cold
HIV and AIDS

endocarditis
primary pulmonary hypertension
sinusitis
sleep apnea

COUGH, BLOOD
edema

COUGH, CHRONIC
gastroesophageal reflux disease

COUGH, INCREASING
pertussis

COUGH, MUCUS OR PUS PRODUCED BY
bronchitis

COUGH, NONPRODUCTIVE
influenza

COUGH, ORTHOPNEIC
congestive heart failure

COUGH, RESIDUAL
pertussis

COUGH, WHILE SWALLOWING
dysphagia, oropharyngeal

COUGH PAROXYSMS
pertussis

CREPITUS
tendinitis

CRYING, INFANT
otitis media

CRYING, INCONSOLABLE
infantile colic

CUSHING'S SYNDROME
amenorrhea

CUTANEOUS DISEASE
candidiasis

CYANOSIS
asthma
bronchitis
chronic obstructive pulmonary disease
herpes simplex virus, neonatal
pericardial effusion
pulmonary edema
Raynaud's phenomenon
seizures

CYSTITIS
Reiter's syndrome

DEATH THOUGHTS
depression-unipolar mood
  disorders

DECLINING SCHOOL PERFORMANCE
seizures

DEFECATION, FREQUENT NEED
diarrhea
ulcerative colitis

DEFECATION, STRAINING
hemorrhoids

DEHYDRATION
diabetes

DELERIUM
hyperthyroidism, thyroid storm
endocarditis

DEMENTIA
HIV and AIDS
hypothyroidism
Parkinson's disease

DENGUE FEVER
insect bites

DEPRESSION
anorexia
HIV and AIDS
hypoglycemia
hypothyroidism
menopause
seizures
sexual dysfunction
sleep apnea
tension headache

DERMAL DISEASE
herpes simplex virus

DERMAL TISSUE NECROSIS
cutaneous drug reactions

DERMATITIS, ATOPIC
food allergy

DERMIS, EPIDERMIS, AND DEEPER LAYERS
burns, third degree

DIAPHORESIS
pulmonary edema

DIAPHRAGM, FLATTENED
asthma

DIARRHEA
allergic rhinitis
dysmenorrhea
food allergy
HIV and AIDS
influenza
insect bites
irritable bowel syndrome
otitis media
roseola
seizures
ulcerative colitis

DIARRHEA, BLOODY
ulcerative colitis

DIARRHEA, MALODOROUS
intestinal parasites

DIARRHEA, VIOLENT
ulcerative colitis

DIGITAL PERIOSITIS
Reiter's syndrome

DISINHIBITED BEHAVIOR
dementia

DISTORTED PERCEPTION OF PHYSICAL SELF
anorexia

DIZZINESS
anxiety
fibromyalgia syndrome
menopause
motion sickness
myocardial infarction

DROWSINESS, DAYTIME
insomnia
sleep apnea

DYSENTERY
intestinal parasites

DYSMENORRHEA
endometriosis

DYSPAREUNIA
endometriosis

DYSPEPSIA
gastritis

DYSPHAGIA
gastroesophageal reflux disease
laryngitis
thyroiditis, Riedel's
thyroiditis, subacute

DYSPNEA
anemia
anxiety
asthma
chronic obstructive pulmonary disease
congestive heart failure
constrictive pericarditis
myocardial infarction
pericardial effusion
pulmonary edema
thyroiditis, Riedel's

DYSPNEA, EXERTIONAL
primary pulmonary hypertension

DYSURIA
herpes simplex virus, genital
prostatitis

EARDRUM, BULGING
otitis media

EAR INFECTIONS
allergic rhinitis

EARLY-MORNING WAKING
insomnia

EAR PAIN
otitis media

EATING, EXTENDED TIME REQUIRED
dysphagia, esophageal

EATING, RELUCTANCE
anorexia

ECZEMATOUS REACTION
cutaneous drug reactions

EDEMA
candidiasis
herpes simplex virus, eye
herpes simplex virus, finger or hand
insect bites

sprains and strains
tendinitis

EDEMA, HANDS AND FACE
preeclampsia

EDEMA, LOWER EXTREMITY
pulmonary edema

EDEMA, LOWER EXTREMITY
pulmonary edema

EDEMA, PERIPHERAL
chronic obstructive pulmonary disease
cirrhosis of the liver
congestive heart failure

EJACULATION, PAINFUL
prostatitis

EJACULATION, PREMATURE OR RETARDED
sexual dysfunction

ELECTROCARDIOGRAM, ABNORMAL
angina

EMACIATION
anorexia

EMBOLUS
atherosclerosis

EMESIS, RECURRENT, INFANTS
gastroesophageal reflux disease

EMOTIONAL EXPRESSION, RESTRAINED
anorexia

EMOTIONAL STRESS
tension headache

ENERGY LOSS
depression-unipolar mood disorders

EPIDERMIS, RED AND PAINFUL
burns, first degree

EPIDERMIS, RED AND PAINFUL WITH BLISTERS
burns, second degree

EPIGASTRIC PAIN
peptic ulcer

EPIGASTRIC PAIN, UPPER RIGHT QUADRANT
gallbladder disease

ERECTION, INABILITY TO MAINTAIN
sexual dysfunction

ERYTHEMA
bursitis
eczema
herpes simplex virus, finger or hand
insect bites

ERYTHEMA, VULVAR
candidiasis

ERYTHEMA MULTIFORME/NODOSUM
cutaneous drug reactions

ERYTHEMATOUS BUCCAL MUCOSA
candidiasis

ERYTHROCYTE SEDIMENTATION RATE, ELEVATED
rheumatoid arthritis

ESOPHAGEAL LESIONS
candidiasis

ESOPHAGUS, SENSATION OF FOOD STUCK
dysphagia, esophageal

EUNUCHOIDISM/GIGANTISM (TALL STATURE)
amenorrhea

EXCORIATIONS
dermatitis

EXECUTIVE FUNCTIONING DISTURBANCE
dementia

EXERCISE INTOLERANCE
congestive heart failure

EXERTION, PAIN BROUGHT ON BY
angina

EXTREMITIES, SWOLLEN
edema

EXTREMITY, LOWER, EDEMA
pulmonary edema

EXTREMITY NUMBNESS
diabetes
Raynaud's phenomenon

EXTREMITY PAIN
endocarditis

EXTREMITY TINGLING
diabetes

EYEBROWS, LOSS OF
hypothyroidism

EYE DISCHARGE
conjunctivitis

EYE ITCHING, TEARING, BURNING
conjunctivitis

EYE PAIN
herpes simplex virus, eye

EYE REDNESS
conjunctivitis

EYES, GRITTY SENSATION
conjunctivitis

EYES, OVERNIGHT CRUSTING
conjunctivitis

EYES, SWELLING
thyroiditis, Hashimoto's

EYES, SWOLLEN, REDDENED, BULGING
hyperthyroidism

FACIAL LESIONS
herpes simplex virus, oral-facial

FACIAL PAIN, LOCALIZED
sinus headache

FACIAL PUFFINESS
edema
hypothyroidism

FACIAL SWELLING
food allergy

FAILURE TO THRIVE, INFANTS
gastroesophageal reflux disease

FATIGUE
allergic rhinitis, severe
anemia
anxiety
bronchitis
congestive heart failure
constrictive pericarditis
depression-unipolar mood
   disorders
diabetes
fibromyalgia syndrome
hepatitis, viral
hyperkalemia
hypoglycemia
endocarditis
influenza
intestinal parasites
motion sickness
osteomyelitis
sleep apnea

FATIGUE, EXCESSIVE
primary pulmonary hypertension

FATIGUE, SEVERE
chronic fatigue syndrome

FATTY FOOD INTOLERANCE
gallbladder disease

FEELINGS OF INEFFECTIVENESS
anorexia
depression

FEELINGS OF UNREALITY
anxiety

FEVER
bronchitis
bursitis
candidiasis
cough
diarrhea
fever of unknown origin
gout
hepatitis, viral
herpes simplex virus, finger
   or hand
herpes simplex virus, genital
herpes simplex virus, neonatal
herpes simplex virus, oral-facial
HIV and AIDS
hyperthyroidism, thyroid storm
endocarditis
laryngitis

osteomyelitis
otitis media
pericarditis
pharyngitis
prostatitis
Reiter's syndrome
roseola
sinus headache
sinusitis
ulcerative colitis
urinary tract infection in women
urolithiasis

FEVER, LOW-GRADE
chronic fatigue syndrome
herpes zoster (varicella-zoster)
pertussis
rheumatoid arthritis
thyroiditis, subacute

FEVER, SUDDEN ONSET
influenza

FEVER (CHILDREN)
common cold

FINGERNAILS/TOENAILS, PITTED AND DISCOLORED
psoriasis

FINGERTIP PAIN (OSLER NODE)
endocarditis

FINGERTIPS, ULCERS
Raynaud's phenomenon

FISSURING, SKIN
dermatitis

FLANK PAIN, SEVERE
urolithiasis

FLATULENCE
food allergy

FLUSHING
pericarditis

FRACTURE, WITHOUT TRAUMA
osteoporosis

GAIT DISTURBANCES
Parkinson's disease

GANGRENE
atherosclerosis

GASSINESS
infantile colic
intestinal parasites
irritable bowel syndrome

GASTRITIS, ANTRAL
peptic ulcer

GASTROESOPHAGEAL REFLUX DISEASE
cough
dysphagia, esophageal

GASTROESOPHAGEAL VARICES, BLEEDING
cirrhosis of the liver

GASTROINTESTINAL BLEEDING
gastritis

GASTROINTESTINAL DISTRESS
cirrhosis of the liver
dysmenorrhea

GASTROINTESTINAL LESIONS
candidiasis

GENITALIA, EXTERNAL, RED AND SWOLLEN
vaginitis

GENITAL LESIONS, EXTERNAL
herpes simplex virus, genital

GINGIVA
herpes simplex virus, oral-facial

GINGIVOSTOMATITIS
herpes simplex virus, oral-facial

GLOBUS SENSATION, NECK
gastroesophageal reflux disease

GLOSSITIS
anemia

GLYCOSURIA
diabetes

GOITER
amenorrhea
iodine deficiency

GROWTH RETARDATION, CHILDREN
hypothyroidism

GUILT, INAPPROPRIATE
depression-unipolar mood
   disorders

GYNECOMASTIA
cirrhosis of the liver

HAIR, DRY, SCALY, THICK, AND COARSE
hypothyroidism

HAIRS, BROKEN OR EASILY REMOVED
alopecia

HALLUCINATIONS
dementia

HAND JOINTS, PAIN
rheumatoid arthritis

HEADACHE
allergic rhinitis
amenorrhea
anemia
chronic fatigue syndrome
dysmenorrhea
fever of unknown origin
fibromyalgia syndrome
food allergy
hepatitis, viral
herpes simplex virus, genital
herpes zoster (varicella-zoster)
HIV and AIDS

hypertension
hypoglycemia
hypothyroidism
endocarditis
influenza
menopause
motion sickness
pharyngitis
seizures
sinusitis

HEADACHE, BIFRONTAL OR OCCIPITAL
tension headache

HEADACHE, FRONTAL
sinus headache

HEADACHE, MORNING
sleep apnea

HEAD FULLNESS, HEAD SHAKING
otitis media

HEAD PAIN, STEADY AND DULL
tension headache

HEARING DIFFICULTY
otitis media

HEARING DISTURBANCES
migraine headache

HEARTBEAT, RAPID
thyroiditis, silent

HEARTBURN
cough
gastroesophageal reflux disease

HEART RATE, RAPID INCREASE
food allergy

HEAVINESS, TIGHTNESS, BURNING IN CHEST
myocardial infarction

HEBERDEN'S NODULES OF DISTAL INTERPHALANGEAL JOINTS
osteoarthritis

HEIGHT, LOSS OF
osteoporosis

HELICOBACTER PYLORI
peptic ulcer

HEMGOLOBINURIA
anemia

HEMIPARESIS
endocarditis

HEMOPTYSIS
congestive heart failure
primary pulmonary hypertension

HEPATIC ENCEPHALOPATHY
cirrhosis of the liver

HEPATOMEGALY
cirrhosis of the liver
herpes simplex virus, neonatal

HERPES
HIV and AIDS

HERPETIC WHITLOW
herpes simplex virus, finger or
hand

HIRSUITISM, FACIAL
menopause

HIVES
allergic rhinitis
food allergy

HOARSENESS
common cold
gastroesophageal reflux disease
hypothyroidism
laryngitis
thyroiditis, Riedel's

HOARSENESS, SUDDEN
food allergy

HOT FLUSHES
amenorrhea
menopause

HYPERACTIVITY
attention-deficit/
  hyperactivity disorder
depression-unipolar mood
  disorders
thyroiditis, silent

HYPERGLYCEMIA
diabetes

HYPERLIPIDEMIA
diabetes

HYPERSALIVATION
motion sickness

HYPERSOMNIA
depression-unipolar mood
  disorders

HYPERTENSION
hyperthyroidism
myocardial infarction
obesity
sleep apnea

HYPERTENSION, PORTAL
cirrhosis of the liver

HYPERVIGILANCE
anxiety

HYPOTENSION
candidiasis
myocardial infarction

HYPOTENSION, RELATIVE
pericardial effusion

**HYPOTENSION, SECONDARY TO
ANAPHYLACTIC SHOCK**
insect bites

HYPOTHERMIA
herpes simplex virus, neonatal

IMPAIRED FUNCTIONING
insomnia

IMPOTENCE
sexual dysfunction
sleep apnea

IMPULSIVITY
attention-deficit/hyperactivity
  disorder

INACTIVITY
depression-unipolar mood
  disorders

INATTENTION
attention-deficit hyperactivity
  disorder

INCONTINENCE
dementia
menopause
Parkinson's disease
seizures

INCOORDINATION
hypoglycemia

INDURATION
eczema

**INFECTION, INCREASED
SUSCEPTIBILITY TO**
diabetes

INFECTIONS, CHRONIC
HIV and AIDS

INFERTILITY
endometriosis

INFLAMMATION
arthritis
burns
candidiasis
gout
insect bites
laryngitis
osteomyelitis
tendinitis
sprains and strains

INFLUENZA
hepatitis, viral

INITIATIVE, RESTRAINED
anorexia

INSOMNIA
anorexia
anxiety
congestive heart failure
depression-unipolar mood
  disorders
tension headache

**INSPIRATIONS, SUDDEN
FORCEFUL**
pertussis

INTERCOURSE, PAIN DURING
sexual dysfunction

INTESTINAL PAIN
endometriosis

IRITIS
Reiter's syndrome

IRRITABILITY
allergic rhinitis, severe
anorexia
anxiety
common cold
depression-unipolar mood
  disorders
herpes simplex virus, oral-facial
hypoglycemia
hypoglycemia
menopause
migraine headache
osteomyelitis
otitis media
seizures
sleep apnea

IRRITABLE BOWEL SYNDROME
fibromyalgia syndrome

ITCHING
eczema
herpes simplex virus, genital
psoriasis
warts

ITCHING, MUCOUS MEMBRANES
allergic rhinitis

ITCHING, PENILE OPENING
urethritis

JAUNDICE
cirrhosis of the liver
hepatitis, viral

JAUNDICE, EPISODIC
anemia

JAUNDICE, PROGRESSIVE
herpes simplex virus, neonatal

**JOINT, SHINY RED OR
PURPLE COLORATION**
gout

JOINT INSTABILITY
sprains and strains

JOINT PAIN
fibromyalgia syndrome
gout
endocarditis
osteoarthritis
psoriasis

**JOINT SWELLING, HEAT, AND
STIFFNESS**
gout

JUGULAR VEIN DISTENSION
constrictive pericarditis

KAPOSI SARCOMA
HIV and AIDS

KERATITIS
Reiter's syndrome

**KERATODERMAL
BLENNORRHAGICA**
Reiter's syndrome

KETOACIDOSIS
diabetes

KOILONYCHIA
anemia

LANGUAGE DETERIORATION
dementia

LARYNGITIS
gastroesophageal reflux disease

LARYNGOEDEMA
insect bites

LEG CRAMPS
atherosclerosis
diabetes

LEG FATIGUE
low back pain

LETHARGY
depression-unipolar mood
  disorders
herpes simplex virus, neonatal
hypothyroidism
seizures

LIBIDO, DIMINISHED
anorexia
depression-unipolar mood
  disorders

LICHENOID
cutaneous drug reactions

LID LAG
hyperthyroidism
hypothyroidism

LIGHTHEADEDNESS
anemia
anxiety

LIP LESIONS
herpes simplex virus, oral-facial

LIPS, SWELLING OR ITCHING
food allergy

LIVER, ENLARGEMENT
hypercholesterolemia

LOUD P2
primary pulmonary hypertension

**LUPUS ERYTHEMATOSUS WITH
MALAR ERYTHEMA**
cutaneous drug reactions

LYME DISEASE
insect bites

LYMPHADENOPATHY
chronic fatigue syndrome
rheumatoid arthritis

**LYMPHADENOPATHY,
AXILLARY**
herpes simplex virus, finger or
hand

LYMPHADENOPATHY, INGUINAL
herpes simplex virus, genital

LYMPHADENOPATHY, PERSISTENT
HIV and AIDS

LYMPH NODE ENLARGEMENT
pharyngitis

MACULOPAPULAR ERUPTIONS
cutaneous drug reactions

MACULOPAPULES
herpes zoster (varicella-zoster)

MALAISE
candidiasis
cirrhosis of the liver
diarrhea
fever of unknown origin
hepatitis, viral
herpes simplex virus, genital
herpes simplex virus, oral-facial
herpes zoster (varicella-zoster)
   virus
endocarditis
laryngitis
motion sickness
osteomyelitis
pericarditis
prostatitis
Reiter's syndrome
rheumatoid arthritis
sinusitis
thyroiditis, subacute
ulcerative colitis

MALARIA
insect bites

MALIGNANCIES
HIV and AIDS

MEMORY IMPAIRMENT
dementia

MEMORY LAPSES
dementia
fibromyalgia

MEMORY LOSS
dementia
Parkinson's disease
sleep apnea

MENSTRUAL DISORDERS
hypothyroidism

MENSTRUAL IRREGULARITIES
cirrhosis of the liver

MENSTRUAL PAIN
dysmenorrhea

MENSTRUATION, ALTERED
hyperthyroidism

MENSTRUATION, HEAVY
dysmenorrhea

MENSTRUATION, PELVIC PAIN CYCLING WITH
endometriosis

MENTAL CONFUSION
dementia
hypoglycemia

MENTAL DEFICIENCY, CHILDREN
hypothyroidism

MENTAL STATUS, SUDDEN CHANGE
edema

MICROABSCESS
candidiasis

MIDEPIGASTRIC PAIN/ TENDERNESS
intestinal parasites

MOOD DISTURBANCES
dementia

MOODINESS
sleep apnea

MOTOR ACTIVITIES, IMPAIRMENT
dementia

MOTOR DISTURBANCES
dementia

MOUTH, DRY
sleep apnea

MOUTH, SWELLING AND ITCHING
food allergy

MOUTH FISSURES
candidiasis

MOUTH INFLAMMATION
Reiter's syndrome

MUCOSAL DISEASE
herpes simplex virus

MUSCLE ACHES
influenza

MUSCLE ATROPHY
atherosclerosis

MUSCLE PAIN
endocarditis

MUSCLES, NECK AND SHOULDERS, TIGHT AND SORE
tension headache

MUSCLE SPASM, TOTAL BODY
seizures

MUSCLE TENSION
anxiety

MUSCLE TONE, POSTURAL, LOSS OF
seizures

MUSCLE WEAKNESS
chronic fatigue syndrome
endocarditis

MUSCULAR PAIN
edema

MYALGIAS
chronic fatigue syndrome
fever of unknown origin
hepatitis, viral

herpes simplex virus, oral-facial
pericarditis

MYIASIS
insect bites

MYOCARDIAL INFARCTION
endocarditis

MYOCLONIC LIMB JERKS
seizures

NASAL CONGESTION
allergic rhinitis
common cold
sinusitis

NASAL DISCHARGE, PURULENT
sinus headache

NASAL MUCOSA, INFLAMMATION
sinusitis

NASAL OBSTRUCTION
allergic rhinitis
influenza

NASAL PASSAGES, RED AND TURGESCENT
sinus headache

NAUSEA
amenorrhea
congestive heart failure
dysmenorrhea
food allergy
gallbladder disease
gastritis
hepatitis, viral
hypertension, severe
influenza
intestinal parasites
migraine headache
motion sickness
myocardial infarction
peptic ulcer
urolithiasis

NECK VEINS, DISTENDED
congestive heart failure

NECROSIS, CUTANEOUS
insect bites

NERVOUSNESS
anxiety
hyperthyroidism
thyroiditis, silent

NEURALGIA
postherpetic
herpes zoster (varicella-zoster)
   virus

NEURALGIA, FACIAL
herpes simplex virus, oral-facial

NEURITIS, ACUTE
herpes zoster (varicella-zoster)

NEUROLOGICAL SIGNS, ABNORMAL
edema

NEUROLOGICAL SYMPTOMS
anemia

NOCTURIA
congestive heart failure
menopause
prostatitis

NOSE, RUNNY AND ITCHING
food allergy

NUMBNESS
endocarditis
Raynaud's phenomenon

OBSESSIVE-COMPULSIVE BEHAVIOR
anorexia

OCULAR ABNORMALITIES
Parkinson's disease

ODYNOPHAGIA
gastroesophageal reflux disease
pericarditis

ORGASM, DIFFICULTY
sexual dysfunction

OSTEOPOROSIS
menopause

PAIN
herpes simplex virus, genital
infantile colic
internal hemorrhoids
Raynaud's phenomenon
Reiter's syndrome
sprains and strains
tendinitis
ulcerative colitis

PAIN, ACUTE ONSET
bursitis
myocardial infarction

PAIN, EXQUISITE
gout

PAIN, LOCALIZED
bursitis

PAIN, THYROID AREA
thyroiditis, suppurative

PAIN FOLLOWING MEALS
gallbladder disease

PAIN REFERRED TO LABIUM
urolithiasis

PAIN REFERRED TO TESTES
urolithiasis

PALATE LESIONS
herpes simplex virus, oral-facial

PALLOR
endocarditis
motion sickness
Raynaud's phenomenon
seizures

PALMAR ERYTHEMA
cirrhosis of the liver

PALPITATIONS
anemia
anxiety
hyperkalemia
hyperthyroidism
hypoglycemia
menopause
primary pulmonary hypertension

PANCREATITIS SYMPTOMS
hypercholesterolemia

PAPULES
eczema

PAPULES, FLESH-TONE
warts

PAPULES, ROUGH, THICKENED, SCARCELY ELEVATED
Plantar warts

PAPULES, TINY AND FLAT
genital warts

PARALYSIS
hyperkalemia
endocarditis
stroke

PARESTHESIA
fibromyalgia
hyperkalemia

PAROTID ENLARGEMENT
cirrhosis of the liver

PELVIC INFLAMMATORY DISEASE
urethritis in women

PELVIC PAIN
endometriosis
pelvic inflammatory disease

PERIANAL INFECTIONS
herpes simplex virus, genital

PERIANAL LUMP
external hemorrhoids

PERICARDITIS
Reiter's syndrome
rheumatoid arthritis

PERINEAL IRRITATION
urinary incontinence

PERIODONTAL DISEASE
osteoporosis

PERIPHERAL EDEMA
constrictive pericarditis
primary pulmonary hypertension

PERLECHE
candidiasis

PERSONAL CONTROL, EXCESSIVE NEED FOR
anorexia

PERSONALITY OR BEHAVIOR CHANGE
sleep apnea

PETECHIAE
endocarditis

PHARYNGEAL MUCUS MEMBRANE INFLAMMATION
pharyngitis

PHARYNGITIS
herpes simplex virus, oral-facial
sinusitis

PHOTOSENSITIVITY
cutaneous drug reactions

PHYSICAL ACTIVITY, PAIN WITH
fibromyalgia
tension headache

PHYSICAL STRESSORS, INCREASED SUSCEPTIBILITY
dementia

PICA
anemia

PLANTAR FASCITIS
Reiter's syndrome

PLEURAL EFFUSION
rheumatoid arthritis

PNEUMONIA
herpes simplex virus

POLYDIPSIA
diabetes

POLYPHAGIA
diabetes

POLYURIA
amenorrhea
diabetes

POSTEXERTIONAL PAIN
fibromyalgia

POSTICTAL CONFUSION
seizures

POSTNASAL DRIP
cough
sinusitis

POSTURAL ABNORMALITIES
osteoporosis
Parkinson's disease

PREMENSTRUAL SYNDROME
dysmenorrhea
tension headache

PREOCCUPATION WITH BODY IMAGE
anorexia

PREOCCUPATION WITH FOOD
anorexia

PROSTATITIS
Reiter's syndrome

PROTEIN, IN URINE
preeclampsia

PROTEINURIA
congestive heart failure

PRURITIC PAPULES
insect bites

PRURITIS
candidiasis
dermatitis
diabetes
external hemorrhoids
herpes zoster (varicella-zoster)
insect bites

PRURITIS, VAGINAL AND VULVAR
vaginitis

PSYCHOLOGICAL DISTURBANCES
Anxiety
dementia
depression-unipolar mood
    disorders
fibromyalgia

PULMONARY CONGESTION
constrictive pericarditis

PULMONARY EDEMA
congestive heart failure

PULMONARY FIBROSIS
gastroesophageal reflux disease

PULMONARY INFARCTION
endocarditis

PULMONIC INSUFFICIENCY
primary pulmonary hypertension

PULSE, LOWERED OR ABSENT
atherosclerosis

PULSE, RAPID
hyperthyroidism, thyroid storm
seizures

PULSE, SLOW
hypothyroidism
thyroiditis, Hashimoto's

PUPILS, DILATED
seizures

PUSTULAR LESIONS
herpes simplex virus, finger or
hand

RALES
pulmonary edema

RANGE OF MOTION, LIMITED
osteoarthritis

RASHES
allergic rhinitis
herpes zoster (varicella-zoster)
HIV and AIDS
roseola

RASHES, DERMATOSOMAL DISTRIBUTION
herpes zoster (varicella-zoster)
    virus

RASHES, PERIRECTAL OR VULVAR
intestinal parasites

RAYNAUD'S PHENOMENON
fibromyalgia

RECOGNITION OF OBJECTS, IMPAIRED
dementia

REFLEXES, SLOW
thyroiditis, Hashimoto's

REGURGITATION
cough
gastroesophageal reflux disease

REGURGITATION, LIQUID THROUGH NOSE
dysphagia, oropharyngeal

RENAL FAILURE
amenorrhea

RESPIRATORY ARREST
pulmonary edema

RESPIRATORY DISTRESS
food allergy
herpes simplex virus, neonatal

RESPIRATORY FAILURE
insect bites

RESPIRATORY SYMPTOMS
roseola

RESPIRATORY TRACT INFECTION, UPPER
cough
pertussis
sinus headache

RESTLESS LEG SYNDROME
fibromyalgia

RESTLESSNESS
common cold
depression-unipolar mood
    disorders
migraine headache

RETINOPATHY
hypertension, severe

RETROSTERNAL BURNING SENSATION
gastroesophageal reflux disease

RETROSTERNAL FULLNESS AFTER SWALLOWING
dysphagia, esophageal

RHEUMATOID NODULES
rheumatoid arthritis

RHINITIS
pertussis

RHINORRHEA
common cold
influenza

RHINORRHEA, YELLOW OR GREEN
sinus headache

RHONCHI
pulmonary edema

RIGHT VENTRICULAR LIFT
primary pulmonary hypertension

RIGHT VENTRICULAR S4
primary pulmonary hypertension

RIGIDITY
Parkinson's disease

RIGID THINKING
anorexia

ROCKY MOUNTAIN FEVER
insect bites

RUBOR
Raynaud's phenomenon

SALIVATION, INCREASED
seizures

SALPINGITIS
urethritis in women

SATELLITE LESIONS, SPREAD TO THIGHS AND ANUS
vaginitis

SCABS
herpes zoster (varicella-zoster)

SCALES
dermatitis
eczema

SCALP ARTERIES, PROMINENT
migraine headache

SCLERITIS
Reiter's syndrome

SEIZURES
dementia
hypertension, severe
hypoglycemia
endocarditis
roseola

SELF-REPROACH
depression-unipolar mood
   disorders

SEMEN, BLOODY
prostatitis

SENSATION, LOSS OF
anemia

SENSATION OF FULLNESS
internal hemorrhoids

SENSE OF IMPENDING DOOM/EXCESSIVE WORRY
anxiety

SENSITIVITY TO LIGHT
conjunctivitis
hyperthyroidism
migraine headache
Reiter's syndrome

SEXUAL DESIRE, LACK OF
sexual dysfunction

SEXUAL DYSFUNCTION
prostatitis

SIGHING RESPIRATION
anxiety

SINUS PAIN AND TENDERNESS
sinusitis

SINUS SYMPTOMS
allergic rhinitis

SITTING DISCOMFORT
hemorrhoids
low back pain

SKIN
erythematous lesions
candidiasis

SKIN, COLOR CHANGES
Raynaud's phenomenon

SKIN, COOL AND DRY
thyroiditis, Hashimoto's

SKIN, INCREASED TEMPERATURE
bursitis, septic

SKIN, LARGE LOCAL REACTION
insect bites

SKIN, MOIST WITH INCREASED PERSPIRATION
hyperthyroidism

SKIN, PALE OR BROWNISH YELLOW AND LEATHERY
burns, third degree

SKIN, RAISED AND THICKENED
hyperthyroidism
hypothyroidism

SKIN, RED
dermatitis

SKIN, STINGING OR BURNING
dermatitis

SKIN, THICKENED AND LICHENIFIED
dermatitis

SKIN, WARMTH AND REDNESS
gout
tendinitis

SKIN CHARRING
burns, third degree

SKIN DARKENING
amenorrhea

SKIN ERUPTIONS, FIXED
cutaneous drug reactions

SKIN LESIONS
eczema
HIV and AIDS

SKIN LESIONS, AFTER INJURIES
psoriasis

SKIN LESIONS, CRUSTING AND INFECTION
insect bites

SKIN LESIONS, RAISED
psoriasis

SKIN LESIONS, VESICULAR
herpes simplex virus, neonatal

SKIN LESIONS (JANEWAY)
endocarditis

SLEEP, DEEP
seizures

SLEEP, IMPAIRED MAINTENANCE
insomnia

SLEEP, IMPAIRED ONSET
insomnia

SLEEP DISORDERS
fibromyalgia

SLEEP DISTURBANCES
anxiety
chronic fatigue syndrome
dementia
hyperthyroidism
menopause
otitis media
Parkinson's disease
sleep apnea

SLEEPINESS, DAYTIME
sleep apnea

SMELL, LOSS OF
sinusitis

SNEEZING
allergic rhinitis
common cold
influenza

SNORING, LOUD AND IRREGULAR
sleep apnea

SOCIAL SPONTANEITY, LIMITED
anorexia

SOCIAL WITHDRAWAL
anorexia

SORES, OPEN
edema

SPATIAL DISORIENTATION
dementia

SPEECH, SLOWED
hypothyroidism

SPEECH, SLURRED
hypoglycemia

SPEECH PROBLEMS
Parkinson's disease

SPINAL DEFORMITY/ HUNCHED BACK
osteoporosis

SPITTING UP AFTER FEEDING
infantile colic

SPLEEN, ENLARGEMENT
hypercholesterolemia

SPLENOMEGALY
cirrhosis of the liver
herpes simplex virus, neonatal

SPLENOMEGALY WITH LEUKOPENIA
rheumatoid arthritis

SPONDYLOARTHROPATHY
Reiter's syndrome

SPUTUM, BLOODY
endocarditis

SPUTUM, EXCESSIVE
chronic obstructive pulmonary
disease

SPUTUM, PINK AND FROTHY
pulmonary edema

STANDING, DIFFICULTY
low back pain

STENOSIS, ARTERIAL
atherosclerosis

STIFFNESS
diabetes
gout
low back pain
osteoarthritis
Reiter's syndrome
rheumatoid arthritis
sprains and strains

STIFFNESS, MORNING
fibromyalgia
Reiter's syndrome

STOMACH, SWOLLEN OR DISTENDED
infantile colic

STOOL, BLOOD AND MUCUS IN
ulcerative colitis

STOOL, COLORLESS
hepatitis, viral

STOOL, DIFFICULT PASSAGE
constipation

STOOL, HARD
constipation

STOOL, LOOSE
diarrhea

STOOL, MUCUS IN
hemorrhoids
irritable bowel syndrome

STOOL, PASSAGE OF WORM
intestinal parasites

STOOL, TARRY OR RED
peptic ulcer

STRAINING DURING DEFECATING
hemorrhoids

SUBLUXATION
osteoarthritis

SUICIDAL BEHAVIOR
dementia
depression

SUICIDAL THOUGHTS
depression-unipolar mood
  disorders

SWALLOWING DIFFICULTY
dysphagia, oropharyngeal
Parkinson's disease

SWALLOWING PAIN
pharyngitis

SWEATING
anxiety

SWEATING, COLD
motion sickness

SWEATING, EXCESSIVE
hypoglycemia

SWEATING, INCREASED
seizures
thyroiditis, silent

SWEATING, NIGHT
cough
HIV and AIDS
endocarditis
menopause
ulcerative colitis

SWELLING
Reiter's syndrome
sprains and strains

SWELLING, BASE OF NECK
hyperthyroidism

SWELLING, LOCALIZED
bursitis

SWELLING, MUSCULAR
edema

SWELLING, PATCHES OF
food allergy

SWELLING, SOFT TISSUE
osteoarthritis

SWELLING AND TENDERNESS, BONE
osteomyelitis

SYNCOPE, EXERTIONAL OR NEAR
primary pulmonary hypertension

SYNCOPE, NEAR
anxiety
migraine headache

TACHYARRHYTHMIA
hyperthyroidism

TACHYCARDIA
anxiety
hyperthyroidism
pericardial effusion

TEETH, ACHING
allergic rhinitis

TEETH GRINDING
tension headache

TENDERNESS, LOCALIZED
bursitis
gout
osteoarthritis
rheumatoid arthritis
tendinitis

TENESMUS, DISTRESSING
ulcerative colitis

TERMINAL FAT PADS, ATROPHY OF
Raynaud's phenomenon

TESTICULAR ATROPHY
cirrhosis of the liver

THIGH PAIN
dysmenorrhea

THIRST
amenorrhea

THROAT, ITCHING OR TIGHTNESS
food allergy

THROAT, SORE
bronchitis
chronic fatigue syndrome
common cold
gastroesophageal reflux disease
influenza
pharyngitis
sleep apnea

THROAT, TICKLING, SCRATCHINESS, RAWNESS
laryngitis

THROAT CLEARING, CONSTANT
laryngitis

THROBBING, SEVERE
migraine headache
Raynaud's phenomenon

THROMBOSIS
atherosclerosis

THRUSH
candidiasis
HIV and AIDS

THYROID GLAND, ASYMMETRICALLY ENLARGED
thyroiditis, Riedel's

THYROID GLAND, ENLARGED AND PAINFUL
thyroiditis, subacute

THYROID GLAND, MODERATELY ENLARGED
thyroiditis, silent

THYROID GLAND, SYMMETRICALLY ENLARGED
thyroiditis, Hashimoto's

TOE TIP PAIN (OSLER NODE)
endocarditis

TONGUE, SWELLING OR ITCHING
food allergy

TONGUE LESIONS
herpes simplex virus, oral-facial

TONIC CONTRACTIONS
seizures

TONSIL ENLARGEMENT
pharyngitis

TOOTHACHE
sinusitis

TOPHI
gout

TREMBLING
anxiety

TREMOR
dementia
hyperthyroidism
Parkinson's disease

TREMULOUSNESS
hypoglycemia

TRICUSPID MURMUR
primary pulmonary hypertension

TRIGLYCERIDES, HIGH LEVELS
hypercholesterolemia

TUBERCULOSIS, PULMONARY
cough

TURNER'S SYNDROME (SHORT STATURE)
amenorrhea

TYMPANIC MEMBRANES, INFLAMED
roseola

ULCER, DUODENAL
peptic ulcer

ULCER, GANGRENOUS, FINGERTIPS
Raynaud's phenomenon

ULCER, GASTRIC
peptic ulcer

ULCERATION
insect bites

URETHRAL DISCHARGE
herpes simplex virus, genital

URETHRAL DISCHARGE, PURULENT OR WHITISH-MUCUS
urethritis, in men

URETHRAL LESIONS
herpes simplex virus, genital

URETHRITIS
Reiter's syndrome

URINARY TRACT ATROPHY
menopause

URINARY TRACT INFECTION
candidiasis

URINARY TRACT INFECTION, RECURRENT
prostatitis

URINATION, BURNING SENSATION
benign prostatic hyperplasia
urethritis in men
urinary tract infection in women

URINATION, COMPLETE INABILITY
benign prostatic hyperplasia

URINATION, DRIBBLING AFTER
benign prostatic hyperplasia

URINATION, FREQUENT
allergic rhinitis
benign prostatic hyperplasia
dysmenorrhea
prostatitis

URINATION, FREQUENT AND UNUSUAL URGE
urinary incontinence
urinary tract infection in women

URINATION, INVOLUNTARY
urinary incontinence

URINATION, PAINFUL
urethritis in women

URINE, BLOOD AND PUS IN
urinary tract infection in women

URINE, BLOOD IN
benign prostatic hyperplasia
endocarditis

URINE, DARK
hepatitis, viral

URINE, DIFFICULTY STARTING STREAM
benign prostatic hyperplasia

URINE, REDUCTION IN AMOUNT
preeclampsia

URINE, STRONG-SMELLING
urinary tract infection in women

URTICARIA
cutaneous drug reactions
food allergy

URTICARIA, GENERALIZED
insect bites

URTICARIAL PAPULES
insect bites

VAGINAL ATROPHY
menopause

VAGINAL DISCHARGE
urethritis in women
vaginitis

VAGINAL DRYNESS
menopause
sexual dysfunction

**VAGINAL MUCOUS
MEMBRANES, RED AND SWOLLEN**
vaginitis

VASCULITIS
cutaneous drug reactions
rheumatoid arthritis

VASOMOTOR SYMPTOMS
menopause

VERTIGO
hypoglycemia
migraine headache

VESICLES
dermatitis
herpes zoster (varicella-zoster)

**VESICLES, OOZING AND
CRUSTING**
eczema

VESICULAR LESIONS
herpes simplex virus, finger
   or hand

VISCERAL DISEASE
herpes simplex virus

VISION DISTURBANCES
migraine headache
preeclampsia

VISUAL FIELD ABNORMALITIES
amenorrhea

VOICE, UNNATURAL CHANGES
laryngitis

VOICE, WEAK
dysphagia, oropharyngeal

VOICE, WEAK
dysphagia, esophageal

VOMITING
congestive heart failure
dysmenorrhea
food allergy
gallbladder disease
gastritis
hepatitis, viral
herpes simplex virus, neonatal
HIV and AIDS
hypertension, severe
influenza
intestinal parasites
migraine headache
motion sickness
myocardial infarction
otitis media
peptic ulcer
pertussis
urolithiasis

VOMITING, BLOOD
peptic ulcer

VULVAR ERYTHEMA
candidiasis

VULVOVAGINITIS
candidiasis

WALKING PROBLEMS
Parkinson's disease

WATER BRASH
gastroesophageal reflux disease

WEAKNESS
chronic fatigue syndrome
cirrhosis of the liver
diabetes
fibromyalgia
hyperkalemia
low back pain
myocardial infarction

WEIGHT GAIN
bronchitis
chronic obstructive
   pulmonary disease
depression-unipolar mood
   disorders
hypothyroidism

**WEIGHT GAIN, SUDDEN AND
EXCESSIVE**
preeclampsia

WEIGHT LOSS
anorexia
chronic obstructive pulmonary
disease, late stages
cirrhosis of the liver
depression-unipolar mood
   disorders
diarrhea
dysphagia, oropharyngeal
HIV and AIDS
hyperthyroidism
intestinal parasites
peptic ulcer
Reiter's syndrome
rheumatoid arthritis
thyroiditis, silent
ulcerative colitis

WEIGHT LOSS, RAPID
diabetes

WHEEZING
asthma
bronchitis
chronic obstructive
   pulmonary disease
cough
gastroesophageal reflux disease

WITHDRAWAL
depression-unipolar mood
   disorders

WORTHLESSNESS, FEELINGS OF
depression-unipolar mood
   disorders

WRIST JOINTS
rheumatoid arthritis

**XANTHOMAS, TENDONS
AND SKIN**
hypercholesterolemia

ZOSTER OPHTHALMICUS
herpes zoster (varicella-zoster) virus

■ **CONDITIONS BY HERB AND
SUPPLEMENT TREATMENT
OPTIONS**

*This extracts the items included in the
Herb and Nutrition sections of each
condition monograph and combines
them to create a collective list of herbs
and supplements, each with a respective
list of conditions where their use may be
considered. Some herbs and supplements listed may not yet have a monograph created in the* Quick Access *system.*

N-ACETYL CYSTEINE
allergic rhinitis
asthma
bronchitis
chronic obstructive
   pulmonary disease
hepatitis, viral
HIV and AIDS
peptic ulcer

ACIDOPHILUS
hepatitis, viral
herpes simplex virus
HIV and AIDS
infantile colic
intestinal parasites
irritable bowel syndrome
osteomyelitis
peptic ulcer
vaginitis

S-ADENOSYLMETHIONINE
osteoarthritis

ALANINE
benign prostatic hyperplasia

ALFALFA
anemia
hypercholesterolemia
hypothyroidism
thyroiditis

ALGAE, BLUE GREEN
alopecia

ALOE
burns
cutaneous drug reactions

ALPHA-LIPOIC ACID
Parkinson's disease

AMINO ACIDS
benign prostatic hyperplasia
Parkinson's disease

ANGELICA
menopause

ANISE SEED
infantile colic
irritable bowel syndrome
pertussis

ANTIMICROBIALS
osteomyelitis

ANTIOXIDANTS
atherosclerosis
cirrhosis of the liver
congestive heart failure
dementia
low back pain
myocardial infarction
Parkinson's disease
Reiter's syndrome
rheumatoid arthritis

ARNICA OIL
sprains and strains

ARTICHOKE LEAVES
edema

ASHWAGANDA
rheumatoid arthritis

ASHWAGANDA ROOT
chronic fatigue syndrome
fibromyalgia

ASPARTATE
osteoporosis

ASTRAGALUS
alopecia
common cold
herpes simplex virus
osteomyelitis
pertussis

ASTRAGALUS ROOT
chronic fatigue syndrome
fibromyalgia
hepatitis, viral

BALM OF GILEAD
cough

BARBERRY
candidiasis
cirrhosis of the liver
diarrhea
intestinal parasites
osteomyelitis
peptic ulcer

BAUME DE CANADA
cough

BEARBERRY
infective endocarditis
prostatitis

BELLADONNA
asthma

BERGAMOT
anxiety

BETA-CAROTENE
bronchitis
burns
chronic fatigue syndrome
common cold
cough
dermatitis
eczema
endometriosis
fever of unknown origin
food allergy
hepatitis, viral
herpes simplex virus

herpes zoster (varicella-zoster) virus
HIV and AIDS
infective endocarditis
influenza
intestinal parasites
myocardial infarction
pertussis
pharyngitis
Reiter's syndrome
roseola
sinus headache
sinusitis
sprains and strains
tension headache
ulcerative colitis
urethritis
urinary tract infection in women
vaginitis
warts

BETAINE
atherosclerosis
congestive heart failure
hypertension

BILBERRY
allergic rhinitis
diabetes mellitus
edema
osteoarthritis
Reiter's syndrome

BIOFLAVONOIDS
allergic rhinitis
dermatitis
eczema
hemorrhoids
migraine headache
sprains and strains
tendinitis

BIOTIN
alopecia
candidiasis
dementia
depression-unipolar mood
    disorders
ulcerative colitis

BISMUTH SUBCITRATE
gastritis
peptic ulcer

BLACKBERRY LEAF
diarrhea

BLACK COHOSH
alopecia
amenorrhea
depression-unipolar mood
    disorders
dysmenorrhea
endometriosis
fibromyalgia
infective endocarditis
menopause
osteoarthritis
osteoporosis
sprains and strains

BLACK HAW
low back pain

BLACK HOREHOUND
motion sickness

BLACK STRAP MOLASSES
anemia

BLACK WALNUT
intestinal parasites

BLADDERWRACK
amenorrhea
hypothyroidism
obesity
osteoporosis
thyroiditis

BLUEBERRIES
urethritis
urinary incontinence
urinary tract infection in women

BLUE FLAG
endometriosis
hypercholesterolemia
osteoporosis
rheumatoid arthritis

BLUE MONKSHOOD
pericarditis

BLUE VERVAIN
hypercholesterolemia

BONESET
bronchitis

BORAGE OIL
amenorrhea
dermatitis
dysmenorrhea
eczema
food allergy

BORON
amenorrhea
osteoarthritis
osteoporosis

BOSWELLIA
osteoarthritis
rheumatoid arthritis

BRAN, RAW
irritable bowel syndrome

BREWER'S YEAST
diabetes mellitus
diarrhea

BROMELAIN
angina
atherosclerosis
burns
bursitis
chronic obstructive pulmonary
    disease
cutaneous drug reactions
dermatitis
eczema
endocarditis
food allergy
gout
hyperthyroidism
insect bites
low back pain
myocardial infarction
Reiter's syndrome
rheumatoid arthritis
sinus headache

sinusitis
sprains and strains
tendinitis
thyroiditis
ulcerative colitis

BROOM
edema
pulmonary edema

BUCHU
edema
urethritis
urinary tract infection in women

BUGLEWEED
hyperthyroidism
thyroiditis

BUPLEURUM
Parkinson's disease

BURDOCK
anemia
constipation
psoriasis

BURDOCK ROOT
eczema
herpes zoster (varicella-zoster) virus
hypercholesterolemia
osteomyelitis

BUTCHER'S BROOM
edema

CALCIUM
amenorrhea
anxiety
attention-deficit/hyperactivity
    disorder
candidiasis
depression-unipolar mood disorders
edema
endometriosis
herpes zoster (varicella-zoster) virus
hyperthyroidism
hypothyroidism
osteoporosis
Raynaud's phenomenon
tension headache
ulcerative colitis

CALCIUM CITRATE
osteoporosis

CALCIUM/MAGNESIUM
dementia
insomnia
low back pain
menopause
tendinitis
tension headache
thyroiditis
urinary incontinence

CALIFORNIA POPPY
burns

CAPRYLIC ACID
candidiasis

CARNITINE
atherosclerosis
cirrhosis of the liver
congestive heart failure

L-CARNITINE
angina
chronic fatigue syndrome
chronic obstructive
  pulmonary disease
HIV and AIDS
myocardial infarction
primary pulmonary hypertension
pulmonary edema

CAROB POWDER
diarrhea

CASCARA SAGRADA
constipation

CASTOR OIL
cough

CATECHIN
cirrhosis of the liver
dermatitis
eczema
hemorrhoids

CATNIP
attention-deficit/hyperactivity disorder
fever of unknown origin
food allergy
infantile colic
peptic ulcer
pertussis
roseola

CAYENNE
diabetes mellitus
tension headache

CELANDINE
food allergy
warts

CERNILTON
prostatitis

CHAMOMILE
attention-deficit/hyperactivity disorder
candidiasis
conjunctivitis
cutaneous drug reactions
dermatitis
diarrhea
eczema
food allergy
herpes simplex virus
herpes zoster (varicella-zoster) virus
insomnia
motion sickness
peptic ulcer
pertussis
roseola

CHAMOMILE OIL
insomnia

CHAMOMILE TEA
dysmenorrhea

CHASTE TREE
alopecia
amenorrhea
dysmenorrhea
endometriosis
menopause
osteoporosis
sexual dysfunction

CHICKWEED
cutaneous drug reactions
dermatitis
eczema

CHICORY
food allergy

CHOLAGOGUE
HIV and AIDS

CHOLINE
cirrhosis of the liver
gallbladder disease
hepatitis, viral
migraine headache
obesity
Parkinson's disease
primary pulmonary hypertension
pulmonary edema

CHROMIUM
atherosclerosis
depression-unipolar mood disorders
hypercholesterolemia
osteoporosis
sleep apnea

CHROMIUM PICOLINATE
diabetes mellitus
fibromyalgia
hypoglycemia
obesity

CITRONELLA OIL
insect bites

CLARY SAGE
fibromyalgia

CLEAVERS
allergic rhinitis
burns
dermatitis
eczema
edema
endocarditis
insect bites
osteomyelitis
otitis media
urethritis

COD LIVER OIL
eczema
otitis media

COENZYME Q10
angina
atherosclerosis
chronic obstructive
  pulmonary disease
congestive heart failure
dementia
diabetes mellitus
edema
endocarditis
fibromyalgia
HIV and AIDS
hypercholesterolemia
hypertension
hyperthyroidism
obesity
pericarditis
primary pulmonary hypertension
pulmonary edema
Raynaud's phenomenon

COLEUS
psoriasis

COLTSFOOT
asthma
chronic obstructive
  pulmonary disease
cough

COMFREY
cutaneous drug reactions
dermatitis
eczema
hemorrhoids
herpes zoster (varicella-zoster) virus
tendinitis

COMFREY ROOT
burns

CONDURANGO
anorexia nervosa

CONEFLOWER
allergic rhinitis
bronchitis
burns
common cold
cutaneous drug reactions
endocarditis
fever of unknown origin
hepatitis, viral
herpes simplex virus
herpes zoster (varicella-zoster) virus
influenza
insect bites
laryngitis
osteomyelitis
otitis media
pertussis
pharyngitis
prostatitis
sinus headache
sinusitis
ulcerative colitis
urethritis
urinary tract infection in women
warts

COPPER
Reiter's syndrome

CORN SILK
endocarditis
prostatitis
urethritis
urinary tract infection in women
urolithiasis

COUCHGRASS
edema
urethritis
urinary tract infection in women

CRAMP BARK
endometriosis
hypertension
pertussis
preeclampsia
sprains and strains
ulcerative colitis
urolithiasis

CRAMP BARK TINCTURES
dysmenorrhea

CRANBERRIES
urethritis
urinary incontinence
urinary tract infection in women

CURCUMA
allergic rhinitis

CURCUMIN
tendinitis

CYANOCOBALAMINE
anemia

DAMIANA
sexual dysfunction

DANDELION
anemia
congestive heart failure
food allergy
HIV and AIDS
obesity

DANDELION LEAF
edema
endocarditis
hypertension
pulmonary edema

DANDELION ROOT
amenorrhea
constipation
edema
endometriosis
gallbladder disease
hypercholesterolemia
osteoporosis
sexual dysfunction

DESSICATED LIVER EXTRACT
cirrhosis of the liver
hepatitis, viral

DEVIL'S CLAW
gout
low back pain
osteoarthritis
rheumatoid arthritis

DIGESTIVE ENZYMES
constipation
intestinal parasites
irritable bowel syndrome
psoriasis

DIMETHYLAMINOETHANOL (DMAE)
Parkinson's disease

DIMETHYL GLYCINE
seizures

ECHINACEA
alopecia
warts

ECLIPTA ALBA
hepatitis, viral

EICOSPENTAENOIC ACID (EPA)
gout

ELDER
edema
fever of unknown origin
influenza
insect bites
roseola

ELDERBERRY
allergic rhinitis
common cold
cough
otitis media

ELECAMPANE
asthma
bronchitis
cough
pertussis

ETHYLENEDIAMINETETRAACETIC ACID (EDTA)
dementia

EUCALYPTUS OIL
chronic obstructive
  pulmonary disease
cough
insect bites
sinus headache
sinusitis

EVENING PRIMROSE
amenorrhea
candidiasis
cirrhosis of the liver
dysmenorrhea
eczema
tension headache

EVENING PRIMROSE OIL
dermatitis
diabetes mellitus
food allergy
hypertension

EYEBRIGHT
allergic rhinitis
conjunctivitis
otitis media
Reiter's syndrome
sinus headache
sinusitis

FATTY ACIDS, ESSENTIAL
alopecia
amenorrhea
angina
atherosclerosis
attention-deficit/hyperactivity
  disorder
benign prostatic hyperplasia
candidiasis
chronic fatigue syndrome
congestive heart failure
dementia
depression-unipolar mood
  disorders
endometriosis
hyperthyroidism
hypothyroidism
migraine headache
obesity
osteoporosis
otitis media
Parkinson's disease
peptic ulcer

prostatitis
psoriasis
Reiter's syndrome
sleep apnea
tendinitis
tension headache
thyroiditis
ulcerative colitis

FENNEL
chronic obstructive pulmonary
  disease
cough
food allergy
roseola

FENNEL SEED
conjunctivitis
constipation
infantile colic
irritable bowel syndrome

FENUGREEK
anorexia nervosa
diabetes mellitus

FERROUS FUMERATE
anemia

FEVERFEW
migraine headache
sprains and strains

FIBER
obesity
ulcerative colitis

FIREWEED
candidiasis

FISH OIL
diabetes mellitus
otitis media

FLAVANOIDS
rheumatoid arthritis

FLAX MEAL
conjunctivitis
constipation
gallbladder disease
hemorrhoids
irritable bowel syndrome
ulcerative colitis

FLAX OIL
hypertension
pericarditis

FLAXSEED
amenorrhea
candidiasis
cirrhosis of the liver
eczema
tension headache

FLAXSEED OIL
cough
cutaneous drug reactions
dermatitis
dysmenorrhea
food allergy

FOLATE
candidiasis
cirrhosis of the liver

depression-unipolar mood
  disorders
diabetes mellitus
psoriasis

FOLIC ACID
anemia
atherosclerosis
congestive heart failure
gout
hepatitis, viral
hypertension
migraine headache
seizures
ulcerative colitis
urolithiasis
warts

FRANKINCENSE
asthma
cough

GAMMA-AMINOBUTYRIC ACID (GABA)
Parkinson's disease

GAMMA-LINOLENIC ACID (GLA)
alopecia

GAMMA-ORYZANOL
menopause

GANA DERMA
rheumatoid arthritis

GARLIC
bronchitis
candidiasis
cough
diabetes mellitus
endocarditis
HIV and AIDS
hypercholesterolemia
intestinal parasites
osteomyelitis
pertussis
primary pulmonary hypertension
pulmonary edema
sinus headache
vaginitis

GARLIC/GINGER TEA
influenza
pharyngitis
roseola
sinusitis

GARLIC OIL
intestinal parasites
otitis media

GELSEMIUM
asthma
burns
endometriosis

GENTIAN
atherosclerosis
HIV and AIDS
obesity

GERANIUM
ulcerative colitis

GINGER
angina
bronchitis

chronic obstructive pulmonary
  disease
constipation
cough
dementia
hypercholesterolemia
laryngitis
migraine headache
rheumatoid arthritis
sinus headache

GINGER ROOT
allergic rhinitis
asthma
burns
dysmenorrhea
endometriosis
hypoglycemia
irritable bowel syndrome
motion sickness
osteoarthritis
pertussis
Raynaud's phenomenon
sexual dysfunction

GINGER ROOT TEA
gastritis

GINKGO
alopecia
angina
asthma
atherosclerosis
dementia
depression-unipolar mood
  disorders
edema
low back pain
menopause
migraine headache
osteomyelitis
Parkinson's disease
primary pulmonary hypertension
Raynaud's phenomenon
sexual dysfunction
tension headache
thyroiditis

GINSENG
rheumatoid arthritis

GINSENG, SIBERIAN
alopecia
anorexia nervosa
chronic fatigue syndrome
dementia
depression-unipolar mood
  disorders
fibromyalgia
HIV and AIDS
hypoglycemia

GLOBE ARTICHOKE
gallbladder disease
hepatitis, viral
Parkinson's disease

GLUCOSAMINE SULFATE
bursitis
osteoarthritis
Reiter's syndrome

GLUTAMIC ACID
benign prostatic hyperplasia
Parkinson's disease

GLUTAMINE
diarrhea
peptic ulcer

L-GLUTAMINE
burns
HIV and AIDS
obesity

GLUTATHIONE
cirrhosis of the liver
hepatitis, viral
Parkinson's disease

GLYCERATE
anemia

GLYCINATE
anemia

GLYCINE
benign prostatic hyperplasia

GLYCYRRHIZIC ACID
herpes simplex virus

GOLDENROD
edema

GOLDENSEAL
anorexia nervosa
burns
candidiasis
common cold
conjunctivitis
cutaneous drug reactions
diarrhea
hepatitis, viral
herpes zoster (varicella-zoster) virus
HIV and AIDS
influenza
intestinal parasites
laryngitis
osteomyelitis
peptic ulcer
pharyngitis
prostatitis
sinus headache
sinusitis
ulcerative colitis
urethritis
urinary tract infection in women
warts

GOLDENSEAL POWDER
insect bites

GOLDENSEAL ROOT
endocarditis
osteomyelitis

GOTU KOLA
burns
chronic fatigue syndrome
dermatitis
fibromyalgia
hypoglycemia
hypothyroidism
Parkinson's disease
rheumatoid arthritis
sexual dysfunction
thyroiditis

GRAPE SEED EXTRACT
diabetes mellitus
Parkinson's disease

GRAVEL ROOT
urolithiasis

GREATER CELANDINE
gallbladder disease
hypercholesterolemia

GREEN TEA
alopecia
asthma
hemorrhoids
hepatitis, viral

GRIFOLD FRONDOSA
rheumatoid arthritis

GRINDELIA
asthma

GUGGUL
hypothyroidism

GUMWEED
cough

HAWTHORN
angina
atherosclerosis
bronchitis
bursitis
congestive heart failure
dementia
edema
endocarditis
hyperkalemia
hypertension
osteoarthritis
Parkinson's disease
pericarditis
primary pulmonary
   hypertension
pulmonary edema
sexual dysfunction
sprains and strains

HAWTHORN BERRIES
hypercholesterolemia
hyperthyroidism
preeclampsia
Raynaud's phenomenon

HESPERIDIN
cutaneous drug reactions
dermatitis
eczema
menopause

**HESPERIDIN METHYL
CHALCONE**
menopause

HOREHOUND
cough

HORSE CHESTNUT
edema

HORSETAIL
alopecia
amenorrhea
edema
hypothyroidism
osteoporosis
Reiter's syndrome
rheumatoid arthritis
thyroiditis

urethritis
urinary incontinence
urinary tract infection
   in women

HORSETAIL HERB
congestive heart failure

HUANG QI
HIV and AIDS

HYDROCHLORIC ACID
eczema

**HYDROCHLORIC ACID
SUPPLEMENTS**
asthma

HYDROXCOBALAMIN
asthma

5-HYDROXYTRYPTOPHAN
fibromyalgia
insomnia
migraine headache
obesity

HYSSOP
pertussis

INDIAN TOBACCO
angina
asthma
bronchitis
congestive heart failure
cough
hypertension
pertussis
preeclampsia
primary pulmonary hypertension
pulmonary edema

INDIAN TOBACCO OIL
otitis media

INOSITOL
primary pulmonary hypertension

IODINE
amenorrhea
thyroiditis

IRISH MOSS
hypothyroidism

IRON
depression-unipolar mood
   disorders
endometriosis

IRON, ELEMENTAL
ulcerative colitis

JAMAICAN DOGWOOD
burns
bursitis
dysmenorrhea
endometriosis
herpes zoster (varicella-zoster)
   virus
insomnia
low back pain
migraine headache
sinus headache
sinusitis
sprains and strains

tension headache
urolithiasis

JASMINE
anxiety

JASMINE OIL
chronic fatigue syndrome
fibromyalgia

JUNIPER
Reiter's syndrome

KAVA KAVA
anxiety
attention-deficit/hyperactivity
   disorder
fibromyalgia
insomnia
sexual dysfunction
tension headache
urethritis
urolithiasis

KELP
amenorrhea
hypothyroidism
obesity
osteoporosis

KHELLA
asthma

LACTOBACILLUS
irritable bowel syndrome

**LACTOBACILLUS
ACIDOPHILUS**
candidiasis

LACTOBACILLUS SPECIES
diarrhea

LADY'S MANTLE
amenorrhea
osteoporosis

LAVENDER
anxiety
asthma
attention-deficit/hyperactivity
   disorder
chronic fatigue syndrome
fibromyalgia
obesity

LAVENDER ESSENCE OIL
candidiasis

LAVENDER OIL
chronic obstructive pulmonary
   disease
insect bites
insomnia
intestinal parasites
sinus headache
sinusitis

LECITHIN
cirrhosis of the liver
gallbladder disease
hepatitis, viral
obesity
Parkinson's disease

LEMON BALM
anorexia nervosa
anxiety
attention-deficit/hyperactivity
   disorder
dementia
depression-unipolar mood
   disorders
fever of unknown origin
fibromyalgia
herpes simplex virus
herpes zoster (varicella-zoster) virus
hyperthyroidism
infantile colic
insomnia
Parkinson's disease
peptic ulcer
sexual dysfunction
ulcerative colitis

LEOPARD'S BANE
low back pain

LICORICE
amenorrhea
anorexia nervosa
candidiasis
chronic obstructive pulmonary
disease
common cold
depression-unipolar mood
   disorders
dysphagia
gastroesophageal reflux disease
HIV and AIDS
hyperthyroidism
influenza
laryngitis
menopause
osteomyelitis
osteoporosis
pharyngitis
Reiter's syndrome
sinus headache
sinusitis
tendinitis

LICORICE,
DEGLYCYRRHIZINATED
gastritis
peptic ulcer

LICORICE ROOT
asthma
bronchitis
chronic fatigue syndrome
constipation
cough
diarrhea
hepatitis, viral
herpes simplex virus
herpes zoster (varicella-zoster)
virus
hypoglycemia
insect bites
pertussis
ulcerative colitis
warts

LILY OF THE VALLEY
congestive heart failure
edema
endocarditis
hyperkalemia
hypertension
pulmonary edema

LINDEN FLOWER
angina
atherosclerosis
attention-deficit/hyperactivity
   disorder
bronchitis
congestive heart failure
cough
dysphagia
edema
endocarditis
gastroesophageal reflux disease
hypertension
infantile colic
pericarditis
primary pulmonary hypertension
pulmonary edema

LIPASE
gallbladder disease

LIPOIC ACID
atherosclerosis

LIPOTROPIC AGENTS
gallbladder disease

LITHIUM
hyperthyroidism

LOBELIA
low back pain

LOMATIUM
bronchitis
herpes simplex virus
osteomyelitis
warts

LOMATIUM ROOT
chronic fatigue syndrome

LUNGWORT
bronchitis

L-LYSINE
herpes simplex virus

MAGNESIUM
alopecia
amenorrhea
anxiety
asthma
atherosclerosis
attention-deficit/hyperactivity
   disorder
candidiasis
chronic obstructive pulmonary
   disease
congestive heart failure
cutaneous drug reactions
depression-unipolar mood
   disorders
diabetes mellitus
dysmenorrhea
edema
fibromyalgia
herpes zoster (varicella-zoster) virus
HIV and AIDS
hypercholesterolemia
hyperkalemia
hypertension
hyperthyroidism
hypoglycemia
endocarditis
irritable bowel syndrome

migraine headache
osteoporosis
preeclampsia
pulmonary edema
seizures
sexual dysfunction
tension headache
ulcerative colitis

MAGNESIUM ASPARTATE
chronic fatigue syndrome
pulmonary edema

MAGNESIUM CITRATE
urolithiasis

MA HUANG
asthma
obesity

MALE FERN
intestinal parasites

MAGNESIUM ASPARTATE
primary pulmonary hypertension

MANGANASE
diabetes mellitus
osteoporosis
tension headache

MANGANESE
Parkinson's disease
seizures

MARIGOLD
burns
candidiasis
conjunctivitis
cutaneous drug reactions
dermatitis
eczema
hemorrhoids
herpes zoster (varicella-zoster) virus
insect bites
laryngitis
otitis media

MARSHMALLOW ROOT
burns
cutaneous drug reactions
diarrhea
gastritis
irritable bowel syndrome
ulcerative colitis
urethritis
urinary incontinence
urinary tract infection in women

MARSHMALLOW ROOT
POWDER
peptic ulcer

MARSHMALLOW ROOT TEA
eczema
food allergy

MAX EPA
hypertension

MEADOWSWEET
bursitis
food allergy
irritable bowel syndrome
migraine headache
osteoarthritis

peptic ulcer
Reiter's syndrome
tension headache
ulcerative colitis

MELATONIN
fibromyalgia
insomnia

METHIONINE
cirrhosis of the liver
hepatitis, viral
obesity

MILK THISTLE
amenorrhea
cirrhosis of the liver
edema
endometriosis
food allergy
gallbladder disease
hepatitis, viral
HIV and AIDS
hypercholesterolemia
hyperthyroidism
irritable bowel syndrome
obesity
osteoporosis
Parkinson's disease
preeclampsia
psoriasis
seizures
sexual dysfunction

MINT
asthma

MISTLETOE
angina
atherosclerosis
congestive heart failure
hypertension

MONKSHOOD
angina
endometriosis

MONKSHOOD OIL
otitis media

MOTHERWORT
angina
congestive heart failure
edema
endocarditis
endometriosis
hypertension
hyperthyroidism
pulmonary edema
thyroiditis

MULLEIN
chronic obstructive pulmonary
   disease
cough
pertussis

MULLEIN FLOWER OIL
otitis media

MUSTARD OIL
cough

MYRRH
endocarditis
laryngitis

NERVINE HERBS
Parkinson's disease

NETTLES
allergic rhinitis
eczema
osteoporosis

NIACIN (see Vitamin B₃)
gout
hypercholesterolemia

NIACINAMIDE
(see Vitamin B₃)
dysmenorrhea
hypoglycemia
insomnia
osteoarthritis

NIGHT-BLOOMING CEREUS
angina
edema
endocarditis
hypertension
pulmonary edema

OATMEAL BATHS
cutaneous drug reactions

OATS
Parkinson's disease

OATSTRAW
amenorrhea
anorexia nervosa
anxiety
depression-unipolar mood
   disorders
edema
hypothyroidism
insect bites
osteoporosis
thyroiditis

OMEGA-3 FATTY ACIDS
anemia
atherosclerosis
attention-deficit/hyperactivity disorder
bursitis
candidiasis
chronic obstructive pulmonary
   disease
cirrhosis of the liver
hypercholesterolemia
migraine headache
osteoarthritis
preeclampsia
psoriasis
Raynaud's phenomenon
rheumatoid arthritis
tension headache

OMEGA-6 FATTY ACIDS
attention-deficit/hyperactivity
   disorder
candidiasis
chronic obstructive pulmonary
disease
cirrhosis of the liver
eczema
psoriasis
tension headache

ONION
cough
diabetes mellitus

OREGANO OIL
cough

OREGON GRAPE
dermatitis
intestinal parasites
peptic ulcer

OREGON GRAPE ROOT
candidiasis

OSHA
warts

PALMITATE
asthma
dermatitis
eczema
food allergy

PANCREATIN
food allergy

PANTHENINE
hypercholesterolemia

PANTOTHENIC ACID
(see Vitamin B₅)
chronic fatigue syndrome
hypoglycemia
ulcerative colitis

PAPAIN
intestinal parasites

PARSLEY
edema
obesity

PASSIONFLOWER
anxiety
attention-deficit/hyperactivity
   disorder
chronic fatigue syndrome
depression-unipolar mood
   disorders
fibromyalgia
food allergy
hypertension
hyperthyroidism
insomnia
irritable bowel syndrome
peptic ulcer
preeclampsia
seizures
sexual dysfunction
thyroiditis
ulcerative colitis

PAU D'ARCO BARK
candidiasis

PAU D'ARCO TEA
vaginitis

PENNYROYAL OIL
insect bites

PEPPERMINT
cutaneous drug reactions
dermatitis
eczema
food allergy
infantile colic
insect bites
laryngitis

motion sickness
obesity
peptic ulcer
roseola

PEPPERMINT LEAF
dermatitis

PEPPERMINT OIL
chronic fatigue syndrome
gallbladder disease
irritable bowel syndrome
tension headache
ulcerative colitis

PETASITES
low back pain

PHOSPHATIDYL CHOLINE
fibromyalgia
Parkinson's disease

PHOSPHATIDYL SERINE
fibromyalgia

PHYLLANTHUS AMARUS
hepatitis, viral

PILL BEARING SPURGE
bronchitis

PINE OILS
cough

PIPSISSEWA
urethritis
urinary tract infection in women
urolithiasis

PLANTAIN
asthma
burns
conjunctivitis
cough
peptic ulcer
urethritis
urinary incontinence
urinary tract infection in women

PLANTAIN LEAVES
insect bites

PLEURISY ROOT
bronchitis

POKE ROOT
endometriosis
sprains and strains

POTASSIUM
peptic ulcer
pulmonary edema
tension headache

POTASSIUM ASPARTATE
edema
primary pulmonary hypertension
pulmonary edema

POTATO, FRESH GRATED
conjunctivitis
hemorrhoids

PRICKLY ASH BARK
alopecia
burns

dermatitis
Raynaud's phenomenon
sexual dysfunction

PRO-FLORA SUPPLEMENTS
food allergy
ulcerative colitis

PROPOLIS
laryngitis
pharyngitis

PSYLLIUM
irritable bowel syndrome
ulcerative colitis

PUMPKIN SEEDS
benign prostatic hyperplasia
prostatitis

PURPLE CONEFLOWER
cough

PYCNOGENOL
diabetes mellitus
Parkinson's disease

PYRIDOXAL-5-PHOSPHATE
asthma

PYRIDOXINE
hypoglycemia
urolithiasis

QUASSIA
intestinal parasites

QUERCETIN
allergic rhinitis
cutaneous drug reactions
dermatitis
diarrhea
eczema
food allergy
hyperthyroidism
insect bites
peptic ulcer
psoriasis
rheumatoid arthritis
sinusitis
sprains and strains
thyroiditis
ulcerative colitis

RAW HEART CONCENTRATE
pulmonary edema

RAW THYMUS GLANDULAR
fibromyalgia

RED ALDER BARK
dermatitis

RED CLOVER
cutaneous drug reactions
dermatitis
eczema
edema
insect bites
osteomyelitis
psoriasis

RED RASPBERRY
dysmenorrhea
endometriosis

RED ROOT
edema
endometriosis

RIBOFLAVIN (see Vitamin B₂)
ulcerative colitis

ROSE HIPS
allergic rhinitis
asthma
dermatitis
dermatitis
eczema
food allergy
hemorrhoids

ROSEMARY
alopecia
atherosclerosis
congestive heart failure
dementia
edema
endocarditis
fibromyalgia
primary pulmonary hypertension
pulmonary edema
Raynaud's phenomenon
sexual dysfunction

ROSEMARY LEAF
chronic fatigue syndrome

ROSEMARY LEAVES
low back pain

ROSEMARY OIL
chronic fatigue syndrome
chronic obstructive pulmonary
disease
insomnia

RUE
edema

RUTIN
dermatitis
eczema

SACROMYCES BOLARDII
diarrhea

SAGE
amenorrhea
asthma
laryngitis

SARSAPARILLA
dermatitis
psoriasis
rheumatoid arthritis

SAW PALMETTO
alopecia
anorexia nervosa
benign prostatic hyperplasia
prostatitis

SCHIZANDRA BERRY
chronic fatigue syndrome
fibromyalgia
hepatitis, viral

SELENIUM
amenorrhea
atherosclerosis
benign prostatic hyperplasia

candidiasis
chronic obstructive pulmonary
disease
cirrhosis of the liver
congestive heart failure
dermatitis
endocarditis
endometriosis
food allergy
hepatitis, viral
herpes simplex virus
HIV and AIDS
hypercholesterolemia
hypothyroidism
Parkinson's disease
primary pulmonary hypertension
prostatitis
psoriasis
pulmonary edema
Reiter's syndrome
rheumatoid arthritis
tension headache
thyroiditis
ulcerative colitis
warts

SKULLCAP
anxiety
asthma
chronic fatigue syndrome
dysphagia
fibromyalgia
gastroesophageal reflux disease
migraine headache
Parkinson's disease
seizures
sexual dysfunction

SKUNK CABBAGE
asthma

SLIPPERY ELM
osteomyelitis

SLIPPERY ELM POWDER
burns
cutaneous drug reactions
diarrhea
dysphagia
gastritis
gastroesophageal reflux disease
herpes zoster (varicella-zoster) virus
irritable bowel syndrome
laryngitis
peptic ulcer
pharyngitis
ulcerative colitis

SOY
menopause

SPEARMINT
fever of unknown origin
infantile colic

SPIRULINA
anemia

SQUAW VINE
amenorrhea
endometriosis
osteoporosis

ST. JOHN'S WORT
anorexia nervosa
anxiety

burns
dementia
depression-unipolar mood
disorders
dysphagia
gastroesophageal reflux disease
herpes simplex virus
herpes zoster (varicella-zoster) virus
HIV and AIDS
influenza
insomnia
low back pain
obesity
osteomyelitis
Parkinson's disease
sexual dysfunction
sinus headache
sinusitis

ST. JOHN'S WORT OIL
otitis media

STINGING NETTLE ROOT
benign prostatic hyperplasia

SULPHUR
peptic ulcer

SUNDEW
bronchitis

SWEET CLOVER
edema
SWEET VIOLET
cough

TANSY
intestinal parasites

TAURINE
congestive heart failure
primary pulmonary hypertension
pulmonary edema
seizures

L-TAURINE
angina
hypercholesterolemia

TEASEL ROOT
osteoarthritis

TEA TREE OIL
candidiasis
intestinal parasites

THIAMINE (see Vitamin B₁)
edema
obesity
ulcerative colitis

THUJA LEAF
warts

THYME
cough
intestinal parasites
pertussis

THYME LEAF
asthma
bronchitis
pulmonary edema
urethritis
urinary tract infection in women

THYME OIL
chronic obstructive pulmonary
disease
cough
intestinal parasites
sinus headache
sinusitis

THYMUS EXTRACT
hepatitis, viral
herpes simplex virus

TURMERIC
burns
bursitis
cutaneous drug reactions
edema
gallbladder disease
hepatitis, viral
hyperthyroidism
insect bites
low back pain
osteoarthritis
rheumatoid arthritis
sprains and strains
thyroiditis

TYROSINE
amenorrhea

L-TYROSINE
hypothyroidism
thyroiditis

USNEA LICHEN
pertussis

UVA URSI
Reiter's syndrome
urethritis
urinary tract infection in women

VALERIAN
anorexia nervosa
asthma
burns
bursitis
depression-unipolar mood
disorders
dysphagia
endometriosis
fibromyalgia
gastroesophageal reflux disease
herpes zoster (varicella-zoster) virus
hypertension
insomnia
irritable bowel syndrome
low back pain
obesity
osteomyelitis
peptic ulcer
pertussis
rheumatoid arthritis
seizures
sprains and strains
tension headache
ulcerative colitis

VANADIUM
diabetes mellitus

VANADYL SULFATE
hypoglycemia

VERVAIN
amenorrhea
endometriosis
osteoporosis
sexual dysfunction

VITAMIN A
allergic rhinitis
amenorrhea
common cold
conjunctivitis
diarrhea
gout
herpes simplex virus
herpes zoster (varicella-zoster) virus
hypothyroidism
endocarditis
influenza
osteoarthritis
osteomyelitis
peptic ulcer
pericarditis
tendinitis
thyroiditis
ulcerative colitis
vaginitis
warts

VITAMIN B$_1$
edema
depression-unipolar mood
   disorders
obesity
ulcerative colitis

VITAMIN B$_2$
depression-unipolar mood
   disorders
hypothyroidism
migraine headache
ulcerative colitis

VITAMIN B$_3$
dysmenorrhea
gout
hypercholesterolemia
hypothyroidism
hypoglycemia
insomnia
osteoarthritis

VITAMIN B$_5$
allergic rhinitis

VITAMIN B$_6$
allergic rhinitis
alopecia
amenorrhea
asthma
atherosclerosis
benign prostatic hyperplasia
congestive heart failure
depression-unipolar mood disorders
edema
hypothyroidism
migraine headache
seizures
sexual dysfunction

VITAMIN B$_{12}$
anemia
asthma
atherosclerosis
congestive heart failure
depression-unipolar mood disorders
herpes zoster (varicella-zoster) virus

HIV and AIDS
hypertension
psoriasis
seizures
ulcerative colitis

VITAMIN B-COMPLEX
anxiety
attention-deficit/hyperactivity
   disorder
candidiasis
chronic fatigue syndrome
cirrhosis of the liver
dementia
diabetes mellitus
dysmenorrhea
fibromyalgia
food allergy
hepatitis, viral
herpes zoster (varicella-zoster) virus
HIV and AIDS
hypercholesterolemia
hypertension
hypoglycemia
hypothyroidism
insect bites
insomnia
laryngitis
low back pain
obesity
osteoporosis
Parkinson's disease
Raynaud's phenomenon
sexual dysfunction
tension headache
thyroiditis
ulcerative colitis
warts

**VITAMIN B-COMPLEX WITH
EXTRA B$_{12}$**
cutaneous drug reactions

VITAMIN C
allergic rhinitis
amenorrhea
anemia
angina
asthma
atherosclerosis
attention-deficit/hyperactivity
   disorder
bronchitis
burns
candidiasis
chronic fatigue syndrome
chronic obstructive pulmonary
   disease
cirrhosis of the liver
common cold
congestive heart failure
conjunctivitis
cough
cutaneous drug reactions
dementia
depression-unipolar mood
   disorders
dermatitis
diabetes mellitus
diarrhea
eczema
edema
endocarditis
endometriosis
fever of unknown origin
fibromyalgia

food allergy
gallbladder disease
gastritis
gout
hemorrhoids
hepatitis, viral
herpes simplex virus
herpes zoster (varicella-zoster) virus
HIV and AIDS
hypercholesterolemia
hyperthyroidism
hypoglycemia
hypothyroidism
influenza
insect bites
intestinal parasites
laryngitis
low back pain
menopause
migraine headache
myocardial infarction
obesity
osteoarthritis
osteomyelitis
otitis media
Parkinson's disease
peptic ulcer
pericarditis
pertussis
pharyngitis
primary pulmonary hypertension
prostatitis
pulmonary edema
Raynaud's phenomenon
Reiter's syndrome
rheumatoid arthritis
roseola
sexual dysfunction
sinus headache
sinusitis
sprains and strains
tendinitis
tension headache
thyroiditis
ulcerative colitis
urethritis
urinary incontinence
urinary tract infection in women
vaginitis
warts

VITAMIN C WITH BIOFLAVONOIDS
bursitis

VITAMIN D
amenorrhea
ulcerative colitis

VITAMIN E
allergic rhinitis
alopecia
amenorrhea
atherosclerosis
burns
candidiasis
chronic obstructive pulmonary disease
cirrhosis of the liver
congestive heart failure
cutaneous drug reactions
dementia
dermatitis
diabetes mellitus
dysmenorrhea
edema
endocarditis
endometriosis

gallbladder disease
hemorrhoids
hepatitis, viral
herpes zoster (varicella-zoster) virus
HIV and AIDS
hypertension
hyperthyroidism
hypoglycemia
low back pain
menopause
migraine headache
myocardial infarction
osteoarthritis
osteomyelitis
Parkinson's disease
peptic ulcer
primary pulmonary hypertension
psoriasis
pulmonary edema
Raynaud's phenomenon
Reiter's syndrome
sexual dysfunction
sprains and strains
tendinitis
tension headache
thyroiditis
vaginitis
warts

VITAMIN K
amenorrhea
cirrhosis of the liver
hepatitis, viral
osteoporosis
ulcerative colitis

WHITE BYRONY
endometriosis

WHITE HOREHOUND
bronchitis

WHITE WILLOW
bursitis

WHITE WILLOW BARK
fever of unknown origin
low back pain
tension headache

WILD CHERRY BARK
asthma
bronchitis
cough

WILD INDIGO
endocarditis
sinus headache
sinusitis

WILD LETTUCE
herpes zoster (varicella-zoster) virus

WILD YAM
amenorrhea
anorexia nervosa
dysmenorrhea
dysphagia
endometriosis
gastroesophageal reflux disease
irritable bowel syndrome
low back pain
osteoporosis
rheumatoid arthritis
ulcerative colitis
urolithiasis

WILLOW
tendinitis

WITCH HAZEL
hemorrhoids
insect bites

WORMSEED
intestinal parasites

WORMWOOD
intestinal parasites

YARROW
alopecia
burns
cutaneous drug reactions
dermatitis
eczema
edema
endometriosis
fever of unknown origin
herpes simplex virus
endocarditis
influenza
osteomyelitis
roseola

YELLOW DOCK
anemia
constipation
eczema
osteomyelitis
psoriasis

YELLOW JASMINE
angina
herpes zoster (varicella-zoster) virus

YOHIMBE BARK
sexual dysfunction

YUCCA
osteoarthritis

ZINC
allergic rhinitis
alopecia
amenorrhea
anorexia nervosa
benign prostatic hyperplasia
bronchitis
burns
common cold
conjunctivitis
cough
cutaneous drug reactions
dementia
dermatitis
diabetes mellitus
eczema
endocarditis
endometriosis
fever of unknown origin
fibromyalgia
food allergy
gastritis
hepatitis, viral
herpes simplex virus
herpes zoster (varicella-zoster) virus
HIV and AIDS
hypertension
hypoglycemia
hypothyroidism
influenza
intestinal parasites

osteomyelitis
osteoporosis
peptic ulcer
pertussis
pharyngitis
prostatitis
psoriasis
Raynaud's phenomenon
Reiter's syndrome
rheumatoid arthritis
roseola
seizures
sinus headache
sinusitis
sprains and strains
tension headache
thyroiditis
ulcerative colitis
urethritis
urinary incontinence
urinary tract infection in women
vaginitis
warts

ZINC LOZENGES
laryngitis

■ HERBS BY USES AND INDICATIONS

This list extracts the items included in the Uses/Indications section of each herb monograph and combines them to create a collection of herbs that may be considered for a particular application or condition.

ABRASIONS
goldenseal

ABSCESS
chamomile, German
echinacea
goldenseal

ACHES AND PAINS
eucalyptus

ACNE
Brewer's yeast
cat's claw
evening primrose

ACNE, INFANT
chamomile, German

ACROCYANOSIS
grape seed extract

ADAPTOGEN
ginseng, American
ginseng, Asian
licorice

ADRENOCORTICAL INSUFFICIENCY, PRIMARY
licorice

AGING-RELATED DISORDERS
evening primrose

AIDS
bromelain
cat's claw
St. John's wort

ALCOHOLISM
evening primrose

ALLERGIES
cat's claw
devil's claw
feverfew
flaxseed oil
ginkgo biloba
licorice
stinging nettle

ALTERATIVE
barberry
echinacea
ginseng, American
ginseng, Asian
stinging nettle

ALZHEIMER'S DISEASE
ginkgo biloba

ANALGESIC
celery seed
devil's claw

ANALGESIC, TOPICAL
cayenne
peppermint

ANEMIA
feverfew
stinging nettle

ANESTHETIC
kava kava

ANGINA PECTORIS
bilberry
bromelain
hawthorn

ANODYNE
ginseng, Asian
valerian root

ANOGENITAL INFLAMMATION
chamomile, German

ANOREXIA
chamomile, Roman
devil's claw
ginseng, Siberian
St. John's wort

ANTIARRHYTHMIAS
hawthorn

ANTIARTERIOSCLEROTIC
green tea

ANTIBACTERIAL
cayenne
chamomile, German
green tea
lemon balm
peppermint

ANTIBIOTICS, POTENTIATION OF
bromelain

ANTICHOLESTEREMIC
garlic
green tea

ANTIDEPRESSANT
ginkgo biloba
ginseng, Asian
St. John's wort

ANTIDIARRHEAL
bilberry

ANTIDOTE TO STINGS
stinging nettle

ANTIEMETIC
ginger root
peppermint

ANTIFUNGAL
green tea

ANTIHELMINITIC
garlic

ANTIHEPATATOXIN
licorice

ANTIHISTAMINE
garlic
stinging nettle

ANTIHYPERTENSIVE
cayenne
garlic

ANTI-INFECTIVE
echinacea

ANTI-INFLAMMATORY
barberry
bilberry
cat's claw
celery seed
chamomile, German
comfrey
echinacea
evening primrose
feverfew
flaxseed
licorice
saw palmetto

ANTILIPIDAEMIC
garlic

ANTIMETASTATIC AGENT
bromelain

ANTIMICROBIAL
chamomile, German
echinacea
garlic
licorice
St. John's wort

ANTIMITOTIC
comfrey

ANTIMUTAGENIC
green tea

ANTIOXIDANT
bilberry
cayenne
green tea

ANTIPARASITIC
peppermint

ANTIPATHOGENIC
goldenseal

ANTIPHOLIGISTIC
chamomile, German

ANTIPYRETIC
devil's claw
licorice

ANTIRHEUMATIC
devil's claw

ANTISEPTIC
barberry
eucalyptus
ginger root

ANTISEPTIC, URINARY
saw palmetto

ANTISPASMODIC
black cohosh
chamomile, German
chamomile, Roman
ginger root
kava kava
licorice

peppermint
valerian root

ANTITHROMBOTIC
ginkgo biloba

ANTITUMOR
licorice

ANTITUSSIVE
flaxseed

ANTIVIRAL
cat's claw
eucalyptus
green tea
licorice

ANXIETY
kava kava
St. John's wort
valerian root

APATHY
St. John's wort

APHRODISIAC
celery seed
ginseng, Asian

APPETITE LOSS
(see anorexia)

APPETITE STIMULANT
barberry
ginseng, Asian

AROMATIC
chamomile, German
peppermint

ARTERIAL WALL PLAQUE DEPOSITS
bilberry
bromelain

ARTERIES, STRENGTHENING OF
cayenne

ARTERIOSCLEROSIS
devil's claw

ARTHRITIS *(see also osteoarthritis, rheumatoid arthritis)*
barberry
burdock
cat's claw
celery seed
devil's claw
evening primrose
feverfew
flaxseed oil
ginger root
licorice

ASTHMA
aloe
cat's claw
evening primrose
flaxseed oil
green tea
licorice

ASTRINGENT
barberry
bilberry

comfrey
eucalyptus
goldenseal
green tea
hawthorn

ATHEROSCLEROSIS
bromelain
cayenne
ginkgo biloba
ginseng, Siberian

ATHEROSCLEROSIS, PREVENTION
green tea

ATTENTION DEFICIT-HYPERACTIVITY DISORDER
ginseng, Siberian

AUTOIMMUNE REACTION
flaxseed oil
licorice

BACTERIAL ILLNESS
licorice

BACTERICIDE
valerian root

BACTERIOSTATIC
chamomile, German

BEDSORES
chamomile, Roman

BENIGN PROSTATIC HYPERPLASIA
saw palmetto
stinging nettle

BILE PRODUCTION
milk thistle

BITTER TONIC
barberry
feverfew
ginseng, American
goldenseal

BLADDER DISORDERS
devil's claw

BLADDER INFLAMMATION
flaxseed

BLOATING AND FULLNESS
chamomile, Roman
lemon balm

BLOOD CHOLESTEROL, LOWERING OF
Brewer's yeast
flaxseed
green tea

BLOOD PRESSURE DISORDERS
ginseng, Siberian

BLOOD PRESSURE REDUCTION
black cohosh
cayenne
evening primrose

BLUNT INJURIES
comfrey

BOILS
echinacea
goldenseal

BONE PAIN
cat's claw

BRONCHIAL INFLAMMATION/ INFECTION
barberry
comfrey
eucalyptus

BRONCHIAL IRRITATION
flaxseed

BRONCHITIS
licorice

BRONCHODILATOR
green tea

BRUISING
comfrey
evening primrose

BURNS
aloe
chamomile, Roman
flaxseed
milk thistle
St. John's wort
stinging nettle

BURSITIS
bromelain

CALCULI *(see also kidney stones)*
celery seed

CANCER
cat's claw
evening primrose
ginseng, American
ginseng, Asian
green tea

CANCER, PREVENTION
celery seed
flaxseed
green tea

CANDIDIASIS, CHRONIC
barberry

CAPILLARY FRAGILITY
bilberry
cayenne
grape seed extract

CAPILLARY WALL FORMATION AND STRENGTH
bilberry

CARBUNCLES
echinacea

CARDIAC INSUFFICIENCY WITH EDEMA
stinging nettle

CARDIAC WEAKNESS
hawthorn

CARDIOTONIC
ginseng, Asian
hawthorn

CARDIOVASCULAR DISEASE
bromelain

CARDIOVASCULAR DISEASE, PREVENTION
flaxseed

CARMINATIVE
cayenne
chamomile, German
ginger root
ginseng, Asian
lemon balm
peppermint
valerian root

CARPAL TUNNEL SYNDROME
cayenne

CATARACTS
bilberry

CATARRH, RESPIRATORY
lemon balm
peppermint
saw palmetto

CEREBRAL VASCULAR INSUFFICIENCY
ginkgo biloba

CHEMOTHERAPEUTIC AGENTS, POTENTIATION OF
bromelain

CHEST CONGESTION
eucalyptus

CHICKEN POX
chamomile, German

CHOLAGOGUE
barberry
ginger root
goldenseal
milk thistle

CHOLANGITIS
milk thistle

CHOLERETIC
milk thistle
peppermint

CHRONIC FATIGUE SYNDROME
evening primrose
ginseng, Siberian

CIRCULATORY DISORDERS
barberry
bilberry
ginkgo biloba

CIRCULATORY STIMULANT
cayenne
ginger root
ginkgo biloba
stinging nettle

CIRRHOSIS
cat's claw
milk thistle

CLAUDICATION, INTERMITTENT
evening primrose
ginkgo biloba

COCHLEAR DEAFNESS
ginkgo biloba

COLD, COMMON
echinacea
eucalyptus
ginger root
ginseng, American
ginseng, Asian
goldenseal
green tea

COLD, COMMON, PREVENTION
garlic

COLD SORES, HERPES SIMPLEX SYMPTOM
lemon balm

COLIC
chamomile, German
chamomile, Roman (folk remedy)

COLIC, INFANTILE
chamomile, Roman

COLIC, INTESTINAL
ginger root

COLLAGEN STABILIZATION
bilberry

COLON, IRRITABLE
peppermint

COLON DISORDERS, LAXATIVE ABUSE
flaxseed

CONCENTRATION, IMPAIRED
ginseng, Asian
ginseng, Siberian

CONGESTIVE HEART FAILURE
evening primrose
hawthorn

CONJUNCTIVITIS
goldenseal

CONSTIPATION
aloe
peppermint

CONSTIPATION, CHRONIC
flaxseed

CONSTIPATION, SPASTIC
chamomile, Roman

CONVALESCENCE, HELP DURING
cat's claw
ginseng, Asian
ginseng, Siberian

CONVULSIONS
valerian root

CORONARY ARTERIOSCLEROSIS
ginseng, Siberian

CORONARY ARTERY DISEASE
hawthorn

COUGH
flaxseed
green tea
licorice

COUGH, DRY
peppermint

COUGH, SPASMODIC
chamomile, German

CRAMPS, NIGHT LEG
valerian root

CRAMPS, STOMACH OR INTESTINAL
valerian root

CYSTITIS
saw palmetto

CYSTITIS, CHRONIC
kava kava

CYSTS
cat's claw

DEBILITY
cat's claw
ginseng, Siberian
saw palmetto

DECONGESTANT
eucalyptus
peppermint

DEMENTIA
ginkgo biloba

DEMULCENT
comfrey
evening primrose
flaxseed
licorice
milk thistle

DEODORANT
chamomile, German
eucalyptus

DEPRESSION
Brewer's yeast
cat's claw
ginkgo biloba
St. John's wort

DEPRESSION (MENOPAUSE)
black cohosh

DEVELOPMENTAL DISORDERS
evening primrose

DIABETES
aloe
bilberry
Brewer's yeast

cat's claw
evening primrose
flaxseed oil
ginseng, American
ginseng, Asian
goldenseal

DIABETES, NON-INSULIN DEPENDENT
stinging nettle

DIABETES, TYPE II
Brewer's yeast

DIABETIC NEUROPATHY
cayenne
evening primrose

DIABETIC RETINOPATHY
bilberry
ginkgo biloba

DIAPHORETIC
barberry
cayenne
chamomile, German
chamomile, Roman
ginger root
lemon balm

DIARRHEA
bilberry
goldenseal
green tea
peppermint

DIARRHEA, CHRONIC
barberry

DIGESTIVE DISORDERS
cat's claw
celery seed
chamomile, German

DIGESTIVE ENZYME
bromelain

DIURETIC
barberry
celery seed
chamomile, German
devil's claw
ginseng, Siberian
hawthorn
kava kava
saw palmetto
stinging nettle

DIVERTICULITIS
flaxseed

DOUCHE
garlic
goldenseal

DRUG RESISTANCE, TUMOR CELL
flaxseed oil

DRUG SIDE EFFECTS
cat's claw

DYSENTERY
barberry
cat's claw
green tea

DYSMENORRHEA
bilberry
flaxseed oil
ginger root
peppermint

DYSMENORRHEA, CONGESTIVE
feverfew

DYSPEPSIA
cayenne
devil's claw

DYSPEPSIA, FLATULENT
cayenne

EAR INFLAMMATION
chamomile, Roman
goldenseal

ECZEMA
chamomile, German
evening primrose
milk thistle

ECZEMA, INFANTILE
evening primrose

EDEMA
ginseng, American
ginseng, Asian

EMMENAGOGUE
black cohosh
celery seed
feverfew
peppermint

EMOLLIENT
comfrey
flaxseed

EMPHYSEMA
cayenne

ENTERITIS
goldenseal

ENTERITIS, MUCILAGE FOR
flaxseed

EPILEPSY, UNCONTROLLED
kava kava

ERYTHEMA
milk thistle

ESOPHAGEAL INFLAMMATION, CHRONIC
licorice

EXPECTORANT
barberry
cayenne
flaxseed
garlic
ginger root
ginseng, Asian
licorice
saw palmetto

EXPECTORANT, RELAXING
comfrey

EYE AILMENTS
barberry

EYE DISORDERS
bilberry

EYE IRRITATION
goldenseal

FATIGUE
Brewer's yeast
ginseng, American
ginseng, Asian
ginseng, Siberian

FATTY ACIDS, ESSENTIAL, DEFICIENCY
evening primrose

FEBRIFUGE
eucalyptus
lemon balm

FEELINGS OF WORTHLESSNESS
St. John's wort

FEVER
barberry
burdock
cayenne
valerian root

FIBROCYSTIC BREAST DISEASE
evening primrose

FIBROMYALGIA
St. John's wort

FIBROSITIS
devil's claw

FISTULAE
cat's claw
chamomile, German

FLATULENCE
chamomile, German
ginger root
lemon balm
peppermint

FOOD SENSITIVITIES
goldenseal

FRACTURES
comfrey

FRONTAL SINUS CATARRH
chamomile, Roman

FUNGAL ILLNESS
echinacea

FUNGUS
cat's claw

FURUNCULOSIS
echinacea

GALACTAGOGUE
celery seed
milk thistle
stinging nettle

GALLBLADDER DISORDERS
chamomile, Roman
devil's claw
milk thistle

GALLSTONES
milk thistle
peppermint

GASTRIC INFLAMMATION, CHRONIC
licorice

GASTRIC MUCUS STIMULATION
bilberry

GASTRITIS
cat's claw
chamomile, Roman
goldenseal

GASTRITIS, CHRONIC
licorice

GASTRITIS, MUCILAGE FOR
flaxseed

GASTROINTESTINAL DISORDERS
devil's claw
lemon balm

GASTROINTESTINAL STIMULANT
cayenne

GASTROINTESTINAL TRACT INFLAM-MATION/INFECTION
barberry
chamomile, German

GASTROINTESTINAL UPSET
bromelain

GINGIVITIS
chamomile, German

GLANDULAR SWELLING
goldenseal

GLAUCOMA
bilberry

GONORRHEA
cat's claw
kava kava

GOUT
celery seed
devil's claw
stinging nettle

HAIR, STRENGTHEN
Brewer's yeast

HAY FEVER
chamomile, Roman

HEADACHE
aloe
devil's claw
ginger root
ginkgo biloba
lemon balm
peppermint

HEADACHE, CLUSTER
cayenne

HEADACHE, MENOPAUSE
black cohosh

HEADACHE, MIGRAINE
cayenne
evening primrose
feverfew
kava kava
valerian root

HEARTBURN
chamomile, German
chamomile, Roman
devil's claw

HEART DISEASE
cat's claw

HEART FAILURE
hawthorn

HELICOBACTER PYLORI
barberry

HEMORRHAGE
barberry

HEMORRHOIDS
aloe
bilberry
cat's claw
chamomile, German
chamomile, Roman
evening primrose
stinging nettle

HEPATITIS
barberry
milk thistle

HEPATORESTORATIVE
milk thistle

HERPES
cat's claw

HERPES SIMPLEX
St. John's wort

HERPES SIMPLEX, COLD SORES
lemon balm

HIRSUTISM
saw palmetto

HIV
aloe
cat's claw

HIVES
aloe
chamomile, German
peppermint

HORMONE RESTORATIVE
ginseng, Asian

HOT FLUSHES (MENOPAUSE)
black cohosh

HYPERCHOLESTEROLEMIA
evening primrose
ginseng, American
ginseng, Asian

HYPERSOMNIA
St. John's wort

HYPERTENSION
cat's claw
celery seed
flaxseed oil

HYPERTENSION, ESSENTIAL
hawthorn

HYPNOTIC, MILD
valerian root

HYPOGLYCEMIC
stinging nettle

HYPOTENSIVE
hawthorn

IMMUNE FUNCTION, NORMALIZATION OF
licorice

IMMUNE SYSTEM DISORDERS
cat's claw

IMMUNE SYSTEM ENHANCEMENT
aloe

IMMUNOSTIMULATION
echinacea

IMPETIGO
chamomile, German

IMPOTENCE
ginkgo biloba

INDIGESTION
barberry
cayenne
ginger root

INFANTILE ERUPTIONS
evening primrose

INFECTION
garlic

INFERTILITY
ginseng, American
ginseng, Asian

INFLAMMATION
flaxseed oil

INFLAMMATION, ARTHRITIS AND RHEUMATISM
black cohosh

INFLUENZA
echinacea
eucalyptus
ginger root
goldenseal
lemon balm
St. John's wort

INFLUENZA, PREVENTION
garlic

INSECT BITES
feverfew
lemon balm
stinging nettle

INSOMNIA
chamomile, German
ginseng, Siberian
kava kava
lemon balm
St. John's wort
valerian root

INTESTINAL INFLAMMATION
goldenseal

INTESTINAL PARASITES
feverfew

INTESTINAL ULCERATION OR EROSION
comfrey

IRRITABILITY
black cohosh
Brewer's yeast

IRRITABLE BOWEL SYNDROME
flaxseed
peppermint

JAUNDICE
barberry

JET LAG
kava kava

JOINT ACHES
ginger root

JOINT INFLAMMATION
bromelain

JOINTS, ARTHRITIC
stinging nettle

KIDNEY DISORDERS
devil's claw
ginseng, Siberian

KIDNEY INFLAMMATION/ INFECTION
barberry

KIDNEY STONES
(see also calculi)
aloe
stinging nettle

LACERATIONS
goldenseal

LACTATION
saw palmetto

LAXATIVE
barberry
goldenseal
licorice

LAXATIVE, BULKING
flaxseed

LAXATIVE ABUSE, COLON PROBLEMS
flaxseed

LEUKOPENIA, RADIOTHERAPY- AND CHEMOTHERAPY-INDUCED
ginseng, Siberian

LIGAMENT STRAINS (see also sprains and strains)
comfrey

LIVER DAMAGE
milk thistle

LIVER DISORDERS
barberry
celery seed
chamomile, Roman
devil's claw
milk thistle

LOCOMOTIVE SYSTEM DISORDERS
devil's claw

LOW BACK PAIN
barberry
ginseng, Siberian

LUMBAGO
devil's claw

LUPUS SCLERODERMA
licorice

LYMPHEDEMA
grape seed extract

MACULAR DEGENERATION
bilberry
ginkgo biloba
grape seed extract

MASTALGIA
evening primrose

MASTECTOMY PAIN
cayenne

MEMBRANE STABILIZATION
bilberry

MEMORY LOSS, SHORT-TERM
ginkgo biloba

MENOPAUSE
black cohosh
ginseng, Asian
kava kava

MENSTRUAL DISORDERS
cat's claw
chamomile, Roman
devil's claw
feverfew
kava kava
lemon balm

MENSTRUAL PAIN
black cohosh
garlic
ginger root
lemon balm

MENSTRUATION, DELAYED
ginger root
lemon balm

MENTAL STAMINA
cat's claw
ginseng, American
ginseng, Asian

METABOLIC DISORDERS
evening primrose

MICTURITION
stinging nettle

MIGRAINE (see headache, migraine)

MILK PRODUCTION (see also lactation)
milk thistle

MONONUCLEOSIS
St. John's wort

MORNING SICKNESS
peppermint

MOTION SICKNESS
ginger root

MOUTH INFLAMMATION
chamomile, German
goldenseal

MOUTH PAIN
cayenne
chamomile, German

MOUTH SORES
barberry

MOUTHWASH
garlic
goldenseal

MUCOUS, EXCESS
goldenseal

MULTIPLE SCLEROSIS
evening primrose
St. John's wort

MUSCLE RELAXANT
bilberry
kava kava

MUSCLE SPASMS
celery seed
valerian root

MUSCLE STRAINS (see also sprains and strains)
comfrey
ginger root

MUSCLE WASTING
saw palmetto

MUSCULOSKELETAL CONDITIONS, DEGENERATIVE
devil's claw

MUSCULOTROPIC
chamomile, German

MYALGIC CONDITIONS
devil's claw
peppermint

MYOCARDIAL INFARCTION, POST
hawthorn

NAILS, STRENGTHEN
Brewer's yeast

NASAL CONGESTION
peppermint

NASAL MUCOSITIS
chamomile, Roman

NASOPHARYNGEAL INFLAMMATION
echinacea

NAUSEA
chamomile, Roman
ginger root
peppermint

NEPHRITIS
flaxseed oil

NERVINE
black cohosh
celery seed
ginseng, Asian
kava kava
valerian root

NERVOUSNESS
valerian root

NERVOUSNESS, MENOPAUSE
black cohosh

NERVOUS UNREST
lemon balm

NEURALGIA
cat's claw
devil's claw
stinging nettle
valerian root

NEURALGIA, POSTHERPETIC
cayenne

NEURALGIA, TRIGEMINAL
cayenne

NEURALGIC CONDITIONS
peppermint

NEUROMUSCULAR INFLAMMATION
St. John's wort

NEWALL PAINFUL ARTHROSES
devil's claw

NICOTINE POISONING
devil's claw

NUTRITION, POOR
evening primrose

NUTRITIVE
stinging nettle

OBESITY
evening primrose

ORAL MUCOSA INFLAMMATION
peppermint

OSTEOARTHRITIS
bromelain
cayenne

PAIN RELIEF
kava kava

PALPITATIONS, MENOPAUSE
black cohosh

PECTORAL TONIC
comfrey

PELVIC CONGESTION
ginger root

PERICHOLANGITIS
milk thistle

PERIPHERAL ARTERIAL INSUFFICIENCY
ginkgo biloba

PEYRONIE'S DISEASE
bromelain

PHARYNGEAL MUCOSITIS
chamomile, Roman

PHYSICAL STAMINA
cat's claw
ginseng, American
ginseng, Asian

PLATELET AGGREGATION, REDUCTION OF
bilberry
bromelain
evening primrose
garlic
green tea

POLYCYSTIC OVARY DISEASE
saw palmetto

PREMENSTRUAL SYNDROME
black cohosh
evening primrose
ginkgo biloba

PSORIASIS
cayenne
chamomile, German
evening primrose
flaxseed oil
milk thistle

PSYCHOLOGICAL DISORDERS
evening primrose

PULMONARY CATTARH
burdock

PYORRHEA
echinacea

RADIATION DAMAGE
evening primrose
green tea

RADIATION SIDE EFFECTS
cat's claw

RASHES
aloe
chamomile, Roman

RASHES, DIAPER
chamomile, German

RASHES, HEAT
chamomile, German

RAYNAUD'S PHENOMENON
evening primrose
ginkgo biloba

RED BLOOD CELL DEPLETION
ginseng, Asian

REHABILITATION
hawthorn

REHABILITATION AFTER ACUTE ILLNESS
ginseng, American

RELAXANT
feverfew
saw palmetto

REPRODUCTIVE SYSTEM, TONIC
saw palmetto

RESPIRATORY INFECTION, CHRONIC
echinacea

RESPIRATORY INFLAMMATION
chamomile, German

RESPIRATORY TRACT CATARRH
eucalyptus

RESPIRATORY TRACT INFECTIONS
bromelain

RESPIRATORY TRACT IRRITATION
chamomile, German

RESTLESSNESS
kava kava

RESTORATIVE
ginseng, American
ginseng, Asian

RHEUMATIC CONDITIONS
burdock
feverfew
stinging nettle

RHEUMATIC PAIN
eucalyptus

RHEUMATISM
barberry
cat's claw
celery seed
devil's claw
licorice
stinging nettle

RHEUMATOID ARTHRITIS
bilberry
bromelain
cayenne
evening primrose
flaxseed oil
ginseng, Siberian

RINGWORM
eucalyptus

ROMEHELD'S SYNDROME
chamomile, Roman

RUBEFACIENT, TOPICAL
cayenne
ginger root
stinging nettle

SALPINGITIS
saw palmetto

SCIATICA
bromelain
stinging nettle

SCLERODERMA
bromelain

SCURVY
burdock

SEBORRHEIC DERMATITIS
Brewer's yeast

SEDATIVE
black cohosh
celery seed
devil's claw
ginseng, Asian
lemon balm
valerian root

SEDATIVE, MILD
chamomile, German

SEPTICEMIA
echinacea

SHINGLES
cat's claw
cayenne

SIALOGOGUE
ginseng, Asian

SJOGREN'S SYNDROME
evening primrose

SKIN, AGING
milk thistle

SKIN, DRY
aloe
evening primrose

SKIN ABRASIONS
chamomile, German

SKIN DISORDERS
flaxseed oil

SKIN ERUPTIONS
goldenseal

SKIN IRRITATION
chamomile, German
flaxseed

SKIN PROBLEMS
burdock

SKIN ULCERATION
echinacea

SLEEP DISORDERS, NERVOUS
lemon balm

SLEEPLESSNESS, CHILDHOOD
chamomile, German

SOPORIFIC
chamomile, Roman

SPASMOLYTIC
lemon balm

SPASMS
barberry

SPLEEN DISORDERS
barberry

SPRAINS AND STRAINS
comfrey
stinging nettle

STIFFNESS
kava kava

STIMULANT
eucalyptus
ginseng, Asian
ginseng, Siberian
peppermint

STOMACHACHE
feverfew

STOMACH BACTERIAL INFECTION
barberry

STOMACHIC
cayenne
chamomile, Roman
evening primrose
ginseng, Asian

STRESS
Brewer's yeast
ginseng, Siberian
kava kava
valerian root

STROKE
ginkgo biloba

STROKE, ISCHEMIC
bilberry

SWELLING REDUCTION
St. John's wort

TELANGIECTASES
grape seed extract

TENDINITIS
bromelain
devil's claw
stinging nettle

THROAT INFLAMMATION
eucalyptus
ginger root
goldenseal

THROMBOPHLEBITIS
bromelain

THROMBOSIS
bromelain
hawthorn

TINNEA
eucalyptus

TINNITUS
feverfew
ginkgo biloba

TINNITUS, MENOPAUSE
black cohosh

TONIC
ginseng, Siberian

TONSILLITIS
echinacea

TRAUMA, INJURIES AND SURGERY
bromelain

TRIGLYCERIDES, ELEVATED
flaxseed
green tea

TUMORS
cat's claw
lemon balm

ULCER
bilberry
bromelain
cat's claw
cayenne
chamomile, German
chamomile, Roman
ginseng, American
ginseng, Asian

ULCER, PEPTIC
aloe
chamomile, German
goldenseal
licorice

ULCERATIVE (BLOOD PURIFIER)
black cohosh

ULCERATIVE COLITIS
flaxseed oil

URETHRITIS
saw palmetto

URINARY TRACT, TONIC
saw palmetto

URINARY TRACT DISORDERS
kava kava

URINARY TRACT INFLAMMATION/INFECTION
barberry
cat's claw
celery seed
flaxseed
stinging nettle

URINARY TRACT INFLAMMATION/INFECTION, IRRIGATION
stinging nettle

VAGINAL DRYNESS
black cohosh

VAGINAL INFLAMMATION
chamomile, German

VARICOSE VEINS
bilberry
bromelain
grape seed extract
hawthorn

VASCULAR DISORDERS
bilberry

VASCULAR FRAGILITY
ginkgo biloba

VASCULAR TONIC
bilberry

VASODILATOR
bilberry
feverfew
garlic
hawthorn

VASODILATOR, PERIPHERAL
ginger root

VEINS, STRENGTHENING OF
cayenne

VENEREAL ERUPTIONS
burdock

VENOUS INSUFFICIENCY, CHRONIC
grape seed extract

VERTIGO
feverfew
ginkgo biloba

VERTIGO, MENOPAUSE
black cohosh

VIRAL ILLNESS
echinacea
ginseng, American
ginseng, Asian
St. John's wort

VIRILITY ENHANCEMENT
ginseng, Siberian

VISUAL FUNCTION, IMPAIRED
grape seed extract

VOMITING
ginger root

VULNERARY *(see wound healing)*

WEIGHT LOSS
Brewer's yeast

WOUND DEBRIDEMENT
bromelain

WOUND HEALING
aloe
cat's claw
chamomile, German
chamomile, Roman
comfrey
echinacea
evening primrose
flaxseed
goldenseal
lemon balm
milk thistle
St. John's wort

■ **HERBS BY WARNINGS, PRECAUTIONS, CONTRAINDICATIONS**

This list extracts the items included in the Warnings, Precautions, Contraindications section of each herb monograph and combines them to create a collection of herbs that must be considered with caution under particular circumstances, or in general due to issues of safety or toxicity.

ABDOMINAL PAIN
aloe

AIDS
burdock

ALLERGIC REACTION
bromelain

ALLERGIC REACTION, RAGWEED
chamomile, German
chamomile, Roman

APPENDICITIS
aloe

ASTHMA
bromelain

BACTERIAL FLORA OF DIGESTIVE TRACT
goldenseal

BILE DUCT INFLAMMATION
eucalyptus

BILIARY TRACT OBSTRUCTION
peppermint oil

BLOOD CLOTTING, SLOW
garlic

BLOOD PRESSURE DISORDERS
ginseng, American
ginseng, Asian

CARDIOVASCULAR DISORDERS
ginseng, American
ginseng, Asian
green tea

CHILDREN UNDER 2 YEARS
cayenne

CHILDREN UNDER 3 YEARS
burdock

CHOLECYSTITIS
peppermint oil

CHOLESTATIC LIVER DISEASE
licorice

CIRRHOSIS
licorice

COAGULATION DISORDERS
bromelain

COLITIS
aloe

CONTACT DERMATITIS
burdock

DERMATITIS
echinacea

DIABETES
ginseng, American
ginseng, Asian

DIET, CALORIE- AND FAT-RESTRICTED
flaxseed oil

DIVERTICULITIS
aloe

DIVERTICULOSIS
aloe

EDEMA
stinging nettle irrigation therapy

ELECTROLYTE IMBALANCE
aloe

EPILEPSY, TEMPORAL LOBE, TRIGGERING OF
evening primrose

ESOPHAGEAL STRICTURE
flaxseed

GALLSTONES
ginger root

GASTROINTESTINAL INFLAMMATION
eucalyptus

GASTROINTESTINAL IRRITATION
aloe
barberry
cayenne

GASTROINTESTINAL SENSITIVITY
green tea

GASTROINTESTINAL STRICTURE
flaxseed

HEART DISORDERS
licorice

HEMORRHAGIC COMPLICATIONS IN SURGERY
garlic

HEMORRHOIDS
aloe

HIV PATIENTS
burdock

HYPERTENSION
bromelain
ginseng, Siberian
goldenseal
licorice

HYPERTONIA
licorice

HYPOKALEMIA
licorice

INFANTS AND YOUNG CHILDREN
eucalyptus
peppermint oil

INTESTINAL INFLAMMATION
flaxseed

INTESTINAL OBSTRUCTION
aloe

IRRITABLE BOWEL SYNDROME
aloe

KIDNEY DISORDERS
bromelain
green tea
licorice

KIDNEY INFLAMMATION
celery seed

LACTATION
aloe
burdock
chamomile, German, excessive use
comfrey
eucalyptus
feverfew
garlic
kava kava
peppermint oil
saw palmetto
St. John's wort
stinging nettle irrigation therapy

LIVER DISEASE, SEVERE
eucalyptus
peppermint oil

LIVER DISORDERS
bromelain
milk thistle

MENSTRUATION
feverfew
garlic
stinging nettle irrigation therapy

ORGAN TRANSPLANT PATIENTS
burdock

OSTEOPOROSIS
Brewer's yeast

PANIC ATTACKS
green tea

PHENOTHIAZINE USE
evening primrose

PREGNANCY
aloe
barberry
black cohosh
burdock
celery seed
chamomile, German, excessive use
comfrey

eucalyptus
feverfew
garlic
ginger root, dried
ginseng, American
ginseng, Asian
ginseng, Siberian
goldenseal
hawthorn
kava kava
lemon balm
licorice
peppermint oil
saw palmetto
St. John's wort
stinging nettle irrigation therapy

SCHIZOPHRENIA
evening primrose

SELF-MEDICATION
hawthorn
saw palmetto

SKIN, BROKEN
comfrey

SKIN GRAFT PATIENTS
burdock

SKIN REACTIONS
bromelain
burdock
cayenne

SPASM
green tea

SYSTEMIC DISEASES
echinacea

TANNING BOOTH
celery seed

THYROID, OVERACTIVE
green tea

TOXICITY
licorice

TUBERCULOSIS PATIENTS
burdock

ULCER
aloe

ULTRAVIOLET THERAPY
celery seed

VITAMIN B
goldenseal, absorption with

YEAST PRODUCTS
Brewer's yeast

■ HERBS BY SIDE EFFECTS

This list extracts the items included in the Side Effects section of each herb monograph and combines them to create a collection of herbs that produce a particular side effect.

ABDOMINAL CRAMPS
aloe

ABDOMINAL PAIN
black cohosh
evening primrose
feverfew
St. John's wort

ABDOMINAL SPASM
green tea

ABORTION
chamomile, Roman

ALLERGIC CONTACT DERMATITIS
garlic

ALLERGIC REACTION
aloe
echinacea
kava kava
stinging nettle

ANXIETY
ginseng, Siberian

APPETITE LOSS
green tea

ATROPINE POISONING
comfrey consumption

BLOATING
St. John's wort

BLOOD PRESSURE, HIGH
ginseng, Siberian
St. John's wort

BRADYCARDIA
black cohosh
peppermint oil

BREATHING DIFFICULTY
barberry
evening primrose toxicity

BURNING SENSATION/ REDNESS
cayenne

CARDIAC ARREST
licorice

CONSTIPATION
St. John's wort

CONTACT URTICARIA
stinging nettle

CONVULSIONS
goldenseal

DIARRHEA
aloe
barberry
cat's claw

eucalyptus leaf
feverfew
goldenseal
green tea

DIZZINESS
black cohosh
ginkgo biloba
kava kava
St. John's wort

EDEMA
stinging nettle

EMESIS
chamomile, German
chamomile, Roman

EXCITABILITY
valerian root

EXTREMITY NUMBNESS
licorice

EYE IRRITATION
barberry

FLATULENCE
feverfew

GASTROINTESTINAL DISTRESS
eucalyptus leaf
garlic
ginkgo biloba
kava kava
saw palmetto
stinging nettle
valerian root

GASTROINTESTINAL IRRITATION
feverfew

HEADACHE
black cohosh
evening primrose
ginkgo biloba
ginseng, Siberian
green tea
kava kava
licorice

HEADACHE, MIGRAINE
hawthorn

HEARTBURN
ginger root
peppermint oil

HIVES
St. John's wort

HYDROQUINONE POISONING
bilberry

HYPERMENORRHEA
bromelain

HYPERSENSITIVITY REACTIONS
peppermint

HYPERTENSION
licorice

ILEUS
flaxseed

INDIGESTION
feverfew

INSOMNIA
ginseng, Siberian
green tea
valerian root

INTRACRANIAL HEMORRHAGE
ginkgo biloba

IRRITABILITY
ginseng, Siberian
green tea

ITCHING
St. John's wort

JOINT PAIN
black cohosh

KIDNEY DAMAGE
eucalyptus leaf

KIDNEY FAILURE, ACUTE
peppermint oil

KIDNEY IRRITATION
barberry

LAXATIVE EFFECT
milk thistle

LETHARGY
barberry
licorice

LIP SWELLING
feverfew

LIVER DAMAGE
eucalyptus leaf

MELANCHOLY
ginseng, Siberian

METRORRHAGIA
bromelain

MOUTH, DRY
St. John's wort

MOUTH IRRITATION
goldenseal

MOUTH ULCERATION
feverfew

MUSCLE TREMORS
peppermint oil

MUSCULAR WEAKNESS
licorice

MYOGLOBINURIA
licorice

NAUSEA
barberry
black cohosh
bromelain
eucalyptus leaf

evening primrose
feverfew
hawthorn
St. John's wort

NEPHRITIS, HEMORRHAGIC
barberry

NEPHRITIS, INTERSTITIAL
peppermint oil

NERVOUSNESS
feverfew
valerian root

NERVOUS SYSTEM OVERSTIMULATION
goldenseal

NOSE BLEED
barberry

OLIGURIA
stinging nettle

PALPITATIONS
ginseng, Siberian
green tea
hawthorn

PERICARDIAL PAIN
ginseng, Siberian

PHOTOSENSITIVITY
St. John's wort

POTASSIUM SECRETION, ELEVATED
licorice

PSEUDOALDOSTERONISM
licorice

RASHES, SKIN
kava kava
peppermint oil
St. John's wort

REFLEX EXCITABILITY, HEIGHTENED
green tea

RESPIRATORY PARALYSIS
barberry

RESTLESSNESS
green tea

SEDATION
evening primrose toxicity

SKIN, BURNING SENSATION
stinging nettle

SKIN IRRITATION
aloe
barberry

SKIN LESIONS, BURN-LIKE
garlic

SLEEP PROBLEMS
St. John's wort

SODIUM RETENTION
licorice

STOOLS, SOFT
evening primrose
hawthorn

TASTE, LOSS OF
feverfew

THROAT IRRITATION
goldenseal

TIREDNESS
St. John's wort

TONGUE SWELLING
feverfew

TREMOR
black cohosh
evening primrose toxicity
green tea

ULCERATION, INTERNAL AND EXTERNAL
goldenseal

VERTIGO
green tea

VISUAL DIMNESS
black cohosh

VOMITING
barberry
black cohosh
bromelain
eucalyptus leaf
feverfew
goldenseal
green tea
St. John's wort

WATER RETENTION
licorice

WEIGHT GAIN
licorice

WHITE BLOOD CELL COUNT, ELEVATED
goldenseal

■ HERBS BY INTERACTIONS WITH OTHER DRUGS, HERBS, SUPPLEMENTS

This list extracts the items included in the Interactions section of each herb monograph and combines them to create a collection of herbs that interact in some way, positively or negatively, with a particular drug, other herb, or supplement.

ALCOHOL
kava kava

ALKALINES
green tea

ANALGESICS
valerian root

ANIMAL PROTEIN DRUGS
cat's claw

ANIMAL SERA
cat's claw

ANTIARRHYTHMICS
aloe

ANTICOAGULANTS
bromelain
garlic
ginger root

ANTICOAGULATION THERAPY
chamomile, German
chamomile, Roman

ANTIDIABETIC DRUGS
ginger root
ginseng, American
ginseng, Asian
St. John's wort

ANTIEPILEPTIC DRUGS
valerian root

ANTIHYPERTENSIVE DRUGS
cayenne
ginseng, American
ginseng, Asian

ANTIPSYCHOTIC DRUGS
ginseng, American
ginseng, Asian
ginseng, Siberian

ANTITHROMBOTIC DRUGS
feverfew

ANXIOLYTIC DRUGS
valerian root

ASPIRIN
feverfew
garlic

BARBITURATES
kava kava

BLOOD PLASMA, FRESH
cat's claw

BLOOD THINNERS
flaxseed oil

CAFFEINE
ginseng, American
ginseng, Asian
ginseng, Siberian

CARDIAC GLYCOSIDES
aloe

CARDIAC MEDICATIONS
ginger root

CENTRAL NERVOUS SYSTEM DEPRESSIVE DRUGS
St. John's wort

CORTICOSTEROIDS
aloe

CRYOPRECIPITATES
cat's claw

DIGITALIS
hawthorn
licorice

DRUG ABSORPTION
flaxseed

EPILEPTOGENICS
evening primrose

ESTROGEN, SYNTHETIC
black cohosh

FLUOXETINE
St. John's wort

FURAZOLIDONE
St. John's wort

GOTU KOLA
goldenseal

GRAVES' DISEASE THERAPY
lemon balm

HOPS
valerian root

HORMONE REPLACEMENT THERAPY
saw palmetto

HORMONES
ginseng, Siberian
saw palmetto

5-HYDROXYTRYPTOPHAN
St. John's wort

HYPERGLYCEMICS
St. John's wort

HYPERIMMUNOGLOBULIN THERAPY, INTRAVENOUS
cat's claw

HYPNOTICS
valerian root

HYPOGLYCEMICS
burdock
eucalyptus extract and oil
St. John's wort

IMMUNIZATIONS
cat's claw

IMMUNOSUPPRESSANT THERAPY
echinacea

INSULIN, BOVINE/PORCINE
cat's claw

ISOCARBOXAZID
St. John's wort

KAVA KAVA
alcohol
barbiturates
valerian root

L-DOPA
St. John's wort

LEMON BALM
valerian root

LICORICE
aloe
thiazide diuretics

MOCLOBEMIDE
St. John's wort

MONOAMINE OXIDASE INHIBITORS (MAOIS)
cayenne
St. John's wort

ORAL CONTRACEPTIVES
black cohosh
saw palmetto

PAROXETINE
St. John's wort

PASSIONFLOWER
valerian root

PEPTIDE HORMONES
cat's claw

PHENELZINE (NARDIL)
ginseng, American
ginseng, Asian

POPPY
valerian root

SELECTIVE SEROTONIN REUPTAKE INHIBITORS (SSRIS)
St. John's wort

SERTRALINE
St. John's wort

SKULLCAP
valerian root

STEROIDS
ginseng, American
ginseng, Asian
ginseng, Siberian

STIMULANTS
ginseng, American
ginseng, Asian
ginseng, Siberian

TETRACYCLINES
bromelain

THIAZIDE DIURETICS
aloe
licorice

THYMIC EXTRACTS, INTRAVENOUS
cat's claw

THYROID TREATMENTS
lemon balm

VALERIAN ROOT
kava kava
lemon balm
passionflower
poppy
skullcap

VITAMIN B
barberry

WARFARIN
feverfew

■ HERBS BY TAXONOMIC CROSS-REFERENCE

This list was produced to facilitate quick location of an herb monograph if only the botanical, pharmacopeial, or plant family name is known. This cross reference of the four names (including English or "common" name) also appears at the beginning of each herb monograph.

ALOE
Aloe vera/Aloe barbadensis/Aloe ferox (Botanical)
Liliaceae (Plant family)
Aloe barbadensis/capensis (Pharmacopeial)

BARBERRY/BARBERRY BARK/ BARBERRY ROOT/ BARBERRY ROOT BARK
Berberis vulgaris (Botanical)
Berberidaceae (Plant family)
Berberis vulgaris/Berberidis cortex/Berberidis radix/Berberidis radicis cortex (Pharmacopeial)

BILBERRY
Vaccinium myrtillus (Botanical)
Ericaceae (Plant family)
Myrtilli fructus/Myrtilli folium (Pharmacopeial)

BLACK COHOSH
Cimicifuga racemosa (Botanical)
Ranunculaceae (Plant family)
Cimicifugae racemosae rhizoma (Pharmacopeial)

BURDOCK
Arctium lappa/Arctium minus/Arctium tomentosum (Botanical)
Asteraceae (Plant family)
Bardanae radix (Pharmacopeial)

CAT'S CLAW
Uncaria tomentosa (Botanical)
Rubiaceae (Plant family)

CAYENNE (PAPRIKA)
Capsicum frutescens/Capsicum spp. (Botanical)
Solanaceae (Plant family)
Capsicum (Pharmacopeial)

CELERY SEED
Apium graveolens (Botanical)
Apiaceae (Plant family)
Apii fructus (Pharmacopeial)

CHAMOMILE, GERMAN
Matricaria recutita (Botanical)
Asteraceae (Plant family)
Matricariae flos (Pharmacopeial)

CHAMOMILE, ROMAN
Chamaemelum nobile (Botanical)
Asteraceae (Plant family)
Chamomillae romanae flos (Pharmacopeial)

COMFREY
Symphytum officinale (Botanical)
Boraginazeae (Plant family)
Symphyti folium/Symphyti radix (Pharmacopeial)

DEVIL'S CLAW *(Devil's Claw root)*
Harpagophytum procubens (Botanical)
Pedaliaceae (Plant family)
Harpagophyti radix (Pharmacopeial)

ECHINACEA *(Echinacea herb-root)*
Echinacea angustifolia herb-root/Echinacea pallida herb-root/Echinacea purpura herb-root (Botanical)
Asteraceae (Plant family)
Echinacea angustofoliae herba-radix/Echinacea pallidae herba-radix/Echinacea purpureae herba-radix (Pharmacopeial)

EUCALYPTUS *(Eucalyptus leaf, Eucalyptus oil)*
Eucalyptus globulus/Eucalyptus fructicetorum/Eucalyptus polybractea/smithii (Botanical)
Myrtaceae (Plant family)
Eucalypti folium/Eucalypti aetheroleum (Pharmacopeial)

EVENING PRIMROSE
Oenothera biennis (Botanical)
Onagraceae (Plant family)

FEVERFEW
Tanacetum parthenium/ Chrysanthemum parthenium (Botanical)
Compositae (Plant family)
Tanaceti parthenii herba (Pharmacopeial)

FLAXSEED
Linum usitatissimum (Botanical)
Linaceae (Plant family)
Lini semen (Pharmacopeial)

GARLIC
Allium sativum (Botanical)
Alliaceae (Plant family)
Allii sativi bulbus (Pharmacopeial)

GINGER
Zingiber officinale (Botanical)
Zingiberaceae (Plant family)
Zingiberis rhizoma (Pharmacopeial)

GINKGO BILOBA
Ginkgo biloba (Botanical)
Ginkgoaceae (Plant family)
Ginkgo folium (Pharmacopeial)

GINSENG, AMERICAN
Panax quinquefolium (Botanical)
Araliaceae (Plant family)
Ginseng radix (Pharmacopeial)

GINSENG, ASIAN
Panax ginseng (Botanical)
Araliaceae (Plant family)
Ginseng radix (Pharmacopeial)

GINSENG, SIBERIAN
Eleutherococcus senticosus/ Acanthopanax senticosus (Botanical)
Araliaceae (Plant family)
Eleutherococci radix (Pharmacopeial)

GOLDENSEAL
Hydrastis canadensis (Botanical)
Ranunculaceae (Plant family)
Hydrastis rhizoma (Pharmacopeial)

GRAPE SEED EXTRACT
Vitis vinifera (Botanical)
Vitaceae (Plant family)

GREEN TEA
Camellia sinensis (Botanical)
(Plant family)
(Pharmacopeial)

HAWTHORN *(Hawthorn Berry/Hawthorn Flower/Hawthorn Leaf/Hawthorn Leaf with Flower)*
Crataegus monogyna/Crataegus laevigata (Botanical)
Rosaceae (Plant family)
Crataegi fructus/crataegi flos/crataegi folium/cratagi folium cum flore (Pharmacopeial)

KAVA KAVA
Piper methysticum (Botanical)
Piperaceae (Plant family)
Piperis methystici rizoma (Pharmacopeial)

LEMON BALM
Melissa officinalis (Botanical)
Lamiaceae (Plant family)
Melissae folium (Pharmacopeial)

LICORICE
Glycyrrhiza glabra (Botanical)
Fabaceae (Plant family)
Liquiritiae radix (Pharmacopeial)

MILK THISTLE *(Milk Thistle fruit/Milk Thistle herb)*
Silybum marianum (Botanical)
Asteraceae (Plant family)
Cardui mariae fructus/Cardui mariae herba (Pharmacopeial)

PEPPERMINT *(Peppermint leaf, Peppermint oil)*
Mentha x piperita (Botanical)
Lamiaceae (Plant family)
Menthae piperitae folium/Menthae piperitae aetheroleum (Pharmacopeial)

SAW PALMETTO *(Saw Palmetto berry)*
Serenoa repens/Sabal serrulata (Botanical)
Aracaceae (Plant family)
Sabal fructus (Pharmacopeial)

ST. JOHN'S WORT
Hypericum perforatum (Botanical)
Hypericaceae (Plant family)
Hyperici herba (Pharmacopeial)

STINGING NETTLE *(Stinging nettle herb, Stinging nettle leaf, Stinging nettle root)*
Urtica dioica/Urtica urens (Botanical)
Urticaceae (Plant family)
Urticae herba/Urticae folium/Urticae radix (Pharmacopeial)

VALERIAN *(Valerian root)*
Valeriana officinalis
Valerianaceae (Plant family)
Valerianae radix (Pharmacopeial)

■ SUPPLEMENTS BY USES AND INDICATIONS

This list extracts the items included in the Uses/Indications section of each supplement monograph and combines them to create a collection of supplements that may be considered for a particular application or condition.

ACNE
selenium
sulfur
vitamin A (retinol)
vitamin B_9 (folic acid)
vitamin B_2 (riboflavin)
vitamin E
zinc

ACRODERMATITIS ETEROPATHICA
zinc

ADOLESCENCE, IRON REQUIREMENT
iron

AGING
dehydroepiandrosterone (DHEA)
gamma-linolenic acid (GLA)
vitamin E

AIDS
dehydroepiandrosterone (DHEA)
glutamine
spirulina
vitamin B_9 (folic acid)

AIRWAY SPASMS
vitamin C

ALCOHOL DETOXIFICATION
vitamin B_5 (pantothenic acid)

ALCOHOLISM
gamma-linolenic acid (GLA)
niacinamide
vitamin B_1
zinc

ALLERGIES
alpha-linolenic acid (ALA)
copper
vitamin B_5 (pantothenic acid)
vitamin C

ALZHEIMER'S DISEASE
ethylenediaminetetraacetic acid (EDTA)
Vitamin E

AMANITA POISONING
alpha-lipoic acid

AMENORRHEA
gamma-linolenic acid (GLA)

ANALGESIC ACTIVITY
creatine

ANEMIA
spirulina

ANEMIA, HEMOLYTIC
vitamin E

ANEMIA, MACROCYTIC
vitamin B_9 (folic acid)

ANEMIA, PERNICIOUS
vitamin B_{12}

ANEMIA, SIDEROBLASTIC
vitamin B_6

ANGINA
magnesium

ANOREXIA NERVOSA
zinc

ANTICLOTTING AGENT
vitamin E

ANTICONVULSANT DRUG THERAPY
vitamin D

ANTIFUNGAL ACTIONS
pau d'arco

ANTI-INFLAMMATORY ACTIONS
creatine
vitamin C

ANTIMICROBIAL ACTIONS
pau d'arco

ANTINEOPLASTIC ACTIONS
pau d'arco

ANTIOXIDANTS, PROTECTION
vitamin C

ANTIVIRAL ACTIONS
pau d'arco

ANXIETY
magnesium
niacinamide

APNEA, RECURRENT IN INFANTS
magnesium

APPETITE SUPPRESSANT
tyrosine

ARSENIC POISONING
ethylenediaminetetraacetic acid (EDTA)

ARTERIOSCLEROSIS, PREVENTION
vitamin D

ARTERIOSCLEROTIC BRAIN DISEASE
vitamin E

ARTHRITIS
cartilage
copper
vitamin C

ASTHMA
lysine
magnesium
pau d'arco
vitamin B_5 (pantothenic acid)
vitamin C

ATHEROSCLEROSIS
manganese
vitamin E

ATHEROSCLEROSIS, PREVENTION
magnesium

ATHLETIC PERFORMANCE
vitamin B_5 (pantothenic acid)

ATOPIC DERMATITIS
gamma-linolenic acid (GLA)

AUTOIMMUNE DISORDERS
alpha-linolenic acid (ALA)
dehydroepiandrosterone (DHEA)
lipase
vitamin D

BENIGN PROSTATIC HYPERPLASIA
zinc

BERI BERI, DRY
vitamin B_1

BERI BERI, INFANTILE
vitamin B_1

BERI BERI, WET
vitamin B_1

BIPOLAR DISORDER
5-hydroxytryptophan (5-HTP)

BLEEDING, EXCESSIVE, PREVENTION
vitamin K

BLEEDING GUMS
vitamin C

BLOATING
spirulina

BLOOD BUILDER
pau d'arco

BLOOD GLUCOSE CONTROL
vitamin H (biotin)

BLOOD LIPID REDUCTION
creatine

BLOOD LOSS, CHRONIC
iron

BLOOD PRESSURE, HIGH
magnesium
vitamin C
vitamin D

BODY BUILDING
vanadium

BODY ODOR
sulfur
vitamin K

BONE FRACTURES
vitamin D

BONE LOSS
calcium

BONE MINERALIZATION
vanadium
vitamin K

ATHEROSCLEROSIS, PREVENTION
magnesium

BRAIN DISORDERS
alpha-lipoic acid

BREAST CANCER
pau d'arco

BREAST CANCER, PREVENTION
vitamin D

BRONCHITIS
pau d'arco

BRUISING
vitamin C

BURNS, SEVERE
vitamin A (retinol)

CADMIUM POISONING
selenium

CADMIUM TOXICITY
manganese

CANCER
alpha-linolenic acid (ALA)
cartilage
dehydroepiandrosterone (DHEA)
gamma-linolenic acid (GLA)
glutamine
manganese
phenylalanine
selenium
spirulina
vitamin E

CANCER, HORMONALLY RELATED
melatonin

CANCER, PREVENTION
vitamin C

CANCER INHIBITOR
psyllium

CANDIDA
spirulina

***CANDIDA ALBICANS* INFECTION**
pau d'arco

CANDIDIASIS
sulfur
vitamin B_9 (folic acid)

CANDIDIASIS, INTESTINAL
vitamin H (biotin)

CAPILLARY FRAGILITY
vitamin C

CARCINOGENESIS, PREVENTION
vitamin E

CARDIAC ARRHYTHMIAS
magnesium
potassium

CARDIOMYOPATHY, ALCOHOLIC
selenium

CARDIOVASCULAR DISORDERS
alpha-linolenic acid (ALA)
calcium
chromium
copper
magnesium
vitamin B_1
vitamin B_3 (niacin)

CARDIOVASCULAR DISORDERS, PREVENTION
vitamin C

CARPAL TUNNEL SYNDROME
vitamin B_2 (riboflavin)

CATARACTS
vitamin B_9 (folic acid)
vitamin B_2 (riboflavin)

CATARACTS, PREVENTION
selenium
vitamin C
vitamin E

CELIAC DISEASE
lipase
vitamin D
vitamin E
zinc

CERVICAL CANCER, PREVENTION
vitamin B_9 (folic acid)

CERVICAL DYSPLASIA
vitamin B_9 (folic acid)
vitamin C

CHEILOSIS
vitamin B_6

CHEMICAL HYPERSENSITIVITY
copper

CHEMOTHERAPY, MOUTH PAIN IN
glutamine

CHOLESTEROL, LOWERING OF
magnesium
psyllium
vanadium
vitamin B_5 (pantothenic acid)
chronic obstructive pulmonary disease
magnesium

CIRRHOSIS OF THE LIVER
selenium

COLITIS
glutamine
spirulina

COLON, CLEANSING AND HEALING OF
psyllium

COLON CANCER, PREVENTION
vitamin B_9 (folic acid)
vitamin D

COMA
vitamin B_1

CONFUSION
vitamin B_6

CONGENITAL DEFECTS
vitamin B_1

CONSTIPATION
phosphorus
psyllium
vitamin B_9 (folic acid)

CORONARY HEART DISEASE
melatonin

COUGH
phosphorus

CRITICAL ILLNESS
glutamine

CROHN'S DISEASE
glutamine

CYSTIC FIBROSIS
vitamin D
vitamin E

CYSTITIS
pau d'arco

DEGENERATIVE BRAIN DISEASE
vitamin E

DEPRESSION
dehydroepiandrosterone (DHEA)
5-hydroxytryptophan (5-HTP)
magnesium
melatonin
niacinamide
phenylalanine
sulfur
tyrosine
vitamin B_6
vitamin B_9 (folic acid)

DERMATITIS
vitamin B_2 (riboflavin)

DIABETES
alpha-lipoic acid
chromium
gamma-linolenic acid (GLA)
magnesium
manganese
niacinamide
potassium
vanadium
vitamin C
vitamin D
zinc

DIABETES, TYPE II
vitamin E

DIABETIC KETOACIDOSIS
phosphorus

DIABETIC NEUROPATHY
alpha-lipoic acid
vitamin H (biotin)

DIALYSIS PATIENTS
zinc

DIARRHEA
psyllium
vitamin B_1

DIARRHEA, CHRONIC
zinc

DIGESTION, IMPAIRED
lipase

DIGESTIVE DISORDERS
sulfur

DIVERTICULAR DISEASE
psyllium

DRUG DETOXIFICATION
tyrosine

DRUG TOXICITY
alpha-lipoic acid

DUCHENNE MUSCULAR DYSTROPHY
vitamin H (biotin)

DYSMENORRHEA
gamma-linolenic acid (GLA)

ECZEMA
alpha-linolenic acid (ALA)
selenium
spirulina
sulfur
vitamin B_2 (riboflavin)
vitamin E

ELDERLY
vitamin B_9 (folic acid)

ELDERLY PATIENTS
vitamin D

ENDURANCE, IMPROVEMENT IN
creatine

ENERGY
vitamin B_5 (pantothenic acid)

ENTERITIS, REGIONAL
cartilage

ENVIRONMENTAL POLLUTANTS, PROTECTION
vitamin E

EPILEPSY
manganese
melatonin

EYE HEALTH
sulfur

EYES, DRY
gamma-linolenic acid (GLA)

EYESIGHT
selenium

FATIGUE
copper
magnesium
melatonin

FATIGUE, CHRONIC
tyrosine

FATIGUE, PMS
magnesium

FAT MALABSORPTION DISORDERS
vitamin D
vitamin E

FAT METABOLISM
vitamin H (biotin)

FECAL ODOR
vitamin K

FIBER SUPPLEMENT
psyllium

FIBROCYSTIC BREAST DISEASE
vitamin E

FIBROMYALGIA
5-hydroxytryptophan (5-HTP)

FOOD ALLERGIES
lipase

FOOD ALLERGIES, HEADACHES
magnesium

FOOD CRAVINGS
glutamine

FORGETFULNESS
sulfur

FREE RADICAL DAMAGE
alpha-lipoic acid
ethylenediaminetetraacetic acid (EDTA)
vitamin B_2 (riboflavin)

GANGRENE
ethylenediaminetetraacetic acid (EDTA)

GAS
spirulina

GASTRIC MUCOSAL METABOLISM
glutamine

GASTRITIS
pau d'arco

GASTROENTERITIS, ACUTE
phosphorus

GASTROINTESTINAL DISORDERS
vitamin B_1

GASTROINTESTINAL DISTURBANCES, CHRONIC
iron

GASTROINTESTINAL HYPOTONIA
vitamin B_1

GENETIC ABNORMALITIES, INFANTS
vitamin H (biotin)

GENITOURINARY INFECTIONS
pau d'arco

GINGIVITIS
calcium

GLAUCOMA
chromium
magnesium

GLOSSITIS
vitamin B$_6$

GLUCOCORTICOID THERAPY
vitamin D

GLUCOSE INTOLERANCE
potassium

GLUCOSE METABOLISM IMPROVEMENT
creatine

GONORRHEA
pau d'arco

HAIR, GRAY
vitamin H (biotin)

HAIR, REJUVENATION
vitamin B$_5$ (pantothenic acid)

HEADACHE
vitamin B$_9$ (folic acid)

HEADACHE, CHILDREN
5-hydroxytryptophan (5-HTP)

HEADACHE, MIGRAINE
5-hydroxytryptophan (5-HTP)
lysine
magnesium

HEADACHE, MIGRAINE, PREVENTION
vitamin B$_2$ (riboflavin)

HEARING
magnesium

HEARING LOSS
manganese

HEART DISEASE
dehydroepiandrosterone (DHEA)
ethylenediaminetetraacetic acid (EDTA)
gamma-linolenic acid (GLA)
selenium
vanadium

HEART DISEASE, PREVENTION
vitamin B$_9$ (folic acid)

HEART IRREGULARITY
calcium

HEART SURGERY
vitamin E

HEAVY METAL DETOXIFICATION
alpha-lipoic acid

HEAVY METAL TOXICITY
selenium

HEMORRHAGE, NEWBORNS
vitamin K

HEMORRHAGE, PREVENTION
vitamin K

HEMORRHOIDS
iron
psyllium
sulfur

HEPATITIS, CHRONIC
alpha-lipoic acid

HERNIA
pau d'arco

HERPES
lysine
pau d'arco

HERPES SIMPLEX VIRUS
spirulina

HIGH-DENSITY LIPOPROTEIN LEVELS
vitamin B$_3$ (niacin)
vitamin C

HODGKINS DISEASE
pau d'arco

HOMOCYSTEINE, HIGH PLASMA LEVELS
vitamin B$_6$
vitamin B$_{12}$

HUMAN CYTOMEGALOVIRUS
spirulina

HYPERCHOLESTEROLEMIA
manganese

HYPERKERATOSIS
vitamin A (retinol)

HYPERTENSION
calcium
potassium

HYPOGLYCEMIA
chromium
niacinamide
spirulina

HYPOKALEMIA
potassium

IMMUNE SUPPORT
spirulina
zinc

IMMUNE SYSTEM ENHANCEMENT
vitamin A (retinol)
vitamin B$_2$ (riboflavin)
vitamin C

IMMUNOCOMPETENCE
manganese

IMMUNODEPRESSION
selenium

INFANCY, IRON REQUIREMENT
iron

INFERTILITY
vitamin B$_9$ (folic acid)

INFLAMMATION
phenylalanine

INFLAMMATORY BOWEL DISEASE
zinc

INFLAMMATORY BOWEL DISEASE, PREVENTION
vitamin D

INFLAMMATORY CONDITIONS
alpha-linolenic acid (ALA)
lipase
selenium

INFLUENZA VIRUS
spirulina

INSOMNIA
5-hydroxytryptophan (5-HTP)
melatonin
niacinamide

INSULIN SECRETION
vitamin D

IRON-DEFICIENT ANEMIA
iron

IRRITABILITY
sulfur
vitamin B$_6$

IRRITABLE BOWEL SYNDROME
psyllium

ISONIAZID OVERDOSE
vitamin B$_6$

JET LAG
melatonin

KIDNEY CALCIUM OXALATE STONES, PREVENTION
vitamin K

KIDNEY DISEASE
zinc

LACK OF APPETITE
spirulina

LACTATE ACIDOSIS, CONGENITAL
vitamin B$_1$

LACTATION
zinc

LAXATIVE, BULK
psyllium

LAXATIVE, MILD
phosphorus

LEAD POISONING
ethylenediaminetetraacetic acid (EDTA)
selenium

LEAKY GUT SYNDROME
glutamine

LEUKEMIA CELLS, INHIBITION
vitamin D

LEUKOPENIA
copper

LIBIDO, STIMULATION OF
tyrosine

LIVER CANCER
pau d'arco
vitamin K

LIVER DISORDERS
pau d'arco
selenium

LONG QT SYNDROME, CONGENITAL
magnesium

LOW-DENSITY LIPOPROTEIN LEVELS
vitamin B$_3$ (niacin)
vitamin E

LUNG CANCER, NON-SMALL CELL
melatonin

LUNG CANCER, PREVENTION
vitamin B$_9$ (folic acid)

LUNG FUNCTION
magnesium

LUPUS
alpha-linolenic acid (ALA)
dehydroepiandrosterone (DHEA)
pau d'arco
selenium
vitamin E

MACULAR DEGENERATION
cartilage
ethylenediaminetetraacetic acid (EDTA)
vitamin E

MACULAR DEGENERATION, PREVENTION
zinc

MALABSORPTION
lipase
spirulina

MALE FERTILITY
selenium
vitamin C
zinc

MALIGNANCY
iron

MANIC DEPRESSION
5-hydroxytryptophan (5-HTP)

MAPLE SYRUP DISEASE
vitamin B$_1$

MEASLES
spirulina

MEASLES, INFANT MORTALITY FROM
vitamin A (retinol)

MEMORY IMPROVEMENT
dehydroepiandrosterone (DHEA)

MENOPAUSE, SYMPTOMS OF
calcium
sulfur

MENSTRUAL BLEEDING
vitamin K

MENSTRUAL CRAMPS
calcium
magnesium

MENTAL HEALTH
magnesium

MENTAL ILLNESS
niacinamide

MERCURY POISONING
ethylenediaminetetraacetic acid (EDTA)
selenium

METAL TOXICITY
ethylenediaminetetraacetic acid (EDTA)

METHYLMALOIC ACIDURIA
vitamin B_{12}

MORNING SICKNESS
vitamin K

MOUTH PAIN
glutamine

MULTIPLE SCLEROSIS
alpha-linolenic acid (ALA)
dehydroepiandrosterone (DHEA)
melatonin
vitamin D

MUMPS
spirulina

MUSCLE CRAMPS
vitamin B_2 (riboflavin)

MUSCLE LOADING
creatine

MUSCLE WASTING
creatine

MUSCLE WEAKNESS
potassium

MUSCULAR CONDITIONS
selenium

MYOCARDIAL INFARCTION
magnesium

MYOCARDIAL INFARCTION, ACUTE
potassium

MYOCARDIAL METABOLISM, INCREASE IN
creatine

MYOTONIC DYSTROPHY
selenium

NAILS, FRAIL, SPLITTING, OR THIN
vitamin H (biotin)

NARCOLEPSY
tyrosine

NASAL POLYPS
lysine

NAUSEA, IN PREGNANCY
vitamin B_6

NECROTIZING ENCEPHALOPATHY, SUBACUTE
vitamin B_1

NERVOUSNESS
magnesium

NEURAL TUBE BIRTH DEFECTS, PREVENTION
vitamin B_9 (folic acid)

NEURITIS OF PREGNANCY
vitamin B_1

NIGHT BLINDNESS
vitamin A (retinol)

OBESITY
chromium
dehydroepiandrosterone (DHEA)
5-hydroxytryptophan (5-HTP)

ORAL CONTRACEPTIVES
zinc

ORAL LEUKOPLAKIA
spirulina

ORAL THRUSH CANDIDIASIS
pau d'arco

OSTEOARTHRITIS
cartilage
niacinamide
sulfur

OSTEOARTHRITIS, CARTILAGE DAMAGE
vitamin D

OSTEOARTHRITIS, PAIN
phenylalanine

OSTEOMALACIA
phosphorus, with calcium
vitamin D

OSTEOPENIA
vitamin D

OSTEOPOROSIS
calcium
chromium
dehydroepiandrosterone (DHEA)
gamma-linolenic acid (GLA)
manganese
melatonin
phosphorus, with calcium
vitamin D
vitamin K

OSTEOPOROSIS, PREVENTION
vitamin B_9 (folic acid)

PAIN, CHRONIC
phenylalanine

PAIN, POSTEPISIOTOMY
lysine

PANCREATIC DISEASE
vitamin D
vitamin E

PARASITES
iron

PARATHYROID, OVERACTIVE
vitamin D

PARENTERAL NUTRITION
vitamin B_1

PARKINSON'S DISEASE
phenylalanine
tyrosine

PERFORMANCE ENHANCEMENT
dehydroepiandrosterone (DHEA)
vanadium

PERIODONTAL DISEASE
calcium

PERIPHERAL NEURITIS
vitamin B_6

PERNICIOUS ANEMIA
vitamin B_{12}

PHENYLKETONURIA (PKU)
tyrosine

PREECLAMPSIA, PREVENTION
calcium
magnesium

PREGNANCY
iron
magnesium
zinc

PREGNANCY, HYPERTENSION INDUCED BY
calcium

PREMENSTRUAL SYNDROME (PMS)
calcium
gamma-linolenic acid (GLA)
magnesium
sulfur
tyrosine
vitamin B_6
vitamin E

PROSTATE CANCER
pau d'arco
zinc

PROSTATE FUNCTION
selenium

PROSTATITIS
pau d'arco
zinc

PROTEIN SOURCE
spirulina

PSORIASIS
alpha-linolenic acid (ALA)
cartilage
selenium
spirulina
vitamin A (retinol)
vitamin B_5 (pantothenic acid)
vitamin E

PSYCHIATRIC SYMPTOMS, ELDERLY
vitamin B_9 (folic acid)

RADIATION DAMAGE, GASTROINTESTINAL
glutamine

RADIATION THERAPY EFFECTS
sulfur

RASHES, DIAPER
sulfur

RECOVERY AFTER SURGERY OR TRAUMA
glutamine

RECOVERY FROM PROLONGED ILLNESS
glutamine

RED BLOOD CELL INTEGRITY
vitamin E

REPRODUCTIVE DISORDERS
vitamin E

RHEUMATISM
pau d'arco
sulfur

RHEUMATOID ARTHRITIS
cartilage
dehydroepiandrosterone (DHEA)
gamma-linolenic acid (GLA)
manganese
phenylalanine
selenium
sulfur
vitamin B_9 (folic acid)
vitamin B_5 (pantothenic acid)
vitamin B_2 (riboflavin)
vitamin D
zinc

RICKETS
phosphorus, with calcium

RICKETS, PREVENTION
vitamin D

RINGWORM
pau d'arco

SCALP, DRY
sulfur

SCHIZOPHRENIA
niacinamide

SEBORRHEIC DERMATITIS
vitamin H (biotin)

SEIZURES, PYRIDOXINE-DEPENDENT
vitamin B6

SEXUAL FUNCTION, MALE
zinc

SHORT BOWEL SYNDROME
vitamin D

SICKLE CELL ANEMIA
vitamin B9 (folic acid)
vitamin B2 (riboflavin)

SJOGREN'S SYNDROME
gamma-linolenic acid (GLA)

SKIN, REJUVENATION
vitamin B5 (pantothenic acid)

SKIN, WOUND TREATMENT
vitamin K

SKIN CANCER, PREVENTION
vitamin D

SKIN DISORDERS
selenium
spirulina
vitamin A (retinol)
vitamin E
vitamin H (biotin)

SKIN PROBLEMS
vitamin B2 (riboflavin)

SLEEP DISTURBANCES
sulfur

SLEEP PATTERNS, RESTORATION OF
melatonin

SMELL, IMPROVEMENT
zinc

SPERM MOTILITY
selenium

STAMINA INCREASE
vitamin B5 (pantothenic acid)

STOMATITIS
pau d'arco
vitamin B6

STOOL SOFTENER
psyllium

STRENGTH, IMPROVEMENT IN
creatine

STRESS
tyrosine
vitamin B2 (riboflavin)

STRESS, EXTREME
glutamine

STROKE
alpha-lipoic acid

STROKE, PREVENTION
magnesium
potassium
vitamin B9 (folic acid)
vitamin D

SUDDEN INFANT DEATH SYNDROME (SIDS)
melatonin
selenium

SUNBURN
vitamin C

TASTE, IMPROVEMENT
zinc

TASTE ALTERATION, CANCER TREATMENT
zinc

TEETH, LOOSE
calcium

TEETH, MINERALIZATION OF
vanadium

TINNITUS
manganese

TONIC
pau d'arco

TORSADE DE POINTES
magnesium

TRANSPLANT REJECTION
vitamin D

TRAUMA
glutamine

TRIGLYCERIDE LEVELS
magnesium
vitamin B3 (niacin)

TUBERCULOSIS, PREVENTION
vitamin D

ULCER
copper
pau d'arco

ULCER, PEPTIC
glutamine

ULCER, PEPTIC, BLEEDING
iron

ULCER, SKIN
vitamin B2 (riboflavin)

ULCERATIVE COLITIS
dehydroepiandrosterone (DHEA)
vitamin B1
zinc

URINE ODOR
vitamin K

VAGINAL CANDIDIASIS
pau d'arco

VASCULITIS
selenium

VEGAN DIET
vitamin D
VIRAL INFECTIONS
vitamin A (retinol)

VITAMIN A DEFICIENCY
spirulina

VITILIGO
copper
phenylalanine

VOMITING, IN PREGNANCY
vitamin B6

WATER RETENTION, PMS
magnesium

WEIGHT LOSS
tyrosine

WEIGHT REDUCTION
psyllium

WERNICKE'S ENCEPHALOPATHY
vitamin B1

WILSON'S DISEASE
zinc

WOUND HEALING
ethylenediaminetetraacetic acid (EDTA)
vitamin B5 (pantothenic acid)
vitamin C
vitamin E
zinc

WOUNDS, SEVERE
vitamin A (retinol)

WOUND TREATMENT
vitamin K

■ **SUPPLEMENTS BY WARNINGS, PRECAUTIONS, CONTRAINDICATIONS**
This list extracts the items included in the Warnings, Precautions, Contraindications section of each supplement monograph and combines them to create a collection of supplements that must be considered with caution under particular circumstances, or in general due to issues of safety or toxicity.

ALCOHOL
vitamin A toxicity

ALCOHOLICS
sulfur

ALLERGIC DERMATITIS
chromium

ALTERED MENTAL STATE
5-hydroxytryptophan (5-HTP)

ANTICOAGULANT DRUGS
vitamin K

ANTIDEPRESSANT DRUGS
5-hydroxytryptophan (5-HTP)

ASTHMA
vitamin B3 (niacin)

ATRIOVENTRICULAR BLOCK, HIGH-GRADE
magnesium

AUTOIMMUNE DISORDERS
melatonin

AUTONOMIC DYSFUNCTION
5-hydroxytryptophan (5-HTP)

BEHAVIORAL PROBLEMS
selenium

BIRTH DEFECTS
vitamin A (retinol)

BLEEDING TIME, PROLONGED
vitamin E

BLOOD-CLOTTING CONDITIONS
pau d'arco

BLOOD COMPOUNDS, MONITORING
ethylenediaminetetraacetic acid (EDTA)

BLOOD PRESSURE, HIGH
tyrosine
vitamin E

BLOOD PRESSURE, MONITORING OF
ethylenediaminetetraacetic acid (EDTA)

BONE MASS, REDUCED
phosphorus

BREAST CANCER
dehydroepiandrosterone (DHEA)

BRONCHOGENIC CARCINOMA
chromium

CALCIFICATION, SOFT TISSUE
calcium

CALCIUM, DRAIN OF
phosphorus

CALCIUM, HIGH BLOOD LEVELS
vitamin D

CANCER, HORMONE-SENSITIVE
dehydroepiandrosterone (DHEA)

CHEMOTHERAPY
vitamin B_1

CHILDREN
psyllium
shark cartilage

CHOLESTEROL, INCREASED LEVEL
lysine

CORTICOSTEROIDS
melatonin

CORTICOSTEROIDS, LONG-TERM USE
sulfur

COUMADIN
vitamin K

CYANOCOBALAMIN
vitamin B_{12} deficiency

DEPRESSION
melatonin

DIABETES
alpha-lipoic acid
vitamin B_3 (niacin)

DROWSINESS
melatonin

ELDERLY PATIENTS
potassium
sulfur

ENDURANCE
creatine

EPILEPSY
Vitamin B_9 (folic acid)

FAT INTAKE
alpha-linolenic acid (ALA)

FERTILITY
melatonin

GALLBLADDER DISORDERS
vitamin B_3 (niacin)

GASTRIC IRRITATION
chromium

GLUCOSE, BLOOD, MONITORING OF
vitamin B_3 (niacin)

GOUT
vitamin B_3 (niacin)

HEART ATTACK PATIENTS
shark cartilage

HEART DISEASE
vitamin D

HEART DISEASE, SEVERE
magnesium

HEMODIALYSIS
copper

HYPERTENSION
vitamin E

HYPOCALCEMIA
calcium chloride

IMMUNE SYSTEM CANCERS
melatonin

KIDNEY DISEASE
magnesium
vitamin D

KIDNEY DISEASE, CHRONIC
vitamin A

KIDNEY DISORDERS
vitamin C

KIDNEY FUNCTION, IMPAIRED
sulfur

KIDNEY FUNCTION, MONITORING
ethylenediaminetetraacetic acid (EDTA)

KIDNEY STONES
calcium

LACTATION
melatonin
phenylalanine
vitamin K

L-DOPA
phenylalanine

LEAD TOXICITY
calcium

LEARNING DISABILITIES
selenium

LEUKEMIA
melatonin

LEVODOPA
vitamin B_6

LIVER DAMAGE
vitamin B_3 (niacin)

LIVER DISEASE, CHRONIC
vitamin A

LIVER FUNCTION, IMPAIRED
sulfur

LUNG IRRITATION
vanadium

LYMPHOMA
melatonin

MALIGNANT MELANOMA
tyrosine

MINERAL DEFICIENCY
magnesium

MOISTURE
glutamine powder

MONOAMINE OXIDASE (MAO) INHIBITORS
tyrosine

MULTIVITAMINS
zinc

NAUSEA
vitamin B_6

NEUROMUSCULAR ABNORMALITIES
5-hydroxytryptophan (5-HTP)

NEUROTOXICITY
vitamin C

ORGAN FUNCTION, MONITORING
ethylenediaminetetraacetic acid (EDTA)

OSTEOPOROSIS
phosphorus

OVARIAN CANCER
dehydroepiandrosterone (DHEA)

PARENTERAL IRON THERAPY
iron

PARKINSON'S DISEASE
vitamin B_6

PATIENTS UNDER 40 YEARS OF AGE
dehydroepiandrosterone (DHEA)

PHENYLKETONURIA
phenylalanine

PHOSPHORUS, HIGH BLOOD LEVELS
vitamin D

PREGNANCY
melatonin
phenylalanine
shark cartilage
sulfur
vitamin A
vitamin B_6
vitamin K

PREMENSTRUAL SYNDROME
vitamin B_6

PROSTATE CANCER
dehydroepiandrosterone (DHEA)

RADIATION
vitamin K

RENAL IMPAIRMENT, SEVERE
potassium

RENAL INSUFFICIENCY
potassium

SCURVY, INFANTS
vitamin C

SKIN ULCER
chromium

SULFITE ALLERGY
sulfur

SURGERY
sulfur

SURGICAL PATIENTS
shark cartilage

TESTICULAR CANCER
dehydroepiandrosterone (DHEA)

TONGUE, GREEN COLOR
vanadium

TOXICITY
chromium
magnesium
manganese
selenium
vitamin A
vitamin B_3 (niacin)

TOXICOSIS
copper

TRANSPLANT PATIENTS
melatonin

TRIGLYCERIDE, INCREASED LEVEL
lysine

ULCER, PEPTIC
vitamin B_3 (niacin)

URINE DISCOLORATION
vitamin B_2 (riboflavin)

VASCULAR FUNCTION, MONITORING
ethylenediaminetetraacetic acid (EDTA)

VITAMIN B_{12} DEFICIENCY
vitamin B_9 (folic acid)

VOMITING
vitamin B_6

WARFARIN
vitamin E
vitamin K

X-RAYS
vitamin K

■ SUPPLEMENTS BY SIDE EFFECTS

This list extracts items included in the Side Effects section of each supplement monograph and combines them to create a collection of supplements that produce a particular side effect.

ABDOMINAL PAIN
vitamin A (retinol)

ACNE
dehydroepiandrosterone (DHEA)

AGGRESSIVE TENDENCIES
dehydroepiandrosterone (DHEA)

ALCOHOL INTOLERANCE
zinc

ALLERGIC REACTIONS
sulfur
vitamin B_1

ALOPECIA
vitamin A (retinol)

ANAPHYLAXIS
iron
psyllium

ANEMIA
zinc

ANEMIA, HEMOLYTIC
vitamin K

ANOREXIA
vitamin A (retinol)

ANXIETY
phenylalanine

ARTHRALGIAS
iron

ARTHRITIS
selenium

ASTHMA
sulfur

ATAXIA
vitamin B_6

BETA CELL DAMAGE
vanadium

BLOOD PRESSURE, LOW
vitamin B_3 (niacin)

BLOOD PRESSURE ELEVATION
dehydroepiandrosterone (DHEA)
manganese
tyrosine
vanadium

BODY ODOR
selenium

BONE FRACTURES
vitamin A (retinol)

BONE PAIN
vitamin D

BRADYCARDIA
potassium

BREATHING, CONSTRICTED
vitamin K

BREATHING DIFFICULTY
potassium

BURNING
vitamin B_2 (riboflavin)

CALCIUM, ABSORPTION
phosphorus

CANCER CELL DIVISION
tyrosine

CARDIAC ARRHYTHMIA
potassium

CARDIOVASCULAR FAILURE
vitamin D

CHEST PAIN
vitamin K

CIRCADIAN RHYTHMS, DISRUPTION
melatonin

CONDUCTION DISTURBANCES
potassium

CONJUNCTIVITIS
vitamin A (retinol)

CONSTIPATION
iron

DEPRESSION
selenium

DIARRHEA
copper poisoning
iron
phosphorus
potassium
vitamin A (retinol)
vitamin B_3 (niacin)
vitamin C
vitamin D
vitamin E

DIARRHEA, BLOODY
iron

DIZZINESS
copper poisoning
zinc

DROWSINESS
zinc

ECZEMA FROM INTRAMUSCULAR INJECTIONS
vitamin K

EPIGASTRIC PAIN
copper poisoning

EYES, DRY
vitamin A (retinol)

EYES, SORE
vitamin D

FAINTING
vitamin B_3 (niacin)

FATIGUE
selenium
sulfur
vitamin A (retinol)
vitamin D

FEELINGS OF FULLNESS
5-hydroxytryptophan (5-HTP)

FEVER
iron
sulfur

FINGERNAIL LOSS
selenium

FLATULENCE
5-hydroxytryptophan (5-HTP)
potassium
vitamin E

FLUSHING
vitamin B_3 (niacin)
vitamin K

GARLICKY BREATH
selenium

GAS
vitamin C

GASTRIC DISTRESS
sulfur
vitamin B_1
vitamin C in excess

GASTRIC HYPOMOTILITY
potassium

GASTRIC IRRITATION
zinc

GASTRIC UPSET, MILD
tyrosine

GASTROINTESTINAL DISORDERS
5-hydroxytryptophan (5-HTP)
iron
selenium
vitamin B_9 (folic acid)

GASTROINTESTINAL IRRITATION
zinc

GASTROINTESTINAL UPSET
vanadium

HAIR GROWTH ON THE FACE
dehydroepiandrosterone (DHEA)

HAIR LOSS
dehydroepiandrosterone (DHEA)
selenium

HALLUCINATIONS
zinc

HEADACHE
copper poisoning
iron
phenylalanine
sulfur
vitamin A (retinol)
zinc

HEADACHE, MIGRAINE
tyrosine

HEARTBURN
5-hydroxytryptophan (5-HTP)
iron
vitamin B_3 (niacin)

HEMOCHROMATOSIS
iron

HEMOLYSIS
vitamin K

HEMORRHAGIC NECROSIS OF THE GASTROINTESTINAL TRACT
iron

HEPATOTOXICITY
dehydroepiandrosterone (DHEA)

HYPERBILIRUBINEMIA
vitamin K

HYPERCALCEMIA
calcium
vitamin D

HYPERKALEMIA
potassium

HYPERPARATHYROIDISM
phosphorus

HYPERTENSION
copper poisoning
phenylalanine

HYPOGLYCEMIA
sulfur

IMMUNE FUNCTION, DEPRESSION OF
zinc

INSULIN, INHIBITION
chromium

INTESTINAL DISTURBANCES
vitamin C

INTRACRANIAL PRESSURE
vitamin A (retinol)

IRON ABSORPTION
phosphorus

IRON TOXICITY
iron

IRRITABILITY
selenium

ITCHING
vitamin B_2 (riboflavin)
vitamin D

JAUNDICE
copper poisoning
vitamin K

JOINT PAIN
vitamin A (retinol)

KIDNEY FAILURE
ethylenediaminetetraacetic acid (EDTA)

LETHARGY
potassium

LEUKOCYTOSIS
vitamin A (retinol)

LIPS, DRY CRACKING
vitamin A (retinol)

LIVER DAMAGE
vitamin K

LIVER MALFUNCTION
vitamin B$_3$ (niacin)

LIVER TOXICITY
vitamin B$_3$ (niacin)

LYMPHADENOPATHY
iron

MAGNESIUM ABSORPTION
phosphorus

MALAISE
iron

MALE PATTERN BALDNESS
dehydroepiandrosterone (DHEA)

MANGANESE TOXICITY
manganese

MANIC DEPRESSION
vanadium

MASCULINIZATION
dehydroepiandrosterone (DHEA)

MEDICATION, INTERFERENCE WITH ABSORPTION
psyllium

METALLIC TASTE
copper poisoning
vitamin D

MUSCLE FUNCTION, IMPAIRED
vitamin D

MUSCLE PAIN
vitamin A (retinol)

MUSCLE WEAKNESS
potassium

MUSCULAR INCOORDINATION
zinc

NAUSEA
cartilage
copper poisoning
5-hydroxytryptophan (5-HTP)
iron
pau d'arco
potassium

vitamin A (retinol)
vitamin B$_3$ (niacin)
vitamin E

NIGHTMARES
melatonin

NUMBNESS
vitamin B$_2$ (riboflavin)

NUTRITIONAL TOXICITY
magnesium

ORGAN CALCIFICATION
phosphorus

ORGAN DAMAGE
ethylenediaminetetraacetic acid (EDTA)
iron

OSTEOPOROSIS
calcium
vitamin D

PAIN FROM INTRAMUSCULAR INJECTIONS
vitamin K

PALPITATIONS
vitamin E

PARALYSIS
potassium

PHLEBITIS
iron

PRICKLING SENSATIONS
vitamin B$_2$ (riboflavin)

PROTEIN SYNTHESIS, INHIBITION OF
vanadium

PSYCHIATRIC ABNORMALITIES
manganese

PULMONARY IRRITATION
vanadium

RASHES
sulfur

RENAL FAILURE
vitamin D

RHEUMATOID ARTHRITIS
iron

RUMBLING SENSATIONS
5-hydroxytryptophan (5-HTP)

SEIZURE
ethylenediaminetetraacetic acid (EDTA)

SENSITIVITY TO LIGHT
vitamin B$_2$ (riboflavin)

SENSORY NEUROPATHY
vitamin B$_6$

SEXUAL AGGRESSIVENESS
dehydroepiandrosterone (DHEA)

SKIN, ALLERGIC REACTIONS
vitamin B$_9$ (folic acid)

SKIN, DRY CRACKING
vitamin A (retinol)

SLEEP PROBLEMS
vitamin B$_9$ (folic acid)

SOFT TISSUE ABSORPTION
phosphorus

STOMACH PAIN
potassium

SWEATING
vitamin K
zinc

SWELLING FROM INTRAMUSCULAR INJECTIONS
vitamin K

TACHYCARDIA
copper poisoning

TASTE, UNPLEASANT
cartilage

TESTICULAR ATROPHY
dehydroepiandrosterone (DHEA)

THIRST, EXCESSIVE
vitamin D

TINGLING SENSATION
vitamin B$_3$ (niacin)

TISSUE NECROSIS
potassium

TOXICITY
vitamin D
zinc

TREMOR
vanadium

ULCERS
vitamin B$_3$ (niacin)

UPPER GASTRIC DISCOMFORT
iron

UREMIA
copper poisoning

URINARY URGENCY
vitamin D

URTICARIA
iron

VIVID DREAMS
melatonin

VOMITING
copper poisoning
iron
potassium
vitamin B$_3$ (niacin)
vitamin D
zinc

WEAKNESS
copper poisoning
potassium

WEIGHT GAIN
creatine

WEIGHT GAIN AROUND THE WAIST
dehydroepiandrosterone (DHEA)

ZINC
phosphorus

■ SUPPLEMENTS BY INTERACTIONS WITH OTHER DRUGS, HERBS, SUPPLEMENTS

This list extracts the items included in the Interactions section of each supplement monograph and combines them to create a collection of supplements that interact, positively or negatively, with a particular drug, herb, or other supplement.

ACE INHIBITORS
potassium

ACETAMINOPHEN
vitamin B_9 (folic acid)

ACETAZOLAMIDE
potassium

ACETYL CARNITINE
melatonin

ADRIAMYCIN
vitamin B_3 (niacin)

ALCOHOL
calcium
copper
dehydroepiandrosterone (DHEA)
magnesium
melatonin
vitamin B_1
vitamin B_9 (folic acid)
vitamin B_3 (niacin)
vitamin B_2 (riboflavin)
vitamin D
vitamin E
vitamin H (biotin)

ALUMINUM-CONTAINING ANTACIDS
calcium

AMILORIDE
potassium

AMINO ACIDS
phenylalanine
sulfur
tyrosine

ANTACIDS
chromium

ANTACIDS, VERY HIGH AMOUNTS
copper

ANTIBIOTICS
vitamin B_2 (riboflavin)
vitamin H (biotin)
vitamin K

ANTICOAGULANT DRUGS
vitamin E

ANTICONVULSANT DRUGS
vitamin B_9 (folic acid)
vitamin H (biotin)

ANTIDEPRESSANT DRUGS
vitamin B_2 (riboflavin)

ANTIHYPERTENSIVE DRUGS
vitamin B_3 (niacin)

ANTI-MALARIAL DRUGS
vitamin B_2 (riboflavin)

ARSENIC POISONING
sulfur

ASCORBIC ACID
vanadium

ASPIRIN
calcium
vitamin B_9 (folic acid)
vitamin K

AVIDIN
vitamin H (biotin)

BARBITURATES
calcium
vitamin B_9 (folic acid)
vitamin B_2 (riboflavin)

BETA-BLOCKERS
melatonin
potassium

BETA-CAROTENE
vitamin C

BILIRUBIN
vitamin C

BRAN, WHEAT
psyllium

BUMETANIDE
potassium

CAFFEINE
calcium
creatine
magnesium
melatonin
phosphorus

CALCIUM
copper
magnesium
manganese
zinc

CALCIUM CARBONATE
chromium

CALCIUM CHANNEL BLOCKERS
melatonin

CATHARTIC AGENTS
vitamin B_2 (riboflavin)

CHEMOTHERAPY DRUGS
vitamin B_9 (folic acid)

CHOLESTYRAMINE
vitamin D
vitamin E
vitamin K

CHOLINE
vitamin B_9 (folic acid)

CHROMIUM
vanadium

CIPROFLOXACIN
iron

COENZYME Q10
vitamin H (biotin)

COLESTIPOL
vitamin E

COPPER
calcium
manganese

COPPER ABSORPTION
vitamin C

COPPER DEFICIENCY
zinc

CYCLOSERINE
vitamin B_6

CYSTEINE
copper

DIGITALIS
magnesium
vitamin D

DIGOXIN
potassium

DISODIUM ETIDRONATE
iron

DIURETICS
magnesium
melatonin
ethylenediaminetetraacetic acid (EDTA)
glutamine
iron
lysine
phenylalanine
selenium
vitamin B_{12}
vitamin B_9 (folic acid)

EGG
copper

EGG WHITE
vitamin H (biotin)

ESTROGENS
vitamin A (retinol)
vitamin B_9 (folic acid)
vitamin B_2 (riboflavin)
vitamin H (biotin)

ETHACYNIC ACID
potassium

ETHYLENEDIAMINETETRAACETIC ACID (EDTA)
vanadium

FAT
magnesium
vitamin A (retinol)

FATTY ACIDS
alpha-linolenic acid (ALA)

FIBER
magnesium
psyllium

FIBER, HIGH
ethylenediaminetetraacetic acid (EDTA)

FIBER DIETARY
zinc

FOLATE ABSORPTION
zinc

FOLIC ACID
magnesium
vitamin H (biotin)

FRUCTOSE
copper

FUROSEMIDE
potassium
vitamin B_1

GLUCOSE
creatine

GLUCOSE TOLERANCE FACTOR (GTF)
chromium

GLUTATHIONE
alpha-lipoic acid

HEPARIN
potassium

H_2 INHIBITORS
iron

HYDRALAZINE
vitamin B_6

IBUPROFEN
vitamin B_9 (folic acid)

INSULIN
magnesium

IODINE
calcium

IRON
calcium
copper
magnesium
manganese
phosphorus
vitamin E
zinc

IRON ABSORPTION
vitamin C

ISONIAZID
vitamin B_6

LEUCINE
vitamin B_3 (niacin)

LEVODOPA
iron

LIPID-REDUCING DRUGS
vitamin B_3 (niacin)

LITHIUM
vanadium

MAGNESIUM
calcium
ethylenediaminetetraacetic acid (EDTA)
5-hydroxytryptophan (5-HTP)
manganese
phosphorus

MAGNESIUM-CONTAINING ANTACIDS
vitamin D

MAGNESIUM SHARK CARTILAGE
cartilage

MAGNESIUM TRISILICATE
iron

MANGANESE
calcium
copper
magnesium

METFORMIN
vitamin B$_{12}$

METHOTREXATE
vitamin B$_2$ (riboflavin)

METHYLENE BLUE
vanadium

MINERAL OIL
vitamin D

MINERAL OIL LAXATIVES
vitamin K

MOLYBDENUM
copper

MONOAMINE OXIDASE INHIBITORS
melatonin
vanadium

NEOMYCIN
calcium

NIACIN
chromium
5-hydroxytryptophan (5-HTP)
vitamin B$_9$ (folic acid)

NIACINAMIDE
melatonin

NORFLOXACIN
iron

NSAIDS
potassium

OFLOXACIN
iron

ORAL CONTRACEPTIVES
vitamin A (retinol)

OXALIC ACID
calcium

PANTOTHENIC ACID
vitamin D
vitamin H (biotin)

PENICILLAMINE
iron
vitamin B$_6$

PHENOBARBITOL
vitamin B$_3$ (niacin)

PHENOTHIAZINES
vanadium
vitamin B$_2$ (riboflavin)

PHENYTOIN
vitamin D
vitamin K

PHOSPHORUS
calcium
magnesium

PHYTATES
copper

PHYTIC ACID
calcium

POTASSIUM SHARK CARTILAGE
cartilage

PRIMIDONE
vitamin B$_3$ (niacin)

PROTEIN
melatonin
vitamin A (retinol)

PROTEIN, HIGH INTAKE
calcium

PROTEINS, MILK
tyrosine

PROTONPUMP INHIBITORS
iron

PYRAZINAMIDE
vitamin B$_6$

(RIBOFLAVIN) IN HIGH DOSAGES
magnesium

SATURATED FATS
calcium
ethylenediaminetetraacetic acid (EDTA)

SEDATIVES, STRONG
calcium

SELENIUM
sulfur
vitamin C
vitamin E

SNAKE VENOMS
vitamin K

SODIUM
calcium
magnesium

SODIUM-POTASSIUM PUMP
vanadium

SPIRONOLACTONE
potassium

ST. JOHN'S WORT
5-hydroxytryptophan (5-HTP)

SUGAR
calcium
magnesium

SULFA DRUGS
vitamin B$_2$ (riboflavin)
vitamin H (biotin)

SULFASALAZINE
vitamin B$_9$ (folic acid)

TETRACYCLINE
iron

THIAZIDE DIURETICS
potassium
vitamin D

TIN
copper

TOBACCO
vanadium

TRANQUILIZERS
vitamin B$_2$ (riboflavin)

TRIAMTERENE
potassium

TRICYCLICS
melatonin

TRIMETHOPRIM
potassium

TRYPTOPHAN
vitamin B$_3$ (niacin)
vitamin B$_2$ (riboflavin)

URONIC ACID
calcium

VALIUM
melatonin

VERAPAMIL
vitamin D

VITAMIN A
vitamin A (retinol)
vitamin E
vitamin K

VITAMIN B$_2$
vitamin B$_3$ (niacin)

VITAMIN B$_6$
copper
glutamine
5-hydroxytryptophan (5-HTP)
melatonin
phenylalanine
tyrosine

VITAMIN B$_{12}$
melatonin
vitamin B$_9$ (folic acid)
vitamin C
vitamin H (biotin)

VITAMIN B$_3$ (NIACIN)
vitamin B$_2$ (riboflavin)

VITAMIN B$_6$ (PYRIDOXINE)
vitamin B$_2$ (riboflavin)

VITAMIN B$_1$ (THIAMINE)
vitamin B$_2$ (riboflavin)

VITAMIN C
alpha-lipoic acid

VITAMIN C HIGH LEVELS
copper

VITAMIN D
phosphorus

VITAMIN E
alpha-lipoic acid
dehydroepiandrosterone (DHEA)
selenium
vitamin A (retinol)
vitamin C
vitamin K

VITAMIN K DEFICIENCY
vitamin E

XANAX
melatonin

ZINC
calcium
copper
magnesium
manganese
selenium
vitamin A (retinol)
vitamin B$_9$ (folic acid)
vitamin H (biotin)

■ COMBINED HERB AND SUPPLEMENT TREATMENT OPTIONS BY CONDITION

This extracts the items included in the Herb and Nutrition sections in each condition monograph and combines them to create a collective list of all conditions in the Quick Access system, with the respective herbs and supplements that may be considered in treating them. Some of the herbs and supplements listed may not yet have a monograph created in the Quick Access system.

ALLERGIC RHINITIS
N-acetyl cysteine
bilberry
bioflavonoids
cleavers
coneflower
curcuma
elderberry
eyebright
ginger root
nettles
quercetin
rose hips
vitamin A
vitamin B_5
vitamin B_6
vitamin C
vitamin E
zinc

ALOPECIA
algae, blue green
astragalus
biotin
black cohosh
chaste tree
echinacea
fatty acids, essential
gamma-linolenic acid (GLA)
ginkgo biloba
ginseng, Siberian
green tea
horsetail
magnesium
prickly ash bark
rosemary
saw palmetto
vitamin B_6
vitamin E
yarrow
zinc

AMENORRHEA
black cohosh
bladderwrack
borage oil
boron
calcium
chaste tree
dandelion root
evening primrose
fatty acids, essential
flaxseed
horsetail
iodine
kelp
lady's mantle
licorice
magnesium
milk thistle

oatstraw
sage
selenium
squaw vine
tyrosine
vervain
vitamin A
vitamin B_6
vitamin C
vitamin D
vitamin E
vitamin K
wild yam
zinc

ANEMIA
alfalfa
black strap molasses
burdock
cyanocobalamine (vitamin B_{12})
dandelion
ferrous fumerate
folic acid
glycerate
glycinate
omega-3 fatty acids
spirulina
vitamin B_{12}
vitamin C
yellow dock

ANGINA
bromelain
L-carnitine
coenzyme Q10
fatty acids, essential
ginger
ginkgo biloba
hawthorn
indian tobacco
linden flower
mistletoe
monkshood
motherwort
night-blooming cereus
L-taurine
vitamin C
yellow jasmine

ANOREXIA NERVOSA
condurango
fenugreek
ginseng, Siberian
goldenseal
lemon balm
licorice
multivitamins
oatstraw
protein supplements
saw palmetto
St. John's wort
valerian
wild yam
zinc

ANXIETY
bergamot
calcium
jasmine
kava kava
lavender
lemon balm
magnesium
oatstraw
passionflower
skullcap

St. John's wort
vitamin B-complex

ASTHMA
N-Acetyl cysteine
belladonna
coltsfoot
elecampane
frankincense
gelsemium
ginger root
ginkgo biloba
green tea
grindelia
hydrochloric acid supplements
hydroxcobalamin
indian tobacco
khella
lavender
licorice root
magnesium
ma huang
mint
palmitate
plantain
pyridoxal-5-phosphate
rose hips
sage
skullcap
skunk cabbage
thyme leaf
valerian
vitamin B_6
vitamin B_{12}
vitamin C
wild cherry bark

ATHEROSCLEROSIS
antioxidants
betaine
bromelain
carnitine
chromium
coenzyme Q10
fatty acids, essential
folic acid
gentian
ginkgo biloba
hawthorn
linden flower
lipoic acid
magnesium
mistletoe
omega-3 fatty acids
rosemary
selenium
vitamin B_6
vitamin B_{12}
vitamin C
vitamin E

ATTENTION-DEFICIT/ HYPERACTIVITY DISORDER
calcium
catnip
chamomile
fatty acids, essential
kava kava
lavender
lemon balm
linden flower
magnesium
omega-3 fatty acids
omega-6 fatty acids
passionflower

vitamin B-complex
vitamin C

BENIGN PROSTATIC HYPERPLASIA
alanine
amino acids
fatty acids, essential
glutamic acid
glycine
pumpkin seeds
saw palmetto
selenium
stinging nettle root
vitamin B_6
zinc

BRONCHITIS
N-acetyl cysteine
beta-carotene
boneset
coneflower
elecampane
garlic
ginger
hawthorn
indian tobacco
licorice root
linden flower
lomatium
lungwort
pill bearing spurge
pleurisy root
sundew
thyme leaf
vitamin C
white horehound
wild cherry bark
zinc

BURNS
aloe
beta-carotene
bromelain
california poppy
cleavers
comfrey root
coneflower
gelsemium
ginger root
L-glutamine
goldenseal
gotu kola
jamaican dogwood
marigold
marshmallow root
plantain
prickly ash bark
slippery elm powder
St. John's wort
turmeric
valerian
vitamin C
vitamin E
yarrow
zinc

BURSITIS
bromelain
glucosamine sulfate
hawthorn
jamaican dogwood
meadowsweet
omega-3 fatty acids
proteolytic enzymes
turmeric
valerian
vitamin C with bioflavonoids
white willow

CANDIDIASIS
antifungal spices
barberry
biotin
calcium
caprylic acid
chamomile
evening primrose
fatty acids, essential
fireweed
flaxseed
folate
garlic
goldenseal
lactobacillus acidophilus
lavender essence oil
licorice
magnesium
marigold
omega-3 fatty acids
omega-6 fatty acids
oregon grape root
pau d'arco bark
selenium
tea tree oil
vitamin B-complex
vitamin C
vitamin E

CHRONIC FATIGUE SYNDROME
ashwaganda root
astragalus root
beta-carotene
L-carnitine
fatty acids, essential
ginseng, Siberian
gotu kola
jasmine oil
lavender
licorice root
lomatium root
magnesium aspartate
pantothenic acid
passionflower
peppermint oil
rosemary leaf
rosemary oil
schizandra berry
skullcap
vitamin B-complex
vitamin C

CHRONIC OBSTRUCTIVE PULMONARY DISEASE
N-acetyl cysteine
bromelain
L-carnitine
coenzyme Q10
coltsfoot
eucalyptus oil
fennel
ginger
hawthorne

lavender oil
licorice
magnesium
mullein
omega-3 fatty acids
omega-6 fatty acids
rosemary oil
selenium
thyme oil
vitamin C
vitamin E

CIRRHOSIS OF THE LIVER
antioxidants
barberry
carnitine
catechin
choline
dessicated liver extract
evening primrose
flaxseed
folate
glutathione
lecithin
methionine
milk thistle
omega-3 fatty acids
omega-6 fatty acids
selenium
vitamin B-complex
vitamin C
vitamin E
vitamin K

COMMON COLD
astragalus
beta-carotene
coneflower
echinacea
elderberry
goldenseal
licorice
vitamin A
vitamin C
zinc

CONGESTIVE HEART FAILURE
antioxidants
betaine
carnitine
coenzyme Q10
dandelion
fatty acids, essential
folic acid
hawthorn
horsetail herb
indian tobacco
lily of the valley
linden flower
magnesium
mistletoe
motherwort
rosemary
selenium
taurine
vitamin B_6
vitamin B_{12}
vitamin C
vitamin E

CONJUNCTIVITIS
chamomile
eyebright
fennel seed
flax meal
goldenseal

marigold
plantain
potato, fresh grated
vitamin A
vitamin C
zinc

CONSTIPATION
burdock
cascara sagrada
dandelion root
digestive enzymes
fennel seed
flax meal
ginger
licorice root
yellow dock

COUGH
balm of Gilead
baume de Canada
beta-carotene
castor oil
coltsfoot
elderberry
elecampane
eucalyptus oil
fennel
flaxseed oil
frankincense
garlic
ginger
gumweed
horehound
indian tobacco
licorice root
linden flower
mullein
mustard oil
onion
oregano oil
pine oils
plantain
purple coneflower
sweet violet
thyme
thyme oil
vitamin C
wild cherry bark
zinc

CUTANEOUS DRUG REACTIONS
aloe
bromelain
chamomile
chickweed
comfrey
coneflower
flaxseed oil
goldenseal
hesperidin
magnesium
marigold
marshmallow root
oatmeal baths
peppermint
quercetin
red clover
slippery elm powder
turmeric
vitamin B-complex with extra B_{12}
vitamin C
vitamin E
yarrow
zinc

DEMENTIA
antioxidants
biotin
calcium/magnesium
coenzyme Q10
ethylenediaminetetraacetic acid (EDTA)
fatty acids, essential
ginger
ginkgo biloba biloba
ginseng, Siberian
hawthorn
lemon balm
rosemary
St. John's wort
vitamin B-complex
vitamin C
vitamin E
zinc

DEPRESSION-UNIPOLAR MOOD DISORDERS
biotin
black cohosh
calcium
chromium
fatty acids, essential
folate
ginkgo biloba
ginseng, Siberian
iron
lemon balm
licorice
magnesium
multivitamins
oatstraw
passionflower
St. John's wort
valerian
vitamin B_1
vitamin B_2 (riboflavin)
vitamin B_6
vitamin B_{12}
vitamin C

DERMATITIS

beta-carotene
bioflavonoids
borage oil
bromelain
catechin
chamomile
chickweed
cleavers
comfrey
evening primrose oil
flaxseed oil
gotu kola
hesperidin
marigold
oregon grape
palmitate
peppermint
peppermint leaf
prickly ash bark
quercetin
red alder bark
red clover
rose hips
rutin
sarsaparilla
selenium
vitamin C
vitamin E
yarrow
zinc

DIABETES MELLITUS

bilberry
brewer's yeast
cayenne
chromium picolinate
coenzyme Q10
evening primrose oil
fenugreek
fish oil
folate
garlic
grape seed extract
magnesium
manganase
onion
pycnogenol
vanadium
vitamin B-complex
vitamin C
vitamin E
zinc

DIARRHEA

barberry
blackberry leaf
brewer's yeast
carob powder
chamomile
glutamine
goldenseal
lactobacillus species
licorice root
marshmallow root
quercetin
sacromyces bolardii
slippery elm powder
vitamin A
vitamin C

DYSMENORRHEA

black cohosh
borage oil
chamomile tea
chaste tree
cramp bark tinctures
evening primrose
flaxseed oil
ginger root
jamaican dogwood
magnesium
niacinamide
red raspberry
vitamin B-complex
vitamin E
wild yam

DYSPHAGIA

licorice
linden flower
skullcap
slippery elm powder
St. John's wort
valerian
wild yam

ECZEMA

beta-carotene
bioflavonoids
borage oil
bromelain
burdock root
catechin
chamomile
chickweed
cleavers
cod liver oil
comfrey
evening primrose
flaxseed
hesperidin
hydrochloric acid
marigold
marshmallow root tea
nettles
omega-6 fatty acids
palmitate
peppermint
quercetin
red clover
rose hips
rutin
vitamin C
yarrow
yellow dock
zinc

EDEMA

artichoke leaves
bilberry
broom
buchu
butcher's broom
calcium
cleavers
coenzyme Q10
couchgrass
dandelion leaf
dandelion root
elder
ginkgo biloba
goldenrod
hawthorn
horse chestnut
horsetail
lily of the valley
linden flower
magnesium
milk thistle
motherwort
night-blooming cereus
oatstraw
parsley
potassium aspartate
red clover
red root
rosemary
rue
sweet clover
thiamine (vitamin B_1)
turmeric
vitamin B_6
vitamin C
vitamin E
yarrow

ENDOCARDITIS

bearberry
beta-carotene
black cohosh
bromelain
cleavers
coenzyme Q10
coneflower
corn silk
dandelion leaf
garlic
goldenseal root
hawthorn
lily of the valley
linden flower
magnesium
motherwort
myrrh
night-blooming cereus
rosemary
selenium
vitamin A
vitamin C
vitamin E
wild indigo
yarrow
zinc

ENDOMETRIOSIS

beta-carotene
black cohosh
blue flag
calcium
chaste tree
cramp bark
dandelion root
fatty acids, essential
gelsemium
ginger root
iron
jamaican dogwood
milk thistle
monkshood
motherwort
poke root
red raspberry
red root
selenium
squaw vine
valerian
vervain
vitamin C
vitamin E
white byrony
wild yam
yarrow
zinc

FEVER OF UNKNOWN ORIGIN

beta-carotene
catnip
coneflower
elder
lemon balm
spearmint
vitamin C
white willow bark
yarrow
zinc

FIBROMYALGIA

ashwaganda root
astragalus root
black cohosh
chromium picolinate
clary sage
coenzyme Q10
ginseng, Siberian
gotu kola
5-Hydroxytryptophan
jasmine oil
kava kava
lavender
lemon balm
magnesium
melatonin
passionflower
phosphatidyl choline
phosphatidyl serine
raw thymus glandular
rosemary
schizandra berry
skullcap
valerian
vitamin B-complex
vitamin C
zinc

FOOD ALLERGY

beta-carotene
borage oil
bromelain
catnip
celandine
chamomile
chicory
dandelion
evening primrose oil
fennel
flaxseed oil
marshmallow root tea
meadowsweet
milk thistle
palmitate
pancreatin
passionflower
peppermint
pro-flora supplements
quercetin
rose hips
selenium
vitamin B-complex
vitamin C
zinc

GALLBLADDER DISEASE
choline
dandelion root
flax meal
globe artichoke
greater celandine
lecithin
lipase
lipotropic agents
milk thistle
peppermint oil
turmeric
vitamin C
vitamin E

GASTRITIS
bismuth subcitrate
ginger root tea
licorice, deglycyrrhizinated
marshmallow root
slippery elm powder
vitamin C
zinc ·

GASTROESOPHAGEAL REFLUX DISEASE
licorice
linden flower
skullcap
slippery elm powder
St. John's wort
valerian
wild yam

GOUT
bromelain
devil's claw
eicospentaenoic acid (EPA)
folic acid (vitamin B_9)
niacin (vitamin B_3)
vitamin A
vitamin C

HEMORRHOIDS
bioflavonoids
catechin
comfrey
flax meal
green tea
marigold
potato, fresh grated
rose hips
vitamin C
vitamin E
witch hazel

HEPATITIS, VIRAL
N-Acetyl cysteine
acidophilus
astragalus root
beta-carotene
chinese thoroughwax
choline
coneflower
dessicated liver extract
eclipta alba
folic acid (vitamin B_9)
globe artichoke
glutathione
goldenseal
green tea
lecithin
licorice root
methionine
milk thistle
phyllanthus amarus

schizandra berry
selenium
thymus extract
turmeric
vitamin B-complex
vitamin C
vitamin E
vitamin K
zinc

HERPES SIMPLEX VIRUS
acidophilus
astragalus
beta-carotene
chamomile
coneflower
glycyrrhizic acid
lemon balm
licorice root
lomatium
L-lysine
selenium
St. John's wort
thymus extract
vitamin A
vitamin C
yarrow
zinc

HERPES ZOSTER (varicella-zoster) virus
beta-carotene
burdock root
calcium
chamomile
comfrey
coneflower
goldenseal
jamaican dogwood
lemon balm
licorice root
magnesium
marigold
slippery elm powder
St. John's wort
valerian
vitamin A
vitamin B_{12}
vitamin B-complex
vitamin C
vitamin E
wild lettuce
yellow jasmine
zinc

HIV AND AIDS
N-Acetyl cysteine
acidophilus
beta-carotene
L-carnitine
cholagogue
coenzyme Q10
dandelion
garlic
gentian
ginseng, Siberian
L-glutamine
goldenseal
huang qi
licorice
magnesium
milk thistle
multivitamins
selenium
St. John's wort
vitamin B_{12}

vitamin B-complex
vitamin C
vitamin E
zinc

HYPERCHOLESTEROLEMIA
alfalfa
blue flag
blue vervain
burdock root
chromium
coenzyme Q10
dandelion root
garlic
ginger
greater celandine
hawthorn berries
magnesium
milk thistle
niacin (vitamin B_3)
omega-3 fatty acids
panthenine
selenium
L-taurine
vitamin B-complex
vitamin C

HYPERKALEMIA
hawthorn
lily of the valley
magnesium

HYPERTENSION
betaine
coenzyme Q10
cramp bark
dandelion leaf
evening primrose oil
flax oil
folic acid (vitamin B_9)
hawthorn
indian tobacco
lily of the valley
linden flower
magnesium
mistletoe
motherwort
night-blooming cereus
passionflower
valerian
vitamin B_{12}
vitamin B-complex
vitamin E
zinc

HYPERTHYROIDISM
bromelain
bugleweed
calcium
coenzyme Q10
fatty acids, essential
hawthorn berries
lemon balm
licorice
lithium
magnesium
milk thistle
motherwort
passionflower
quercetin
Rehmania glutinosa
Stephania tetranda
turmeric
vitamin C
vitamin E

HYPOGLYCEMIA
chromium picolinate
ginger root
ginseng, Siberian
gotu kola
licorice root
magnesium
niacinamide (vitamin B_3)
pantothenic acid (vitamin B_5)
pyridoxine (vitamin B_6)
vanadyl sulfate
vitamin B-complex
vitamin C
vitamin E
zinc

HYPOTHYROIDISM
alfalfa
bladderwrack
calcium
coleus foreskohlii
fatty acids, essential
gotu kola
guggul
hawthorne
horsetail
irish moss
kelp
oatstraw
selenium
L-tyrosine
vitamin A
vitamin B_2 (riboflavin)
vitamin B_3
vitamin B_6
vitamin B-complex
vitamin C
zinc

INFANTILE COLIC
acidophilus
anise seed
catnip
fennel seed
lemon balm
linden flower
peppermint
spearmint

INFLUENZA
beta-carotene
coneflower
elder
garlic/ginger tea
goldenseal
licorice
St. John's wort
vitamin A
vitamin C
yarrow
zinc

INSECT BITES
bromelain
citronella oil
cleavers
coneflower
elder
eucalyptus oil
goldenseal powder
lavender oil
licorice root
marigold
oatstraw
pennyroyal oil
peppermint
plantain leaves
quercetin
red clover
turmeric
vitamin B-complex
vitamin C
witch hazel

INSOMNIA
calcium/magnesium
chamomile
chamomile oil
5-HTP (5-Hydroxytryptophan)
jamaican dogwood
kava kava
lavender oil
lemon balm
melatonin
niacinamide
passionflower
rosemary oil
St. John's wort
valerian
vitamin B-complex

INTESTINAL PARASITES
acidophilus
barberry
beta-carotene
black walnut
digestive enzymes
garlic
garlic oil
goldenseal
lavender oil
male fern
oregon grape
papain
quassia
tansy
tea tree oil
thyme
thyme oil
vitamin C
wormseed
wormwood
zinc

IRRITABLE BOWEL SYNDROME
acidophilus
anise seed
bran, raw
digestive enzymes
fennel seed
flax meal
ginger root
lactobacillus
magnesium
marshmallow root
meadowsweet
milk thistle

passionflower
peppermint oil
psyllium
slippery elm powder
valerian
wild yam

LARYNGITIS
coneflower
ginger
goldenseal
licorice
marigold
myrrh
peppermint
propolis
sage
slippery elm powder
vitamin B-complex
vitamin C
zinc lozenges

LOW BACK PAIN
antioxidants
black haw
bromelain
calcium/magnesium
devil's claw
ginkgo biloba
jamaican dogwood
leopard's bane
lobelia
petasites
rosemary leaves
St. John's wort
turmeric
valerian
vitamin B-complex
vitamin C
vitamin E
white willow bark
wild yam

MENOPAUSE
angelica
black cohosh
calcium/magnesium
chaste tree
gamma-oryzanol
ginkgo biloba
hesperidin
hesperidin methyl chalcone
licorice
soy
vitamin C
vitamin E

MIGRAINE HEADACHE
bioflavonoids
choline
fatty acids, essential
feverfew
folic acid (vitamin B$_9$)
ginger
ginkgo biloba
5-Hydroxytryptophan
jamaican dogwood
magnesium
meadowsweet
omega-3 fatty acids
skullcap
vitamin B$_2$ (riboflavin)
vitamin B$_6$
vitamin C
vitamin E

MOTION SICKNESS
black horehound
chamomile
ginger root
peppermint

MYOCARDIAL INFARCTION
antioxidants
beta-carotene
bromelain
L-carnitine
vitamin C
vitamin E

OBESITY
bladderwrack
choline
chromium picolinate
coenzyme Q10
dandelion
fatty acids, essential
fiber
gentian
L-glutamine
hawthorne
5-HTP (5-Hydroxytryptophan)
kelp
lavender
lecithin
ma huang
methionine
milk thistle
multivitamins
parsley
peppermint
St. John's wort
thiamine (vitamin B$_1$)
valerian
vitamin B-complex
vitamin C

OSTEOARTHRITIS
S-Adenosylmethionine
bilberry
black cohosh
boron
boswellia
devil's claw
ginger root
glucosamine sulfate
hawthorn
meadowsweet
niacinamide
omega-3 fatty acids
teasel root
turmeric
vitamin A
vitamin C
vitamin E
yucca

OSTEOMYELITIS
acidophilus
analgesics
antimicrobials
astragalus
barberry
burdock root
cleavers
coneflower
garlic
ginkgo biloba
goldenseal
goldenseal root
licorice
lomatium

red clover
slippery elm
St. John's wort
valerian
vitamin A
vitamin C
vitamin E
yarrow
yellow dock
zinc

OSTEOPOROSIS
aspartate
black cohosh
bladderwrack
blue flag
boron
calcium citrate
chaste tree
chromium
dandelion root
fatty acids, essential
horsetail
kelp
lady's mantle
licorice
magnesium
manganase
milk thistle
nettles
oatstraw
squaw vine
vervain
vitamin B-complex
vitamin K
wild yam
zinc

OTITIS MEDIA
cleavers
cod liver oil
coneflower
elderberry
eyebright
fatty acids, essential
fish oil
garlic oil
indian tobacco oil
marigold
monkshood oil
mullein flower oil
St. John's wort oil
vitamin C

PARKINSON'S DISEASE
alpha-lipoic acid
amino acids
antioxidants
choline
dimethylaminoethanol (DMAE)
fatty acids, essential
gamma-aminobutyric acid (GABA)
ginkgo biloba
globe artichoke
glutamic acid
glutathione
gotu kola
grape seed extract
hawthorn
lecithin
lemon balm
manganese
milk thistle
nervine herbs
oats
phosphatidyl choline
pycnogenol
selenium
skullcap
St. John's wort
vitamin B-complex
vitamin C
vitamin E

PEPTIC ULCER
N-Acetyl cysteine
acidophilus
barberry
bismuth subcitrate
catnip
chamomile
fatty acids, essential
glutamine
goldenseal
lemon balm
licorice, deglycyrrhizinated
marshmallow root powder
meadowsweet
oregon grape
passionflower
peppermint
plantain
potassium
quercetin
slippery elm powder
sulphur
valerian
vitamin A
vitamin C
vitamin E
zinc

PERICARDITIS
blue monkshood
coenzyme Q10
flax oil
hawthorn
linden flower
vitamin A
vitamin C

PERTUSSIS
anise seed
astragalus
beta-carotene
catnip
chamomile
coneflower
cramp bark
elecampane

garlic
ginger root
hyssop
indian tobacco
licorice root
mullein
thyme
usnea lichen
valerian
vitamin C
zinc

PHARYNGITIS
beta-carotene
coneflower
garlic/ginger tea
goldenseal
licorice
propolis
slippery elm powder
vitamin C
zinc

PREECLAMPSIA
cramp bark
hawthorn berries
indian tobacco
magnesium
milk thistle
omega-3 fatty acids
passionflower

PRIMARY PULMONARY HYPERTENSION
L-carnitine
choline
coenzyme Q10
garlic
ginkgo biloba
hawthorn
indian tobacco
inositol
linden flower
manesium aspartate
potassium aspartate
rosemary
selenium
taurine
vitamin C
vitamin E

PROSTATITIS
bearberry
cernilton
coneflower
corn silk
fatty acids, essential
goldenseal
pumpkin seeds
saw palmetto
selenium
vitamin C
zinc

PSORIASIS
burdock
coleus
digestive enzymes
fatty acids, essential
folate
milk thistle
omega-3 fatty acids
omega-6 fatty acids
quercetin
red clover
sarsaparilla

selenium
vitamin B_{12}
vitamin E
yellow dock
zinc

PULMONARY EDEMA
broom
L-carnitine
choline
coenzyme Q10
dandelion leaf
garlic
hawthorn
indian tobacco
lily of the valley
linden flower
magnesium
magnesium aspartate
motherwort
night-blooming cereus
potassium
potassium aspartate
raw heart concentrate
rosemary
selenium
taurine
thyme leaf
vitamin C
vitamin E

RAYNAUD'S PHENOMENON
calcium
coenzyme Q10
ginger root
ginkgo biloba
hawthorn berries
omega-3 fatty acids
prickly ash bark
rosemary
vitamin B-complex
vitamin C
vitamin E
zinc

REITER'S SYNDROME
antioxidants
beta-carotene
bilberry
bromelain
copper
eyebright
fatty acids, essential
glucosamine sulfate
horsetail
juniper
licorice
meadowsweet
selenium
uva ursi
vitamin C
vitamin E
zinc

RHEUMATOID ARTHRITIS
antioxidants
ashwaganda
blue flag
boswellia
bromelain
devil's claw
flavanoids
gana derma
ginger
ginseng
gotu kola

grifold frondosa
horsetail
nightshades
omega-3 fatty acids
quercetin
sarsaparilla
selenium
turmeric
valerian
vitamin C
wild yam
zinc

ROSEOLA
beta-carotene
catnip
chamomile
elder
fennel
garlic/ginger tea
peppermint
vitamin C
yarrow
zinc

SEIZURES
dimethyl glycine
folic acid (vitamin B_9)
magnesium
manganese
milk thistle
passionflower
skullcap
taurine
valerian
vitamin B_6
vitamin B_{12}
zinc

SEXUAL DYSFUNCTION
chaste tree
damiana
dandelion root
ginger root
ginkgo biloba
gotu kola
hawthorn
kava kava
lemon balm
magnesium
milk thistle
passionflower
prickly ash bark
rosemary
skullcap
St. John's wort
vervain
vitamin B_6
vitamin B-complex
vitamin C
vitamin E
yohimbe bark

SINUS HEADACHE
beta-carotene
bromelain
coneflower
eucalyptus oil
eyebright
garlic
ginger
goldenseal
jamaican dogwood
lavender oil
licorice
St. John's wort
thyme oil
vitamin C
wild indigo
zinc

SINUSITIS
beta-carotene
bromelain
coneflower
eucalyptus oil
eyebright
garlic/ginger tea
goldenseal
jamaican dogwood
lavender oil
licorice
quercetin
St. John's wort
thyme oil
vitamin C
wild indigo
zinc

SLEEP APNEA
chromium
fatty acids, essential

SPRAINS AND STRAINS
arnica oil
beta-carotene
bioflavonoids
black cohosh
bromelain
cramp bark
feverfew
hawthorn
jamaican dogwood
poke root
quercetin
turmeric
valerian
vitamin C
vitamin E
zinc

TENDINITIS
bioflavonoids
bromelain
calcium/magnesium
comfrey
curcumin
fatty acids, essential
licorice
vitamin A
vitamin C
vitamin E
willow

TENSION HEADACHE
beta-carotene
calcium
calcium/magnesium
cayenne

evening primrose
fatty acids, essential
flaxseed
ginkgo biloba
jamaican dogwood
kava kava
magnesium
manganase
meadowsweet
omega-3 fatty acids
omega-6 fatty acids
peppermint oil
potassium
selenium
valerian
vitamin B-complex
vitamin C
vitamin E
white willow bark
zinc

THYROIDITIS
alfalfa
bladderwrack
bromelain
bugleweed
calcium/magnesium
fatty acids, essential
ginkgo biloba
gotu kola
horsetail
iodine
motherwort
oatstraw
passionflower
quercetin
selenium
turmeric
L-tyrosine
vitamin A
vitamin B-complex
vitamin C
vitamin E
zinc

ULCERATIVE COLITIS
beta-carotene
biotin
bromelain
calcium
coneflower
cramp bark
fatty acids, essential
fiber
flax meal
folic acid (vitamin B_9)
geranium
goldenseal
iron, elemental
lemon balm
licorice root
magnesium
marshmallow root
meadowsweet
pantothenic acid (vitamin B_5)
passionflower
peppermint oil
pro-flora supplements
psyllium
quercetin
vitamin B_2 (riboflavin)
selenium
slippery elm powder
thiamine (vitamin B_1)
valerian
vitamin A

vitamin B_{12}
vitamin B-complex
vitamin C
vitamin D
vitamin K
wild yam
zinc

URETHRITIS
beta-carotene
blueberries
buchu
cleavers
coneflower
corn silk
couchgrass
cranberries
goldenseal
horsetail
kava kava
marshmallow root
plantain
thyme leaf
uva ursi
vitamin C
zinc

URINARY INCONTINENCE
blueberries
calcium/magnesium
cranberries
horsetail
marshmallow root
plantain
vitamin C
zinc

URINARY TRACT INFECTION IN WOMEN
beta-carotene
blueberries
buchu
coneflower
corn silk
couchgrass
cranberries
goldenseal
horsetail
marshmallow root
plantain
thyme leaf
uva ursi
vitamin C
zinc

UROLITHIASIS
corn silk
cramp bark
folic acid (vitamin B_9)
gravel root
jamaican dogwood
kava kava
magnesium citrate
pyridoxine
wild yam

VAGINITIS
acidophilus
beta-carotene
garlic
pau d'arco tea
vitamin A
vitamin C
vitamin E
zinc

WARTS
beta-carotene
celandine
coneflower
echinacea
folic acid (vitamin B_9)
goldenseal
licorice root
lomatium
osha
selenium
thuja leaf
vitamin A
vitamin B-complex
vitamin C
vitamin E
zinc

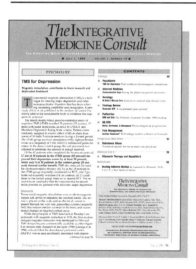